THE KIDNEY IN LIVER DISEASE

FOURTH EDITION

THE KIDNEY IN LIVER DISEASE

FOURTH EDITION

Edited by

MURRAY EPSTEIN, MD, FACP

Professor of Medicine
Division of Nephrology
University of Miami School of Medicine
Attending Physician
Veterans Affairs Medical Center
Miami, Florida

HANLEY & BELFUS, INC./ Philadelphia

Publisher: HANLEY & BELFUS, INC.
            210 S. 13th Street
            Philadelphia, PA 19107
            (215) 546-7293
            FAX (215) 790-9330

Library of Congress Cataloging-in-Publication Data

The kidney in liver disease / edited by Murray Epstein.—4th ed.
        p.   cm.
    Includes bibliographical references and index.
    ISBN 1-56053-166-5 (hardcover : alk. paper)
    1. Hepatorenal syndrome.   2. Liver—Diseases—complications.
    3. Kidneys—Diseases.   I. Epstein, Murray, 1937–   .
    [DNLM: 1. Liver Diseases—complications.   2. Liver Diseases—
    pathophysiology.   3. Hepatorenal Syndrome—pathophysiology.
    4. Hepatorenal Syndrome—therapy.   5. Renin-Angiotensin System—
    physiology.   WI 700 K45 1995]
    RC848.H46K53   1996
    616.3′62-dc20
    DNLM/DLC
    for Library of Congress   95-46921
                                                                   CIP

THE KIDNEY IN LIVER DISEASE   ISBN 1-56053-166-5

Last digit is the print number: 9 8 7 6 5 4 3 2 1

To Nina,
and David, Susanna, and Jonathan

CONTENTS

SECTION 1   CLINICAL DISORDERS OF RENAL FUNCTION

1. Renal Sodium Handling in Liver Disease 1
   Murray Epstein, M.D., F.A.C.P.

2. Renal Water Handling in Liver Disease 33
   Carlos A. Vaamonde, M.D.

3. Hepatorenal Syndrome 75
   Murray Epstein, M.D., F.A.C.P.

4. Derangements of Acid-Base Homeostasis in Liver Disease 109
   James R. Oster, M.D., and Guido O. Perez, M.D.

5. Glomerular Abnormalities in Liver Disease 123
   Garabed Eknoyan, M.D.

6. The Significance of Hepatitis C Virus Infection in the Care of Patients
   with Renal Disease 151
   David Roth, M.D.

7. Venoocclusive Disease of the Liver Following Bone Marrow Transplantation 167
   Robert Sackstein, M.D., Ph.D., and Nelson J. Chao, M.D.

SECTION 2   ASCITES

8. Pathophysiology of Ascites Formation 179
   Mortimer Levy, M.D., F.R.C.P.(C)

9. Hepatic Circulation in Homeostasis 221
   W. Wayne Lautt, Ph.D., and Clive V. Greenway, M.D.

SECTION 3   HEMODYNAMIC DERANGEMENTS

10. Hemodynamics, Distribution of Blood Volume, and Kinetics of
    Vasoactive Substances in Cirrhosis 241
    Jens H. Henriksen, M.D., and Soren Møller, M.D.

11. Low-Pressure Baroreceptors II—New Perspectives: The Phrenic Nerve
    as a Visceral Reflex Pathway 259
    David R. Kostreva, Ph.D.

SECTION 4   RENIN-ANGIOTENSIN-ALDOSTERONE

12. Renin-Angiotensin System in Liver Disease 267
    Murray Epstein, M.D., F.A.C.P.

13. Aldosterone in Liver Disease 291
    Murray Epstein, M.D., F.A.C.P.

SECTION 5   HORMONAL AND NEURAL ALTERATIONS OTHER
               THAN RENIN-ANGIOTENSIN-ALDOSTERONE

     14.   Lipid-Derived Autacoids and Renal Function in Liver Cirrhosis.................. 307
            *Giacomo Laffi, M.D., Giorgio La Villa, M.D., Massimo Pinzani, M.D.,
            and Paolo Gentilini, M.D.*

     15.   Atrial Natriuretic Factor and Liver Disease 339
            Murray Epstein, M.D., F.A.C.P.

     16.   Natriuretic Hormone 359
            Vardaman M. Buckalew, Jr., M.D.

     17.   Nitric Oxide and Renal Function: The Control of Blood Pressure 373
            under Normal Conditions and During Cirrhosis
            J.C. Romero, M.D., Joaquin Garcia-Estañ, M.D., and Noemi M. Atucha, M.D.

     18.   Endothelin and Renal Dysfunction in Liver Disease 387
            Michael S. Goligorsky, M.D., and Edward P. Nord, M.D.

     19.   Renal Sympathetic Nervous System in Hepatic Cirrhosis 405
            Edward J. Zambraski, Ph.D., and Gerald DiBona, M.D.

     20.   Jaundice and the Kidney 423
            Arieh Bomzon, M.D., Giris Jacob, M.D., and Ori S. Better, M.D.

SECTION 6   THERAPEUTICS

     21.   Diuretic Therapy in Liver Disease 447
            Murray Epstein, M.D., F.A.C.P.

     22.   Pharmacokinetics and Pharmacodynamics in Cirrhosis 459
            D. Craig Brater, M.D

     23.   Paracentesis in the Management of Cirrhotics with Ascites 479
            *Ramón Planas, M.D., Pere Ginès, M.D., Angels Ginès, M.D.,
            and Vicente Arroyo, M.D.*

     24.   Peritoneovenous Shunt in the Management of Ascites
            and the Hepatorenal Syndrome 491
            Murray Epstein, M.D., F.A.C.P.

     25.   Transjugular Intrahepatic Portosystemic Shunt in the Treatment of
            Refractory Ascites and Hepatorenal Syndrome 507
            Kenneth A. Somberg, M.D.

     26.   Dialysis, Hemofiltration, and other Extracorporeal Techniques
            in the Treatment of the Renal Complications of Liver Disease 517
            *Guido O. Perez, M.D., Thomas A. Golper, M.D.,
            Murray Epstein, M.D., F.A.C.P., and James R. Oster, M.D.*

     27.   Liver Transplantation and Renal Function: Results in Patients
            With and Without Hepatorenal Syndrome 529
            Thomas A. Gonwa, M.D., F.A.C.P., and Alan H. Wilkinson, M.D.

INDEX   543

CONTRIBUTORS

VICENTE ARROYO, M.D.
Professor of Medicine, Liver Unit, University of Barcelona School of Medicine, Barcelona, Catalunya, Spain

NOEMI M. ATUCHA, M.D.
Research Assistant, Department of Physiology, University of Murcia, Murcia, Spain

ORI S. BETTER, M.D.
Professor, Dr. R. Chutick Crush Syndrome Center, Bruce Rappaport Faculty of Medicine, Technion, Israel Institute of Technology, Haifa, Israel

ARIEH BOMZON, Ph.D., F.R.C.U.S.
Associate Professor of Pharmacology, Bruce Rappaport Faculty of Medicine, Technion-Israel Institute of Technology, Haifa, Israel; Associate Professor of Medicine, University of Calgary Faculty of Medicine, Calgary, Alberta, Canada

D. CRAIG BRATER, M.D.
Chairman, Department of Medicine, Indiana University School of Medicine, Indianapolis, Indiana

VARDAMAN M. BUCKALEW, JR., M.D.
Professor of Internal Medicine and Physiology, and Chief of Nephrology, Bowman Gray School of Medicine of Wake Forest University, Winston-Salem, North Carolina

NELSON J. CHAO, M.D.
Assistant Professor of Medicine, Division of Bone Marrow Transplantation, Stanford University Medical School, Stanford, California

GERALD F. DIBONA, M.D.
Professor and Chairman, Department of Internal Medicine, University of Iowa College of Medicine, Iowa City, Iowa

GARABED EKNOYAN, M.D.
Professor of Medicine, Section of Nephrology, Baylor College of Medicine, Houston, Texas

MURRAY EPSTEIN, M.D., F.A.C.P.
Professor of Medicine, Division of Nephrology, University of Miami School of Medicine; Attending Physician, Veterans Affairs Medical Center, Miami, Florida

JOAQUIN GARCIA-ESTAÑ, M.D.
Professor of Physiology, University of Murcia, Murcia, Spain

PAOLO GENTILINI, M.D.
Professor of Medicine, Istituto di Medicina Interna, Universita Degli Studi di Firenze, Florence, Italy

ANGELS GINÈS, M.D.
Research Fellow, Liver Unit, University of Barcelona School of Medicine, Barcelona, Catalunya, Spain

PERE GINÈS, M.D.
Faculty Member, Liver Unit, University of Barcelona School of Medicine, Barcelona, Catalunya, Spain

MICHAEL S. GOLIGORSKY, M.D., Ph.D.
Associate Professor of Medicine and Physiology, Division of Nephrology and Hypertension, State University of New York at Stony Brook, Stony Brook, New York

THOMAS A. GOLPER, M.D.
Professor of Medicine, Division of Nephrology, University of Arkansas for Medical Sciences, Little Rock, Arkansas

THOMAS A. GONWA, M.D., F.A.C.P.
Alan Hull Professor of Transplant Medicine, Department of Transplantation Services, Baylor University Medical Center, Dallas, Texas

CLIVE V. GREENWAY, M.D.
Professor of Pharmacology, Department of Pharmacology and Therapeutics, University of Manitoba Faculty of Medicine, Winnipeg, Manitoba, Canada

CARLOS GUARNER, M.D.
Associate Professor of Medicine, Department of Gastroenterology, Autonomous University, Barcelona, Spain

JENS HENRIK HENRIKSEN, M.D.
Professor of Clinical Physiology, Hvidovre Hospital, University of Copenhagen, Hvidovre, Denmark

GIRIS JACOB, M.D., Ph.D.
Rambam Medical Center, Haifa, Israel

DAVID R. KOSTREVA, Ph.D.
Senior Scientist and Associate Manager, New Business Development, Procter & Gamble Pharmaceuticals, Cincinnati, Ohio

GIACOMO LAFFI, M.D.
Associate Professor of Gastroenterology, Istituto di Medicina Interna, Universita Degli Studi di Firenze, Florence, Italy

W. WAYNE LAUTT, Ph.D.
Professor, Department of Pharmacology and Therapeutics, University of Manitoba, Faculty of Medicine, Winnipeg, Manitoba, Canada

GIORGIO LA VILLA, M.D.
Associate Professor of Medicine, Istituto Di Medicina Interna, University of Florence School of Medicine, Florence, Italy

MORTIMER LEVY, M.D., F.R.C.P.(C)
Professor of Medicine and Physiology, McGill University Faculty of Medicine, Montreal, Quebec, Canada

SOREN MØLLER, M.D.
Research Fellow, Department of Clinical Physiology, Hvidovre Hospital, University of Copenhagen, Hvidovre, Denmark

EDWARD P. NORD, M.D.
Associate Professor of Medicine, and Chief, Division of Nephrology and Hypertension, State University of New York at Stony Brook, Stony Brook, New York

JAMES R. OSTER, M.D.
Professor of Medicine, University of Miami School of Medicine; Associate Chief, Medical Service, Veterans Affairs Medical Center; Miami, Florida

GUIDO O. PEREZ, M.D.
Professor of Medicine, University of Miami School of Medicine, Miami, Florida

MASSIMO PINZANI, M.D., Ph.D.
Assistant Professor of Medicine, Istituto di Medicina Interna, Universita Degli Studi di Florence, Firenze, Italy

RAMON PLANAS, M.D.
Medical Director and Head, Liver Section, Department of Gastroenterology, Hospital Universitari Germans Trias, Barcelona, Catalunya, Spain

J. CARLOS ROMERO, M.D.
Professor of Physiology and Biophysics, Mayo Medical School, Rochester, Minnesota

DAVID ROTH, M.D.
Medical Director, Renal Transplant Unit; Professor, Department of Medicine, University of Miami School of Medicine, Miami, Florida

ROBERT SACKSTEIN, M.D., Ph.D.
Assistant Professor, Department of Internal Medicine, University of South Florida School of Medicine, Tampa, Florida

KENNETH A. SOMBERG, M.D.
Assistant Professor of Medicine, Associate Medical Director, Liver Transplantation Program, Department of Gastroenterology, University of California, San Francisco, San Francisco, California

CARLOS A. VAAMONDE, M.D., F.A.C.P.
Professor of Medicine, University of Miami School of Medicine, Miami; Chief, Nephrology Section, Veterans Affairs Medical Center, Miami, Florida

ALAN H. WILKINSON, M.B., B.Ch., M.R.C.P.
Professor of Medicine, University of California, Los Angeles, Los Angeles, California

EDWARD J. ZAMBRASKI, Ph.D.
Professor of Physiology, Department of Biological Sciences, Rutgers University, New Brunswick, New Jersey

PREFACE

I have long felt that there is a need for a comprehensive, up-to-date text focusing on the renal functional abnormalities that complicate advanced liver disease. In 1978, I undertook to edit the first edition of *The Kidney in Liver Disease*. The book was intended to meet this need by bringing into sharp focus the present knowledge about this highly important area and to provide nephrologists, gastroenterologists, hepatologists, endocrinologists, physiologists, internists, and surgeons with ready reference information that might otherwise be difficult to retrieve. In so doing, I strove to avoid merely cataloging this diverse information. Instead, each author was asked to inject a personal flavor either by providing original research data or by elaborating on personal and published clinical observations. The favorable comments that attended publication of each of the three editions of the book indicated that I was correct in my perception. There is now a need for a fourth edition.

In the 18 years since the publication of the first edition of the book, the explosive growth of literature pertaining to the physiology and diseases of the kidney in the setting of liver disease continues unabated. Few major breakthroughs have occurred to lessen the incidence of these complications, but a large amount of new experimental and clinical information has become available. Major advances have occurred in the areas of increasing experience with large volume paracentesis, increasing awareness of the participation of additional humoral mediators in the pathogenesis of renal dysfunction, and the maturation and success of liver transplantation.

In this fourth edition of *The Kidney in Liver Disease*, the contributors once again have attempted to review critically the available literature dealing with specific facets of renal functional alterations in liver disease. Much-needed chapters have been added on a wide range of new subjects, including hepatitis C virus infection and veno-occlusive liver disease after bone marrow transplantation. Moreover, the scope of hormonal and neural aspects has been broadened to include discussions on endothelin and the effect of nitric oxide on renal function in cirrhosis. Of course, chapters that appeared in the previous edition have been revised and updated. The focus of some of the repeating chapters has been broadened or changed to keep abreast of new developments, reflecting in part the special talents and interests of new authors. The prostaglandin chapter has been rewritten by Drs. Laffi, Gentilini, and coworkers, and has been expanded to include more aspects of this important subject and to highlight new information derived from the application of newer technologies, including cloning and gene sequence analysis of the major enzymes involved in arachidonic acid metabolism.

The fifth section is devoted to an examination of the role of hormonal systems other than renin-angiotensin since the importance of these systems in the modulation of renal function is becoming increasingly apparent. Dr. Buckalew critically examines the possible contribution of natriuretic hormones, including digitalis-like factors. The explosive interest in endothelin has prompted several investigations of the possibility that this vasoconstrictor peptide may contribute to the pathogenesis of renal dysfunction. Drs. Goligorsky and Nord provide an in-depth review of this important subject, which is complemented by Drs. Henriksen and Møller. Finally, the possible role of nitric oxide as a putative mediator of both the hyperdynamic circulation and renal dysfunction is examined by Drs. Romero and coworkers.

The final section discusses treatment modalities of many of the renal complications of liver disease enumerated above. In view of the continuing widespread interest in the role of paracentesis, Drs. Arroyo and associates from the University of Barcelona draw from their vast experience with this procedure to provide an update of the attributes and disadvantages of paracentesis in the management of the patient with ascites.

The limitations and drawbacks of currently available therapies for refractory ascites have prompted interest in and investigation of the transjugular intrahepatic portosystemic shunt (TIPS) as a possible alternative treatment. Dr. Somberg draws on his wide experience to provide a critical review of this emerging technique.

The final chapter by Drs. Gonwa and Wilkinson reviews the increasingly important and indeed pivotal role of liver transplantation. Over the past decade liver transplantation has moved from the realm of experimentation to the clinical arena, and now constitutes a successful and accepted treatment for almost all patients with end-stage liver disease. The authors share their extensive experience with orthotopic liver transplantation by providing an in-depth review of pivotal issues, including (1) the intraoperative and postoperative changes that occur in renal function and fluid and electrolyte status, and (2) the effect of the post-liver transplantation course on native renal function.

I wish to express my gratitude to all the contributors for their excellent and willing cooperation. I have considered it good fortune indeed to have been associated with them in this undertaking. Finally, I would like to express my deep gratitude to my wife for her continuing support and encouragement in seeing this undertaking through to fruition.

Murray Epstein, M.D.
Miami, Florida

Chapter 1

RENAL SODIUM HANDLING IN LIVER DISEASE

MURRAY EPSTEIN, M.D., F.A.C.P.

Clinical Features
  Prevalence of Abnormal Renal Sodium Handling
  Do Compensated Cirrhotic Patients Have an
    Abnormality in Renal Sodium Handling?
  Etiology of Hepatic Disease as a Determinant of
    Renal Sodium Retention
Pathogenesis
Afferent Events
  Diminished Effective Volume (Traditional Underfill
    Theory)
  Peripheral Arterial Vasodilation (Revised Underfill
    Theory)
  Overflow Theory
Efferent Factors
  Sites of Sodium Reabsorption
  Hyperaldosteronism
  Renin-Angiotensin System
  Renal Prostaglandins

Kallikrein-Kinin System
Humoral Natriuretic Factor
Atrial Natriuretic Peptides (Auriculin, ANF, ANP)
Renal Natriuretic Peptide (Urodilatin)
Brain Natriuretic Peptide
Sympathetic Nervous System Activity
Endothelins
Nitric Oxide
Redistribution of Renal Blood Flow
Endogenous Opioids
Estrogen
Prolactin
Vasoactive Intestinal Peptide
Why Ascites Predominates in Liver Disease
**Recommendations for Medical Therapy of Ascites
  and Edema**
Basic Management
Conclusion

*When the liver is full of fluid and this overflows into the peritoneal cavity, so that
the belly becomes full of water, death follows.*

Hippocrates, ca. 400 B.C.[1]

The clinical course of patients with decompensated Laënnec's cirrhosis is complicated frequently by progressive impairment of renal sodium handling, leading to the formation of ascites and peripheral edema. Such involvement of the kidney in cirrhosis has been known for many years. As early as 1685, John Brown recorded the association of edema and ascites in a patient with nodular cirrhosis.[2] Although interest in this defect was evinced sporadically during the subsequent 250 years, it was reawakened in the 1940s and 1950s. Initially, several groups of investigators documented the avid sodium retention and resultant positive sodium balances encountered in many cirrhotic patients.[3–5] Subsequently, attempts were made to delineate further the abnormalities of renal sodium handling by assessing the renal excretory response to an acutely administered sodium chloride load.[6,7] It was demonstrated that many cirrhotic patients were unable to excrete such a load at a normal rate,[6] although this finding is not universal.[7] Finally, additional investigations succeeded in documenting the absence or frank reversal of the normal diurnal excretory rhythm for sodium in decompensated cirrhosis.[8,9]

Despite extensive studies delineating the derangement in renal sodium handling, the mediating mechanisms remain incompletely defined. Until recently the majority of investigations have focused on the importance of hyperaldosteronism in mediating the sodium retention of cirrhosis, largely to the exclusion of other hormonal effectors. The past decade has witnessed a resurgence of interest in the investigation of renal sodium handling in liver disease, reassessing the putative predominance of hyperaldosteronism in mediating this abnormality. Furthermore, increased attention has been devoted to nonmineralocorticoid factors, including the role of renal prostaglandins, renal sympathetic activity, and other vasoactive substances. This chapter reviews the role of renal sodium handling in liver disease and the reappraisal of our thinking with regard to this abnormality in the light of recent findings from several laboratories.

A brief consideration of the clinical features of deranged sodium homeostasis is followed by a review of the pathophysiology of sodium retention. This review is organized into two major sections: the first deals with "afferent" events and the second with "efferent" mechanisms. This arbitrary approach does not presuppose that either the afferent or efferent events responsible for the deranged sodium homeostasis of liver disease are completely defined. Rather, the intention is to provide an organizational framework to permit the reader to approach more easily the numerous and seemingly isolated events that characterize cirrhosis and that may contribute to the sodium retention encountered clinically. Finally, although my original intent was to survey the aberrations of sodium homeostasis in liver disease of diverse etiology, it became readily apparent that the review must be limited largely to cirrhosis because of the paucity of information about this subject in other hepatic conditions in humans.

CLINICAL FEATURES

Patients with Laënnec's cirrhosis manifest a remarkable capacity for sodium chloride retention; indeed, they frequently excrete urine that is virtually free of sodium.[3-5] The result is excessive accumulation of extracellular fluid that eventually becomes evident as clinically detectable ascites and edema. Cirrhotic patients who are unable to excrete sodium continue to gain weight and accumulate ascites and edema as long as the dietary sodium content exceeds maximal urinary sodium excretion. If access to sodium is not curtailed, the relentless retention of sodium may lead to the accumulation of vast amounts of ascites (on occasion up to 28 L) (Fig. 1.1). By contrast, weight gain and ascites formation cease when sodium intake is markedly limited.

Prevalence of Abnormal Renal Sodium Handling

Determining the prevalence of renal functional abnormalities in liver disease is extremely difficult.

For the most part, we lack detailed or complete epidemiologic information and, in other instances, available data are fragmentary and reflect a particular interest of a group of investigators. In the absence of adequate denominator data, and with variable definitions of the numerator, one can only surmise the frequency with which deranged sodium homeostasis occurs. Nevertheless, recent reports have suggested that renal sodium retention in liver disease is a frequent occurrence. It has been suggested that renal failure may occur in 50–75% of patients dying of cirrhosis. Since ascites is thought to precede the development of hepatorenal syndrome, extrapolation of these data suggests that renal sodium retention constitutes a frequent complication of cirrhosis.

Do Compensated Cirrhotic Patients Have an Abnormality in Renal Sodium Handling?

Whether patients with well-compensated cirrhosis have an abnormality in renal sodium handling before the development of cirrhosis has been investigated only recently in a systematic fashion. These studies have focused on interventions that could unmask abnormalities in renal function and their vasoactive hormones.

Initially, Naccarato et al.[10] assessed this defect in early cirrhosis. The investigators assessed the natriuretic response to acute saline administration in cirrhotic patients who had manifested no evidence of ascites or edema. The absence of ascites was confirmed by laparoscopic examination. Following extracellular volume expansion (ECVE), both absolute and fractional sodium excretion was diminished compared with the values of normal subjects undergoing an identical study. Thus it is apparent that the defect in renal sodium handling may occur early in the course of cirrhosis.

Recently, Simón et al.[11] assessed whether dietary sodium restriction could unmask changes in vasoactive hormones and systemic hemodynamics. They investigated the renal, circulatory, and hormonal responses to dietary sodium restriction in patients with compensated cirrhosis. Mean arterial pressure (MAP), sympathetic nervous activity, and proximal sodium reabsorption were evaluated in 16 healthy control subjects and 21 nonazotemic cirrhotic patients under two experimental conditions: after 4 days on an unrestricted sodium diet and after 4 days on a restricted sodium diet (40 mmol/day). Cirrhotic patients without ascites did not differ from controls under basal conditions. In contrast, cirrhotic patients with ascites manifested lower basal MAP and higher basal levels of plasma norepinephrine and fractional proximal sodium reabsorption than control subjects. In response to sodium restriction, however, nonascitic patients differed from controls by manifesting an elevation in plasma norepinephrine and in fractional proximal sodium reabsorption. In addition, the nonascitic cirrhotic patients became hypotensive compared with controls when subjected to the low sodium diet. The investigators interpreted their studies as indicating (1) that cirrhotic patients without ascites have an enhanced sensitivity to sodium restriction, presumably as a consequence of reduction in effective arterial volume, and (2) that this response can be unmasked only by interventions such as sodium restriction.

Wood et al.[12] assessed the response to acute saline loading in 14 well-compensated, cirrhotic patients and 6 normal controls. The cirrhotic patients had biopsy-proven alcoholic cirrhosis but no evidence of ascites, edema, or encephalopathy. Following equilibration on a 100-mmol sodium diet, an intravenous infusion of 2 L of normal saline was administered over 1 hour. Glomerular filtration rate (GFR) and renal plasma flow (RPF) were assessed by [^{3}H]inulin clearance and p-aminohippurate clearance, respectively, at hourly intervals over the entire study period. At 3 hours after infusion urinary sodium excretion in cirrhotic patients (199 ± 141 pmol/min) was significantly lower than in controls (387 ± 104 pmol/min; p < 0.01). In contrast to controls, renal plasma flow and glomerular filtration rate did not increase in the cirrhotics in response to acute saline loading. Cirrhotic subjects with impaired functional liver cell mass, as assessed by antipyrine clearance, were unable to modulate proximal tubular reabsorption. Whereas the natriuresis in the control group was accompanied by a significant increase in GFR and RPF by the second hour after infusion, cirrhotic patients were unable to augment GFR or RPF in response to saline administration.

Wood et al.[12] also measured hepatic vein pressure gradient, indocyanine green extraction ratio, indocyanine green clearance, and antipyrine clearance as indices of portal pressure, intrahepatic shunting, hepatic blood flow, and functional hepatocellular mass, respectively. Urinary sodium

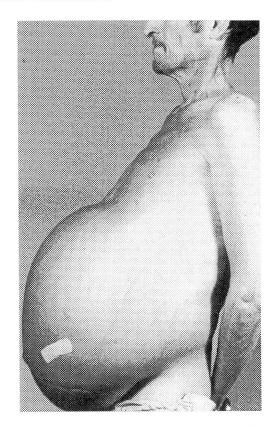

FIGURE 1.1.   An example of marked ascites in a patient with advanced cirrhosis of the liver.

excretion in cirrhotic patients correlated strongly with antipyrine clearance (r = 0.839, p < 0.0001) and weakly with portal pressure (r = 0.562, p = 0.037). No correlation was seen with the other indices of hepatic blood flow and shunting.

The abnormality of renal sodium handling in cirrhosis is not a static and unalterable condition. Rather, cirrhotic patients may undergo a spontaneous diuresis followed by a return to avid salt retention.[13,14] Although a considerable number of patients who are maintained on a sodium-restricted diet may demonstrate a spontaneous diuresis, information about the frequency with which this occurs is inadequate. A report by Bosch et al.[15] has suggested that a spontaneous diuresis occurs in one-third of patients with cirrhosis and ascites in response to bed rest and dietary sodium restriction. The severity and reversibility of the liver disease appear to be determinants of such a favorable response. Patients who have *reversible* liver disease, such as those with alcohol-induced fatty liver, also tend to respond favorably to abstinence from alcohol, bed rest, and a nutritious diet low in sodium.

Although ascites is often viewed as an indicator of decompensated hepatic disease, this caveat is not always true. The onset of ascites often is related directly to increased sodium intake and is more a reflection of salt loading than of progressive alterations in hepatic function with consequent renal changes. Occasionally a history of increased intake of salted foods in the period before the development of ascites can be elicited, whereas other patients resort to the use of sodium-containing remedies such as antacids. If a history of recent increased sodium intake is elicited, spontaneous natriuresis often occurs when dietary sodium intake is restricted. Female patients with liver disease who develop significant ascites and edema premenstrually may undergo a significant diuresis following the prescription of a sodium-restricted diet, the onset of which coincides with the onset of menstrual flow.

Finally, it cannot be overemphasized that the primary renal excretory abnormality causing fluid retention is a disturbance of sodium rather than of water excretion. Many sodium-retaining patients with ascites and edema can excrete urine of low osmolality when given excessive amounts of water without sodium.[13,16,17] Nevertheless, when sodium is administered, it is not excreted.

Like other chronic diseases, cirrhosis of the liver has an evolutionary, alternating pattern with differing manifestations during different stages of the pathologic process. We were fortunate to have had the opportunity to follow prospectively the clinical status, renal sodium handling, plasma renin activity (PRA), and plasma aldosterone (PA) levels in several patients with advanced liver disease for a prolonged period. During this time their clinical course waxed and waned and was characterized by periods of transition from decompensation (presence of ascites and/or edema) to compensation and return to decompensation. Renal sodium handling, assessed by the peak natriuretic response to a volume expansive maneuver, i.e., water immersion, did not correlate closely with the magnitude of ascites. Such observations underscore the potential futility of prognosticating or drawing definite inferences from the patient's clinical status alone at any single point in time. Implicit in such a formulation is the poor relationship between the presence or absence of "compensation", as defined clinically, and the impairment of renal sodium handling, as measured functionally. It is not possible to predict the presence or magnitude of the impairment of renal sodium handling in the cirrhotic patient merely on the basis of the absence of ascites or edema or both.

Etiology of Hepatic Disease as a Determinant of Renal Sodium Retention

In contrast to patients with Laënnec's cirrhosis in whom renal sodium retention is common, patients with primary biliary cirrhosis (PBC) do not appear to manifest this abnormality. Chaimovitz et al.[18] assessed the natriuretic and diuretic response to extracellular volume expansion (ECVE) in five patients with PBC. Despite conspicuous evidence of portal hypertension, ascites and edema were absent. The investigators demonstrated that the natriuretic and diuretic response exceeded that observed in both healthy normal volunteers and in edema-free patients with Laënnec's cirrhosis. The authors suggested that a common mechanism may underlie both the augmented natriuretic response to volume expansion in patients with PBC and the rarity of fluid retention in this type of cirrhosis.[18] The reasons why PBC and Laënnec's cirrhosis, with comparable portal hypertension, manifest markedly different responses to volume expansion require additional study.

PATHOGENESIS

Despite extensive study, the mechanisms mediating the sodium retention of cirrhotic patients remain incompletely defined. Until recently the focus has been mainly on the importance of hyperaldosteronism, largely to the exclusion of other hormonal effectors. The past several years have witnessed a resurgence of interest in the reassessment of the putative predominance of hyperaldosteronism in mediating this abnormality. Increased attention has been devoted to nonmineralocorticoid factors, including alterations of renal prostaglandins and other vasoactive substances. The following section reviews the reappraisal of current thinking about deranged renal sodium handling in the light of recent findings.

An examination of the pathogenetic events leading to the deranged sodium homeostasis of cirrhosis is simplified by a consideration of afferent and efferent events. A discussion of afferent events usually includes consideration of the detector element responsible for the recognition of the degree of volume alterations as well as a consideration of the extracellular fluid translocations

Theories of Ascites Formation in Cirrhosis

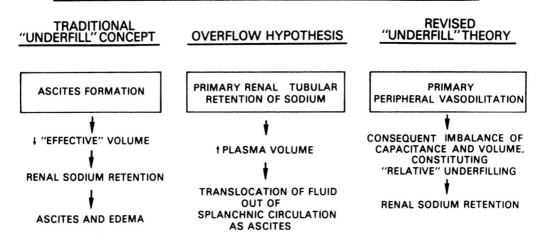

| TRADITIONAL "UNDERFILL" CONCEPT | OVERFLOW HYPOTHESIS | REVISED "UNDERFILL" THEORY |

FIGURE 1.2. Presumed sequence of events eventuating in ascites formation, according to three alternative theories: the traditional underfill theory, the overflow theory, and the revised underfill theory. The primary events are shown within the *rectangular boxes*. According to the traditional underfill theory, the primary event is a diminution in effective volume attributable to the development of abnormal Starling forces in the portal circulation with a maldistribution of circulating volume. This diminished effective volume constitutes an afferent signal to the renal tubule to augment renal salt and water reabsorption. In contrast, the overflow theory holds that retention of excessive sodium by the kidneys is the primary event. In the setting of abnormal Starling forces in the portal venous bed, the expanded plasma volume is sequestered preferentially in the peritoneal sac with ascites formation. The most recent theory, which has been termed the peripheral arterial vasodilation theory, holds that the diminished effective volume is attributable to primary peripheral vasodilitation with a consequent imbalance of capacitance and volume.

or sequestration into serous spaces or interstitial fluid compartments that characterize advanced liver disease. Because the afferent perturbations that supervene in advanced liver disease have been reviewed in depth,[19–21] this discussion reviews only briefly the concepts of a diminished effective volume and the overflow theory of ascites formation. Greater emphasis is placed on the efferent events that mediate sodium retention.

AFFERENT EVENTS

Diminished Effective Volume (Traditional Underfill Theory)

The concept of effective volume was proposed by John Peters in 1935.[22] Peters suggested not only that the volume of the circulating blood was an important determinant of urinary sodium excretion, but specifically that the *distribution* of this volume was important. This concept of a diminished effective volume constitutes a linchpin for the traditional underfill theory.

Traditionally, ascites formation in cirrhotic patients is considered to begin when a critical

imbalance of Starling forces (i.e., increased portal pressure, decreased colloid oncotic pressure) develops in the hepatic sinusoids and splanchnic capillaries. As a result of this imbalance, the amount of lymph formation exceeds the capacity that the thoracic duct can return to the circulation.[23,24] Consequently, lymph accumulates in the peritoneal space as ascites. As ascites increases, there is progressive redistribution of plasma volume with subsequent contraction of the effective plasma volume (i.e., the part of total circulating volume that appears to stimulate volume receptors).

Regardless of cause, the diminution of effective plasma volume is believed to constitute an afferent signal to the renal tubule to augment salt and water reabsorption. Thus, the traditional underfill formulation suggests that the renal retention of sodium is a *secondary* rather than primary event (Fig. 1.2).

Peripheral Arterial Vasodilation (Revised Underfill) Theory

The principal distinguishing feature of a newly proposed revision of the underfill theory is that the decrease in effective blood volume is attributable

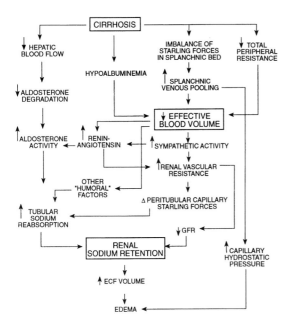

FIGURE 1.3. Factors operative in the traditional or underfill theory of sodium retention in cirrhosis. As can be seen, an imbalance of Starling forces in the hepatosplanchnic microcirculation is not the sole mechanism. Acting in concert, these factors promote a reduction in effective plasma volume.

primarily to an early increase in vascular capacitance.[25] Thus, peripheral vasodilation is the initial determinant of intravascular underfilling, and an imbalance between the expanded capacitance and available volume constitutes a diminished effective volume (see Fig. 1.2). This concept brings the hypothesis into accord with experimental observations that were not consistent with the original postulate. For example, recent careful balance studies in animals with experimental cirrhosis have shown clearly that sodium retention precedes ascites formation.[26,27]

Primary systemic hemodynamic changes characterized by peripheral vasodilation with a secondary increase in cardiac output occur early in experimental cirrhosis and in humans with compensated cirrhosis.[26–30] The decrease in effective volume induced by these hemodynamic alterations is compounded further by an impaired pressor response to vasoactive agents, including exogenous angiotensin II and noradrenaline.[31] Even in patients who eventually develop an increase in total plasma volume, the relative fullness of the arteriovenous tree is decreased.

Total peripheral resistance is diminished significantly in most edematous cirrhotic patients

and in animals with toxic cirrhosis[26,27] or with bile duct ligation[30] (Fig. 1.3). There is no doubt that the diminution of total peripheral resistance in cirrhotic patients is related partially to vasodilation and a consequent increase in vascular capacity. Indeed, when widely developed, such vascular changes may assume the proportion of arteriovenous shunts.[28,29] It has been proposed that some undefined endogenous vasodilator (either produced by or not inactivated by the diseased liver) plays a role.

Both underfill theories provide a possible explanation of why fluid retention often fails to attenuate the stimulus for neurohormonal activation and the continuing sodium and water retention. Despite a progressive increase in total extracellular fluid volume, fluid is sequestered into one or more of the other fluid compartments without normalizing effective blood volume. Because the capacity of the interstitial fluid (ISF) and its associated spaces—for example the peritoneum—is largely limitless, the kidneys encounter great difficulty in filling such a space and the sodium retention becomes relentless. Only correction of the disturbance in the forces governing fluid distribution and reversing the peripheral arterial vasodilatation will permit a reexpansion of effective blood volume to normal. Importantly, the peripheral arterial vasodilation theory highlights the florid systemic hemodynamic disturbances and the importance of attempting to correct not only the renal hemodynamic disturbances but also the concomitant systemic hemodynamic derangements.

An alternate formulation has emphasized that the renal vasoconstriction is attributable to unique events independent of a contracted volume, i.e., a primary cause. According to this theory, advanced liver damage, in conjunction with some other unknown abnormality, induces a primary disorder in one or more of the modifiers that regulate renal vascular tone. The renal ischemia, it is argued, is not an expression of the normal neural and hormonal response to liver damage; rather, it represents either an alteration in the synthesis, degradation, or potency of a vasoactive substance or a malfunction of the normal feedback regulation of its release. Such abnormalities might result from impaired hepatic degradative or excretory capacity, portosystemic shunting of blood, or altered neural connections between the liver and the kidney.

The mechanisms mediating the peripheral vasodilation remain incompletely defined. Recent studies[32] have suggested that peripheral vasodilation may be attributable in part to a potential derangement of α_1-adrenoreceptors with decreased sensitivity to pressors such as norepinephrine. Alternatively, the arteriolar vasodilation and hyperdynamic circulation may be attributable to an overproduction of nitric oxide (NO) by the vascular endothelium (see chapter 17).

Overflow Theory

Twenty-five years ago, Lieberman and associates[33,34] proposed an alternative hypothesis to the two underfill theories: the overflow theory of ascites formation, which postulates that the initial *primary* event is the inappropriate retention of excessive amounts of sodium by the kidneys (see Fig. 1.2). In the setting of abnormal Starling forces in the portal venous bed and hepatic sinusoids (both portal venous hypertension and a reduction in plasma colloid osmotic pressure), the expanded plasma volume is sequestered preferentially in the peritoneal space, with ascites formation. Thus, renal sodium retention and plasma volume expansion *precede rather than follow* the formation of ascites (see Fig. 1.2).

The overflow theory of ascites formation has engendered much controversy. Demonstrations that plasma volume is increased in cirrhosis with ascites and that a spontaneous diuresis and natriuresis have occurred independently of measurable changes in the volume of the nonsplanchnic vascular compartment have been cited as supportive evidence. Additional support derives from a series of elegant investigations by Levy[27,35,36] in dogs with portal cirrhosis produced by the feeding of dimethylnitrosamine. Levy demonstrated in sequential studies that renal sodium retention is the initial event that precedes ascites formation. Also, elimination of ascites in cirrhotic dogs with the LeVeen shunt did not prevent sodium retention during liberal sodium intake.[36] Together these studies support the view that the initiating event in the renal sodium retention of cirrhosis is not related to underfilling. A cautionary note has been sounded, however; an important, albeit undetectable, increase in vascular capacity (i.e., peripheral vasodilatation) may have initiated the early sodium retention.[37]

To assess the relative importance of the underfilling vs. the overflow hypothesis in mediating the sodium retention of cirrhosis, Decaux et al.[38,39] recently studied the relationship between fractional excretion (FE) of sodium, urea, and uric acid. Their initial study demonstrated a significant increase in the clearance of urea and uric acid, which they attributed to an increase in effective vascular volume.[38] Subsequently, they investigated 60 cirrhotic patients without azotemia.[39] Like patients with the syndrome of inappropriate secretion of antidiuretic hormone (SIADH), cirrhotic patients with high FE uric acid have raised FE urea only when salt excretion is low. It is believed that the low salt excretion is not caused by a decrease in effective intravascular volume and that this is increased in cirrhotic patients with raised FE uric acid. Although their interpretation may be correct, it is also possible that the changes in clearances represented, at least in part, primary defects of renal tubular function.

Although the above observations collectively support the overflow theory of ascites formation, a number of clinical observations in humans are inconsistent with such a theory. Thus, rapid volume expansion with exogenous solutions (including saline, mannitol, and albumin) and ascitic fluid frequently results in a transient improvement in renal sodium and water handling.[26,40,41] Similarly, infusion of metaraminol to counteract the peripheral vasodilatation induces natriuresis.[42] Finally, normalization of Starling forces by surgical decompression of the portal bed in certain patients with cirrhosis may be associated with mobilization of ascites, improvement in renal function, and natriuresis.[43] Of note, all of these maneuvers may overcome the circulatory disturbance without improving the function of the cirrhotic liver.

Nevertheless, the fact that several of the utilized maneuvers nonspecifically increase the volume of all fluid compartments—and the presumed concomitant alterations in plasma composition—has precluded definitive statements about the etiologic role of a diminished effective plasma volume. Thus the results of many earlier studies must be considered inconclusive because of the confounding effects of the experimental designs.

Studies from our laboratory over the past 27 years have circumvented many of the experimental problems by applying a unique investigative tool, the water immersion model, to the assessment of renal function and volume hormonal relationships in diverse edematous disorders.[44–47] It may be useful to describe briefly the salient features of the model (Table 1.1) and to underscore

TABLE 1.1. Salient Features of the Model of Head-out Water Immersion

1. Immersion produces a *prompt* redistribution of circulating blood volume with a relative central hypervolemia.

2. Cardiac output is increased by 25–33% and central blood volume by approximately 700 ml.

3. The alterations in central hemodynamics are *sustained* throughout a 4-hr immersion period and promptly reversible after cessation of immersion.

4. Immersion-induced central hypervolemia is associated with profound and progressive natriuresis and diuresis. These alterations are promptly reversible after cessation of immersion.

5. The central hemodynamic and renal effects of immersion are equal in magnitude to those induced by acute saline administration (2 L of saline/2 hr).

6. The alterations in renal sodium, potassium, and water handling in the sodium-replete state (the only condition as yet studied) occur in the absence of changes in renal plasma flow and glomerular filtration rate.

7. Immersion is associated with prompt and profound (approximately two-thirds) suppression of plasma renin activity (PRA) and plasma aldosterone (PA). Cessation of immersion is associated with prompt return of both PRA and PA to prestudy levels.

8. Immersion induces prompt, marked, and sustained augmentation of atrial natriuretic factor (ANF). Cessation of immersion is associated with prompt return of ANF to prestudy levels.

9. The above alterations in renal function, renin-aldosterone, and ANF responsiveness occur in the absence of changes in plasma composition.

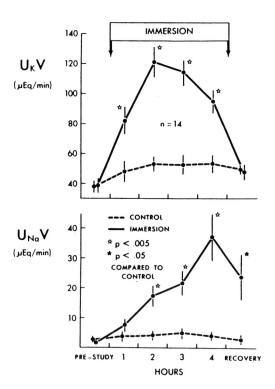

FIGURE 1.4. Effect of water immersion to the neck following 1 hr of quiet sitting (prestudy) on rate of sodium excretion ($U_{Na}V$) and potassium excretion (U_KV) in 14 normal subjects in balance on a 10 mEq Na/100 mEq K diet. Immersion was associated with prompt and progressive increase in $U_{Na}V$ throughout immersion. Recovery was associated with a return toward prestudy levels, although $U_{Na}V$ continued to exceed both control and prestudy values. The natriuresis was accompanied by a profound kaliuresis throughout immersion.

the differences between water immersion and more traditional attempts to achieve ECVE, such as saline administration.

Head-out water immersion of a patient in the seated posture results in a prompt redistribution of blood volume with a sustained increase in central blood volume.[44–48] Furthermore, studies of the efferent limb of immersion have demonstrated a marked natriuretic and kaliuretic response during immersion (Fig. 1.4). It also has been demonstrated that the natriuretic and kaliuretic response is indistinguishable from that of saline administration (2 L/120 min) in normal subjects, assuming an identical seated posture.[46] Although water immersion constitutes a potent means of inducing central volume expansion comparable with infusion of isotonic saline, it is capable of circumventing many of the problems associated with the infusion of exogenous volume expanders:

1. Water immersion is associated with a decrease in body weight rather than the increase that attends saline infusion.

2. The volume stimulus of immersion is promptly reversible after cessation of immersion, whereas the hypervolemia that follows saline administration is relatively sustained and thus helps to minimize risk to the patient.

3. The volume stimulus of immersion occurs in the absence of changes in plasma composition.[44–47]

The delineation of the immersion model and the demonstration that it constitutes a potent central volume stimulus without the necessity of infusing exogenous volume expanders commended

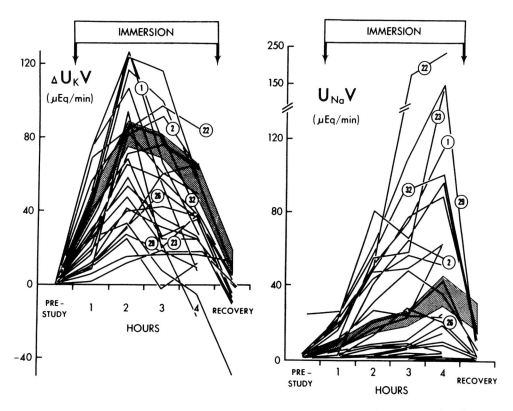

FIGURE 1.5 Effects of water immersion after 1 hr of quiet sitting (prestudy) on rate of sodium excretion ($U_{Na}V$) and potassium excretion (U_KV) in a large group of patients with alcoholic liver disease. The *circled numbers* represent individual patients. Data for U_KV are expressed in terms of absolute changes from prestudy hour (ΔU_KV). The *shaded area* represents the mean ± SE for 14 normal control subjects undergoing an identical immersion study while ingesting an identical 10 mEq Na/100 mEq K/day diet. Over half of the cirrhotic patients manifested an appropriate or exaggerated natriuretic response. In general, the increase in $U_{Na}V$ was associated with a concomitant increase in ΔU_KV.

its use in assessing the role of alterations of effective plasma volume in the derangements of renal sodium homeostasis in cirrhosis.

Studies in 32 patients with decompensated cirrhosis demonstrated a striking normalization of renal sodium handling after water immersion, which resulted in marked natriuresis and kaliuresis in the majority of patients. (Fig. 1.5) During the final hour of immersion, the rate of sodium excretion ($U_{Na}V$) was 20-fold greater than it was during the prestudy hour. Thus, the marked antinatriuresis of cirrhosis was reversed promptly by a manipulation that merely altered the distribution of plasma volume without increasing (and often decreasing) total plasma volume. Indeed, in many instances the natriuresis of such patients exceeded markedly the response manifested by normal subjects to the same procedure. Together these studies strongly support the concept that a diminished effective

intravascular volume is a major determinant of the enhanced tubular reabsorption of sodium in cirrhosis.

Further evidence that the immersion-induced natriuretic response is indeed supportive of a role for diminished effective volume and not merely an appropriate response comparable to that of normal subjects can be adduced from the concomitant changes in creatinine clearance (C_{Cr}) during immersion.[19,48] In marked contrast to the findings in normal controls,[44] immersion was associated with significant increments in C_{Cr} in a majority of cirrhotic patients.[19] Two-thirds of the cirrhotic patients manifested increments in C_{Cr} (3- to 5-fold) that exceeded markedly the increments observed in sodium-depleted normal subjects. These observations suggest that immersion tends to normalize the diminished effective volume of cirrhotic humans with a resultant normalization of renal vascular tone.

Studies by Henriksen et al.[48a,48b] have provided further support for the concept of a reduced effective blood volume. The authors demonstrated that the estimated central blood volume (ECBV; i.e., blood volume in the heart cavities, lungs and central arterial tree) is decreased in patients with cirrhosis.[48a] More recently they assessed the relationship between ECBV, systemic and portal hemodynamics, and markers of overall and renal sympathetic nervous activity.[48b] They measured the ECBV and the circulating and renal venous levels of norepinephrine, arterial epinephrine, and atrial natriuretic factor (ANF) before and after β-adrenergic blockade in patients with cirrhosis and esophageal varices who were undergoing hemodynamic investigation. They observed that the arterial norepinephrine level, an index of overall sympathetic nervous activity, was negatively correlated with ECBV. Similarly, renal venous norepinephrine level (an index of renal sympathetic tone) was inversely correlated with ECBV. They proposed the following formulation to explain their findings: reduced ECBV probably "unloads" volume receptors and baroreceptors, thus enhancing overall and renal sympathetic nervous activity and contributing to increased renal salt and water retention in cirrhosis. During β-adrenergic blockade ECBV changes correlated with alterations in preload and afterload. These findings indicate that central circulatory and arterial underfilling is a key element of the hemodynamic derangement in patients with decompensated cirrhosis.

Although the presently available evidence favors a prominent role for diminished effective volume in mediating the avid sodium retention of many cirrhotic patients, the theories of diminished effective volume and overflow may not be mutually exclusive. As noted above, cirrhosis is not a static disease, but rather a constantly evolving clinical disorder. Yet virtually all of the available clinical studies of deranged sodium homeostasis were carried out at a single stage of the disease—when decompensation was well established. Little information was gathered during the incipient stage of sodium retention. In contrast, the studies with the canine cirrhosis model deal with the relatively early stage of sodium retention. Any formulation that suggests that the same antinatriuretic forces are operative throughout the evolution of sodium retention in cirrhotic humans is probably a marked oversimplification. Rather, one should adopt a more global view of

the pathogenesis of abnormal sodium retention in cirrhosis in which differing forces participate in varying degrees as the derangement in sodium homeostasis evolves.

EFFERENT FACTORS

The initial attempts to explain the abnormalities of renal sodium handling focused on the decrement in glomerular filtration rate (GFR) that occurs frequently in patients with advanced liver disease. A number of observations indicate, however, that a decrease in GFR cannot constitute the major determinant of the abnormalities in renal sodium handling. Sodium retention occurs often despite preserved GFR. Furthermore, avid sodium reabsorption has been observed even in the face of supranormal GFR.[13,19,49]

Sites of Sodium Reabsorption

Although the weight of evidence demonstrates that the renal sodium retention accompanying cirrhosis is attributable primarily to enhanced tubular reabsorption rather than to alterations in the filtered load of sodium, the precise nephron sites that are operative remain controversial. Most available evidence has suggested that the avid reabsorption of filtrate along the proximal tubule is largely responsible for the sodium retention of cirrhosis.[13,40,41,50] Subsequently, however, several investigators have emphasized the importance of excessive sodium reabsorption at more distal sites.[49,51]

We carried out additional studies in 18 cirrhotic patients to elucidate further the nephron sites responsible for enhanced tubular reabsorption of sodium.[51] Because changes in phosphate clearance may provide an index of proximal sodium reabsorption, we undertook to characterize the effects of an immersion-induced volume expansion on renal sodium and phosphate handling. Cirrhotic patients manifested a wide continuum of responses characterized by either a sluggish or barely discernible natriuretic response (group I) or an appropriate natriuretic response (group II) (Fig. 1.6). Despite widely varying natriuretic responses, group I patients manifested a phosphaturic response to immersion that was virtually identical to that of group II patients. We believe that our findings are consistent with the formulation that alterations of distal sodium reabsorption contribute importantly to the sodium content of the final urine in cirrhotic patients with sodium retention. Such observations, however, do not militate against a major role for enhanced proximal tubular reabsorption of sodium; rather, they suggest that enhanced reabsorption at both sites contributes to varying degrees in most decompensated cirrhotic patients.

Because both traditional clearance methods and phosphate clearances have inherent pitfalls,[52] several investigators have used lithium clearances as a means of assessing the tubular sites that mediate sodium reabsorption. As detailed in several reviews,[53,54] lithium clearances have been used as an index of proximal tubular sodium handling. Micropuncture studies have disclosed that lithium is reabsorbed in parallel with sodium and water in the proximal tubule and that it is not reabsorbed in the distal tubule when fractional sodium excretion exceeds 0.4%, thus confirming the validity of lithium clearance as a marker of proximal tubular function.[55]

Angeli et al.[56] used lithium clearances to evaluate renal tubular sodium handling in 27 nonazotemic cirrhotic patients with ascites and positive sodium balance and in 17 controls. Lithium clearance was used as an index of fluid delivery to the distal tubule. There was a correlation between lithium clearance and sodium clearance only in cirrhotic patients (r = 0.62; p < 0.01). Distal sodium reabsorption evaluated as a percent of filtered sodium load was lower in cirrhotics than in controls (19.1 ± 1.0 vs. 22.4 ± 1.2%; p < 0.05). The investigators interpreted their findings as indicating that a decrease in filtered sodium load and an increase in proximal sodium reabsorption play a major role in the impairment of renal sodium handling in nonazotemic cirrhotic patients with ascites.

Díez et al.[57] also used lithium clearance to calculate proximal and distal sodium reabsorption in a large group of normal control subjects (n = 21) and cirrhotic patients with ascites (n = 24). Patients were studied following 4 days on a sodium-restricted diet. Fractional lithium clearance was lower in the cirrhotic patients than in controls (7.4 ± 0.9 vs. 18.1 ± 1.8%; p <0.001). Fractional proximal sodium reabsorption was increased in cirrhotic patients compared with controls. Although no differences were found in fractional distal sodium reabsorption between the entire group of cirrhotic patients and controls, a subanalysis disclosed changes. When patients were separated into two subgroups according to

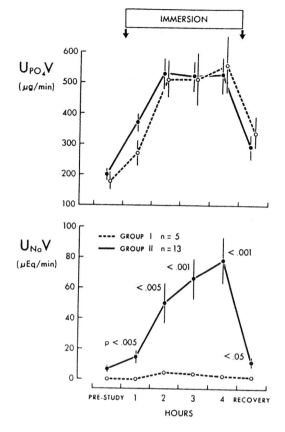

FIGURE 1.6. Effect of water immersion on the rate of phosphate excretion ($U_{PO_4}V$, *upper panel*) and sodium excretion ($U_{Na}V$, *lower panel*) in 18 cirrhotic patients. Immersion resulted in a marked and progressive phosphaturia in group I patients that was virtually identical with that in group II patients. In contrast to the identical phosphaturic responses, groups I and II manifested marked difference in renal sodium handling. Group I patients manifested a sluggish and barely discernible natriuretic response, whereas group II patients manifested a profound natriuretic response that exceeded that of normal control subjects undergoing an identical immersion study. Results are mean ± SE. (Reproduced with permission from Epstein M, Ramachandran M, DeNunzio AG: Interrelationships of renal sodium and phosphate handling in cirrhosis. Miner Electrolyte Metab 1982;7:305–315.)

their sodium balance, it was found that fractional distal sodium reabsorption was increased in patients whose balance remained positive compared with patients in a negative sodium balance. The authors concluded that proximal sodium reabsorption is increased in cirrhotics with ascites. In addition, distal sodium reabsorption is enhanced only in patients who exhibit avid sodium retention.

TABLE 1.2 Factors Influencing the Sodium
Retention of Liver Disease

Hormonal
   Hyperaldosteronism
   Possible role of renin-angiotensin system
   Alterations in renal prostaglandins
   Alterations in kallikrein-kinin system
   Humoral natriuretic factor
   Atrial natriuretic peptides
   Endothelins
   Nitric oxide
   Possible effects of estrogens
   Prolactin
   Vasoactive intestinal peptide
Neural and hemodynamic
   Alterations in intrarenal blood flow distribution
   Increase in sympathetic nervous system activity

The mediators of the enhanced tubular reabsorption of sodium in cirrhosis and their relative participation in the avid sodium retention have not been elucidated completely. Several hormonal, neural, and hemodynamic mechanisms have been suggested (Table 1.2). Mechanisms for which there is some evidence and their interrelationships are summarized schematically in Figure 1.7.

Hyperaldosteronism

Cirrhosis often is associated with increased levels of aldosterone in urine and plasma.[48,58–62]

The elevation of plasma aldosterone (PA) is attributable to increased adrenal secretion and decreased metabolic degradation of the hormone. The rate of hepatic degradation is related directly to hepatic blood flow, which is markedly decreased in patients with decompensated cirrhosis.

Nevertheless, the etiologic relationship between hyperaldosteronism and sodium retention is uncertain. Initially, many observers seized on this observation and proposed that aldosterone is a major determinant of sodium retention.[63] In contrast to this longheld traditional view, many lines of evidence have challenged the etiologic role of elevated PA levels in mediating the sodium retention of cirrhosis. First, the widely held view that PA levels are usually elevated in advanced liver disease is probably an oversimplification [61] (Fig. 1.8). Furthermore, increasing evidence demonstrates a dissociation between sodium excretion and PA in diverse clinical and experimental conditions, thereby challenging the predominance of elevated PA levels in mediating sodium retention in cirrhosis.[60–62]

Additional studies utilizing the immersion model complemented this formulation. Immersion studies were carried out during chronic aldosterone blockade.[64] We proposed that the

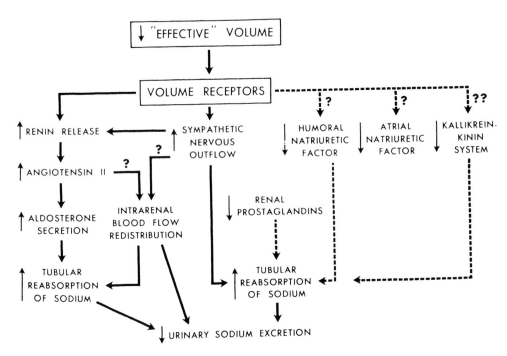

FIGURE 1.7.   Possible mechanisms whereby a diminished effective volume results in sodium retention. The *solid arrows* indicate pathways for which evidence is available. The *dashed lines* represent proposed pathways, the existence of which remains to be established.

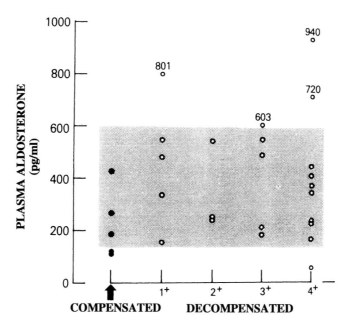

FIGURE 1.8. An assessment of the relationship between plasma aldosterone (PA) levels and degree of ascites accumulation in 28 cirrhotic patients. *Closed circles* indicate compensated (absence of ascites and edema) patients. *Open circles* indicate patients with varying degrees of ascites and/or edema. The *shaded area* subtends the mean ± 2 SD for 14 normal subjects studied under identical conditions of sodium and potassium intake, posture, and time of day. As can be seen, relatively few patients manifested increments in PA despite advanced liver disease and ascites accumulation. (Reproduced with permission from Epstein M: The Kidney in Liver Disease, 2nd ed. New York: Elsevier Biomedical, 1983, p 385.)

administration of spironolactone to patients undergoing both control and immersion studies would permit an assessment of the relative contribution of aldosterone to the changes in renal sodium, potassium, and water handling. It was demonstrated that spironolactone administration without immersion resulted in only a modest increase in sodium excretion (Fig. 1.9). If the encountered sodium retention was attributable to elevated aldosterone levels per se, one would have anticipated a significant natriuresis with spironolactone administration alone. In contrast, there was a marked increase in sodium excretion when immersion was carried out during chronic spironolactone administration, thereby indicating that the major contribution to the natriuresis was an enhanced distal delivery of filtrate. This explanation was supported by the documentation of a concomitant kaliuresis and an increase in free-water clearance.[64]

Finally, Epstein carried out immersion studies following acute desoxycorticosterone (DOCA) administration (10 mg intramuscularly) in a number of cirrhotic patients with ascites and edema (unpublished studies). Immersion induced a significant increase in sodium excretion despite the acute administration of pharmacologic doses of mineralocorticoid (Fig. 1.10), supporting the concept that the enhanced sodium reabsorption can occur independently of elevated circulating aldosterone levels.

More compelling evidence against a predominant role for aldosterone derives from immersion studies kinetically assessing the relationship of PA responsiveness to renal sodium handling.[48] Despite suppression in PA to comparable nadir levels in 16 cirrhotic patients, half of the patients manifested absent or blunted natriuretic responses during immersion.[48] This demonstration of a dissociation between the suppression of circulating aldosterone and the absence of a natriuresis lends strong support to the interpretation that aldosterone is not the primary determinant of impaired sodium excretion in cirrhosis.

To the extent that differences in distal delivery of filtrate may account for the discrepancies between the magnitude of PA suppression and that of sodium excretion, a study by Nicholls et al.[65] is of interest. The investigators carried out water immersion studies with or without norepinephrine (NE) administration. The rationale of admin-

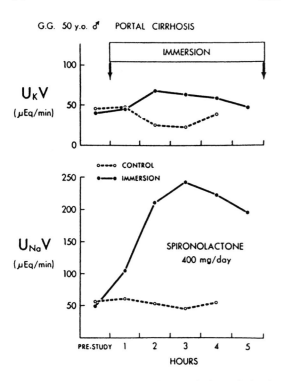

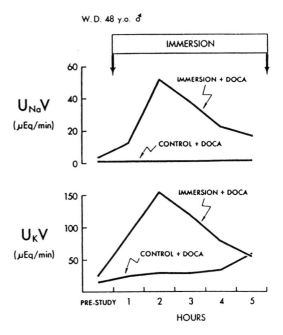

FIGURE 1.9. Representative study in a cirrhotic patient during chronic spironolactone administration (400 mg/day). The administration of spironolactone resulted in a modest increase in the rate of sodium excretion ($U_{Na}V$) during seated control (control + spironolactone) from 2 to 45–60 µEq/min. When the patient subsequently underwent immersion, there was a profound increase in $U_{Na}V$ from a prestudy value of 49 to a peak value of 242 µEq/min. Of note, the natriuresis was associated with a maintained or slightly increased rate of potassium excretion (U_KV) rather than the anticipated decrease. (Reprinted by permission from Epstein M, et al: Determinants of deranged sodium and water homeostasis in decompensated cirrhosis. J Lab Clin Med 1976;87: 822–839.)

istering the vasoconstrictor was to avoid a further diminution in peripheral vascular resistance in cirrhotic patients who are already vasodilated. They observed that the natriuresis of immersion varied inversely with the degree of PA suppression. Based on these observations, the authors proposed that aldosterone constitutes an important modulator of sodium excretion in cirrhotic patients with diminished effective blood volumes.

In summary, current evidence appears to favor the postulate that the hyperaldosteronism of cirrhosis may be a permissive factor only and that the major component of the abnormal renal sodium handling in many patients is a diminished distal

FIGURE 1.10. Representative study of a cirrhotic patient undergoing immersion after acute desoxycorticosterone (DOCA) administration (10 mg intramuscularly). During a seated control study after DOCA administration, the rate of sodium excretion ($U_{Na}V$) was approximately 1 µEq/min throughout the study. Immersion after DOCA administration resulted in a significant increase in $U_{Na}V$ from a prestudy value of 3 to 52 µEq/min by hour two. Concomitantly, the rate of potassium excretion (U_KV) rose progressively to 153 µEq/min during hour two of immersion, exceeding the preimmersion value of 25 µEq/min.

delivery of filtrate. Although it is apparent that additional studies correlating PA with sodium excretion during diverse experimental manipulations are indicated, caution in the interpretation of such data is necessary. The determinants of sodium excretion include not only the aldosterone levels acting at distal nephron sites, but also the extent of the delivery of filtrate to these sites. To interpret adequately the role of aldosterone, it is necessary to correlate aldosterone levels with sodium excretion corrected for distal delivery. The demonstration that hyperaldosteronism cannot account completely for sodium retention in cirrhosis has prompted a search for other hormonal mediators.

Renin-Angiotensin System

An attractive possibility to account in part for the sodium retention of cirrhosis is increased activity of the renin-angiotensin system in influencing renal sodium handling, which is independent of its ability to stimulate aldosterone secretion.

It is well established that the renin-angiotensin system is of major importance in the control of sodium homeostasis and extracellular fluid volume.[66] In addition to its effects on the peripheral circulation, the adrenal glands, and the nervous system, angiotensin II can directly influence renal hemodynamics and tubular reabsorptive function.[67,68] The ultimate sodium-conserving effect of angiotensin II appears to be orchestrated by a sequence of synergistic actions that include direct effects on tubular reabsorption rate as well as the more generally recognized actions on the microvasculature.

Even very low concentrations of angiotensin II stimulate proximal reabsorption rate. Elevated angiotensin II levels in the renal interstitium, effected either through increased delivery of angiotensin II via the circulation or through conversion of angiotensin I generated locally, can also enhance proximal reabsorption rate. With greater increases in interstitial angiotensin II concentration, reductions in glomerular pressure have been observed, demonstrating a powerful action on preglomerular arterioles that predominates over the well-known effects on efferent arterioles. At such higher doses, the hemodynamic actions of angiotensin II, together with the effects on the glomerular filtration coefficient, directly reduce filtered sodium load. Through synergistic effects on both tubular reabsorptive and hemodynamic function, angiotensin II can elicit sustained decreases in distal nephron sodium delivery that contribute greatly to its efficacy as a regulator of sodium excretion.[69]

Compelling evidence for the role of intrarenal angiotensin in mediating enhanced sodium reabsorption is derived from studies utilizing an inhibitor of angiotensin-converting enzyme in humans. Hollenberg et al.[70] demonstrated that the administration of teprotide (an inhibitor of angiotensin-converting enzyme) to patients with essential hypertension induced a significant natriuresis in every patient. Since the natriuresis occurred within as little as 20 minutes of teprotide administration, and since the offset in aldosterone's renal action is measured in hours, the natriuresis clearly occurred independently of a suppression in aldosterone.

If such a mechanism applies to cirrhotic humans, it is conceivable that the stimulated renin-angiotensin system in many patients with cirrhosis may contribute directly to impaired renal sodium handling. The subject of the renin-angiotensin system, its characterization utilizing pharmacological blockade, and its possible pathogenetic role in mediating abnormal renal function in liver disease are reviewed elsewhere in chapter 12.

Renal Prostaglandins and Renal Sodium Handling

The possibility that prostaglandins (PGs) participate in mediating the sodium retention of cirrhosis must be considered. Since several studies suggest the possibility that alterations in prostaglandin release may constitute a determinant of the natriuretic response to extracellular fluid volume expansion,[71] alterations in renal prostaglandin synthesis may contribute to derangements in renal sodium handling. Several studies demonstrate that the administration of inhibitors of prostaglandin synthetase to patients with decompensated cirrhosis results in profound decrements of renal hemodynamics, GFR, and sodium excretion.[72–74]

Since the above-cited studies have examined the effect of inhibiting endogenous production of renal prostaglandins, it was of great interest to assess an opposite experimental manipulation, i.e., augmentation of endogenous prostaglandins.[75] We utilized water immersion to the neck, which redistributes blood volume with concomitant central hypervolemia and enhances prostaglandin E (PGE) excretion in normal humans.[71] It was demonstrated that decompensated cirrhotic patients manifested an increase in mean PGE excretion that is 3-fold greater than that observed in normal subjects under identical conditions.[75] This is attended by a marked natriuresis and an increase in creatinine clearance. Thus, derangements in renal PGE production appear to contribute to the renal dysfunction of cirrhosis, including sodium retention. It is tempting to postulate that in the setting of cirrhosis of the liver, enhancement of PG synthesis is a compensatory or adaptive response to incipient renal ischemia. An important clinical corollary of this formulation is that the administration of agents that inhibit PG synthesis often results in clinically significant sodium retention and deterioration of renal function.[76]

It has been suggested that sulindac differs from other nonsteroidal antiinflammatory drugs by sparing renal but inhibiting systemic PGs.[77] This is reflected by the lack of an effect on urinary PGE_2 excretion and on other putative endpoints of renal PG synthesis such as renin release and response to furosemide, whereas inhibition of systemic PGs is reflected by the decreased production of thromboxane by platelets.[77] If such findings are extrapolated to cirrhotic patients, one might anticipate that sulindac would be associated with the lowest incidence of sodium retention. Despite impressive preliminary results, it is unsettled whether sulindac is indeed renal-sparing in cirrhotic patients. Indeed, Brater et al.[78] reported that sulindac did not differ from ibuprofen in its ability to decrease urinary PGE_2 and that both decreased the pharmacodynamics of response to furosemide. Daskalopoulos et al.[79] compared the effects of sulindac and indomethacin on furosemide-induced augmentation of PGE_2 and on renal sodium and water handling. Although only indomethacin reduced creatinine clearance, urinary volume, sodium, and PGE_2 prior to furosemide, these differences were virtually abolished following furosemide administration. That is, indomethacin appeared only slightly more potent in reducing the diuresis (55% vs. 38%), natriuresis (67% vs. 52%), and PGE_2 release (81% vs. 74%). Thus, under conditions of furosemide-enhanced prostaglandin activity, sulindac does affect renal function. To the extent that the ability to augment renal prostaglandin synthesis constitutes an important adaptive response in disorders characterized by decreased renal perfusion, the observations of Daskalopoulos et al.[79] merit attention. Additional studies are necessary to define the differences between sulindac and indomethacin in patients with cirrhosis, both under basal conditions and during maneuvers that alter (i.e., augment) renal PG production (see chapter 14).

Kallikrein-Kinin System

The possibility that the kallikrein-kinin system may contribute to the mediation of sodium retention of liver disease is raised by several preliminary reports of abnormalities of the plasma kallikrein system.[81] Since bradykinin has been suggested as a physiologic renal vasodilator,[80] it is possible that failure of bradykinin formation may contribute to the renal cortical vasoconstriction documented in patients with decompensated cirrhosis. The data so far are sparse but provocative.

Studies of the renal kallikrein-kinin system in cirrhosis have been few, and their results have been contradictory. Greco et al.[82] found increased levels of urinary kallikrein in nonazotemic cirrhotic patients with and without ascites. Zipser et al.,[83] however, reported low urinary kallikrein in such patients. More recently, Pérez-Ayuso et al.[84] reported that urinary kallikrein activity is increased in cirrhotic patients with ascites but without renal failure. In addition, renal plasma flow and glomerular filtration rate correlated with urinary kallikrein activity. Based on these findings, the authors suggested that the renal kallikrein-kinin system is involved in the maintenance of renal hemodynamics in cirrhosis.

The interpretation of the above results is confounded by methodologic and conceptual issues with respect to urinary kallikrein.[80,85] In most published investigations, the activity of the renal kallikrein-kinin system is inferred from the measurement of urinary kallikrein. At present, however, there is no clear proof that urinary kallikrein parallels the intrarenal generation of kinins.[85] Finally, the above studies use differing assays (i.e., kininogenase assay, steriolitic assay, and assay of kallikrein's amidolytic effect on synthetic substrate) that measure only active kallikrein but not the absolute amount of kallikrein in the urine. Because approximately 50% of urinary kallikrein is in inactive form in humans, such indices of urinary kallikrein may be misleading. Moreover, the urine normally contains kallikrein inhibitors that may interfere with indirect techniques of measuring kallikrein.[85] Therefore, the different kallikrein activity observed in the present study in normal subjects and cirrhotic patients with and without renal failure may be related to differences in the amount of kallikrein inhibitors or in the proportion between active and inactive kallikrein present in their urine.

Humoral Natriuretic Factor

Several lines of evidence suggest that a circulating natriuretic factor may constitute a component part of the biologic control system regulating sodium excretion in humans.[86–89] It is conceivable, therefore, that deficiencies of this hormone could mediate, at least in part, sodium retention in cirrhosis, i.e., that sodium retention results from a failure to elaborate natriuretic hormone when extracellular fluid volume increases in response to renal sodium retention.

Several preliminary observations using bioassay systems are consistent with such a formulation.[10,90] The search for endogenous inhibitors of the sodium pump that specifically bind to the cardiac glycoside-binding site on Na-K-ATPase and affect its activity has occupied many investigators. Evidence for circulating inhibitors of the pump first came from cross-circulation studies of volume-expanded animals. Since at least 50% of renal sodium reabsorption depends on the basolateral Na-K-ATPase of renal tubular cells, a hormonal inhibitor of the sodium pump may regulate sodium reabsorption. DeWardener and Clarkson[86] reviewed the evidence for circulating Na-K-ATPase inhibitors and noted that atrial natriuretic peptides are not digitalis-like factors because they do not inhibit Na-K-ATPase and cannot explain data supporting the existence of sodium pump inhibitors measured during volume expansion. Evidence to date indicates that certain lipids account for most of what has been termed "cardiac glycosidelike activity," at least in plasma. Although the physiologic importance of this inhibitory activity is unclear, it is hoped that further characterization will delineate the role of such a natriuretic factor in the pathogenesis of sodium retention in cirrhosis (see chapter 16).

Atrial Natriuretic Peptides (Auriculin, ANF, ANP)

In contrast to cardiac glycosidelike compounds, additional circulating natriuretic factors can be differentiated by virtue of their failure to inhibit Na-K-ATPase. These mediators have been called atrial natriuretic factors or peptides.[91] It has recently been shown that mammalian atria contain potent natriuretic and vasoactive peptide(s), which have been referred to as atrial natriuretic factor (ANF) and auriculin[92] Several laboratories have purified, sequenced, and synthesized atrial peptides that have the natriuretic vasoactive properties of crude atrial extract.[93,94] Maack and colleagues[95,96] characterized the renal hemodynamic and hormonal effects of ANF by investigating the effects of a continuous infusion of synthetic auriculin on blood pressure, renal hemodynamics, GFR, and renal excretory functions in intact dogs. The results demonstrate that this peptide of atrial origin decreases blood pressure and increases GFR and sodium excretion without a sustained increase in renal plasma flow. In addition, synthetic auriculin decreased renin secretory

rate, plasma renin levels, and PA levels.[96] Together these observations suggest an important potential role for auriculin in the regulation of blood pressure, renal function, and sodium-volume homeostasis.

In light of several lines of evidence suggesting that stretch receptors residing in the atria may participate in regulating volume homeostasis,[44,45,97] it is tempting to attribute a cardinal role to this peptide in modulating renal sodium handling in both normal states and edematous disorders. Specifically, the sodium retention and activation of the renin-angiotensin-aldosterone system in patients with cirrhosis may result from a failure to elaborate ANF when extracellular fluid volume increases in response to renal sodium retention. In light of active investigations in many laboratories with these peptides, it is hoped that the role for this putative effector in mediating sodium retention in cirrhotic humans will be delineated.

Observations by Jiménez et al.[98] are of interest. In studies of rats with experimental cirrhosis, they investigated whether cirrhosis with ascites is associated with altered tissue content of ANF. They demonstrated that the diuretic and natriuretic potency of atrial extracts from cirrhotic rats was markedly lower than that of control rats, suggesting that the atrial content of ANF was reduced in cirrhotic rats.

Despite such theoretical considerations, recent evidence indicates that a deficiency of circulating ANF levels per se does not account for the sodium retention. Most studies have demonstrated that plasma ANF levels in cirrhotic patients with ascites are either appropriate or occasionally elevated[99,100] (see chapter 15).

Renal Natriuretic Peptide (Urodilatin)

The demonstration that the 32-amino acid peptide [ANP-(95-126)], known as urodilatin, possesses natriuretic and diuretic properties in humans[101–103] raises the possibility that a diminution of urodilatin may contribute to the sodium retention. Recently, Norsk et al.[104] used the water immersion model to investigate the relationship between urodilatin and renal sodium and water handling in normal subjects. Immersion induced an increase in renal urodilatin and guanosine 3',5'-cyclic monophosphate (cGMP) excretion. Because they demonstrated a correlation between renal urodilatin excretion and both urine flow and sodium excretion, the investigators concluded that urodilatin may be one of the mechanisms mediating the natriuresis and diuresis of water immersion in humans. Such studies suggest that a systematic investigation of alterations in urodilatin in patients with decompensated liver disease is warranted.

Brain Natriuretic Peptide

Brain natriuretic peptide (BNP) is a novel natriuretic peptide first isolated in the brain of pigs; subsequently, it was isolated from the hearts of experimental animals and humans. BNP is a cardiac hormone with natriuretic activity that is involved in the regulation of cardiovascular and volume homeostasis.[105] It possesses a spectrum of pharmacological activities quite similar to those of ANP, including diuretic, natriuretic, hypotensive, and smooth muscle relaxant activities.

La Villa et al.[106] measured plasma levels of BNP in 11 normal subjects, 13 cirrhotic patients without ascites, 18 nonazotemic cirrhotic patients with ascites, and 6 cirrhotic patients with ascites and functional renal failure. Plasma levels of BNP were similar in normal subjects and cirrhotic patients without ascites. In contrast, cirrhotic patients with ascites, with and without functional renal failure, had plasma concentrations of brain natriuretic peptide that exceeded those of normal subjects and patients without ascites. Fifteen of the 18 nonazotemic cirrhotic patients with ascites and all of the patients with ascites and functional renal failure had plasma BNP values that exceeded the upper normal limit of BNP in healthy subjects. BNP levels did not differ between the two groups of cirrhotic patients with ascites. The demonstration that levels are increased in cirrhotic patients with ascites suggests that sodium retention in cirrhosis is not due to deficiency of BNP.

Sympathetic Nervous System Activity

An increase in sympathetic nervous system activity also may contribute to the sodium retention in cirrhosis. Thus, the decrease in central blood volume as well as the increase in renal sympathetic activity.[107–109] Furthermore, studies have demonstrated that an increase in sympathetic tone promotes antinatriuresis by altering intrarenal hemodynamics and by a direct tubular effect.[107,109]

There are differing formulations as to what constitutes the predominant afferent limb for increased renal sympathetic tone in cirrhosis. It is of interest that proponents of both the underfill and overflow theories invoke neural reflex mechanisms that elicit increases in efferent renal sympathetic nerve activity (ERSNA). The predominant afferent limb, however, differs according to the respective theory. According to the underfill theory, a decrease in central blood volume elicits increased ERSNA. The pathways whereby decreased effective blood volume would result in a stimulation of ERSNA include perception of the decrease by both high-pressure sinoaortic as well as low-pressure cardiopulmonary baroreceptors.[107–110] In contrast, according to the overflow theory, intrahepatic receptors constitute the afferent limb. Compelling evidence supports the formulation that elevated intrahepatic pressure results in reflex stimulation of ERSNA.[111] Regardless of the initiating event, it is apparent that the increase in renal sympathetic nerve activity results in renal sodium retention.

The mechanisms whereby renal sympathetic nerves modulate renal sodium reabsorption are multiple. Increases in ERSNA produce renal vasoconstriction with decreases in renal blood flow and GFR. In addition, increased ERSNA favors sodium retention by possibly altering intrarenal hemodynamics with a preferential redistribution toward the inner cortical nephrons.[112] Much attention has been directed to the ability of increased ERSNA to promote an antinatriuresis without eliciting changes in GFR, renal blood flow, or intrarenal distribution of blood flow.[113,114] In contrast to earlier formulations, it is now thought that the direct renal tubular effect of increased ERSNA acts at several differing loci in the nephron.

Several studies have provided an anatomic basis for the influence of the renal nerves in modulating renal sodium and water handling. Although micropuncture methods have localized the proximal tubule as a site responsible for the changes in sodium and water reabsorption resulting from alterations in neural activity,[114] recent studies have suggested that neural activity may modulate sodium reabsorption in other nephron segments as well. Thus, Barajas et al.[115] quantitatively assessed the innervation of the different portions of the cortical tubular nephron in the rat and demonstrated innervations of the thick ascending limb of Henle (TALH), the distal convoluted tubule, and the collecting duct. DiBona and

Sawin[116] reported that low-frequency renal nerve stimulation has a direct effect on sodium and chloride absorption in Henle's loop. Thus, the observations of Barajas provide an anatomic basis for the functional effects of the renal nerves on multiple segments of the nephron.

Despite such theoretical considerations, only recently have rigorous data supported the importance of alterations in the sympathetic nervous system in cirrhotic humans. Over 25 years ago, studies by Epstein et al.[117] raised the possibility that adrenergic activity may be enhanced in cirrhosis. In the course of assessing intrarenal hemodynamics in cirrhotic patients, the investigators observed that the intrarenal infusion of the α_1-adrenergic blocker phentolamine failed to increase renal blood flow significantly in cirrhotic patients.[117] Although the failure of phentolamine to enhance renal perfusion was interpreted initially as indicating the absence of increased renal adrenergic tone, caution is required in reaching such a conclusion. A majority of patients who received an intrarenal infusion of phentolamine manifested transient hypotension. It is conceivable, therefore, that such concomitant alterations in systemic hemodynamics might have masked a phentolamine-induced enhancement of renal perfusion.

Lunzer et al.[118] observed that cardiovascular responsiveness to reflex autonomic stimulation may be impaired in patients with cirrhosis. Thus, the observers noted impaired vasoconstrictor responses to diverse stimuli, including ice on the forehead, mental arithmetic, lower body negative pressure, and the Valsalva maneuver. One possible interpretation for such widespread interference in the peripheral and central autonomic nervous system in cirrhotic patients is an increased occupancy of endogenous catecholamine receptors.

Several groups of investigators have attempted to assess the activity of the sympathetic nervous system in cirrhotic humans by measuring plasma catecholamine levels during basal conditions and following postural manipulations.[119–123] Ring-Larsen et al.[119] determined plasma NE and epinephrine concentrations in differing vascular beds of cirrhotic patients at the time of hepatic venous catheterization. Based on differences in regional NE levels, they concluded that the elevated NE levels in patients with cirrhosis were attributable to enhanced sympathetic nervous system activity rather than decreased metabolism.

Bichet et al.[110] examined the potential role of increased sympathetic activity in mediating the impaired sodium and water excretion in cirrhosis. They reported that patients with advanced cirrhosis manifest elevated concentrations of plasma NE. In addition to documenting an increase in NE, they correlated plasma NE levels with the ability to excrete an acute water load in 26 patients with cirrhosis.

Although most observers agree that mean peripheral NE levels are elevated in cirrhotic patients,[119–123] it may be an oversimplification to suggest that such alterations in catecholamine metabolism affect all cirrhotic patients with deranged sodium and water homeostasis. We have examined the relationship between plasma NE levels and renal sodium and water handling during immersion-induced central blood volume expansion.[123] Although mean NE levels were elevated for the group as a whole, more than half of the patients with decompensated cirrhosis manifested appropriate (nonelevated) NE levels. Furthermore, NE levels did not correlate with alterations in renal sodium or water excretion[123] (Fig. 1.11).

A more relevant consideration is not whether peripheral NE levels are elevated but whether they are appropriate indices of renal sympathetic activity. As detailed in several recent reviews,[124–127] however, the plasma concentrations of norepinephrine are an inadequate guide to either total or regional sympathetic activity. Global measures of sympathetic activity, such as plasma norepinephrine, fail to identify sources of norepinephrine release and cannot delineate regional patterns of sympathetic nervous activation. Recently, Esler et al.[126] conducted a physiologic and neurochemical evaluation of patients with cirrhosis, applying tracer kinetic techniques with radiolabeled norepinephrine, thereby allowing a more precise description of the regional pattern of the sympathetic nervous derangement in cirrhosis. They demonstrated that the elevated plasma norepinephrine concentration in patients with cirrhosis is attributable to higher overall rates of spillover of the neurotransmitter to plasma and not to reduced plasma clearance caused by liver disease. The administration of clonidine reduced previously elevated norepinephrine overflow rates for the whole body, kidneys, and hepatomesenteric circulation. This sympathetic inhibition was accompanied by several potentially clinically beneficial effects: the

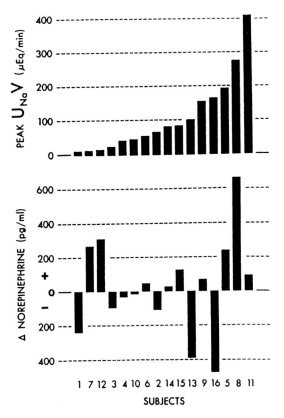

FIGURE 1.11. Relationship of renal sodium excretion *(upper panel)* to alterations in plasma norepinephrine (NE) *(lower panel)* during immersion in 16 cirrhotic patients. The numbers along the horizontal axis designate the individual patients. As can be seen, the magnitude of the natriuresis, as assessed by peak rate of sodium excretion ($U_{Na}V$), varied independently of ΔNE ("nadir" minus prestudy NE) during immersion (r = 0.256; not significant). (Reproduced with permission from Epstein M, et al: Effects of water immersion on plasma catecholamines in decompensated cirrhosis. Miner Electrolyte Metab 1985;11:25–34.)

lowering of renal vascular resistance, an augmentation of GFR, and the reduction of portal venous pressure.[126]

In summary, the available data indicate that the sympathetic nervous system is activated in cirrhosis, both in the kidney and in other regional vascular beds, consequently contributing to the renal vasoconstriction and sodium retention of cirrhosis.[124,126]

Endothelins

In the past 15 years endothelins (ET) have emerged as an important new peptide family in the hormonal regulation of body fluid and cardiovascular homeostasis.[128,129] The ET family comprises ET-1, ET-2, and ET-3, peptides that have 21 amino acids and two disulfide bridges and are synthesized primarily by vascular endothelial cells but also by epithelial and other cells. Stimuli for synthesis and release (constitutive pathway) include various growth factors, shear forces, hypoxia, and, in the kidney, increased medullary osmolality.[128,130,131]

ETs are the most potent vasoconstrictors known to date. They release Ca^{2+} and also potentiate Ca^{2+} release stimulated by other vasoconstrictors, including AVP and angiotensin II. The renal ET system appears to modulate renal perfusion and attenuates the action of AVP at the inner medullary collecting duct (IMCD) by direct interference with cAMP synthesis. Increasing evidence suggests that ET plays a role in the pathogenesis of diverse disorders, contributing to hypertensive disease and mediating renal injury via its vascular effects—i.e., in acute renal failure due to cyclosporine, contrast media, or endotoxemia and in chronic forms of renal impairment.[128]

Rabelink et al.[132,133] recently demonstrated that exogenous infusion of endothelin-1 in normal human volunteers induced not only a major increase in renal vascular resistance but also a decrease in sodium excretion. These findings suggest an important role for endothelin in human renal pathophysiology.

Uchihara et al.[134] investigated changes in plasma endothelin concentration in patients with chronic liver disease of differing etiologies. Plasma endothelin concentrations were more than two-fold higher in patients with cirrhosis and ascites than in normal controls. In contrast, endothelin levels in cirrhotic patients without ascites and in patients with chronic hepatitis did not differ from those in normal controls. Furthermore, plasma endothelin levels were two-fold higher in patients with endotoxemia than in those without endotoxemia. Because endotoxin has been reported to stimulate endothelin synthesis,[135] the investigators speculated that endotoxin may be responsible for the elevated plasma endothelin concentrations with consequent renal dysfunction.

Uemasu et al.[136] also demonstrated increased plasma endothelin levels in patients with cirrhosis. Of interest, they observed that patients both with and without ascites had elevations in endothelin.

Endothelin levels were two-fold higher in compensated cirrhotic patients than in controls. The compensated cirrhotic patients tended to have a further elevation, although the differences did not attain statistical significance.

The extent to which elevated endothelin levels may contribute to the deranged sodium and water homeostasis of cirrhosis remains to be defined. The physiology of endothelin and its role in sodium and water homeostasis are reviewed in detail in chapter 18.

Nitric Oxide

A more recent approach to investigating the pathogenesis of sodium retention has focused on the florid systemic hemodynamic disturbances that invariably accompany the syndrome, including hyperdynamic circulation, increased heart rate and cardiac output, and decreased blood pressure and systemic vascular resistance.[27,29] These observations have suggested the likelihood of excessive production of a vasodilator.[137]

Recently, attention has focused on the role of nitric oxide (NO) as a mediator of both the hyperdynamic circulation and renal failure.[138] NO, a vasodilator synthesized from L-arginine, accounts for the biologic activity of endothelium-derived relaxing factor.[139–141] In animals, the agonist-induced release of NO from the vascular endothelium leads to peripheral vasodilation, a fall in blood pressure, and tachycardia.[141] Such effects are short-lived, however, and vascular tone returns to normal once the agonist infusion is stopped. On the other hand, a second, distinct, inducible NO synthase occurs in response to bacterial lipopolysaccharide endotoxin.[142] Once induced, this enzyme releases NO for many hours without the need for further stimulation.

On the basis of several considerations, Vallance and Moncada[138] have postulated that endotoxemia induces an NO synthase in peripheral blood vessels and that increased NO synthesis and release accounts for the associated hyperdynamic circulation. This theory does not posit that renal vasoconstriction is directly related to NO but rather suggests that renal hypoperfusion and sodium retention are secondary to a diversion of blood away from the kidney.

If this hypothesis is correct, the inhibition of nitric oxide synthesis should restore sensitivity to vasoconstrictors and reverse the hemodynamic abnormalities. Specific inhibitors of either the constitutive or the inducible NO synthase theoretically should facilitate a more precise manipulation of NO synthesis and help to establish the pathophysiologic importance of nitric oxide in endotoxemia and cirrhosis.

Recently, Clâria et al.[143] investigated the pressor and renal effects of intravenous Nw-nitro-L-arginine (NNA), a competitive inhibitor of NO biosynthesis, in conscious control rats and cirrhotic rats with ascites. The aim of the study was to assess whether the arteriolar vasodilation and secondary arterial hypotension in cirrhosis with ascites is related to increased activity of NO. Cirrhosis was induced by inhalation of carbon tetrachloride. Arterial pressure, estimated renal plasma flow, glomerular filtration rate, and sodium excretion were measured in 12 cirrhotic rats with ascites and 10 control rats before and during the sequential infusion of increasing doses of NNA. NNA produced a significantly greater increase in arterial pressure than in 17 conscious control rats. In control rats, NNA caused a decrease in estimated renal plasma flow without affecting glomerular filtration rate or sodium excretion. In contrast, NNA administration to cirrhotic animals produced no appreciable renal vasoconstrictor effect and increased glomerular filtration rate and sodium excretion. These results, which indicate that cirrhotic rats show enhanced sensitivity to the pressor effect of NO inhibition, support the postulate that an increased systemic release of nitric oxide in experimental cirrhosis with ascites contributes to the complication of arterial hypotension. In addition, they suggested that NO does not play a major role in the maintenance of renal hemodynamics in cirrhosis.

Is this formulation valid in patients with cirrhosis? A preliminary report indicated that serum nitrite and nitrate levels, an index of NO production, were elevated in a group of cirrhotic patients.[144] The patients with ascites manifested higher nitrite and nitrate levels than did cirrhotic patients without ascites. Furthermore, there was a direct correlation between serum nitrite and nitrate levels and endotoxemia. Additional studies are required to substantiate this hypothesis in humans with liver disease.

Redistribution of Renal Blood Flow

The redistribution of blood flow within the kidneys may also enhance net tubular sodium reabsorption in cirrhosis. The results of studies using diverse methods of measurement in both animal and human kidneys have demonstrated different regional rates of blood flow.[145-147] It has become increasingly apparent that changes in intrarenal hemodynamics may influence renal sodium handling through mechanisms other than a change in the overall GFR. Several lines of evidence have suggested that regional flow rates in the cortex and outer medulla are largely determined by salt intake in normal humans.[148,149] A high salt intake increases the flow rate to the cortex. Conversely, dietary sodium restriction reduces outer cortical flow while concomitantly increasing perfusion in the inner cortex and outer medulla. Such reciprocal changes in intrarenal perfusion may well constitute a major contributing factor to the kidney's capacity to modulate sodium excretion in both health and disease.

There are at least three major alternative mechanisms through which changes in intrarenal perfusion may influence sodium handling: increased perfusion of juxtamedullary nephrons, preferential decline in GFR per nephron in outer cortical nephrons, and enhanced net tubular reabsorption in superficial cortical nephrons.

Originally, it was postulated that juxtamedullary nephrons might have an intrinsically greater capacity for sodium reabsorption than superficial nephrons.[147] A shift of a greater proportion of the renal blood flow to the juxtamedullary nephron population would thereby result in increased sodium reabsorption. However, the assumption that the various nephrons differ in their ability to transport sodium has not yet been critically tested.

Alternatively, it has been proposed that the GFR of single nephrons in the two nephron populations changes in response to altered intrarenal blood-flow distribution and that such changes affect the net amount of sodium reabsorbed by the kidney.[150] A reduction in the single nephron GFR of nephrons in the larger cortical nephron population, occurring in response to intrarenal blood flow redistribution in cirrhosis, may result in increased total net sodium reabsorption by the kidney, even if the fraction of filtrate reabsorbed in both nephron populations remained unchanged.

A third hypothesis relates the alterations in sodium reabsorption—induced by intrarenal blood flow distribution—to alterations in the Starling forces in superficial and juxtamedullary nephrons.[151] Reductions in capillary hydrostatic pressure and increases in colloid osmotic pressure

in the peritubular capillaries of the superficial cortical nephrons, which occurred in response to a preferential reduction of the blood-flow rate in the outer cortical region, might be a plausible explanation for the alterations in sodium reabsorption observed in cirrhosis.

The application of tracer techniques, including the xenon-washout method, has provided an index of mean and cortical blood flow in both normal and various disease states, including cirrhosis. Epstein et al.[117,152] used the xenon-washout technique to assess intrarenal hemodynamics in cirrhosis and demonstrated a decrease in mean renal blood flow with a concomitant striking reduction in the early or cortical component of renal blood flow ($C_1\%$) in cirrhotic patients with sodium retention. Kew et al.[153] confirmed these findings in patients with cirrhosis.

In summary, despite the attractiveness of invoking abnormalities of intrarenal perfusion as a major contributing factor to the pathologic sodium retention of cirrhosis, this hypothesis has not been tested critically. Furthermore, since intrarenal hemodynamics in cirrhotic humans are characterized by marked vasomotor instability,[117,152] caution must be exercised in the interpretation of intrarenal hemodynamic studies in this patient population.

Endogenous Opioids

Several lines of evidence suggest that endogenous opioids may participate in the regulation of cardiovascular homeostasis, fluid and electrolyte excretion, and AVP release[154-157]; they also may contribute to renal sodium and water retention in patients with liver cirrhosis and ascites. This hypothesis is supported by the following observations:

1. Opioid peptides such as "β-endorphin and enkephalins, have vasodilator[158,159] and antinatriuretic and antidiuretic properties[160,161]; systemic vasodilation is believed to initiate renal sodium and water retention in cirrhosis (vide supra).

2. Increased levels of plasma enkephalins have been reported in patients with cirrhosis of the liver.[161,162]

To examine this hypothesis, Leehey et al.154 administered the opioid antagonist naloxone (5 mg bolus followed by a 0.06 mg/min infusion) to 8 male patients with alcoholic cirrhosis and ascites and to 5 healthy age- and sex-matched control subjects and determined the effects of naloxone on fluid and electrolyte excretion after a nonsustained water load (20 ml/kg). In comparison with saline vehicle infusion, naloxone administration in patients with cirrhosis resulted in a 50% increase in urine output and creatinine clearance and two-fold increases in sodium and potassium excretion. Additional studies are warranted to assess the possible role of endogenous opioids in mediating sodium retention.

Estrogen

In the search for other sodium-retaining factors in cirrhosis, it has been suggested that an impaired hepatic inactivation of estrogens with a resultant increase in circulating estrogen participates in mediating the sodium retention. Thus estrogens have been shown to exert a moderate sodium-retaining effect in humans independently of their ability to stimulate aldosterone.[163] Furthermore, much evidence indicates that estrogens are inactivated normally by the liver.[164] Finally, male alcoholics frequently manifest stigmata of feminization, including gynecomastia, testicular atrophy, decreased libido and potency, and spider angiomata.[165,166] Over three decades ago, a number of studies demonstrated elevated urinary estrogen levels in cirrhosis.[165–167] Subsequent studies with radioimmunoassay techniques confirmed the presence of elevated estradiol levels in cirrhosis,[168,169] although this finding is not universal.[170]

Elevated estradiol levels per se do not establish an etiologic role for elevated estrogen activity in the sodium retention of cirrhosis. In an attempt to assess this possibility, Preedy and Aitken[171] determined the effect of daily administration of 10 mg of estradiol benzoate on sodium and water balance. The authors demonstrated significant retention of sodium and water in cirrhotic patients without ascites and edema compared with normal controls. In contrast, the resultant retention of sodium and water in cirrhotic patients with ascites was less marked, although it exceeded retention in normal controls given estradiol. Additional studies are necessary to assess the functional significance of elevated estradiol levels in cirrhotic patients in mediating the concomitant sodium retention.

Prolactin

Apart from the obvious role of prolactin (PRL) in lactation, it is unclear whether human PRL exerts additional effects in normal subjects. Nevertheless, several lines of evidence have raised the possibility that PRL may constitute one of the factors responsible for the sodium retention of liver disease. Although the effects of PRL are numerous,[172] several are worthy of consideration. PRL administration to humans may cause sodium and potassium retention.[173] In animals, PRL administration may potentiate the sodium- and fluid-retaining effects of aldosterone and antidiuretic hormone and thus cause edema.[174,175] Finally, PRL has been demonstrated to potentiate the vasoconstrictor effects of angiotensin and NE in rats.[176] Unanimity about the physiologic role of prolactin in humans, however, is lacking. Carey et al.[177] suggested that the effects of ovine prolactin on water and electrolyte excretion in humans may be attributable to vasopressin contamination and that prolactin may not exert a physiologic role in the acute regulation of renal function in humans.

That such observations about the physiologic effects of PRL may be relevant to cirrhotic humans is supported by two reports suggesting the occurrence of hyperprolactinemia in patients with liver disease. Wernze and Schmitz[178] reported a significant increase in basal plasma PRL levels in a large group of patients with liver cirrhosis and noted that the incidence of hyperprolactinemia was greater in cirrhosis of alcoholic etiology (54%) than in the nonalcoholic type (11%). In contrast, Morgan et al.[179] noted that only 12% of patients with liver disease of varying etiology manifested hyperprolactinemia.

Panerai et al.[180] examined both basal and stimulated PRL levels in patients with liver disease. They reported that mean baseline PRL values were not significantly higher in patients with liver disease than in corresponding control subjects. Nevertheless, they demonstrated that the administration of thyrotropin-releasing hormone to patients with advanced liver disease resulted in an exaggerated and sustained increase in PRL. Unfortunately, concomitant changes in renal function were not reported. Although several reports suggest that PRL levels may be elevated in some patients, the possibly confounding role of estrogens must be considered in evaluating PRL concentration in patients with chronic liver disease. PRL concentrations are elevated by hyperestrogenemia, which may account for the results. Although the above considerations merely raise the possibility that PRL may contribute in part to the sodium retention of liver disease, such a possibility is worthy of investigation since hyperprolactinemia can be managed successfully. At present, it is possible to suppress PRL secretion in humans by the administration of either L-dopa or more completely by bromoergocryptine.

Vasoactive Intestinal Peptide

Twenty-five years ago, Said and Mutt[181] isolated from the small bowel a polypeptide that was capable of reproducing some of the common hemodynamic changes of cirrhosis, including increased cardiac output, peripheral vasodilation, pulmonary shunting, and hyperventilation. Since vasoactive intestinal peptide (VIP) has been demonstrated to be inactivated during its passage through the liver,[182] it is conceivable that in patients with liver failure the peptide escapes hepatic inactivation and reaches the peripheral circulation. Indeed, Hunt et al.[183] reported that patients with cirrhosis and those with acute and chronic liver disease manifest VIP levels that exceed those of normal individuals and patients with chronic illness but without liver involvement.

The pathophysiologic significance of increased VIP levels has been investigated subsequently. Calam et al.[184] examined the effects of VIP infusion on renal hemodynamics and excretory function in 6 normal subjects and 3 patients with liver disease. The administration of VIP to normal subjects did not alter the clearance rates of either para-aminohippurate or creatinine. In contrast, urine flow rate fell to one-third and electrolyte excretion to one-half of the control values. Patients with liver disease responded similarly. Based on these observations, the authors proposed that the elevated plasma VIP levels may contribute to salt and water retention in liver disease. In contrast, several investigators have recently focused attention on the natriuretic properties of VIP. VIP has been reported to have natriuretic effects when administered intravenously to conscious rabbits[185] and intrarenally to anesthetized rats.[186] This natriuresis was presumed to be tubular in origin because of the accompanying decrease in renal plasma flow and GFR in the intravenous study.

Duggan and MacDonald[187] attempted to ascertain whether VIP acts directly on the kidney and also to define renal responses. They compared the natriuretic and hemodynamic responses to intravenous infusion of VIP with responses to direct infusion into the renal artery in conscious male rabbits. VIP induced a significant fall in effective renal plasma flow and GFR without changing systemic arterial pressure or pulse rate. Despite the significant decline in filtered sodium load, there was a significant log dose-related increase in fractional sodium excretion with intrarenal infusion of VIP.

Such observations confound attempts to infer a pathophysiologic role for VIP in the sodium retention of cirrhotic humans; additional studies are required to establish its precise role.

Summary

The above 16 sections exemplify the mechanisms that may contribute to the deranged sodium homeostasis of cirrhosis. It is apparent that the renal sodium retention of advanced liver disease is a complex pathophysiologic constellation with numerous and diverse causes. Fig 1.7 attempts to integrate diverse findings and to summarize some of the mechanisms whereby diverse hormonal mediators may act in concert to induce sodium retention.

WHY ASCITES PREDOMINATES IN LIVER DISEASE

The hormonal and neural mechanisms that mediate the abnormal salt retention in cirrhosis may be similar to mechanisms that are operative in other edematous states, such as congestive heart failure and nephrosis. Why, then, do cirrhotic patients manifest fluid retention so frequently as ascites? Various factors appear to play a role in determining why the peritoneal sac constitutes the site of accumulation of retained fluid, including portal hypertension, hypoalbuminemia, and abnormalities of the peritoneal membrane. Such factors, which may retard the normal cycling of fluid between the peritoneal cavity and the vascular compartment, are considered in chapters 8 and 9.

RECOMMENDATIONS FOR MEDICAL THERAPY OF ASCITES AND EDEMA

The general principles for the medical therapy of hospitalized patients with ascites are outlined in Table 1.3. The initial goal should be weight loss due to spontaneous diuresis in association with consistent and scrupulous adherence to a

TABLE 1.3. General Principles in the Treatment of Ascites

1. Daily measurement of the patient's weight and careful clinical monitoring are mandatory.
2. Biochemical parameters (i.e., blood urea nitrogen, serum creatinine, serum electrolytes) should be monitored at appropriate intervals.
3. Make sure that liver and renal functions are stable before instituting diuretic therapy.
4. Attempt to mobilize ascites and edema initially via rest and restriction of dietary sodium before instituting diuretic therapy.
5. Aim for a daily weight loss of 0.5–1.0 kg in patients who have ascites with edema and 0.3 kg in those who have ascites without edema.
6. Maintain as the endpoint of therapy the greatest degree of patient comfort possible with the minimum of drug-induced complications.

well-balanced diet with rigid dietary sodium restriction (250 mg/day or about 10 mEq).

In patients with liver disease and ascites, the assumption of upright posture is associated with marked activation of the renin-angiotensin-aldosterone and sympathetic nervous systems, a reduction of glomerular filtration rate and sodium excretion, and a diminished response to loop diuretics.[188,189] Theoretically, therefore, bed rest should be a useful adjunct for treatment of ascites.

The sodium intake prescribed for cardiac patients (1200–1500 mg/day) is not sufficiently restrictive for cirrhotic patients, who often continue to gain weight on such a regimen. Because cirrhotic patients frequently excrete less than 5–10 mEq of sodium/day, it is evident that a 1500-mg sodium diet (i.e., 65 mEq of sodium) may result in a net positive sodium balance exceeding 400 mEq/week with an attendant potential weight gain of approximately 3 kg. Although the frequency with which dietary management successfully relieves ascites is unsettled, a sodium-restricted diet should be prescribed if feasible to all hospitalized patients because it is impossible to predict which patients will respond.

In occasional symptomatic patients, however, less rigid sodium restriction may be advisable for several reasons. First, as a consequence of anorexia, such patients will eat only part of the meals offered to them and thus only a fraction of the daily sodium allowance. Second, in malnourished patients, nutrition must have priority over rigid sodium restriction.

Although most clinicians adhere to the important role of dietary sodium restriction in the management of cirrhotic ascites, others have suggested that it may be more practical to liberalize dietary sodium intake and to offset this maneuver with diuretics. Reynolds et al.[190] proposed that a normal sodium diet would tend to prevent

diuretic-induced acute electrolyte disorders and azotemia. To examine this possibility, a multicenter study was undertaken in France by the ENTAC Group (National Inquiry for the Treatment of Cirrhotic Ascites).[191] Cirrhotic patients with ascites were randomized into two treatment groups: (1) a low sodium diet (21 mmol/day) or (2) unrestricted sodium intake. Both groups received effective doses of diuretics (spironolactone or, if necessary, spironolactone and furosemide); 140 patients from 12 liver units were included according to well-defined criteria. After an initial 4- to 7-day period of bed rest and salt restriction (21 mmol sodium/day), randomization was carried out in each center. The investigators observed no significant differences between the two groups with respect to (1) clinical and biochemical data; (2) mortality or withdrawal (definitive or temporary) because of biochemical disturbances (group 1, 34%; group 2, 22%); (3) actuarial survival (curves plotted to the 120th day), which was not statistically different (p = 0.18); and (4) hospitalization time and costs, which were identical in both groups. On the other hand, the time for complete disappearance of ascites was significantly shorter (p = 0.014) for the salt-restricted patients. I agree with the ENTAC investigators that a normal salt diet has no advantage over a sodium-restricted diet.

BASIC MANAGEMENT

Although the mainstay of therapy for sodium retention is careful restriction of sodium and fluid intake together with rational diuretic therapy, several specific therapeutic measures appear to be of practical value in some patients. Examples include large-volume paracentesis, peritoneovenous shunt, dialytic intervention in carefully selected patients, and, most recently, transjugular intrahepatic portosystemic shunt (TIPS). These newer and more specific approaches are discussed in chapters 23, 24, 25, and 26.

CONCLUSION

Renal sodium retention in patients with advanced liver disease constitutes a fascinating constellation with numerous and diverse causes and an elusive pathophysiology. The dissociation between hyperaldosteronism and the attendant changes in renal sodium handling and the demonstration of an impairment in natriuretic hormone release despite the absence of overt signs of sodium retention underscore the complex nature of the derangement. It is probable that the development of sodium retention necessitates the participation of several hormonal and/or neural effectors, acting in concert. Additional insight must await further biochemical characterization of some of the mediators and a delineation of their pathophysiologic role.

Acknowledgment. The author is grateful to Elsa V. Reina for her expert preparation of the manuscript.

REFERENCES

1. Hippocrates. Cited in Atkinson M: Ascites in liver disease. Postgrad Med J 1956;32:482–485.
2. Brown J: The philosophical transaction of the Royal Society. 1685;111:248.
3. Farnsworth EB, Krakusin JS: Electrolyte partition in patients with edema of various origins: Qualitative and quantitative definition of cations and anions in hepatic cirrhosis. J Lab Clin Med 1948;33:1545–1554.
4. Eisenmenger WJ, Blondheim SH, Bongiovanni AM, Kunkel HG: Electrolyte studies on patients with cirrhosis of the liver. J Clin Invest 1950;29:1491–1499.
5. Faloon WW, Eckhardt RD, Cooper AM, Davidson CS: The effect of human serum albumin, mercurial diuretics, and a low sodium diet on sodium excretion in patients with cirrhosis of the liver. J Clin Invest 1949; 28:595–602.
6. Goodyer AVN, Relman AS, Lawrason FD, Epstein FH: Salt retention in cirrhosis of the liver. J Clin Invest 1950;29:973–981.
7. Papper S, Saxon L: The influence of intravenous infusions of sodium chloride solutions on the renal excretion of sodium in patients with cirrhosis of the liver. J Clin Invest 1956;35:728.
8. Goldman R: Studies in diurnal variation of water and electrolyte excretion: Nocturnal diuresis of water and sodium in congestive failure and cirrhosis of the liver. J Clin Invest 1951;30:1191–1199.
9. Jones RA, McDonald GO, Last JH: Reversal of diurnal variation in renal function in cases of cirrhosis with ascites. J Clin Invest 1952;31:326–334.
10. Naccarato R, Messa P, D'Angelo A, et al: Renal handling of sodium and water in early chronic liver disease. Gastroenterology 1981;81:205–210.
11. Simón MA, Díez J, Prieto J:Abnormal sympathetic and renal responses to sodium restriction in compensated cirrhosis. Gastroenterology 1991;101:1354–1360.
12. Wood LJ, Massie D, McLean AJ, Dudley FJ: Renal sodium retention in cirrhosis: Tubular site and relation to hepatic dysfunction. Hepatology 1988;8:831–836.
13. Klingler EL Jr, Vaamonde CA, Vaamonde LS, et al: Renal function changes in cirrhosis of the liver. Arch Intern Med 1970;125:1010–1015.
14. Gabuzda GJ: Cirrhosis, ascites, and edema. Clinical course related to management. Gastroenterology 1970; 58:546–553.
15. Bosch J, Arroyo V, Rodés J, et al: Compensación espontanea de la ascitis en la cirrosis hepatica. Rev Clin Esp 1974;133:441–446.
16. Papper S, Saxon L: The diuretic response to administered water in patients with liver disease. II. Laënnec's cirrhosis of the liver. Arch Intern Med 1959;103:750–757.
17. Vaamonde CA: Renal water handling in liver disease. In Epstein M (ed): The Kidney in Liver Disease, 3rd ed. Baltimore: Williams & Wilkins, 1988;31–72.
18. Chaimovitz C, Rochman J, Eidelman S, Better OS: Exaggerated natriuretic response to volume expansion in patients with primary biliary cirrhosis. Am J Med Sci 1977;274:173–178.
19. Epstein M: Renal sodium handling in liver disease. In Epstein M (ed): The Kidney in Liver Disease, 3rd ed. Baltimore: Williams & Wilkins, 1988;3–30.
20. Epstein M: Renal sodium handling in cirrhosis: a reappraisal. Nephron 1979;23:211–217.
21. Epstein M: Deranged sodium homeostasis in cirrhosis. Gastroenterology 1979;76:622–635.
22. Peters JP: Body Water in the Exchange of Fluids in Man. Springfield, IL: Charles C Thomas, 1935;288.
23. Conn HO: The rational management of ascites. In Popper H, Schaffner F (eds): Progress in Liver Disease, Vol. 4. New York: Grune & Stratton, 1972;269–288.
24. Witte MH, Witte CL, Dumont AE: Progress in liver disease: physiological factors involved in the causation of cirrhotic ascites. Gastroenterology 1971;61: 742–750.
25. Schrier RW, Arroyo V, Bernardi M, et al: Peripheral arterial vasodilation hypothesis: A proposal for the initiation of renal sodium and water retention in cirrhosis. Hepatology 1988;8:1151–1157.
26. Levy M: Sodium retention in dogs with cirrhosis and ascites: efferent mechanisms. Am J Physiol 1977;233: F586–F592.
27. Levy M: Pathogenesis of sodium retention in early cirrhosis of the liver: Evidence for vascular overfilling. Semin Liver Dis 1994;14:4–13.
28. Tristani FE, Cohn JN: Systemic and renal hemodynamics in oliguric hepatic failure: Effect of volume expansion. J Clin Invest 1967;46:1894–1906.
29. Cohn JN: Renal hemodynamic alterations in liver disease. In Suki WN, Eknoyan G (eds): The Kidney in Systemic Disease, 2nd ed. New York: John Wiley & Sons, 1981;509–519.

30. Shasha SM, Better OS, Chaimovitz C, Doman J, Kishon Y: Haemodynamic studies in dogs with chronic bile duct ligation. Clin Sci 1976;50:533–537.

31. Ames RP, Borkowski AJ, Sicinski AM, Laragh JH: Prolonged infusions of angiotensin II and norepinephrine and blood pressure, electrolyte balance, and aldosterone and cortisol secretion in normal man and in cirrhosis with ascites. J Clin Invest 1965;44:1171–1186.

32. Pinzani M, Marra F, Fusco BM, et al: Evidence for α_1-adrenoreceptor hyperresponsiveness in hypotensive cirrhotic patients with ascites. Am J Gastroenterol 1991; 86:711–714.

33. Lieberman FL, Denison EK, Reynolds TB: The relationship of plasma volume, portal hypertension, ascites and renal sodium retention in cirrhosis: The overflow theory of ascites formation. Ann NY Acad Sci 1970; 170:202–212.

34. Lieberman FL, Ito S, Reynolds TB: Effective plasma volume in cirrhosis with ascites. Evidence that a decreased value does not account for renal sodium retention, a spontaneous reduction in glomerular filtration rate (GFR) and a fall in GFR during drug-induced diuresis. J Clin Invest 1969;48:975–981.

35. Levy M: Observations on renal function and ascites formation in dogs with experimental portal cirrhosis. In Epstein M (ed): The Kidney in Liver Disease. New York: Elsevier/North-Holland, 1978;131–142.

36. Levy M, Wexler MJ, McCaffrey C: Sodium retention in dogs with experimental cirrhosis following removal of ascites by continuous peritoneovenous shunting. J Lab Clin Med 1979;94:933–946.

37. Better OS, Schrier RW: Disturbed volume homeostasis in patients with cirrhosis of the liver. Kidney Int 1983; 23:303–311.

38. Decaux G, Dumont I, Naeije N, et al: High uric acid and urea clearance in cirrhosis secondary to increased "effective vascular volume." Am J Med 1982;73:328–334.

39. Decaux G, Prospert F, Namias B, et al: Raised urea clearance in cirrhotic patients with high uric acid clearance is related to low salt excretion. Gut 1992;33:1105–1108.

40. Schedl HP, Bartter FC: An explanation for and experimental correction of the abnormal water diuresis in cirrhosis. J Clin Invest 1960;39:248–261.

41. Vlahcevic ZR, Adam NF, Jick H, et al: Renal effects of acute expansion of plasma volume in cirrhosis. N Engl J Med 1965;272:387–391.

42. Gornel DL, Lancestremere RG, Papper S, Lowenstein LM: Acute changes in renal excretion of water and solute in patients with Laënnec's cirrhosis induced by the administration of the pressor amine, metaraminol. J Clin Invest 1962;41:594–603.

43. Schroeder ET, Anderson GH, Smulyan H: Effect of peritoneovenous shunt on renin in the hepatorenal syndrome. Kidney Int 1979;15:54–61.

44. Epstein M: Renal effects of head-out water immersion in man: Implications for an understanding of volume homeostasis. Physiol Rev 1978;58:529–581.

45. Epstein M: Renal effects of head-out water immersion in humans: A 15-year update. Physiol Rev 1992;72:563–621.

46. Epstein M, Pins DS, Arrington R, et al: Comparison of water immersion and saline infusion as a means of inducing volume expansion in man. J Appl Physiol 1975; 39:66–70.

47. Epstein M, Re R, Preston S, Haber E: Comparison of the suppressive effects of water immersion and saline administration on renin-aldosterone in normal man. J Clin Endocrinol Metabol 1979;49:358–363.

48. Epstein M, Levinson R, Sancho J, et al: Characterization of the renin-aldosterone system in decompensated cirrhosis. Circ Res 1977;41:818–829.

48a. Henriksen JH, Bendtsen F, Gerbes AL, et al: Estimated central blood volume in cirrhosis: Relationship to sympathetic nervous activity, β-adrenergic blockade and atrial natriuretic factor. Hepatology 1992;16:1163–1170.

48b. Henriksen JH, Bendtsen F, Sörensen TIA, et al: Reduced central blood volume in cirrhosis. Gastroenterology 1989;97:1506–1513.

49. Chaimovitz C, Szylman P, Alroy G, Better OS: Mechanism of increased renal tubular sodium reabsorption in cirrhosis. Am J Med 1972;52:198–202.

50. Chiandusi L, Bartoli E, Arras S: Reabsorption of sodium in the proximal renal tubule in cirrhosis of the liver. Gut 1978;19:497–503.

51. Epstein M, Ramachandran M, DeNunzio AG: Interrelationship of renal sodium and phosphate handling in cirrhosis. Miner Electrolyte Metab 1982;7:305–315.

52. Schuster VL, Seldin DW: Renal clearance. In Seldin DW, Giebisch G (eds): The Kidney, Physiology and Pathophysiology. New York: Raven Press, 1985;1:365–395.

53. Thomsen K: Lithium clearance: A new method for determining proximal and distal reabsorption of sodium and water. Nephron 1984;37:217–223.

54. Strazzullo P, Iacoviello I, Iacone R, Giorgione N: Use of fractional lithium clearance in clinical and epidemiological investigation: A methodological assessment. Clin Sci 1988;74:651–657.

55. Thomsen K, Holstein-Rathlou NH, Leyssac PP: Comparison of three measures of proximal tubular sodium reabsorption: Lithium clearance, occlusion time and micropuncture. Am J Physiol 1981;241:F348–F355.

56. Angeli P, Gatta A, Caregaro L, et al: Tubular site of renal sodium retention in ascitic liver cirrhosis evaluated by lithium clearance. Eur J Clin Invest 1990;20:111–117.

57. Díez J, Simón MA, Antón F, et al: Tubular sodium handling in cirrhotic patients with ascites as analysed by the renal lithium clearance method. Eur J Clin Invest 1990;20:266–271.

58. Coppage WS Jr, Island DP, Cooner AE, Liddle GW: The metabolism of aldosterone in normal subjects and in patients with hepatic cirrhosis. J Clin Invest 1962; 41:1672–1680.

59. Vecsei P, Dusterdieck G, Jahnecke J, et al: Secretion and turnover of aldosterone in various pathological states. Clin Sci 1969;36:241–256.

60. Rosoff L Jr, Zia P, Reynolds T, Horton R: Studies of renin and aldosterone in cirrhotic patients with ascites. Gastroenterology 1975;69:698–705.

61. Epstein M: Aldosterone in liver disease. In Epstein M (ed): The Kidney in Liver Disease, 3rd ed. Baltimore: Williams & Wilkins, 1988;356–373.

62. Chonko AM, Bay WH, Stein JH, Ferris TF: The role of renin and aldosterone in the salt retention of edema. Am J Med 1977;63:881–889.

63. Wilkinson SP, Jowett TP, Slater JDH, et al: Renal sodium retention in cirrhosis: Relation to aldosterone and nephron site. Clin Sci 1979;56:159–177.

64. Epstein M, Pins DS, Schneider N, Levinson R: Determinants of deranged sodium and water homeostasis in decompensated cirrhosis. J Lab Clin Med 1976;87: 822–839.

65. Nicholls KM, Shapiro MD, Kluge R, et al: Sodium excretion in advanced cirrhosis: Effect of expansion of central blood volume and suppression of plasma aldosterone. Hepatology 1986;6:235–238.

66. Navar LG: Renal regulation of body fluid balance. In Staub NC, Taylor AE (eds): Edema. New York: Raven Press, 1984;319–352.

67. Navar LG, Rosivall L: Contribution of the renin-angiotensin system to the control of intrarenal hemodynamics. Kidney Int 1984;25:857–868.

68. Harris PJ, Navar LG: Tubular transport responses to angiotensin. Am J Physiol 1985;248:F621–F630.

69. Navar LG, Saccomani G, Mitchell KD: Synergistic intrarenal actions of angiotensin on tubular reabsorption and renal hemodynamics. Am J Hypertens 1991; 4:90–96.

70. Hollenberg NK, Swartz SL, Passan DR, Williams GH: Increased glomerular filtration rate after converting–enzyme inhibition in essential hypertension. N Engl J Med 1979;301:9–12.

71. Epstein M, Lifschitz M, Hoffman DS, Stein JH: Relationship between renal prostaglandin E and renal sodium handling during water immersion in normal man. Circ Res 1979;45:71–80.

72. Boyer TD, Zia P, Reynolds TB: Effect of indomethacin and prostaglandin A$_1$ on renal function and plasma renin activity in alcoholic liver disease. Gastroenterology 1979;77:215–222.

73. Zipser RD, Hoefs JC, Speckart PF, et al: Prostaglandins: Modulators of renal function and pressor resistance in chronic liver disease. J Clin Endocrinol Metab 1979;48:895–900.

74. Planas R, Arroyo V, Rimola A, et al: Acetylsalicylic acid suppresses the renal hemodynamic effect and reduces the diuretic action of furosemide in cirrhosis with ascites. Gastroenterology 1983;84:247–252.

75. Epstein M, Lifschitz M, Ramachandran M, Rappaport K: Characterization of renal PGE responsiveness in decompensated cirrhosis: Implications for renal sodium handling. Clin Sci 1982;63:555–563.

76. Epstein M: Renal prostaglandins and the control of renal function in liver disease. Am J Med 1986;80 (Suppl 1A):46–55.

77. Ciabottoni G, Cinotti GA, Pierucci A, et al: Effects of sulindac and ibuprofen in patients with chronic glomerular disease. Evidence for the dependence of renal function on prostacyclin. N Engl J Med 1984;310: 279–283.

78. Brater DC, Anderson S, Baird B, et al: Effects of ibuprofen, naproxen, and sulindac on prostaglandins in men. Kidney Int 1985;27:66–73.

79. Daskalopoulos G, Kronborg I, Katkov W, et al: Sulindac and indomethacin suppress the diuretic action of furosemide in patients with cirrhosis and ascites: Evidence that sulindac affects renal prostaglandins. Am J Kidney Dis 1985;6:217–221.

80. Carretero OA, Scicli AG: The kallikrein–kinin system as a regulator of cardiovascular and renal function. In Laragh JH, Brenner BM (eds): Hypertension: Pathophysiology, Diagnosis, and Management,. 2nd ed. New York: Raven Press, 1995;983–999.

81. O'Connor DT, Stone RA: The renal kallikrein-kinin system: Description and relationship to liver disease. In Epstein M (ed): The Kidney in Liver Disease, 2nd ed. New York: Elsevier Biomedical, 1983;469–477.

82. Greco AV, Porcelli G, Ghirlanda G: L'escrezione di callicreina urinaria nella cirrosi epatica. Minerva Med 1975;66:1504–1508.

83. Zipser RD, Kerlin P, Hoefs JC, et al: Renal kallikrein excretion in alcoholic cirrhosis. Am J Gastroenterol 1981;75:183–187.

84. Pérez-Ayuso RM, Arroyo V, Camps J, et al: Renal kallikrein excretion in cirrhotics with ascites: Relationship to renal hemodynamics. Hepatology 1984;4:247–252.

85. Levinsky NG: The renal kallikrein-kinin system. Circ Res 1979;44:441–451.

86. DeWardener HE, Clarkson EM: Concept of a natriuretic hormone. Physiol Rev 1985;65:658–759.

87. Epstein M, Bricker NS, Bourgoignie JJ: The presence of a natriuretic factor in urine of normal men undergoing water immersion. Kidney Int 1978;13:152–158.

88. Haddy FJ, Buckalew VM Jr: Endogenous digitalis-like factors in hypertension. In Laragh JH, Brenner BM (eds): Hypertension: Pathophysiology, Diagnosis, and Management, 2nd ed. New York: Raven Press, 1995; 1055–1067.

89. Hamlyn JM, Manunta P, Hamilton BP: Endogenous ouabain in the pathogenesis of hypertensive and cardiovascular disorders. In Laragh JH, Brenner BM (eds): Hypertension: Pathophysiology, Diagnosis, and Management, 2nd ed. New York: Raven Press, 1995;1069–1081.

90. Favre H: Role of the natriuretic factor in the disorders of sodium balance. In Hamburger J, Crosnier J, Maxwell MH (eds): Advances in Nephrology. Chicago: Year Book, 1981;11:3–23.

91. Lewicki JA, Protter AA: Physiological studies of the natriuretic peptide family. In Laragh JH, Brenner BM (eds): Hypertension: Pathophysiology, Diagnosis, and Management, 2nd ed. New York: Raven Press, 1995; 1029–1053.

92. De Bold AJ, Borenstein HR, Veress AT, Sonnenberg H: A rapid and potent natriuretic response to intravenous injection of atrial myocardial extracts in rats. Life Sci 1981;28:89–94.

93. Atlas SA, Kleinert HD, Camargo MJF, et al: Purification, sequencing and synthesis of natriuretic and vasoactive rat atrial peptides. Nature 1984;309:717–719.

94. Currie MG, Geller DM, Cole BR, et al: Purifications and sequence analysis of bioactive atrial peptides (atriopeptins). Science 1984;223:67–69.

95. Camargo MJF, Kleinert HD, Atlas SA, et al: Ca-dependent hemodynamic and natriuretic effects of atrial extract in isolated rat kidney. Am J Physiol 1984;246: F447–F456.

96. Maack T, Marion DN, Camargo MJF, et al: Effects of auriculin (atrial natriuretic factor) on blood pressure, renal function, and the renin–aldosterone system in dogs. Am J Med 1984;77:1069–1075.

97. Gauer OH: Mechanoreceptors in the intrathoracic circulation and plasma volume control. In Epstein M (ed): The Kidney in Liver Disease. New York: Elsevier/North-Holland, 1978;3–17.

98. Jiménez W, Martínez-Pardo A, Arroyo V, et al: Atrial natriuretic factor: Reduced cardiac content in cirrhotic rats with ascites. Am J Physiol 1986;250:F749–F752.

99. Epstein M, Loutzenhiser R, Norsk P, Atlas S: Relationship between plasma ANF responsiveness and renal sodium handling in cirrhotic humans. Am J Nephrol 1989;9:133–143.

100. Epstein M, Loutzenhiser R, Friedland E, et al: Stimulation of plasma atrial natriuretic factor in cirrhotic humans by immersion-induced central hypervolemia. In Brenner B, Laragh J (eds): Biologically Active Atrial Peptides. New York: Raven Press, 1987;1:552–555.

101. Epstein M, Gerzer R: Natriuretic peptides and the kidney. In Massry SG, Glassock RJ (eds): Textbook of Nephrology, 3rd ed. Baltimore: Williams & Wilkins, 1995;1:227–231.

102. Abassi ZA, Golomb E, Klein H, Keiser HR: Urodilatin: A natriuretic peptide of renal origin. Cardiovasc Drug Rev 1992;10:199–210.

103. Goetz KL, Drummer C, Zhu JL, et al: Evidence that urodilatin, rather than ANP, regulates renal sodium excretion. J Am Soc Nephrol 1990;1:867–874.

104. Norsk P, Drummer C, Johansen LB, Gerzer R: Effect of water immersion on renal natriuretic peptide (urodilatin) excretion in humans. J Appl Physiol 1993;74:2881–2885.

105. Mukoyama M, Nakao K, Hosoda K, et al: Brain natriuretic peptide as a novel cardiac hormone in humans: Evidence for an exquisite dual natriuretic peptide system, atrial natriuretic peptide and brain natriuretic peptide. J Clin Invest 1991;87:1402–1412.

106. La Villa G, Romanelli RG, Casini Raggi V, et al: Plasma levels of brain natriuretic peptide in patients with cirrhosis. Hepatology 1992;16:156–161.

107. DiBona GF: The functions of the renal nerves. Rev Physiol Biochem Pharmacol 1982;94:75–181.

108. Thames MD: Neural control of renal function: Contribution of cardiopulmonary baroreceptors to the control of the kidney. Fed Proc 1977;37:1209–1213.

109. DiBona GF: Renal neural activity in hepatorenal syndrome. Kidney Int 1984;25:841–853.

110. Bichet DG, Van Putten VJ, Schrier RW: Potential role of increased sympathetic activity in impaired sodium and water excretion in cirrhosis. N Engl J Med 1982; 307:1552–1557.

111. Unikowsky B, Wexler MJ, Levy M: Dogs with experimental cirrhosis of the liver but without intrahepatic hypertension do not retain sodium or form ascites. J Clin Invest 1983;72:1594–1604.

112. Stein JH, Boonjarern S, Wilson CB, Ferris TF: Alterations in intrarenal blood flow distribution: Methods of measurement and relationship to sodium balance. Circ Res 1973;32–33:61–72.

113. DiBona GF: Neurogenic regulation of renal tubular sodium reabsorption. Am J Physiol 1977;233:73–81.

114. Gottschalk CW: Renal nerves and sodium excretion. Annu Rev Physiol 1979;41:229–240.

115. Barajas L, Powers K, Wang P: Innervation of the renal cortical tubules: A quantitative study. Am J Physiol 1984;247:50–60.

116. DiBona GF, Sawin LL: Effect of renal nerve stimulation on NaCl and H_2O transport in Henle's loop of the rat. Am J Physiol 1982;11:576–580.

117. Epstein M, Berk DP, Hollenberg NK, et al: Renal failure in the patient with cirrhosis: The role of active vasoconstriction. Am J Med 1970;49:175–185.

118. Lunzer MR, Newman SP, Bernard AG, et al: Impaired cardiovascular responsiveness in liver disease. Lancet 1975;2:382–385.

119. Ring-Larsen H, Hesse B, Henriksen JH, Christensen NJ: Sympathetic nervous activity and renal and systemic hemodynamics in cirrhosis: Plasma norepinephrine concentration, hepatic extraction and renal release. Hepatology 1982;2:304–310.

120. Henriksen JH, Ring-Larsen H, Kanstrup I-L, Christensen NJ: Splanchnic and renal elimination and release of catecholamines in cirrhosis: Evidence of enhanced sympathetic nervous activity in patients with decompensated cirrhosis. Gut 1984;25:1034–1043.

121. Henriksen JH, Ring-Larsen H, Christensen NJ: Sympathetic nervous activity in cirrhosis: A survey of plasma catecholamine studies. J Hepatol 1984;1:55–65.

122. Arroyo V, Planas R, Gaya J, et al: Sympathetic nervous activity, renin-angiotensin system and renal excretion of prostaglandin E_2 in cirrhosis: Relationship to functional renal failure and sodium and water excretion. Eur J Clin Invest 1983; 13:271–278.

123. Epstein M, Larios O, Johnson G: Effects of water immersion on plasma catecholamines in decompensated cirrhosis: Implications for deranged sodium and water homeostasis. Miner Electrolyte Metab 1985;11:25–34.

124. Kopp UC, Dibona GF: The neural control of renal function. In Seldin DW, Giebisch G (eds): The Kidney: Physiology and Pathophysiology, 2nd ed. New York: Raven Press, 1992;1157–1204.

125. Folkow B, DiBona G, Hjemdahl P, et al: Measurements of plasma norepinephrine concentration in human primary hypertension—a word of caution concerning their applicability for assessing neurogenic contribution. Hypertension 1983;5:399–403.

126. Esler M, Dudley F, Jennings G, et al: Increased sympathetic nervous activity and the effects of its inhibition with clonidine in alcoholic cirrhosis. Ann Intern Med 1992;116:446–455.

127. Willett I, Esler M, Burke F, et al: Total and renal sympathetic nervous system activity in alcoholic cirrhosis. J Hepatol 1985;1:639–648.

128. Lüscher TF, Bock HA, Yang Z, Diederich D: Endothelium-derived relaxing and contracting factors: Perspectives in nephrology. Kidney Int 1991;39:575–590.

129. Rubanyi GM: Endothelin in cardiovascular homeostasis. In Laragh JH and Brenner BM (eds): Hypertension: Pathophysiology, Diagnosis, and Management, 2nd ed. New York: Raven Press, 1995;1109–1124

130. Michel H, Bäcker A, Meyer–Lehnert H, et al: Rat renal, aortic and pulmonary endothelin-1 receptors: Effects of changes in sodium and water intake. Clin Sci 1993;85:593–597.

131. Migas I, Bäcker A, Meyer-Lehnert H, et al: Characteristics of endothelin (ET)l receptors and intracellular signaling in porcine inner medullary collecting duct (IMCD) cells. Am J Hypertens 1993;6:611–618.

132. Rabelink AJ, Kaasjager KAH, Boer P, et al: Effects of endothelin-1 on renal function in humans: Implications for physiology and pathophysiology. Kidney Int 1994; 46:376–381.

133. Bijlsma JA, Rabelink AJ, Kaasjager KAH, Koomans HA: L-Arginine does not prevent the renal effects of endothelin in humans. J Am Soc Nephrol 1995;5: 1508–1516.

134. Uchihara M, Izumi N, Sato C, Marumo F: Clinical significance of elevated plasma endothelin concentration in patients with cirrhosis. Hepatology 1992;16:95–99.

135. Sugiura M, Inagami T, Kon V: Endotoxin stimulates endothelin release in vivo and in vitro as determined by radioimmunoassay. Biochem Biophys Res Commun 1989;161:1220–1227.

136. Uemasu J, Matsumoto H, Kawasaki H: Increased plasma endothelin levels in patients with liver cirrhosis. Nephron 1992;60:380.

137. Epstein M: Hepatorenal syndrome: Emerging perspectives of pathophysiology and therapy. J Am Soc Nephrol 1994;4:1735–1753.

138. Vallance P, Moncada S: Hyperdynamic circulation in cirrhosis: A role for nitric oxide? Lancet 1991;337: 776–784.

139. Palmer RMJ, Ferrige AG, Moncada S: Nitric oxide release accounts for the biological activity of endothelium-derived relaxing factor. Nature 1987;327:524– 526.

140. Palmer RMJ, Ashton DS, Moncada S: Vascular endothelial cells synthesize nitric oxide from L-arginine. Nature 1988;333:664–666.

141. Umans JS, Levi R: The nitric oxide system in circulatory homeostasis and its possible role in hypertensive disorders. In Laragh JH and Brenner BM (eds): Hypertension: Pathophysiology, Diagnosis, and Management, 2nd ed. New York: Raven Press, 1995;1083– 1095.

142. Radlomski MW, Palmer RMJ, Moncada S: Glucocorticoids inhibit the expression of an inducible, but not the constitutive, nitric oxide synthase in vascular endothelial cells. Proc Natl Acad Sci USA 1990;87: 10043–10047.

143. Clària J, Jiménez W, Ros J, et al: Pathogenesis of arterial hypotension in cirrhotic rats with ascites: Role of endogenous nitric oxide. Hepatology 1992;15:343–349.

144. Tomás A, Soriano G, Guarner C, et al: Increased serum nitrite and nitrate in cirrhosis: Relationship to endotoxemia [abstract]. J Hepatol 1992;16(Suppl 1):4.

145. Aukland K, Bower BF, Berliner RW: Measurement of local blood flow with hydrogen gas. Circ Res 1964; 14:164–187.

146. Thurau K: Renal hemodynamics. Am J Med 1964; 36:698–719.

147. Barger AC: Renal hemodynamic factors in congestive heart failure. Ann NY Acad Sci 1966;139:276–284.

148. Hollenberg NK, Epstein M, Guttmann RD, et al: Effect of sodium balance on intrarenal distribution of blood flow in normal man. J Appl Physiol 1970;28: 312–317.

149. Epstein M, Hollenberg NK, Guttmann RD, et al: Effect of ethacrynic acid and chlorothiazide on intrarenal hemodynamics in normal man. Am J Physiol 1971;220: 482–487.

150. Horster M, Thurau K: Micropuncture studies on the filtration rate of single superficial and juxtamedullary glomeruli in the rat kidney. Pfluegers Arch 1968;301: 162–181.

151. Kilcoyne MM, Cannon PJ: Influence of thoracic caval occlusion on intrarenal blood flow distribution and sodium excretion. Am J Physiol 1971;220:1220–1230.

152. Epstein M, Schneider NS, Befeler B: Relationship of systemic and intrarenal hemodynamics in cirrhosis. J Lab Clin Med 1977;89:1175–1187.

153. Kew MC, Varma RR, Williams HS, et al: Renal and intrarenal blood flow in cirrhosis of the liver. Lancet 1971;2:504–510.

154. Leehey DJ, Gollapudi P, Deakin A, Reid RW: Naloxone increases water and electrolyte excretion after water loading in patients with cirrhosis and ascites. J Lab Clin Med 1991;118:484–491.

155. Holaday JW: Cardiovascular effects of endogenous opioid systems. Ann Rev Pharmacol Toxicol 1983;23: 541–594.

156. Johnson MW, Mitch WE, Wilcox CS: The cardiovascular actions of morphine and the endogenous opioid peptides. Prog Cardiovasc Dis 1985;27:435–450.

157. Kamoi K, Robertson GL: Opiates and vasopressin secretion. In Schrier RW (ed): Vasopressin. New York: Raven Press, 1985;259–264.

158. Grossman A, Clement-Jones V: Opiate receptors: Enkephalins and endorphins. Clin Endocrinol Metab 1983;12:31–56.

159. Pasanini F, Sloan L, Rubin PC: Cardiovascular properties of metkephamid, a delta-opioid receptor agonist, in man. Clin Sci 1985;68:209–213.

160. Danesh S, Walker LA: Effects of central administration of morphine on renal function in conscious rats. J Pharmacol Exp Ther 1988;244:640–645.

161. Thornton JR, Dean H, Losowsky MS: Is ascites caused by impaired hepatic inactivation of blood borne endogenous opioid peptides? Gut 1988;29:1167–1172.

162. Thornton JR, Losowsky MS: Plasma leucine enkephalin is increased in liver disease. Gut 1989;30: 1392–1395.

163. Christy NP, Shaver JC: Estrogens and the kidney. Kidney Int 1974;6:366–376.

164. Pearlman WH: The chemistry and metabolism of the estrogens. In Pincus G, Thimann KV (eds): The Hormones. New York: Academic Press, 1948;1:351– 405.

165. Lloyd CW, Williams RH: Endocrine changes associated with Laënnec's cirrhosis of the liver. Am J Med 1948;4:315–327.

166. Rupp J, Cantarow A, Rakoff AE, Paschkis KE: Hormone excretion in liver disease and in gynecomastia. J Clin Endocrinol Metab 1952;11:688–699.

167. Dohan FC, Richardson EM, Bluemle LW Jr, Gyorgy P: Hormone excretion in liver disease. J Clin Invest 1952; 31:481–498.

168. Chopra IJ, Tulchinsky D, Greenway FL: Estrogen-androgen imbalance in hepatic cirrhosis: Studies in 13 male patients. Ann Intern Med 1973;79:198–203.

169. Kley HK, Nieschlag E, Wiegelmann W, et al: Steroid hormones and their binding in plasma of male patients with fatty liver, chronic hepatitis and liver cirrhosis. Acta Endocrinol 1975;78:275–285.

170. Galvao-Teles A, Burke CW, Anderson DC, et al: Biologically active androgens and oestradiol in men with chronic liver disease. Lancet 1973;1:173–177.

171. Preedy JRK, Aitken EH: The effect of estrogen on water and electrolyte metabolism. II. Hepatic disease. J Clin Invest 1956;35:430–442.

172. Horrobin DF: Prolactin: Physiology and Clinical Significance. Lancaster, England: Medical and Technical Publishing, 1973.

173. Horrobin DF, Lloyd IJ, Lipton A, et al: Actions of prolactin on human renal function. Lancet 1971;2:352–354.

174. Burstyn PG, Horrobin DF, Manku MS: Saluretic action of aldosterone in the presence of increased salt intake and restoration of puerperal action by prolactin or by oxytocin. J Endocrinol 1972;55:369–376.

175. Horrobin DF, Manku MS, Robertshaw D: Water-losing action of antidiuretic hormone in the presence of excess cortisol: Restoration of normal action by prolactin or by oxytocin. J Endocrinol 1973;58:135–136.

176. Manku MS, Nassar BA, Horrobin DF: Effects of prolactin on the responses of rat aortic and arteriolar smooth muscle to noradrenaline and angiotensin. Lancet 1973; 2:991–994.

177. Carey RM, Johanson AJ, Seif SM: The effects of ovine prolactin on water and electrolyte excretion in man are attributable to vasopressin contamination. J Clin Endocrinol Metab 1977;44:850–858.

178. Wernze H, Schmitz E: Plasma prolactin and prolactin release in liver cirrhosis. Acta Hepatogastroenterol 1977;24:97–101.

179. Morgan MY, Jakobovits AW, Gore MBR, et al: Serum prolactin in liver disease and its relationship to gynaecomastia. Gut 1978;19:170–174.

180. Panerai AE, Salerno F, Manneschi M, et al: Growth hormone and prolactin responses to thyrotropin releasing hormone in patients with severe liver disease. J Clin Endocrinol Metab 1977;45:134–140.

181. Said SE, Mutt V: Polypeptide with broad biological activity: Isolation from small intestine. Science 1970; 169:1217–1218.

182. Kitamura S, Yoshida T, Said SI: Vasoactive intestinal polypeptide: Inactivation in liver and potentiation in lung of anesthetized dogs. Proc Soc Exp Biol Med 1975;148:25–29.

183. Hunt S, Vaamonde CA, Rattazzi T, et al: Circulating levels of vasoactive intestinal polypeptide in liver disease. Arch Intern Med 1979;139:994–996.

184. Calam J, Unwin RJ, Singh J, et al: Renal function during vasoactive intestinal peptide (VIP) infusions in normal man and patients with liver disease. Peptides 1984;5:441–443.

185. Dimaline R, Peart WS, Unwin RJ: Effects of vasoactive intestinal polypeptide (VIP) on renal function in the conscious rabbit. J Physiol (London) 1983;344:379–388.

186. Rossa R, Stoff JS, Silva P, Epstein FH: Tubular diuresis induced by vasoactive intestinal peptide (VIP) in the isolated perfused rat kidney. Clin Res 1977;25:669A.

187. Duggan KA, MacDonald GJ: Vasoactive intestinal peptide: A direct renal natriuretic substance. Clin Sci 1987; 72:195–200.

188. Ring-Larsen H, Henriksen JH, Wilken C, et al: Diuretic treatment in decompensated cirrhosis and congestive heart failure: Effects of posture. BMJ 1986;292:1351–1353.

189. Bernardi M, Santini C, Trevisani F, et al: Renal function impairment induced by change in posture in patients with cirrhosis and ascites. Gut 1985;26:629–635.

190. Reynolds TB, Lieberman FL, Goodman AR: Advantages of treatment of ascites without sodium restriction and without complete removal of excess fluid. Gut 1978;19:549–553.

191. Gauthier A, Levy VG, Quinton A, et al: The Entac Group: Salt or no salt in the treatment of cirrhotic ascites: A randomized study. Gut 1986;27:705–709.

Chapter 2

RENAL WATER HANDLING IN LIVER DISEASE

CARLOS A. VAAMONDE, M.D., F.A.C.P.

Role of the Liver in Water Metabolism
  Hepatic Osmoreceptors
  Hepatic Metabolism of Antidiuretic Hormone
Effect of Alcohol Ingestion on Renal Water Excretion
  Hyponatremia of Beer Drinkers
Renal Response to Water Administration in Cirrhosis
Pathogenesis of Impaired Water Excretion in Cirrhosis
  Increased Activity of Antidiuretic Hormone
  Decreased Delivery of Filtrate to Distal Nephron
    Diluting Segments

Enhanced Non–ADH-Mediated Back-Diffusion of
  Water
Water Excretion in Hepatitis and Biliary Cirrhosis
  Hepatitis
  Postnecrotic Cirrhosis
  Primary Biliary Cirrhosis
Clinical Consequences of Abnormalities of Water Excretion in Cirrhosis
  Hyponatremia
  Hypernatremia
Renal Water Conservation in Cirrhosis
Summary

That patients with cirrhosis have some impairment in the capacity for water excretion has been known for many years.[1,2] Indeed, salt and water retention leading to ascites and edema is the renal abnormality most commonly observed in patients with cirrhosis. Hyponatremia, the expression of the impaired capacity to excrete water, is a common clinical problem well-known to all physicians caring for cirrhotic patients.[3] The recognition that some patients with decompensated cirrhosis also develop hypernatremia has become a subject of new interest. A basic understanding of the pathophysiologic mechanisms leading to water retention and hyponatremia is required for rational treatment.

This chapter reviews renal water handling in liver disease, with particular emphasis on clinical aspects. Detailed exposition of the sodium renal handling in cirrhosis is presented in chapter 1. Despite the wealth of information obtained in many experimental studies, the actual relevance of animal models to human cirrhosis or other liver diseases remains unknown and largely conjectural, particularly with models of acute portal hypertension and extrahepatic obstruction of the bile conduits.

Because minor abnormalities in water excretion have been reported only occasionally in acute hepatic disease not complicated by renal failure[4] and in primary biliary cirrhosis,[5] the following description is related largely to findings in patients with cirrhosis of the liver. Since alcoholic liver disease constitutes the most common cause of cirrhosis of the liver in the United States, a brief description of the effects of alcohol on the kidney also is included.

ROLE OF THE LIVER IN WATER METABOLISM

Although a large body of information about abnormalities of renal water excretion in liver disease is available, it is less certain what role the liver itself may play in the renal handling of water. Two aspects are of particular interest: hepatic osmoreceptors and hepatic metabolism of antidiuretic hormone.

Hepatic Osmoreceptors

The existence of intrahepatic sodium or volume sensor mechanisms for detection of changes in the extracellular compartment has been described,[6–9] and their possible role in sodium retention in liver disease has been suggested.[10] The possibility that the liver also may possess some osmoreceptor function was raised by Haberich et al.[11,12] and Lydtin[13] almost 30 years ago. Sawchenko and Friedman[6] later reviewed this subject. The hypothesis was intriguing for two reasons: first, the critical location of the liver between the gut (the normal route of acquisition of water) and the systemic circulation; second, the possibility of hepatic osmoreceptor dysfunction in liver disease. When water was infused directly into the portal vein of conscious rats, reduction in portal vein osmolality was rapid and marked, without simultaneous changes in systemic blood osmolality.[11,12] The diuresis that followed was more rapid and greater than that observed when the same amount of water was infused into the inferior vena cava. On the other hand, the infusion of hypertonic sodium chloride into the portal vein resulted in antidiuresis. The "hepatogeneous" diuresis or antidiuresis was abolished by cutting the small branch of the vagal nerve from the stomach to the liver. Similar results were obtained by Lydtin[13] in experiments conducted in dogs. Investigators also reported that normal subjects had a more rapid diuretic response to water given intragastrically than to water injected into a peripheral vein.[12,14]

Although the concept of hepatic portal osmoreceptors was subsequently supported by neurophysiologic studies,[15–17] the findings of Haberich et al.[11,12] and Lydtin[13,14] were not reproduced by other investigators.[18–20] Subsequent data obtained in unanesthetized chronically cannulated dogs, however, have added further support to the hypothesis that intrahepatic osmoreceptors may be important in the physiologic regulation of water metabolism.[21] Intraportal infusions of hypertonic saline rapidly increased plasma antidiuretic hormone (ADH) activity (in this chapter the terms ADH, vasopressin, and arginine vasopressin [AVP] are used as synonyms) in the absence of significant changes in systemic plasma osmolality. That this plasma antidiuretic activity was indeed related to changes in ADH release is supported by observations that the activity was lost by incubation of the plasma with sodium thioglycolate and that the intraportal hypertonic saline infusion was temporally associated with the decrease in the diuresis of hydrated animals. The section of hepatic vagal afferent fibers abolished the ADH increase. Furthermore, plasma ADH levels did not change when isotonic saline was infused intraportally or when a similar hypertonic solution was given in a peripheral vein. The

observed increases in plasma ADH activity were related to changes in portal blood osmolality rather than to sustained hypertonicity per se. Of importance, portal vein blood sampled during the hour following a standard meal showed a significant increase in osmolality from the value prior to feeding.[21] The role of the putative hepatic osmoreceptors under normal conditions may be to provide a mechanism whereby potential osmotic challenges to the extracellular compartment may be rapidly tempered.[6,12] Indeed, it was shown that hepatic vagotomy affects neither overall water intake nor urine output in freely fed and watered rats, but it does limit the ability of the animal to adjust its urine output rapidly in response to intragastric water load or water deprivation.[16] The interrelationships between the suggested hepatic osmotic, volume, and pressor sensor systems have not been studied so far. Thus, the possibility that the liver may have some influence on renal water handling remains a fascinating and attractive idea awaiting more critical evaluation.

Hepatic Metabolism of Antidiuretic Hormone

Because plasma ADH concentration is determined by the difference between production and removal of the hormone from the circulation, it follows that the role of the liver in the metabolism of ADH is probably an important determinant of water homeostasis in liver disorders. It is known that ADH is largely metabolized in the liver, kidney, and, to some extent, small intestine.[22–26] Although it is generally accepted that the liver and kidney inactivate approximately equal amounts of ADH, through the years their relative contributions have been controversial.[24] This may be explained in part by the use of different animal species and experimental designs and by assessment of ADH activity with bioassay methods of unproved accuracy.[22,24,26] The state of hydration of the animal or subject prior to and during the study may be of particular importance, since dehydration increases and overhydration decreases the total metabolic clearance of ADH.[25,27] In the normal conscious rat undergoing a water diuresis, for example, no evidence was obtained to support any degradation by the liver of administered AVP.[24,28] On the other hand, hepatic clearance of AVP was present in the isolated perfused liver preparations of guinea pigs[29] and rats,[30] was not dependent on aerobic metabolism or glucose as a source of exogenous fuel, and was not saturated by high AVP concentrations.[30] Aziz and Schmidt[28] suggested that disturbances of liver cell function induced by alcohol, narcotics, thioacetamide, or isolation of the organ[29,30] might lead to liberation of ADH-destroying enzymes (vasopressinases) into the hepatic sinusoids and enhance the metabolism of circulating ADH.[28] The authors further suggested that the destruction of liver cells by CCl_4 may lead to a decrease in and finally cessation of production of this enzyme, resulting in a decrease in the hepatic clearance of ADH.[29,31] The report that the metabolic clearance of AVP, measured by a sensitive radioimmunoassay (RIA) technique, is not delayed in anephric humans indicates that AVP removal must occur predominantly at nonrenal sites (liver, small intestine).[25,32] One thus may speculate that the liver in the absence of kidney tissue and function may be capable of adequately handling the metabolism of ADH. The nature of the hepatic and renal enzymatic processes that inactivate AVP are not completely known but involve as a first step reduction of the disulfide bridge followed by cleavage of the bond between amino acids one and two by aminopeptidases.[25] The factors that influence the rate of metabolism of AVP and thus contribute to the modulation of its plasma levels in health and disease remain largely undetermined. It is thus conceivable that abnormalities of ADH metabolism in liver disease might play some role in the observed perturbations of water metabolism in patients with hepatic disorders.[33] The data at hand, however, do not permit a definitive answer to this important question.

EFFECT OF ALCOHOL INGESTION ON RENAL WATER EXCRETION

Alcohol ingestion induces a variety of electrolyte and acid-base disturbances that have been recently reviewed elsewhere.[34–36] The fact that ethyl alcohol ingestion results in increased urine excretion is a well-known and familiar experience to most readers. The ability of ethanol to induce in humans a diuresis was described by Miles over 70 years ago.[37] Earlier studies attributed the diuresis to a direct effect of alcohol on the kidney. The alcohol-induced water diuresis was accompanied by a moderate retention of sodium, chloride, and potassium.[38,39] Although plasma AVP concentrations could not be measured years ago, many investigators attributed the water diuresis to an alcohol-induced inhibition of ADH release by the posterohypophysis.[40–42] Many of these earlier experiments now have only historical value, but their physiologic soundness and importance should not be forgotten.

The alcohol-induced water diuresis is approximately proportional to the rising blood ethanol levels and can be prevented or inhibited by administration of pitressin[41,42] or nicotine, a potent stimulus for AVP release.[43] Once the diuresis is established, however, it cannot be maintained even when ethanol levels are kept constant or continue rising.[43] Furthermore, when alcohol was given during the declining phase of the diuresis, urine output did not increase (or urine osmolality decrease), indicating that the fading diuresis was not mediated by ADH release.[44] It was also shown that the diuresis was not due to an increase in glomerular filtration rate (GFR)[39,42,45] or renal prostaglandin E_2 (PGE_2) production.[46] Finally, ethanol did not increase urine flow when given under experimental conditions suggestive of very low or absent AVP levels, which in themselves make it impossible to demonstrate the inhibitory effect of alcohol on ADH release. The conditions included dogs with experimental diabetes insipidus,[47] normal humans at the height of a water diuresis,[48] and a cirrhotic patient who also had diabetes insipidus[49] (see Table 2.6).

With the development of accurate RIA methods for AVP measurement,[25] a better characterization of ADH levels during alcohol-induced diuresis was obtained. Ethanol ingestion is associated with a rapid decline in AVP levels.[50] Alcohol inhibits AVP release in humans by decreasing the response of AVP to changes in plasma osmolality.[50] This response is affected by age. Elderly subjects exhibited only a transient suppression of AVP levels despite a continuing increase in blood alcohol concentration in contrast to the AVP suppression found in young adults.[51] This may relate in part to an increased osmoreceptor sensitivity in the elderly.[51] Other factors that influence the release of ADH (discomfort, pain, posture, vomiting, dehydration) may interfere with the effect of ethanol on AVP levels and water excretion.[52] An example is found in the study of Linkola and coworkers in alcohol-intoxicated humans.[53] The authors found that AVP levels were higher at the time of peak ethyl alcohol levels and during the following hangover period than at baseline. Dehydration and, most likely, nausea and vomiting[52] probably acted as AVP-stimulatory factors, masking the effect of alcohol. Patients with edematous states, panhypopituitarism, adrenal insufficiency, and the syndrome of inappropriate secretion of ADH do not exhibit the inhibitory effect of ADH after alcohol administration.[35,54,55]

Studies on the effect of chronic alcohol intake on water excretion and fluid balance are scarce. Body fluid expansion was reported in dogs[56] and alcoholic humans[57] after chronic ethanol administration. Decreased diuresis, enhanced sodium reabsorption, and augmented voluntary intake of fluids were responsible for the expansion of body fluids. Conversely, renal water, sodium, and chloride excretion were augmented during acute withdrawal from ethyl alcohol in chronic alcoholic patients, normalizing the expanded body fluids within a few days.[57]

Ethanol readily elevates the plasma osmolality measured by freezing-point depression osmometry because of its lower molecular weight. On the other hand, if a vapor pressure osmometer is used, changes are negligible because of the low boiling point of ethanol and its insignificant contribution to the vapor pressure measurements of aqueous solutions.[58] Ethanol concentration can be accurately estimated by calculating an elevation in the osmolar gap, that is, when measured plasma osmolality appreciably exceeds the osmolality predicted on the basis of plasma glucose, urea, and electrolyte concentration.[59,60] However, the ethanol-induced increase in plasma osmolality does not stimulate AVP secretion, presumably because ethanol penetrates cells, including osmoreceptors, with ease and thus does not cause an "effective" osmotic pressure gradient.[61]

In recent years, considerable interest has developed in the central effects of ethanol and their relationship to endogenous opioids (endorphins).[61] Dunn and coworkers[62] studied the effects of the potent opioid antagonist naloxone on the ethanol-induced suppression of vasopressin in the stimulated (dehydrated or hypertonic saline-injected) rat. Without naloxone, the inhibitory effect of ethanol on AVP secretion appeared to be due largely to an elevation of the set point of the osmostat that regulates AVP secretion.[25] Treatment with naloxone partially reversed this effect, suggesting that the actions of ethanol on AVP are partially mediated by endogenous opioids.[62] Since AVP release may be influenced by several opioid pathways (both stimulatory and inhibitory) acting at different levels on both osmotic and nonosmotic stimuli, a word of caution is needed in the interpretation of these studies.[63] The potential use of endogenous opioid antagonists in the treatment of hyponatremia of cirrhosis is discussed below.

Hyponatremia of Beer Drinkers

The ingestion of large amounts of beer by alcoholics whose diet contains little solute obligated for excretion into the urine (urea) results in severe hyponatremia and water intoxication.[34,64–67] The majority of such patients consume several liters (2–5 or more) per day of beer, are usually malnourished, and may have very low blood urea nitrogen and serum creatinine levels.[67] Serum sodium can reach levels close to 100 mEq/L, and urine is often moderately hypertonic and contains little urea. Patients occasionally present with the central nervous system (CNS) manifestations of water intoxication.

Beer is a hyperosmolar fluid (600–800 mOsm/kg H_2O) with little sodium content (usually less than 2–4 mEq/L). The hyperosmolality is due to its alcohol and carbohydrate content; thus after metabolism, beer drinking equals water drinking. *The beer drinker's hyponatremia is due to an excessive ingestion of free water.* In addition, because of the low protein intake the only obligatory solutes excreted in the urine represent obligatory protein catabolism, which in such patients is diminished by the protein-sparing effect of the high carbohydrate content of beer.[34] We have shown that young, healthy volunteers ingesting a normal diet (generating about 1100 mOsm of urinary solute per day) were capable of drinking up to 12 liters daily of water without appreciable changes in serum sodium concentration, because their urine volume rose appropriately to match the forced water intake.[68] Indeed, Gill et al.[69] demonstrated the effects of a beer binge on normal young healthy volunteers, who ingested 3.3 liters of beer (612 mOsm/kg H_2O, 2 mEq/L of sodium and 7.6 mEq/L of potassium) in 3 hours at night. A typical water diuresis ensued (increased urine volume and free water clearance with low urine osmolality) and was accompanied by normal suppression of plasma AVP and no discernible changes in serum sodium concentration. On the other hand, chronic alcoholic patients may excrete little urinary solute (urea and sodium chloride), facilitating the appearance of this syndrome by combining large fluid intake (free-water–generating beer), poor protein intake, inhibition of endogenous protein catabolism (carbohydrate-sparing effect), and low sodium intake. Any level of ADH present under such conditions (discomfort, pain, dehydration, vomiting, upright posture, smoking) may confound water retention and aggravate the hyponatremia. Treatment depends on the severity of the hyponatremia and ranges from simple water restriction combined with increased protein intake to administration of hypertonic saline solution.

Considering the large consumption of beer throughout the world and the relative rarity of this syndrome, it is safe to conclude that chronic wasted alcoholic patients consuming diets with little protein content are probably at higher risk of developing severe hyponatremia when ingesting huge amounts of beer.

RENAL RESPONSE TO WATER ADMINISTRATION IN CIRRHOSIS

Most studies examining the characteristics of water excretion in liver disease have used the technique of water loading. In evaluating the response to water administration, consideration should be given to the maximal urine flow (V max)

and solute-free water generation (CH_2O max) rates and to the minimal urine osmolality (UOsm min). In cirrhotic patients a continuum of responses has been described. Figure 2.1 (right panel) illustrates a normal response to water administration in a cirrhotic patient with ascites and edema and normal GFR. In response to a standard oral water load (20 ml/kg of body weight), the patient rapidly increased urine flow to about 10 ml/min despite the presence of severe fluid retention. He excreted little sodium (< 5 µEq/min)—an expression of avid sodium retention—and produced dilute urine (U_{OSM} 32 mOsm/kg H_2O). Indeed, some of the lowest urine osmolalities following water administration are observed in patients with decompensated cirrhosis. If such patients are given or drink water, they are able to handle the load normally and thus maintain a serum sodium concentration within the normal range. The left panel of Figure 2.1, on the other hand, shows the other end of the spectrum of responses in liver disease. A severely decompensated cirrhotic patient with a decreased GFR and a low rate of excretion of sodium (comparable, however, to that of the previous patient) was unable to increase urine output in response to an intravenously administered water load and excreted consistently hypertonic urine. If such patients ingest or receive water in excess of their markedly

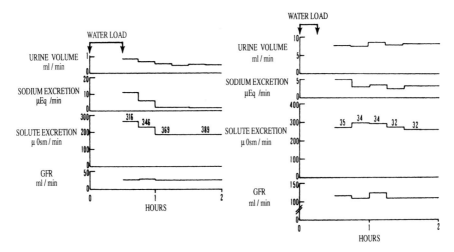

FIGURE 2.1.   Response to oral or intravenous water loading in decompensated cirrhotic patients. *Right,* Normal response to a sustained oral water load (20 ml/kg of body weight given in 15 min) in a 45-year-old cirrhotic patient with ascites and edema. From top to bottom the urine volume, rate of sodium and solute excretion and glomerular filtration rate (GFR) are depicted. The numbers on top of the lines representing solute excretion are the corresponding urine osmolalities. *Left,* Lack of diuretic response to sustained intravenous 4% invert sugar in water (20 ml/kg of body weight) given to a 63-year-old cirrhotic patient with ascites and edema. Both patients received a diet containing 10 mEq of sodium daily. Note that the range of units in the vertical scales are different.

Table 2.1. Response to Water Administration in Cirrhotic Patients*

	Compensated (n = 5)		Decompensated (n = 5)
Maximal urine flow (ml/min)[a]	14.1 ± 4.0^b	$p < 0.01$	5.7 ± 3.2
Maximal CH_2O (ml/min)[a]	12.0 ± 3.5	$p < 0.02$	4.4 ± 2.8
Minimal UOsm (mOsm/kg H_2O)[c]	42 ± 4	$p < 0.05$	71 ± 25
$U_{Na}V$ (µEq/min)[d]	32 ± 25	$p < 0.05$	2 ± 1
C_{Cr} (ml/min)[d]	131 ± 34	$p < 0.02$	84 ± 18
$\dfrac{CH_2O + C_{Na}}{CH_2O}$/GFR (ml/min)[e] /GFR[f]	9.6 ± 1.0	$p < 0.01$	5.4 ± 2.8
$CH_2O + C_{Na}$	98.2 ± 1.3	NS	98.5 ± 1.9

* Patients received a diet containing 10 mEq of sodium daily for at least 5 days prior to studies.
[a] Highest urine volume or free-water clearance (CH_2O) following oral water loading (20 ml/kg of body weight).
[b] Data are mean ± SD, evaluated by unpaired t-test.
[c] Lowest urine osmolality after water loading.
[d] Average value of urinary sodium excretion ($U_{Na}V$) or endogenous creatinine clearance (C_{Cr}).
[e] Maximal fractional distal delivery of sodium during water loading.
[f] Maximal fractional sodium reabsorption in the distal nephron during water loading.
From Vaamonde CA, et al: The role of vasopressin and urea in the renal concentrating defect of patients with cirrhosis of the liver. Clin Sci Mol Med 1971;41:441–452, with permission.

reduced capacity for water excretion, water retention and hyponatremia will rapidly ensue. Indeed, the patient's serum sodium concentration decreased by 11 mEq/L, reaching 124 mEq/L, 2 hours after the water load; whereas in the first patient, who exhibited no limitation in water excretion, the change in serum sodium concentration was less than 3 mEq/L, and 3 hours after completion of the water load the serum sodium concentration had returned to baseline. Note that both patients received the water load under ideal controlled conditions: low sodium diet, recumbency, minimal stress, no smoking, and absence of medications that may interfere with AVP. Under normal living circumstances such controlled conditions rarely exist, potentiating the clinical effects of impaired water excretion in patients with cirrhosis.

The frequency of abnormalities in water excretion in cirrhosis is difficult to assess. Most reported observations relate to groups of patients studied once at a given clinical stage of cirrhosis; very few include repeated renal function studies as the clinical course of the disease unfolds. Patients are usually grouped as decompensated (with various degrees of ascites or edema or both) or compensated (without clinical evidence of ascites or edema).

When patients are grouped according to the results of a single evaluation, it appears that decompensated patients have abnormal responses to water administration, whereas patients without ascites or edema excrete water normally (Table 2.1).[70–74] This generalization, however, should be considered carefully because exceptions are not uncommon (Table 2.2). Not all decompensated cirrhotic patients excrete water abnormally (see below), and some patients without ascites and edema (early cirrhosis) may exhibit a mild impairment in water excretion.[75] Thus, a spectrum of responses to water administration is commonly found in patients with cirrhosis.

Some years ago we performed sequential studies of the response to water administration in cirrhotic patients as the disease evolved.[71] The results are summarized in Table 2.2. Patients 1–10 were studied first when they were in a decompensated state and subsequently when they achieved compensation. Patients 11–13 were studied in reverse order. The patients, none of whom had the renal failure of cirrhosis (GFR > 60 ml/min),[2] were followed for weeks or months; the data shown in Table 2.2 detail only the most striking changes, excluding many of the intermediate studies. In terms of V max, compensated patients, with perhaps one exception, excreted water normally (9.3 to 27.6 ml/min). On average, the patients studied during the decompensated state had a lower V max after water loading (10.5 ± 2.1 [SE] ml/min) than when studied during the compensated state (15.4 ± 1.9 ml/min; p > 0.05). However, in examining the individual data it is apparent that some patients with decompensated cirrhosis had clear impairments (patients 1, 4, 5,

TABLE 2.2. Response to Water Administration in Cirrhotic Patients Studied Sequentially When Ascites and/or Edema Were Present (Decompensated, D) or Absent (Compensated, C)

Patient[a]	Weeks Between Studies	Serum Na[b] (mEq/L)		Vmax[c] (ml/min)		UOsm[d] (mOsm/kg H$_2$O)		CH$_2$O[c] (ml/min)		UNa[e] (mEq/L)		UNaV[f] (µEq/min)		C$_{IN}$[f] (ml/min)	
		D	C	D	C	D	C	D	C	D	C	D	C	D	C
1	30	138	136	5.4	–	82	–	3.9	–	1	–	4	–	96	80
2	13	139	137	12.5	12.5	65	103	9.1	6.4	8	39	71	482	58	110
3	1	134	133	20.8	17.2	63	73	16.1	12.8	10	15	201	203	164	127
4	10	133	127	5.7	7.9	69	47	4.0	6.2	1	1	6	4	109	81
5	25	130	142	3.0	27.6	243	39	2.6	23.5	1	3	11	161	204	191
6	10	133	132	14.8	22.6	44	55	12.7	17.9	9	18	211	363	105	121
7	7	138	132	2.4	12.2	145	50	1.0	9.9	1	8	2	91	111	131
8	35	136	127	14.2	10.1	58	59	10.9	7.8	12	7	224	66	110	107
9	3	133	132	19.8	20.7	62	74	15.4	15.0	15	15	219	210	135	111
10	23	137	138	10.3	–	40	–	8.7	–	7	–	61	–	118	105
11	12	136	136	1.2	9.3	328	44	0.02	7.9	33	4	23	18	79	66
12	29	141	141	7.0	17.9	68	45	6.0	15.0	1	11	4	189	97	149
13	10	142	123	14.1	11.2	43	40	11.7	9.4	4	2	49	12	123	136

[a] Patients 1–10 were studied initially during decompensation (presence of ascites/edema; patients 11–13 were first evaluated when compensated (no clinical evidence of ascites or edema). Patients received a diet containing 10 mEq of sodium daily for at least 5 days prior to the studies.
[b] Values obtained before water administration.
[c] Represents highest urine flow rate (V max) or free-water clearance (CH$_2$O) following water loading.
[d] Represents the lowest value following water loading.
[e] Values for urinary sodium concentration (UNa) and urine sodium excretion rate (UNaV) at the time of V max.
[f] C$_{IN}$ represents inulin clearance and is the average of at least four collection periods following water loading.
From Klingler EL, Jr, et al: Renal function changes in cirrhosis of the liver: A prospective study. Arch Intern Med 1970;125: 1010–1015.

7, and 11), whereas others excreted water normally (patients 2, 3, 6, 8, 9, 10, and 13). It is also evident that some patients did not show appreciable changes in their responses, regardless of clinical state or direction of change (patients 2, 3, 8, 9, and 13). In general, changes in CH$_2$O followed, with few exceptions, the change in maximal urine flow.

Almost all patients with compensated cirrhosis excreted markedly hypotonic urines (10 of 11 had minimal urine osmolalities less than 75 mOsm/kg H$_2$O, and 6 had values between 50 and 39 mOsm/kg H$_2$O). On the other hand, although the majority of decompensated patients were able to excrete a urine hypotonic to plasma (11 of 13), fewer achieved very low urine osmolalities.

Since in these patients,[71] as well as those reported elsewhere[70–74,76,77] no measurements of circulating ADH levels were available, it was difficult to exclude completely the possibility that a minimal amount of ADH was present in some of the decompensated patients. Equally important, in some decompensated patients (Table 2.2,

patients 4 and 12; Table 2.4, patients 14 and 16) the subnormal excretion of water could not be attributed to the presence of ADH because of the low urine osmolalities, suggesting that other mechanisms were responsible. It is, therefore, important to emphasize that although the excretion of urine of low osmolality (less than 100 to 75 mOsm/kg H$_2$O) after water loading may give assurance of an appropriate physiological inhibition of ADH, the rate of water excretion still may be subnormal and hyponatremia may result (Table 2.3). Low solute (sodium and urea) excretion in decompensated cirrhotics, as we demonstrated,[70] probably explains this dissociation between the variables traditionally used to evaluate water excretion. Furthermore, the presence of a supernormal GFR (defined as an inulin and/or creatinine clearance consistently elevated to more than 3 SD above the mean of control subjects) was not necessarily associated with a normal V max[71] (Table 2.2, patient 5).

More recently, measurements of AVP in decompensated patients with cirrhosis during water

TABLE 2.3. Dissociation between Minimal Urine Osmolality (UOsm min) and the Rate of Water Excretion (V max, CH₂O max, and % of Water Load Excreted) after Water Loading in Patients with Decompensated Cirrhosis without Initial Hyponatremia*

	Patient A	Patient B	Patient C
Ccr (ml/min)	97	87	31
UOsm (mOsm/kg H_2O)	65	78	77
V max (ml/min)	7.0	5.4	3.3
CH_2O (ml/min)	5.3	3.9	2.3
H_2O load excreted (% in 4 hr)	66	44[†]	49
UNaV (μEq/min)	5	1	7
UOsm V (μEq/min)	428	359	250
Serum Na (mEq/L)			
Baseline	135	136	135
End of study	132	133	124

* All patients received a 20 ml/kg water load given intravenously as 4% invert sugar in water.
† % of water load excreted in 2 hr.

administration have shown a relationship between high plasma AVP levels and the inability to excrete water.[78,79] Even some compensated patients without ascites or edema who have baseline plasma AVP levels within the normal range have been shown not to suppress AVP levels normally following an oral water load,[75] although most compensated patients are capable of doing so.[80]

Solute excretion is characteristically very low in many such patients, with virtually no sodium and little urea in the urine.[2,70,81] In terms of urinary sodium excretion, although compensated cirrhotic patients excreted more sodium than decompensated patients, there was great variability among them and it was clear that not all subjects retaining sodium avidly had impaired water excretion (Fig. 2.1, Table 2.2).

A subgroup of decompensated cirrhotic patients who developed renal failure (hepatorenal

syndrome) weeks or months after the initial observations was also studied (Table 2.4). When renal failure developed, they exhibited a uniform pattern characterized by the complete inability to excrete solute-free water, associated with excretion of a hypertonic urine almost devoid of sodium. When these patients were first studied in the decompensated stage, they exhibited the same variability in the ability to excrete water alluded to (Table 2.2). Thus the response to water administration was not a useful index for predicting the evolution of the severely decompensated cirrhotic patient into the hepatorenal syndrome (HRS).

The contribution of urea to urine osmolality is decreased in cirrhotic patients. Throughout a wide range of urine flow (0.4–15 ml/min) the cirrhotic patients studied by Vaamonde et al.[70] consistently excreted less urea than controls. When diluted urine of cirrhotic and control patients was compared at similar flow rates and lower sodium

TABLE 2.4 Response to Water Administration in Four Decompensated (D) Cirrhotic Patients who Subsequently Developed the Hepatorenal Syndrome (RF)*

Patient*	Weeks Between Studies	Serum Na (mEq/L)		V max (ml/min)		UOsm (mOsm/kg H_2O)		CH_2O (ml/min)		UNa (mEq/L)		UNaV (mEq/min)		C_{IN} (ml/min)		C_{PAH}[†] (ml/min)	
		D	RF	D	RF	D	RF	D	RF	D	RF	D	RF	D	RF	D	RF
14	19	139	124	4.1	0.2	70	305	3.0	−0.01	1	17	1	2	63	7	317	–
15	4 days	131	122	3.5	1.5	64	155	2.6	0.6	1	3	3	3	131	23	–	210
16	9	132	130	1.8	0.6	109	332	1.1	−0.01	1	6	1	3	58	5	377	63
17	6	121	121	10.0	1.9	66	407	7.2	−0.4	1	1	1	1	148	42	–	–

* See Table 2.2 for explanations of column heads.
† Represents clearance of paraaminohippurate.
From Klingler EL Jr, et al: Renal function changes in cirrhosis of the liver: A prospective study. Arch Intern Med 1970;125:1010–1015, with permission.

content, the cirrhotic group had a slightly lower urine osmolality than controls; this difference can be explained entirely by their lower urinary concentration of urea[70] (Fig. 2.2).

The correlation in decompensated cirrhosis between the rate of sodium excretion and urine flow during water loading is depicted in Figure 2.3.[81] Although a good correlation between urinary flow and sodium excretion was observed throughout a wide range of sodium excretion, there was no correlation between both variables at very low rates of sodium excretion (< 10 µEq/min). Therefore, under conditions of intense and almost complete renal sodium reabsorption, the rate of sodium appearing in the urine is not a sensitive index of delivery of sodium to the distal diluting sites.

It is difficult to correlate the capacity for water diuresis with specific clinical features.[2,71,81] The poorest diuretic response tends to occur in the most severely ill patients, but some patients who are equally ill in terms of general appearance may have reasonably good water diuresis. In addition, maximal water diuresis does not correlate well with degree of ascites or level of jaundice.[71] Other investigators, however, have found good correlation between some clinical and laboratory

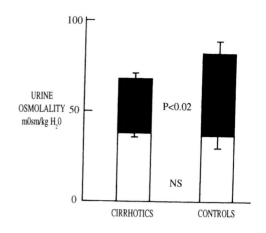

FIGURE 2.2. Composition of dilute urine in 9 cirrhotic and 9 chronically ill (control) patients compared at a urine flow of 6–8 ml/min. Patients received a diet containing 10 mEq of sodium, 80–100 mEq of potassium, and 1.5 gm of protein/kg of body weight and were studied during a standard oral water load. Urine osmolality was lower in the cirrhotic patients (p < 0.05) and the difference was due to the lower concentration of urea (p < 0.02) (*shaded columns*), whereas nonurea solute concentration was similar (*white columns*). (Adapted from Vaamonde CA, et al: The role of vasopressin and urea in the renal concentrating defect of patients with cirrhosis of the liver. Clin Sci Mol Med 1971;41:441–452.)

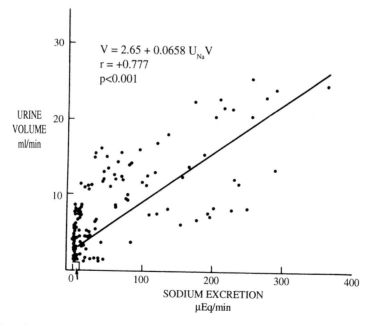

FIGURE 2.3. Correlation between urine volume and rate of sodium excretion in decompensated cirrhotic patients during water administration. In the area indicated by the *arrow* there were 75 points. The correlations (not illustrated) between urine flow and rate of solute excretion (r = 0.81) and between V and CH_2O (r = 0.58) were also significant (p < 0.01 for both). (Adapted from Lancestremere RJ: Some aspects of renal function in patients with cirrhosis. M.D. thesis. University of Buenos Aires School of Medicine, Buenos Aires, 1962.)

findings of liver disease and impaired water excretion,[78] including high plasma renin activity and aldosterone levels, low urinary sodium and serum albumin, and elevated serum bilirubin levels. Experimentally, however, short-term exposure of toad hemibladders to bilirubin did not alter basal or vasopressin-stimulated urea or water transepithelial transport.[82] Perhaps impaired water excretion correlates better with the severity of liver disease in general than with specific clinical or laboratory features.[71] The detailed relationships of plasma ADH levels with water excretion in cirrhosis are discussed in the next section.

PATHOGENESIS OF IMPAIRED WATER EXCRETION IN CIRRHOSIS

Although the pathogenesis of the impairment in water diuresis in cirrhosis is not fully established, three mechanisms acting solely or in combination are known to be involved: (1) increased ADH activity, (2) decreased delivery of filtrate to the diluting nephron segments, and (3) enhanced non–ADH-mediated back-diffusion of water in the distal nephron (Table 2.5).

TABLE 2.5.   Pathogenesis of Impaired Water Excretion in Cirrhosis of the Liver

Increased antidiuretic hormone (ADH) activity
Enhanced nonosmotic release of ADH*
Enhanced adrenergic activity*
Enhanced RAS activity
Altered renal prostaglandins modulation*
Atrial natriuretic factor
Other possible influences†
Endothelin
Nitric oxide
Abnormal osmoreceptor function
Resetting of systemic osmoreceptors
Abnormal liver osmoreceptors
Decreased hepatic metabolism of ADH
Enhanced sensitivity of the distal nephron of ADH†
Drug-induced ADH-like activity
Decreased delivery of glomerular filtrate to diluting nephron segments*
Decreased filtrate volume*
Decreased solute (sodium chloride, urea) availability*
Enhanced non–ADH-mediated back-diffusion of water in distral nephron
Combination of any of the above mechanisms*

RAS = Renin angiotensin system
* Most important.
† Remain unproved.

Although evidence for the contributions of the second and third mechanisms, particularly of decreased distal delivery of filtrate, is convincing, the role of enhanced ADH activity in the genesis of subnormal dilution capacity most recently has received strong support. The recent development of sensitive and specific RIA techniques for ADH permitted the precise measurement of hormone levels at physiologic concentrations under most common clinical or well-defined experimental conditions.[25]

Increased Activity of Antidiuretic Hormone in Cirrhosis

The distortion of fluid volume and the hypoosmolality commonly observed in cirrhosis and the possibility that the liver disease itself interferes with the hormonal degradation of ADH suggest a role for ADH in the abnormal water handling in cirrhosis.

Indirect Assessment of Activity of Antidiuretic Hormone in Cirrhosis

Before the era of reliable ADH measurements, a number of workers approached the assessment of the ADH status in cirrhosis in various indirect ways:

1. Classically, UOsm was measured under controlled conditions for diet and posture following a standard water load (20 ml/kg) and interpreted as an indirect index of the circulating levels of ADH. The basic assumption was that a very low UOsm (75 or less mOsm/kg H_2O) excluded with certainty the presence of elevated levels of ADH, particularly in the presence of subnormal V max and CH_2O values[70,71] (Tables 2.1, 2.2, and 2.3).

2. About 40 years ago, Strauss and coworkers[55] demonstrated that the ingestion of 100 gm of alcohol increased urine flow and decreased urine osmolality in severely decompensated cirrhotic patients with normal GFR and virtually complete sodium reabsorption. Before alcohol ingestion the patients had failed to respond to a water load maintained for 6 hr (V max ranging from 0.6–2 ml/min and UOsm from 142–960 mOsm/kg H_2O). This observation was interpreted by the authors as strongly suggesting that alcohol had inhibited the release of ADH,[48] as subsequently demonstrated in noncirrhotic patients by other investigators[50–52] (see section on alcohol ingestion), implying that circulating blood levels of

ADH were elevated in cirrhotic patients. The authors, however, pointed out that the magnitude of the alcohol-induced diuresis was subnormal, indicating that factors other than ADH were limiting the V max.

3. Subsequently, De Troyer and coworkers[83] reported increases in urine output with concomitant decreases in urine osmolality after giving demeclocycline to patients with decompensated cirrhosis. Other investigators[84–87] have also confirmed this observation. Because this tetracycline derivative appears to interfere with the renal tubular action of ADH[88,89] specifically by interacting with calmodulin-dependent enzymes,[90] the data were offered also as indirect evidence for enhanced ADH activity in cirrhotic patients. Since some of these patients also exhibited an increase in sodium excretion, the mechanism of the increased urine output remains undefined.[83,91] The therapeutic implications of the use of demeclocycline in cirrhosis is discussed later.

4. Of some interest are studies in which liver disease or ascites exists in the absence of ADH. Laragh and coworkers[92] demonstrated in 1956 that dogs with experimentally induced diabetes insipidus maintained polyuria and polydypsia despite the accumulation of ascites and edema following thoracic inferior vena caval occlusion. This finding suggests a role for ADH in mediating the oliguria observed in this model of hepatic congestion when the anterior hypothalamus is intact.

Over 20 years ago we studied a 44-year-old man with longstanding diabetes insipidus (20 years) and severe alcoholic cirrhosis (5 years)[49] on two occasions: first when he was compensated and later at a time when he had ascites and edema (Table 2.6). His GFR was normal on both occasions, and he conserved sodium avidly on a 10-mEq/day sodium intake. Pitressin was discontinued a few days in advance of each study, and with a high fluid intake, stable body weight and renal function were maintained throughout the study periods. The responses to a standard oral water load during compensation or a combined oral/intravenous water load plus 50 gm of 5% alcohol given intravenously during decompensation were entirely normal on both occasions. The patient's urine became highly diluted, and following the administration of exogenous vasopressin, he was able to increase urine osmolality to or above plasma osmolality. Alcohol did not improve the already normal water diuresis, suggesting further

TABLE 2.6. Water Excretion in Patient with Alcoholic Cirrhosis and Central Diabetes Insipidus*

Patient Characteristics	Compensated	Decompensated	
Body weight (kg)	72.5	79.5	
Ascites	0	++	
Edema	0	+	
Baseline[†]			
C_{IN}	136	123	
C_{PAH} (ml/min)	691	572	
V (ml/min)	6	3.6	
UOsm (mOsm/kg H_2O)	47	92	
UNaV (µEq/min)	8	1	
Water load (20 ml/kg of body weight)			
V max (ml/min)	11.2	14.1[‡]	15.1[§]
UOsm (mOsm/kg H_2O)	40	38[‡]	36[§]
CH_2O max (ml/min)	9.4	11.7[‡]	12.9[§]
UNaV (µEq/min)	13	19	10[§]
Response to exogenous vasopressin[∥]			
UOsm max (mOsm/kg H_2O)	475	281	

* Pitressin tannate in oil was discontinued a few days in advance and body weight and renal function were maintained stable prior to studies by giving sufficient fluid intake. The patient was maintained on a 10 mEq/day sodium intake. See text for details.
† Values prior to water loading.
‡ Part of H_2O load given intravenously.
§ After infusion of 50 gm of 5% alcohol.
∥ 200 mU of aqueous vasopressin followed by 200 mU/hr intravenously.

that ADH was not present. Of interest, his baseline urine flow was lower and the osmolality higher prior to water loading in the decompensated state than after water administration, perhaps in part as the consequence of intravenous water loading. Such results suggest that at baseline a decreased distal delivery of filtrate to the distal nephron may have counterbalanced the effect of the lack of ADH, resulting in the excretion of a concentrated urine and resembling the classical observations of Berliner and Davidson in dogs.[93] The absence of ADH resulted in a normal response to water administration. A similar patient with partial central diabetes insipidus has been recently reported.[94]

Measurements of Antidiuretic Hormone in Cirrhosis

Throughout the 1950s and 1960s a number of investigators using various bioassay systems reported the presence or absence of ADH-like activity in serum and urine of patients with liver disease. Such conflicting data, however, are not evaluated here because of the uncertainty about the validity of the methods and the inadequacy of controls. Readers with an interest in the historical development of the field are referred elsewhere.[33,95–100]

Measurements of plasma vasopressin levels with highly sensitive RIA techniques have been performed recently in numerous patients with cirrhosis[78–80,86,101–110] The assessment of AVP plasma levels and the analysis of its relationships with plasma osmolality or plasma sodium concentration constitute fundamental aspects of all modern experimental and clinical studies of water excretion in liver disease. Clinically, this powerful approach permits the unmasking of nonosmotic influences by eliminating confounding variables due to small concurrent changes in osmotic stimulation.[25] Elevated AVP values have been reported by most investigators.[78–80,86,101,104,106,107,109,110] Padfield and Morton,[101] for example, found normal or elevated plasma AVP values in 10 cirrhotic patients, with no apparent association between elevated AVP values and presence of ascites or hyponatremia. Increased AVP plasma levels were reported in patients without ascites or hyponatremia,[104] and values similar to those of normal controls were recorded in decompensated patients.[86,101,110] One group documented plasma AVP levels lower than normal in cirrhotic patients.[105] The reports of lack of correlation between plasma AVP levels and serum sodium concentration in cirrhotic patients are not surprising if one considers that elevated AVP may result from nonosmotic stimulation of ADH release.

Bichet et al.[78,106] reported their cumulative experience with 26 patients with alcoholic liver disease and variable degrees of ascites and edema. The authors measured plasma AVP levels before and during the 5 hours after intravenous infusion of a water load of 20 ml/kg of body weight. Seventy-three percent (19 of 26) of the patients had an abnormal response to water administration (excreted less than 80% of the water load) and had elevated mean plasma AVP levels (2.1 ± 0.5 pg/ml vs. 0.7 ± 0.1 pg/ml; p < 0.01). All had ascites, low GFR and urinary sodium excretion, and low serum albumin and plasma sodium concentrations. The higher concentrations of AVP were present despite plasma hypoosmolality, which was not found in the patients with normal water excretion and lower AVP levels. Unfortunately, the authors did not provide individual

values to permit detailed assessment of the interrelationships between plasma levels of AVP, sodium, osmolality, and response to water administration. Pérez Ayuso et al.[79] also studied AVP levels before and after intravenous water loading in 27 cirrhotic patients. Before water loading, most (11 of 14) patients with severely impaired water excretion had elevated AVP plasma levels compared with controls. After water administration, all failed to suppress AVP to the levels achieved by controls. Cirrhotic patients with subnormal responses to water had intermediate basal and postload AVP. As a group, however, their values were higher than controls but lower than those of patients with the poorest responses. More recently, Castellano et al.[80] reported the results of a controlled study in 35 cirrhotic patients and 15 controls. Normal baseline plasma AVP levels were found in the subgroups of compensated (n = 15) and decompensated cirrhotic patients without hyponatremia (n = 15) (2.9 ± 0.7 [$\bar{x}$ ± SD] and 3.4 ± 1.5 vs. 2.7 ± 0.7 pg/ml for controls, respectively). In contrast, AVP was significantly elevated at baseline in the 10 decompensated patients with hyponatremia (serum sodium below 135 mEq/L) (4.5 ± 0.9 pg/ml; p < 0.05–0.01 vs. other groups). As expected, the decompensated cirrhotic patients exhibited an abnormal response to oral water administration; this was particularly severe in the subgroup with hyponatremia, who exhibited essentially no free-water formation and excretion of hypertonic urine. Of importance, all patients had a decrease in plasma AVP levels following the water load (nadir between 90 and 120 minutes), but the levels of the hyponatremic decompensated cirrhotic patients always remained above all others, indicating a poor suppressibility of ADH in the presence of hyponatremia. The authors concluded that in decompensated cirrhotic patients without hyponatremia, impaired excretion of water cannot be ascribed to high levels of ADH; rather it appears to be related to reduced delivery of filtrate to the diluting segment of the nephron.[80] Technical problems with RIA, uncontrolled experimental conditions, and use of different protocols may be largely responsible for the apparent conflicting results of AVP plasma levels reported in patients with cirrhosis.

Evidence of enhanced ADH activity and its possible causative mechanism(s) also has been obtained in various experimental models of liver disease,[111–119] as described in detail elsewhere.[120]

In brief, a chronologic relationship has been shown in longitudinal studies in rats with experimental cirrhosis and ascites between the elevation of AVP levels and the impaired ability to excrete administered water.[113,115] Rats with apparently early compensated cirrhosis induced by CCl$_4$, on the other hand, do not exhibit elevated AVP levels.[116] Hypophysectomy abolishes the antidiuresis induced by acute portal hypertension in anesthetized dogs.[111] Furthermore, rats with congenital defect in ADH secretion that caused hereditary diabetes insipidus (Brattleboro strain) and liver disease induced by chronic bile duct ligation[113] or CCl$_4$[114] did not develop abnormal water excretion[114] in comparison to chronic bile duct-ligated or cirrhotic animals with intact ADH mechanism. The ability to respond appropriately to water administration is restored in cirrhotic rats by the administration of a V$_2$-receptor antagonist (d[CH$_2$] 5 Tyr [Et] VAVP (SKF 100398),[117] which unfortunately possesses agonistic activities in humans. Nevertheless, Tsuboi et al.[118] recently reported that the acute administration of a new nonpeptide V$_2$-receptor antagonist (OPC-31260)[119] to rats with experimental cirrhosis improved their ability to excrete water.

Of great interest is the recent report of Kim et al.[121] of increased hypothalamic synthesis and pituitary release of AVP in rats with experimental cirrhosis. The authors demonstrated increased levels of plasma AVP in the CCl$_4$-phenobarbital model of cirrhosis, concomitantly with elevated levels of hypothalamic AVP messenger RNA and normal hypothalamic and pituitary AVP contents. The data taken as a whole suggest increased ADH hypothalamic production and enhanced pituitary release of the hormone. Hypothalamic oxytocin messenger RNA in cirrhotic animals was not different from that in controls, a finding that supports the possibility that stimuli for enhanced ADH hypothalamic synthesis were of nonosmotic origin.[122]

Mechanisms of Increased Activity of ADH in Cirrhosis

The possible mechanisms for increased ADH activity in patients with liver disease (Table 2.5) include (1) enhanced nonosmotic release of ADH, (2) abnormal osmoreceptor function, (3) decreased hepatic metabolism of ADH, (4) enhanced tubular sensitivity to ADH, (5) drug-induced ADH-like activity, and (6) a combination of any of the above.

Increased Nonosmotic Release of Antidiuretic Hormone. Under normal circumstances, the development of hyponatremia and hypotonicity indicates that the enhanced hormonal secretion occurs in response to a stimulus other than extracellular fluid osmolality (nonosmotic ADH stimulation). Although total plasma volume may be increased in cirrhosis, it is known that, perhaps by virtue of its unique distribution, the physiologic circumstances may mimic reduction in plasma volume (reduced effective plasma volume[2]). The concept of the traditional underfilling theory of ascites formation or its revised version (early peripheral arterial vasodilatation) is discussed in detail elsewhere.[123–125] In brief, portal hypertension induces splanchnic arteriolar vasodilatation causing underfilling of the arterial vascular compartment (the traditional reduced effective plasma volume,[2] since measured plasma volume in cirrhosis is usually increased). The arterial underfilling is sensed by the high-pressure baroreceptors and stimulates the renin angiotensin-aldosterone and sympathetic nervous systems, resulting in a decrease in afferent parasympathetic activity, an increase in ADH release,[78,126,127] and secondary salt and water retention. Early in cirrhosis, when the splanchnic arterial vasodilatation is moderate and the lymphatic system compensates for the tendency of pooling blood by returning the increased lymph formation into the systemic circulation, the arterial underfilling is minimized by transient (secondary) salt and water retention by the kidney. This retention suppresses the increase in vasoactive activity and ADH, but at the cost of an increased total body sodium and water balance status. Progressive liver disease is characterized by increased splanchnic blood pooling (particularly in the venous side of the system), further arterial underfilling, decreased venous return to the heart secondary to development of tense ascites, and hypoalbuminemia, all of which stimulate the renin-angiotensin-aldosterone and adrenergic systems and further the release of ADH. Water and sodium retention become permanent and intense, and severe ascites and edema characterize the decompensated clinical phase of cirrhotic patients.

Because alterations in systemic hemodynamics frequently alter parasympathetic tone in both low- and high-pressure cardiovascular sites[128] the above-mentioned pathways may be activated in cirrhosis and result in elevated ADH levels.

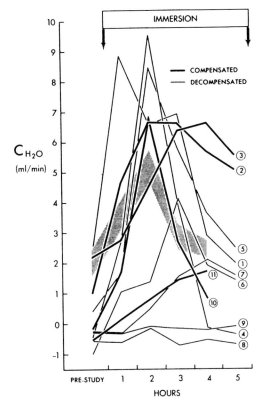

FIGURE 2.4. Effect of water immersion follow-ing 1 hr of quiet sitting (prestudy) on free-water clearance (CH_2O) in 11 patients with alcoholic liver disease receiving a diet containing 10 mEq of sodium and 100 mEq of potassium. *Shaded area* represents the mean ± SE for CH_2O for 18 normal control subjects undergoing immersion while in balance on a 150-mEq sodium diet.[134] These con-trols received a water load (1700 ml) twice as great as that utilized in the present study. Immer-sion resulted in a significant increase in CH_2O (p < 0.01) that equaled or exceeded that of the controls on the higher sodium and water intake. All patients diluted their urine impressively, attaining levels of minimal UOsm that were equal to or less than that of the controls (129 ± 99 [SE] mOsm/kg H_2O; p < 0.01). (Reprinted by permission of the C.V. Mosby Company from Epstein, M, et al: Determinants of deranged sodium and water homeostasis in de-compensated cirrhosis. J Lab Clin Med 1976;87: 822–839.)

Bichet et al.[78,106] and Pérez Ayuso et al.[79] con-cluded that the lack of appropriate ADH sup-pressibility in decompensated cirrhotic patients during water diuresis indicated nonosmotic (baroreceptor) stimulation of ADH release. As noted before, others[80] have concluded that in the absence of hyponatremia the impaired water

excretion in decompensated cirrhotics cannot be attributed solely to enhanced ADH levels, sug-gesting that other mechanisms (e.g., decreased distal delivery of filtrate) may have a predomi-nant role.

Recent studies performed in cirrhotic patients undergoing water immersion to the neck are of particular interest.[108,131] Since redistribution of central blood volume[132] and suppression of plasma AVP levels[133] have been shown in normal humans upon water immersion, a similar expla-nation is plausible in immersed patients with cir-rhosis, who previously were shown to respond to immersion with enhanced free-water clearance[134] (Fig. 2.4). By inference, one may assume that central volume depletion in decompensated cir-rhosis induces ADH release.

Bichet and coworkers[131] in Denver reported the effect of central volume expansion induced by water immersion in 8 decompensated cirrhotic patients studied during the administration of a water load of 20 ml/kg of body weight. Control studies,[132–134] as usual, consisted of the same pro-tocol used outside the immersion tank. Head-out water immersion was associated with suppres-sion of AVP levels and improvement in water ex-cretion (from 36% to 63% of water load). In contrast, Epstein et al.[108] in Miami failed to demonstrate plasma AVP suppression with im-mersion in the majority of 17 patients (15 had de-compensated cirrhosis) (Fig. 2.5). The authors concluded that alterations in water handling in some decompensated cirrhotic patients may occur independently of changes in plasma AVP concen-trations; therefore, other concomitantly operating mechanisms may be responsible. Such data, never-theless, cannot exclude completely a role for ADH release in mediating the impaired water ex-cretion in cirrhosis because the patients—unlike those illustrated in Figure 2.4—were hydropenic at the time of immersion. Indeed, within the con-text of the experimental maneuvers, the data may suggest either the possibility of impairment of ADH metabolism or an altered (blunted) sensitiv-ity to water immersion-induced central volume expansion in cirrhotic patients.

The results of the two immersion studies cannot be compared because of their different protocols. Of necessity, both groups studied pa-tients in the sitting position. This, incidentally, may explain why Bichet et al.[131] did not observe suppression of AVP during the control study (water loading outside the immersion tank); their

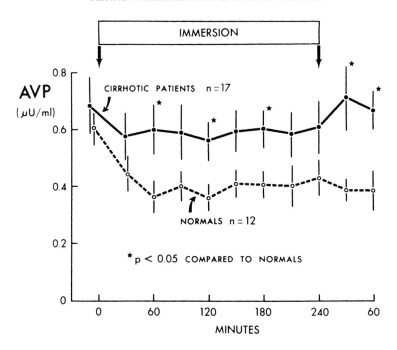

FIGURE 2.5. Comparison of the effects of immersion on plasma arginine vasopressin (AVP) in hydropenic cirrhotic patients (n = 17) and in normal subjects (n = 12). The cirrhotic patients undergoing immersion failed to suppress AVP despite that more exhibited a diuresis, and 7 of 14 increased CH_2O from -0.2 ± 2.2 ml/min to 1.1 ± 1.8 ml/min. In contrast, normal subjects undergoing an identical study manifested a persistent suppression of AVP. Results are mean ± SE; p < 0.05 compared to normal controls. Data for normal hydropenic subjects are from Epstein et al.[133] (Reprinted by permission of S. Karger AG, Basel, from Epstein M, et al: Relationship between plasma arginine vasopressin and renal water handling in decompensated cirrhosis. Miner Electrolyte Metab 1984;10:155–165.)

previous study was presumably carried out in recumbent patients.[78] Furthermore, as already pointed out, whereas the Miami patients were dehydrated, the Denver patients were undergoing an intravenous water load. Thus, even assuming that patients were clinically similar, the physiologic conditions at the time of immersion were dissimilar. Patients studied by Bichet et al.[131] received a stronger stimuli (immersion plus intravenous water load), which resulted in more effective suppression of AVP. Furthermore, unexplained higher AVP levels were recorded at baseline in the study of Bichet et al. on the day of immersion, perhaps suggesting that the AVP status of their patients might not have been stable.

When a peritoneovenous shunt was placed for the control of intractable ascites[107] or ascitic fluid was reinfused,[135] the elevated AVP levels were not suppressed, despite centrally induced hypervolemia and associated diuresis. However, Solis-Herruzo et al.[136] used paracentesis to remove 3 liters of ascites to decrease the intrathoracic and intraabdominal pressures (by 61% and 39%, respectively; both p < 0.001) in 20 cirrhotic patients with tense ascites and demonstrated a 32% suppression of the elevated levels of AVP (p < 0.001). The authors suggested that the high concentration of AVP in the ascitic fluid either returned to the circulation[135] or removed[137] most likely explains the opposite results observed by others.[107,135]

When one considers the different physiologic conditions under which the above studies were done,[78,79,106–108] their results are not surprising and should not be interpreted as contradictory. *On the whole, clinical data strongly support the activation of nonosmotic stimuli for ADH release in decompensated cirrhotics.* It is also clear that in some patients mechanisms other than high ADH levels are also responsible for the abnormal water excretion ability.

Finally, a recent study in rats with CCl_4-phenobarbital-induced cirrhosis[138] demonstrated that the administration of a selective antagonist of the vascular effects of AVP (blockade of V_1-receptor) (d[CH_2]5 Tyr [Me] AVP [SKF100273]) produced arterial hypotension in rats with ascites, impaired water excretion, and hyponatremia. The authors suggested that AVP hypersecretion in cirrhosis not only contributes to impaired water excretion, but also maintains arterial pressure. Thus, arterial hypotension may be the initial nonosmotic stimuli for ADH release in cirrhosis (see comment on the modified filling theory of ascites formation).

Mediators of Nonosmotic Release of Antidiuretic Hormone. Recent evidence supports the role of mediators of the nonosmotic stimulation of ADH release in cirrhosis. According to the traditional underfilling view or its modified version,[123] the low effective volume results in enhanced adrenergic activity with possible stimulation of ADH release and enhanced renin-angiotensin activity. The possible roles of both vasodilator and vasoconstrictor prostaglandins, atrial natriuretic peptide, and other less well studied substances (endothelin, nitric oxide) are also reviewed.

ENHANCED ADRENERGIC SYSTEM ACTIVITY. Plasma norepinephrine (NE) levels have been suggested as an index of sympathetic activity,[139] particularly of baroreceptor function.[140] Using a sensitive RIA, several investigators have reported elevated plasma NE values in patients with cirrhosis,[79,106,131,141–147] particularly in those with decompensated cirrhosis (for a full review of this subject the reader is referred elsewhere[145]). Elevated renal venoarterial ratios of NE also have been reported, suggesting increased renal production rather than decreased NE metabolism in cirrhosis.[143,146] Epstein et al.,[145] however, found basal NE levels increased in only 9 of 16 patients and reported that the magnitude of the elevation in NE varied independently of the degree of ascites. Bichet et al.[102,131] reported that intravenous water loading in cirrhotic patients with or without water immersion resulted in suppression of NE levels, that a negative correlation between NE levels and the ability to excrete water could be shown, and that a positive correlation was established between high levels of NE and AVP. Similarly, in another study,[79] patients with the poorest responses to water loading had the highest NE values. In addition, Blendis and coworkers[146] demonstrated normalization of the elevated NE values 2 weeks after placement of a peritoneovenous shunt in 6 patients with massive refractory ascites. A word of caution in the interpretation of the above described studies, however, has been

raised by Epstein et al.[145] In response to water immersion, the majority of the 16 patients showed no relationship between changes in NE levels and peak urine flow rate (Fig. 2.6). Measurements of the difference in renal venoarterial concentration of plasma NE during water immersion are necessary to define more precisely the contribution of enhanced adrenergic activity to impaired dilution in cirrhosis.

In recent years, it has become apparent that an increase in efferent renal sympathetic nerve activity can influence water excretion in ways not involving ADH release.[149,150] The most important effect appears to be a decrease in distal delivery of filtrate secondary to enhanced proximal tubular reabsorption of sodium[149,151] Other mechanisms include renal vasoconstriction and possibly activation of the renin-angiotensin system. Evidence, however, suggests that the adrenergic nerve effect on tubular function is independent of renin-angiotensin or prostaglandins.[148,149]

RENIN-ANGIOTENSIN SYSTEM. Cirrhotic patients frequently have elevated plasma renin activity and angiotensin levels,[80,152–156] which possibly constitute another pathway for the stimulation of ADH release in cirrhosis.[157] Such a possibility seems unlikely, however, for three reasons: (1) neither intravenous nor intracarotid infusions of angiotensin II interfere with water excretion in anesthetized[158] or conscious[159] dogs; (2) experiments in normal humans suggest little, if any, direct effect of angiotensin II on plasma AVP levels under physiologic conditions;[160] and (3) angiotensin II infusion, even at nonpressor dosages, causes marked natriuresis and diuresis in some cirrhotic patients with ascites.[161] For further information see chapter 12.

RENAL PROSTAGLANDINS. Renal prostaglandins (PGs), particularly prostaglandin E_2 (PGE$_2$; see chapter 14), are important in maintaining water homeostasis[162,163] It is not surprising, therefore, that the contribution of PGs to the abnormal excretion of water in cirrhosis has received increased attention in recent years.[79,164–171] The major action of PGs appears to be inhibition of the tubular effects of ADH, which favors generation of water clearance.[162,163] Additional effects include the washout of medullary tonicity secondary to increases in medullary renal blood flow and distal delivery of filtrate.[172] The first mechanism interferes with the cellular hydroosmotic effect of ADH, whereas the increases in blood flow and filtrate delivery are independent of

ADH. The three actions, however, favor water excretion. Thus, if renal PG levels are suppressed, decreased, or not increased appropriately (in response, for example, to renal vasoconstrictive stimuli), water excretion may be impaired.

In one study,[79] PGE_2 excretion was significantly elevated in decompensated cirrhotics with a subnormal response to water excretion. Despite high levels of plasma AVP, patients who were capable of increasing free-water formation following the water load had higher PGE_2 urinary excretion. In contrast, urinary PGE_2 did not increase in the patients unable to dilute the urine. Pérez-Ayuso et al.[79] interpreted the results to indicate that in the first group, the elevated PGE_2 levels probably contributed to more normal water excretion by interfering with the tubular effect of ADH, as assumed from the high levels of AVP along with an almost normal response to water administration. In the cirrhotic group with normal or low urinary PGE_2 values and complete failure to dilute the urine, the absence of an increase in urinary PGE_2 excretion could not counteract the higher plasma AVP levels, adding to the markedly impaired dilution.[79] Others have also shown elevated basal values of PGE_2 excretion in cirrhotic patients.[165–167] $PGE_{2\alpha}$ values were not elevated.[75,166] Epstein et al.[167] demonstrated an increase in PGE excretion during water immersion that was 3-fold greater in decompensated patients than in normal subjects.[173] A careful analysis of the data suggested that the observed increase in PGE excretion was not solely the result of an increase in urine flow rate but also reflected an increase in renal PGE production.[167]

Other studies that focused on the effects of inhibition of PG synthesis in cirrhosis reported impaired water excretion, associated with decreased GFR and renal blood flow.[79,164,165,168,169] Of particular interest are studies in which low doses of cyclooxygenase inhibitors were acutely given in an attempt to dissociate the renal hemodynamic from the water handling effects of PG inhibition[79,169] Markedly reduced water clearance was found in patients with cirrhosis and ascites but not in cirrhotic patients without ascites or in normal subjects. Such effects occurred in the absence of changes in AVP levels or were independent of changes in renal hemodynamics. Furthermore, the same investigators observed that the improved water excretion that followed demeclocycline administration was also associated with increased urinary PGE_2 excretion.[87]

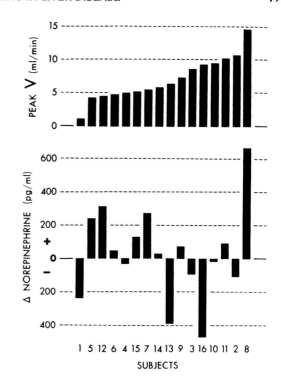

FIGURE 2.6. Relationship of renal water handling to alterations in plasma norepinephrine (NE) (*lower panel*) during immersion in 16 cirrhotic patients. The numbers along the horizontal axis designate the individual patients. As can be seen the magnitude of the diuresis, as assessed by peak V (*top panel*), varied independently of ΔNE ("nadir" minus prestudy NE) during immersion (r = 0.24; not significant). (Reprinted by permission of S. Karger AG, Basel, from Epstein M, et al: Effects of water handling on plasma catecholamines in decompensated cirrhosis. Implications for deranged sodium and water homeostasis. Miner Electrolyte Metab 1985;11:25–34.)

Attempts at improving renal water handling in cirrhosis with administration of PGs have given contradictory results. Gines et al.[174] were unable to confirm the results of Fevery et al.,[175] indicating a possible effect of the oral PGE_1 analogue misoprostol in improving water excretion in patients with early HRS. Gines et al. attributed their negative results to the fact that neither the oral administration of misoprostol nor the intravenous administration of PGE_2 was associated with prior or concomitant volume expansion, as in the study of Fevery et al.

The role of increased renal production of thromboxane A_2[176] in the abnormal water excretion of cirrhosis remains unclear. However, a recent study of the effects of an antagonist (0N0-3708) of thromboxane A_2 in cirrhotic patients reported a mild improvement in the diluting capacity with increased urine flow and free-water formation,[177] suggesting the possibility of an interference with the tubular action of ADH.[178]

Thus the overwhelming current information supports a role for PG in renal water handling. The accepted hypothesis is that renal PGs modulate renal water excretion by antagonizing the tubular action of endogenous ADH. Patients with cirrhosis thus may be highly sensitive to spontaneous changes or interference with renal capacity to synthesize PG.

ATRIAL NATRIURETIC FACTOR.   In recent years, considerable interest has developed in the physiologic role of atrial natriuretic factor (ANF), a peptide thought to be essential in the regulation of circulating blood volume.[179,180] Because atrial release and plasma concentration of ANF increase in response to extracellular fluid volume expansion or elevations in right atrial pressure,[179] it is conceivable that ANF may play some role in the abnormal water excretion of cirrhosis. Indeed, recent experimental evidence indicates that ANF inhibits the central release of ADH and thus participates in water homeostasis.[181–185] Of note, the intracerebroventricular infusion of ANF in normally hydrated conscious sheep decreased plasma ANF levels and increased water clearance without inducing sodium or potassium diuresis or an increase in mean arterial pressure.[185] Inhibition by ANF of the hydroosmotic action of ADH in the medullary collecting duct has also been described.[186]

The atrial content of ANF in cirrhotic rats with ascites was found to be lower than that in noncirrhotic animals by Jiménez et al.[187] Whether the low atrial ANF levels were due to decreased synthesis or increased release was not investigated. In a subsequent preliminary report, Valdivieso et al.[187a] found decreased ANF binding sties in the renal medulla of cirrhotic rats. Atrial peptide extract concentrations were higher in hearts obtained at autopsy from cirrhotic patients,[188] suggesting the possible existence of species differences in ANF pathophysiology. The extracts proved to have diuretic and hypotensive activities when infused to rats.[188]

Elevated basal plasma ANF values have been recently reported in patients with decompensated cirrhosis.[189–192] Other investigators, however, reported normal[193,194] or lower than normal plasma values.[195] Preliminary results on the effects of water immersion on plasma ANF were reported after standard (4 hours)[193] or short (1 hour) immersion procedures.[189,194] Such studies showed various degrees of increase in ANF with immersion-induced hypervolemia. Subsequently, Vesely and coworkers[196–199] demonstrated a prompt and marked increase of ANF, N-terminus of the ANF, and kaliuretic stimulator (a new atrial natriuretic peptide with the most potent kaliuretic properties of this class of hormones[199]) in response to water immersion in normal subjects[196] and patients with cirrhosis.[197,198] Finally, it was also shown that ANF levels increase appropriately in response to intravascular volume loading, with right atrial filling resulting from peritoneovenous shunting in cirrhosis.[200] Together such data suggest that circulating levels of ANF are not deficient in patients with decompensated cirrhosis. Alterations in ANF structure or an effect of elevated ANF values in modulating other vasoconstrictive influences in cirrhosis (angiotensin, NE) has not been excluded. The effect of ANF on water excretion in cirrhosis remains to be defined; its known effect on sodium excretion, however, makes this task difficult (see chapter 15).

ENDOTHELIN.   Endothelin is a potent endothelium-derived vasoconstrictor peptide.[201] Elevated values of endothelin-1 and endothelin-3 have been recently reported in patients with cirrhosis and renal failure (HRS),[202,203] whereas other investigators reported values lower than normal in cirrhotics without HRS.[204] The significance of abnormal plasma endothelin values in cirrhosis, particularly in the HRS, remains unknown. Endothelin inhibits the hydroosmotic action of AVP, particularly in the inner medullary[205,206] and cortical collecting duct segments.[207] No information is available about a possible role of the endothelins in water excretion in cirrhosis, although one would expect any effect to be masked by the consequences of their powerful vasoactive action. For further information see chapter 18.

NITRIC OXIDE.   It is currently accepted that nitric oxide (NO) is a potent endogenous endothelium-derived vasodilator[208,209] and that the endothelium plays an important role in the intrinsic modulation of vascular tone by elaborating potent vasoactive substances. In normal animals[209] and rats with cirrhosis induced by bile duct ligation,[210] or CCl_4,[210a] NO produces diuresis and natriuresis. Increased levels of circulating vasodilatory substances have been implicated in the pathogenesis of the vasodilatation associated with portal hypertension,[211,212] including hyporeactivity to AVP, norepinephrine, angiotensin II, and potassium chloride.[213,214] Furthermore, it has recently been suggested that NO mediates vascular hyporeactivity to vasopressors in the mesenteric vessels of rats with portal hypertension[215,216] and may be a factor in the arterial vasodilatation of cirrhosis (see comments on the modified underfilling theory). Indeed, a recent preliminary report by Martin et al.[210a] indicates that normalization of vascular NO production with the NO synthesis inhibitor L-NAME corrected the arterial vasodilatation and the hyperdynamic circulation in rats with cirrhosis and ascites. No direct evidence links NO to the observed abnormalities in water excretion in cirrhosis. For further information, see chapter 17.

Abnormal Osmoreceptor Function. The possibility exists of a resetting of the osmoreceptors to an abnormally low level in cirrhosis; that is, decompensated cirrhotic patients may be unable to produce an appropriately dilute urine despite marked plasma hypoosmolality. Indeed, Earley and Sanders[217] reported that patients with decompensated cirrhosis demonstrated adequate sensitivity to further changes in tonicity induced by water diuresis or hypertonic saline infusion, suggesting that the release of ADH was regulated in a qualitatively normal fashion but was based on a lower than normal level of osmolality. Furthermore, in a study of dogs with chronic bile duct ligation (BDL), a similar resetting of the osmostat was subsequently described.[112] The osmotic threshold for AVP release was lower in dogs with chronic BDL than in control animals. Thus, for any given value of plasma osmolality, AVP concentration was higher in animals with chronic BDL. More recently, however, Ardaillou et al.[110] demonstrated that following hypertonic saline infusion, AVP levels rapidly increased in 15 cirrhotic patients. The maximal AVP level in the 9 patients with ascites was similar to that in the 6 patients without ascites. The authors concluded that the release of ADH in response to hypertonicity was not altered by decompensation. Thus, resetting of the osmoreceptors in cirrhosis seems unlikely.

As discussed above, impaired function of the putative hepatic osmoreceptors might be expected in chronic liver disease.[11-13,21] However attractive this hypothesis may seem, proof of its relevance remains elusive.

Impaired Metabolic Clearance of Antidiuretic Hormone. Abnormalities in the metabolic clearance of ADH are an obvious and important consideration in patients with liver disease. Earlier experiments suggested no decrease in capacity to inactivate either endogenous or exogenous ADH in cirrhosis.[55,218-221] In such studies[218-220] the time to attain peak urine flow rates after a standard water load was determined in cirrhotic patients and compared with that of controls. In addition, small amounts of ADH were injected, and the time required to achieve and recover from maximal antidiuresis were also recorded. No appreciable differences were found between cirrhotic and control patients. Similar conclusions were reached by Strauss and coworkers[55] in studies of alcohol diuresis in patients with cirrhosis. Delayed inactivation of ADH by the liver was excluded by Hör et al.[221] when levels of plasma ADH were assessed by bioassay in cirrhotic patients after rather large doses of vasopressin. Likewise, no significant difference was detected between the ability of the normal and cirrhotic human liver to inactivate exogenous vasopressin in vitro.[222] On the other hand, other investigators have suggested that experimental destruction of liver cells (CCl_4 model) may decrease the hepatic clearance of ADH.[29,31]

Using modern ADH measurement techniques,[25] attention again has been called to the possibility of impaired inactivation of AVP in human liver disease.[109,110,223] Skowsky et al.[109] reported in preliminary studies that the metabolic clearance rate of AVP was decreased in 6 cirrhotic patients to about 10–15% of normal, resulting in prolongation of AVP half-life. Because some of their patients had impaired renal function, the relative contributions of the kidney and liver to the AVP clearance were unknown. Ardaillou and coworkers[110] obtained evidence of decreased hepatic clearance of AVP in decompensated cirrhotics by demonstrating a slower decline of elevated plasma AVP levels induced by hypertonic saline than in patients without ascites or edema. Furthermore, the half-life of AVP measured after rapid intravenous administration of 2 μg of synthetic AVP was significantly slower in patients with ascites. Whereas the volume of distribution was not different, the calculated metabolic clearance rate was also slower in the decompensated patients (185 ± 37 ml/min/m² vs. 367 ± 49 ml/min/ m²; $p < 0.05$). Because the patients did not have decreased renal function, the authors concluded that severe liver disease may be accompanied by decreased AVP catabolism. Likewise, the metabolic clearance of infused AVP was also significantly reduced and the AVP half-life was prolonged in a recent study of 43 patients with cirrhosis by Solís-Herruzo and coworkers.[223] Such changes correlated with the degree of liver dysfunction, prothrombin activity, and levels of serum albumin and bilirubin but not with creatinine clearance.[223] To what extent the observed decreased hepatic catabolism of AVP affects the abnormalities of water excretion in patients with cirrhosis remains unclear; it can be argued that the resultant water retention, hyponatremia, and hypoosmolality should suppress AVP release (see previous section on the role of AVP).

Enhanced Sensitivity of the Distal Nephron to Antidiuretic Hormone.   No evidence whatsoever suggests enhanced sensitivity of the distal nephron to ADH in cirrhosis.[219,220]

Drug-induced ADH-like Activity.   The concomitant use of drugs with ADH-like activity in patients with decompensated cirrhosis may confound water retention and induce hyponatremia (see section below on clinical consequences and treatment).

Combination of Mechanisms.   Any combination of mechanisms throughout the clinical course of the disease is possible, considering the wide spectrum of patients with cirrhosis. However, increased nonosmotic release of ADH and impaired metabolic clearance of ADH with the occasional contribution from drug-induced ADH-like activity are the most likely combinations responsible for enhanced ADH activity in cirrhosis.

In summary, strong clinical and experimental evidence suggests the presence of enhanced ADH activity in patients with decompensated cirrhosis. Although the mechanism remains incompletely defined, the evidence points to nonosmotic stimulation of ADH release by the adenohypophysis, mediated primarily by a critical decrease in the effective circulating blood volume. ADH responsiveness in patients with decompensated cirrhosis appears to be modulated by the perturbed adrenergic activity and the response of the renal prostaglandins. The exact roles of other influences (atrial natriuretic factor, endothelin, nitric oxide) and of the putative impairment of the hepatic clearance of ADH in liver disease remain to be clarified.

Further studies of renal water handling in cirrhosis are necessary. Such studies should control for the other major factors capable of impairing water excretion. It is particularly important to define the circadian and day-to-day variations (including the effect of posture and daily activities) of AVP plasma levels in patients with decompensated cirrhosis and the appropriateness of AVP levels in response to perturbations of extracellular fluid tonicity and volume.

Decreased Delivery of Filtrate to Distal Nephron Diluting Segments

A well-recognized and important mechanism limiting water excretion in cirrhosis is the decreased delivery of filtrate to the distal nephron. This may occur when the volume of filtrate (low GFR) is so reduced or the proximal reabsorption of sodium chloride is so increased (reduced effective plasma volume) that less filtrate reaches the loop of Henle and distal tubule.[224] Free-water generation has been shown to improve in some cirrhotic patients following volume expansion with infusions of hypotonic saline,[55] isotonic mannitol[225] or saline,[225] or saline plus albumin;[226] after administration of norepinephrine[161] or aminophylline;[227] after infusion of ascitic fluid;[228] after peritoneovenous shunting;[107,229] or during water immersion.[132,134] Such observations strongly suggest the importance of distal delivery of filtrate in improving water excretion in cirrhosis.

We usually assume that in most decompensated cirrhotic patients, because of the combination of a decrease in GFR and an enhanced proximal tubular reabsorption of sodium, the delivery of filtrate to the distal nephron must be reduced (see Table 2.1), thus imposing a quantitative limitation on maximal urine flow and water clearance. Many decompensated patients with a low GFR are capable, however, of eliminating water normally, which raises the possibility that distal delivery of filtrate may not be critically reduced in all patients or at all times during the course of the disease. On the other hand, even the presence of a supernormal GFR (on the average above 200 ml/min[70,71]) in some decompensated cirrhotic patients does not exclude the possibility of decreased fractional water clearance due to decreased distal delivery of filtrate, as measured at the peak of water diuresis (Fig. 2.7).

Chaimovitz et al.[231] reported that, in 4 decompensated cirrhotic patients undergoing moderate salt restriction, maximal urine flow, water clearance, and calculated absolute and fractional distal delivery of sodium during hypotonic saline infusion were not decreased in comparison with normal subjects. Because 3 of the 4 patients had impaired capacity to dilute the urine after a standard oral water load (prior to hypotonic saline loading), measures that enhanced the distal sodium load (above the lower levels during water diuresis alone) ostensibly normalized water clearance. Furthermore, the investigators noted that the intense avidity for distal tubular sodium reabsorption resulted in higher water clearance at similar distal sodium loads in cirrhotic patients than in normal subjects.[231] The latter difference, however, was not apparent in our compensated and decompensated cirrhotic patients during water diuresis (see Table 2.1); both groups exhibited the same high maximal distal fractional sodium reabsorption.[70] Similarly, we noted no differences in distal fractional sodium reabsorption between the decompensated hyponatremic cirrhotic patients with supernormal GFR and control subjects (Fig. 2.7).

Of interest are the studies by Epstein and coworkers[134] of cirrhotic patients during head-out water immersion (see Fig. 2.4). Controls exhibited an increase in free-water generation in response to immersion. Compensated subjects and most decompensated cirrhotic patients (with the exception of two patients who did not exhibit immersion-induced natriuresis) were capable of increasing free-water generation and lowering urine osmolality (not illustrated) during immersion, despite receiving only one-half of the amount of water given to controls. These and more recent data were interpreted as evidence of an immersion-induced enhancement of delivery of filtrate to the distal nephron.[108,132,134] Nevertheless, the possibility of inhibition of ADH release during immersion cannot be excluded completely, because AVP levels were not measured.

As noted, the major problem in interpreting the above studies is that maneuvers leading to expansion of extracellular fluid volume enhance the distal delivery of filtrate to the diluting sites and concomitantly suppress ADH release by the pituitary gland. Such limitations make separation of the two important factors difficult.

Enhanced Non–ADH-Mediated Back-Diffusion of Water

When tubular urine flow rate is very slow, the possibility exists that water leaves the most distal segments of the nephron, even in the absence of circulating ADH levels, by approaching osmotic

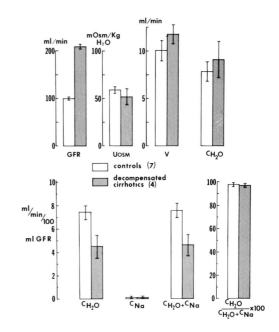

FIGURE 2.7. Maximal response to administration of water in decompensated cirrhotic patients with supernormal glomerular filtration rate (GFR) and adequate suppression of antidiuretic hormone (ADH). Data have been obtained and recalculated from Papper and Saxon,[73] Earley and Sanders,[217] and Birchard et al.[230] The controls were hospitalized patients with chronic disorders other than renal or liver disease studied by Vaamonde et al.[70] in a similar fashion. All but one patient[217] received water orally. Three of the cirrhotic patients were hyponatremic (117, 128, 134 mEq/L). Mean sodium excretion at time of study was 42 ± 6 μEq/min in the cirrhotic and 30 ± 6 μEq/min in the control patients. In the cirrhotic patients urine osmolality at V max was less than 77 (76–41) mOsm/kg H_2O, reasonably excluding the presence of ADH. Despite a GFR in the cirrhotic patients twice the value of that of the controls (over 200 ml/min), fractional CH_2O was lower, resulting from a decreased distal delivery of filtrate ($CH_2O + C_{Na}/100$ GFR). There were no differences, however, in the maximal fractional sodium reabsorption in the distal nephron ($CH_2O/[CH_2O + C_{Na} \times 100]$). Another cirrhotic patient (not included in the figure) with supernormal GFR (inulin clearance [C_{IN}] 191 ml/min and normal serum sodium concentration (142 mEq/L) was similarly evaluated during the compensated state and had values not different from those of controls.[71]

equilibration with the papillary interstitium.[93] The low tubular flow occurs when GFR is reduced or filtrate reabsorption is intensely enhanced through the length of the nephron, but most likely along the collecting duct.

TABLE 2.7. Response to Water Administration in 10 Male Patients during the Acute Phase of Viral Hepatitis*

V max (ml/min)	16.3 ± 1.2	(12.7–23.2)
UOsm (mOsm/kg H_2O)[†]	58 ± 4	(36–77)
CH_2O (ml/min)[†]	12.9 ± 1.0	(10.0–17.8)
$U_{Na}V$ (µEq/min)[†]	100 ± 25	(36–290)
Creatinine clearance (ml/min)[†]	169 ± 12	(124–232)
Total bilirubin (mg/100 ml)	9.1 ± 1.8	(2.4–18.0)

* Patients were 21–34 years old and the studies were performed within 2–4 weeks of the beginning of symptoms. The results (mean ± SE and range of values) represent the maximal response after a sustained oral or intravenous water load (20 ml/kg of body weight) given while receiving a normal NaCl intake. Because only slightly better values were obtained with intravenous than oral water administration, the data have been pooled.

[†] Values obtained at V max.

Adapted from Papper S, et al: The diuretic response to administered water in patients with liver disease. 1. Acute infectious hepatitis. Arch Intern Med 1959;103:746–749.

This mechanism may be operative in many edematous patients and may be more important than is usually appreciated in the day-to-day regulation of water balance in decompensated cirrhotic patients. For example, if one considers that many such patients pass only 300 or 400 ml of urine in 24 hours, which on the average represents a urine flow of less than 0.3 ml/min—a very low flow rate indeed—one can easily imagine the effect on urine osmolality of sluggish tubular flow rate and increased back-diffusion of water.

Schrier and coworkers[232] improved urinary dilution in edematous patients with the administration of furosemide in the presence of vasopressin and without volume expansion. The lowering effects on urinary osmolality were more striking in patients with nephrotic syndrome and congestive heart failure than in patients with decompensated cirrhosis. The authors attributed the improvement in dilution to the increased tubular fluid flow rate in the distal nephron (a consequence of the diuretic-induced solute diuresis), making less likely the possibility of osmotic equilibration of the collecting-duct urine with the interstitium and thus producing urine that was hypotonic to plasma.

WATER EXCRETION IN HEPATITIS AND BILIARY CIRRHOSIS

Information on renal water handling in patients with hepatitis and biliary cirrhosis is limited.

Hepatitis

Acute Viral Hepatitis. Some investigators have reported impaired diluting ability in patients with acute infectious hepatitis.[233,234] These earlier observations are difficult to evaluate, because the patients were not a homogenous group and were assessed under uncontrolled conditions and without adequate measurements of renal function. On the other hand, in a careful study of the diuretic response to a standard water load, Papper and coworkers[4] found normal values in 10 patients during the early stages of acute viral hepatitis (Table 2.7; compare with Tables 2.1 and 2.2).

Of interest are the reports that during acute liver injury there may be release into the liver sinusoids of vasopressinases, which may accelerate the destruction of ADH;[28,29,31] with chronic damage the opposite may occur, resulting in decreased hepatic clearance of ADH.[28] The relevance of this finding to the normal renal water handling observed by Papper et al.[4] during the acute phase of moderate-to-severe viral hepatitis is unknown. One may speculate, however, that the hepatic clearance of ADH is enhanced in such patients and thus counteracts the effects of increased central release of ADH or other mechanisms known to disturb water balance in liver disease. The kinetics of ADH release and metabolism have not been studied in patients with acute liver disease, including hepatitis.

At the other extreme, patients with fulminant hepatitis secondary to severe viral or toxic disease may develop acute renal failure (acute tubular necrosis or HRS)[234] and exhibit marked alterations of renal water handling.

Chronic Hepatitis. Urinary renal PGs have been recently studied in patients with chronic hepatitis by Uemura et al.[166] PGE_2 levels were moderately increased but less so than in patients with chronic cirrhosis. There were no differences in PGE_2 excretion between patients with chronic persistent and chronic active hepatitis. After acute administration of indomethacin, renal hemodynamics decreased by one-third; this decrease, however, was less pronounced than in patients with cirrhosis (for further information, see chapter 5).

Postnecrotic Cirrhosis

Patients who develop postnecrotic cirrhosis (Table 2.8) show perturbations in renal water excretion similar to those described for patients with alcoholic cirrhosis (see Table 2.8).

Primary Biliary Cirrhosis

In patients with primary biliary cirrhosis (PBC), edema and ascites are rare and may appear only as late manifestations of the disease.[236] Rochman et al.[5] suggested that the enhanced natriuresis exhibited by patients with PBC in response to volume expansion with hypotonic saline may account for the lack of salt retention and the rarity of edema and ascites. The only available study on renal water excretion in PBC is that of Rochman et al.[5] Although the authors did not present detailed data, one may assume that the response of patients to a standard oral water load given prior to saline administration was normal. UOsm was less than 75 mOsm/kg H_2O, and urine flow was greater than 15 ml/min/100 ml GFR. During hypotonic saline loading, no difference in water clearance at similar rates of distal delivery of filtrate was detected between patients and controls.[5] Thus, the renal diluting mechanism appears to function appropriately in patients with PBC. A detailed review of the effects of jaundice on the kidney is found in chapter 20.

CLINICAL CONSEQUENCES OF ABNORMALITIES OF WATER EXCRETION IN CIRRHOSIS

Hyponatremia

Clinical Manifestations

Whatever its pathogenesis, the inability to elaborate dilute urine and to excrete water normally results in hyponatremia. In hospitalized chronic patients with decompensated cirrhosis, hyponatremia is a common finding; it is present on admission or develops while the patient is in the hospital. The degree of hyponatremia is usually mild to moderate (serum sodium concentration: around 130 mEq/L), but not infrequently serum sodium values are less than 125 mEq/L. Indeed, hyponatremia probably represents the single most common electrolyte abnormality that confronts the physician treating patients with cirrhosis of the liver. For example, 20 of 50 (40%) patients with cirrhosis admitted to a liver unit in 1 year by Arroyo et al.[237] were found to have a serum sodium concentration below 130 mEq/L.

A crucial point to remember is that hyponatremia usually results from the patient's inability to reduce water intake or from administration of hypotonic fluids in excess of the limited renal

TABLE 2.8. Maximal Response to Intravenous Water Administration in Patient with Postnecrotic Cirrhosis*[†]

V max (ml/min)	4.1
UOsm (mOsm/kg H_2O)	70
CH_2O (ml/min)	3.0
$U_{Na}V$ (µEq/min)	1
Serum Na (mEq/L)	130
Creatinine clearance (ml/min)[†]	97

* A 57-year-old woman with postnecrotic cirrhosis was studied while receiving a 10-mEq/day sodium intake. She had no ascites or edema at time of study (compensated state). She received a 20-mg/kg of body weight sustained water load given intravenously as 4% invert sugar in water.
[†] Values were obtained at V max.
From Vaamonde CA, et al: The role of vasopressin and urea in the renal concentrating defect of patients with cirrhosis of the liver. Clin Sci Mol Med 1971;41:441–452, with permission.

capacity to excrete water. The former occurs with equal frequency at home and in the hospital and results from lack of prescription of fluid restriction by the attending physician or the patient's lack of compliance with the physician's instructions. Indeed, it is rather common to witness the development of hyponatremia during hospitalization in patients with decompensated cirrhosis who had normal serum sodium on admission. Such hospital-induced hyponatremia is multifactorial in origin (sodium-restricted diet, diuretics, unsuspected administration of drugs with ADH-like activity, deambulation, smoking), but ingestion and/or administration of water in excess of the patient's limited capacity for excretion is always the dominant factor. Thus, hyponatremia in decompensated cirrhotics almost universally represents dilutional hyponatremia.

Figure 2.8 emphasizes this important point. Decompensated cirrhotic patients, as expected, developed mild-to-moderate hyponatremia 2 hours after receiving a standard water load (mean decrease in serum sodium = 3.1 ± 1.3 mEq/L; $p < 0.05$), whereas controls exhibited an insignificant increase (0.4 ± 0.9 mEq/L). In contrast, when cirrhotic and control patients were subjected to overnight water restriction for 16 hours, the increase in serum sodium concentration above baseline was not different (cirrhotics, 3.6 ± 0.9 mEq/L; controls, 4.1 ± 2.6 mEq/L). Furthermore, the mean serum sodium concentration achieved by the cirrhotic patients after hydropenia was normal (138 ± 0.8 mEq/L), and the value of only one patient was slightly below 135 mEq/L. In

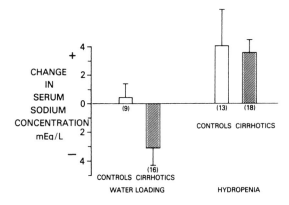

FIGURE 2.8. Changes in serum sodium concentration following water administration (water loading) or water restriction (hydropenia) in decompensated cirrhotic and control patients. Cirrhotic and control patients received a diet containing 10 mEq of sodium, 100 mEq of potassium, and 1.5 gm of protein/kg of body weight daily for 5 to 7 days prior to study. Diuretics were discontinued 1 week before. *Left,* Changes in serum sodium concentration occurring 2 hr after completion of a 20 ml/kg of body weight water load. *Right,* Changes after 16 hr of overnight hydropenia (before vasopressin administration). Both values were compared with their respective baselines (without water loading, without hydropenia). Studies were separated by 3 days or more. Numbers in parentheses represent number of patients studied (Source: Vaamonde CA: Renal water handling in liver disease. In Epstein M (ed): The Kidney in Liver Disease, 3rd ed. Baltimore: Williams & Wilkins, 1988, pp 31–72. Unpublished data recalculated from Vaamonde et al.[70,292,293])

contrast, 2 hours after water loading, 12 of 16 patients had hyponatremia. Thus, water restriction increases or normalizes serum sodium concentration in decompensated cirrhosis.

Hyponatremia usually develops slowly, with serum sodium decreasing by a few mEq/L over several days. Nevertheless, on occasions cirrhotic patients with ascites and edema present with hyponatremia of rapid onset. In such circumstances one should look for causes that may have aggravated the already limited mechanism for renal water excretion, including the following (not in order of importance or frequency):

1. Development of renal failure or urinary tract obstruction.

2. Severe diarrhea or vomiting with salt and fluid loss and further stimulation of ADH release via contraction of effective extracellular fluid volume.

3. Extreme (and overly successful) diuretic-induced diuresis,[238,239] particularly in patients with ascites but no edema.[240] Spontaneous natriuresis associated with improvement of liver disease is not accompanied by development of low serum sodium levels unless fluids are not restricted or are forced into the patient.

4. Rapid removal of several liters of ascitic fluid by paracentesis.[241]

5. Concomitant use of drugs that, by enhancing the release or potentiating the effect of ADH, may add to the already enhanced renal tubular water reabsorption (e.g., vasopressin, oxytocin, narcotics, barbiturates, nicotine, chlorpropamide)[242–244] (Table 2.9), particularly if a relative excess of water is given.

The assumption that moderate sodium restriction and diuretics—particularly loop-type diuretics—will correct retention and maldistribution of excessive fluid and therefore the hyponatremia in cirrhotic patients is simplistic if not erroneous. Diuretic agents alone do not increase free-water clearance and thus cannot correct hyponatremia without concomitant correction of decreased distal delivery of filtrate, attainment of negative fluid balance by coupling insensible losses with fluid restriction, or both. Indeed, the careless use of diuretics in cirrhosis often results in severe hyponatremia.

The mechanism of diuretic-induced hyponatremia is multifactorial and includes stimulation of ADH release secondary to hypovolemia (which may not be readily apparent in patients with marked fluid retention[239]). Furthermore, diuretics attenuate the normally hypotonic tubular fluid reaching the distal nephron by impairing sodium chloride reabsorption in the water-impermeable medullary and cortical segments of the ascending limb of the loop of Henle. In addition, diuretics may facilitate the development of hyponatremia by further decreasing distal delivery of filtrate through enhancement of proximal tubular sodium chloride reabsorption as a consequence of reduced GFR. Finally, diuretic-induced potassium depletion may result in an intracellular shift of extracellular sodium or in the stimulation of ADH release.

When renal failure appears in cirrhosis, the patient's ability to excrete water is markedly suppressed. In response to a water load the patient's urine osmolality remains hypertonic to plasma, and hyponatremia appears rapidly (see Fig. 2.1). Diluting ability is difficult to study in many patients with HRS. Some are so uncomfortable that ADH release may be stimulated for reasons unrelated to liver disease. A number of observations have been made under controlled conditions, and, with only rare exceptions, such patients cannot elaborate dilute urine and are hyponatremic (see Table 2.4).[2,71,77,237,245,246] Serum sodium concentration may be normal or modestly decreased in early renal failure, but it usually declines as the disease evolves, invariably as a consequence of water administered in excess of water excreted.[2,247] As already mentioned, such patients are particularly prone to the rapid development of hyponatremia.

The spontaneous development of severe hyponatremia (< 125 mEq/L) is considered a poor prognostic sign in decompensated cirrhosis.[238,248–251] This assumption, however, is not supported by all investigators[2,237] and may depend to a great extent on the presence of markedly decreased GFR.[71,237] Although it has been suggested that the inability to excrete water may herald renal failure in decompensated cirrhosis,[76] we have observed that this finding, although common, is not invariable.[71]

The symptoms of hyponatremia associated with severe liver disease are not different from those found in dilutional hyponatremia of other etiologies: difficulty in mental concentration, anorexia, headache, apathy, nausea, vomiting, and occasionally, seizures. The same symptoms can be found in patients with hepatic coma or precoma but with normal serum sodium concentration. Thus, not infrequently, it is difficult to ascertain whether symptoms relate to hyponatremia or to severe liver disease; one may observe an increase in serum sodium levels without significant changes in symptoms. If the patient is not receiving diuretics or undergoing spontaneous diuresis, the hyponatremia is accompanied by a low urinary sodium concentration, usually less than 10 mEq/L.

Central Nervous Dysfunction

Disturbances of the central nervous system (CNS) are responsible in great measure for the morbidity and mortality associated with severe hyponatremia.[251] Although it is commonly accepted that the movement of water from the extracellular fluid into the brain cells causes cerebral edema, it is now also appreciated that several steroid (gonadal) and peptide hormones (vasopressin, angiotensin) enhance water movement into the CNS in the absence of hyponatremia.[251]

TABLE 2.9.   Drugs that Impair Renal Water Excretion and May Contribute to Antidiuresis and Hyponatremia in Cirrhosis

Stimulation of thirst	
Antihistamines	Phenothiazines
Anticholinergics	Tricyclic antidepressants
Release of antidiuretic hormone (ADH)	
Nicotine	Clofibrate
Vincristine*	Isoproterenol
Bromocriptine*	Carbamazepine
Barbiturates	Ifosfamide*
Morphine	
Potentiation of ADH-like activity	
Oxytocin	Biguanides (phenformin,
Vasopressin*	metaformin)
Vasopressin analogues	Nonsteroidal antiinflam-
(dDAVP)	matory agents (aspirin,
Chlorpropamide*	indomethacin)
Tolbutamide	Acetaminophen
Interference with renal NaCl transport	
Diuretics*	
Solute diuretics (mannitol, glucose, glycerol, urea)	
Unknown mechanisms	
Cyclophosphamide*	Fluphenazine
Amitriptyline	Thioridazine
Haloperidol*	

* Of clinical importance, i.e., capable of producing water retention and hyponatremia.
Modified from Vaamonde CA: Maintenance of body fluid tonicity. In Froelich ED (ed): Pathophysiology—Altered Regulatory Mechanisms in Disease, 3rd ed. Philadelphia: J.B. Lippincott, 1984, pp 271–298.

The adaptation of the brain to chronic hyponatremia results from its capacity to extrude sodium, potassium, amino acids, and osmotically inactive intracellular anions, thereby minimizing brain swelling.[252,253] The activity of the Na+, K+-ATPase pump, which is responsible for cation extrusion in the brain, appears to be influenced by sex hormones and to be less in female animals.[251] Furthermore, AVP in rats may increase water permeability of brain capillaries, thereby favoring brain edema.[254]

In the chronic hyponatremia of cirrhosis, the brain and plasma osmolalities are assumed to be similarly low because of loss of osmotically active cations (sodium, potassium, and amino acids).[252,253] Several factors in patients with cirrhosis may increase the risk of CNS dysfunction. Plasma androgen levels are decreased, whereas estrogen and AVP levels are increased,[251] although the responsiveness of the V_2 receptors to AVP is unknown. Furthermore, the downside of the brain's adaptive phenomenon to hypoosmolality is that the loss of cations and amino acids may inhibit brain energy metabolism and interfere with neurotransmitter amino acid release at the synaptic function, thus leading to decreased brain function and encephalopathy.[255] Perhaps the above factors may explain the hormonal (less androgen, more estrogen and AVP) and biochemical basis for the apparent predilection of cirrhotic patients to brain edema and encephalopathy associated with hyponatremia.[251] However, because of coexisting hepatic failure, renal failure, hyponatremia, hyperventilation with potential respiratory alkalosis,[256] and the effects of numerous therapeutic agents (see Table 2.9), it is likely that the hyponatremic encephalopathy of cirrhosis has a multifactorial origin and a varied and sometimes confusing symptomatology.

In 1959 Adams et al.[257] described central pontine myelinosis (CPM) in alcoholic and/or malnourished patients with liver disease. By 1990 over 200 patients had been reported, all with either chronic debilitating illness (cancer), malnutrition, or chronic alcoholism.[251] According to Arieff, less than 25% had a history of hyponatremia, whereas 10% had hypernatremia.[258] The clinical expression of CPM is extremely variable, ranging from minimal findings to inability to speak and swallow, impaired response to painful stimuli, facial weakness, and flaccid quadriplegia.[257] The morphologic findings of CPM include destruction of medullary myelin sheets, usually in the center of the basilar portion of the pons, with frequent extension to nerves in the lower pons. The nerve cells and vessels are typically preserved.[251,.257] Many reported cases exhibit extrapontine demyelination resembling hypoxia-anoxia lesions.[258,259] Whether the demyelinating lesions are pontine or extrapontine in location, they require confirmation by computed tomography, magnetic resonance imaging, or autopsy before they are assumed to be the cause of hyponatremic encephalopathy. The etiology of CPM remains unclear. Originally it was attributed to rapid correction of hyponatremia,[259] but the prevalent current opinion is that correction to hypernatremic levels—rather than the rapidity of correction—may be the critical factor in patients with liver disease.[260]

Despite the continued controversy,[261] it appears reasonable to follow the recommendations of Arieff et al.[251] and Ayus et al.[260] in the few symptomatic cirrhotic patients in whom active correction of hyponatremia is deemed necessary. Adequate studies are not yet available to assess the clinical impact of hyponatremic encephalopathy in patients with cirrhosis in terms of morbidity, prognosis, and mortality.

Prevention

The discussion of pathogenesis suggests that the prevention of hyponatremia in patients with cirrhosis (Table 2.10) is based on the following factors: (1) maintenance of fluid intake that matches the current status of the patient's sodium intake and limited ability for water excretion (preventive restriction of about 1 liter [or less] of total fluid ingestion suffices in most patients; of course, excessive renal [diuretic-induced] or extrarenal losses should be appropriately repaired); (2) enforcement of sodium restriction; (3) careful use of diuretics to avoid diuretic-induced hyponatremia; (4) avoidance of drugs that may impair water excretion (see Table 2.9); and (5) cessation of smoking.

Treatment

Fluid Restriction. The treatment of hyponatremia in decompensated cirrhosis is straightforward; it consists simply of water restriction. In practical terms, however, achievement of this simple goal is rather difficult, and one may have to accept a moderate degree of hyponatremia in many patients. Although the basis for this classic recommendation should be evident from the previous discussion, some authors suggest that this approach should not be applied to all decompensated patients.[237]

The magnitude of fluid restriction may be a source of problems. Patients with mild hyponatremia (135–130 mEq/L) usually do not require fluid restriction. Many patients with moderate-to-severe hyponatremia may require a marked reduction in total daily fluid intake, i.e., 400–500 ml/day or even no fluid intake for 24 hours. Fixing water intake to the "magic" level of 1000 ml per day is not a great enough reduction in many patients; this relatively high intake, which caused the hyponatremia in the first place, will contribute to it maintenance.

Sodium Restriction. As noted above, sodium restriction should be enforced.

Diuretics. Diuretics should be discontinued in patients with severe hyponatremia; they may be reinstituted together with sodium restriction for the control of sodium retention under careful control and when serum sodium concentration approaches 135 mEq/L.

There are no detailed reports of the success and safety of rapidly correcting hyponatremia in cirrhotic patients with the syndrome of inappropriate ADH secretion.[262] Rapid correction involves induction of a negative water balance with a loop diuretic as urinary electrolyte losses are quantitatively replaced with hypertonic solutions. As mentioned, in preliminary studies with this technique, Schrier et al.[232] achieved only modest improvement in diluting ability in some cirrhotic patients.

Pockros and Reynolds[240] have recently shown that only decompensated patients without edema developed renal failure, severe hyponatremia (serum sodium: 126 ± 4 mEq/L [mean $\pm$ SD]), and hyperkalemia after rapid diuresis with large doses of oral furosemide plus either amiloride or spironolactone. Although the authors concluded that cirrhotic patients with peripheral edema appear to be protected from such adverse effects, presumably because of preferential mobilization of edema, a word of caution is appropriate. Indeed, in this study, water intake was fixed at 1000 ml/day, and even the patients with ascites and edema developed mild hyponatremia. In view of the risk of rapid correction of hyponatremia in cirrhotic patients[251-261] (see previous section), we believe that it has no benefits. Intermittent ingestion of urea concomitant with fluid restriction was of some help in hyponatremic patients with ascites resistant to diuretics and with low or normal blood urea concentration.[263]

Circumstances to Avoid

Large-volume Paracentesis. Large-volume paracentesis used without plasma volume expansion for treatment of cirrhotic patients with tense ascites produced no changes in serum or creatinine concentration and plasma volume.[264] Others, however, have recently reported contradictory results[265] (see chapter 23 for further information).

Drugs that Interfere with Water Excretion. If hyponatremia is to be avoided in cirrhotic patients, special care should be exercised when using drugs that may interfere with water excretion.[242-244] Table 2.9 lists the drugs currently thought to induce antidiuresis, their clinical relevance, and their suggested mechanisms of action. Of interest, bromocriptine (a dopaminergic agonist known to induce release of ADH in normal subjects), which has been used to treat chronic portosystemic encephalopathy

TABLE 2.10. Prevention and Treatment of Hyponatremia in Cirrhosis

Prevention
- Maintain a fluid intake that is adequate to the current status of the patient's sodium intake and limited ability for water excretion. This requires preventive fluid restriction (usually 1 L of total fluid intake or less).
- Sodium restriction
- Use diuretic agents carefully. Avoid diuretic-induced hyponatremia.
- Avoidance of drugs that may impair renal water excretion (see Table 2.9); refrain from smoking

Treatment
- Fluid restriction. This is the cornerstone of treatment. In general, less than 500–600 ml/day. Rarely, no fluid intake for brief periods (12 to 36 hours).
- Sodium restriction, should be enforced
- Diuretics. Should be discontinued during treatment of symptomatic hyponatremia (see text for details).
- Avoid:
  Large volume paracentesis without volume replacement
  Drugs that interfere with water excretion (see Table 2.9)
  Excessive deambulation
- Other measures
  Removal of free-water by dialytic/ultrafiltration procedures
  Pharmacologic modulation of release or tubular action of ADH
    Demeclocycline—should not be used
    Vasopressin analogues
    Opioid antagonists (naloxone)

in selected cirrhotic patients, may produce profound hyponatremia.[266]

Dialytic Ultrafiltration Procedures. Water removal by dialysis has also been used for correction of severe hyponatremia in cirrhosis. Ring-Larsen and coworkers[267] treated 16 patients with decompensated cirrhosis, hepatic coma, renal failure (in 8), and hyponatremia with peritoneal dialysis. Serum sodium averaged 119 mEq/L before dialysis and remained above 130 mEq/L for the week following dialysis. Ultrafiltration by means of continuous arteriovenous hemofiltration (CAVH) represents another dialytic choice for the treatment of severe intractable hyponatremia when appropriate changes are made in the substitution fluid.[268,269] The application of such techniques solely for the purpose of correcting severe hyponatremia in decompensated cirrhosis probably has no indication in practical management unless extreme symptoms attributable to hyponatremia are present: even then, they probably should be used only to raise the plasma sodium concentration by several mEq/L to a safer level and not to achieve complete correction to "normal" levels (for further information see chapter 26).

Pharmacologic Modulation of Antidiuretic Hormone

Demeclocycline. Various investigators[83–87] have suggested the use of agents such as demeclocycline, which block the hydroosmotic effect of ADH, for correction of hyponatremia in cirrhotic patients. In view of the numerous reports of renal failure in cirrhotic patients treated with demeclocycline,[83,84,86,87,91,270,271] however, it should not be used.

Vasopressin Analogs. The discovery of vasopressin antagonists that specifically block vasopressin (V_1) receptors in the distal nephron has raised expectations for their clinical application in patients with hyponatremia and edematous states.[272] The most recently tested analogs produced a dose-dependent increase in water excretion with marked urine hypoosmolality in conscious water-loaded monkeys.[273] The compounds also antagonized in a competitive fashion the antidiuresis induced by exogenous vasopressin.[272,274] Clinical studies in patients with cirrhosis or in animals with experimental liver diseases, ascites, and hyponatremia have not yet been published.

Endogenous Opioids. Endogenous opioids may be involved in the release of AVP,[275] and experimental evidence suggests an effect on salt and water retention as well.[276,277] Increased plasma levels of methionine-enkephalin and leucine-enkephalin have been found in patients with cirrhosis and ascites,[278] probably as a result of impaired hepatic metabolism.[279] Leehey et al.[280] recently studied the effects of the opioid antagonist naloxone in patients with cirrhosis and ascites. Naloxone induced an increase in urine output and sodium excretion in cirrhotic patients without altering renal function in controls. The action of naloxone was due to an increase in GFR and solute excretion without changes in renal diluting ability and with a concomitant appropriate suppression of AVP plasma levels. Thus, endogenous opioids—at least in the small number of patients evaluated—appear to have no important role in the diluting mechanism.

Correction of Volume Depletion. Only in rare circumstances, such as severe vomiting or diarrhea, does hyponatremia in cirrhotic patients result from absolute or relative losses in extracellular fluid volume. Under such conditions, volume should be replaced with normal saline and water intake should be restricted.

Hypernatremia

In view of the frequency of hyponatremia in cirrhosis, the recent recognition of the development of hypernatremia (serum sodium concentration > 145 mEq/L) and its consequences in patients with decompensated liver disease associated with hepatic failure, gastrointestinal hemorrhage, or HRS is of considerable interest.[235,281]

In 1974 Wilkinson et al.[235] found hypernatremia in 11 of 48 patients with fulminant hepatic failure and encephalopathy; all 11 patients died. Subsequently, Warren et al.[281] found hypernatremia in 15 of 25 patients with decompensated liver disease (the majority had alcoholic cirrhosis); 13 of the 15 patients with hypernatremia died.

Hypernatremia appears to be confined largely to cirrhotic patients with ascites and edema. We seldom have seen its appearance in compensated cirrhosis. The real prevalence of hypernatremia is unknown, but it has been estimated as high as one-third of hospitalized patients with liver disease.[235,251,281,282] Typically, the hypernatremia was not present on admission to the hospital but appeared later, usually within a few days of the patient's death, suggesting that hypernatremia is primarily an iatrogenic phenomenon. In some patients, however, hyponatremia was diagnosed on admission.[281] Table 2.11 summarizes the course of a cirrhotic patient with chronic renal failure who developed reversible hypernatremia of multifactorial origin.

Although the mechanism of hypernatremia is not clear, increased insensible water losses coupled with decreased water intake due to encephalopathy and use of osmotic cathartics (lactulose, mannitol) have been implicated.[282] In other cirrhotic patients, hypernatremia appeared after an acute important upper gastrointestinal bleed[283,284] and was attributed to the increased solute diuresis promoted by the enhanced urea load. In patients with fulminant hepatic failure the osmotic diuresis was caused by intravenous administration of hypertonic glucose.[285] In a few reports necrosis of the posterior pituitary in patients with fulminant hepatitis led to diabetes insipidus.[285]

The appearance of hypernatremia is gradual and associated with a high mortality (92%). The clinical features include fever, intense thirst, irritability, twitching, convulsions, and coma. There are no studies of the renal handling of water in cirrhotic patients with hypernatremia. Whether correction of hypernatremia with hypotonic solutions improves survival is conjectural and remains to be shown.

RENAL WATER CONSERVATION IN CIRRHOSIS

Although the abnormalities of renal water handling in cirrhosis relate to impairment in water excretion with development of hyponatremia or, less frequently, hypernatremia, studies of renal concentrating ability have been helpful in understanding some of the pathogenetic mechanisms involved in abnormal renal water excretion. Information about the kidney's ability to concentrate the urine in cirrhosis is limited.[286–291] Because most early studies were uncontrolled for dietary salt intake, had questionable experimental designs, or focused on patients with unknown degrees of malnutrition, we undertook a systematic assessment of the mechanism of renal concentration in patients with cirrhosis.[70,292,293] Of particular interest was the observation that patients with cirrhosis exhibited a low maximal urine osmolality (UOsm max) but had normal solute-free water reabsorption (T^cH_2O) during mannitol diuresis,[289] an observation similar to findings in patients with sickle-cell anemia.[294] Jick et al.[289] suggested that the data were consistent with increased medullary blood flow and washout of medullary hypertonicity due to increased shunting of blood in cirrhosis. Because of the relevance of salt and protein restriction to the kidney's ability to concentrate the urine maximally,[290,295–298] in our studies we compared the results with those of chronically ill patients without liver disease under similar dietary conditions.

Our studies revealed consistent decreases in UOsm max during hydropenia and vasopressin administration,[292,293] or during vasopressin infusion in the hydrated state.[70] The magnitude of this concentrating defect, however, was modest. After hydropenia and vasopressin, UOsm max was 560 ± 38 mOsm/kg H_2O, a value significantly lower than that of age- and diet-matched controls (825 ± 64 mOsm H_2O; $p < 0.001$).[293] Compensated patients had UOsm max values higher than those of cirrhotic patients studied during decompensation.[70,292] More recently, other investigators have

TABLE 2.11. Hypernatremia in Patient with Decompensated Cirrhosis and Chronic Renal Failure*

Days	Serum Sodium (mEq/L)	Serum Creatinine (mg/dl)
–360	137	2.0
–180	139	3.4
– 30	140	6.0
1 (admission) Ascites, edema, infection, diarrhea	145	5.7
11	143	7.5
13	144	8.0
14 Lactulose	152	8.7
16	167	–
17	163	7.3
18	154	–
19	150	–
20	141	7.4

* A 49-year-old man with cirrhosis of the liver secondary to chronic alcoholism and chronic renal failure, who had normal serum sodium concentrations during the prior year (137–140 mEq/L). He was admitted (day 1) with decompensated cirrhosis, fever, watery diarrhea, urinary tract infection, and a serum sodium of 145 mEq/L. Oral lactulose was started on day 11 (60 gm/day) and given for 6 days. The patient developed encephalopathy and required intubation. When his serum sodium had risen to 167 mEq/L on day 16, lactulose was discontinued, and hydration with hypotonic solutions normalized the serum sodium in four days without changing the renal failure. Subsequently, the patient was placed on maintenance hemodialysis.

reported UOsm max values in cirrhotic patients similar to those in our earlier observations.[79,108] The distal nephron appears to respond normally to exogenous vasopressin, and there was no difference in the rapidity and magnitude of the response to vasopressin between compensated and decompensated cirrhotics[70] (Fig. 2.9).

The UOsm max defect can be attributed almost entirely to decreased availability of urea necessary for the concentrating process.[70] Patients with cirrhosis excreted significantly less urea than controls under the studied conditions: water diuresis, vasopressin administration following water diuresis or during hydropenia. Furthermore, urea infusion in one patient resulted in an increase in UOsm max; increased urea excretion accounted for the entire increase.[70] We concluded that in addition to salt restriction,[290,295] a decrease in the medullary and papillary urea content contributes largely to decreased interstitial osmolality and explains the defect in UOsm max in decompensated cirrhotics at low urine flow rates. The exact nature of the defect, however, remains

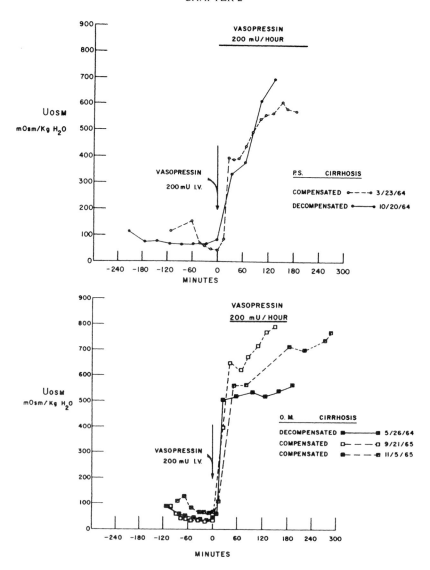

FIGURE 2.9. Changes in urine osmolality (UOsm) following the administration of aqueous vasopressin during a sustained water diuresis in two patients with cirrhosis receiving a 10-mEq sodium diet studied during the course of the disease (compensation, decompensation). A 20 ml/kg of body weight oral water load was given at –260 to –240 min, and when the response to water was maximal and stable, 200 mU of aqueous vasopressin was injected intravenously as indicated by the arrows, and the infusion sustained at a rate of 200 mU/hr. Water was provided to match urine output during the study. Note that on all occasions both patients diluted the urine below 100 mOsm/kg H_2O, that the response to exogenous vasopressin was very rapid (within 15 min), and that there was no difference in the highest UOsm achieved during compensation or decompensation. (Adapted from Vaamonde CA, et al: The role of vasopressin and urea in the renal concentrating defect of patients with cirrhosis of the liver. Clin Sci Mol Med 1971;41:441–452.)

speculative. Increased medullary blood flow has been suggested as a cause of the washout of medullary solute.[290] Decreased delivery of filtrate to the distal concentrating site or a defect in the transport of urea to the water-permeable segments of the nephron also may be implicated. The fact that patients with cirrhosis excrete significantly less urea at low (< 1 ml/min) and relatively high (4–10 ml/min) rates of urine flow militates against the latter possibility.[70]

The following evidence suggests that decreased availability of urea for the concentrating process was largely responsible for the observed UOsm max defect in cirrhosis. Cirrhotic patients had a decreased filtered load of urea (mostly the consequence of low plasma urea levels). Yet during water diuresis prior to vasopressin administration, when collecting duct permeability to urea should be low, they also had a higher overall fractional tubular reabsorption of urea than controls, a finding that resembles the renal response associated with protein depletion.[299] Finally, less urea was removed from the collecting-duct urine and presumably less accumulated in the papillary interstitium during vasopressin antidiuresis. We calculated that in changing from maximal water diuresis to maximal antidiuresis, cirrhotic patients accumulated a maximum of 83 ± 64 μmol of urea per minute in the renal medullary interstitium, whereas control patients more than doubled that amount (183 ± 72 μmol/min; p < 0.01). A large part of the difference was explained by the dissimilar filtered loads of urea (p < 0.005). The decreased availability of urea in cirrhosis can be attributed most likely to protein depletion or to decreased synthesis of urea.[300]

No experimental data support a role for increased medullary blood flow in determining the UOsm max defect in cirrhosis; they suggest that it may occur.[70,289,292,293,301] In the past we attempted to approach this question with the simplistic view that large doses of vasopressin, because of their presumed vasoactive effect on medullary vessels,[302,303] may decrease the assumed medullary vasodilation in cirrhosis and thus improve the decreased UOsm max.[49] Paired measurements of UOsm max were performed in age-matched decompensated cirrhotic patients and chronically ill controls who received two dosages of vasopressin; the degree of hydropenia was comparable. On two separate occasions each patient received either the standard dosage (200 mU prime and 200 mU/hr of aqueous vasopressin) or a high dosage (10 U of pitressin tannate in oil given 12 hr before the study, plus in some patients 1000 mU of aqueous vasopressin in addition to the standard dosage). In all decompensated cirrhotic patients, UOsm increased with a mean rise of 110 ± 5 mOsm/kg H_2O (a 20% increase; p < 0.005), whereas the change in controls was 34 ± 3 mOsm/kg H_2O (a 4.6% increase; p < 0.005). The difference between the two groups was statistically significant (p < 0.05). To control for spontaneous variation in measurements of UOsm max, we determined the change in UOsm max in 9 decompensated cirrhotic patients and 6 chronically ill controls receiving the

standard dosage of vasopressin. The mean ± SEM change in UOsm max between the first and second measurement was 9 ± 23 mOsm/kg H_2O in cirrhotic patients, and 13 ± 20 mOsm/kg H_2O in controls—values that were not significantly different.[49] These results were not different from the spontaneous variation in UOsm max values observed by Vaamonde et al.[68] in replicate studies of healthy young volunteers. There were no untoward effects or changes in blood pressure, GFR, urine flow, osmolar clearance, or urea excretion between groups. Thus, it appears that the increase in UOsm max after high-dose vasopressin clearly exceeded the spontaneous change expected in replicate studies. The interpretation of such results, however, is more difficult. Despite the recently described hyporeactivity of splanchnic vessels in response to vasopressin and other vasoactive agents,[214,216] whether the results represent a vasoactive action of vasopressin influencing medullary blood flow or some other action of vasopressin cannot be elucidated from the above preliminary studies, although the data at least were consistent with the postulated premise.

Because PG activity my be increased in patients with cirrhosis,[79,164,169] one may speculate that prostaglandins also have some role in the determination of the UOsm max defect in cirrhosis. PGs are known to influence the renal concentrating mechanism by interfering with the cellular mechanism of action of ADH.[162,163,304] Thus, it is conceivable that the high doses of vasopressin used to increase UOsm max[49] somehow balanced the hypothetical effect of prostaglandins on UOsm max in cirrhosis. The recent results obtained by Pérez-Ayuso et al.[79] in hydropenic patients, however, cast some doubts on this suggestion. Decompensated cirrhotics with low UOsm max after overnight hydropenia had lower PGE_2 excretion rates than controls. Further studies are necessary to clarify the role of factors other than availability of urea in the determination of abnormal concentrating ability in cirrhosis.

Tubular reabsorption of water (T^cH_2O) measured during hypertonic mannitol diuresis was decreased in the decompensated patients that we studied (cirrhotic patients, 2.5 ± 0.4 ml/min/GFR; controls, 5.6 ± 0.2 ml/min/GFR; p < 0.001)[292,293] and improved with clinical compensation (Fig. 2.10). Compensated cirrhotics had less marked impairment of T^cH_2O (3.3 ± 0.4 ml/min GFR).

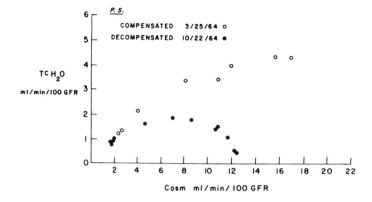

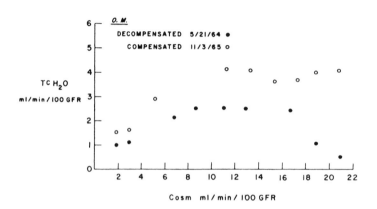

FIGURE 2.10. Solute-free tubular reabsorption of water (T^{c}H$_2$O) during compensated or decompensated liver disease. The patients received a diet containing 10 mEq of sodium, 80 mEq of potassium, and 1.5 gm of protein/kg of body weight daily. The T^{c}H$_2$O formation was measured during hydropenia, vasopressin, and 10% mannitol infusion. There was improvement in T^{c}H$_2$O values during clinical compensation to the levels observed in control patients receiving the same low-sodium diet. (Reprinted by permission from Vaamonde CA, et al: Renal concentrating ability in cirrhosis. 1. Changes associated with the clinical status and course of the disease. J Lab Clin Med 1967;70: 179–194.)

Our results are contrary to those reported by Jick and associates.[290] We have discussed elsewhere[292] why we believe salt restriction is not the major factor explaining this difference. Perhaps the results may be explained by differences in patient population or experimental design.

When the distal delivery and tubular concentration of sodium were increased by infusing hypertonic saline in hydropenic patients with reduced T^{c}H$_2$O, there was no correction of T^{c}H$_2$O generation, despite the appearance of large amounts of sodium in the urine[293] (Fig. 2.11). Furthermore, we found no correlation between diluting and concentrating capacities in paired studies of cirrhotic patients.[70] Some cirrhotic patients during water diuresis apparently delivered filtrate to the distal nephron in amounts sufficient for normal water clearance and far in excess of that needed to correct impaired T^{c}H$_2$O during hydropenia.[70] Although the reason for the abnormally low T^{c}H$_2$O formation in cirrhosis is not apparent, we concluded that neither decreased delivery of filtrate to nor low concentration of sodium chloride at the distal nephron concentrating site appears to be responsible.[293] The possibility that

increased medullary blood flow may be involved in the T^{c}H$_2$O defect has not been excluded.

Although the abnormalities in renal concentrating ability observed in patients with cirrhosis are of modest magnitude and of no apparent clinical significance, their study has contributed to our understanding of the effects that perturbations of intrarenal circulation and urea handling may have on the renal concentration process.

SUMMARY

Most compensated cirrhotic patients can excrete water without limitations. Many decompensated cirrhotic patients show a normal or moderately subnormal capacity to handle water; others exhibit a decreased capacity (low V max and CH$_2$O). In general, cirrhotic patients excrete dilute urine (< 100 mOsm/kg H$_2$O) in response to water loading. Low rates of sodium and urea excretion are for the most part responsible. Only in cirrhotic patients with renal failure is derangement of this homeostatic function complete. There is a gross correlation between clinical severity and impairment of renal diluting capacity.

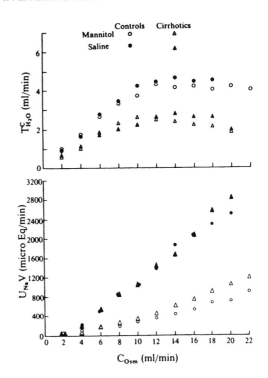

FIGURE 2.11. Relationships between solute-free tubular water reabsorption (T^cH_2O; *top panel*) and urinary sodium excretion ($U_{Na}V$; *bottom panel*) and osmolal clearance (COsm) in five cirrhotic (*triangles*) and five noncirrhotic control (*circles*) patients during 10% mannitol (*open symbols*) and 3% saline (*closed symbols*) diuresis. All cirrhotic and control patients received a diet containing 10mEq of sodium, 100 mEq of potassium, and 1.5 gm of protein/kg of body weight daily. A 2–7 day interval separated the studies. Note that the decreased T^cH_2O values in the cirrhotic patients did not increase toward the values of the control subjects despite comparable rates of sodium excretion throughout the range of COsm studied. (Reprinted with permission from Vaamonde CA, et al: Renal concentrating ability in cirrhosis. III. Failure of hypertonic saline to increase T^cH_2O formation. Kidney Int 1972;1:55–64.)

Dilutional hyponatremia is the consequence of impaired renal water handling in liver disease and results from the ingestion of water in excess of the limited renal ability to excrete water. Water restriction is the treatment of choice for hyponatremia of cirrhosis.

Decreases in distal delivery of filtrate coupled with enhanced ADH activity are the most important mechanisms limiting water excretion in severely oliguric patients. ADH levels appear to be elevated in many patients. Strong evidence implicates increased ADH release via nonosmotic stimulation, whereas the role of impaired hepatic metabolism of ADH remains to be established. Catecholamines and renal prostaglandins (PGE_2) appear to contribute most to the impaired water homeostasis in cirrhosis. A modest impairment in renal concentrating ability can be demonstrated in most decompensated cirrhotic patients.

Finally, renal handling of water in cirrhotic patients is commonly evaluated under experimental conditions (acute water or hypotonic saline loading in the recumbent position, diet, time of day) that are quite different from conditions determining the fluid-balance status of patients during their usual activities (e.g., ambulation, seated posture, absolute or relative high intake of water, dietary salt and protein content, use of pharmacologic agents capable of releasing or mimicking ADH action). Thus, the role of some of the mechanisms under assessment may be obscured by the experimental design of the studies.

Acknowledgments. Throughout the years the original work of the author cited in the chapter has been supported by research grants from the National Institutes of Health and the Department of Veterans Affairs. The author thanks Esther Márquez for her invaluable secretarial assistance.

REFERENCES

1. Flint A: Clinical report on hydroperitoneum, based on an analysis of forty-six cases. Am J Med Sci 1963;45: 306–339.
2. Vaamonde CA, Papper S: The kidney in liver disease. In Earley LE, Gottschalk CW (eds): Diseases of the Kidney, 3rd ed. Boston: Little, Brown, 1979;1289–1317.
3. Papper S, Vaamonde CA: Renal and electrolyte abnormalities in liver disease: A listing. In Epstein M (ed): The Kidney in Liver Disease. New York: Elsevier/North Holland, 1978;33–34.
4. Papper S, Seifer HW, Saxon L: The diuretic response to administered water in patients with liver disease. I. Acute infectious hepatitis. Arch Intern Med 1959;103: 746–749.
5. Rochman J, Chaimowitz C, Eidelman S, Better OS: Renal handling of sodium, water and divalent ions in patients with primary biliary cirrhosis. In Massry SG, Ritz E (eds): Phosphate Metabolism. New York: Plenum, 1977;121–129.

6. Sawchenko PE, Friedman MI: Sensory functions of the liver—a review. Am J Physiol 1979;236:R5–R20.

7. Passo SS, Thornborough JR, Rothballer AB: Hepatic receptors in control of sodium excretion in anesthetized cats. Am J Physiol 1972;224:373–375.

8. Kostreva DR, Castaner A, Kampine JP: Reflex effects of hepatic baroreceptors on renal and cardiac sympathic nerve activity. Am J Physiol 1980;238:R390–R394.

9. Valdivieso AJ, Perez GO: Renal response to isotonic saline infusion into portal and jugular vein in sodium-loaded, conscious rats. Proc Soc Exp Biol Med 1981; 167:261–266.

10. Lopez-Novoa JM, Martinez-Maldonado M: Impaired renal response to splanchnic infusion of hypertonic saline in conscious cirrhotic rates. Am J Physiol 1982; 242:F390–F394.

11. Haberich F, Aziz O, Nowacki PE: Über einen osmoreceptorisch tätigen Mechanismus in der Leber. Pflüegers Arch 1965;285:73–89.

12. Haberich FJ: Osmoreception in the portal circulation. Fed Proc 1968;27:1137–1141.

13. Lydtin H: Untersuchungen über Mechanismen der Osmo-und Volumen regulation. II. Untersuchungen uber den Einfluss intravenös, intraportal und oral zugeführten hypotoner Kochsalzlösungen auf die Diurese des Hundes. Z Gesamte Exp Med 1969;149:193–210.

14. Lydtin H: Untersuchungen über Mechanismen der Osmo-und Volumen regulation. III. Untersuchungen am Menschen über die Wirkung von oral und intravenös zugeführten Kochsalzlosungen auf die Harnausscheidung. Z Gesamte Exp Med 1969;149:211–225.

15. Andrews WHH, Orbach I: Sodium receptors activating some nerves of perfused rabbit livers. Am J Physiol 1974;227:1273–1275.

16. Adachi A, Niijima A, Jacobs HL: A hepatic osmoreceptor mechanism in the rat: Electrophysiological and behavioral studies. Am J Physiol 1976;231:1043–1049.

17. Perlmutt JH, Kao C-C, Hill PK: Concentration and dilution of the urine in partially hepatoectomized, conscious rats. Pflüegers Arch 1977;369:233–238.

18. Schneider EG, Davis JO, Robb CA, et al: Lack of evidence for a hepatic osmoreceptor mechanism in conscious dogs. Am J Physiol 1970;218:42–45.

19. Glasby MA, Ramsay DJ: Hepatic osmoreceptors? J Physiol (Lond) 1974;243:765–776.

20. Bennett WM, Hennes D, Elliot D, Porter GA: In search of a hepatic osmoreceptor in man. Am J Dig Dis 1974; 19:143–148.

21. Chwalbinska-Moneta J: Role of hepatic portal osmoreception in the control of ADH release. Am J Physiol 236:E603–E609, 1979.

22. Lauson HD: Metabolism of antidiuretic hormones. Am J Med 42:713–744, 1967.

23. Walter R, Bowman RH: Mechanism of inactivation of vasopressin and oxytocin by the isolated perfused rat kidney. Endocrinology 1973;92:189–193.

24. Lauson HD: Metabolism of the neurohypophyseal hormones. In Knobil E, Sawyer WH (eds): Handbook of Physiology, vol. 4. Washington, DC: American Physiological Society, 1974;287–393.

25. Robertson GL: The use of vasopressin assays in physiology and pathophysiology. Semin Nephrol 1994;14: 368–383.

26. Rabkin R, Share L, Payne PA, Young J, Crofton J: The handling of immunoreactive vasopressin by the isolated perfused rat kidney. J Clin Invest 1979;63:6–13.

27. Kleeman CR, Berl T: The neurohypophyseal hormones: Vasopressin. In De Groot LJ, Cahill GF Jr. Odell WD, et al (eds): Endocrinology, vol. 1. New York: Grune & Stratton, 1979;253–275.

28. Aziz O, Schmidt W: Elimination of vasopressin by the normal and the damaged liver. Experiments on unanesthetized normal and thioacetamide treated rats, with a note on the influence of ethanol. Pflüegers Arch 1976; 367:165–168.

29. Eser S, Tüzünkam P: Le foie et l'hormone antidiurétique. Ann Endocr (Paris) 1950;11:124–130.

30. Rabkin R, Ghazeleh S, Share L, et al: Removal of immunoreactive arginine vasopressin by the perfused rat liver. Endocrinology 1980;106:930–934.

31. Schnieden H: Comparison between the effects of intravenous and intraportal vasopressin in normal rats, malnourished rats, and rats treated with carbon tetrachloride. J Endocr 1962;24:397–402.

32. Maxwell D, McMurray S, Szwed J, et al: The effect of distribution and clearance on plasma vasopressin in man. Clin Res 1976;24:407A.

33. Wolff HP, Koczorek KR, Buchborn E: Aldosterone and antidiuretic hormone (adiuretin) in liver disease. Acta Endocrinol 1958;27:45–58.

34. Blachley J, Knochel JP: Alcohol-induced disturbances in electrolyte and acid-base homeostasis. In Kokko JP, Tanner RL (eds): Fluids and Electrolytes. Philadelphia: W.B. Saunders, 1986;515–547.

35. Schaefer RM, Teschner M, Heidiand A: Alterations of water, electrolyte and acid-base homeostasis in the alcoholic. Miner Electrolyte Metab 1987;13:1–6.

36. Eiser AR: The effects of alcohol on renal function and excretion. Alcohol Clin Exp Res 1987;11:127–138.

37. Miles WR: The comparative concentrations of alcohol in human blood and urine at intervals after ingestion. J Pharmacol Exp Ther 1922;20:265–319.

38. Nicholson WM, Taylor HM: The effect of alcohol on the water and electrolyte balance in man. J Clin Invest 1938;17:279–285.

39. Rubini ME, Kleeman CR, Lamdin E: Studies on alcohol diuresis. 1. The effect of ethyl alcohol ingestion on water, electrolyte balance in man. J Clin Invest 1955; 34:439–447.

40. Murray MM: The diuretic action of alcohol and its relation to pituitrin. J Physiol (Lond) 1932;76:379–386.

41. Eggleton MG: The diuretic action of alcohol in man. J Physiol (Lond) 1942;101:172–191.

42. Strauss MB, Rosenbaum JD, Nelson WT: The effect of alcohol on the renal excretion of water and electrolyte. J Clin Invest 1950;29:1053–1058.

43. Eggleton MG: The effect of nicotine on the diuresis induced by ethyl alcohol. J Physiol (Lond) 1949;108: 482–490,

44. Rosenbaum JD, Papper S, Cohen HW, McLean R: The influence of ethanol upon maintained water diuresis in man. J Clin Invest 1957;36:1202–1207.

45. Kalbfleish JM, Lindeman RD, Ginn HE, Smith WO: The effects of ethanol administration on urinary excretion of magnesium and other electrolytes in alcoholic and normal subjects. J Clin Invest 1963;42:1471–1475.

46. Zawada ET, Johnson M, Sica D: Ethanol-induced water diuresis is not prostaglandin dependent. Nephron 1985; 40:149–151.

47. van Dyke HB, Ames RG: Alcohol diuresis. Acta Endocrinol (Copenh) 1951;7:110–121.

48. Kleeman CR, Rubini ME, Lamdin E, Epstein FH: Studies on alcohol diuresis. II. The evaluation of ethyl alcohol as an inhibitor of the neurohypophysis. J Clin Invest 1955;34:448–455.

49. Vaamonde CA: Renal water handling in liver disease. In Epstein M: The Kidney in Liver Disease. New York: Elsevier/North Holland, 1978;76–77.

50. Eisenhofer G, Johnson RH: Effect of ethanol ingestion on plasma vasopressin and water balance in humans. Am J Physiol 1982;242:R522–R527.

51. Heiderman JH, Vestal RE, Rowe JW, et al: The response of arginine vasopressin to intravenous ethanol and hypertonic saline in man: The impact of aging. J Gerontol 1978;33:39–47.

52. Rowe JW, Shelton RL, Heiderman JH, et al: Influence of the emetic reflex on vasopressin release in man. Kidney Int 1979;16:729–735.

53. Linkola J, Ylikahri R, Fyhrquist F, Wallenius M: Plasma vasopressin in ethanol intoxication and hangover. Acta Physiol Scand 1978;104:180–187.

54. Knochel JP, Osborn JR, Cooper EB: Excretion of aldosterone in inappropriate secretion of antidiuretic hormone following head trauma. Metabolism 1965;14:715–725.

55. Strauss MB, Birchard WH, Saxon L: Correction of impaired water excretion in cirrhosis of the liver by alcohol ingestion or expansion of extracellular fluid volume: The role of the antidiuretic hormone. Trans Assoc Am Physicians 1956;69:222–228.

56. Beard JD, Barlow G, Oberman RR: Body fluids and blood electrolytes in dogs subjected to chronic alcohol administration. J Pharmacol Exp Ther 1965;148: 348–355.

57. Beard JD, Knott DH: Fluid and electrolyte balance during acute withdrawal in chronic alcoholic patients. JAMA 1968;204:135–139.

58. Lund ME, Banner WF, Finley PR, et al: Effect of alcohols and selected solvents on serum osmolality measurements. J Toxicol Clin Toxicol 1983;20:115–132.

59. Robinson AG, Loeb JN: Ethanol ingestion. Commonest cause of an elevated plasma osmolality? N Engl J Med 1971;284:1253–1255.

60. Tzamaloukas AH, Jackson JE, Long DA, Gallegos JC: Serum ethyl alcohol levels and osmolal gaps. J Toxicol Clin Toxicol 1982–1983;19:1045–1050.

61. Oiso Y, Robertson GL: Effect of ethanol on vasopressin secretion and the role of endogenous opioids. In Schrier RW (ed): Vasopressin. New York: Raven Press, 1985; 265–269.

62. Dunn FL, Brennan TJ, Nelson AE, Robertson GL: The role of blood osmolality and volume in regulating vasopressin in the rat. J Clin Invest 1973;52:3212–3219.

63. Forsling ML: Opioid peptides and vasopressin release. In Schrier RW (ed): Vasopressin. New York: Raven Press, 1985;425–434.

64. Demanet JD, Bonnyns M, Bleiberg H, Stevens-Rocmans C: Coma due to water intoxication in beer drinkers. Lancet 1971;2:1115–1117.

65. Gwinup G, Chelvam R, Jabola R, Meister L: Beer drinkers hyponatremia. Calif Med 1972;116:78–81.

66. Hilden P, Svendsen TL: Electrolyte disturbances in beer drinkers: A specific "hypo-osmolality syndrome." Lancet 1975;2:245–246.

67. Kessler RK, Channick BJ, Kessler WB, Metzger MD: Beer drinker's hyponatremia: A hypo-osmolality syndrome. Del Med J 1984;56:625–628.

68. Vaamonde CA, Presser JI, Clapp W: Effect of high fluid intake on the renal concentrating mechanism of normal man. J Appl Physiol 1974;36:434–439.

69. Gill GV, Baylis PH, Flear GTG, et al: Acute biochemical responses to moderate beer drinking. BMJ 1982; 285:1770–1773.

70. Vaamonde CA, Vaamonde LS, Presser JI, et al: The role of vasopressin and urea in the renal concentrating defect of patients with cirrhosis of the liver. Clin Sci Mol Med 1971;41:441–452.

71. Klingler EL Jr, Vaamonde CA, Vaamonde LS, et al: Renal function changes in cirrhosis of the liver: A prospective study. Arch Intern Med 1970;125:1010–1015.

72. Papper S, Rosenbaum JD: Abnormalities in the excretion of water and sodium in "compensated" cirrhosis of the liver. J Lab Clin Med 1952;40:523–530.

73. Papper S, Saxon L: The diuretic response to administered water in patients with liver disease. II. Laennec's cirrhosis of the liver. Arch Intern Med 1959;103: 750–757.

74. Caregaro L, Lauro S, Angeli P, et al: Renal water and sodium handling in compensated liver cirrhosis: Mechanism of the impaired natriuresis after saline loading. Eur J Clin Invest 1985;15:360–364.

75. Jespersen B, Pedersen EB, Madsen M, et al: Disturbed relationship between urinary prostaglandin E2 excretion, plasma arginine vasopressin and renal water excretion after oral water loading in early hepatic cirrhosis. Eur J Clin Invest 1988;18:202–206.

76. Baldus WP, Feichter RN, Summerskill WHJ, et al: The kidney in cirrhosis. II. Disorders of renal function. Ann Intern Med 1964;60:366–377.

77. Shear L, Hall PW, Gabuzda GJ: Renal failure in patients with cirrhosis of the liver. II. Factors influencing maximal urinary flow rate. Am J Med 1965;39:199–209.

78. Bichet D, Szatalowicz V, Chaimovitz C, Schrier RW: Role of vasopressin in abnormal water excretion in cirrhotic patients. Ann Intern Med 1982;96:413–417.

79. Pérez-Ayuso RM, Arroyo V, Camps J, et al: Evidence that renal prostaglandins are involved in renal water metabolism in cirrhosis. Kidney Int 1984;26:72–80.

80. Castellano G, Sólis-Herruzo JA, Morillas JD, et al: Antidiuretic hormone and renal function after water loading in patients with cirrhosis of the liver. Gastroenterology 1991;26:49–57.

81. Lancestremere RG: Algunos aspectos de la función renal en los cirróticos. M.D. thesis, University of Buenos Aires School of Medicine, Buenos Aires, 1962.

82. Brem AS, Cashore WJ, Pacholski M, et al: Effects of bilirubin on transepithelial transport of sodium, water, and urea. Kidney Int 1985;27:51–57.

83. De Troyer A, Pilloy W, Broeckaert I, Demanet J-C: Demeclocycline treatment of water retention in cirrhosis. Ann Intern Med 1976;85:336–337.

84. Poupon R, Gustot P, Damis F: La déméclocycline: un nouveau traitement de la reténtion hydrosodée des cirrhoses et des ascites refractaires? Nouv Presse Med 1976;5:1993–1994.

85. Delavelle F, Becchio J, Freis D: Utilisation de la déméclotétracycline pour le traitement de l'hyponatremie des ascites cirrhotiques. Nouv Presse Med 1977;6:101–104.

86. Martin J, Codinach N, Conte-Devolx B, Gauthier A: Traitement des ascites cirrhotiques avec hyponatremie par déméthychlortétracycline. Nouv Presse Med 1977; 6:4066.

87. Perez-Ayuso RM, Arroyo V, Camps J, et al: Effect of demeclocycline on renal function and urinary prostaglandin E2 and kallikrein in hyponatremic cirrhotics. Nephron 1984;36:30–37.

88. Singer I, Rotenberg D: Demeclocycline-induced nephrogenic diabetes insipidus. In vivo and in vitro studies. Ann Intern Med 1973;79:679–683.

89. Feldman HA, Singer I: Comparative effects of tetracyclines on water flow across toad urinary bladders. J Pharmacol Exp Ther 1974;190:358–364.

90. Schlondorf D: Interactions of vasopressin with calmodulin and protein kinase C. In Schrier RW (ed): Vasopressin. New York: Raven Press, 1985;113–123.

91. Miller PD, Linas SL, Schrier RW: Plasma demeclocycline levels and nephrotoxicity. Correlation in hyponatremic cirrhotic patients. JAMA 1980;243:2513–2515.

92. Laragh JH, Van Dyke HB, Jacobson J, et al: The experimental production of ascites in the dog with diabetes insipidus. J Clin Invest 1956;35:897–903.

93. Berliner RW, Davidson DG: Production of hypertonic urine in the absence of pituitary antidiuretic hormone. J Clin Invest 1957;36:1416–1427.

94. Radó JP, Taller A: Simultaneous occurrence of diabetes insipidus and ascites due to liver cirrhosis: Clinical and pathophysiological studies. Exp Clin Endocrinol 1990; 95:369–373.

95. Ralli EP, Robson IS, Clark DH, Hoagland CL: Factors influencing ascites in patients with cirrhosis of the liver. J Clin Invest 1945;24:316–325.

96. Van Dyke JB, Ames RG, Plough IC: The excretion of antidiuretic hormone in the urine of patients with cirrhosis of the liver. Trans Assoc Am Physicians 1950; 63:35–38.

97. Mitchell GL Jr, Fitzhugh FW Jr, Freeman OW, Merril AJ: Antidiuretic substances in blood and plasma of patients with congestive heart failure and cirrhosis. Am J Med 1953;14:755–756.

98. Stein M, Schwartz R, Mirsky IA: The antidiuretic activity of plasma of patients with hepatic cirrhosis, congestive heart failure, hypertension and other clinical conditions. J Clin Invest 1954;33:77–81.

99. Chaudhury RR, Chuttani HK, Ramalingaswami V: The antidiuretic hormone and liver damage. Clin Sci 1961; 21:199–203.

100. Lee J, Kerr DNS: The concentration of vasopressin in the blood and the rate of urinary excretion of the hormone by patients with cirrhosis of the liver. Clin Sci 1963;25:375–384.

101. Padfield PL, Morton JJ: Application of a sensitive radioimmunoassay for plasma arginine vasopressin to pathological conditions in man. Clin Sci Mol Med 1974;47:16P–17P.

102. Beardwell CG, Geelen G, Palmer HM, Roberts D, et al: Radioimmunoassay of plasma vasopressin in physiological and pathological states in man. J Endocr 1975; 67:189–202.

103. Wagner H, Maier V, Franz HE: Improved method and its clinical application of a radioimmunoassay of arginine vasopressin in human serum. Horn Metab Res 1977;9:223–227.

104. Guillemant S, Vitoux J-F, Desgrez P, et al: Dosage radio-immunologique de l'arginine-vaso-pressine plasmatique chez le cirrhotique. Nouv Presse Med 1978; 7:3048–3049.

105. Le Bihan G, Bourreille J, Brunelle PH, Basuyau JP: Hormone antidiuretique an cours des cirrhosis decompensees. Nouv Presse Med 1979;8:700.

106. Bichet D, Van Putten VJ, Schrier RW: Potential role of increased sympathetic activity in impaired sodium and water excretion in cirrhosis. N Engl J Med 1982;307: 1552–1557.

107. Reznick RK, Langer B, Taylor BR, et al: Hyponatremia and arginine vasopressin secretion in patients with refractory hepatic ascites undergoing peritoneovenous shunting. Gastroenterology 1983;84:713–718.

108. Epstein M, Weitzman RE, Preston S, DeNunzio AG: Relationship between plasma arginine vasopressin and renal water handling in decompensated cirrhosis. Miner Electrolyte Metab 1984;10:155–165.

109. Skowsky R, Riestra J, Martinez I, et al: Arginine vasopressin (AVP) kinetics in hepatic cirrhosis. Clin Res 1976;24:101A.

110. Ardaillou R, Benmansour M, Rondeau E, Caillens H: Metabolism and secretion of antidiuretic hormone in patients with renal failure, cardiac insufficiency, and liver insufficiency. Adv Nephrol 1984;13:35–49.

111. Anderson RJ, Cronin RE, McDonald KM, Schrier RW: Mechanisms of portal hypertension-induced alterations in renal hemodynamics, renal water excretion, and renin secretion. J Clin Invest 1976;58:964–970.

112. Melman A, Robertson GL: Alteration of osmotic threshold for vasopressin release in chronic bile duct ligated dogs. Clin Res 1977;25:139A.

113. Better OS, Aisembrey GA, Berl T, et al: Role of antidiuretic hormone in impaired urinary dilution associated with chronic bile-duct ligation. Clin Sci 1980;58: 493–500.

114. Linas SL, Anderson RJ, Guggenheim SJ, et al: Role of vasopressin in impaired water excretion in conscious rats with experimental cirrhosis. Kidney Int 1981; 20:173–180.

115. Camps J, Solá J, Arroyo V, Pérez-Ayuso RM, et al: Temporal relationship between the impaired of free water excretion and antidiuretic hormone hypersecretion in rats with experimental cirrhosis. Gastroenterology 1987;93:498–505.

116. Elias AN, Vaziri ND, Domurat ES, et al: Atrial natriuretic peptide, arginine vasopressin, aldosterone and plasma renin activity in carbon-tetrachloride-induced cirrhosis. J Pharmacol Exp Ther 1990;252:438–441.

117. Cláriá J, Jiménez W, Arroyo V, et al: Blockade of the hydroosmotic effect of vasopressin normalizes water excretion in cirrhotic rats. Gastroenterology 1989;97: 1294–1299.

118. Tsuboi Y, Ishikawa S, Fugisawa G, et al: Therapeutic efficacy of the non-peptide AVP antagonist OPC-31260 in cirrhotic rats. Kidney Int 1994;46:237–244.

119. Yamamura Y, Ogawa H, Yamashita H, et al: Characterization of a novel aquaretic agent, OPC-31260, as an orally effective, nonpeptide vasopressin V2-receptor antagonist. Br J Pharmacol 1992;105:787–791.

120. Lopez-Novoa JM: Pathophysiological features of the carbon tetrachloride/phenobarbital model of experimental liver cirrhosis in rats. In Epstein M (ed): The Kidney in Liver Disease, 3rd ed. Baltimore: Williams & Wilkins, 1988;309–327.

121. Kim JK, Summer SN, Howard RL, Schrier RW: Vasopressin gene expression in rats with experimental cirrhosis. Hepatology 1993;17:143–147.

122. Van Tol HHM, Voorhuis DAM, Burbach JPH: Oxytoxin gene expression in discrete hypothalamic magnocellular cell group is stimulated by prolonged salt loading. Endocrinology 1987;120:71–76.

123. Schrier RW, Arroyo V, Bernardi M, et al: Peripheral arterial vasodilatation hypothesis: A proposal for the initiation of renal sodium and water excretion in cirrhosis. Hepatology 1988;89:1151–1157.

124. Epstein M: Renal sodium handling in liver disease. In Epstein M (ed): The Kidney in Liver Disease, 3rd ed. Baltimore: Williams & Wilkins, 1988;3–30.

125. Gines P, Humphreys MH, Schrier RW: Edema. In Massry SG, Glassock RJ (eds): Textbook of Nephrology, 3rd ed. Baltimore: Williams & Wilkins, 1995;582–599.

126. Schrier RW, Berl T: Mechanism of the antidiuretic effect associated with interruption of parasympathetic pathways. J Clin Invest 1972;51:2613–2620.

127. Anderson RJ, Cadnapaphornchai P, Harbottle JA, et al: Mechanism of effect of thoracic inferior vena cava constriction on renal water excretion. J Clin Invest 1974;54:1473–1479.

128. Gupta PD, Henry JP, Sinclair R, Von Baumgarten R: Responses of atrial and aortic baroreceptors to nonhypotensive hemorrhage and to transfusion. Am J Physiol 1966;211:1429–1437.

129. Tristani FE, Cohn JN: Systemic and renal hemodynamics in oliguric hepatic failure: Effect of volume expansion. J Clin Invest 1967;46:1894–1906.

130. Cohn JN: Renal hemodynamic alterations in liver disease. In Suki WN, Eknoyan G (eds): The Kidney in Systemic Disease. New York: John Wiley & Sons, 1976;225–234.

131. Bichet DG, Groves BM, Schrier RW: Mechanisms of improvement of water and sodium excretion by immersion in decompensated cirrhotic patients. Kidney Int 1983;24:788–794.

132. Epstein M: Cardiovascular and renal effects of head-out water immersion in man. Applications of the model in the assessment of volume homeostasis. Circ Res 1976;39:619–628.

133. Epstein M, Preston S, Weitzman RE: Isosmotic central blood volume expansion suppress plasma arginine vasopressin in normal man. J Clin Endocrinol Metab 1981;52:256–262.

134. Epstein M, Pins DS, Schneider N, Levinson R: Determinants of deranged sodium and water homeostasis in decompensated cirrhosis. J Lab Clin Med 1976; 87:822–839.

135. Burmeister P, Scholmerich J, Diener W, Gerok W: Renin, aldosterone and arginine vasopressin in patients with liver cirrhosis: The influence of ascites retransfusion. Eur J Clin Invest 1986;16:117–123.

136. Solís-Herruzo JA, Moreno D, Gonzalez A, et al: Effect of intrathoracic pressure on plasma arginine vasopressin levels. Gastroenterology 1991;101:607–617.

137. Gentile S, Angelico M, Bologna E, Capocaccia L: Clinical, biochemical, and hormonal changes after a single, large volume paracentesis in cirrhosis and ascites. Am J Gastroenterol 1988;84:279–284.

138. Clária J, Jiménez W, Arroyo V, et al: Effect of V_1-vasopressin receptor blockade on arterial pressure in conscious rats with cirrhosis and ascites. Gastroenterology 1991;100:494–501.

139. Lake CR, Ziegler MG, Kopin IJ: Use of plasma norepinephrine for evaluation of sympathetic neuronal functions in man. Life Sci 1976;18:1315–1325.

140. Grossman SH, Davis D, Gunnells JC, Shand DG: Plasma norepinephrine in the evaluation of baroreceptor function in humans. Hypertension 1982;4: 566–571.

141. Henriksen JH, Christensen NJ, Ring-Larsen H: Noradrenaline and adrenaline concentrations in various vascular beds in patients with cirrhosis. Relation to hemodynamics. Clin Physiol 1981;1:293–304.

142. Ring-Larsen H, Hesse B, Henriksen JH, Christensen NJ: Sympathetic nervous activity and renal and systemic hemodynamics in cirrhosis: Plasma norepinephrine concentration, hepatic extraction, and renal release. Hepatology 1982;2:304–310.

143. Ring-Larsen H, Henriksen JH, Christensen NJ: Increased sympathetic activity in cirrhosis. N Engl J Med 1983;308:1029–1030.

144. Bernardi M, Trevisani F, Santini C, et al: Plasma norepinephrine, weak neurotransmitters and renin activity during active tilting in liver cirrhosis: Relationship with cardiovascular homeostasis and renal function. Hepatology 1983;3:56–64.

145. Epstein M, Larios O, Johnson G: Effects of water immersion on plasma catecholamines in decompensated cirrhosis. Implications for deranged sodium and water homeostasis. Miner Electrolyte Metab 1985; 11:25–34.

146. Blendis LM, Sole MJ, Campbell P, et al: The effect of peritoneovenous shunting on catecholamine metabolism in patients with hepatic ascites. Hepatology 1987; 7:143–148.

147. Shapiro MD, Nicholls KM, Groves BM, et al: Interrelationship between cardiac output and vascular resistance as determinants of effective arterial blood volume in cirrhotic patients. Kidney Int 1985;28: 206–211.

148. Zambraski EJ, DiBona GF: Sympathetic nervous system in hepatic cirrhosis. In Epstein M (ed): The Kidney in Liver Disease, 3rd ed. Baltimore: Williams & Wilkins, 1988;469–485.

149. DiBona GF: Renal nerve activity in hepatorenal syndrome. Kidney Int 1984;25:841–853.

150. Better OS, Schrier RW: Disturbed volume homeostasis in patients with cirrhosis of the liver. Kidney Int 1983;23:303–311.

151. Gottschalk CW: Renal nerves and sodium excretion. Annu Rev Physiol 1979;41:229–240.

152. Ayers CR: Plasma renin activity and renin-substrate concentration in patients with liver disease. Circ Res 1967;20:594–598.

153. Schroeder ET, Eich RH, Smulyan H, et al: Plasma renin level in hepatic cirrhosis. Relation to functional renal failure. Am J Med 1970;49:186–191.

154. Chonko AM, Bay WH, Stein JH, Ferris TF: The role of renin and aldosterone in the salt retention of edema. Am J Med 1977;63:881–889.

155. Epstein M, Norsk P: Renin-angiotensin system in liver disease. In Epstein M (ed): The Kidney in Liver Disease, 3rd ed. Baltimore: Williams & Wilkins, 1988; 331–355.

156. Saruta T, Kondo K, Saito I, Nakamura R: Characterization of the components of the renin-angiotensin system in cirrhosis of the liver. In Epstein M (ed): The Kidney in Liver Disease. New York: Elsevier/North-Holland, 1978;207–223.

157. Bonjour JP, Malvin RL: Stimulation of ADH release by the renin-angiotensin system. Am J Physiol 1970;218: 1555–1559.

158. Cadnapaphornchai P, Boykin J, Harbottle JA, et al: Effect of angiotensin II on renal water excretion. Am J Physiol 1975;228:155–159.

159. Heinrich W, Handelman W, Erickson A, et al: Effect of angiotensin II (AII) on renal water excretion. Clin Res 1979;27:74A.

160. Padfield PL, Morton JJ: Effects of angiotensin II on arginine-vasopressin in physiological and pathological situations in man. J Endocr 1977;74:251–259.

161. Laragh JH, Cannon PJ, Bentzel CJ, et al: Angiotensin II, norepinephrine, and renal transport of electrolytes and water in normal man and in cirrhosis with ascites. J Clin Invest 1963;42:1179–1192.

162. Stokes JB: integrated actions of renal medullary prostaglandins in the control of water excretion. Am J Physiol 1981;240:F471–F480.

163. Gross PA, Schrier RW, Anderson RJ: Prostaglandins and water metabolism: A review with emphasis on in vivo studies. Kidney Int 1981;19:839–850.

164. Boyer TD, Zia P, Reynolds TB: Effects of indomethacin and prostaglandins A_1 on renal function and plasma renin activity in alcoholic liver disease. Gastroenterology 1979;77:215–222.

165. Zipser RD, Hoefs JC, Speckart PF, et al: Prostaglandins. Modulators of renal function and pressor resistance in chronic liver disease. J Clin Endocrinol Metab 1979;48:895–900.

166. Uemura M, Tswii T, Fukui H, et al: Urinary prostaglandins and renal function in chronic liver disease. Scand J Gastroenterol 1986;21:75–81.

167. Epstein M, Lifschitz M, Ramachandran M, Rappaport K: Characterization of renal PGE responsiveness in decompensated cirrhosis. Implications for renal sodium handling. Clin Sci 1982;63:555–563.

168. Mirouze D, Zipser RD, Reynolds TB: Effect of inhibitors of prostaglandin synthesis on induced diuresis in cirrhosis. Hepatology 1983;3:50–55.

169. Arroyo V, Gines P, Rimola A, Gaya J: Renal function abnormalities, prostaglandins, and effects of nonsteroidal anti-inflammatory drugs in cirrhosis with ascites. An overview with emphasis on pathogenesis. Am J Med 1986;81(Suppl 2B):104–122.

170. Moore K, Ward PS, Taylor GW, Williams R: Systemic and renal production of thromboxane A_2 and prostacyclin in decompensated liver disease and hepatorenal syndrome. Gastroenterology 1991;100:1069–1077.

171. Wong F, Massie D, Hsu P, Dudley F: Indomethacin-induced renal dysfunction in patients with well-compensated cirrhosis. Gastroenterology 1993;104:869–876.

172. Berl T, Schrier RW: Mechanism of effect of prostaglandin E1 on renal water excretion. J Clin Invest 1973; 52:463–471.

173. Epstein M, Lifschitz M, Hoffman DS, Stein JH: Relationship between renal prostaglandin E and renal sodium handling during water immersion in normal man. Circ Res 1979;45:71–80.

174. Ginés A, Salmerón JM, Ginés P, et al: Oral misoprostol or intravenous prostaglandin E_2 do not improve renal function in patients with cirrhosis and ascites with hyponatremia or renal failure. J Hepatol 1993;17:220–226.

175. Fevery J, Van Cutsen E, Nevens F, et al: Reversal of hepatorenal syndrome in four patients by peroral misoprostol (prostaglandin E_1 analogue) and albumin administration. J Hepatol 1990;11:153–158.

176. Rimola A, Ginés P, Arroyo V, et al: Urinary excretion of 6-keto-$PGF_{1\alpha}$, thromboxane B_2, and prostaglandin E_2 in cirrhosis with ascites: Relationship to functional renal failure (hepatorenal syndrome). J Hepatol 1986;3: 111–117.

177. Laffi G, Marra F, Carloni V, et al: Thromboxane receptor blockade increases water diuresis in cirrhotic patients with ascites. Gastroenterology 1992;103:1017–1021.

178. Escalante B, Reyes JL: Intracellular mechanisms of the effects of thromboxane A_2 on water transport. Adv Prostaglandin Thromboxane Leukotriene Res 1989;19: 229–232.

179. Maak T, Camargo MJF, Lleinert HD, et al: Atrial natriuretic factor: Structure and functional properties. Kidney Int 1985;27:607–615.

180. Warner L, Skorecki K, Blendis LM, Epstein M: Atrial natriuretic factor and liver disease. Hepatology 1993; 17:500–513.

181. Samson WK: Atrial natriuretic factor inhibits dehydration and hemorrhage-induced vasopressin release. Neuroendocrinology 1985;40:277–279.

182. Obana K, Naruse M, Inagami T, et al: Atrial natriuretic factor inhibits vasopressin secretion from rat posterior pituitary. Biochem Biophys Res Commun 1985;132: 1088–1094.

183. Iitake K, Share L, Crofton JT, et al: Central atrial natriuretic factor reduces vasopressin secretion in the rat. Endocrinology 1986;119:438–440.

184. Yamada T, Nakao K, Morii N, et al: Central effect of natriuretic polypeptide on angiotensin II-stimulated vasopressin secretion in conscious rats. Eur J Pharmacol 1986;125:453–456.

185. Lee J, Malvin RL, Claybaugh JR, Huang BS: Atrial natriuretic factor inhibits vasopressin secretion in conscious sheep. Proc Soc Exp Biol Med 1987;185: 272–276.

186. Dillingham MH, Anderson RJ: Inhibition of vasopressin action by atrial natriuretic factor. Science 1986; 231:1572–1573.

187. Jiménez W, Martinez-Pardo A, Arroyo V, et al: Atrial natriuretic factor: Reduced cardiac content in cirrhotic rats with ascites. Am J Physiol 1986;250:F749–F752.

187a. Valdivieso A, Ortíz M, Salas SP, et al: Decreased atrial natriuretic peptide (ANP) binding sites in renal medulla of cirrhotic rats. J Am Soc Nephrol 1993;4: 448A.

188. Croxatto H, Rozas R, Villalon R, Valdivieso A: Effects of cirrhotic human atrial extracts on blood pressure, diuresis, natriuresis and kaliuresis in the rat. Clin Res 1986;34:593A.

189. Fernandez-Cruz L, Marco J, Cuadrado LM, et al: Plasma levels of atrial natriuretic peptide in cirrhotic patients. Lancet 1985;2:1439–1440.

190. Gerbes AL, Arendt RM, Ritter D, et al: Plasma atrial natriuretic factor in patients with cirrhosis. N Engl J Med 1985;313:1609–1610.

191. Wernze H, Burghardt W: Atrial natriuretic peptide, the sympathetic nervous system, and decompensated cirrhosis (letter). Lancet 1986;1:331.

192. Morgan T, Imada T, Inagami T: Atrial natriuretic protein (ANP) in the hepatorenal syndrome (HRS). Hepatology 1986;6:1215.

193. Epstein M, Preston R, Aceto R, et al: Dissociation of plasma irANF and renal sodium handling in cirrhotic humans undergoing water immersion. Kidney Int 1987; 31:269A.

194. Gerbes AL, Wernze H, Arendt R, et al: Effect of water immersion (WI) on renal sodium handling in cirrhosis: Relation to atrial natriuretic factor (ANF) and sympathetic nervous activity. Hepatology 1986;6:1159.

195. Bonkovsky H, Hartle D, Simon D, et al: Decreased plasma atrial natriuretic peptides in cirrhotic ascitic patients. Hepatology 1986;6:1213.

196. Vesely DL, Norsk P, Gower WR Jr, et al: Release of kaliuretic stimulator during immersion-induced central hypovolemia in healthy humans. Proc Soc Exp Biol Med 1995;209:20–26.

197. Vesely DL, Preston R, Winters CJ, et al: Increased release of the N-terminal and C-terminal portions of the atrial natriuretic factor prohormone during immersion-induced central hypervolemia in cirrhotic humans. Am J Nephrol 1991;11:207–216.

198. Vesely DL, Preston R, Gower WR Jr, et al: Increased release of kaliuretic peptide during immersion-induced central hypervolemia in cirrhotic humans. Am J Nephrol (in press).

199. Vesely DL, Douglass MA, Dietz JR, et al: Three peptides from the atrial natriuretic factor prohormone aminoterminus lower blood pressure and produce diuresis, natriuresis, and/or kaliuresis in humans. Circulation 1994;90:1129–1140.

200. Campbell P, Blendis LM, Skorecki K, et al: The effect of peritoneovenous shunting (PVS) on plasma immunoreactive atrial natriuretic peptide (ANP) levels in hepatic ascites. Hepatology 1986;6:1120.

201. Yamagisawa M, Kurihara H, Kimura H, et al: A novel vasoconstrictor peptide produced by vascular endothelial cells. Nature 1988;332:411–415.

202. Moore K, Wendon J, Frazer M, et al: Plasma endothelin immunoreactivity in liver disease and the hepatorenal syndrome. N Engl J Med 1992;327:1774–1778.

203. Uchihara M, Izumi N, Sato C, Marumo F: Clinical significance of elevated plasma endothelin concentration in patients with cirrhosis. Hepatology 1992;16: 95–99.

204. Veglio F, Pinna G, Melchio R, et al: Plasma endothelin levels in cirrhotic subjects. J Hepatol 1992;15:85–87.

205. Oishi R, Nonoguchi H, Tomita K, Marumo F: Endothelin-1 inhibits AVP stimulated osmotic water permeability in rat inner medullary collecting duct. Am J Physiol 1991;261:F951–F956.

206. Naddler SP, Zimpelmann J, Hebert RC: Pertussis toxin sensitive signalling pathway for endothelin in rat inner medullary collecting duct. J Am Soc Nephrol 1991;2: 410A.

207. Takemoto F, Uchida S, Katagiri H, et al: Desensitization of endothelin-1 binding by vasopressin via a cAMP-mediated pathway in rat CCD. Am J Physiol 1995;268:F385–F390.

208. Moncada S, Palmer RMJ, Higgs EA: The discovery of nitric oxide as the endogenous nitrovasodilator. Hypertension 1988;12:365–372.

209. Romero JC, Lahera V, Salom MG, Biondi ML: Role of endothelium-depending relaxing factor nitric oxide on renal function. J Am Soc Nephrol 1992;2:1371–1387.

210. Ramírez AM, Atucha NM, Quesdada T, et al: Efectos de la inhibición de la sintesis de óxido nitrico en la hemodinámica y excreción renal de ratas con cirrhosis biliar crónica. Nefrologia 1994;14:656–662.

210a. Martin P-Y, Niederberger M, Morris K, et al: Normalization of vascular nitric oxide (NO) production corrects arterial vasodilatation and hyperdynamic circulation in rats with cirrhosis and ascites. J Am Soc Nephrol 1994;5:585A.

211. Vallance P, Moncada S: Hyperdynamic circulation in cirrhosis: A role for nitric oxide? Lancet 1991;337: 776–777.

212. Stark ME, Szurskewki JH: Role of nitric oxide in gastrointestinal and hepatic function and disease. Gastroenterology 1992;103:1928–1949.

213. Murray BM, Paller MS: Pressor resistance to vasopressin in sodium depletion, potassium depletion, and cirrhosis. Am J Physiol 1986;251:R525–R530.

214. Mesh CL, Joh T, Korthuis RJ, et al: Intestinal vascular sensitivity to vasopressin in portal hypertensive rats. Gastroenterology 1991;100:916–921.

215. Pizcueta P, Pique JM, Bosch J, et al: Effects of endogenous nitric oxide inhibition on the hemodynamic changes of portal hypertensive rats. Gastroenterology 1991;100:785A.

216. Sieber CC, Groszman RJ: Nitric oxide mediates hyporeactivity to vasopressors in mesenteric vessels of portal hypertensive rats. Gastroenterology 1992;103: 235–239.

217. Earley LE, Sanders CA: The effect of changing serum osmolality on the release of antidiuretic hormone in certain patients with decompensated cirrhosis of the liver and low serum osmolality. J Clin Invest 1959;38: 545–550.

218. White AG, Rubin G, Leiter L: Studies in edema. III. The effect of pitressin on the renal excretion of water and electrolytes in patients with and without liver disease. J Clin Invest 1951;30:1287–1297.

219. Nelson WP III, Welt LG: The effects of pitressin on the metabolism and excretion of water and electrolytes in normal subjects and patients with cirrhosis and ascites. J Clin Invest 1952;31:392–400.

220. Bernstein SH, Weston RE, Ross G, et al: Studies on intravenous water diuresis and nicotine and pitressin antidiuresis in normal subjects and patients with liver disease. J Clin Invest 1953;32:422–427.

221. Hör G, Avenhaus H, Buchborn E: ADH-Plasmaspiegel und-Verteilungsraum nach exogener Zufuhr von ADH am Menschen. Untersuchungen zum Problem der hepatischem ADH-Inaktivierung bei Gesunden und bei Lebercirrhose. Klin Wochenschr 1963;41:366–371.

222. Miller GE, Townsend CE: The in vitro inactivation of pitressin by normal and cirrhotic human liver. J Clin Invest 1954;33:549–554.

223. Solís-Herruzo JA, González-Gamarra A, Castellano G, Muñoz-Yagüe MT: Metabolic clearance rate of arginine vasopressin in patients with cirrhosis. Hepatology 1992;16:974–979.

224. Van Giesen G, Reese M, Kill F, et al: The characteristics of renal hypoperfusion in dogs with acute and chronic reductions in glomerular filtration rate as disclosed by the pattern of water and solute excretion after hypotonic saline infusions. J Clin Invest 1964;43:416–423.

225. Schedl HP, Bartter FC: An explanation for experimental correction of the abnormal water diuresis in cirrhosis. J Clin Invest 1960;39:248–261.

226. Vlahcevic ZR, Adham NF, Jick H, et al: Renal effects of acute expansion of plasma volume in cirrhosis. N Engl J Med 1965;272:387–390.

227. Milani L, Merkel C, Gatta A: Renal effects of aminophylline in hepatic cirrhosis. Eur J Clin Pharmacol 1983;24:757–760.

228. Yamahiro HS, Reynolds TB: Effects of ascitic fluid infusion on sodium excretion, blood volume, and creatinine clearance in cirrhosis. Gastroenterology 1961;40:497–503.

229. Blendis LM, Greig PD, Langer B, et al: The renal and hemodynamic effects of the peritoneovenous shunt for intractable hepatic ascites. Gastroenterology 1979;77:250–257.

230. Birchard WH, Prout TE, Williams TF, Rosenbaum JD: Diuretic response to oral and intravenous water loads in patients with hepatic cirrhosis. J Lab Clin Med 1956;48:26–35.

231. Chaimovitz C, Szylman P, Alroy G, Better OS: Mechanism of increased renal tubular sodium reabsorption in cirrhosis. Am J Med 1972;52:198–202.

232. Schrier RW, Lehman D, Zacherle B, Earley LE: Effect of furosemide on free water excretion in edematous patients with hyponatremia. Kidney Int 1973;3:30–34.

233. Adlersberg D, Fox OL Jr: Changes of the water tolerance test in hepatic disease. Ann Intern Med 1943;19:642–650.

234. Labby DH, Hoagland CL: Water storage and movement of body fluids and chlorides during acute liver disease. J Clin Invest 1947;26:343–353.

235. Wilkinson SP, Blendis LM, Williams R: Frequency and type of renal and electrolyte disorders in fulminant hepatic failure. BMJ 1974;1:186–189.

236. Sherlock S, Scheuer PJ: The presentation and diagnosis of 100 patients with primary biliary cirrhosis. N Engl J Med 1973;289:674–678.

237. Arroyo V, Rodés J, Gutiérrez-Lizárraga MA, Revert L: Prognostic value of spontaneous hyponatremia in cirrhosis with ascites. Dig Dis 1976;21:249–256.

238. Sherlock S, Senewiratne B, Scott A, Walker JG: Complication of diuretic therapy in hepatic cirrhosis. Lancet 1966;1:1049–1053.

239. Fichman MP, Vorherr H, Kleeman CR, Telfer N: Diuretic-induced hyponatremia. Ann Intern Med 1971;75:853–863.

240. Pockros PJ, Reynolds TB: Rapid diuresis in patients with ascites from chronic liver disease: The importance of peripheral edema. Gastroenterology 1986;90:1827–1833.

241. Nelson WP III, Rosenbaum JD, Strauss MB: Hyponatremia in hepatic cirrhosis following paracentesis. J Clin Invest 1951;30:738–744.

242. Schrier RW, Berl T, Anderson RJ: Osmotic and nonosmotic control of vasopressin release. Am J Physiol 1979;236:F321–F332.

243. Vaamonde CA: Maintenance of body fluid tonicity. In Frohlich ED (ed): Pathophysiology—Altered Regulatory Mechanisms in Disease, 3rd ed. Philadelphia: Lippincott, 1984;271–298.

244. Vaamonde CA: Selected renal and electrolyte abnormalities in liver disease. AKF Nephrol Lett 1992;9:13–28.

245. Lancestremere RG, Davidson PL, Earley LE, et al: Renal failure in Laennec's cirrhosis: III. Diuretic response to administered water. J Lab Clin Med 1962;60:967–975.

246. Ralli EP, Leslie SH, Stueck GH Jr, Laken B: Studies of serum and urine constituents in patients with cirrhosis of the liver during water tolerance tests. Am J Med 1951;11:157–169.

247. Papper S, Belsky JL, Bleifer KH: Renal failure in Laennec's cirrhosis of the liver. I. Description of clinical and laboratory features. Ann Intern Med 1959;51:759–773.

248. Leaf A: The clinical and physiological significance of serum sodium concentration. N Engl J Med 1962;267:77–83.

249. Ring-Larsen H: The significance of hyponatremia in liver failure. Postgrad Med J 1975;51:542–543.

250. Summerskill WHJ: Pathogenesis and treatment of disorders of water and electrolyte metabolism in hepatic disease. Proc Mayo Clin 1960;35:89–97.

251. Papadakis MA, Fraser CL, Arieff AI: Hyponatremia in patients with cirrhosis. Q J Med 1990;279:675–688.

252. Melton JE, Patlak CS, Pettigrew KD, Cserr HF: Volume regulatory loss of Na, Cl and K from rat brain during acute hyponatremia. Am J Physiol 1987;252:F661–F669.

253. Thurston JF, Hanhart RE, Nelson JS: Adaptive decrease in amino acids (taurine in particular), creatine, and electrolytes prevent cerebral edema in chronically hyponatremic mice: Rapid correction (experimental model of central pontine myelinosis) causes dehydration and shrinkage of brain. Metabol Brain Dis 1987;2:223–241.

254. D'oczi T, Jo'o F, Szerdayelyi P, Bodosi M: Regulation of brain water and electrolyte contents: The opposite actions of central vasopressin and atrial natriuretic factor (ANF). Acta Neurochir 1988;43(Suppl):186–188.

255. Arieff A, Papadakis MA: Hyponatremia and hypernatremia in liver disease. In Epstein M (ed): The Kidney in Liver Disease, 3rd ed. Baltimore: Williams & Wilkins, 1988;73–88.

256. Wilder CE, Morrison RS, Tyler JM: Relationship between serum sodium and hyperventilation in cirrhosis. Ann Rev Respir Dis 1967;96:971–976.

257. Adams RD, Victor M, Mancall EL: Central pontine myelinosis: A hitherto undescribed disease occurring in alcoholic and malnourished patients. Arch Neurol Psychiatry 1959;81:154–172.

258. Arieff AI: Hyponatremia associated with permanent brain damage. Adv Intern Med 1987;32:325–344.

259. Norenberg MD, Leslie KO, Robertson AS: Association between rise in serum sodium and central pontine myelinosis. Ann Neurol 1982;11:128–135.

260. Ayus JC, Krathapalli R, Arieff AI: Treatment of symptomatic hyponatremia and relationship to brain damage: A prospective study. N Engl J Med 1987;317:1190–1195.

261. Narins RG: Therapy of hyponatremia. Does haste make waste? N Engl J Med 1986;314:1573–1575.

262. Hantman D, Rossier B, Zohlman R, Schrier R: Rapid correction of hyponatremia in the syndrome of inappropriate secretion of antidiuretic hormone: An alternative treatment to hypertonic saline. Ann Intern Med 1973;78:870–875.

263. Decaux G, Mols P, Cauchic P, et al: Treatment of hyponatremic cirrhosis with ascites resistant to diuretics by urea. Nephron 1986;44:337–343.

264. Kao HW, Rakov NE, Sabage F, Reynolds TB: The effect of large volume paracentesis on plasma volume—a cause of hypovolemia? Hepatology 1985;5:403–407.

265. Gines P, Arroyo V, Quintero E, et al: Comparison of paracentesis and diuretics in the treatment of cirrhotics with tense ascites. Results of a randomized study. Gastroenterology 1987;93:234–241.

266. Marshall AW, Jakobovits AW, Morgan MY: Bromocriptine-associated hyponatremia in cirrhosis. BMJ 1982;285:1534–1535.

267. Ring-Larsen H, Clausen E, Ranek L: Peritoneal dialysis in hyponatremia due to liver failure. Scand J Gastroenterol 1973;8:33–40.

268. Larnier AJ, Vickers CR, Adu D, et al: Correction of severe hyponatremia by continuous arteriovenous hemofiltration before liver transplantation. BMJ 1988;297:1514–1515.

269. Sigler MH, Teehan BP: Continuous hemofiltration. In Massry SG, Glassock RJ (eds): Textbook of Nephrology, 3rd ed. Baltimore: Williams & Wilkins, 1995;1588–1596.

270. Oster JR, Epstein M, Ulano HB: Deterioration of renal function with demeclocycline administration. Curr Ther Res 1976;20:794–801.

271. Carrilho F, Bosch J, Arroyo V, et al: Renal failure associated with demeclocycline in cirrhosis. Ann Intern Med 1977;87:195–197.

272. Sawyer WH, Pang PKT, Seto J, et al: Vasopressin analogs that antagonize antidiuretic responses by rats to the antidiuretic hormone. Science 1981;212:49–51.

273. Kinter LB, Dubb J, Huffman W, et al: Potential role of vasopressin antagonists in the treatment of water-retaining disorders. In Schrier RW (ed): Vasopressin. New York: Raven Press, 1985;553–561.

274. Stassen FL, Heckman GD, Schmidt DB, et al: Actions of vasopressin antagonist: Molecular mechanism. In Schrier RW (ed): Vasopressin. New York: Raven Press, 1985;145–154.

275. Kamoi K, Robertson GL: Opiates and vasopressin secretion. In Schrier RW (ed): Vasopressin. New York: Raven Press, 1985;259–264.

276. Huidobro-Toro JP, Huidobro F, Croxatto R: Effects of beta-endorphin and D-alanine, eukephalinamide on urine production and urine electrolyte excretion in the rat. Life Sci 1980;24:697–704.

277. Kapusta DR, Jones SY, Kopp UC, DiBona GF: Role of renal nerves in excretory responses to exogenous and endogenous opioid peptides. J Pharmacol Exp Ther 1989;251:230–237.

278. Thornton JR, Losowksy MS: Plasma leucine encephalin is increased in liver disease. Gut 1989;30:1392–1395.

279. Thorton JR, Dean H, Losowsky MS: Is ascites caused by impaired hepatic inactivation of blood borne endogenous opioid peptides? Gut 1988;29:1167–1172.

280. Leehey DJ, Gollapudi P, Deakin A, Reid RW: Naloxone increases water and electrolyte excretion after water loading in patients with cirrhosis and ascites. J Lab Clin Med 1991;118:484–491.

281. Warren SE, Mitas JA II, Swerdin AHR: Hypernatremia in hepatic failure. JAMA 1980;243:1257–1260.

282. Kaupke C, Sprague T, Gitnick G: Hypernatremia after the administration of lactulose. Ann Intern Med 1977;86:745–746.

283. Vesin P, Roberti A, Kac J, Viginé R: Coma avec azotemie, hypernatrémie et hyperchlorémie chez un cirrhotique. Sem Hôp Paris 1965;41:1220–1223.

284. Rodés J, Arroyo V, Brodas JM, Bruguera M: Hypernatremia following gastrointestinal bleeding in cirrhosis with ascites. Am J Dig Dis 1975;20:127–133.

285. Wilkinson SP: Hypernatremia. In Hepatorenal Disorders. New York: Marcel Dekker, 1982;138.

286. Gigli G, Giovanneti S: La funzione renale nella cirrosi epatica. Riv Gastro Enterol 1951;3:79–94.

287. Rivera A, Peña JC, Barcena C, et al: Renal excretion of water, sodium and potassium in cirrhosis of the liver. Metabolism 1961;10:1–17.

288. MacGaffey K, LeZotte LA Jr, Snyder JG, et al: Ethacrynic acid: A drug which abolishes the concentrating ability of kidney. Proc Soc Exp Biol Med 1964;116:11–16.

289. Jick H, Kamm DE, Snyder JG, et al: On the concentrating defect in cirrhosis of the liver. J Clin Invest 1964;43:258–266.

290. Jick H, Sweet RH, Smith W, et al: The effect of dietary sodium restriction on the urine concentrating mechanism of cirrhosis. Clin Sci 1964;26:397–403.

291. Perri T, Rubegni DiM, Pucetti F, Corconi S: Azione dell'ormone antidiuretico postipofisario sulla diuresi osmotica da mannitolo nelia cirrosi epatica. Minerva Nefrol 1965;12:240.

292. Vaamonde CA, Vaamonde LS, Morosi HJ, et al: Renal concentrating ability in cirrhosis. I. Changes associated with the clinical status and course of the disease. J Lab Clin Med 1967;70:179–194.

293. Vaamonde CA, Presser JI, Vaamonde LS, Papper S: Renal concentrating ability in cirrhosis. III. Failure of hypertonic saline to increase reduced TcH$_2$O formation. Kidney Int 1972;1:55–64.

294. Vaamonde CA, Oster JR, Strauss J: The kidney in sickle cell disease. In Suki WN, Eknoyan G (eds): The Kidney in Systemic Disease, 2nd ed. New York: John Wiley & Sons, 1981;159–195.

295. Stein RM, Levitt BH, Goldstein MH, et al: The effects of salt restriction on renal concentrating operation in normal, hydropenic man. J Clin Invest 1962;41:2101–2111.

296. Epstein FH, Kleeman CR, Pursel S, Hendrikx A: The effect of feeding protein and urea on the renal concentrating process. J Clin Invest 1957;36:635–641.

297. Klahr S, Tripathy K, Garcia FT, et al: On the nature of the renal concentrating defect in malnutrition. Am J Med 1967;43:84–96.

298. McCance RA, Crowne RS, Halt TS: The effect of malnutrition and food habits on the concentrating power of the kidney. Clin Sci 1969;37:471–490.

299. Clapp JR: Renal tubular reabsorption of urea in normal and protein-depleted rats. Am J Physiol 1966;210:1304–1308.

300. Rudman D, Difulco TJ, Galambos JT, et al: Maximal rates of excretion and synthesis of urea in normal and cirrhotic subjects. J Clin Invest 1973;52:2241–2249.

301. Whang R, Papper S: The possible relationship of renal cortical hypoperfusion and diminished renal concentrating ability in Laennec's cirrhosis. J Chronic Dis 1974;27:263–265.

302. Fourman J, Kennedy GC: An effect of antidiuretic hormone on the flow of blood through the vasa recta of the rat kidney. J Endocr 1966;35:173–176.

303. Fourman J, Moffat DB: The Blood Vessels of the Kidney. Oxford: Blackwell, 1971;129–139.

304. Anderson RJ, Berl T, McDonald KD, Schrier RW: Evidence for an in vivo antagonism between vasopressin and prostaglandin in the mammalian kidney. J Clin Invest 1975;56:420–426.

Chapter 3

HEPATORENAL SYNDROME

MURRAY EPSTEIN, M.D., F.A.C.P.

Clinical Features
Pathogenesis
  Afferent Events
  Efferent Events
Acute Renal Failure
Hepatorenal Syndrome vs. Acute Tubular
  Necrosis: Different Diseases or a Continuum?

Diagnostic Considerations
Treatment
  Basic Management
  Other Treatment Modalities
Conclusion

The hepatorenal syndrome (HRS) is a unique form of acute renal failure occurring in patients with liver disease for which a specific cause cannot be elucidated. Despite intense clinical and investigative interest, until recently relatively little progress had been made in the understanding and management of HRS. The past several years have witnessed newer insights in both pathophysiology and therapeutics. The application of newer methodology such as tracer kinetics has delineated more rigorously the role of a number of pathogenic mechanisms, including activation of the sympathetic nervous system. The characterization of endothelin and the nitric oxide (NO)-arginine pathway and their roles in biology and medicine has provided additional insights into the pathogenesis of hepatorenal syndrome. Finally, recently initiated therapeutic approaches, including the maturation of orthotopic liver transplantation and transjugular intrahepatic portosystemic shunt (TIPS), lend a note of optimism to the future management of a syndrome that so often is incompatible with recovery.

Progressive oliguric renal failure commonly complicates the course of advanced hepatic disease.[1-4] This condition has been designated by many names, including functional renal failure, hemodynamic renal failure, hepatic nephropathy, renal failure of cirrhosis, and others, but the most commonly used is HRS, a more appealing, albeit less specific term. For the purpose of this discussion, HRS is defined as unexplained renal failure in patients with liver disease in the absence of clinical, laboratory, or anatomic evidence of other known causes of renal failure.

When confronted with a patient who has concomitant renal and hepatic disease, the clinician should consider not only HRS but also a number of potentially treatable disorders that simultaneously involve the liver and the kidney.[3,4] Such disorders, termed pseudohepatorenal syndromes, include toxic, hematologic, neoplastic, genetic, hemodynamic, and infectious processes (Table 3.1). The importance of recognizing these disorders lies in the fact that they may be reversible if detected early and treated appropriately.

CLINICAL FEATURES

The essential features of HRS were first described by Austin Flint[5] in a surprisingly up-to-date report published over a century ago. Then Professor of the Principles and Practice of Medicine at the Bellevue Hospital Medical College in Manhattan, Flint wrote a classic paper based on the analysis of 46 cases.[5] He concluded that cirrhotic liver disease related to alcohol was the cause of ascites in most patients. Of interest, in the light of things to come, he also observed "a little lymph . . . on the convex surface of the organ." Flint noted the presence of oliguria and the absence of albuminuria. He commented further that in 11 of the autopsied patients in whom the condition of the kidneys was noted, the kidneys were considered to be normal in 5 and

TABLE 3.1. Conditions Causing Simultaneous Liver and Renal Failure

Infections
   Sepsis
   Leptospirosis
   Reye's syndrome

Toxins
   Methoxyflurane
   Carbon tetrachloride
   Tetracyclines (especially in third trimester of pregnancy)
   Acetaminophen
   Elemental phosphorus (contained in some rodent poisons)

Circulatory
   Congestive heart failure
   Shock

Neoplasms
   Metastatic
   Hypernephroma

Collagen vascular disease
   Systemic lupus erythematosus
   Polyarteritis nodosa

Genetic
   Polycystic kidney disease

Miscellaneous
   Amyloidosis

"diseased" in 6. Detailed descriptions of the diseased kidneys are not presented, except that one kidney was noted to be "granular." Flint recommended therapy as follows:

> To sum up in a few words, the management of hydroperitoneum, . . . the first object generally being to effect the removal or diminution of the peritoneal effusion, we may make cautious trial of diuretics and hydragogue cathartics. If these means do not prove promptly efficacious (as they will very rarely do), it is useless to persist in the former (diuretics) and injurious to consider the latter (hydragogues).

The clinical features of HRS have been detailed in several recent reviews[1–4] and are summarized in Table 3.2. In brief, HRS usually occurs in cirrhotic patients who are alcoholic, although cirrhosis is not a sine qua non for the development of HRS. HRS may complicate other liver diseases, including acute hepatitis, fulminant hepatic failure, and hepatic malignancy.[4,6,7] Although renal failure may develop in patients in whom normal serum creatinine levels have been documented within a few days of onset of HRS, this finding does not imply that the patients had a normal glomerular filtration rate (GFR). The serum creatinine level has been shown to be a poor index of renal function in patients with chronic liver disease, often masking markedly

reduced GFRs.[8] Implicit in such a formulation is the concept that patients with HRS may have a low GFR for weeks to months before coming to medical attention. We are therefore dealing with kidneys that almost certainly are susceptible to further insult by hemodynamic or other stimuli.

Numerous reports have emphasized the development of renal failure after events that reduce effective blood volume, including abdominal paracentesis, vigorous diuretic therapy, and gastrointestinal bleeding, although renal failure can occur in the absence of an apparent precipitating event. Several careful observers have noted that patients with HRS seldom arrive in the hospital with preexisting renal failure; rather, HRS seems to develop in the hospital, indicating that iatrogenic events might precipitate the syndrome.[1,4]

The development of renal failure in the course of Laënnec's cirrhosis is of grave prognostic significance.[1,4,9] The majority of patients die within 3 weeks of the onset of azotemia. In his series of 200 patients, Papper[1] observed only 2 patients who recovered spontaneously. On the other hand, some investigators have reported a higher incidence of spontaneous recovery.[9–11] Reynolds[10] reported 13% spontaneous recovery in a series of 62 patients. Gordon and Anderson[11] estimated that "perhaps as many as 20–30% of patients will attain peak serum creatinine values of 2–5 mg/dl (177–442 mmol/L), which later decline." Although the exact figures may depend on a number of factors, including severity at the time of diagnosis, spontaneous recovery occurs in a minority of patients. In most instances, the carefully documented recoveries have appeared to follow a

TABLE 3.2. Major Clinical Features of Hepatorenal Syndrome

1. Usually occurs in patients after they have been admitted to the hospital.
2. No apparent precipitating factor.
3. Renal failure usually occurs in patients with moderate to tense ascites.
4. There is no consistent relationship to jaundice.
5. Some degree of hepatic encephalopathy is present in most patients.
6. The blood pressure is often lower than usual for that specific patient.
7. There is marked oliguria, almost complete absence of sodium, and usually hyponatremia.
8. Urinary indices are similar to those of prerenal azotemia and contrast with those seen in acute tubular necrosis.
9. Spontaneous recovery is unusual.

dramatic and rapid improvement in the condition of the liver.

Despite the bleak prognosis, it is difficult to attribute the poor outcome directly to renal failure in patients in whom azotemia is moderate. Such observations suggest that the renal failure may be more of a reflection of a broader lethal event and that, in most instances, it is not in itself the major determinant of survival. A truly uremic death is a rarity.

PATHOGENESIS

A substantial body of evidence lends strong support to the concept that the renal failure in HRS is functional in nature. Despite the severe derangement of renal function, pathologic abnormalities are minimal and inconsistent.[1,4,12] Furthermore, tubular functional integrity is maintained during the renal failure, as manifested by a relatively unimpaired sodium reabsorptive capacity and concentrating ability. Finally, more direct evidence is derived from (1) the demonstration that kidneys transplanted from patients with HRS are capable of resuming normal function in the recipient[13] (Fig. 3.1) and (2) the return of renal function when the patient with HRS successfully receives a liver transplant (Fig. 3.2).[14]

Despite extensive study, the precise pathogenesis of HRS has not been delineated. Many studies using diverse hemodynamic techniques have documented a significant reduction in renal perfusion.[15–17] Because a similar decrement of renal perfusion is compatible with urine volumes exceeding 1 liter in many patients with chronic renal failure, it is unlikely that a decrease in mean blood flow per se is responsible for the oliguria.[18]

Using the ^{133}xenon washout technique and selective renal arteriography to study HRS, our laboratories demonstrated a significant reduction in calculated mean blood flow as well as a preferential reduction in cortical perfusion.[16] In addition, cirrhotic patients manifested marked vasomotor instability that was characterized not only by variability between serial xenon washout studies but also by instability within a single curve.[16] This phenomenon has not been encountered in renal failure of other etiologies. In addition, Epstein and coworkers[16] performed simultaneous renal arteriography to delineate further the nature

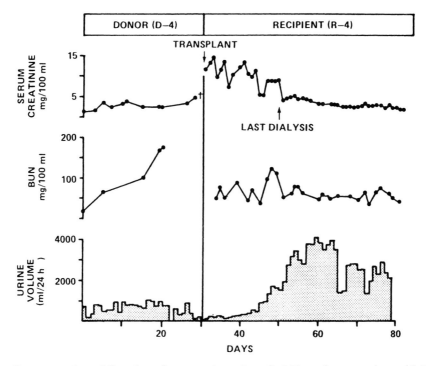

FIGURE 3.1. Recovery of renal function after transplantation of a kidney from a patient with HRS. Course of a donor (D-4) before death, indicated by cross (†), and that of the recipient (R-4) after renal transplantation. (Reproduced with permission from Koppel M, et al: Transplantation of cadaveric kidneys from patients with hepatorenal syndrome. Evidence for the functional nature of renal failure in advanced liver disease. N Engl J Med 1969;280:1367–1371.)

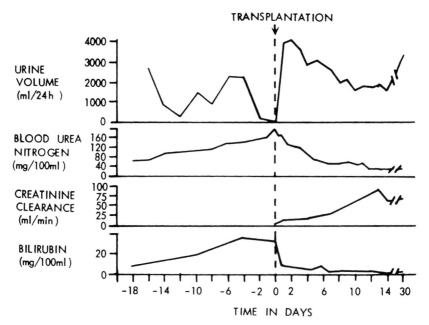

FIGURE 3.2. Changes in renal function in a patient before and after orthotopic liver transplantation. (Reproduced with permission from Iwatsuki S, et al: Recovery from hepatorenal syndrome after orthotopic liver transplantation. N Engl J Med 1973;289:1155–1159.)

of the hemodynamic abnormalities. Selective renal arteriograms disclosed marked beading and tortuosity of the interlobar and proximal arcuate arteries and an absence of distinct cortical nephrograms and vascular filling of the cortical vessels (Fig. 3.3A). Postmortem angiography performed on the kidneys of 5 patients studied during life disclosed a striking normalization of the vascular abnormalities with a reversal of all vascular abnormalities in the kidneys (Fig. 3.3B). The peripheral vasculature filled completely, and the previously irregular vessels became smooth and regular. Such findings provide additional evidence for the functional basis of the renal failure, operating through active renal vasoconstriction.[16]

Although renal hypoperfusion with preferential renal cortical ischemia has been shown to underlie the renal failure of HRS,[16,19] the factors responsible for sustaining reduction in cortical perfusion and suppression of filtration in HRS have not been elucidated. The pathogenetic events leading to intrarenal hemodynamic derangements and decrease in GFR may be classified as afferent and efferent. The discussion of afferent events focuses on extracellular fluid translocations or sequestration into serous spaces or interstitial fluid compartments, which characterize advanced liver disease. The discussion of efferent events encompasses a survey of the

hormonal and neural mechanisms proposed or implicated in the pathogenesis of renal failure. Emphasis is placed on recent studies characterizing the sympathetic nervous system, renal thromboxanes, nitric oxide-arginine pathway, and the possible contribution of endothelin.

Afferent Events

Traditionally, it has been proposed that contraction of the effective blood volume constitutes a pivotal event in patients predisposed to HRS.[1–4,20–22] The term effective plasma volume refers to the part of the total circulating volume that is effective in stimulating volume receptors. The concept is somewhat elusive because the actual volume receptors remain incompletely defined. A diminished effective volume may reflect subtle alterations in systemic hemodynamic factors, such as decreased filling of the arterial tree, diminished central blood volume, or both. Despite massive retention of salt and water, effective blood volume remains functionally contracted because of a disturbance in the Starling forces, which govern the distribution of fluid within the extracellular fluid (ECF) compartment.

Studies by Henriksen et al.[23,24] have provided further support for the concept of a reduced effective blood volume. They demonstrated that the

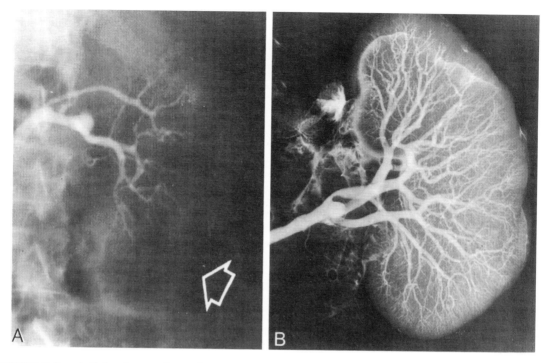

FIGURE 3.3. *A,* Selective renal arteriogram in a patient with oliguric renal failure and cirrhosis (T.L.). Note the extreme abnormality of the intrarenal vessels, including the primary branches off the main renal artery and the interlobar arteries. The arcuate and cortical arterial system is not recognizable, nor is a distinct nephrogram present. The arrow indicates the edge of the kidney. *B,* Postmortem angiogram of the same kidney with the intraarterial injection of micropaque in gelatin as the contrast agent. Note filling of the renal arterial system throughout the vascular bed to the periphery of the cortex. The vascular attenuation and tortuosity are no longer present. The vessels were also histologically normal. (Reproduced with permission from Epstein M, et al: Renal failure in the patient with cirrhosis. The role of active vasoconstriction. Am J Med 1970;49:175–185.)

estimated central blood volume (ECBV; i.e., blood volume in the heart cavities, lungs, and central arterial tree) is decreased in patients with cirrhosis.[23] More recently the same authors assessed the relationship among ECBV, systemic and portal hemodynamics, and markers of overall and renal sympathetic nervous activity.[24] They measured the ECBV and the circulating and renal venous levels of norepinephrine and arterial epinephrine in patients with cirrhosis and esophageal varices who were undergoing hemodynamic investigation. They observed that arterial norepinephrine levels, an index of overall sympathetic nervous activity, was negatively correlated with ECBV. Similarly, renal venous norepinephrine levels (an index of renal sympathetic tone) was inversely correlated with ECBV. The authors proposed the following explanation of their findings: reduced ECBV probably "unloads" volume receptors and baroreceptors, thus enhancing overall and renal sympathetic nervous

activity and contributing to renal vasoconstriction, azotemia, and renal salt and water retention in cirrhosis. Such findings indicate that central circulatory and arterial underfilling is a key element of the renal hemodynamic derangements in patients with decompensated cirrhosis.

The mechanisms contributing to diminished effective volume are multiple. Traditionally, it has been proposed that ascites formation in cirrhotic patients begins when a critical imbalance of Starling forces in the hepatic sinusoids and splanchnic capillaries causes an excessive amount of lymph formation that exceeds the capacity of the thoracic duct to return this excessive lymph to the circulation.[1,20–22] Consequently, excessive lymph accumulates in the peritoneal space as ascites, with a subsequent contraction of circulating plasma volume. Thus, as ascites develops, there is a progressive redistribution of plasma volume.

Although an imbalance of Starling forces in the hepatosplanchnic microcirculation is thought to contribute significantly to the relative decrease in effective blood volume, it is not the sole mechanism. An additional determinant is the significant diminution of total peripheral resistance in most cirrhotic patients who retain sodium and water.[4,25,26] This decrease in peripheral vascular resistance is no doubt partially related to anatomic arteriovenous shunts and possibly to some undefined vasodilator (either produced by or not inactivated by the diseased liver). Thus, despite an increase in total plasma volume, the relative "fullness" of the arteriovenous tree is diminished. In summary, several hemodynamic events act in concert to diminish effective volume, thereby activating the mechanisms that promote a decrease in renal perfusion and GFR. Regardless of cause, the resultant diminution of effective volume is thought to constitute an afferent signal to the renal tubule to augment salt and water reabsorption and to decrease GFR. Thus, the traditional underfill formulation suggests that the renal retention of sodium is a *secondary* rather than primary event.

Peripheral Arterial Vasodilation Theory (Revised Underfill Theory)

The principal distinguishing feature of a newly proposed revision of the underfill theory is that the decrease in effective blood volume is attributable primarily to an early increase in vascular capacitance.[26,27] Thus, peripheral vasodilation is the initial determinant of intravascular underfilling, and an imbalance between the expanded capacitance and available volume constitutes a diminished effective volume. This concept brings the hypothesis into accord with experimental observations that were not consistent with the original postulate. For example, careful balance studies in animals with experimental cirrhosis have shown clearly that sodium retention precedes ascites formation.[28]

Primary systemic hemodynamic changes characterized by peripheral vasodilation occur very early in experimental cirrhosis and in humans with compensated cirrhosis.[25,27–29] The decrease in effective volume induced by these hemodynamic alterations is compounded further by an impaired pressor response to vasoactive agents, including exogenous angiotensin II and noradrenaline.[4,26] Even in patients who eventually develop an increase in total plasma volume, the relative fullness of the arteriovenous tree is decreased.

According to the peripheral arterial vasodilation hypothesis, the hepatorenal syndrome constitutes an extreme extension of underfilling of the arterial circulation, with the most extreme elevations of vasoactive hormones, including plasma renin activity (PRA), norepinephrine (NE), and vasopressin, and the most extreme degree of renal vasoconstriction.[26]

Overflow Theory

An alternative hypothesis to the two underfill theories is the overflow theory of ascites formation.[28,30] In contrast to the underfill formulation, the overflow theory postulates that the initial *primary* event is the inappropriate retention of excessive amounts of sodium by the kidneys, which is unrelated to defense of plasma volume (and thought to be due to intrahepatic hypertension). In the setting of abnormal Starling forces in the portal venous bed and hepatic sinusoids (both portal venous hypertension and a reduction in plasma colloid osmotic pressure), the expanded plasma volume is sequestered preferentially in the peritoneal space, with ascites formation. Thus, renal sodium retention and plasma volume expansion *precede rather than follow* the formation of ascites.

In summary, both underfill theories provide a possible explanation of why fluid retention often fails to attenuate both the stimulus for neurohormonal activation and the continuing sodium and water retention. Despite a progressive increase in total ECF volume, fluid is sequestered into one or more of the other fluid compartments without normalizing effective blood volume. Because the capacity of the interstitial fluid (ISF) and its associated spaces—for example, the peritoneum—is largely limitless, the kidneys encounter great difficulty in filling such a space and the sodium retention becomes relentless. Only correction of the disturbance in the forces governing fluid distribution and reversing the peripheral arterial vasodilatation will permit a reexpansion of effective blood volume to normal. Of importance, the peripheral arterial vasodilation theory highlights the florid systemic hemodynamic disturbances and the importance of attempting to correct not only the renal hemodynamic disturbances but also the concomitant systemic hemodynamic derangements.

An alternate formulation has emphasized that the renal vasoconstriction is attributable to unique events independent of a contracted volume, i.e., a primary cause. According to this theory, advanced liver damage, in conjunction with some other unknown abnormality, induces a primary disorder in one or more of the modifiers that regulate renal vascular tone. The renal ischemia, it is argued, is not an expression of the normal neural and hormonal response to liver damage but rather represents either an alteration in the synthesis, degradation, or potency of a vasoactive substance or a malfunction of the normal feedback regulation of its release. Such abnormalities might result from impaired hepatic degradative or excretory capacity, portosystemic shunting of blood, or altered neural connections between the liver and the kidney.

Although many investigators have focused on a contraction of effective arterial blood volume (EABV) as a major etiologic factor in the pathogenesis of HRS, there is lack of unanimity on this point. Some authors have proposed that because a diminished EABV causes the typical syndrome of prerenal failure (easily reversible with volume replacement) and sometimes leads to acute tubular necrosis (ATN), it cannot be considered as the prepotent etiologic factor for HRS. Although HRS is induced primarily by a unique cause of renal ischemia that does not necessitate contracted EABV, a contributory role for contracted EABV need not be excluded. A contracted EABV or the concomitant activation of neurohormonal mediators that attends such hypovolemia may amplify the renal vasoconstrictive effects of the putative, as yet undefined, mediators.[4] Indeed, because the majority of studies have reported that reduction of EABV is a typical feature of patients with HRS, this alteration in volume status may be a necessary but not sufficient factor predisposing patients to HRS.

An alternate formulation to reconcile the presence of contracted EABV in both prerenal azotemia and HRS posits that they represent differences in degree and occupy disparate points on a continuum.[4,26] Conceivably, patients with moderate contraction of EABV develop prerenal azotemia, which is reversible by volume depletion. With advancing liver disease, the magnitude of the contraction becomes greater and at some point is no longer reversible by volume expansive maneuvers. Presumably this point marks the transition from prerenal azotemia to HRS.

Cardiac Output

Myocardial dysfunction often attends the renal failure of liver disease.[25,31] Diminished venous return due to tense ascites,[32] alcohol myopathy, and malnutrition can interfere with myocardial performance. Although many patients with HRS manifest a decrease in cardiac output,[22,25] the HRS is not merely another "cardiorenal syndrome," comprising prerenal failure secondary to diminished performance of the heart. Most available evidence suggests that a diminution in cardiac output is not an important factor in the renal ischemia underlying HRS. Tristani and Cohn[31] studied 21 patients with oliguric hepatic failure, of whom 13 had a low or normal cardiac index and 8 had an increased cardiac output. The patients with low cardiac output responded to volume expansion with isooncotic dextran with an increase in cardiac output, an even greater increase in renal blood flow (148%), and a rise in the proportion of cardiac output delivered to the kidney (renal fraction). Renal vasoconstriction, however, often persisted—and often required local infusion of a potent renal vasodilator (dopamine) to restore renal blood flow to normal.[33] Moreover, the magnitudes of the diuretic responses to various maneuvers (e.g., raising arterial blood pressure, reinfusion of ascites) varied greatly among patients who were oliguric, even when renal perfusion had been restored toward normal.

Epstein and colleagues[34] studied the relationship of systemic and intrarenal hemodynamics in 20 patients with advanced alcoholic cirrhosis, of whom 10 had increased cardiac output (7–14 L/min), 7 had normal cardiac output (5–7 L/min), and 3 had depressed values (3.7–4.1 L/min). Of interest was the observation that renal blood flow did not correlate with the level of cardiac output (Fig. 3.4). Comparable reductions in total renal blood flow, as well as cortical flow, were observed in the low- and high-output groups. In congestive heart failure, on the other hand, cardiac output directly correlates with cortical flow (as determined by ^{133}Xe washout techniques).[35] Such findings suggest that local renal vasoconstrictor influences are extremely important as a final determinant for intrarenal vascular resistance.

Ring-Larsen and associates[36] measured mean renal blood flow in 6 patients with cirrhosis requiring an end-to-side portacaval anastomosis. Although portal decompression caused a significant increase in cardiac output, renal perfusion either declined or remained unaltered. Collectively, these observations emphasize that the renal vasoconstriction of HRS varies independently of changes in cardiac output.

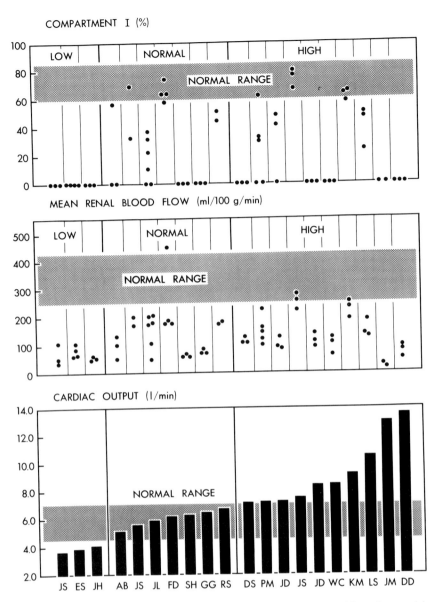

FIGURE 3.4. Relationship of cardiac output and renal hemodynamics in 20 patients with cirrhosis. The *upper panel* depicts the percent flow to the rapid flow components ($C_1\%$). The *middle panel* depicts mean renal blood flow, and the *lower panel* depicts cardiac output. Each point represents a single xenon washout study. The *shaded area* in the *upper* and *middle panels* represents mean $\pm$ SE of seven normal subjects. The *shaded area* in the *lower panel* represents the normal range for cardiac output in this laboratory. The degree of renal hypoperfusion and cortical ischemia was independent of cardiac output. (Reproduced with permission fom Epstein M, et al: Relationship of systemic and intrarenal hemodynamics in cirrhosis. J Lab Clin Med 1977;89:1175–1187.)

Finally, the hypotension of liver disease merits comment. Although jaundice interferes with cardiac performance, the major cause of hypotension is peripheral vasodilation. The pathogenesis of the vasodilation is complex and in part may be attributable to vasodilatory hormones from the intestines, such as glucagon, vasoactive intestinal peptide (VIP), and substance P, that bypass the liver or are inadequately degraded by the diseased liver and escape into the circulation. Recent studies have suggested that generation of NO by circulating endotoxin accounts for the severe intractable hypotension associated with septic shocks and decompensated liver failure.

Presumably milder forms of liver failure are associated with more modest activation of NO and more modest hypotension.[37] Chapter 17 reviews the important role of the nitric oxide system in cirrhosis in renal failure. Thus, the systemic circulation is exposed to enhanced vasodilator activity.

Jaundice

In light of the constellation of jaundice and renal failure, several investigators have proposed that jaundice may play an important role in mediating the renal failure. A number of bile constituents have been investigated. Dawson[38] postulated that conjugated hyperbilirubinemia sensitizes the kidneys to anoxic damage. In contrast, Aoyagi and Lowenstein[39] proposed that bile salts rather than bilirubin aggravate the ischemic damage in the rat kidney. Alon et al.[40] and Finestone et al.[41] demonstrated that the direct intrarenal infusion of bile does not impair GFR or renal plasma flow in dogs. Indeed, acute bile duct ligation actually increases GFR and renal blood flow in dogs.[42]

An additional mechanism whereby bile salts may contribute to renal dysfunction relates to their ability to interfere with the action of sodium-potassium ATPase.[43] Theoretically, interference with sodium-potassium ATPase activity in heart muscle and kidney may explain the cardiac and renal dysfunction of cirrhosis. Although it has been suggested that such a mechanism does not apply,[44] the possibility has not been rigorously excluded. Green and Better[45] have considered the growing body of evidence that bile constituents (e.g. bile acids, bilirubin, cholesterol) do not exert a direct nephrotoxic effect.

Increased Abdominal and Renal Venous Pressure

Mullane and Gliedman[46] suggested that pressure on the renal venous system, because of the presence of ascites, interferes with the renal circulation and causes renal ischemia. Indeed, they suggested that such increments in renal venous pressure may occur in the absence of ascites. Direct measurements of renal venous pressure in cirrhotic patients do not support this hypothesis. In any event, many patients with tense ascites, in whom the pressure exerted on the renal veins exceeds the pressure attributable to the column of fluid because of muscular elasticity, show perfectly normal renal function.[46,48]

Controversy has attended the question of whether or not removal of ascites by paracentesis improves renal function. Gordon[49] observed a transient improvement in renal function in patients with HRS following removal of ascites by paracentesis. Cade et al.[50] examined the contribution of altered intraperitoneal pressure by measuring GFR, renal plasma flow and pressure in the vena cava, hepatic vein free flow, and hepatic vein wedged pressure before, during, and after paracentesis to reduce the intraperitoneal pressure from 30–40 cm H_2O to 12–17 cm H_2O. Venous pressures moved parallel to ascitic fluid pressures, and GFR, renal plasma flow, and urine flow improved sharply; as the formation of ascitic fluid continued to reduce vascular volume, however, urine flow, GFR, and renal plasma flow decreased slowly.

In contrast to the above findings, several other observations militate against a major etiologic role for increased renal venous pressure. Relieving the pressure on the renal veins in ascitic patients by placing them in the prone position on a Stryker frame has produced only transient improvement in renal function. Perhaps more to the point is the fact that the pressures required to impair renal function in patients with HRS far exceed the pressures observed even in patients with the most tense ascites. In summary, it appears that increased renal venous pressure is not a major determinant of the renal ischemia of HRS.

Efferent Events

The effectors that promote renal ischemia and a decrease in GFR remain incompletely defined. Several major hypotheses have been suggested: (1) alterations of the renin-angiotensin system; (2) an increase in sympathetic nervous system activity; (3) alterations in renal eicosanoids, including a relative decrease in renal vasodilatory prostaglandins and an increase in vasoconstrictor thromboxanes; (4) enhanced nitric oxide production with peripheral vasodilation; (5) elevated plasma endothelin levels; (6) a relative impairment of renal kallikrein production; and (7) endotoxemia (Table 3.3). These proposed mechanisms and their interrelationships are summarized schematically in Figure 3.5.

Renin-Angiotensin System

Several lines of evidence suggest a role for the renin-angiotensin axis in sustaining the vasoconstriction in HRS. Patients with decompensated

TABLE 3.3. Known and Postulated Mechanisms
That May Contribute to the Renal Failure
of Liver Disease

Hormonal
    Activation of the renin-angiotensin system
    Alterations in renal eicosanoids
        Diminished vasodilatory prostaglandins
        Increased vasoconstrictor Tx
    Enhanced NO production
    Elevated plasma endothelin levels
    Endotoxemia
    Relative impairment of renal kallikrein production
    Diminished atrial natriuretic peptides
    Vasoactive intestinal peptide
    Glomerulopressin deficiency
Neural and Hemodynamic
    An increase in sympathetic nervous system activity
    Alterations in intrarenal blood flow distribution

---

cirrhosis frequently manifest marked elevations of plasma renin levels.[4,51–54] An examination of the relationship between renal function and plasma renin levels has disclosed that cirrhotic patients with impaired renal function manifested the most profound elevations in plasma renin levels. Although the elevation of plasma renin is attributable in part to the decreased hepatic inactivation

of renin, it is evident that the major determinant is increased renin secretion by the kidney. Of note, the elevation of plasma renin often occurs despite diminished hepatic synthesis of the α_2-globulin, renin substrate.[55]

There are at least two reasonable explanations for the increased renin secretion in cirrhosis: (1) renal hypoperfusion may be the primary event, with a resultant activation of the renin-angiotensin system, and (2) activation of the renin-angiotensin system may be a secondary response to a diminished effective blood volume.

The observations of Barnardo et al.[54] have been interpreted as supporting the former hypothesis. The authors infused dopamine into 10 patients whose cirrhosis was associated with various degrees of renal functional impairment. Dopamine caused a consistent increase in effective renal plasma flow but little change in GFR or sodium and water excretion. Concomitantly, dopamine suppressed plasma renin activity (PRA). One might object that increases in arterial pressure or cardiac output during dopamine administration could confound the interpretation of the results. Such a possibility did not pertain to this study, however, because dopamine was administered in

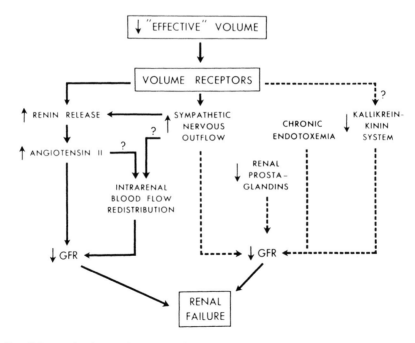

FIGURE 3.5. Possible mechanisms whereby a diminished effective volume might modulate a number of hormonal effectors, eventuating in renal failure. The *heavy arrows* indicate pathways for which evidence is available. The *dashed lines* represent proposed pathways, the existence of which remains to be established. (Modified from Epstein M: Hepatorenal syndrome. In Berk JE (ed): Bockus Gastroenterology, 4th ed. Philadelphia: W.B. Saunders, 1985, pp 3138–3149.)

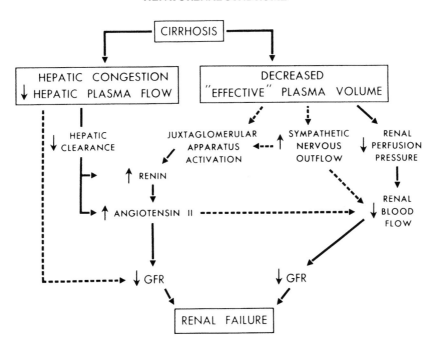

FIGURE 3.6. Probable mechanisms whereby the renin-angiotensin system and the sympathetic nervous system interact to produce renal failure. Both a diminished effective volume and impaired hepatic clearance of renin-angiotensin result in a marked enhancement of circulating plasma renin activity with a resultant decrease in glomerular filtration rate (GFR). An increase in sympathetic nervous system activity (possibly attributable to effective volume) decreases GFR both by diminishing renal perfusion and by activating the renin-angiotensin system.

subpressor doses and the changes in cardiac output were slight and inconsistent. Furthermore, it had been shown previously that dopamine given intravenously to normal subjects or directly into the renal artery of normal dogs does not reduce PRA.[54] It is therefore unlikely that dopamine reduced renin secretion by directly affecting the juxtaglomerular apparatus. Rather, the ability of dopamine to reduce PRA is most probably attributable to its ability to increase primarily renal plasma flow. The authors interpreted their findings as indicating that the increased PRA of cirrhosis is secondary to impaired renal perfusion rather than its cause.[54]

Regardless of mechanism(s), the activation of the renin-angiotensin system has profound implications for renal function (Fig. 3.6). In light of compelling experimental evidence that angiotensin plays an important role in the control of the renal circulation,[56,57] it is tempting to speculate that enhanced angiotensin levels contribute to the renal vasoconstriction and reduction in filtration rate associated with renal failure in cirrhosis. Observations by Cade et al.[50] underscored the role of angiotensin II in mediating the reduction in

renal perfusion and GFR in patients with HRS. The infusion of angiotensin II caused a marked reduction of renal plasma flow and GFR, with a marked increase in filtration fraction.

In addition to activation of the renin-angiotensin system, attention has focused on the possibility that the depletion of renin substrate may be the principal etiologic factor for the hemodynamic abnormalities that accompany HRS.[58,59] Iwatsuki et al.[14] demonstrated that renin substrate levels rose significantly after hepatic transplantation and preceded the improvement in renal function by several days. Subsequently, Berkowitz et al.[59] infused renin substrate-rich fresh frozen plasma into 2 patients with HRS and noted a prompt increase in creatinine clearance and urine output coincident with a significant rise in renin substrate and in suppression of peripheral renin concentration.[60] After termination of the infusion, both urine flow and creatinine clearance decreased progressively over the next 5 days as renin substrate concentrations declined toward preinfusion levels.

Cade et al.[50] have extended these observations. They administered either 750 ml of stored plasma or 750 ml of fresh frozen plasma in random order on successive days. The infusion of fresh frozen plasma improved function more than did stored plasma and in addition returned a very low filtration fraction toward normal. Plasma renin substrate concentration was uniformly low and was increased by an infusion of fresh frozen plasma. Arterial blood pressure, initially low, was improved by the infusion of stored plasma but increased far more when fresh frozen plasma was infused. The low filtration fraction observed in all patients was depressed even more by expansion with stored plasma but returned toward normal when fresh frozen plasma was infused.[50] Additional studies are needed to establish the significance of these provocative observations.

The availability of pharmacologic agents that interrupt the renin-angiotensin axis has suggested a possible approach for defining further the role of angiotensin as a determinant of the state of the renal vasculature.[61] Unfortunately, attempts to block the renin-angiotensin system in cirrhotic humans have been complicated by a striking fall in blood pressure and by the intrinsic activity of the partial agonists in use, which may have blunted the influence on GFR.[62,63] The synthesis of more specific angiotensin antagonists that act preferentially at the level of the renal vascular bed without inducing concomitant hypotension may contribute to further characterization of the pathogenesis of HRS (see chapter 12).[61]

Renal Prostaglandins

Alterations of renal prostaglandins also participate in mediating the renal failure of cirrhosis. Attempts to investigate the role of renal prostaglandins in modulating renal hemodynamics and mediating the sodium retention in cirrhosis have encompassed two manipulations: (1) the administration of exogenous prostaglandins and (2) the alteration of the endogenous production of prostaglandins by inhibition of prostaglandin synthesis. Initially, the problem was approached by examining the renal hemodynamic response to administration of exogenous prostaglandins.[64] Unfortunately, the relevance of such studies in cirrhotic humans is tenuous because any action of prostaglandins on the kidney must be as a local tissue hormone.[65,66] Thus, any evaluation of the physiologic role of prostaglandins in renal function necessitates an experimental design in which endogenous production of the lipids is altered.

Several investigators have demonstrated that administration of inhibitors of prostaglandin synthetase (both indomethacin and ibuprofen) resulted in significant decrements in GFR and effective renal plasma flow (ERPF) in patients with alcoholic liver disease and ascites.[67,68] Of interest, the decrement in renal hemodynamics varied directly with the degree of sodium retention, i.e., the patients with the most avid sodium retention manifested the largest decrements in GFR.[68–70]

Because the above studies examined the effect of inhibiting the endogenous production of renal prostaglandins, it was of great interest to assess an opposite experimental manipulation—the effects on renal function of augmentation of endogenous prostaglandins. Epstein and associates[71] used water immersion to the neck, an experimental maneuver that redistributes blood volume, with concomitant central hypervolemia, and enhances prostaglandin E (PGE) excretion in normal humans. They demonstrated that decompensated cirrhotic patients manifested an increase in mean PGE excretion that was three-fold greater than that observed in normal subjects under identical conditions.[72] This was attended by a marked natriuresis and an increase in creatinine clearance. When interpreted in concert with the earlier studies using prostaglandin synthetase inhibitors, such findings suggest that derangements in renal PGE production contribute to the renal dysfunction of cirrhosis. Specifically, it is tempting to postulate that, in the setting of cirrhosis of the liver, the ability to enhance prostaglandin synthesis constitutes a compensatory or adaptive response to incipient renal ischemia. The corollary of this formulation is that the administration of agents that impair such an adaptation may induce a clinically important deterioration of renal function.

The above findings are not isolated observations. One may conceive of renal prostaglandins as constituting critical modulators of renal function during conditions or disease states involving volume contraction.[70] The findings that synthetase inhibition affected renal function only in decompensated patients (with ascites and/or edema) and not in compensated cirrhotic patients and that the effects of synthetase inhibition vary as a function of the degree of renal sodium avidity are consistent with this formulation.[69,70]

Additional studies have suggested that alterations of thromboxanes may contribute to the renal dysfunction. Thromboxane A_2 (TxA_2), a potent proaggregatory and vasoconstrictor substance, is synthesized by platelets and a large number of other cell types and tissues, including the kidney.[73,74] Renal TxA_2 production is thought to be involved in the regulation of glomerular hemodynamics by acting on glomerular capillary filtration surface area[73,74] and by modulating the tone of afferent and efferent arterioles.[74] It has been proposed that the ratio of the vasodilator PGE_2 to the vasoconstrictor TxA_2 (i.e., PGE_2/TxA_2, rather than absolute levels of PGE_2) may determine the degree of renal vasoconstriction of HRS. Zipser et al.[75] determined the urinary excretion of PGE_2 and TxB_2 (the nonenzymatic metabolite of TxA_2) in 14 patients with HRS. They observed that, whereas PGE_2 levels were decreased in comparison with healthy controls as well as patients with acute renal failure, TxB_2 levels were markedly elevated. The authors concluded that an imbalance of vasodilator and vasoconstrictor metabolites of arachidonic acid contribute to the pathogenesis of HRS.

The findings of an increase in TxB_2 by other researchers are somewhat different. Rimola et al.[76] studied 18 normal subjects, 49 cirrhotic patients with ascites (but without renal failure), and 20 patients with HRS. Cirrhotic patients without HRS had a significantly higher urinary excretion of 6-keto-$PGF_{1\alpha}$, TxB_2, and PGE than did normal subjects. In contrast to the findings of Zipser et al.,[75] patients with HRS failed to manifest increases in urinary PGE_2, 6-keto-PGF_{1a}, and TxB_2. Rimola et al.[76] speculated that the discrepancy between their findings and those of Zipser et al.[75] may be attributable to differences in the patient population. Thus, Rimola et al.[76] studied patients with moderate impairment of hepatic and renal function, whereas the patients in the studies of Zipser et al.[75] had hepatic failure and severe renal insufficiency. Additional studies are required to assess alterations in the differing eicosanoids with progressive renal functional impairment (see chapter 14).

Because such findings suggest that thromboxanes may contribute to the development of HRS, attempts have been made to modify the course of HRS by the administration of selective inhibitors of thromboxane synthesis and thromboxane receptor antagonists.[77–79] Such interventions either have been negative or have failed to augment GFR substantively. Additional studies with thromboxane receptor antagonists in patients with widely varying degrees of acute renal insufficiency are required to define further the role of TxA_2 as a major determinant of the renal vasoconstriction in HRS (see chapter 14).

Kallikrein-Kinin System

The possibility that the kallikrein-kinin system may contribute to the pathogenesis of renal failure of liver disease is raised by several preliminary reports of abnormalities of the plasma kallikrein system.[80] Since bradykinin has been suggested to be a physiologic renal vasodilator,[81] it is possible that failure of bradykinin formation may contribute to the renal cortical vasoconstriction in patients with decompensated cirrhosis. The data so far are sparse but provocative.

Studies of the renal kallikrein-kinin system in cirrhosis have been few, and the results have been contradictory. Greco et al.[82] found increased levels of urinary kallikrein in nonazotemic cirrhotic patients with and without ascites. On the contrary, Zipser et al.[83] reported low urinary kallikrein in such patients. More recently, Pérez-Ayuso et al.[84] reported that urinary kallikrein activity is increased in cirrhotic patients with ascites but without renal failure; renal plasma flow and glomerular filtration rate correlated with urinary kallikrein activity. Based on such findings, the authors suggested that the renal kallikrein-kinin system is involved in the maintenance of renal hemodynamics in cirrhosis.

The interpretation of the above results is confounded by methodological and conceptual issues with respect to urinary kallikrein.[81,85] In most published investigations, the activity of the renal kallikrein-kinin system is inferred from the measurement of urinary kallikrein. At present, however, there is no clear proof that urinary kallikrein parallels the intrarenal generation of kinins.[85] Finally, the above studies use differing assays (i.e., kininogenase assay, steriolitic assay, and assay of kallikrein's amidolytic effect on synthetic substrate) that measure only active kallikrein but not the absolute amount of kallikrein in urine. Since approximately 50% of urinary kallikrein is in inactive form in humans, such indices may be misleading. Moreover, urine normally contains kallikrein inhibitors that may interfere with indirect techniques of measuring kallikrein.[85] Therefore, the different kallikrein activity observed in normal subjects and cirrhotic patients with and without renal failure may be related to differences in the amount of kallikrein inhibitors or in the proportion between active and inactive kallikrein in the urine.

Increase in Sympathetic Nervous System Activity

An increase in sympathetic nervous system activity also contributes to the renal failure of cirrhosis. It is now well established that alterations in the input of cardiopulmonary receptors induce changes in renal sympathetic activity.[86-89] Thus, a decrease in effective blood volume is sensed as a decrease in left atrial pressure (the sensor of the low pressure vascular system). This "unloads" the left atrial mechanoreceptors, which in turn discharge into afferent vagal fibers that have appropriate central nervous system representation.

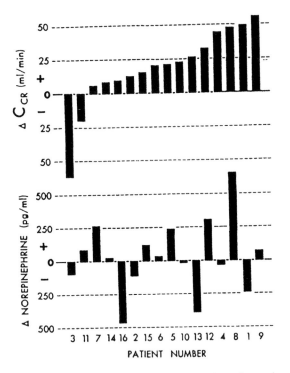

FIGURE 3.7. Relationship of alterations in Δcreatinine clearance (C_{Cr}) *(upper panel)* to alterations in plasma norepinephrine (NE) *(lower panel)* during immersion in 16 cirrhotic patients. The numbers along the *horizontal axis* designate the individual patients. As can be seen, the magnitude of the increase in C_{Cr} as assessed by ΔCr (mean of 2 highest values minus prestudy C_{Cr}) varied independently of NE (nadir minus prestudy NE) during immersion (r = 0.178; p > 0.5). (Reproduced with permission from Epstein M, et al: Effects of water immersion or plasma catecholamines in decompensated cirrhosis. Implications for deranged sodium and water homeostasis. Miner Electrolyte Metab 1985;11:25–34.)

As a consequence, efferent renal sympathetic nerve activity (ERSNA) is augmented.[87,88] Such an increase in sympathetic tone tends to produce renal vasoconstriction and to decrease GFR.

Although such theoretical considerations suggest a role for the sympathetic nervous system in the renal vasoconstriction and sodium retention of cirrhosis, only recently has this possibility been tested. Studies to assess the activity of the sympathetic nervous system in cirrhotic humans have measured plasma catecholamine levels during basal conditions and after postural manipulations.[88,90-94] Most observers agree that mean peripheral norepinephrine levels are elevated in cirrhotic patients (Fig. 3.7).[91-94] Ring-Larsen et al.[91] have determined plasma norepinephrine (NE) and epinephrine concentrations in differing vascular beds of cirrhotic patients at the time of hepatic venous catheterization. On the basis of differences in regional norepinephrine levels, they concluded that the elevated norepinephrine levels in patients with cirrhosis were attributable to enhanced sympathetic nervous system activity rather than to decreased metabolism.

As detailed in several recent reviews,[95-97] however, plasma concentrations of norepinephrine are an inadequate guide to either total or regional sympathetic activity. Global measures of sympathetic activity, such as plasma norepinephrine, fail to identify sources of norepinephrine release and cannot delineate regional patterns of sympathetic nervous activation. Recently, Esler et al.[97] conducted a physiologic and neurochemical evaluation of patients with cirrhosis by using tracer kinetic techniques with radiolabeled norepinephrine, which allow a more precise description of the regional pattern of the sympathetic nervous derangement in cirrhosis. The authors demonstrated that the elevated plasma norepinephrine concentration in patients with cirrhosis is attributable to higher overall rates of spillover of the neurotransmitter to plasma and not to reduced plasma clearance caused by liver disease. The administration of clonidine reduced previously elevated norepinephrine overflow rates for the whole body, kidneys, and hepatomesenteric circulation. This sympathetic inhibition was accompanied by several potentially beneficial effects: lowering of renal vascular resistance, augmentation of GFR, and reduction of portal venous pressure.[97]

In summary, the available data indicate that the sympathetic nervous system is activated in cirrhosis, both in the kidney and in other regional vascular beds and thus contributes substantively to the renal vasoconstriction and dysfunction of cirrhosis (see chapter 19).

Endotoxins

Systemic endotoxemia may participate in the pathogenesis of the renal failure of cirrhosis. Endotoxins, the lipopolysaccharide constituents of the cell wall of certain bacteria, are potent renal vasoconstrictors.[98,99] It has been hypothesized that enteric endotoxin is liberated into the systemic circulation through naturally or surgically created portosystemic shunts, thus bypassing the hepatic Kupffer cells, the major site of endotoxin removal. Recent studies that measured endotoxin by the limulus lysate technique have reported that endotoxin is present in the portal and systemic circulation of many cirrhotic patients, particularly those with ascites. Because several investigators have demonstrated a high frequency of positive limulus assays in cirrhotic patients with renal failure but not in those without renal failure, endotoxins may contribute to the pathogenesis of renal failure. Endotoxemia is appealing as a possible humoral agent not only because it may cause renal vasoconstriction, but also because it may produce vasodilatation in other circulatory beds and may be a treatable condition.[98,99] Indeed, Vallance and Moncada[37] have proposed that endotoxemia induces nitric oxide synthase in peripheral blood vessels with resultant vasodilation (vide infra). In vivo studies in dogs and rats have demonstrated that the vasodilation and decreased vascular responsiveness that occur in response to endotoxin or cytokines are mediated by NO synthesis.[100,101] Furthermore, the induction of NO synthase with increased production of NO also may explain the peripheral vasodilation in response to endotoxin infusion in humans[102] or in patients with septic shock.[103]

Although endotoxemia is frequently observed in patients with chronic liver disease, its role in contributing to the development of renal failure is unclear. Attempts to correlate the occurrence of renal failure with the presence of endotoxemia are conflicting. On the one hand, Clemente et al.[104] observed endotoxemia in 9 of 22 patients with HRS, but not in cirrhotic patients with a normal GFR. On the other hand, Gatta et al.[105] demonstrated that in patients with cirrhosis without overt renal failure, renal vasoconstriction did not seem to be related to endotoxemia. Coratelli et al.[106] have observed two patients before and

after the development of HRS and demonstrated the appearance of endotoxemia coincident with the development of HRS.

Despite the ostensible appeal of this hypothesis, much additional study is required for its confirmation. As pointed out in several reviews,[98,99] the limulus tests for endotoxin have variations, and their individual accuracy is controversial. A correlation with renal failure in cirrhosis may reflect the retention of endotoxins rather than a causal relationship of endotoxins to HRS.[99]

Nitric Oxide

More recent investigations of pathogenesis have focused on the florid systemic hemodynamic disturbances that invariably accompany HRS, including hyperdynamic circulation, increased heart rate and cardiac output, and decreased blood pressure and systemic vascular resistance.[4,25–28] Such observations suggest the likelihood of excessive production of a vasodilator.[107] A number of vasodilators have been postulated, including prostacyclin, bradykinin, substance P, and atrial natriuretic peptide (ANP), but clear evidence is lacking.[107]

Recent attention has focused on the role of nitric oxide as a mediator of both the hyperdynamic circulation and renal failure.[37] Nitric oxide, a vasodilator synthesized from L-arginine, accounts for the biologic activity of endothelium-derived relaxing factor.[108–110] In animals, the agonist-induced release of nitric oxide from the vascular endothelium leads to peripheral vasodilation, fall in blood pressure, and tachycardia.[111,112] These effects are short-lived, however, and vascular tone returns to normal once the agonist infusion is stopped. On the other hand, a second, distinct, inducible nitric oxide synthase occurs in response to bacterial lipopolysaccharide endotoxin.[113] Once induced, this enzyme releases nitric oxide for many hours without the need for further stimulation (see chapter 17).

The in vitro incubation of vascular rings with endotoxin or cytokines leads to the induction of nitric oxide synthase in both the endothelium and the smooth muscle and to progressive vascular relaxation with diminished responsiveness to vasoconstrictors.[114,115] When induced by endotoxin, these effects can be prevented by cycloheximide (an inhibitor of protein synthesis), polymyxin B (an antagonist of endotoxin), and NG-monomethyl-L-arginine (an inhibitor of nitric oxide synthase).[113,114] Once nitric oxide synthase is induced and the vascular rings are relaxed, however, only NG-monomethyl-L-arginine will reverse the changes.[114] On the basis of these considerations, Vallance and Moncada[37] postulated that endotoxemia induces a nitric oxide synthase in peripheral blood vessels and that this increased nitric oxide synthesis and release accounts for the associated hyperdynamic circulation. This theory does not posit that renal vasoconstriction is directly related to NO but rather suggests that renal hypoperfusion and insufficiency are secondary to a diversion of blood away from the kidney. If this hypothesis is correct, the inhibition of nitric oxide synthesis should restore sensitivity to vasoconstrictors and reverse the hemodynamic abnormalities. Specific inhibitors of either the constitutive or the inducible nitric oxide synthase theoretically should facilitate a more precise manipulation of nitric oxide synthesis and help to establish the pathophysiologic importance of nitric oxide in endotoxemia and cirrhosis.

In a recent preliminary communication, the investigators reported that serum nitrite and nitrate levels, an index of nitric oxide production, were elevated in a group of cirrhotic patients.[116] Patients with ascites manifested higher nitrite and nitrate levels than cirrhotic patients without ascites. Furthermore, there was a direct correlation between serum nitrite and nitrate levels and endotoxemia. Additional studies are required to substantiate this hypothesis.

Endothelin

In the past 15 years endothelins (ET) have emerged as an important new peptide family in the hormonal regulation of body fluid and cardiovascular homeostasis.[117,118] ETs are the most potent vasoconstrictors known to date. They release Ca^{2+} and also potentiate Ca^{2+} release stimulated by other vasoconstrictors, including AVP and angiotensin II. Increasing evidence suggests that ET plays a role in the pathogenesis of diverse disorders, contributing to hypertensive disease and mediating renal injury via its vascular effects— i.e., in acute renal failure due to cyclosporine, contrast media, or endotoxemia as well as in chronic forms of renal impairment.[119,119a]

Rabelink et al.[120,121] recently demonstrated that exogenous infusion of endothelin-1 in normal human volunteers induced a major increase in renal vascular resistance. Such findings suggest an important role for endothelin in human renal pathophysiology.

Uchihara et al.[122] investigated changes in plasma endothelin concentration in patients with chronic liver disease of differing etiologies. Plasma endothelin concentrations were more than two-fold higher in patients with cirrhosis and ascites than in normal controls. In contrast, endothelin levels in cirrhotic patients without ascites and in patients with chronic hepatitis did not differ from those in normal controls. Furthermore, plasma endothelin levels were two-fold higher in patients with endotoxemia than in those without endotoxemia. Because endotoxin has been reported to stimulate endothelin synthesis,[123] the investigators speculated that endotoxin may be responsible for the elevated plasma endothelin concentrations with consequent renal dysfunction.

Uemasu et al.[124] also demonstrated increased plasma endothelin levels in patients with cirrhosis. Of interest, they observed that both patients with and without ascites had elevated levels of endothelin. Endothelin levels were two-fold higher in compensated cirrhotic patients than in controls. The compensated cirrhotic patients tended to have a further elevation, although the differences did not attain statistical significance.

Recently, Moore et al.[125] suggested the possibility that alterations in endothelin may play a pathogenetic role in the renal failure of the hepatorenal syndrome. They reported that patients with hepatorenal syndrome had markedly elevated plasma endothelin-1 and endothelin-3 concentrations compared with normal subjects, patients with acute or chronic renal failure, and patients with liver disease without renal dysfunction. The investigators concluded that ETs play a role in the pathogenesis of HRS.

Moller et al.[126] confirmed and extended earlier observations. They characterized concentrations of ET-1 in various vascular beds, including the hepatic artery/vein, the right renal artery/vein, and the right femoral artery/vein, and related the findings to clinical status and hemodynamic alterations. Median brachial venous ET-1 concentrations were more than two-fold higher in patients with cirrhosis than in controls. In patients with cirrhosis, ET-1 was directly correlated to serum creatinine.

As noted in a recent editorial, it is equally possible if not probable that the results merely represent pari passu events.[127] Thus, elevated plasma endothelin concentrations might be attributable to decreased renal disposal of endothelin.The recent availability of several chemically diverse endothelin antagonists, including agents that block the generation of endothelin and agents that antagonize its binding to cellular receptors, provides an opportunity for using such pharmacologic probes in delineating the pathogenetic role of endothelin.

Biologically Active Atrial Peptides

Another hormone that should be included in any consideration of the pathogenetic mechanisms of HRS is atrial natriuretic factor (ANF) or atriopeptin. Since the demonstration by DeBold et al.[128] in 1981 that saline extracts of rat heart atria (but not ventricles) caused a marked natriuresis and diuresis when injected into normal rats, there has been much interest in the role of ANF as a mediator of volume homeostasis.[129] Micropuncture studies in rats have shown that ANF, given by either bolus injection or continuous infusion, causes a significant increase in GFR[130,131] as well as natriuresis and diuresis.[132]

Because ANF has thus been shown to be of importance in volume homeostasis and because volume homeostasis is of critical importance in patients with cirrhosis and portal hypertension, a number of investigators have sought a role for ANF in severe hepatic disease.

Despite proposals that ANF deficiency may contribute to the renal dysfunction of liver disease, the available data fail to support this formulation. Most investigators have found ANF levels in plasma to be either normal[133,134] or increased[135,136] in cirrhotic patients with ascites. Morgan et al.[137] compared circulating ANF levels in 7 patients with hepatorenal syndrome and 7 patients with advanced alcoholic liver disease and ascites but normal serum creatinine levels. They demonstrated that ANF levels were two-fold higher in the patients with hepatorenal syndrome, indicating that a deficiency of ANF does not contribute to the renal failure (see chapter 15).

Adenosine

Adenosine, an endogenous nucleoside derived mainly from the intracellular catabolism of ATP, also may contribute to the development of HRS. Although adenosine is a vasodilator in most vascular territories, in the kidney it induces marked vasoconstriction and reduces GFR by increasing the responsiveness of afferent arterioles to angiotensin II.[138–141] That adenosine may play a pathogenic role is underscored by the realization that the intrarenal synthesis and tissue levels of adenosine increase in settings of enhanced oxygen demand (e.g., increased sodium reabsorption) or of reduced supply (e.g., renal hypoperfusion)[138]; both circumstances are common in patients with advanced cirrhosis.

To assess this possibility, Llach et al.[142] investigated the sensitivity of the renal circulation to endogenous adenosine in cirrhotic patients with normal GFR and different degrees of sodium retention. Renal function and vasoactive hormone levels were evaluated before and after administration of dipyridamole, a drug that blocks the cellular uptake of adenosine, resulting in an increase in extracellular levels. The authors demonstrated that in patients with ascites and increased PRA, dipyridamole induced marked reductions in renal plasma flow, GFR, urine volume, free water clearance and sodium excretion (in the absence of changes in arterial pressure), PRA and aldosterone levels, norepinephrine and antidiuretic hormone. In patients without ascites and in patients with ascites and normal PRA, renal plasma flow and GFR did not change significantly after dipyridamole administration, whereas excretion of sodium and free water was reduced. The authors concluded that in cirrhotic patients with ascites and overactivity of the renin-angiotensin system, dipyridamole induces renal vasoconstriction in the absence of changes in systemic hemodynamics, suggesting that such patients are particularly sensitive to the renal vasoconstrictor effect of endogenous adenosine.

Insulin-like Growth Factor-1

Insulinlike growth factor-1 (IGF-1) is a single-chain polypeptide that is 70 aminoacids in length. More than 90% of the total circulating IGF-1 is synthesized and secreted by the liver under the control of growth hormone.[143] During physiologic conditions almost all circulating IGF-1 is associated with several specific, high-affinity binding proteins of hepatic origin (IGFBP) that influence the access of IGF-1 to the tissues.[143] Administration of IGF-1 to rats and humans increases glomerular filtration rate and renal plasma flow.[144,145]

Several reports have suggested that hepatic synthesis and secretion of IGF-1 is diminished in patients with liver cirrhosis.[146,147] In addition, alterations in the different forms of circulating IGFBP have been described recently in patients with different forms of chronic liver disease.[148] Whether IGF-1 influences renal function in patients with liver cirrhosis has not been established. It has been postulated, however, that renal function in patients with liver disease might be influenced by the tissue availability of IGF-1 and that the development of HRS in cirrhotic patients may be attributable in part to a reduction in the kidney availability of this hormone.

Calcitonin Gene-Related Peptide

Recently it has been suggested that calcitonin gene-related peptide (CGRP) may constitute a possible mediator of the peripheral vasodilatation of the hepatorenal syndrome.[149] CGRP, which contains 37 amino acid residues, is produced by alternative processing of the primary calcitonin gene transcript.[150] Its extensive distribution in neural, vascular and endocrine systems as well as within the circulation suggests that CGRP is physiologically active in hemodynamic regulation.[150,151] It has pronounced effects on vascular smooth muscle and appears to be the most potent vasodilator known.[152]

Recently, Gupta et al.[149] determined plasma CGRP levels in 8 patients with alcoholic cirrhosis and hepatorenal syndrome, 7 patients with alcoholic cirrhosis and ascites without hepatorenal syndrome, and 10 healthy controls. Plasma CGRP levels were higher in patients with alcoholic cirrhosis and hepatorenal syndrome than in healthy controls. Patients with cirrhosis and ascites but without hepatorenal syndrome tended to have elevated CGRP levels, although the levels did not differ significantly from normal controls.

Although Gupta et al.[149] speculated that CGRP may contribute to the hemodynamic derangements, their study involves three major problems: (1) relatively few patients were studied; (2) the authors did not ascertain whether CGRP was elevated simply because of impaired hepatic clearance in diseased livers; and (3) it is difficult to reconcile this postulate with the observation that CGRP dilates norepinephrine-constricted afferent glomerular arterioles in a dose-dependent manner and increases renal blood flow.[153,154]

Platelet-activating Factor

Over the past two decades, an increasing body of evidence has accrued regarding a new lipid mediator, usually termed platelet-activating factor (PAF). This mediator, characterized as 1-alkyl-2-acetyl-*sn*-glycero-3-phosphocholine,[155] has been identified in urine,[156] amniotic fluid,[157] saliva,[158] and blood (after specific experimental interventions, such as the venous effluent after removal of a constriction of the renal artery[159]).

PAF exhibits an impressive spectrum of biologic activities. In addition to platelet activation, it stimulates polymorphonuclears, contracts smooth muscle from ileum and pulmonary strips,[160] and induces hypotension and massive permeability when infused intravenously into rats.[161] These effects suggest that alterations of PAF may contribute to the pathogenesis of the deranged systemic hemodynamics and renal failure of HRS.

Caramelo et al.[162] determined the levels of platelet-activating factor in blood and ascitic fluid from cirrhotic patients and in blood from a group of controls, using a recently described technique for extraction and measurement. They reported increased concentrations in the blood and ascitic fluid of cirrhotic patients, with the highest concentrations in patients with decompensated cirrhosis. The demonstration that BN 52021, a specific antagonist of PAF, reversed the low peripheral vascular resistance in rats with experimental cirrhosis of the liver raises the possibility that PAF may mediate some of these hemodynamic derangements.[163] Additional studies are necessary to assess the possible role of PAF in the pathogenesis of some of the clinical manifestations of hepatic cirrhosis.

Glomerulopressin

A decade ago, Alvestrand and Bergstrom[164] proposed an intriguing hypothesis to explain the pathophysiology of HRS. They suggested that in normal individuals, the liver produces a hormone (termed glomerulopressin or GP) that is involved in the normal regulation of GFR. The investigators speculated that hepatic failure might result in decreased synthesis of all proteins, including GP. This would eventuate in the relatively unopposed action of vasoconstrictor substances, including angiotensin II, NE, and vasoactive amines, a resultant decrease in GFR, and development of HRS. Unfortunately, no published studies in the subsequent decade have substantiated this hypothesis.

ACUTE RENAL FAILURE

Although much attention has been directed to HRS, cirrhotic patients are as vulnerable as non-cirrhotic patients to the development of acute renal failure due to acute tubular necrosis (ATN). Among patients with liver disease who developed renal failure, the etiology of renal failure is more commonly ATN than HRS.[1-4] The increased frequency of ATN may relate to the hypotension, bleeding dyscrasias, infection, and multiple metabolic disorders that complicate the clinical course of such patients.

As mentioned earlier in this chapter, several investigators have proposed that jaundice may play an important role in mediating the renal failure. Over 30 years ago, Dawson[38] postulated that conjugated hyperbilirubinemia sensitizes the kidneys to anoxic damage. Several reports indicate a strong association between postsurgical renal failure and obstructive jaundice. Acute renal failure occurs in approximately 8–10% of patients requiring surgery for relief of obstructive jaundice and contributes to eventual mortality in 70–80% of patients who develop it. Despite advances in perioperative care, the figures have changed little over the past 25 years.[165] The incidence of postoperative acute renal failure in patients with obstructive jaundice seems to be directly related to the degree of jaundice. A large series of 2,358 biliary tract operations performed on nonjaundiced patients[166] reported only 3 deaths from renal failure. All deaths were in patients with preexisting renal disease. In another series the incidence of postoperative renal failure was 6.8% in 103 jaundiced patients contrasted with an incidence of renal failure of only 0.1% in 2,353 emergency partial gastrectomies for perforated peptic ulcer. This low incidence of postoperative renal failure in nonjaundiced patients occurred despite the fact that many patients were in shock before resuscitation and despite the greater extent of surgery compared with biliary surgery on the jaundiced patients.[167] The close link between high bilirubin levels and postsurgical renal failure has been substantiated by other investigators.[168]

In a recent review, Green and Better[45] considered the growing body of evidence indicating that bile constituents (e.g., bile acids, bilirubin, cholesterol) do not exert a direct nephrotoxic effect. Rather they proposed that retention of bile during cholestatic jaundice has deleterious effects on cardiovascular function and blood volume. This, in turn, sensitizes the kidney to prerenal failure and acute tubular necrosis in postsurgical patients with obstructive jaundice. Consequently, institution of prophylactic measures, including maintenance of adequate extracellular fluid volume and avoidance of NSAIDs, may improve the overall prognosis of jaundiced patients undergoing surgery. Finally, it has been postulated that endotoxemia caused by the absence of bile salts in the intestine is at least partially responsible for the high incidence of renal failure and mortality associated with obstructive jaundice. Several reports showing that preoperative administration of sodium deoxycholate to jaundiced patients prevents systemic and portal endotoxemia as well as postoperative renal dysfunction are consistent with this theory.[169,170] At present, the use of one or more antiendotoxin therapeutic measures (biliary drainage, bile acids, antibiotics, lactulose) remains an unresolved issue and awaits further confirmation by well-designed, controlled studies.[171,172]

There have been several attempts to develop diagnostic tests to discriminate reliably between acute renal failure and HRS.[173-179] To date, such tests, which rely on enzymuria or electrolyte excretory patterns, are often suggestive but lack sufficient selectivity to be reliable (see below).

HEPATORENAL SYNDROME VS. ACUTE TUBULAR NECROSIS: DIFFERENT DISEASES OR A CONTINUUM?

Renal function in HRS is fundamentally different from that in ATN. In ATN, the reduction in GFR is generally much more severe, and the accompanying decrease in tubular reabsorption is generally regarded as evidence of intrinsic tubular dysfunction. In HRS, on the other hand, the reduction in GFR is usually not as severe, and the avid tubular reabsorption of sodium and water attests to normal intrinsic tubular function, which appears to be responding to extrinsic stimuli.

It is immediately evident to the experienced clinician that patients do not necessarily read textbooks. Often, the urinary indices are confusing and fall in the gray zone, which spans the different presentations of HRS and ATN (see below). Furthermore, patients with HRS often develop classic ATN as their condition deteriorates. Although rigorous data are lacking, I believe that HRS can evolve into ATN; in many cases, the natural history appears to be a continuum between the two. In terms of management, however, it is often confusing to be faced with a pattern of renal function that does not clearly fit into the categories outlined above. Under such circumstances, the only practical approach is to consider the patient as "prerenal"

TABLE 3.4. Differential Diagnosis of Acute Azotemia in Patients with Liver Disease

Biochemical Characteristics	Important Differential Urinary Findings		
	Prerenal Azotemia	Hepatorenal Syndrome	Acute Renal Failure (Acute Tubular Necrosis)
Urine sodium concentration (mEq/L)	< 10	< 10	> 30*
Urine to plasma creatinine ratio	< 30:1	> 30:1	< 20:1
Urine osmolality	At least 100 mOsm > plasma osmolality	At least 100 mOsm > plasma osmolality	Equal to plasma osmolality
Urine sediment	Normal	Unremarkable	Casts, cellular debris

* It has recently been appreciated that radiocontrast agents and sepsis may lower urinary sodium concentration in patients with acute tubular necrosis.

and to search diligently for reversible causes of prerenal azotemia.

Diagnostic Considerations

The abrupt onset of oliguria in a cirrhotic patient does not necessarily imply the presence of HRS. Prerenal causes are important to differentiate, particularly because they constitute reversible conditions if recognized and treated in the incipient phase. Volume contraction or cardiac pump failure may appear as a pseudohepatorenal syndrome. Furthermore, as already emphasized, it is not uncommon for patients with alcoholic cirrhosis to develop classic ATN. In many instances, the differentiation from HRS can be made readily by recognition of the precipitating event and by characteristic laboratory findings that are helpful in differentiating the three principal causes of acute azotemia in patients with liver disease (Table 3.4). The most uniform urinary finding in patients with HRS is a strikingly low sodium concentration, usually less than 10 mEq/L, and occasionally as low as 2–5 mEq/L. Unfortunately, prerenal azotemia is associated with similarly low urinary sodium concentrations. In contrast, patients with oliguric ATN frequently have urinary sodium concentrations exceeding 30 mEq/L and usually even higher.

Although avid renal sodium retention is evident in the majority of patients with HRS, in occasional patients with HRS the urinary sodium concentration [U_{Na}] is consistently greater than 10 mEq/L. In some of these patients, [U_{Na}] is initially low but increases to levels of approximately 40 mEq/L as renal impairment progresses; it has been suggested that the late increase in urinary sodium concentration may represent the possible transition to ATN. In other patients HRS has developed and progressed in the presence of a [U_{Na}] persistently in the range of 20–30 mEq/L.[1,4]

Dudley et al.[173] studied a small group of patients in the latter group. They found no increase in [U_{Na}] as the serum creatinine increased, suggesting that the high [U_{Na}] did not represent transition to ATN, and no histologic evidence of tubular necrosis or other forms of renal disease in the 3 patients on whom autopsies were performed.

A similar caveat applies to the test based on fractional excretion of filtered sodium (FE_{Na}).[174] In general, the FE_{Na} has been demonstrated to be a reliably discriminating test between prerenal azotemia and ATN. However, increasing clinical use has brought numerous recent reports of low FE_{Na} (less than 1%). The clinical settings of these reports include oliguric and nonoliguric ATN, urinary tract obstruction, acute glomerulonephritis, HRS, and sepsis.[174] Clearly, no single urinary index can be expected to discriminate reliably between prerenal azotemia and acute renal failure in all cases. The utility of the FE_{Na} test in the differential diagnosis of acute renal failure must be interpreted in conjunction with the patient's clinical course and additional urinary and serum tests.

Sherman and Eisinger[175] suggested that, in a substantial number of cases, the measurement of urinary sodium or chloride alone fails to detect renal salt retention. A disparity characterized by a urinary sodium concentration exceeding that of chloride may be associated with the necessity for urinary excretion of substantial quantities of poorly reabsorbed anions (penicillin, ketones, or diatrizoate), a rapidly falling serum bicarbonate level (due to resolving metabolic or developing respiratory alkalosis), or substantial renal insufficiency (serum creatinine greater than 3 mg/dl). In such instances, the [U_{Na}] is misleading as an index of the underlying sodium retentive state.

Based on their observations, the authors concluded that both urinary sodium and chloride should be determined for evidence of renal salt retention.

A confounding factor in the interpretation of urinary diagnostic indices is the prior administration of natriuretic agents, which tends to augment FE_{Na}. Recently Kaplan and Kohn[176] proposed that the fractional excretion of urea (FE_{Ur}) may serve as a useful guide for the clinical evaluation of renal hypoperfusion even when natriuretic agents have been administered. Under conditions of normal renal function and adequate hydration, the mean FE_{Ur} is between 50 and 65%. In contrast, azotemia associated with $FE_{Ur} \leq 35$ % suggests a component of diminished renal perfusion or possibly HRS.

Both HRS and prerenal azotemia manifest well-maintained urinary concentrating ability characterized by a urine-to-plasma osmolality ratio (U/P_{Osm}) exceeding 1.0, whereas patients with ATN excrete a relatively isoosmotic urine (i.e., neither concentrated nor dilute). The urine-to-plasma creatinine ratio is greater than 30:1 (and at times 40:1) in both prerenal failure and HRS, whereas the urine-to-plasma creatinine ratio is 20:1 or less in ATN. Proteinuria is absent or minimal in HRS.

Another clinical setting that may mimic HRS is myoglobinuric acute renal failure. In the setting of renal insufficiency, myoglobin is converted extensively to bilirubin.[177] Furthermore, myoglobinuric ATN is one of the settings of ATN associated with a low $[U_{Na}]$. Thus, the clinician may fall into the trap of falsely diagnosing myoglobinuric ATN as HRS.

In light of the dilemma surrounding attempts to differentiate ATN from HRS, the continuing efforts to find a marker that differentiates the two disorders are not surprising. One such substance might be β_2-microglobulin.[178] Although it has been suggested recently that the renal tubular handling of β_2-microglobulin is intact in patients with HRS and not in patients with acute renal failure of other etiologies,[178] this observation should be considered preliminary; additional experience is necessary to define the role of this test.

In contrast, Rector et al.[179] suggested that β_2-microglobulin excretion cannot be used to differentiate between patients with HRS and patients with acute tubular injury, such as that due to aminoglycosides. They demonstrated that urine β_2-microglobulin was significantly higher in patients with HRS than in control patients with normal serum creatinine concentrations. The degree of β_2-microglobulin elevation correlated directly with the serum bilirubin; the more deeply jaundiced the patient, the greater the probability of an elevated urinary β_2-microglobulin value.

In summary, the finding of a low urinary sodium concentration in the presence of oliguric acute renal failure usually precludes the diagnosis of ATN. Only when prerenal failure and ATN are excluded can one establish the diagnosis of HRS.

TREATMENT

The management of HRS has been discouraging; there is no reproducible effective treatment. Because knowledge about the pathogenesis of HRS is inferential and incomplete, therapy to the present time has been supportive (Table 3.5). Because iatrogenic events often precipitate HRS and because therapy is difficult once the syndrome is established, prevention constitutes the linchpin of management.

The initial step in the management of a cirrhotic patient with acutely reduced renal function is not to equate decreased renal function with HRS, but rather to search diligently for and treat

TABLE 3.5. Principles of Management of Patients with Hepatorenal Syndrome

1. General measures
   Try not to make the diagnosis
      Attempt to rule out other likely diagnoses
      - Acute renal failure
      - Prerenal azotemia
      - Use of central venous pressure or Swan-Ganz catheter
      - Volume challenge
   Primum non nocere
2. Specific therapeutic considerations
   General
      - Sodium and fluid restriction
      - Correct acid-base disturbances
      - Correct severe anemia
      - Treat encephalopathy
   Ascites reinfusion
   Infusion of vasodilators
      - Acetylcholine
      - Phentolamine
      - Prostaglandins A_1 and E
      - Dopamine
   Portacaval shunting
   Dialysis
   Continuous arteriovenous ultrafiltration (CAVU)
   LeVeen (peritoneovenous) shunting
   Hepatic transplantation

TABLE 3.6. Drugs and Procedures that
Adversely Affect Patients with Liver
Disease and Ascites

Drugs
  Nonsteroidal antiinflammatory drugs
  Demeclocycline
  Lactulose
Procedures
  Overly vigorous or inordinately rapid diuresis

correctable causes of azotemia, such as volume contraction, cardiac decompensation, and urinary tract obstruction. The diagnosis of ATN clearly should be considered because ATN occurs commonly in cirrhotic patients, who may be expected to recover if supported with dialytic therapy.

Although we commonly invoke the caveat of primum non nocere, it takes on greater meaning in the patient with HRS. As noted previously, nonsteroidal anti-inflammatory drugs, which inhibit prostaglandin synthetase activity, often adversely influence renal function in the patient with liver disease and ascites.[67,68,70] Similarly, the broad-spectrum antibiotic demeclocycline may induce acute azotemia in the patient with cirrhosis and ascites.[180,181] Finally, drugs that may be indicated for the management of complications of liver disease (i.e., lactulose for the treatment of hepatic encephalopathy) are capable of inducing profound hypovolemia (secondary to diarrhea) with resultant azotemia (Table 3.6).

β-Blockers have achieved widespread acceptance as effective agents in the prophylaxis of recurrent variceal bleeding.[182] Because propranolol reduces both renal plasma flow and GFR by 10–20% in patients with essential hypertension,[183,184] one might be concerned that β-blockers also contribute to renal functional impairment in cirrhosis. In other words, the administration of some β-blockers may increase the risk of ATN or HRS in patients with advanced liver disease. Recent information indicates, however, that in contrast to findings in patients with essential hypertension, β-blockers (at least nadolol and propranolol) do not appear to alter renal function in patients with cirrhosis. Thus, Bataille et al.[185] studied 13 patients with cirrhosis without overt ascites within 1 hour after the oral administration of 40 mg of propranolol and then 1 month later. Throughout this interval, the patients received propranolol in doses sufficient to decrease heart rate by 25% (the mean daily dose was 186 ± 106 mg). Despite a marked reduction in cardiac output and an increase in calculated systemic vascular resistance, both renal blood flow (measured by a thermodilution catheter advanced into the right renal vein) and renal vascular resistance were unaltered.[185] These findings suggest that β-blockers (at least propranolol) probably do not enhance the likelihood of renal failure in cirrhotic patients.

An additional consideration for prevention of acute renal failure relates to the synergism between gentamicin and endotoxin. Zager and Prior[186] demonstrated that gram-negative sepsis may enhance the nephrotoxicity of gentamicin.[186] This effect was shown to be mediated in part by endotoxin and in part by increased renal gentamicin uptake. Implicit in these findings is the notion that gram-negative bacteremia, a prime indication for gentamicin treatment, may dramatically predispose to the drug's nephrotoxic potential.

In excluding reversible prerenal azotemia, there are several management considerations (Fig. 3.8). Because HRS and prerenal azotemia have similar urinary diagnostic indices, one often must use a functional maneuver—e.g., the administration of volume expanders—to differentiate between the two entities. The frame of reference for cirrhotic patients may be quite different from that pertaining to other disease states. The degree of volume expansion necessary to replete the cirrhotic patient at times may be marked, occasionally requiring the infusion of massive amounts of colloid.

No defined regimen allows one to predict the amount of volume expanders necessary to replete the cirrhotic patient suspected of hypovolemia. I recommend infusion of expanders when alterations in clinical status (blood pressure, urine flow rate, creatinine clearance) and central hemodynamics (central venous pressure [CVP], data derived from Swan-Ganz catheter) are monitored. Furthermore, the change in CVP often is more important than the absolute level; for example, although a CVP reading may not be extremely low, it may not increase until large amounts of expanders are administered. Such guidelines do not presuppose a correlation between central hemodynamics and volume deficit. Rather, manometric determinations are used as a guideline to assist in assessing when to discontinue volume expansion to avoid overt fluid overload. Of note, volume expansion carries the risk of opening up fragile esophageal varices with secondary bleeding, although in my experience this complication is infrequent.

Many patients with HRS manifest myocardial dysfunction. Although the pathogenesis and characteristics of this complication are considered elsewhere,[187,188] a few comments about the management of cardiac dysfunction are warranted. Studies by Gould et al.[187] and Limas et al.[188] suggest that some patients with cirrhosis have latent congestive heart failure that may be ameliorated by the decrease in afterload due to peripheral vasodilation. On the other hand, at least theoretically, correction of hypotension with vasopressors, thereby increasing the afterload of the heart, may precipitate pulmonary edema in patients with cirrhosis.[188] Similarly, the infusion of colloid solutions, which increases CVP, also may precipitate pulmonary edema, if the patient is not monitored and if excessive volume is administered.

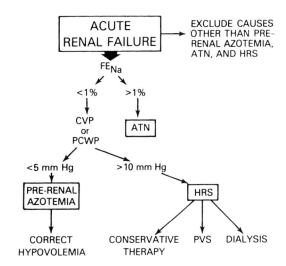

FIGURE 3.8. Algorithm for the evaluation and management of a cirrhotic patient with acute renal failure.

Basic Management

Once correctable causes of renal functional impairment are excluded, the mainstay of therapy for HRS is to prevent clinical deterioration by careful restriction of sodium and fluid intake. A number of specific therapeutic measures have been attempted, but only a few have proved to be of practical value. Attempts at volume expansion with different agents have resulted in only transient improvement in renal hemodynamics without significant alteration of outcome. Similarly, attempts at reinfusion of concentrated ascitic fluid have provided no lasting improvement. Below are the major new approaches that have attracted investigative attention and may warrant future considerations.

Paracentesis

The role of paracentesis in the treatment of HRS, with or without simultaneous plasma volume expansion, has not been established. The potential renal benefit of reduction of ascitic fluid volume includes diminished intraabdominal pressure with possible relief of inferior vena caval obstruction and augmentation of cardiac output. Improvement in renal function, when it occurs, is transient, because the abnormal hydraulic pressures that sustain ascites formation are not altered by paracentesis. Continued fluid removal is necessary and may result in progressive depletion of intravascular volume with subsequent deterioration in cardiac function and renal perfusion.

Nevertheless, over the past several years, the Barcelona group has marshaled evidence that paracentesis may induce a more favorable renal excretory and hormonal response than was previously thought.[189–191]

Dialysis

Dialysis was previously reported to be ineffective in the management of HRS.[192,193] Our recent experience, however, suggests that such a sweeping condemnation should be qualified (see chapter 26). Although most of the literature indeed suggests a dismal prognosis for patients who are dialyzed, such early reports have dealt with patients with chronic end-stage liver disease. In a few instances, we have undertaken dialysis in patients with HRS and acute hepatic disease and have been gratified by the ultimately favorable outcome. Our experience suggests that in selected patients—i.e., those with acute hepatic dysfunction in whom there is reason to believe that renal failure may reverse with resolution of the acute hepatic insult—dialytic therapy is indicated.

With the recent maturation and refinement of orthotopic liver transplantation and its acceptance as the treatment of choice for end-stage liver disease, dialysis has assumed an important ancillary role. Dialysis is now widely used as a supportive measure in the management of many patients awaiting liver transplantation.

In addition to stabilizing renal function, it is often necessary to remove fluid, either to prevent life-threatening emergencies such as acute pulmonary edema or to permit the administration of requisite fluids such as bicarbonate solutions or hyperalimentation. Although hemodialysis often constitutes the therapeutic modality of choice for this purpose, it is not feasible in many patients with severe liver disease and associated hemodynamic instability. Unfortunately, patients with decompensated cirrhosis frequently become hypotensive in response to the institution of hemodialysis. To circumvent this problem, we have used continuous arteriovenous hemofiltration (CAVH) as an alternative maneuver in a few patients with HRS and have been successful in mobilizing fluid without concomitant hemodynamic instability.[194,195] Additional experience is required to clarify the role of this approach in managing patients with HRS (see chapter 26).

Peritoneovenous (LeVeen) Shunt

An advance that has engendered major controversy in the management of HRS is the development of peritoneovenous (PV) shunting[196-198] (see chapter 24). The past 20 years have witnessed a flurry of enthusiasm for the use of PV (LeVeen) shunting in the management of HRS. Because the underlying abnormality is thought to be a maldistribution of extracellular fluid (ECF) with a resultant diminished effective blood volume, attention has focused on developing procedures to redistribute body fluids between compartments, so that the central compartment is replenished despite decreasing ascites. Unfortunately, despite a few well-documented "successes"[197] (see chapter 24), the majority of reports have been anecdotal with insufficient details to allow critical assessment. Even when sufficient data were available, the majority of putative successes occurred in patients who were not clearly documented to have HRS; rather, many patients probably had reversible azotemia secondary to diminished effective blood volume.[198]

Only two prospective, randomized studies of the role of the peritoneovenous shunt (PVS) in the treatment of HRS have been performed.[199,200] Linas et al.[199] prospectively compared the effects of the PVS (n = 10) or medical therapy (n = 10) on renal function and mortality in 20 patients with HRS associated with alcoholic liver disease. After 48–72 hours, body weight and serum creatinine were increased with medical therapy and decreased (from 3.6 ± 0.4 to 3.0 ± 0.5 mg/dl; p < 0.05) in patients with the shunt. Despite the improvement of renal function, only 1 patient with the PV shunt had prolonged survival (210 days). In the remainder, survival was 13.8 ± 2.2 days compared with 4.1 ± 0.6 days with medical therapy. The investigators concluded that, whereas PV shunting often stabilizes renal function, it does not prolong life in patients with HRS. Additional studies are currently underway in patients with less advanced disease.

In the VA Cooperative Study,[200] although there were 7 long-term survivors in a group of 14 patients treated with PV shunting, the results were not statistically significant compared with those of a group of 19 patients undergoing medical therapy. The mean survival of patients treated with the shunt did not differ significantly from that of controls. Of note, the group of patients with HRS was carefully selected, and patients with severe complications of chronic liver disease were excluded.

Available data have not established a beneficial role for the PV shunt in the treatment of the HRS. Although some patients exhibit improved renal function, further controlled studies with larger number of patients are necessary to delineate the effect of the PV shunt on long-term survival, quality of life, and incidence of complications.

Orthotopic Liver Transplantation

Orthotopic liver transplantation (OLTX) has recently become the accepted treatment for end-stage liver disease201 (see chapter 27). Of interest, many patients are admitted with varying degrees of concomitant renal dysfunction, including HRS. OLTX has been reported to reverse HRS acutely.[14,202,203] Four years ago, Gonwa et al.[201] reviewed the extensive experience of the Baylor University transplant group and reported good long-term survival with return of acceptable renal function for prolonged periods. They retrospectively reviewed the first 308 patients undergoing OLTX. The incidence of HRS was 10.5%. Patients with HRS manifested an increase in GFR from a baseline of 20 ± 4 ml/min to a mean of 33 ± 3 ml/min at 6 weeks, with a further increase to 46 ± 6 ml/min at 1 year. GFR remained stable at 2 years postoperatively (38 ± 6 ml/min). There was no difference in perioperative (90-day) mortality between HRS and non-HRS patients, despite a worse preoperative status and a more unstable postoperative course. The actuarial 1- and 2-year survival rate for patients with HRS was 77% (no different from that of non-HRS patients).

The investigators concluded that with aggressive pretransplant and posttransplant management, one can anticipate excellent results after OLTX in patients with HRS. Gonwa and Wilkinson have updated the extensive Baylor experience (see chapter 27).

Transjuglar Intrahepatic Portosystemic Shunt

Recently, a few anecdotal reports have described improved renal function in patients with HRS after insertion of a transjugular intrahepatic portosystemic shunt (TIPS).[204–206] The rationale for this procedure is similar to that for the establishment of a side-to-side portacaval shunt; it creates a portal to systemic vascular pathway that serves to decompress the portacaval system.[207] Although TIPS obviates the need for performing major vascular surgery, it is not nearly so simple and innocuous as some of its adherents propose. It is operator-dependent, requiring skilled and experienced interventional radiologists for successful insertion. The reported experience is quite preliminary, and the available data consist in great part of a few preliminary and anecdotal reports. Chapter 25 offers an in-depth review of the rationale and experience with TIPS, as well as considerations about its potential future in the therapeutic armamentarium.

Newer Experimental Modalities

As noted previously, nonsteroidal anti-inflammatory drugs (NSAIDs) have been shown to induce reversible decrements in renal perfusion and renal function in patients with decompensated cirrhosis.[67–70] Conversely, we have shown that the augmentation of renal prostaglandins induced by water immersion is associated with marked increments in creatinine clearance.[71,72] The infusion of vasodilator prostaglandins to correct a possible renal prostaglandin deficiency has been unrewarding.[64] The widest experience has been with prostaglandin A (PGA) and prostaglandin E (PGE). Although such therapeutic manipulations have occasionally resulted in salutary effects on renal function, the benefits have not been sustained.

Fevery et al.[208] recently attempted to extend these observations by investigating the effects of the administration of a PGE_1 analog (misoprostol) on renal function in 4 patients with alcoholic cirrhosis and HRS. In response to misoprostol administration (0.4 mg orally 4 times daily) and albumin infusions, urine volume increased three- to four-fold. Concomitantly, serum creatinine levels diminished. All patients had hyponatremia, which normalized with misoprostol administration. Although the experience is preliminary, it suggests that the provision of exogenous prostaglandins may have a salutary role in the management of hepatorenal syndrome. Enthusiasm must be tempered, however, by the subsequent failure of the investigators and other groups to confirm initial observations.

Thromboxane Inhibitors

As detailed above, several investigators have proposed that alterations of thromboxanes may contribute to the development of renal dysfunction.[75,77,79] Consequently, there have been attempts to modify the course of HRS by administration of selective inhibitors of thromboxane synthesis.[77,78] Whereas nonspecific cyclooxygenase inhibitors, such as indomethacin and aspirin, reduce both thromboxane and prostaglandin synthesis to varying degrees in different biologic systems, selective inhibitors of thromboxane synthesis preserve or possibly increase the production of other metabolites of arachidonic acid, such as the potent vasodilator prostacyclin. Zipser et al.[77] administered the thromboxane synthetase inhibitor dazoxiben to patients with alcoholic hepatitis and progressive azotemia. Although the administration of dazoxiben reduced the urinary excretion of the thromboxane metabolite TxB_2 by approximately 50%, excretion of PGE_2 and 6-keto $PGF_{1\alpha}$ was essentially unaltered. Despite the reduction in thromboxane excretion, there was no consistent reversal of the progressive renal deterioration.[77]

Gentilini et al.[78] also investigated the effects of a thromboxane-synthase inhibitor in cirrhotic patients. They administered OKY 046, a selective TxA_2 synthase inhibitor, 200 mg thrice daily for 5 days, to 9 nonazotemic cirrhotic patients with ascites and avid sodium retention. OKY 046 increased inulin clearance by 19%, whereas renal blood flow was unchanged. Drug administration did not alter the avid sodium retention and did not affect PRA or plasma aldosterone levels.

Unfortunately, the administration of Tx-synthase inhibitors is associated with a number of confounding factors that render the results difficult to interpret. Indeed, these drugs may lead to the accumulation of the prostaglandin endoperoxides PGG_2 and PGH_2, which mimic the renal effects of TxA_2 by interacting with the same receptors. As an example, arachidonic acid-induced vasoconstriction in rat kidneys is only partially reduced by pretreatment with a Tx-synthase inhibitor, whereas it is completely abolished by administration of a Tx-receptor antagonist.[209]

In an attempt to obviate such problems, Laffi et al.[79] recently conducted a randomized, double-blind, crossover trial to characterize the effects of the thromboxane-receptor antagonist ONO-3708 on renal hemodynamics and excretory function in 15 nonazotemic cirrhotic patients with ascites. Urinary TxB_2 excretion was three-fold higher than in healthy subjects. The administration of ONO-3708 significantly blocked TxA_2 receptors; bleeding time showed a twofold increase, and platelet aggregation to the Tx-receptor agonist U-46619 was abolished in all patients. ONO-3708 induced an 86% increase in free water clearance compared with placebo (p < 0.001), which was associated with significant diuresis. Renal plasma flow, as measured by P-aminohippurate (PAH) clearance, increased 14% during Tx-receptor blockade (p < 0.05), whereas glomerular filtration rate, as assessed by inulin, was unchanged. Additional studies with thromboxane-receptor antagonists in patients with widely varying degrees of acute renal insufficiency are required to define further their possible utility in the treatment of hepatorenal syndrome.

Other Treatment Modalities

In view of the prominent role assigned to renal cortical ischemia in the pathogenesis of HRS, numerous attempts have been made to treat HRS with vasodilators. The intrarenal infusion of nonspecific vasodilators, such as acetylcholine and papaverine, improves renal blood flow but does not augment GFR.[210] Similarly, the blockade of vasoconstrictor α-adrenergic nerves by the intrarenal infusion of phentolamine or phenoxybenzamine or the stimulation of vasodilator β-adrenergic nerves with isoproterenol has no significant effect on GFR.[16]

The direct stimulation of renal dopaminergic receptors by the infusion of nonpressor doses of dopamine produces renal vasodilation; again, however, GFR and urine flow are virtually unaffected, despite infusions for as long as 24 hours.[53,211,212]

Finally, various other treatment modalities have been proposed, including prednisone, exchange transfusion, charcoal hemoperfusion, xenobiotic cross-circulation, and ex vivo baboon liver perfusion.[4,213] None is of demonstrated benefit, and the actual and potential complications are of sufficient magnitude to dictate great hesitation in clinical use.

Water Immersion

We are often asked in consultation if water immersion might be tried as a therapeutic maneuver for a patient who has been diagnosed with HRS. As noted above, the underlying abnormality in patients with decompensated cirrhosis is not solely an excess of total body fluid; to a greater extent, the problem is maldistribution of extracellular fluid. Consequently, much attention has been focused on developing procedures to redistribute body fluids, not only between compartments, as with PVS, but also within the vascular compartment.

Studies from our laboratory have provided substantial evidence that head-out water immersion markedly augments central blood volume.[89,214] To the extent that diminished effective blood volume constitutes a major determinant of renal sodium retention in established liver disease, one might justifiably speculate on the use of water immersion as a means of replenishing the contracted effective volume. Although at first glance such a proposal appears attractive, several arguments have been marshaled in opposition: (1) the repeated use of water immersion is a time-consuming and costly procedure requiring the continuous attendance of paramedical personnel; (2) exposure of clinically fragile patients to the marked hemodynamic alterations that attend immersion requires close medical monitoring; and (3) a patient can reasonably be immersed for only a small percentage of the day, and it is unknown if this confers a lasting beneficial effect.

The long-term effect of water immersion on central blood volume is unknown. Certainly, water immersion constitutes a powerful and highly productive means of investigating deranged volume homeostasis in many edematous disorders, especially cirrhosis.[20,52,89] We believe, however, that at this time, pending carefully controlled investigative pilot studies, immersion should not be used uniformly as therapy for patients with decompensated cirrhosis.

Calcium Antagonists

An additional investigative approach that has not been undertaken but that merits consideration is the possible role of calcium antagonists. Studies from several laboratories, including our own, have demonstrated profound effects of calcium antagonists on renal vascular smooth muscle and concomitant alterations in renal function.[215,216] Specifically, calcium antagonists have been shown to augment and restore GFR in diverse experimental settings characterized by renal vasoconstriction. This effect is due, in part, to the selective reduction of afferent arteriolar resistance. In essence, calcium antagonists may constitute selective renal vasodilators that reverse or attenuate renal ischemia.[217] Indeed, studies from several laboratories have recently demonstrated that calcium antagonists are effective in the prophylaxis of acute renal insufficiency in diverse clinical settings, including cadaveric kidney transplantation and radiocontrast-induced renal dysfunction.[217] Because patients with hepatorenal syndrome manifest a more extreme degree of preferential renal cortical ischemia, it appears reasonable to anticipate that calcium antagonists can induce a similar salutary effect on renal hemodynamics. If calcium antagonists can be safely administered to patients with decompensated cirrhosis without inducing concomitant hypotension, they may constitute an additional therapeutic approach to the management of HRS.

Vasoconstrictor Therapy

A final therapeutic approach that warrants consideration is the administration of vasoactive agents that preferentially reverse the decreased systemic vascular resistance without increasing renal vascular resistance. As discussed previously, there has been a resurgence of interest in the role of peripheral vasodilation as the primary determinant of intravascular underfilling. The resultant imbalance between the expanded capacitance and the available volume eventuates in a diminished effective volume. Such a formulation dictates that therapy should be directed toward correction of the diminished systemic vascular resistance in patients with HRS. Such an approach is not novel. Thirty years ago Gornel et al.[218] demonstrated that the administration of the pressor amine metaraminol in cirrhotic patients is often followed by an increase in GFR and urine flow and elaboration of a more dilute urine. Although the use of metaraminol was fraught with problems, the general approach of administering pressor agents may be valid.

Twenty-seven years ago Cohn et al.[219] demonstrated that a synthetic analogue of lysine vasopressin (octapressin; PLV-2) had the unique property of producing renal vasodilation combined with systemic vasoconstriction and thereby redistributing blood flow to the kidney. The investigators studied the systemic and renal hemodynamic effects of PLV-2 in patients with decompensated cirrhosis of the liver. Low doses (0.004–0.02 U/min) increased renal blood flow (indicator–dilution technique), reduced renal vascular resistance, and produced a slight increase in arterial pressure and systemic vascular resistance. The fraction of the cardiac output delivered to the kidney was increased at all dose levels. The increased renal blood flow was accompanied by a more rapid intrarenal dye transit time and a slight increase in the renal extraction ratio of P-aminohippurate, suggesting a rise in cortical blood flow. The authors concluded that PLV-2 produced renal vasodilation in small doses and preferential extrarenal vasoconstriction in larger doses, resulting in redistribution of blood flow to the kidney. On the basis of these findings, Cohn et al.[219] proposed a possible role for PLV-2 in the management of HRS. Unfortunately, additional studies were not undertaken.

Recently, interest in the hemodynamic derangements and attempts to improve renal function by countervailing this hyperdynamic state have been renewed. Lenz et al.[220] investigated the effects of the infusion of ornipressin on renal and circulatory function. Their preliminary report observed that ornipressin reversed the hyperdynamic state. Concomitantly, renal function was improved, as assessed by a more than 70% increase in creatinine clearance and a doubling in urine flow. Preliminary observations support the concept that the peripheral vasodilation of liver disease contributes importantly to renal dysfunction. Consequently, maneuvers that counter the vasodilation may improve renal function. In this regard, clinical trials attempting to reverse HRS should be undertaken with additional vasoactive agents that selectively increase systemic vascular resistance.

CONCLUSION

Despite considerable progress in the past three decades, we still lack a comprehensive understanding of the pathogenetic cascade that produces HRS, and therapy is largely empirical. The intrarenal hemodynamic alterations that underlie the HRS are understood more clearly, but the numerous attempts at treating HRS empirically with vasodilators have not resulted in important therapeutic innovations. The failure of many patients with HRS to survive despite partial correction of renal hemodynamic abnormalities reflects the precarious state of the patient with liver failure; hemorrhage, infection, and hepatic coma are the usual causes of death.

Any future breakthroughs in providing definitive treatment of HRS must be predicated on a greater clarification of the mechanisms and a delineation of the mediators. Recent reappraisal makes clear that dialysis has a role in supporting patients awaiting hepatic transplantation. Dialysis also may be warranted as a supportive measure in some patients with apparently reversible hepatic dysfunction. Hepatic transplantation has evolved over the past decade to the point that it constitutes definitive therapy for patients with hepatic dysfunction and concomitant renal failure. Although anecdotal information suggests that PV shunting has a role in the management of selected patients with HRS, the results of prospective studies have failed to confirm such an approach. Finally, the advent of the peripheral vasodilation theory and its focus on the generalized hemodynamic perturbations in patients with HRS have refocused attention on the florid extrarenal hemodynamic derangements. Pharmacologic interventions that counter the peripheral vasodilation may improve both systemic hemodynamics and renal function. It is hoped that future clinical trials will establish the precise contribution of these treatment modalities and their respective roles in the therapeutic armamentarium.

Acknowledgment. The author thanks Elsa V. Reina for her expert secretarial help. Portions of this chapter have been adapted with permission from earlier reviews by the author: The hepatorenal syndrome. In Epstein M (ed): The Kidney in Liver Disease, 3rd ed. Baltimore: Williams & Wilkins, 1988, pp 89–118, and Hepatorenal syndrome: Emerging perspectives of pathophysiology and therapy. J Am Soc Nephrol 1994;4:1735-1753.

REFERENCES

1. Papper S: Hepatorenal syndrome. In Epstein M (ed): The Kidney in Liver Disease, 2nd ed. New York: Elsevier Biomedical, 1983;87–106.
2. Epstein M: Functional renal abnormalities in cirrhosis: Pathophysiology and management. In Zakim D, Boyer TD (eds): Hepatology: A Textbook of Liver Disease, 2nd ed. Philadelphia: W.B. Saunders, 1990;493–512.
3. Epstein M: Liver disease. In Massry SG, Glassock RJ (eds): Textbook of Nephrology. Baltimore: Williams & Wilkins, 1990;6.304–6.313.
4. Epstein M: The hepatorenal syndrome. Emerging perspectives of pathophysiology and therapy. J Am Soc Nephrol 1994;4:1735–1753.
5. Flint A: Clinical report on hydro-peritoneum, based on an analysis of forty-six cases. Am J Med Sci 1863;45:306–339.
6. Ritt DJ, Whelan G, Werner DJ, et al: Acute hepatic necrosis with stupor or coma. Medicine 1969;48:151–172.
7. Epstein M, Oster JR, DeVelasco RE: Hepatorenal syndrome following hemihepatectomy. Clin Nephrol 1976;5:128–133.
8. Papadakis MA, Arieff AJ: Unreliability of clinical evaluation of renal function in cirrhosis: A prospective study. Am J Med 1987;82:945–952.
9. Goldstein H, Boyle JD: Spontaneous recovery from the hepatorenal syndrome. Report of four cases. N Engl J Med 1965;272:895–898.
10. Reynolds TB: The hepatorenal syndrome. In Schaffner F. Sherlock S, Leevy CM (eds): The Liver and Its Diseases. New York: Intercontinental Medical Book Corp., 1974;307–313.
11. Gordon JA, Anderson RJ: Hepatorenal syndrome. Semin Nephrol 1981;1: 37–41.
12. Shear L, Kleinerman J, Gabuzda GJ: Renal failure in patients with cirrhosis of the liver. I. Clinical and pathologic characteristics. Am J Med 1965;39:184-198.
13. Koppel MH, Coburn JW, Mims MM, et al: Transplantation of cadaveric kidneys from patients with hepatorenal syndrome. Evidence for the functional nature of renal failure in advanced liver disease. N Engl J Med 1969;280:1367–1371.
14. Iwatsuki S, Popovtzer MM, Corman JL, et al: Recovery from hepatorenal syndrome after orthotopic liver transplantation. N Engl J Med 1973;289:1155-1159.
15. Schroeder ET, Shear L, Sanceta SM, Gabuzda GJ: Renal failure in patients with cirrhosis of the liver. III. Evaluation of intrarenal blood flow by para amino-hippurate extraction and response to angiotensin. Am J Med 1967;43:887–896.
16. Epstein M, Berk DP, Hollenberg NK, et al: Renal failure in the patient with cirrhosis: The role of active vasoconstriction. Am J Med 1970;49:175–185.
17. Epstein M, Schneider N, Befeler B: Relationship of systemic and intrarenal hemodynamics in cirrhosis. J Lab Clin Med 1977;89:1175–1187.
18. Hollenberg NK, Epstein M, Basch RI, et al: Acute oliguric renal failure im man: Evidence for preferential renal cortical ischemia. Medicine 1968;47:455–474.
19. Kew MC, Varma RR, Williams HS, et al: Renal and intrarenal blood flow in cirrhosis of the liver. Lancet 1971;2:504–510.
20. Epstein M: Determinants of abnormal renal sodium handling in cirrhosis: A reappraisal. Scand J Clin Lab Invest 1980;40:689–694.
21. Witte CL, Witte MH, Dumont AE: Lymph imbalance in the genesis and perpetuation of the ascites syndrome in hepatic cirrhosis. Gastroenterology 1980;78:1059–1066.
22. Better OS, Schrier RW: Disturbed volume homeostasis in patients with cirrhosis of the liver. Kidney Int 1983;23:303–311.

23. Henriksen JH, Bendtsen F, Sørensen TIA, et al: Reduced central blood volume in cirrhosis. Gastroenterology 1989;97:1506–1513.

24. Henriksen JH, Bendtsen F, Gerbes AL, et al: Estimated central blood volume in cirrhosis: Relationship to sympathetic nervous activity, β-adrenergic blockade and atrial natriuretic factor. Hepatology 1992;1163–1170.

25. Cohn JN: Renal hemodynamic alterations in liver disease. In Suki WN, Eknoyan G (eds): The Kidney in Systemic Disease, 2nd ed. New York: John Wiley & Sons, 1981;509–519.

26. Schrier RW, Arroyo V, Bernardi M, et al: Peripheral arterial vasodilation hypothesis: A proposal for the initiation of renal sodium and water retention in cirrhosis. Hepatology 1988;8:1151–1157.

27. Schrier RW, Niederberger M, Weigert A, Gines P: Peripheral arterial vasodilation: Determinant of functional spectrum of cirrhosis. Semin Liver Dis 1994; 14:14–22.

28. Levy M: Pathogenesis of sodium retention in early cirrhosis of the liver: Evidence for vascular overfilling. Semin Liver Dis.1994;14:4–13.

29. Tristani FE, Cohn JN: Systemic and renal hemodynamics in oliguric hepatic failure: Effect of volume expansion. J Clin Invest 1967;46:1894–1906.

30. Lieberman FL, Denison EK, Reynolds TB: The relationship of plasma volume, portal hypertension, ascites and renal sodium retention in cirrhosis: The overflow theory of ascites formation. Ann NY Acad Sci 1970; 170:202–212.

31. Tristani FE. Cohn JN: Systemic and renal hemodynamics in oliguric hepatic failure: Effect of volume expansion. J Clin Invest 1967;46:1894–1906.

32. Guazzi M, Polese A, Magrini F, et al: Negative influences of ascites on cardiac function in cirrhotic patients. Am J Med 1975;59:165–170.

33. Cohn JN, Tristani FE, Khatri M: Renal vasodilator therapy in the hepatorenal syndrome. Med Ann DC 1970;39:1–7.

34. Epstein M, Schneider N, Befeler B: Relationship of systemic and intrarenal hemodynamics in cirrhosis. J Lab Clin Med 1977;89:1175–1187.

35. Fluck DC, Evans TR, Siggers DC, et al: Distribution of blood flow in patients with heart disease. Clin Sci 1972;42:627–634.

36. Ring-Larsen H, Hesse B, Stigsby B: Effect of portal-systemic anastomosis on renal hemodynamics in cirrhosis. Gut 1976;17:865–870.

37. Vallance P, Moncada S: Hyperdynamic circulation in cirrhosis: A role for nitric oxide? Lancet 1991;337: 776–778.

38. Dawson JL: Jaundice and anorexic renal damage: Protective effect of mannitol. Br Med J 1964;1:810–811.

39. Aoyagi T, Lowenstein L: The effect of bile acid and renal ischemia on renal function. J Lab Clin Med 1968;71:686–691.

40. Alon U, Berant M, Mordechovitz D, Better OS: The effect of intrarenal infusion of bile on the kidney function in the dog. Clin Sci 1982;62:431–433.

41. Finestone H, Fechner C, Levy M: Effects of bile and bile salt infusions on renal function in dogs. Can J Physiol Pharmacol 1984;62:762–768.

42. Levy M, Finestone H: Renal response to four hours of biliary obstruction in the dog. Am J Physiol 1983;244: F516–F525.

43. Harries JT, Sladen GE: Effects of bile acids on small intestinal absorption of glucose, water and sodium. Gut 1971;12:855.

44. Better OS: Renal and cardiovascular dysfunction in liver disease. Kidney Int 1986;29:598–607.

45. Green J, Better OS: Systemic hypotension and renal failure in obstructive jaundice—mechanic and therapeutic aspects. J Am Soc Nephrol 1995;5:1853–1871.

46. Mullane JR, Gliedman ML: Elevation of the pressure of the abdominal inferior vena cava as a cause for hepatorenal syndrome in cirrhosis. Surgery 1966;59: 1135–1146.

47. Baldus WP: Etiology and management of renal failure in cirrhosis and portal hypertension. Ann NY Acad Sci 1969;170:267–278.

48. Maxwell MH, Breed ES, Schwartz IL: Renal venous pressure in chronic congestive heart failure. J Clin Invest 1950;29:342–348.

49. Gordon ME: The acute effects of abdominal paracentesis in Laennec cirrhosis upon exchanges of electrolytes and water, renal function and hemodynamics Am J Gastroenterol 1960;33:15–37.

50. Cade R, Wagemaker H, Vogel S, et al: Hepatorenal syndrome: Studies of the effect of vascular volume and intraperitoneal pressure on renal and hepatic function. Am J Med 1987;82:427–438.

51. Schroeder ET, Eich RH, Smulyan H, et al: Plasma renin level in hepatic cirrhosis. Am J Med 1970;49: 186–191.

52. Epstein M, Levinson R, Sancho J, et al: Characterization of the renin-aldosterone system in decompensated cirrhosis. Circ Res 1977;41:818–829.

53. Barnardo DE, Summerskill WHJ, Strong CB, Baldus WP: Renal function, renin activity and endogenous vasoactive substances in cirrhosis. Am J Dig Dis 1970; 15:419–425.

54. Barnardo DE, Baldus WP, Maher FT: Effects of dopamine on renal function in patients with cirrhosis. Gastroenterology 1970;58:524–531.

55. Ayers CR: Plasma renin activity and renin-substrate concentration in patients with liver disease. Circ Res 1967;20:594–598.

56. Levens NR, Peach MJ, Carey RM: Role of the intrarenal renin-angiotensin system in the control of the renal function. Circ Res 1981;48:157–167.

57. Mitchell KD, Navar LG: Intrarenal actions of angiotensin II in the pathogenesis of experimental hypertension. In Laragh JH, Brenner BM (eds): Hypertension: Pathophysiology, Diagnosis and Management, 2nd ed. New York: Raven Press, 1995;1437–1450.

58. Berkowitz HD: Renin substrate in the hepatorenal syndrome. In Epstein MF (ed): The Kidney in Liver Disease. New York: Elsevier/North Holland, 1978; 251–270.

59. Berkowitz HD, Calvin C, Miller LD: Significance of altered renin substrate in the hepatorenal syndrome. Surg Forum 1972;23:342–343.

60. McCombs PR, Berkowitz HD, Miller LD, Rosato EF: Renin substrate infusions in hepatorenal syndrome. Surg Forum 1975;26:419–421.

61. Hollenberg NK: Renin, angiotensin, and the kidney: Assessment by pharmacological interruption of the renin-angiotensin system In Epstein M (ed): The Kidney in Liver Disease, 3rd ed. Williams & Wilkins: Baltimore, 1988;375–389.

62. Pariente EA, Bataille C, Bercoff E, Lebrec D: Acute effects of captopril on systemic and renal hemodynamics and on renal function in cirrhotic patients with ascites. Gastroenterology 1985;88:1255–1259.

63. Schroeder ET, Anderson GH, Goldman SH, Streeten DHP: Effects of angiotensin II (AII) blockade with 1–Sar-8-Ala AII (saralasin) in patients with cirrhosis and ascites. Kidney Int 1976;9:511–519.

64. Arieff AI, Chidsey CA: Renal function in cirrhosis and the effects of prostaglandin A$_1$. Am J Med 1974;56: 695–703.

65. McGiff JC, Miller MJS: Renal functional aspects of eicosanoid- dependent mechanisms. In Fisher JW, (ed): Kidney Hormones. New York: Academic Press, 1986; 363–395.

66. Quilley J, Bell-Quilley CP, McGiff JC: Eicosanoids and hypertension. In Laragh JH, Brenner BM (eds): Hypertension: Pathophysiology, Diagnosis and Management, 2nd ed. New York: Raven Press, 1995;963–982.

67. Boyer TD, Zia P, Reynolds TB: Effect of indomethacin and prostaglandin A$_1$, on renal function and plasma renin activity in alcoholic liver disease. Gastroenterology 1979;77:215–222.

68. Zipser RD, Hoefs JC, Speckart PF, et al: Prostaglandins. Modulators of renal function and pressor resistance in chronic liver disease. J Clin Endocrinol Metab 1979; 48:895–900.

69. Epstein M, Lifschitz MD: Volume status as a determinant of the influence of renal PGE on renal function. Nephron 1980;25:157–159.

70. Epstein M: Renal prostaglandins and the control of renal function in liver disease. Am J Med 1986; 80(Suppl 1A):46–55.

71. Epstein M, Lifschitz M, Hoffman DS, Stein JH: Relationship between renal prostaglandin E and renal sodium handling during water immersion in normal man. Circ Res 1979;45:71–80.

72. Epstein M, Lifschitz M, Ramachandran M, Rappaport K: Characterization of renal PGE responsiveness in decompensated cirrhosis: Implications for renal sodium handling. Clin Sci 1982;63:555–563.

73. Mené P, Dunn MJ: Contractile effects to TxA$_2$ and endoperoxide analogues on cultured rat glomerular mesangial cells. Am J Physiol 1986;251:F1029–F1035.

74. Loutzenhiser R, Epstein M, Horton C, Sonke P: Reversal of renal and smooth muscle actions of the thromboxane mimetic U-44069 by diltiazem. Am J Physiol 1986;250:F619–F626.

75. Zipser RD, Radvan GH, Kronborg KJ, et al: Urinary thromboxane B$_2$ and prostaglandin E$_2$ in the hepatorenal syndrome: Evidence for increased vasoconstrictor and decreased vasodilator factors. Gastroenterology 1983;84:697–705.

76. Rimola A, Ginés P, Arroyo V, et al: Urinary excretion of 6-keto-prostaglandin F$_1$ alpha, thromboxane B$_2$ and prostaglandin E$_2$ in cirrhosis with ascites. Relationship to functional renal failure (hepatorenal syndrome). J Hepatol 1986;3:111–117.

77. Zipser RD, Kronborg I, Rector W, et al: Therapeutic trial of thromboxane synthesis inhibition in the hepatorenal syndrome. Gastroenterology 1984;87:1228–1232.

78. Gentilini P, Laffi G, Meacci E, et al: Effects of OKY 046, a thromboxane-synthase inhibitor, on renal function in non-azotemic cirrhotic patients with ascites. Gastroenterology 1988;94:1470–1477.

79. Laffi G, Marra F, Carloni V, et al: Thromboxane-receptor blockade increases water diuresis in cirrhotic patients with ascites. Gastroenterology 1992;103:1017–1021.

80. O'Connor DT, Stone RA: The renal kallikrein-kinin system: description and relationship to liver disease. In Epstein M (ed): The Kidney in Liver Disease, 2nd ed. New York: Elsevier Biomedical, 1983;469–477.

81. Carretero OA. Scicli AG: The kallikrein-kinin system as a regulator of cardiovascular and renal function. In Laragh JH, Brenner BM (eds): Hypertension: Pathophysiology, Diagnosis and Management, 2nd ed. New York: Raven Press, 1995;983–1000.

82. Greco AV, Porcelli G, Ghirlanda G: L'escrezione di calicreina urinaria nella cirrosi epatica. Minerva Med 1975;66:1504–1508.

83. Zipser RD, Kerlin P, Hoefs JC, et al: Renal kallikrein excretion in alcoholic cirrhosis. Am J Gastroenterol 1981;75:183–187.

84. Pérez-Ayuso RM, Arroyo V, Camps J, et al: Renal kallikrein excretion in cirrhotics with ascites: Relationship to renal hemodynamics. Hepatology 1984;4:247–252.

85. Levinsky NG: The renal kallikrein-kinin system. Circ Res 1979;44:441–451.

86. Thames MD: Neural control of renal function: Contribution of cardiopulmonary baroreceptors to the control of the kidney. Fed Proc 1977;37:1209–1213.

87. DiBona GF: The functions of the renal nerves. Rev Physiol Biochem Pharmacol 1982;94:75–181.

88. DiBona GF: Renal neural activity in hepatorenal syndrome. Kidney Int 1984;25:841–853.

89. Epstein M: Renal effects of head-out water immersion in humans: A 15 year update. Physiol Rev 1992; 72: 563–621.

90. Bichet DG, VanPutten VJ, Schrier RW: Potential role of increased sympathetic activity in impaired sodium and water excretion in cirrhosis. N Engl J Med 1982;307: 1552–1557.

91. Ring-Larsen H, Hesse B, Henriksen JH, Christensen NJ: Sympathetic nervous activity and renal and systemic hemodynamics in cirrhosis: Plasma norepinephrine concentration, hepatic extraction and renal release. Hepatology 1982;2:304–310.

92. Henriksen JH, Ring-Larsen H, Christensen NJ: Sympathetic nervous activity in cirrhosis: A survey of plasma catecholamine studies. J Hepatol 1984;1:55–65.

93. Epstein M, Larios O, Johnson G: Effects of water immersion on plasma catecholamines in decompensated cirrhosis. Implications for deranged sodium and water homeostasis. Miner Electrolyte Metab 1985;11:25–34.

94. Bichet DG, Groves BM, Schrier RW: Mechanisms of improvement of water and sodium excretion by immersion in decompensated cirrhotic patients. Kidney Int 1983;24:788–794.

95. Kopp UC, Dibona GF: The neural control of renal function. In Seldin DW, Giebisch G (eds): The Kidney: Physiology and Pathophysiology, 2nd ed. New York: Raven, 1992;1157–1204.

96. Folkow B, DiBona G, Hjemdahl P, et al: Measurements of plasma norepinephrine concentration in human primary hypertension—a word of caution concerning their applicability for assessing neurogenic contribution. Hypertension 1983;5:399–403.

97. Esler M, Dudley F, Jennings G, et al: Increased sympathetic nervous activity and the effects of its inhibition with clonidine in alcoholic cirrhosis. Ann Intern Med 1992;116:446–455.

98. Liehr H, Jacob AI: Endotoxin and renal failure in liver disease. In Epstein M (ed): The Kidney in Liver Disease, 2nd ed. New York: Elsevier Biomedical, 1983; 535–551.

99. Bourgoignie JJ, Valle GA: Endotoxin and renal dysfynction in liver disease. In Epstein M (ed): The Kidney in Liver Disease, 3rd ed. Baltimore: Williams & Wilkins, 1988;486–507.

100. Gray GA, Schott C, Julou-Schaeffer G, et al: The effect of inhibitors of the L-arginine/nitric oxide pathway on endotoxin-induced loss of vascular responsiveness in anaesthetized rats. Br J Pharmacol 1991;103:1218–1224.

101. Fleming I, Julou-Schaeffer G, Gray GA, et al: Evidence that an L-arginine/nitric oxide dependent elevation of tissue cyclic GMP is involved in depression of vascular reactivity by endotoxin. Br J Pharmacol 1991;103:1047–1052.

102. Suffredini AF, Fromm RF, Parker MM, et al: The cardiovascular response of normal humans to the administration of endotoxin. N Engl J Med 1989;321:280–287.

103. Petros A, Bennett D, Vallance P: Effect of nitric oxide synthase inhibitors on hypotension in patients with septic shock. Lancet 1991;338:1557–1558.

104. Clemente C, Bosch J, Rodés J, et al: Functional renal failure and haemorrhagic gastritis associated with endotoxaemia in cirrhosis. Gut 1977;18:556–560.

105. Gatta A, Milani L, Merkel C, et al: Lack of correlation between endotoxemia and renal hypoperfusion in cirrhotics without overt renal failure. Eur J Clin Invest 1982;12:417–422.

106. Coratelli P. Passavanti G, Munno I, et al: New trends in hepatorenal syndrome. Kidney Int 1985;28:S143–S147.

107. Bosch J, Ginés P, Arroyo V, et al: Hepatic and systemic hemodynamics and the neurohumoral systems in cirrhosis. In Epstein M (ed): The Kidney in Liver Disease, 3rd ed. Baltimore: Williams & Wilkins, 1988;286–305.

108. Umans JG, Levi R: The nitric oxide system in circulatory homeostasis and its possible role in hypertensive disorder. In Laragh JH, Brenner BM (eds): Hypertension: Pathophysiology, Diagnosis and Management, 2nd ed. New York: Raven Press, 1995;1083–1096.

109. Palmer RMJ, Ferrige AG, Moncada S: Nitric oxide release accounts for the biological activity of endothelium-derived relaxing factor. Nature 1987;327:524–526.

110 Palmer RMJ, Ashton DS, Moncada S: Vascular endothelial cells synthesize nitric oxide from L-arginine. Nature 1988;333:664–666.

111. Rees DD, Palmer RMJ, Moncada S: The role of endothelium-derived nitric oxide in the regulation of blood pressure. Proc Natl Acad Sci USA 1989;86:3375–3378.

112. Aisaka K, Gross SG, Griffith OW, Levi R: L-arginine availability determines the duration of acetylcholine-induced systemic vasodilation in vivo. Biochem Biophys Res Commun 1989;163:710–717.

113. Radlomski MW, Palmer RMJ, Moncada S: Glucocorticoids inhibit the expression of an inducible, but not the constitutive, nitric oxide synthase in vascular endothelial cells. Proc Natl Acad Sci USA 1990;87:10043–10047.

114 Rees DD, Cellek S, Palmer RMJ, Moncada S: Dexamethasone prevents the induction by endotoxin of a nitric oxide synthase and the associated effects on vascular tone. An insight into endotoxin shock. Biochem Biophys Res Commun 1990;173:541–547.

115. Busse R, Mulsch A: Induction of nitric oxide synthase by cytokines in vascular smooth muscle cells. FEBS Lett 1990;275:87–90.

116. Tomás A, Soriano G, Guarner C, et al: Increased serum nitrite and nitrate in cirrhosis: Relationship to endotoxemia [abstract]. J Hepatol 1992;16(Suppl 1):4.

117. King AJ: Endothelins: Multifunctional peptides with potent vasoactive properties. In Laragh JH, Brenner BM (eds): Hypertension: Pathophysiology, Diagnosis, and Management, 2nd ed. New York: Raven Press, 1995;631–672.

118. Rubanyi GM: Endothelin in cardiovascular homeostasis. In Laragh JH, Brenner BM (eds): Hypertension: Pathophysiology, Diagnosis and Management, 2nd ed. New York: Raven Press, 1995;1109–1124.

119. Tomita K, Ujiie K, Nakanashi T, et al: Plasma endothelin levels in patients with acute renal failure. N Engl J Med.1989;321:1127.

119a. Deray G, Carayon A, Maistre G, et al: Endothelin in chronic renal failure. Nephrol Dial Transplant 1992;7:300–305.

120. Rabelink AJ, Kaasjager KAH, Boer P, et al: Effects of endothelin-1 on renal function in humans: Implications for physiology and pathophysiology. Kidney lnt 1994;46:376–381.

121. Bijlsma JA, Rabelink AJ, Kaasjager KAH, Koomans HA: L-Arginine does not prevent the renal effects of endothelin in humans. J Am Soc Nephrol 1995;5:1508–1516.

122. Uchihara M, Izumi N, Sato C, Marumo F: Clinical significance of elevated plasma endothelin concentration in patients with cirrhosis. Hepatology 1992;16:95–99.

123. Sugiura M, lnagami T, Kon V: Endotoxin stimulates endothelin release in vivo and in vitro as determined by radioimmunoassay. Biochem Biophys Res Commun 1989;161:1220–1227.

124. Uemasu J, Matsumoto H, Kawasaki H: Increased plasma endothelin levels in patients with liver cirrhosis. Nephron 1992;60:380.

125. Moore K, Wendon J, Frazer M, et al: Plasma endothelin immunoreactivity in liver disease and the hepatorenal syndrome. N Engl J Med 1992;327:1774–1778.

126. Moller S, Emmeluth C, Henriksen JH: Elevated circulating plasma endothelin-1 concentrations in cirrhosis. J Hepatol 1993;19:285–290.

127 Epstein M: The hepatorenal syndrome: Newer perspectives [editorial]. N Engl J Med 1992;327:1810–1811.

128. DeBold AJ, Borestein HR, Veress AT, Sonnenberg H: A rapid and potent natriuretic response to intravenous injection of atrial myocardial extracts in rats. Life Sci 1981;28:89–94.

129. Lewicki JA, Protter AA: Physiological studies of the natriuretic peptide family. In Laragh JH, Brenner BM (eds): Hypertension: Pathophysiology, Diagnosis and Management, 2nd ed. New York: Raven Press, 1995; 1029–1054.

130. Maack T. Marion DN, Camargo MJF, et al: Effects of auriculin (atrial natriuretic factor) on blood pressure, renal function, and the renin-aldosterone system in dogs. Am J Med 1984;77:1069–1075.

131. Cantin M, Genest J: The heart and the atrial natriuretic factor. Endocr Rev 1985;6:107–127.

132. Needleman P, Adams SP, Cole BR, et al: Atriopeptins as cardiac hormones. Hypertension 1985;7: 469–482.

133. Fyhrquist F, Totterman KJ, Tikkanen I: Infusion of atrial natriuretic peptide in liver cirrhosis with ascites. Lancet 1985;2:1439.

134. Epstein M, Loutzenhiser R, Norsk P, Atlas S: Relationship between plasma ANF responsiveness and renal sodium handling in cirrhotic humans. Am J Nephrol 1989;9:133–143.

135. Epstein M: Atrial natriuretic factor in patients with liver disease. Am J Nephrol 1989;9:89–100.

136. Gerbes AL, Arendt RM, Ritter D, et al: Plasma atrial natriuretic factor in patients with cirrhosis. N Engl J Med 1985;313:1609–1610.

137. Morgan TR, Imada T, Hollister AS, Inagami T: Plasma human atrial natriuretic factor in cirrhosis and ascites with and without functional renal failure. Gastroenterology 1988;95:1641–1647.

138. Anderson RJ: Adenosine: Mechanism of renal action. In Stein JH, Goldfarb S, Ziyadeh F (eds): Hormones, Autacoids, and the Kidney. New York: Churchill Livingstone, 1991;281–296.

139. Collis MG: The vasodilator role of adenosine. Pharmacol Ther 1989;41:143–162.

140. Fredholm BB, Sollevi A: Cardiovascular effects of adenosine. Clin Physiol 1986;6:1–21.

141. Spielman WS, Thompson CI: A proposed role for adenosine in the regulation of renal hemodynamics and renin release. Am J Physiol 1982;242:F423–F425.

142. Llach J, Ginés P, Arroyo V, et al: Effect of dipyridamole on kidney function in cirrhosis. Hepatology 1993;17: 59–64.

143. Cohick WS, Clemmons DR: The insulin-like growth factors. Annu Rev Physiol 1993; 55:131–153.

144. Hirschberg R, Kopple JD: Evidence that insulin-like growth factor 1 increases renal plasma flow and glomerular filtration rate in fasted rats. J Clin Invest 1989; 83:326–330.

145. Hirschberg R, Brunori G, Kopple JD, Guler HP: Effects of insulin-like growth factor 1 on renal function in normal men. Kidney Int 1993;43:387–397.

146. Schimpff RM, Lebrec D, Donnadieu M: Somatomedin production in normal adults and cirrhotic patients. Acta Endocrinol 1977;88:355–362.

147. Mendenshall CL, Chernansek SD, Ray MB: The interactions of insulin-like growth factor 1 (IGF-1) with protein-calorie malnutrition in patients with alcoholic liver disease. V.A. Cooperative Study on Alcoholic Hepatitis. Alcohol 1989;24:319–329.

148. Chang A. Firek AF, Nelson JC Mohan S, Balasubramaniam K: Hepatic disease differentially affects insulin like growth factors (IGF) and their binding proteins [abstract]. Gastroenterology 1993;105:A817.

149. Gupta S, Morgan TR, Gordan GS: Calcitonin gene-related peptide in hepatorenal syndrome: A possible mediator of peripheral vasodilation? J Clin Gastroenterol 1992;4:22–26.

150. Rosenfeld MG, Mermod JJ, Amara SG, et al: Production of a novel neuropeptide encoded by the calcitonin gene via tissue-specific RNA processing. Nature 1983;304:129–135.

151. Girgis SI, MacDonald DWR, Stevenson JC, et al: Calcitonin gene-related peptide: Potent vasodilator and major product of calcitonin gene. Lancet 1985;2:14–16

152. Brain SD, Williams TJ, Tippins JR, et al: Calcitonin gene-related peptide is a potent vasodilator. Nature 1985;313:54–56.

153. Villareal D, Freeman RH, Verberg KM, Brando MW: Effects of calcitonin gene-related peptide on renal blood flow in the rat. Proc Soc Exp Biol Med 1988; 188:316–322.

154. Edwards RM, Trizna W: Calcitonin gene-related peptide: Effects on renal arteriolar tone and tubular cAMP levels. Am J Physiol 1990;258:F121–F125

155. Blank ML, Snyder F, Byers LW, et al: Antihypertensive activity of an alkyl ether analog of phosphatidylcholine. Biochem Biophys Res Commun 1979;90:1194–1200.

156. Sanchez Crespo M, Iñarrea P, Alvarez V, et al: Presence in normal urine of a hypotensive and platelet-activating phospholipid. Am J Physiol 1983;244:F706–711.

157. Billah MM, Johnston JM: Identification of a phospholipid platelet activating factor (1-alkyl-2acetyl-sn-glycero-3-phosphocholine). Biochem Biophys Res Commun 1983;113:51–58.

158. Cox P, Warlow ML, Jorgensen R, Farr RS: The presence of platelet activating factor (PAF) in normal human mixed saliva. J Immunol 1983;127:46–50.

159. Muirhead EE: Depressor functions of the kidney. Semin Nephrol 1983;3:14–29.

160. Pinkard RN, McManus L, Hanahan DS: Chemistry and biology of acetyl-glycerol ether phosphorylcholine (platelet activating factor). In Weismann G (ed): Advances in inflammation research. New York: Raven Press, 1982;147–179.

161. Sanchez-Crespo M, Alonso F, Alvarez V, Egido J: Vascular actions of synthetic PAF-acether (platelet activating factor) in the rat. Incidence of a platelet independent mechanism. Immunopharmacology 1979;4: 173–185.

162. Caramello C, Fernández-Gallardo S, Santos JC, et al: Increased levels of platelet-activating factor in blood from patients with cirrhosis of the liver. Eur J Clin Invest 1987;17:7–11.

163. Villamediana LM, Sanz E, Fernández-Gallardo S, et al: Effects of the platelet- activating factor antagonist BN52021 on the hemodynamics of rats with experimental cirrhosis of the liver. Life Sci 1986;39:201–205.

164. Alvestrand A, Bergstrom J: Glomerular hyperfiltration after protein ingestion, during glucagon infusion, and in insulin-dependent diabetes is induced by a liver hormone: Deficient production of this hormone in hepatic failure causes hepatorenal syndrome. Lancet 1984; 1:195–197.

165. Wait RB, and Kahng KV: Renal failure complicating obstructive jaundice. Am J Surg 1989;157:256–263.

166. Glenn F, McSherry CK: Etiological factors in fatal complications following operations upon the biliary tract. Ann Surg 1963;157:695.

167. Dawson JL: Acute postoperative renal failure in obstructive jaundice. Ann R Coll Surg.1968;42:163–181.

168. Dixon J M, Armstrong CP, Duffy SW, Davies GC: Factors affecting morbidity and mortality after surgery for obstructive jaundice: A review of 373 patients. Gut 1985;24:845–852.

169. Cahill CJ: Prevention of postoperative renal failure in patients with obstructive jaundice. The role of bile salts. Br J Surg 1983;70:590–595.

170. Cahill CJ, Pain JA, Bailey ME: Bile salts, endotoxin and renal function in obstructive jaundice. Surg Gynecol Obstet 1987;165:519–522.

171. Pain JA, Cahill CJ, Bailey ME: Perioperative complications in obstructive jaundice: Therapeutic considerations. Br J Surg 1985; 72:942–945.

172. Thompson JN, Cohen J, Blenkhorn JI, et al: A randomized clinical trial of oral ursodeoxycolic acid in obstructive jaundice. Br J Surg 1986;73:634–636.

173. Dudley FJ, Kanel GC, Wood LJ, Reynolds TB: Hepatorenal syndrome without avid sodium retention. Hepatology 1986;6:248–251.

174. Zarich S, Fang LS, Diamond JR: Fractional excretion of sodium. Exceptions to its diagnostic value. Arch Intern Med 1985;145:108–112.

175. Sherman RA, Eisinger RP: Urinary sodium and chloride during renal salt retention. Am J Kidney Dis 1983;3:121–123.

176. Kaplan A, Kohn OF: Fractional excretion of urea as a guide to renal dysfunction. Am J Nephrol 1992;12: 49–54.

177. Daly JSF, Little JM, Troxler RF, Lester R: Metabolism of ^{3}H-myoglobin. Nature 1967;216:1030.

178. Cabrera J, Arroyo V, Ballesta AM, et al: Aminoglycoside nephrotoxicity in cirrhosis. Value of urinary β2-microglobulin to discriminate functional renal failure from acute tubular damage. Gastroenterology 1982;82: 97-105.

179. Rector WG Jr, Kanel GC, Rakela J, Reynolds TB: Tubular dysfunction in the deeply jaundiced patient with hepatorenal syndrome. Hepatology 1985;5:321-326.

180. Oster JR, Epstein M, Ulano HB: Deterioration of renal function with demeclocycline administration. Curr Ther Res 1976;20:794–801.

181. Carrilho F, Bosch J, Arroyo V, et al: Renal failure associated with demeclocycline in cirrhosis. Ann Intern Med 1977;87:195–197.

182. Lebrec D, Poynard T, Hillon P, Benhamou J-P: Propranolol for prevention of recurrent gastrointestinal bleeding in patients with cirrhosis. A controlled study. N Engl J Med 1981;305:1371–1374.

183. Epstein M, Oster JR: Beta-blockers and the kidney. Miner Electrolyte Metab 1982;8:237–254.

184. Epstein M, Oster JR: Beta blockers and renal function: A reappraisal. J Clin Hypertens 1985;1:85–99.

185. Bataille C, Bercoff E, Pariente E, et al: Effects of propranolol on renal blood flow and renal function in patients with cirrhosis. Gastroenterology 1984;86:129–153.

186. Zager RA, Prior RB: Gentamicin and gram-negative bacteremia: A synergism for the development of experimental nephrotoxic acute renal failure. J Clin Invest 1986;78:196–204.

187. Gould L. Shariff M, Zahir M, DiLieto M: Cardiac hemodynamics in alcoholic patients with chronic liver disease and a presystolic gallop. J Clin Invest 1969;48: 860–864.

188. Limas CJ, Guiha NH, Lekagul O, Cohn JN: Impaired left ventricular function in alcoholic cirrhosis with ascites. Circulation 1974;69:755–759.

189. Ginés P, Arroyo V, Vargas V, et al: Paracentesis with intravenous infusion of albumin as compared with peritoneovenous shunting in cirrhosis with refractory ascites. N Engl J Med 1991;325:829–835.

190. Planas R, Ginés P, Arroyo V, et al: Dextran-70 versus albumin as plasma expanders in cirrhotic patients with tense ascites treated with total paracentesis. Results of a randomized study. Gastroenterology 1990;99:1736–1744.

191. Ginés P, Arroyo V, Quintero E, et al: Comparison of paracentesis and diuretics in the treatment of cirrhotics with tense ascites. Results of a randomized study. Gastroenterology 1987;93:234–241.

192. Pérez GO, Oster JR: A critical review of the role of dialysis in the treatment of liver disease. In Epstein M (ed): The Kidney in Liver Disease. New York: Elsevier; 1978;325–336.

193. Wilkinson SP, Weston MJ, Parsons V, Williams R: Dialysis in the treatment of renal failure in patients with liver disease. Clin Nephrol 1977;8:287–292.

194. Epstein M, Pérez GO: Continuous arterio-venous ultrafiltration in the management of the renal complications of liver disease. Int J Artif Organs 1986;9:217–218.

195. Epstein M, Pérez GO, Bedoya LA, Molina R: Continuous arterio-venous ultrafiltration in cirrhotic patients with ascites or renal failure. Int J Artif Organs 1986;9:253–256.

196. Epstein M: The peritoneovenous shunt in the management of ascites and the hepatorenal syndrome. Gastroenterology 1982;82:790–799.

197. Pladson TR, Parrish RM: Hepatorenal syndrome: Recovery after peritoneovenous shunt. Arch Intern Med 1977;157:1248–1249.

198. Epstein M: The LeVeen shunt for ascites and hepatorenal syndrome. N Engl J Med 1980;302:628–630.

199. Linas SL, Schaffer JW, Moore EE, et al: Peritoneovenous shunt in the management of the hepatorenal syndrome. Kidney Int 1986;30:736–740.

200. Stanley MM, Ochi S, Lee KK, et al: Peritoneovenous shunting as compared with medical treatment in patients with alcoholic cirrhosis and massive ascites. New Engl J Med 1989;321:1632–1638.

201. Gonwa TA, Morris CA, Goldstein RM, et al: Long-term survival and renal function following liver transplantation in patients with and without hepatorenal syndrome—experience in 300 patients. Transplantation 1991;51:428–430 .

202. Wood RP, Ellis D, Starzl TE: The reversal of the hepatorenal syndrome in four pediatric patients following successful orthotopic liver transplantation. Ann Surg 1987;205:415–419.

203. Gunning TC, Brown MR, Swygert TH, et al: Perioperative renal function in patients undergoing orthotopic liver transplantation. Transplantation 1991;51: 422–427.

204. Conn H: Transjugular intrahepatic portal-systemic shunts: The state of the art. Hepatology 1993;17: 148–158.

205. Somberg K, Lake J, Tomlanovich S, et al: Transjugular intrahepatic portosystemic shunt for refractory ascites: Assessment of clinical and humoral response and renal function [abstract]. Gastroenterology 1994; 104:A998.

206. Lake J, Ring E, LaBerge J, et al: Transjugular intrahepatic portacaval stent shunt in patients with renal insufficiency. Transplant Proc 1992;25:1766–1767.

207. Orloff MJ: Effect of side-to-side portacaval shunt in intractable ascites, sodium excretion, and aldosterone metabolism in man. Am J Surg 1966;112:287–298.

208. Fevery J, Van Cutsem E, Nevens F, et al: Reversal of hepatorenal syndrome in four patients by peroral misoprostol (prostaglandin E_1 analogue) and albumin administration. J Hepatol 1990;11:153–158.

209. Quilley J, McGiff JC, Nasjletti A: Role of endoperoxides in arachidonic acid-induced vasoconstriction in the isolated perfused kidney of the rat. Br J Pharmacol 1989;96:111–116.

210. Cohn JN, Tristani FE, Khatri M: Renal vasodilator therapy in the hepatorenal syndrome. Med Ann DC 1970;39:1–7.

211. Bennett WM, Keeffe E, Melnyk C, et al: Response to dopamine hydrochloride in the hepatorenal syndrome. Arch Intern Med 1975;135:964–971.

212. Wilson JR: Dopamine in the hepatorenal syndrome. JAMA 1977;238:2719–2720.

213. Horisawa M, Reynolds TB: Exchange transfusion in hepatorenal syndrome with liver disease. Arch Intern Med 1976;136:1135–1137.

214. Begin R, Epstein M, Sackner MA, et al: Effects of water immersion to the neck on pulmonary circulation and tissue volume in man. J Appl Physiol 1976;40: 293–299.

215. Loutzenhiser RD, Epstein M: The effects of calcium antagonists on renal hemodynamic [editorial review]. Am J Physiol 1985;249:F619–F629.

216. Loutzenhiser RD, Epstein M, Horton C, Sonke P: Reversal of renal and smooth muscle actions of the thromboxane mimetic U-44069 by diltiazem. Am J Physiol 1986;250:F619–F626.

217. Epstein M: Calcium antagonists and renal protection: Current status and future perspectives. Arch Intern Med 1992;152:1573–1584.

218. Gornel DL, Lancestremere RG, Papper S, Lowenstein LM: Acute changes in renal excretion of water and solute in patients with Laennec's cirrhosis induced by the administration of the pressor amine, metaraminol. J Clin Invest 1962;41:594–605.

219. Cohn JN, Tristani FE, Khatri IM: Systemic vasoconstrictor and renal vasodilator effects of PLV-2 (octapressin) in man. Circulation 1968;38:151–157

220. Lenz K, Hortnagl H, Druml W, et al: Beneficial effect of 8-ornithin vasopressin on renal dysfunction in decompensated cirrhosis. Gut 1989;30:90–96.

Chapter 4

DERANGEMENTS OF ACID-BASE HOMEOSTASIS IN LIVER DISEASE

JAMES R. OSTER, M.D.
GUIDO O. PEREZ, M.D.

**Role of the Liver in Normal and Abnormal
  Acid-Base Balance**
  Ureagenesis
  Lactate Metabolism
  Ketogenesis
Abnormalities of Acid-Base Status in Liver Disease
  Acute Liver Disease
  Chronic Liver Disease
  Acid-base Abnormalities in Patients Undergoing
    Hepatic Transplantation

**Pathophysiology of Acid-Base Disorders
  Associated with Liver Disease**
  Respiratory Alkalosis
  Metabolic Alkalosis
  Metabolic Acidosis
Therapy
  Severe Metabolic Alkalosis
  Lactic Acidosis
Conclusion

There are several important associations between liver function and acid-base balance.[1,2] First, primarily because of its metabolism of organic acid anions,[3,4] the liver has an important influence on normal acid-base homeostasis. Second, under some conditions, such as ketoacidosis and certain types of lactic acidosis, the liver may become a major net producer of hydrogen ions (H^+). Third, patients with various types of liver disease often develop complicating acid-base disturbances. Finally, acid-base abnormalities may occur as complications of the management of liver disease, as when diuretic therapy results in metabolic alkalosis.[5,6] This chapter briefly reviews these associations, with emphasis on controversial and newer developments, including whether the process of hepatic ureagenesis serves a primary acid-base function and the syndrome of D-lactic acidosis. We have reviewed the acid-base disorders associated with gastrointestinal disease elsewhere.[7]

ROLE OF THE LIVER IN NORMAL AND ABNORMAL ACID-BASE BALANCE

According to the metabolic process analysis used by Halperin and associates, when a nutrient is metabolized to a product that contains a greater net anionic charge than the parent compound, there is a release of H^+.[3,4] Conversely, the formation of a compound with a net anionic charge less than that of the parent molecule consumes protons.[3] Thus, formation of urea from the positively charged NH_4 ion liberates protons, whereas the conversion of neutral (uncharged) amino acids to glucose and/or urea has no acid-base impact. Similarly, the conversion of the neutral sulphur-containing dietary amino acids methionine and cysteine into glucose, urea, and sulfate is accompanied by H^+ release.[3,4] Metabolism of the cationic (basic) amino acids arginine, lysine, and some histidine residues constitutes a proton-generating process. On the other hand, metabolism of dietary constituents, such as the anionic (dicarboxylic) amino acids glutamate and aspartate or the dietary organic anions acetate, lactate, malate, and citrate, removes H^+. In contrast, the hepatic metabolism of glutamine and asparagine is a metabolically neutral process because the liver rapidly converts the liberated ammonium to urea (a proton-releasing process[4]).

If the usual daily amount of protein (predominantly from meat) in the typical American diet is ingested, metabolic oxidation results in the production of about 1000–1400 mmol of ammonium.[3,4,8,9] The amount of bicarbonate generated, however, is somewhat less, because of the hepatic metabolism of cysteine, methionine, lysine, arginine, and histidine (offset in part by the removal of protons by virtue of hepatic metabolism of anionic amino acids and organic acid anions[3,4]). The net daily hepatic production of H^+ ions related to components of a typical diet appears to be approximately 60–70 mEq (about 30–40 mEq H^+ as H_2SO_4 and 30 mEq as $H^+ + HPO_2^=$).[3,4,8] A fundamental tenet of the conventional understanding of acid-base homeostasis is that the kidney's role is to offset the formation of these 60–70 mEq of H^+. This is accomplished to a lesser extent by excretion of titratable acid and more importantly by the renal tubules when they simultaneously generate NH_4 and HCO_3 ions from metabolism of glutamine extracted from peritubular blood and from the glomerular filtrate.[3,4] This NH_4 is excreted in the urine, whereas the HCO_3 enters the systemic circulation in the renal venous blood. Although urinary NH_4 excretion per se is no longer believed to remove protons from the body (accomplished by the oxidation of 2-oxoglutarate, the carbon skeleton of glutamine), it does obviate its hepatic metabolism, which would regenerate protons.[4]

Ureagenesis

According to the traditional concept, the teleologic role of hepatic ureagenesis (2 NH_4 + 2 $HCO_3 \rightarrow CO(NH_2)_2 + CO_2 + 3 H_2O$) is the removal of the ammonium ion.[3,4,8–12] More recently, some investigators have promulgated the viewpoint that an important role for ureagenesis is to modulate the regulation of HCO_3 consumption, i.e., to prevent metabolic alkalosis.[13–21] Figure 4.1 illustrates schematically the principal differences between the traditional and the alternative concepts of ureagenesis.[8]

From their study using an isolated perfused rat liver model, Häussinger and Gerok concluded that there is a pH-dependent component of urea synthesis, which they believe is predominantly modulated by mitochondrial carbonic anhydrase-catalyzed changes in the supply of HCO_3 for carbamoyl phosphate (and thus citrulline) synthesis.[16] According to this hypothesis, when acidosis inhibits ureagenesis relatively more NH_4 is converted into glutamine (rather than urea), which fosters acid-base homeostasis because glutamine synthesis does not result in proton formation.[21] Nissim et al. reported recently that ureagenesis in

isolated hepatocytes is limited by chronic metabolic acidosis, perhaps because of decreased formation of aspartate from glutamine.[15] On the other hand, the data obtained by Halperin and associates[8] indicate that, in the absence of changes in the exogenous nitrogen load, the rate of urea synthesis in experimental rats is neither augmented by HCO_3 administration nor attenuated by acid-loading. These observations support the classical view that the rate of hepatic ureagenesis is not primarily related to acid-base status but rather to the availability of excess nitrogen. This viewpoint is also supported by the recent findings of Boon et al.,[21a] who proposed that urea synthesis is directly regulated by neither pH nor HCO_3. The investigators observed that the reduced urea formation in rats with experimentally induced metabolic acidosis resulted from inhibition of amino acid transport across the hepatocyte plasma membrane rather than from inhibtion within the ornithine (urea) cycle. A primary role for the liver in acid-base homeostasis implies that inhibition of urea synthesis in acidosis must occur after the release of HCO_3 (whereas amino acid transport in hepatocytes occurs before release of HCO_3). Because this finding indicates that HCO_3 would not be spared in the liver, the data of Boon et al. militate against an important role for the ornithine cycle in regulation of acid-base homeostasis.

Although the possible role of ureagenesis in the regulation of acid-base balance remains controversial, we favor the conventional point of view.[3,4,8–12] In 1986 Walser[22] also concluded that "a significant role of the liver in the regulation of acid-base balance has yet to be demonstrated." Halperin and associates believe that because, taken in sum, protein is converted to urea plus CO_2, ureagenesis is essentially "a neutral process placing no demands on acid-base regulation."[8] They also believe that NH_4 and HCO_3 should not be considered as endproducts of protein (nitrogen) metabolism.[9,11] Although in humans both NH_4 and HCO_3 are produced from protein, NH_4 is generated first from glutamate via mitochondrial glutamate dehydrogenase.[23,24] Throughout the process, the intramitochondrial compartment may be considered to be at risk of severe acidosis,[9] not alkalosis, because bicarbonate is generated later in the hepatocyte cytoplasm.[9,12,23,24] If this is true, an increasing plasma HCO_3 subsequent to protein catabolism cannot be the driving force for ureagenesis because of an initial deficit in HCO_3 (due to HCO_3 consumption during the metabolism of NH_4). Furthermore, if the concentration of HCO_3 were an important modulator of ureagenesis via enhancement of the supply of carbamoyl phosphate, its level within mitochondria would have to be less than saturating (i.e., close to the range of the K_m for HCO_3, which is approximately 5 mmol/L[11]). Instead, its usual intramitochondrial concentration probably is considerably higher than that of plasma.[10,11] Thus, the level of HCO_3 in vivo cannot be rate-limiting for ureagenesis.[10]

Lactate Metabolism

The liver acts as the major organ disposing of lactate, by its metabolism either to glucose or to CO_2.[21,25] In normal humans, the daily rate of lactate and H^+ production has been estimated to be as high as approximately 20 mmol/kg body weight.[25] Hepatic metabolism is believed to account for about 50–70% of total lactate disposal.[21,25] A much greater percentage of lactate is converted to glucose than to CO_2 and H_2O. The overall pathway that involves conversion of glucose by glycolysis to lactate plus H^+ and reconversion of lactate (with concomitant utilization of H^+) is called the Cori cycle. Dysfunction of this cycle, with an increase in lactate formation, a decrease in its disposal, or both, may produce lactic acidosis.[12,25]

Whether increased lactate production or decreased lactate utilization is the predominant factor in causing most forms of lactic acidosis remains controversial. It is likely that in most instances both factors are important. When hepatic perfusion and intracellular pH are very low, the liver may become a source rather than a consumer of lactate and H^+. In fact, Halperin and Fields have speculated that in most acute situations, lactate formation from hepatic glycogen or exogenous glucose is required to produce life-threatening lactic acidosis.[26] Of interest is the report by Goodgame et al. of a patient with cancer who developed lactic acidosis during the infusion of hypertonic glucose.[27]

Patients with stable chronic liver disease exhibit marked impairment of lactate utilization.[28] Many causes of reduced hepatic lactate utilization may contribute to the induction of lactic acidosis,[29] including various unusual congenital enzymatic defects in gluconeogenesis and/or pyruvate oxidation,[30,31] defects of the respiratory

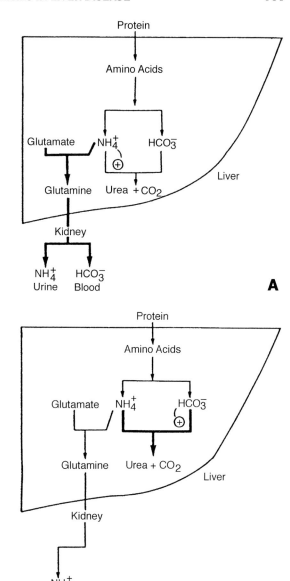

FIGURE 4.1. *A*, The traditional role of the liver and kidney in acid-base homeostasis. Synthesis of urea is not principally involved in acid-base balance. *B*, The alternative role of ureagenesis wherein its principal role is considered to be the consumption of bicarbonate. In both panels, the pH-sensitive steps and principal reactions are indicated by heavy arrows and heavy lines. (Reprinted with permission from Halperin ML, Chen CB, Cheema-Dhadli S, et al: Is urea formation regulated primarily by acid-base balance in vivo? Am J Physiol 1986;250: F605–F612.)

chain,[32] or, rarely, severe deficiency of thiamine (a cofactor for hepatic pyruvate dehydrogenase) in patients with beriberi. Medications and toxins may produce lactic acidosis by impairing hepatic and/or renal lactate utilization.[33–36] Such impairment may result from massive hepatic injury or from interference with gluconeogenesis,[35,36] as has been postulated with acetaminophen toxicity or possibly with the disordered mitochondrial electron transport attributed to chloramphenicol.[34]

Ketogenesis

Catabolism of any fuel may generate H+, but complete oxidation of fat and carbohydrate has no effect on acid-base status.[37] Ketogenesis represents the incomplete oxidation of fatty acids; every molecule of hydroxymethylglutaryl coenzyme A synthesized during ketogenesis results in a net production of one proton .[38] The acidosis associated with abnormal ketogenesis is due principally to depletion of extracellular HCO_3 by generated H+.

The mitochondria of hepatocytes are by far the most important source of ketones.[39,40] Ketone bodies are released by hepatocytes against a concentration gradient; the process is favored by an increase in plasma HCO_3.[41] Ketones are disposed of by oxidation of acetoacetate, primarily in kidney, muscle, and brain; unlike lactate and several other organic anions, acetoacetate is not oxidized to any important extent in the liver.[39,40] Ketoanion oxidation utilizes H+; this in effect represents HCO_3 generation.

Obviously, hepatic ketone overproduction may exert an adverse influence on acid-base homeostasis. Appreciable ketone production ordinarily occurs during the fasting state; except during prolonged starvation,[12,38–40] the effect on acid-base balance is trivial. Conversely, the various ketoacidotic states are associated with a markedly exaggerated rate of ketone formation and, apparently, a decreased rate of ketoanion utilization.[12,40] In prolonged starvation and diabetic ketoacidosis (DKA), ketogenesis may be accelerated to levels of the order of 1200 to 1600 mMol/1.73 m²/24hr or greater.[12,39,40] An important concept is that ketone production is limited by the rate of hepatic turnover of adenosine triphosphate (ATP).[39]

Insulin deficiency, either absolute or relative, appears to be the principal abnormality underlying all states of ketoacidosis.[42] It not only results in markedly enhanced rates of ketone production but also appears to impair peripheral ketone utilization.

It has been shown recently that the livers of rats with experimentally induced DKA are relatively resistant to inhibition of gluconeogenesis by acidosis.[21,43] Acetyl coenzyme A-modulated activation of pyruvate carboxylase with subsequent enhancement of gluconeogenesis,[21,43] which thereby protects hepatic intracellular pH, may explain this phenomenon. Indeed, Cohen postulated that, if hepatic lactate uptake matches ketone body production precisely, DKA can be considered as a form of peripheral lactic acidosis.[21]

Hood has shown that net ketogenesis is modulated in part by changes in systemic pH so that ketoacid production and/or release is reduced by acid-loading and enhanced by alkali-loading.[44] To some extent, it appears that this teleologically appropriate feedback regulatory system may not be confined only to ketoacids and under some circumstances may involve lactate (plus H+) production as well.[44]

ABNORMALITIES OF ACID-BASE STATUS IN LIVER DISEASE (Table 4.1)

Acute Liver Disease

Fulminant hepatic failure (FHF) is most commonly noted in patients with severe acute viral hepatitis, Reye's syndrome, or ingestion of toxins such as carbon tetrachloride and paracetamol.[45] In such conditions (as for all types of severe liver disease), the prevalence of alkalosis is great. In one study of 11 patients, 27 of 42 measurements revealed either respiratory, metabolic, or mixed respiratory-metabolic alkalosis.[46] Alkalemia (pH > 7.45) was present in 21 measurements. In another report, alkalemia was found in 49 of 65 observations in 28 patients with FHF.[47] Respiratory alkalosis predominated over metabolic alkalosis in a ratio of approximately 2:1. Serum lactate concentrations were often moderately elevated, but the levels did not correlate well with the type of acid-base disturbance; in the absence of circulatory failure, lactic acidosis was rare.[47] Frank lactic acidosis was reported in only 4 patients, of whom 3 had ingested toxic doses of paracetamol.[48]

The observations of Bihari and colleagues are somewhat different.[45,49] In contrast to the findings of several other workers, they observed an abnormal elevation of mixed venous lactate levels (mean = 5.0 mmol/L; range = 0.8–21.0 mmol/L) in 26 of 32 (81%) patients with FHF, the majority of whom had taken overdoses of paracetamol.[45]

Metabolic acidosis was present in 53% of patients, but pure respiratory alkalosis was observed in only 22% (31% had mixed metabolic acidosis-respiratory alkalosis). There was a statistically significant inverse correlation of blood lactate level with the oxygen extraction ratio.[45] The authors speculated that the lactic acidosis resulted, at least in part, from covert tissue hypoxia (secondary to arteriovenous shunting), despite apparently adequate blood pressure, blood flow, and systemic oxygenation.[45,49] Such findings suggest that whereas lactic acidosis associated with severe liver disease is usually considered to be an example of a type B (nonhypoxic) lactic acidosis, it may represent in part a mixture of type A and type B abnormalities (probably as do many other conditions).

Reye's syndrome is often associated with respiratory alkalosis or mixed respiratory-metabolic alkalosis, frequently severe; hyperventilation sometimes correlates well with blood ammonia levels. Metabolic acidosis (probably lactic acidosis) may coexist with respiratory alkalosis in fatal cases.

Of interest, preliminary data in only 3 patients raise the possibility that, in patients with acute hepatic failure waiting for hepatic transplantation, devascularization of the liver pending transplantation appeared to diminish the degree of metabolic acidosis.[50] The authors concluded that in this regard a totally failing liver may be more hazardous than no liver at all.

Chronic Liver Disease

The prevalence of acid-base abnormalities is high in patients with chronic liver disease.[1] In one study, blood gas values were normal in only a few of 32 patients,[51] and in two other studies the frequency of abnormalities among 70 and 55 patients was approximately 96%[52] and 50%,[53] respectively.

Alkalosis is the most common disturbance. In fact, of 884 separate measurements in 631 cirrhotic patients (11 studies), alkalosis was present in 71%.[1] Isolated respiratory alkalosis was approximately three times more common than isolated metabolic alkalosis (38% vs. 13%) and was the most frequent abnormality in seven of the 11 studies.[1] The degree of hyperventilation and resulting alkalemia is usually modest. In patients with metabolic alkalosis, the association between the presence of hypokalemia and metabolic alkalosis is very strong.

TABLE 4.1. Acid-Base Disorders Associated with Severe Liver Disease

Type of Liver Disease	Usual Acid-Base Disorder(s)
Acute liver disease	
Fulminant hepatic failure	Respiratory alkalosis
	Lactic acidosis (uncommon)
Chronic liver disease	
Alcoholic liver disease	Respiratory alkalosis
	Metabolic alkalosis of iatrogenic (e.g., diuretic) or extrarenal origin*
	Lactic acidosis, renal tubular acidosis (RTA) (rare)
	Drug-induced (in addition to diuretic-induced alkalosis):
	Hyperkalemic hyperchloremic acidosis— by potassium-sparing diuretic
	Hypokalemic hyperchloremic metabolic acidosis—by lactulose
	Respiratory acidosis (very rare)
Autoimmune liver disease	Same as for alcoholic liver disease, but RTA with hyperchloremic metabolic acidosis is not uncommon

* As discussed in the text, according to the controversial formulation espoused by Häussinger and associates,[17,18] liver failure may lead to metabolic acidosis directly by reduced ureagenesis—a process that consumers HCO_3.

Acidosis is far less prevalent than alkalosis (13% vs. 71% of the measurements reviewed); respiratory acidosis is rare (only 2% of measurements) and is often an ominous preterminal finding.[1] Acidosis occurs typically in the setting of hypotension or renal insufficiency and often is due to lactic acidosis. In the series of critically ill patients with liver disease reported by Kruse et al., frank lactic acidosis was found only in patients with clinical evidence of circulatory shock.[54] The mortality rate correlated closely with the peak lactate level. The more recent findings of Moreau et al. in cirrhotic patients with septic shock were similar, showing severe hepatic dysfunction, lactic acidosis, and a mortality rate of 100% in the intensive care unit.[55] Lactate levels were higher in patients with cirrhosis than in patients without cirrhosis.[55] Except in chronic autoimmune liver disease (vide infra), the complete form of distal renal tubular acidosis (RTA) is rare.

The acid-base status of patients with hepatic encephalopathy reflects the complexity of the abnormalities frequently found in patients with severe liver disease. This complexity is related to (1) the numerous biochemical perturbations that may occur, (2) the prevalence of multiorgan failure, and (3) the influence of therapeutic maneuvers. Nevertheless, the distribution of abnormalities is similar to that in portal cirrhosis, and alkalosis appears to be the most common disorder. For example, in one study, 13 of 19 encephalopathic patients were alkalemic (mean pH = 7.49) compared with only 5 of 20 patients without encephalopathy.[56] Respiratory alkalosis occurs more frequently than metabolic alkalosis, but diuretic therapy resulting in potassium depletion, vomiting, and massive blood transfusion may cause metabolic alkalosis. Metabolic acidosis is considerably less common and is usually attributable to lactic acidosis, renal insufficiency (when the hepatorenal syndrome supervenes), or, rarely, to RTA. Respiratory acidosis is extremely uncommon in patients with liver disease but may occur in the presence of extreme ascites and pleural effusions, when either severe hypokalemia or hypophosphatemia impairs respiratory muscle strength, or as a terminal event.

Mixed acid-base disturbances occur frequently in patients with chronic decompensated severe liver disease. Indeed, such disorders were observed in 10 of 14 studies reviewed.[1] By far the most common complex disturbance is respiratory plus metabolic alkalosis.

Acid-Base Abnormalities in Patients Undergoing Hepatic Transplantation

There are relatively few data regarding acid-base status during and following hepatic transplantation. In a report of 86 patients, Fortunato et al. found that prior to surgery 9 patients had metabolic acidosis and 12 had metabolic alkalosis;[57] 39 patients had moderate to severe metabolic acidosis (demonstrated in at least one blood sample) during surgery. Metabolic acidosis occurred immediately after reperfusion in 30 of 79 patients. During the first few days postoperatively, 56 patients (64%) demonstrated pronounced metabolic alkalosis in at least one blood sample, but the investigators did not believe that this finding was related to the large amounts of $NaHCO_3$ or of citrated blood administered intraoperatively. Of note, no patient with postoperative metabolic acidosis survived, but 38 of the 53 survivors manifested metabolic alkalosis in the postoperative period. Not surprisingly, the

acid-base changes associated with hepatic transplantation depend in part on surgical technique. Thus, for example, in their studies in dogs, Jakab et al. reported that the use of active venovenous bypass considerably decreases (without preventing) metabolic acidosis during the anhepatic phase.[58]

PATHOPHYSIOLOGY OF ACID-BASE DISORDERS ASSOCIATED WITH LIVER DISEASE

Respiratory Alkalosis

As mentioned, respiratory alkalosis is common in patients with severe clinical manifestations of liver disease; its pathogenesis remains uncertain. Hypoxemia, attributed to ventilation-perfusion imbalance secondary to ascites and to venous admixture due to portopulmonary or intrapulmonary shunts, has been suggested as a leading cause.[59,60] Nevertheless, the hypoxemia is frequently mild, and there may be no correlation between the degree of hypoxemia and the arterial blood P_{CO_2}.

Hyperammonemia has been considered a possible cause of hyperventilation.[56,61] Although a lack of correlation in some studies between plasma ammonia levels and the degree of alveolar ventilation casts some doubt on the importance of the association, both hyperammonemia and hyperventilation are common clinical manifestations in patients with Reye's syndrome[62] or ornithine carbamyl transferase deficiency.[63] Finally, increased plasma progesterone levels, hyponatremia, intracellular acidosis, and physical stimuli are other possible causes of hyperventilation in such patients.[64]

Metabolic Alkalosis

Metabolic alkalosis in patients with chronic liver disease almost always may be attributed to either extrarenal or iatrogenic factors.[5] Secondary aldosteronism probably causes metabolic alkalosis only rarely unless diuretics are administered. This is because, for the patient with peripheral edema and ascites, the delivery of sodium to the collecting tubule is limited by its reabsorption more proximally. Therefore, although the avidity for sodium reabsorption in the cortical collecting tubule is high, limited availability of the sodium ion attenuates the voltage-related enhancement of

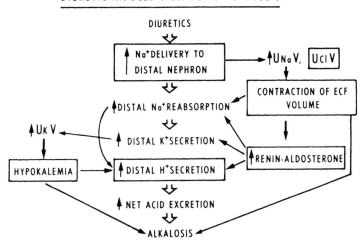

FIGURE 4.2. The pathogenesis of diuretic-induced metabolic alkalosis. The interrelationship between increased delivery of sodium to the distal nephron (and its subsequent reabsorption there) and the resultant facilitation of distal potassium and H^+ secretion is emphasized. The putative roles of potassium depletion, volume contraction, and hyperaldosteronism are also indicated. (Reprinted with permission from Oster JR: The binge-purge syndrome: A common albeit unappreciated cause of acid-base and fluid-electrolyte disturbances. South Med J 1987;80:58–67.)

potassium and H^+ secretion resulting from sodium reabsorption (vide infra).[5] Thus, alkalosis and potassium depletion[65] of renal origin are rare in untreated patients with decompensated cirrhosis. Once diuretics are given, however, a higher rate of sodium delivery to the most distal nephron is ensured, and renal potassium wasting, hypokalemia, and hypochloremic alkalosis often ensue (Fig. 4.2). The mechanism of increased acid excretion in this setting in part may involve enhanced activity of H-ATPase or H-K-ATPase, with stimulation of the former enzyme by aldosterone excess and of the latter by hypokalemia.[66,67] Of course, in addition to diuretic administration, the cause of metabolic alkalosis in decompensated cirrhosis may be of extrarenal origin (e.g., vomiting).

Alkalosis of any cause tends to be maintained (bicarbonaturia prevented) not only by a decrease in effective plasma volume but also by mineralocorticoid excess, hypokalemia, chloride deficiency, and reduction in glomerular filtration rate.[5,6]

Because the cause of metabolic alkalosis in cirrhotic patients is almost always either extrarenal or iatrogenic, therapy is usually rather straightforward.[5] Thus, if it is due to vomiting or chronic diarrhea, the principal effort should be to correct these processes. If the alkalosis relates to diuretics or to mineralocorticoid administration, the physician should try, unless it is inappropriate,

to reduce the dose of such agents or to stop them. In terms of specific therapy, reversal of hypokalemia with potassium chloride, or of frank volume contraction with sodium chloride, tends to correct the alkalosis. The therapeutic administration of acetazolamide (an inhibitor of carbonic anhydrase) to patients with severe liver disease involves the risk of inducing hepatic encephalopathy.[1]

Metabolic Acidosis

Lactic Acidosis

Despite the importance of the liver in lactate metabolism, frank lactic acidosis is not common in patients with chronic liver disease. Basal lactate levels are usually either within normal limits or only modestly increased, that is, usually less than 4 mmol/L. When lactic acidosis occurs, it usually is in association with additional factors, such as sepsis, shock, bleeding, and decreased blood flow, that either further depress hepatic or renal lactate utilization or increase lactate generation.[5] Other potential factors include ethanol abuse, medications such as phenformin, fructose (ethanol, fructose, and biguanides cause a reduction of the hepatic redox state), or sorbitol; hypotension; hyperventilation; and possibly acidemia (which reduces hepatic lactate uptake).

Although the role of hyperventilation is controversial, several lines of evidence suggest that it may be important in the pathogenesis of lactic acidosis. First, functional exclusion of the liver may transform primary respiratory alkalosis into progressive and irreversible lactic acidosis.[68] Second, an apparent progressive transformation of primary respiratory alkalosis to severe lactic acidosis has been reported in at least 4 patients, including 2 with hepatic metastases (in whom marginal hepatic reserve also may have played a role).[69] The authors of one carefully performed study stressed that PCO_2 reduction was the common denominator in almost all of their patients with lactic acidosis.[70] Hyperventilation may produce hyperlactatemia by enhancement of glycolysis through activation of the pH-dependent enzyme phosphofructokinase, which is stimulated by alkalemia. Additionally, hypocapnia has been shown to result in a reduction of hepatic blood flow. Despite the above-mentioned considerations, hyperventilation in both humans and experimental animals is usually associated with only small increases in plasma lactate.

Finally, the entity of D-lactic acidosis is a good (but rare) example of how the putative inability of the liver (or kidney) to consume the D-isomer of lactate may cause or contribute to severe lactic acidosis. D-lactic acidosis is an uncommon metabolic disturbance that has been reported only recently in humans.[71–74] It occurs in patients with a short bowel and/or blind loop syndrome, typically several months or a few years subsequent to a jejunoileostomy for treatment of massive obesity. Patients suffer from poorly understood neurologic abnormalities (possibly due to various bacteria-produced aldehydes and alcohols[74a]), including ataxia, weakness, slurred speech, somnolence, memory loss, and confusion, in association with metabolic acidosis that is often, but not necessarily, of the high anion gap type.[71,72]

Normally, carbohydrate undergoes complete digestion in a relatively sterile part of the gastrointestinal tract. In patients with D-lactic acidosis, however, incompletely digested carbohydrate apparently undergoes fermentation by anaerobic gram-positive bacteria, either in the colon or in the blind loop itself. These bacteria are capable of producing both L-lactic acid (the usual form of lactic acid in humans and other mammals) and D-lactic acid. Some, but not all, investigators claim that D-lactic acid is slowly metabolized in mammals[74]; if so, it may be the principal cause of the

acidosis. By providing substrate for the responsible bacteria, carbohydrate loading appears to exacerbate the condition.[73] Whether liver disease predisposes to or unmasks instances of D-lactic acidosis is unknown.

The preliminary diagnosis of D-lactic acidosis must be based on the clinical setting. Routine clinical laboratory studies detect only L-lactate. Because the level of L-lactate is not elevated in patients with this syndrome, the total lactate level will be erroneously reported as normal. Mass spectrometry permits the diagnosis because it measures the level of total lactate (i.e., D-lactate plus L-lactate). The definitive tests include specific enzymatic assay for D-lactate and analyses using nuclear magnetic resonance spectroscopy.[73] Treatment of D-lactic acidosis involves either dietary restriction of carbohydrate, temporary fasting with hyperalimentation, oral administration of an appropriate broad-spectrum antibiotic such as vancomycin, or taking down of the jejunoileostomy.[71–74]

In summary, although severe lactic acidosis complicates the terminal course of only a small percentage of patients with liver disease, it is important because of its ominous prognosis. Lactic acidosis generally occurs in the presence of severe hepatic damage and in conjunction with other metabolic insults. Owing to multiple influences on lactate homeostasis, which increase the formation of lactate and impede its disposal, persistent hyperventilation may play a pivotal pathogenic role in some patients. Patients with D-lactic acidosis need not have liver disease; it is alleged that the normal liver is able to metabolize only at a slow rate the D-lactate produced by certain abnormally proliferating intestinal anaerobic bacteria.

Renal Tubular Acidosis

Renal tubular acidosis (RTA) includes a group of clinical syndromes in which one of the principal functions of the renal acidification process is impaired disproportionately to any decrement of the glomerular filtration rate. Renal acidification may be considered to subsume the processes of bicarbonate reabsorption, formation of urine of appropriately low pH, and acid excretion. Recently, great emphasis has been placed on the important roles of two proton ATPases (an H-ATPase and an H-K-ATPase), both in normal terminal nephron acidification and in development of various types of distal RTA.[67,75,76] The most important diagnostic feature of RTA is an abnormally low rate of production and/or urinary excretion of NH_4.[77] Indeed, by definition NH_4 excretion is low in every type of distal RTA.[77,78] Even in instances of proximal RTA, wherein the steady state urine pH may be appropriately low, NH_4 excretion is inappropriately reduced in view of the fact that the patient is acidotic.[79] The reader if referred to current reviews of normal and abnormal renal ammonia metabolism and RTA for further information.[76–83]

RTA in Patients with Autoimmune Liver Disease. RTA has been described in association with both autoimmune liver disease (ALD) and ethanol-induced chronic liver disease; it is a common and sometimes important feature of patients with various types of chronic ALD, e.g., chronic active hepatitis (CAH), primary biliary cirrhosis (PBC), and cryptogenic cirrhosis.[1] Most patients with RTA and ALD have either chronic PBC or CAH.[1] The association of RTA and ALD seems to be strongest in patients with PBC[84] and appears to be weaker in cryptogenic cirrhosis. Almost always, the acidification defect appears to be of the distal (type 1) form. Nevertheless, "maximal" tubular bicarbonate reabsorption may also be decreased, raising the possibility of an additional abnormality in the proximal tubule. Puig et al.[85] described 3 patients with CAH and an isolated proximal tubular acidifying defect, possibly on the basis of somewhat incomplete data.[85] Multiple proximal defects characteristic of the Fanconi syndrome do not occur.

The clinical manifestations of patients with RTA and ALD are similar to those of patients with RTA in the absence of liver disease. Very rarely, patients with CAH complicated by distal RTA may present with hypokalemic paralysis, which in one report resulted in respiratory failure.[86] Evidence for hepatic dysfunction and vasculitic manifestations is common. No correlation has been found between the severity of hepatic disease and the presence or absence of RTA. As expected, many of the patients are young, and most are female. Owing to hypokalemia, acidemia, and, less commonly, osteomalacia, patients may complain of polydipsia, polyuria, muscular weakness, and bone pain. Nephrocalcinosis and nephrolithiasis are infrequent. The incomplete syndrome of distal RTA is far more common than spontaneous hyperchloremic acidosis.[1] Although the pathogenesis of RTA in ALD is uncertain, cell-mediated immunologic perturbations appear to

play a major role in mediating not only the hepatic lesions but also the renal tubular defects.[1]

In PBC as well as Wilson's disease, copper-induced tubular lesions appear to play an important pathogenic role.[84] Significantly higher plasma and urinary copper levels have been observed in patients with CAH and RTA and correlated with the minimal urinary pH after an ammonium chloride load. Perhaps failure of biliary excretion of copper leads to abnormal urine and plasma levels and to deposition of copper in the renal tubules.[84] Of interest, Izumi et al. reported that patients with biliary cirrhosis may manifest hypouricemia (another indicator of renal tubular damage) resulting from increased renal urate clearance.[87] The underlying mechanism in a single carefully studied patient with distal RTA and hypouricemia appeared to be decreased postsecretory reabsorption of urate (the same defect believed to account for the hypouricemia in Wilson's disease).

Alcoholic Cirrhosis. The frequency and pathogenesis of RTA in alcoholic cirrhosis differs to a great extent from that in patients with ALD. In 15 reports involving a total of 255 patients, there were 98 instances (38%) of incomplete distal RTA, but only 8 instances of the complete syndrome.[1] Thus, the finding of a low plasma HCO_3, together with an elevated plasma Cl should raise the suspicion of an acid-base disorder other than RTA, such as secretory diarrhea[6] or respiratory alkalosis.[88] Some investigators,[88] but not others, believe that RTA is somewhat more likely in patients with severe liver disease. The tubular defect does not appear to be related to the renal or intrarenal hemodynamic alterations[89] Ascites and peripheral edema are commonly noted in patients with RTA, but abnormal acidification may occur in the absence of such findings. In one study, 2 of 9 patients with incomplete RTA had no ascites, and 5 of the 9 were without edema[90] In another study, a lower minimal urine pH after NH_4Cl was observed in patients without ascites than in patients with ascites.[91] There is no evidence of an association between hyperglobulinemia and RTA in cirrhotic patients.

A recent report[92] demonstrating that 28% of 61 alcoholic patients without cirrhosis had abnormal renal acidification (which disappeared almost completely after 4 weeks of abstinence from ethanol) is of considerable interest and importance. This observation indicates that recent alcohol abuse, not controlled for in the above-mentioned studies, may account for some instances of abnormal renal acidification previously attributed to cirrhosis.

The question of whether RTA increases the risk of encephalopathy remains unanswered. Either the acidosis or the hypokalemia associated with RTA might facilitate renal ammoniagenesis; the increased urine pH might divert some of this "extra" ammonia into the renal venous blood. To our knowledge, however, only one group of investigators reported a correlation between RTA and a history of repeated episodes of hepatic encephalopathy.[93]

Despite some data to the contrary,[88] decreased delivery of sodium to the most distal nephron appears to play an important pathogenic role in the impaired acidification of patients with alcoholic cirrhosis. Several investigators have observed intense avidity for sodium reabsorption in patients with RTA. Furthermore, the administration of diuretics, sodium sulfate, or sodium phosphate, which increases distal sodium delivery, often results in a marked lowering of urine pH. Several lines of evidence link distal sodium delivery and reabsorption to H^+ secretion.[94] Renal acidification is less efficient in the presence of sodium depletion, and a modest sodium deficiency impairs the ability to lower urine pH maximally. In several varieties of incomplete distal RTA, increasing sodium delivery with sodium sulfate leads to reduction of urine pH. Finally, several studies have linked the impaired acidification induced by amiloride and lithium to defective distal tubular sodium reabsorption[84,85] (voltage-dependent RTA[94]). Nevertheless, whether decreased distal delivery of sodium is the sole cause of abnormal acidification in alcoholic cirrhosis or a factor that merely unmasks another underlying defect remains unknown. Although potassium deficiency may interfere with renal acidification, enough normokalemic cirrhotic patients with RTA have been described to eliminate potassium deficiency as the major cause of the defect.

In summary, an incomplete syndrome of distal RTA is a common complication of alcoholic liver disease. A low distal delivery of sodium, possibly by limiting the transtubular potential difference, might be partially responsible. The clinical importance of this incomplete RTA remains unknown. A small number of patients appear to have clinically important renal potassium wasting as a related or associated defect; perhaps by facilitating renal ammoniagenesis, this defect

may predispose to the development of hepatic encephalopathy.

Respiratory Acidosis

Although respiratory acidosis is extremely uncommon in patients with liver disease, it may occur in the presence of severe restrictive lung disease secondary to massive ascites and/or pleural effusions. In addition, respiratory muscle weakness secondary to hypokalemia or hypophosphatemia and respiratory center depression from narcotics and other medications usually detoxified by the liver may lead to acute respiratory failure.

THERAPY

A detailed discussion of therapy is beyond the scope of this chapter. Furthermore, for the most part, the treatment of acid-base disorders in patients with liver disease does not differ substantially from that for the same disturbances in other types of patients. This section, therefore, comments briefly on acid-base abnormalities for which the presence of underlying liver disease sometimes mandates special considerations or for which therapy is controversial.

Severe Metabolic Alkalosis

By definition, the mainstay of therapy for the saline-responsive type of metabolic alkalosis is administration of isotonic saline. For the patient with severe liver disease and associated hypoalbuminemia, clinicians must be alert to the possibility of markedly exacerbating edema and ascites by overenthusiastic infusion of saline. Rarely, one might consider temporarily correcting any decrease in effective extracellular fluid volume with a colloid in the form of salt-poor albumin. Another related caveat regarding the therapy of life-threatening metabolic alkalosis is in order. The administration of either the carbonic anhydrase-inhibiting diuretic acetazolamide or ammonium chloride is occasionally called for in the patient with severe alkalemia. Both agents, however, are contraindicated in the presence of end-stage liver disease because both may induce hyperammonemia and hepatic encephalopathy. According to conventional thinking, acetazolamide does so because the marked increase in urine pH retards the urinary excretion of ammonium, and ammonium chloride raises the blood ammonia level directly.[1] On the other hand, in accordance with their controversial concept of the role of the liver in acid-base homeostasis discussed earlier, Häussinger and colleagues believe that the hyperammonemic effect of carbonic anhydrase inhibition in patients with advanced liver disease is attributable to its suppression of ureagenesis in the face of the diminished capacity of perivenous hepatic scavenger cells to synthesize glutamine.[17]

Lactic Acidosis

Recently, there has been considerable controversy regarding the appropriate therapy for severe lactic acidosis.[95–98] Unfortunately, no form of therapy has much success, and mortality is extremely high, particularly in patients with liver failure ,in whom lactic acidosis often represents a preterminal finding. The controversy revolves around the value vs. the risk of giving large amounts of HCO_3.[95–98] Although studies in experimental animals have demonstrated that HCO_3 fails to improve the dismal prognosis,[97] possibly because it may exacerbate intracellular acidosis, Narins and Cohen[97] have argued that the administration of alkali should remain an important component of therapy.

Determination of whether the alkalinizing agent Carbicarb (an experimental buffer composed of sodium bicarbonate and disodium carbonate that avoids the generation of CO_2[98]) will prove useful in patients with lactic acidosis (with or without liver disease) remains under investigation. In rats rendered acidotic with NH_4Cl, alkalinization therapy with $NaHCO_3$ caused increases in P_{CO_2}, transient severe decrements in blood pressure and cardiac output, and statistically significant transient decreases in hepatic intracellular pH, whereas alkalinization of the extracellular fluid with Carbicarb was associated with no major changes in mean blood pressure, cardiac output, or P_{CO_2}.[98] Furthermore, Carbicarb increased rather than decreased intrahepatocyte pH. In some other animal models, such encouraging results have not been observed.

Present data are insufficient to judge whether dichloroacetate (DCA—an unmarketed experimental intravenous medication) will prove to be helpful in the management of life-threatening lactic acidosis in patients with severe liver disease. DCA exerts diverse effects on intermediary metabolism. It facilitates the metabolism of pyruvate

and lactate at least in part by inhibiting PDH kinase and thereby stimulating the activity of the PDH enzyme complex.[99] Aside from its metabolic effects, evidence suggests that it improves cardiac output and systemic hemodynamics, probably by facilitating myocardial metabolism of carbohydrate and lactate.[100] Thus, DCA is believed to decrease net lactate production by directly facilitating aerobic lactate metabolism as well as by increasing the perfusion and oxygenation of peripheral tissues.[99] Despite theoretical considerations and the results of initial studies, DCA has proved to be beneficial not only in type B lactic acidosis but also in patients and experimental animals with type A lactic acidosis.[100,101] DCA has been reported to decrease lactate production in experimental animals given biguanides[102] and to reduce fructose-induced hyperlactatemia in galactosamine-treated rats.[103] In rats with experimental DKA, DCA decreases the net release of lactate, pyruvate, and alanine from extrasplanchnic tissues and inhibits ketogenesis.[104]

In a study comparing the effects of DCA and NaCl in dogs with experimentally induced hypoxic lactic acidosis, Graf et al. demonstrated an increase in hepatic lactate extraction, a decrease in tissue lactate levels in liver and skeletal muscle, and an increase in muscle intracellular pH only in DCA-treated animals.[101]

SUMMARY

The liver has an important role in acid-base metabolism both in the normal state and in many acid-base disorders. Specifically, hepatic metabolism of amino acids, lactate, ketoanions, and ammonium is associated with important changes in either H^+ generation or utilization. In patients with liver disease, respiratory and metabolic alkalosis are the most prevalent acid-base disorders. Metabolic acidosis may be due to lactic acidosis or RTA. Respiratory acidosis is rare.

REFERENCES

1. Oster JR: Acid-base homeostasis and liver disease. In Epstein M (ed): The Kidney in Liver Disease, 2nd ed. New York: Elsevier Science Publishing Co., 1983; 147–182.
2. Oster JR, Perez GO: Acid-base disturbances in liver disease. J Hepatol 1986; 2:299–306.
3. Halperin ML, Jungas RL: The metabolic production and renal disposal of hydrogen ions: An examination of the biochemical processes. Kidney Int 1983;24: 709–713.

4. Halperin ML, Kamel KS, Ethier JH, et al: Biochemistry and physiology of ammonium excretion. In Seldin DW, Giebisch G (eds): The Kidney: Physiology and Pathophysiology, 2nd ed. New York: Raven Press, 1992;2645–2679.

5. Oster JR, Vaamonde CA: Metabolic alkalosis. In Massry SG, Glassock RJ (eds): Textbook of Nephrology. Baltimore: Williams & Wilkins, 1983;3.130–3.138.

6. Luke RG, Galla JH: Metabolic alkalosis. In Glassock RJ (ed): Current Therapy in Nephrology and Hypertension, 3rd ed. St. Louis: Mosby, 1992;45–50.

7. Perez GO, Oster JR, Rogers A: Acid-base disturbances in gastrointestinal disease. Digest Dis Sci 32:1987; 1033–1043.

8. Halperin ML, Chen CB, Cheema-Dhadli S, et al: Is urea formation regulated primarily by acid-base balance in vivo? Am J Physiol 1986;250:F605–F612.

9. Jungas RL, Halperin ML, Brosnan JT: Quantitative analysis of amino acid oxidation and related gluconeogenesis in humans. Physiol Rev 1992;72:419–448.

10. Cheema-Dhadli S, Jungas RL, Halperin ML: Regulation of urea synthesis by acid-base balance in vivo: Role of NH_3 concentration. Am J Physiol 1987;F221–F225.

11. Halperin ML, Jungas RL, Cheema-Dhadli S, Brosnan JT: Disposal of the daily acid load: An integrated function of the liver, lungs and kidneys. Trends Biochem Sci 1987;197–199.

12. Halperin ML, Rolleston FS: Biochemical Detective Stories: A Problem-based Approach to Clinical Cases. Burlington, NC: Neil Patterson, 1990.

13. Atkinson DE, Bourke E: Metabolic aspects of the regulation of systemic pH. Am J Physiol 1987;252:F947–F956.

14. Bean ES, Atkinson DE: Regulation of the rate of urea synthesis in liver by extracellular pH: A major factor in pH homeostasis in mammals. J Biol Chem 1984;259: 1552–1559.

15. Nissim I, Cattano C, Lin Z, Nissim I: Acid-base regulation of hepatic glutamine metabolism and ureagenesis: Study with ^{15}N. J Am Soc Nephrol 1992;3:1416–1427.

16. Häussinger D, Gerok W: Hepatic urea synthesis and pH regulation: Role of CO_2, HCO_3^-, pH and the activity of carbonic anhydrase. Eur J Biochem 1985;152:381–386.

17. Häussinger D: Liver and systemic pH- regulation. Zeitschr Gastroenterol 1992;30:147–150.

18. Häussinger D, Steeb R, Gerok W: Metabolic alkalosis as driving force for urea synthesis in liver disease: Pathogenetic model and therapeutic implications. Clin Invest 1992;70:411–415.

19. Almond MK, Flynn G, Smith A, Cohen RD: The liver as an organ of acid-base regulation: The role of glutamine synthesis. Clin Sci 1989;77(Suppl 21):37P.

20. Häussinger D, Steeb R, Gerok W: Ammonium and bicarbonate homeostasis in chronic liver disease. Klin Wochenschr 1990;68:175–182.

21. Cohen RD: Roles of the liver and kidney in acid-base regulation and its disorders. Br J Anaesth 1991;67: 154–164.

21a. Boon L, Blommaart PJE, Meijer AJ, et al: Acute acidosis inhibits liver amino acid transport: No primary role for the urea cycle in acid-base balance. Am J Physiol 1994; 267:F1015–F1020.

22. Walser M: Roles of urea production, ammonium excretion, and amino acid oxidation in acid-base balance. Am J Physiol 1986;250:F181–F188.

23. Stryer L: Biochemistry. San Francisco: W.H. Freeman and Company, 1975 432–455.

24. Lehninger AL: Biochemistry, 2nd ed. New York: Worth Publishers, 1975;579–586.

25. Kreisberg RA: Lactate homeostasis and lactic acidosis. Ann Intern Med 1980;92:227–237.

26. Halperin ML, Fields ALA: Review: Lactic acidosis—emphasis on the carbon precursors and buffering of the acid load. Am J Med Sci 1985; 289:154–159.

27. Goodgame JT, Pizzo P, Brennam MF: Iatrogenic lactic acidosis. Association with hypertonic glucose administration in a patient with cancer. Cancer 1978;42: 800–803.

28. Woll PJ, Record CO: Lactate elimination in man: Effects of lactate concentration and hepatic dysfunction. Eur J Clin Invest 1979;9:397–404.

29. Madias NE: (principal discussant): Lactic acidosis. Kidney Int. 1986;29:752–774.

30. Matsuo M, Ookita K, Takemine H, et al: Fatal case of pyruvate dehydrogenase deficiency. Acta Paediatr Scand 1985;74:140–142.

31. Asano K, Miyamoto I, Matsushita T, et al: Succinic acidemia: A new syndrome of organic acidemia associated with congenital lactic acidosis and decreased NADH-cytochrome c reductase activity. Clin Chim Acta 1988;173:305–312.

32. Parrot-Rouland F, Carre M, Lamirau T, et al: Fatal neonatal hepatocellular deficiency with lactic acidosis: A defect of the respiratory chain. J Inher Metab Dis 1991;14:289–292.

33. Krapf R, Schaffner T, Iten PX: Abuse of germanium associated with fatal lactic acidosis. Nephron 1992; 62:351–356.

34. Evans LS, Kleiman MB: Acidosis as a presenting feature of chloramphenicol toxicity. J Pediatr 1986;108: 475–477.

35. Zabrodski RM: Anion gap acidosis with hypoglycemia in acetaminophen toxicity. Ann Emer Med 1984;13: 956–959.

36. Gray TA, Buckley BM, Vale JA: Hyperlactatemia and metabolic acidosis following paracetamol overdose. Q J Med 1987;65:811–821.

37. Owen OE, Schramm JL: Lipid metabolism during starvation: Hepatic energy balance and ketogenesis. Biochem Soc Trans 1981;9:342–344.

38. Owen OE, Caprio S, Reichard GA Jr, et al: Ketosis of starvation: A revisit and new perspectives. Clin Endocrinol Metab 1983;12:359–379.

39. Halperin ML, Cheema-Dhadli S: Renal and hepatic aspects of ketoacidosis: A quantitative analysis based on energy turnover. Diabetes/Metab Rev 1989;5:321–336.

40. Oster JR, Epstein M: Acid-base aspects of ketoacidosis. Am J Nephrol 1984;4:137–151.

41. Fafournoux P, Demigné C, Rémésy C: Mechanisms involved in ketone body release by rat liver cells: Influence of pH and bicarbonate. Am J Physiol 1987;252:G200–G208.

42. Foster DW, McGarry JD: The metabolic derangement and treatment of diabetic ketoacidosis. N Engl J Med 1983;309:159–169.

43. Beech JS, Williams SR, Cohen RD, Iles RA: Gluconeogenesis and the protection of hepatic intracellular pH during diabetic ketoacidosis in the rat. Biochem J 1989;263:737–744.

44. Hood VL, Tannen RL: pH control of lactic acid and keto acid production: A mechanism of acid-base regulation. Miner Electrolyte Metab 1983;9:317–325.

45. Bihari D, Gimson AES, Lindridge J, William R: Lactic acidosis in fulminant hepatic failure: Some aspects of pathogenesis and prognosis. J Hepatol 1985;1:405–416.

46. Kosaka Y, Tanaka K, Sawa H, et al: Acid-base disturbance in patients with fulminant hepatic failure. Gastroenterol Jpn 1979;14:24-30.

47. Record CO, Iles RA, Cohen RD, Williams R: Acid-base and metabolic disturbances in fulminant hepatic failure. Gut 1975;16:144–449.

48. Proudfoot AT, Wright N: Acute paracetamol poisoning. Br Med J 1970;3:557–558.

49. Bihari D, Gimson AES, Waterson M, Williams R: Tissue hypoxia during fulminant hepatic failure. Crit Care Med 1985;13:1034–1039.

50. Husberg BA, Goldstein RM, Klintman GB, et al: A totally failing liver may be more harmful than no liver at all: Three cases of total hepatic devascularization in preparation for emergency liver transplantation. Transplant Proc 1991;23:1533–1535.

51. Kardel T, Rasmussen SN: Blood gases and acid-base disturbances of arterial blood in chronic liver diseases. Scand J Clin Lab Invest 1973;31:307–309.

52. Mincev M, Valkov J. Acid-base balance of the blood in patients with hepatic cirrhosis. Folia Med 1971;13:298–303.

53. Prytz H, Thomsen AC: Acid-base status in liver cirrhosis. Disturbances in stable, terminal and portal-caval shunted patients. Scand J Gastroenterol 1976;11:249–256.

54. Kruse JA, Zaidi SAJ, Carlson RW: Significance of blood lactate levels in critically ill patients with liver disease. Am J Med 1987;83:77–82.

55. Moreau R, Hadengue A, Soupison T, et al: Septic shock in patients with cirrhosis: Hemodynamic and metabolic characteristics and intensive care unit outcome. Crit Care Med 1992;20:746–750.

56. Casey TH, Summerskill WHJ, Bickford RG, Rosevear JW: Body and serum potassium in liver disease. II. Relationships to arterial ammonia, blood pH, and hepatic coma. Gastroenterology 1965;48:208–215.

57. Fortunato FL Jr, Kang Y, Aggarwal S, et al: Acid-base status during and after orthotopic liver transplantation. Transplant Proc 1987;9:59-60.

58. Jakab F, Závodszky Z, Sugár I, et al: Changes in pH and acid-base equilibrium during experimental liver transplantation by active and passive veno-venous bypass. Acta Chir Hung 1988;29:107–116.

59. Williams MH Jr: Hypoxemia due to venous admixture in cirrhosis of the liver. J Appl Physiol 1960;33:71–74.

60. Karetzky MS, Mithoefer JC: The cause of hyperventilation and arterial hypoxemia in patients with cirrhosis of the liver. Am J Med Sci 1967;254:797–804.

61. Wichser J, Kazemi H: Ammonia and ventilation: Site and mechanism of action. Respir Physiol 1974;20:393–406.

62. Shannon DC, De Long R, Bercu B, et al: Studies on the pathophysiology of encephalopathy in Reye's syndrome: Hyperammonemia in Reyes's syndrome. Pediatrics 1975;56:999–1004.

63. Campbell AGM, Rosenberg LE, Snodgrass PJ, Nuzum CT: Ornithine transcarbamylase deficiency: A cause of lethal neonatal hyperammonemia in males. N Engl J Med 1973;288:1–6.

64. Kaehny WD: Respiratory acid-base disorders. Med Clin North Am 1983;67:915–928.

65. Perez GO, Oster JR: Altered potassium metabolism in liver disease. In Epstein M (ed): The Kidney in Liver Disease, 2nd ed. New York: Elsevier Science Publishing Co., 1983;183–201.

66. Eiam-Ong S, Lonis B, Kurtzman NA, Sabatini S: The biochemical basis of hypokalemic metabolic alkalosis. Trans Assoc Am Physicians 1992;105:157–164.

67. Eiam-Ong S, Kurtzman NA, Sabatini S: Effect of furosemide-induced metabolic alkalosis on renal transport enzymes. Kidney Int 1993;43:1015–1020.

68. Perret CL, Poli S, Enrico JF: Lactic acidosis and liver damage. Helv Med Acta 1969/1970;35:377–406.

69. Spechler SJ, Esposito AL, Koff RS, Hong WK: Lactic acidosis in oat cell carcinoma with extensive hepatic metastases. Arch Intern Med 1978;138:1663–1664.

70. Mulhausen R, Eichenholz A, Blumentals A: Acid-base disturbances in patients with cirrhosis of the liver. Medicine 1967;46:185–189.

71. Oh M, Phelps KR, Traube M, et al: D-lactic acidosis in a man with a short-bowel syndrome. N Engl J Med 1979;301:249–252.

72. Stolberg L, Rolfe R, Gitilin N, et al: D-lactic acidosis due to abnormal gut flora. Diagnosis and treatment of two cases. N Engl J Med 1982;306:1344–1348.

73. Ramakrisham T, Stokes P: Beneficial effects of fasting and low carbohydrate diet in D-lactic acidosis associated with short-bowel syndrome. J Parenteral Enteral Nutr 1985;9:361–363.

74. Cammack R: Assay, purification and properties of mammalian D-2 hydroxy acid dehydrogenase. Biochem J 1969;115:55–64.

74a. Halperin ML: Personal communication, 1994.

75. Eiam-Ong S, Kurtzman NA, Sabatini S: Regulation of collecting tubule adenosine triphosphatases by aldosterone and potassium. J Clin Invest 1993;91:2385–2392.

76. Sabatini S, Kurtzman NA: Pathophysiology of the renal tubular acidoses. Semin Nephrol 1991;11:202–211.

77. Carlisle EJF, Donnelly SM, Halperin ML: Renal tubular acidosis (RTA): Recognize The Ammonium defect and pHorget the urine pH. Pediatr Nephrol 1991;5:242–248.

78. DuBose TD Jr, Good DW, Hamm LL, Wall SM: Ammonium transport in the kidney: New physiological concepts and their clinical implications. J Am Soc Nephrol 1991;1:1193–1203.

79. Caruana RJ, Buckalew VM Jr: The syndrome of distal (type 1) renal tubular acidosis: Clinical and laboratory findings in 58 cases. Medicine 1988;67:84–99.

80. Rocher LL, Tannen RL: The clinical spectrum of renal tubular acidosis. Ann Rev Med 1986;37:319–331.

81. Goldstein MG, Levin A: Insights derived from the urine in acid-base disturbances. KF Nephrol Lett 1989;6:19–26.

82. Kurtz I, Dass PD, Cramer S: The importance of renal ammonia metabolism to whole body acid-base balance: A reanalysis of the pathophysiology of renal tubular acidosis. Miner Electrolyte Metab 1990;16:331–340.

83. Buckalew VM Jr: Calcium nephrolithiasis and renal tubular acidosis. In Coe FL, Favus MJ (eds): Disorders of Bone and Mineral Metabolism. New York: Raven Press, 1992;729–756.

84. Pares A, Rimola A, Bruguera M, et al: Renal tubular acidosis in primary biliary cirrhosis. Gastroenterology 1981;80:681–686.

85. Puig JG, Anton FM, Gomez ME, et al: Complete proximal tubular acidosis (type 2, RTA) in chronic active hepatitis. Clin Nephrol 1980;13:267–292.

86. Koul PA, Saleem SM: Chronic active hepatitis with renal tubular acidosis presenting as hypokalemic periodic paralysis with respiratory failure. Acta Paediatr 1992;81:568–569.

87. Izumi N, Sakai H, Shinokara S, et al: Hypouricemia and renal tubular acidosis in primary biliary cirrhosis. Gastroenterol Jpn. 1985;20:374–379.

88. Paré P, Reynolds TB: Impaired renal acidification in alcoholic liver disease. Arch Intern Med 1984;144:941–944.

89. Caregaro L, Lauro S, Ricci G, et al: Distal renal tubular acidosis in hepatic cirrhosis: Clinical and pathogenetic study. Clin Nephrol 1981;15:143–147.

90. Oster JR, Hotchkiss JL, Carbon M, Vaamonde CA: Abnormal renal acidification in alcoholic liver disease. J Lab Clin Med 1975;85:987–1000.

91. Charmes JP, Nicot G, Valette JP, et al: Acidose tubulaire renale latente du cirrhotique. Nouv Presse Med 1976;5:1731–1734.

92. DeMarchi S, Cecchin E, Basile A, et al: Renal tubular dysfunction in chronic alcohol abuse—effects of abstinence. N Engl J Med 1993;329:1927–1934.

93. Shear L, Bonkowsky HL, Gabuzda GL: Renal tubular acidosis in cirrhosis: A determinant of susceptibility to recurrent hepatic precoma. N Engl J Med 1969;280:1–7.

94. Kurtzman NA (principal discussant): Acquired distal renal tubular acidosis. Kidney Int 1983;24:807–819.

95. Graf H, Leach WJ, Arieff AL: Metabolic effects of sodium bicarbonate in hypoxic acidosis in dogs. Am J Physiol 1985;249:F630–F635.

96. Stacpoole PW: Lactic acidosis: The case against bicarbonate therapy. Ann Intern Med 1986;105:276-279.

97. Narins RG, Cohen JJ: Bicarbonate therapy for organic acidosis: The case for its continued use. Ann Intern Med 1987;106:615–618.

98. Shapiro JI, Whalen M, Chan L: Hemodynamic and hepatic pH responses to sodium bicarbonate and Carbicarb during systemic acidosis. Magn Reson Med 1990; 16:403–410.

99. Stacpool PW, Lorenz AC, Thomas RG, Harman EM: Dichloroacetate in the treatment of lactic acidosis. Ann Intern Med 1988;108:58–63 .

100. Abu Romen S, Tannen RL: Therapeutic benefit of dichloroacetate in experimentally induced hypoxic lactic acidosis. J Lab Clin Med 1986;107:378–383.

101. Graf H, Leach W, Arieff AI: Effects of dichloroacetate in the treatment of hypoxic lactic acidosis in dogs. J Clin Invest 1985;76:919–925.

102. Park R, Arieff AI: Treatment of lactic acidosis with dichloroacetate in dogs. J Clin Invest 1982;70:853–862.

103. Johnson GAH, Alberti KG: The metabolic effects of sodium dichloroacetate in experimental hepatitis in the rat. Biochem Soc Trans 1977;5:1387–1389.

104. Blackshear PJ, Holloway PA, Alberti KG: Metabolic interactions of dichloroacetate and insulin in experimental diabetic ketoacidosis. Biochem J 1975;146: 447–456.

Chapter 5

GLOMERULAR ABNORMALITIES IN LIVER DISEASE

GARABED EKNOYAN, M.D.

Cirrhosis of the Liver
Infectious Diseases
    Hepatitis B Virus Infection
    Human Immunodeficiency Virus Infection
    Schistosomiasis
    Malaria
    Infectious Mononucleosis
    Other Infectious Diseases

Systemic Diseases
    Amyloidosis
    Hemochromatosis
    Sickle-Cell Disease
    Collagen Diseases
    Toxemia
    Acute Fatty Liver of Pregnancy
    Congenital diseases

An association between disorders of the liver and the kidney in a variety of conditions, which span a wide spectrum of congenital and acquired diseases, has long been recognized.[1,2] The principal impetus for the quest of such a relationship came from attempts to explain renal insufficiency in cases of advanced liver failure. This so-called hepatorenal syndrome (HRS), which captured the fancy of hepatologists and nephrologists alike, initially became a catchall term into which were dumped several entities.[3] Since then, careful studies by a number of investigators—coupled with advances in experimental and clinical nephrology, basic and clinical immunology, and correlative electron and immunofluorescent microscopy of renal tissue with studies using new techniques in molecular biology—have led to a clearer definition of the functional changes of the kidney that actually characterize HRS and to the recognition and clearer description of other conditions that may simultaneously cause injury to the liver and the kidney (also see chapters 3, 6, and 7). This chapter focuses on the latter category, with special emphasis on the glomerular abnormalities that develop in the kidneys of patients with liver disease. Specifically, it considers the glomerular alterations observed in cirrhosis of the liver; infectious diseases, especially those caused by hepatitis B virus (HBV) and human immunodeficiency virus (HIV); systemic diseases, such as amyloidosis and sickle-cell disease; pregnancy; and congenital diseases (Table 5.1).

CIRRHOSIS OF THE LIVER

The changes in renal function that develop in the course of progressive cirrhosis of the liver have been the subject of considerable investigation and are detailed elsewhere (see chapters 4, 5, and 21). Because of the failure to identify consistent and specific structural changes of the glomeruli, to which the often profound changes in glomerular filtration rate (GFR) could be attributed, much of the older literature focused on the more obvious tubular alterations noted at postmortem examination of the kidney.[4,5] However, over the past several decades increasing evidence supports the presence of glomerular abnormalities in the kidneys of patients with cirrhosis. Many of the earlier reports consist of postmortem studies; as such, they suffer from several limitations, including autolysis that may have set in prior to examination of the specimens, agonal changes that may be induced in the kidneys of dying patients with serious hemodynamic changes, the retrospective nature of such studies and therefore the bias in selecting cases, the absence of controls, the thickness of the sections examined, and the failure of most authors to provide functional data. Since the mid 1960s, reports of kidney tissue obtained by needle biopsy and

TABLE 5.1. Conditions in which Diseases of the Liver Are Associated with Glomerular Abnormalities

Cirrhosis of the liver

Infectious diseases
  Hepatitis B virus
  Human immunodeficiency virus
  Schistosomiasis
  Malaria
  Infectious mononucleosis
  Other infectious diseases

Systemic diseases
  Amyloidosis
  Hemochromatosis
  Sickle-cell disease
  Collagen diseases

Pregnancy
  Toxemia
  Acute fatty liver

Congenital diseases
  Polycystic kidney disease
  Miscellaneous

examined by light, electron, and immunofluorescent microscopy have provided more thorough information on the glomerular changes that may occur in patients with cirrhosis of the liver. Despite differences in the terminology used by different authors over the years, a distinct, though not necessarily specific, glomerular lesion of various gradations of severity seems to occur in some patients. The basic histologic pattern is one of glomerular hypertrophy with an increase in mesangial matrix, varying degrees of sclerotic changes with thickening of the capillary walls, a modest increase in cell size and number, and deposits of immunoglobulins and electrondense material in the mesangium and capillary walls.

The incidence of glomerular changes reported in autopsy series varies from 11.7% to 100%. Of the 1,000 cases reported, an abnormality seems to have been detected in about 45% (Table 5.2). This figure is higher in biopsy studies (Table 5.3), which reported an abnormality in over 98.5% of patients. The higher incidence of changes in biopsy specimens may reflect the better preservation of the tissue specimens and the higher resolution provided by electron microscopy; the changes may be minor and go undetected when viewed by light microscopy alone; more importantly, however, biopsied cases are selected on the basis of clinical and laboratory evidence of renal dysfunction.

Initial reference to mesangial changes of the glomerular tuft in cirrhosis of the liver was made following the description of intercapillary glomerulosclerosis by Kimmelstiel and Wilson,[6] in the quest for evidence of this lesion in diseases other than diabetes mellitus.[7,8] Morphologic changes in the glomeruli of cirrhotics were first described in some detail by Baxter and Ashworth in 1946.[4] In 10 of 25 patients with relatively uncomplicated portal cirrhosis, they noted periglomerular fibrosis and hyaline thickening of the basement membrane. They attributed such changes to arterial and arteriolar sclerosis, which was present in every patient in whom the glomerular changes were seen. Following sporadic subsequent reports,[9–11] Bloodworth and Sommers in 1959[12] were the first to suggest that specific glomerular changes occur in cirrhosis. In a series of 100 consecutive autopsy cases, a glomerular lesion of varying severity was noted to be present in 78. In its mild form, the lesion consisted of hypercellularity of both endothelial and epithelial cells (predominantly epithelial) and a mild thickening of the mesangium by period acid Schiff (PAS)-positive material. In its fully developed form, the lesion consisted of marked PAS-positive fibrillar thickening of the mesangium and capillary walls, giving them a "wire loop" appearance. The endothelial cells were swollen and vacuolated and stained positive for lipid. The increase in cellularity and swelling of endothelial cells obliterated the lumen of some glomeruli. This lesion, which was most frequent and more severe in cases of portal cirrhosis, was also seen in cases of postnecrotic and biliary cirrhosis.

Bloodworth and Sommers labeled such changes "cirrhotic glomerulosclerosis." The term "hepatic glomerulosclerosis" was suggested when similar glomerular changes were observed in kidney biopsies from patients with various forms of liver disease, including portal, postnecrotic, and biliary cirrhosis as well as alcoholic and acute viral hepatitis.[131,14] Electron microscopy demonstrated changes in all patients, regardless of the duration, severity, or nature of the hepatic disease. The changes that were more severe in patients with chronic rather than acute liver disease consisted of electron-dense deposits in the capillary wall and mesangium, thickening of the basement membrane, and increase in the basement membranelike material in the mesangium. The electron-dense osmophilic deposits were present in the mesangial matrix, in the subendothelial aspect

TABLE 5.2. Autopsy Findings in the Kidney of Patients with Cirrhosis of the Liver

Ref.	Year	No. of Cases	Hepatic Lesions	Proteinuria	No. with Lesions	GS	GBM Thickening	Hyper-cellularity	Mesangial Matrix Thickening	Comments by Authors
1	1863	11	Cirrhosis		6	NR	NR	NR		Kidneys enlarged, "granular"
5	1938	26	Cirrhosis	NR	15	+	−	−	−	Congestion in 11
7	1942	1	Cirrhosis	NR	1	+	−	−	+	Intercapillary sclerosis
4	1946	25	Cirrhosis	+ in 60%	10	−	+	−	−	Periglomerular fibrosis
9	1951	60	Cirrhosis	NR	7	+	−	+	−	Intercapillary GS
11	1955	50	Cirrhosis	NR	50	−	−	+	−	Glomerulotubular nephrosis (also in 50% of controls)
8	1958	33	Fatty metamorphosis	NR	6	+	−	−	+	Kimmelstiel-Wilson-like lesions
		23	Cirrhosis	NR	4	+	−	−	+	
12	1959	65	Cirrhosis	NR	57	+	+	+	+	Cirrhotic GS, proliferation of endothelial cells
		16	Postnecrotic cirrhosis	NR	11	+	+	+	+	
		11	Biliary cirrhosis	NR	5	+	+	+	+	
		8	Miscellaneous	NR	5	+	+	+	+	
10	1959	100	Cirrhosis	NR	25	+	+	+	+	
70	1961	100	Cirrhosis	NR	28	+	+	+	−	Same lesions in 10% of controls
31	1965	50	Cirrhosis	+	13	+	NR	+	NR	Miscellaneous renal lesions
	1968	60	Cirrhosis	+ in 18 Massive in 11	60	+	−	−	+	Intercapillary GS of varying degree
62	1968	85	Cirrhosis	+	52	+	+	−	+	Minimal in 44, advanced in 8
70	1973	30	Cirrhosis	NR	30	+	−	−	+	
21	1978	90	Cirrhosis	NR	30	+	+	+	+ (3/30)	IgA deposits in 61, IgG or IgM in 41, complement in 7
		2	Postnecrotic							
		2	Hemochromatosis							
		6	Miscellaneous							
22	1978	3	Cirrhosis	NR	3	+	+	−	+	
134	1979	62	Cirrhosis		56	+	+	+	+	IgG in 42%, IgM in 77%, IgA in 62%, C_1q in 71%, C_3 in 77%, C_4 in 41%
29	1982	79	Cirrhosis (7 alcoholic, 12 postnecrotic, 55 posthepatitis, 5 biliary)	+	51	+	+	+	+	IgA deposits in 34, IgM in 24, IgG in 21, complement in 37
30	1983	50	Cirrhosis Alcoholic and posthepatitis	+ in 11 >1 gm/day in 7	46	+	+	+	+	IgA deposits in 35, IgM in 27 IgG in 16, complement in 32

GS = glomerulosclerosis, GBM = glomerular basement membrane; NR = not recorded.

of the basement membrane, and within the basement membrane. Irregular black particles surrounded by a clear zone or halo were found mainly in the mesangial matrix.

These findings were confirmed by Fischer and Perez-Stable[15] in a prospective study correlating renal function studies with ultrastructural changes of renal biopsies from 12 patients with portal cirrhosis. Glomeruli from 5 of 8 subjects with normal renal function exhibited increased cellularity, mesangial thickening, focal electron-dense deposits within the mesangium and in the subendothelial spaces, and wrinkling and occasional longitudinal splitting of the lamina densa. Such alterations were qualitatively similar but more pronounced in 4 of the cirrhotic patients with abnormal renal function (GFR of 32–42 ml/min and proteinuria of 1.3, 1.9, 3.2, and 5.1 g/24 hr). The duration and severity of the cirrhosis were greater in patients with impaired renal function. In 1 patient the changes were more pronounced in a second biopsy 1 year after the initial examination. Appropriately, the lesions were termed cirrhotic "glomerulonephritis" rather than "glomerulosclerosis." The progressive nature of this lesion, at least in some cases, was also suggested by Nochy and coworkers.[16] In a study of 34 patients with overt glomerulonephritis and chronic liver disease, 8 patients had repeat biopsies. In 4 patients, the lesions remained unchanged. In

TABLE 5.3.   Renal Biopsy Findings in Patients with Cirrhosis of the Liver*

Ref.	Year	No. of Cases	Hepatic Lesions	Proteinuria	NS	No. with Lesions	GS	GBM Thickening	Hyper-cellularity	Mesangial Matrix Thickening	IgG	IgA	Com
13,61	1965	3	Alcoholic hepatitis	+ to 4+	2	3	+	+	−	+	NR	NR	NR
		4	Postnecrosis	Trace to 4+		4							
		10	Cirrhosis	Trace to 4+		10							
		1	Biliary	+		1							
15	1968	12	Cirrhosis	1.3, 1.9 gm/day	2	12	+	+	+	+	+	NR	NR
17	1969	3	Cirrhosis	+	—	3	+	+	+(1)	−	NR	NR	NR
18	1970	14	Cirrhosis	+ in 3	1	14	+	+	+(3)	+	+	+	+
		6	Fatty metamorphosis			6							
19	1974	7	Cirrhosis	+	NR	7	+	−	−	+	+	+	+
20	1975	10	Cirrhosis	NR	NR	10	+	+	−	+	+	+	+
16	1976	22	Cirrhosis	+	11	22	+	+	+(1)	+	+	NR	NR
		12	Fatty metamorphosis			12	+	+	−	+	+	NR	NR
21	1978	11	Cirrhosis	NR	NR	10	+	+	+(6)	+	+	+	+
22	1978	1	Cirrhosis	NR	NR	1	+	+	−	+	NR	NR	NR
24	1983	3	Cirrhosis	+0.5,2.2, 3 gm/day	1	3	+	+	+	+	NR	+	+
25	1984	6	Cirrhosis	+0.8, 1.5 gm/day	2	5	−	−	+	+	NR	+(1)	+(2)
26	1985	1	Cirrhosis	+2.7 gm/day		1	+	+	−	+	NR	NR	NR
27	1986	12	Cirrhosis	+0.8–8.8 gm/day	5	12	+	+	+	+	+	+(2)	+(8)
28	1987	2	Cirrhosis	+0.8, 1.5 gm/day		2	−	−	+	+	NR	+(2)	−

* Numbers in parentheses indicate number of cases showing lesion.
NS = nephrotic syndrome, GBM = glomerular basement membrane, Com = complement, NR = not recorded.

1 patient with glomerulosclerosis and mesangial deposits, membranoproliferative glomerulonephritis was found 6 years after the initial biopsy; another patient revealed changes typical of end-stage kidney disease.

Immunoglobulin deposits were detected by immunofluorescence in the two latter studies, but complement was not present and immunoglobulin G (IgG) could not be eluted at acid pH, suggesting that the globulin is trapped rather than deposited by an antigen-antibody reaction. However, over the past two decades, reports by different groups of studies of biopsy specimens from patients with fatty and cirrhotic livers (see Table 5.3) have called attention to the association of the mesangial changes with mesangial and subendothelial deposits of IgA as well as of IgG and complement.[16–27]

On the basis of their study of kidneys from 100 autopsies and 11 biopsies, Berger and associates[21] proposed a classification of the glomerular lesions into two types, depending on the presence or absence of cellular proliferation. In the first type without proliferation, the deposits are mainly mesangial but frequently extend into the subendothelial space. IgA nearly always is the main immunoglobulin detected in the deposits, but it is often accompanied by IgG, IgM, or both. The complement component C3 is not prominent and Clq is present in about one-third of the cases. Such cases do not usually have abnormalities of the urine sediment. In the second type, associated with proliferative changes, IgA is again the main, and sometimes only, immunoglobulin present, but the deposits are intramembranous and the glomerular basement thickness is increased. Proteinuria, sometimes in the nephrotic range, and hematuria, either microscopic or macroscopic, occurs in this group. In one patient with endothelial and epithelial cell proliferation, the course was one of rapidly progressive crescentic glomerulonephritis. The immunoglobulin deposits were as prominent in cases without proliferative changes as they were in cases with proliferation. Similar results have since been reported by others (see Tables 5.2 and 5.3), both in biopsy[24–28] and autopsy studies.[29–31]

Further evidence on the prevalence of the glomerular lesions has been forthcoming from prospective studies of the renal morphology and function in patients with end-stage liver disease awaiting or undergoing orthotopic liver transplantation. In a study of 17 nonalcoholic adults with well-preserved renal function, glomerular abnormalities were present in all.[32] The lesions were minor in 8 patients, glomerulosclerotic in 7, membranoproliferative in 1, and mesangioproliferative in another. Immunofluorescent studies revealed the presence of IgM in all patients and of IgA in 11. In another study of 6 children with hematuria and proteinuria, membranoproliferative glomerulonephritis was present in all patients, with evidence of deposition of IgG and IgM in various combinations with complement; only 2 patients had IgA.[33] The frequency with which IgA has been detected in such studies is variable,[27] but it seems to be more prominent in cases with hematuria and proteinuria.[24,28]

The frequent presence of IgA in patients with hepatic cirrhosis certainly provides evidence for an immune-mediated injury. Although this usually goes unsuspected in asymptomatic cases, in patients with proteinuria or hematuria most recent studies note principally a membranoproliferative or mesangioproliferative glomerulonephritis, with mesangial expansion or sclerosis. Mesangial and subendothelial IgA deposits are present in most but not all such cases.[27] Complement, IgG, and IgM deposits are also present and may be the only deposits detected in some cases.[32,33] The pathogenesis of the renal lesions in cases that do not demonstrate IgA deposits remains unexplained, but clearly it is also associated with immune complex deposition.[23,27] Intriguing in this regard is the presence of antimitochondrial antibodies, usually found in primary biliary cirrhosis, in the sera of patients with antiglomerular basement (GBM) disease, and its cross-reactivity with anti-GBM.[34] Although the significance of this observation remains to be determined, its clinical relevance may be gleaned from the report of a case of life-threatening pulmonary hemorrhage and focal proliferative glomerulonephritis in a patient with primary biliary cirrhosis.[35]

The pathogenesis of the immunoglobulin deposits in the kidneys of such patients remains undefined. The deposits could be the result of precipitation in the glomeruli of either aggregated immunoglobulins or circulating complexes. Hypocomplementemia and cryoglobulinemia are found in patients with cirrhosis[36–39] and, when measured, have been shown to be present in a significant number of patients with glomerular lesions.[16,24,27] The hypocomplementemia could be due to activation of complement components, reduced hepatic synthesis, or a combination of both. Cryoglobulinemia, present in one-third of the cases in one series[16] but much less in others,[25,27] could be construed as evidence of circulating immune complexes. Although neither the hypocomplementemia nor the cryoglobulinemia is invariably present in such cases, their presence in others, together with the demonstration of complement and immunoglobulin deposits by immunofluorescence (see Table 5.3), may be construed as evidence in favor of an immune complex-mediated pathogenesis. A more consistent finding is the elevation of serum IgA. The cryoprecipitate and circulating immune complexes have been shown to contain IgA.[16,23,38] There is a strong correlation between IgA deposits in the kidney and the increased circulating levels of IgA. The circulating levels of IgA are increased in well over 75% of cases showing mesangial IgA deposits.[39] In a brief report of 24 patients with cirrhosis, circulating dimeric IgA levels were increased 7.28-fold compared with controls, whereas monomeric IgA levels were increased 2.41-fold.[37]

With failure of the hepatic reticuloendothelial cell function, increased portacaval shunting, or both, as liver disease progresses, either IgA originating from the gut or IgA from its complexes with antigenic components of intestinal bacterial, viral, or dietary antigens could be increased in the circulation with subsequent deposition in the glomeruli and initiation of the lesions observed.[23,24,37,40] Rate of deposition, amount of deposits, genetic differences, or other undefined additional factors may then account for the differences in response and for the variability in the severity of the lesion. A relationship between a gluten-containing diet and high levels of IgA immune complexes has been demonstrated in cases of primary IgA nephropathy.[41] Whether a similar relationship exists in cases of cirrhosis of the liver with IgA deposits remains to be examined. Dietary discrepancies might provide an explanation for the different geographical distribution of IgA deposits reported from different countries.[24,27–30] A role for alcohol ingestion also has been proposed.[42,43] In rats given a continuous infusion of a liquid diet and alcohol, mesangial IgA deposits were noted in 60% at 6 weeks and in 100% at 16 weeks.[44]

Cutaneous purpuric lesions that on biopsy reveal a leukocytoclastic vasculitis have been a feature of some cases of cirrhosis of the liver associated with rapidly progressive renal failure manifested by proteinuria and hematuria.[25,27] The etiology of the vasculitis in these cirrhotic patients, all of whom tested negative for hepatitis B surface antigen (HBsAg), is unknown, but it is likely immune complex-mediated. Indeed, the IgA deposits are not limited to the glomeruli. They have been detected in the vasculature of the skin, jejunum, choroid plexus, and perisinusoidal spaces of the liver[45] and may account for some of the unexplained systemic manifestations.

Glomerular changes, the structural features of which are similar to those seen in humans, have been shown to develop in experimental animals with hepatic injury induced by dietary deficiency and hepatotoxic agents.[46–49] Lewis rats rendered cirrhotic by the administration of carbon tetrachloride develop mesangial and subendothelial deposits of immunoglobulins, especially IgA and complement.[49,50] They also develop circulating immune complexes and markedly elevated serum IgA concentrations. Bile-duct ligation has been shown to enhance the mesangial deposition of IgA in rats immunized to give rise to IgA.[51] Such experimental models suggest that defective hepatic sequestration of circulating IgA polymers and immune complexes may be responsible for the glomerular deposits. Circulating immune complexes are cleared by the mononuclear phagocytic system in the liver and spleen.[52]

Experimental studies have shown that the hepatic Kuppfer cells are important in the uptake and metabolism of the insoluble immune complexes and the endothelial cells of the soluble immune complexes.[53] Any compromise in this essential clearing function, due either to cellular injury secondary to cirrhosis or to shunting of the portal circulation from the liver secondary to portal hypertension, would result in increased circulating complexes.[40,54–56]

Supporting evidence that such a mechanism may be operative comes from the report of resolution of cirrhotic glomerulonephritis following successful liver transplantation.[57] In a 38-year-old man with cirrhosis of the liver who presented with hematuria and massive proteinuria, kidney biopsy revealed membranoproliferative glomerulonephritis with positive staining for IgA and complement. Following orthotopic liver transplantation proteinuria and hematuria rapidly resolved.

Although the improvement of glomerular abnormalities may be attributed to immunosuppressive therapy instituted following transplantation, it also could have resulted from restored hepatic function. This does not seem to be a uniform finding; persistent glomerular abnormalities following orthotopic liver transplantation appear to be more common.[58] However, the persistent or new development of renal dysfunction after transplantation may be due to immunosuppressive therapy rather than progression or persistence of the glomerular lesions.[59] A response to immunosuppressive therapy has been seen after treatment with steroids in patients with chronic active hepatitis.[32] Although the renal lesions associated with the latter are different in morphology and pathogenesis, this finding buttresses the argument that the favorable response reported in some cases following hepatic transplantation may have been due to immunosuppressive therapy instituted to prevent rejection.

Of further interest in the pathogenesis of the glomerular lesions is the report of 4 patients with advanced liver disease whose plasma had low lecithin-cholesterol acyltransferase (LCAT) activity, markedly reduced concentration of cholesterol esters, and increased content of polar lipids and the large molecular fraction of low-density lipoproteins.[22] In the renal biopsy from 1 patient and in the autopsy specimen from another, deposition of osmophilic material was found in the glomerular basement membrane, mesangium, and subendothelial regions. The deposits were similar to those previously described in patients with LCAT deficiency and were thought to represent cholesterol and phospholipids. The deposited particles had a diameter of approximately 1000–2000Å and were present in vacuoles of obliquely transected endothelial cells, subendothelial regions, and the basement membrane. With light microscopy, the changes observed in all 4 cases were similar to those described in patients with cirrhosis: widening of the mesangial region, irregularly thickened capillary basement membrane, and occasionally pronounced glomerulosclerotic alterations.

The possibility that this lipid deposition may be responsible for the glomerulosclerotic changes is intriguing, particularly in light of current evidence for a role of glomerular lipid deposits as a cause of renal injury.[60] In dogs with choledochocaval shunts, lipid deposition occurs within a few weeks and is associated with slight glomerulosclerotic lesions.[22] The initial article by

Bloodworth and Sommers[12] points to the proliferation of endothelial cells that sometimes contained lipid. In addition, the deposited particles and surrounding vacuolization referred to in earlier studies using electron microscopy[13,14] appear to be similar to those described with LCAT deficiency.[22]

There is limited information on the functional changes that accompany the glomerular structural changes described in patients with liver cirrhosis and their clinical course. However, the glomerular lesions may be accompanied by clinical manifestations and biochemical abnormalities indicating renal dysfunction. Massive proteinuria, sufficient to be in the nephrotic range, has been noted in about 17% of the cases reported in biopsy studies (see Table 5.3). Undoubtedly, this finding could represent some bias in obtaining biopsies in patients who had urinary abnormalities in the first place. In any case, the fact that massive proteinuria and nephrotic syndrome occur with some frequency is worthy of note.

In patients who develop massive proteinuria and have microscopic hematuria, the course of the disease is usually one of progressive renal failure. Less severe proteinuria, reported as 1+ to 4+ on urinalysis, is present in the majority of biopsied cases.[4,13,15,17,18,20,24–28,61,62] Hematuria, both gross and microscopic, also occurs.[14,17,20,28] Episodes of macroscopic hematuria may be associated with reversible acute renal failure that may require supportive dialytic therapy.[28] As suggested by Berger and colleagues[21] and confirmed by others,[24–28,63] the abnormalities in urine sediment are more frequent in patients having proliferative changes in addition to mesangial sclerosis and IgA deposits. It is probably safe to conclude that patients with minimal degrees of renal glomerular changes, limited to sclerosis and mesangial deposits of IgA, appear to be asymptomatic, whereas in the presence of distinct proliferative changes, hematuria or proteinuria and nephrotic syndrome may develop.

Massive proteinuria is more common in patients with advanced membranoproliferative lesions. Given the hypoalbuminemia and massive edema of liver cirrhosis, the renal lesions may go unsuspected even in the presence of abnormalities in the urine sediment. Modest elevations of blood pressure are another clue to the presence of renal parenchymal disease, since low blood pressure is characteristic of the generalized vasodilatation and reduced vascular resistance of cirrhotics.[64,65] The prevalence of renal lesions in the general population with cirrhosis of the liver is unknown. The frequency with which they are encountered depends on the vigilance with which they are sought. In a combined biopsy and autopsy series from one center, 89 of 202 patients (44%) with chronic liver disease had overt signs of glomerular disease.[63]

Two other morphologic changes deserve comment. The first concerns changes in juxtaglomerular apparatus, particularly when electrolyte changes are present.[66] An increase in thickness of the macula densa cells is seen in association with low serum sodium or high serum potassium. The juxtaglomerular cell count is raised when the serum sodium concentration is low, and the number of granulated juxtaglomerular cells shows a direct relationship with serum creatinine and potassium.[66] Given the hemodynamic changes associated with advanced cirrhosis and demonstrated elevations in plasma renin, such changes in the juxtaglomerular apparatus are not unexpected. Angiotensin II receptor density has been shown to be higher in cirrhotic than in control rats, with consequent increased total angiotensin II binding in rats with cirrhosis.[67] However, no functional differences were detected between the control and cirrhotic animals, suggesting a postreceptor blockade of the angiotensin II signal in cirrhotic rats.

The second change of note is the increased kidney weight observed by several investigators.[10,12,68] The recorded weights range from 175–207 g per kidney. In one study, kidney weight was found to be directly proportional to the degree of hepatomegaly.[68] Glomerular diameter, measured by an ocular micrometer, is increased in proportion to the change in kidney weight.[68,69] Experimental studies in rats reveal that the cross-sectional area of glomeruli from cirrhotic rats is 42% greater than that of glomeruli from control animals.[67] Assay of renal tissue fluid, protein, lipid, and carbohydrate content has revealed no disproportionate accumulation of any of these substances, suggesting that the nephromegaly was the result of added tissue mass best explained by cellular hypertrophy and hyperplasia. Immunofluorescent studies reveal an increase in type IV collagen, laminin, and fibronectin in the expanded glomerular mesangial areas and along the glomerular capillary walls in cirrhosis compared with normal renal tissue.[69]

Relevant to changes in glomerular size are recent experimental and clinical studies either early in the course of cirrhosis or in patients with well-compensated cirrhosis.[71,72] Contrary to findings in severe decompensated liver disease, in well-compensated alcoholic cirrhosis the renal vascular resistance was significantly reduced (8629 ± 612 vs 11315 ± 1287) and accompanied by a significant and proportional increase in glomerular filtration rate (151 ± 11 vs. 105 ± 11 ml/min) and renal plasma flow (525 ± 23 vs. 420 ± 53 ml/min).[71] Such changes are accentuated after protein intake.[73] The oral administration of 50 mg indomethacin results in a transient but significant decrease in glomerular filtration rate and renal plasma flow, indicating a role of prostaglandins in the pathogenesis of hyperfiltration in such patients.[74]

A similar increase in glomerular filtration rate and a higher renal plasma flow have been shown in cirrhotic rats compared with control animals.[63] Thus, whereas there is no question that in decompensated liver disease the renal vascular resistance is increased and the renal blood flow and glomerular filtration are decreased, it appears that the endogenous vasodilators, which account for the reduced systemic vascular resistance and lower blood pressure throughout the course of cirrhosis, also may reduce the renal vascular resistance early in the course of disease.[71–75] The resultant glomerular hyperfiltration and hypertrophy could contribute to the pathogenesis of hepatic glomerulosclerosis by a hemodynamic mechanism or growth-related local factors.[76–78] As liver disease progresses, there is a gradual increase in renal vascular resistance with consequent reduction of renal perfusion[79,80] that may contribute to glomerulosclerosis by an ischemic mechanism,[81] postulated to be operative in initial reports of renal lesions of cirrhotic patients.[4]

Coupling the hemodynamic mechanisms of injury with those of immune-mediated injury, it is possible to formulate a probable model for the glomerular changes that have been described in cirrhosis of the liver (Fig. 5.1). On the one hand, glomerulosclerosis could be initiated by the early hyperfiltration and hypertrophy and then perpetuated by the subsequent ischemia that characterizes renal hemodynamic changes later in the course of progressive liver cirrhosis. On the other hand, the reduced capacity of the diseased liver cells to clear immune complexes, coupled by shunting away of blood from the liver due to

portal hypertension, results in increased levels of circulating IgG, IgM, and IgA immune complexes. Their deposition in the mesangium and subendothelium of the glomerular capillaries initiates varying degrees of mesangial and membranoproliferative changes. Depending on the extent and severity of such changes, varying degrees of abnormalities of urine sediment, reduction in glomerular filtration rate, and increments in blood pressure may result in patients with liver cirrhosis.

Certain generalities about glomerular lesions reported in patients with cirrhosis of the liver can be made:

1. The severity of the renal lesions appears to be influenced by the chronicity of the liver disease, diffuseness of hepatic cell damage, and magnitude of portal hypertension.[14,56]

2. The incidence of renal lesions increases with advancing age of the patient[82] and is higher in women.[70]

3. There is an association with hyperglobulinemia and more specifically with elevated serum IgA levels.[20]

4. Cryoglobulinemia, hypocomplementemia, or cutaneous vasculitis may be present in some cases.[25]

5. The glomerular lesions noted at autopsy are usually those of glomerulosclerosis, whereas lesions detected on renal biopsy of patients with urinary abnormalities are those of a proliferative glomerulonephritis, either mesangioproliferative or membranoproliferative, with IgA deposits detected, in most but not all cases, on immunofluorescent study.[28] The pathogenesis of the sclerotic and proliferative changes may be different (see Fig. 5.1), but their coexistence in the same individual may adversely affect the progress of the lesions.

6. Although most patients with mild glomerulonephritis may remain asymptomatic, both nephritic and nephrotic sediments with reduced glomerular filtration rate are present in about one-third of patients in whom the proliferative glomerular lesions are more severe.[39]

INFECTIOUS DISEASES

Hepatitis B Virus Infection

Convincing evidence that infection with hepatitis B virus (HBV) may initiate an immunologic process responsible for the development of

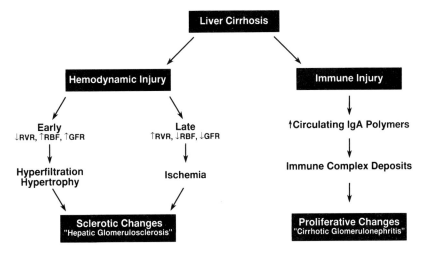

FIGURE 5.1. Likely pathogenesis of glomerular changes in cirrhosis of the liver. RVR = renal vascular resistance, RBF = renal blood flow, GFR = glomerular filtration rate.

glomerular changes and chronic renal disease has accrued over the past two decades. In fact, information about this issue antedates the discovery and identification of HBV and its antigens.

Interest in renal involvement in hepatitis was aroused in the mid 1950s when attention was drawn to a group of young patients with chronic active hepatitis who developed an unusually florid multisystemic disease characterized by arthritis, skin rash, pleurisy, thrombocytopenia, and "glomerulonephritis."[83] The etiology of the liver disease was unknown. Some authors favored a viral origin.[84] Others regarded it as an unusual manifestation of systemic lupus erythematosus (SLE), because some patients had an occasional positive LE cell test,[83] and therefore termed it "lupoid hepatitis." However, liver involvement in SLE is rare, and this terminology was not universally accepted. Different authors labeled the disease "active juvenile cirrhosis," "subacute hepatitis," "autoimmune hepatitis," "liver disease in young women with hyperglobulinemia," and "subacute hepatic necrosis."[83–86] It is now evident that most of these cases were probably clinical variants of an identical process: chronic active hepatitis.[84] Because specific tests for HBV had not yet been developed, it was impossible to determine whether some of the cases were in fact due to the virus. Nevertheless, renal involvement was frequent, and abnormalities of the urinary sediment and proteinuria, with or without the nephrotic syndrome, were often recorded.[83,86–90] When noted, the glomerular changes were described as consisting of membranous and proliferative changes.[83,85,90]

In a study of the kidney biopsies from 12 patients with so-called "active juvenile cirrhosis," membranous glomerulonephritis was present in 7 (58%).[85] All 7 had irregular focal thickening of the glomerular basement membrane and proliferative changes considered by the authors as similar to those of "early lupus nephropathy." The endogenous creatinine clearance (C_{Cr}) was less than 70 ml/min in 4 of the 12, and the protein excretion was 200–400 mg/day in another 4. In an early study of tissue-bound immunoglobulins, two patients diagnosed with "chronic liver disease with positive LE cell test" demonstrated nodular deposits of IgG, IgM, and complement in their glomeruli.[91] In another study, serum from 25 patients with "autoimmune lupoid hepatitis" was shown to react with cells of rat kidney glomerulus.[92] This "antibody" was demonstrated in the serum of a patient with membranous glomerulonephritis, whose glomeruli were shown to contain IgG by immunofluorescence.[92] Of interest, the authors suggested that in autoimmune hepatitis "globulin in the glomeruli is deposited as a result of a reaction in situ, whereas in SLE it is part of an antigen-antibody complex formed remotely and lodged accidentally in the renal glomerulus." Thus, by the beginning of the 1970s about 70 cases of renal involvement in patients with chronic active hepatitis had been reported. An association with HBV was first made in 1971,[93] and its possible pathogenesis as part of the natural course of infection with HBV began to be formulated. Of interest is the now reported occurrence of HBV-associated

TABLE 5.4. Clinical Summary of Patients with Hepatitis B Virus-associated Nephropathy

Ref.	Year	No. of Patients	Age (years)	Sex	Blood Pressure (mmHg)	Creatinine (mg/100 ml)	Urea Nitrogen (mg/100 ml)	Albumin Total Protein (gm/100 ml)
93	1971	1	53	M	NR	1.3	35	1.7/NR
100	1973	1	30	F	↑	2.2–2.8	NR	1.4–2.4/5.7
101	1974	3	24	M	140/100	0.8	12	NR
			18	F	NR	25	90	3.0/6.2
			22	M	190/120	3.6	38	2.5/5.5
106	1974	1	53	M	NR	1.7	NR	3.2/NR
107	1974	1	42	M	185/135	1.1	10	3.4/6.6
102	1975	1	33	NR	170/100	NR	NR	NR
103	1975	2	Child	NR	NR	0.9	NR	NR
			Child	NR	NR	0.4	NR	NR
115	1975	9	9–42	6M, 3F	NR	NR	NR	NR
108	1975	1	19	M	NR	NR	NR	1.5/6.1
104	1976	1	68	M	145/100	1.5	34–59	2.7/6.6
109	1976	1	35	F	250/130	0.6	30	2.1/5.7
110	1976	1	8	M	NR	NR	10	NR
111	1977	1	26	M	NR	1.2	20	2.8/NR
112	1977	1	45	M	200/100	0.9	NR	1.9/4.2
113	1978	1	9	F	140/90	0.8	NR	2.9/NR
117	1978	11	3–15	9M, 2F	NR	NR	NR	NR
118	1979	15	2–13	13M, 2F	NR	NR	NR	1.2–2.8/4–4.9
97	1979	2	5	M	116/70	0.6	24	1.4/3.9
			8	M	150/90	1.0	26	1.9/5
125	1982	1	37	M	120/90	0.9	19	1.8/4.6
126	1985	2	6, 27	M	NR	0.7, 1.1	7,19	2.4, 2.7
133	1985	16	2–12	13M, 3F	N	NR	NR	NR

HBsAG = hepatitis B surface antigen, N = normal, NR = not recorded, ANA = antinuclear antibody.

glomerulonephropathy in patients with systemic lupus erythematosus.[94]

Infection with HBV nearly always produces some immune reaction. Antibodies may be formed to any of its known antigenic particles: anti-HBc, anti-HBs, and anti-HBe. Using different methods of detection, circulating immune complexes have been demonstrated in the acute and chronic forms of infection with the virus; HBsAg is the more commonly identified inciting agent.[95–97] This immune complex phenomenon has been incriminated as the causative mechanism of the extrahepatic manifestations of viral hepatitis in skin, joints, small arteries and arterioles, and renal glomeruli.[98,99]

The suggestion that HBV through one of its antigens, HBsAg, was involved in the formation of immune complexes whose glomerular deposition initiated a pathologic process leading to development of membranous glomerulonephritis was first made in 1971.[93] The suggestion was based on studies of kidney tissue obtained at renal biopsy from a 53-year-old man who had developed HBs-Ag-positive chronic active hepatitis from a complication of transfusion therapy and subsequently presented with massive proteinuria and reduced renal function[93] (Table 5.4). Since this first report of the association between HBV and membranous nephropathy, several other cases have been reported, strongly suggesting that HBV, through the immune response elicited by one of its antigens, is causally related to the development of glomerular changes in humans.[93,97–134] The clinical and laboratory data of 73 patients culled

TABLE 5.4. Clinical Summary of Patients with Hepatitis B Virus-associated Nephropathy (*Cols. cont.*)

Complement Level	Creatinine Clearance (ml/min)	Proteinuria (gm/24 hr)	Urinalysis	HBsAg	Anti-HBS	Comments
N	76	1.3–3.8	RBCs, WBCs, casts	+	–	Steroid Rx, unsuccessful
↓	20–30	4–6	Many RBC casts	+	NR	Progressive renal failure over 6 years
NR	130	2.9	NR	+	NR	Steroid and cyclophosphamide Rx, unsuccessful
NR	5	4.3	NR	–	+	Drug addict, kidney transplant
N	40	4.7	NR	+	–	Steroid and azathioprine Rx
N	55	(Massive)	NR	+	NR	
N	130	1.8	RBCs, casts	+	–	
↓	70	2.0	RBCs	+	–	Drug addict
↓	NR	(Massive)	NR	+	NR	
↓	NR	(Massive)	NR	+	NR	
NR	NR	NR	NR	+	+	
NR	NR	4–11	NR	+	NR	Drug addict
N	42	(Massive)	NR	+	–	Died, ANA positive, latex positive
NR	NR	(3+)	NR	–	–	Anti-DNA, ANA positive
NR	NR	NR	Proteinuria	+	NR	
N	100	4.9–9	RBCs, WBCs	+	NR	Steroid Rx, no response
↓	NR	4–6	RBCs, RBC casts	+	–	Eosinophilia
N	100	5	RBCs	+	NR	
NR	NR	NR	RBCs, proteinuria	+	NR	
NR	NR	1.8	NR	+	NR	1 on dialysis, 11 remissions
N	112	4	RBCs, casts	–	–	Anti-HBs
N	95	5	RBCs, casts	–	–	Anti-HBs
N	106–150	5.6	RBCs, casts	+	NR	Anti-HBs
N ↓	107	15.6, 1.6	RBCs	+	NR	HBsAG, anti-HBs
N ↓	N	(Massive)	RBCs	+	–	HBsAg in 11

from reports with sufficient detail to permit extraction of relevant information are shown in Table 5.4. The kidney biopsy findings in these and an additional 24 patients,[122] for whom no clinical data were presented, are shown in Table 5.5.

Of the 70 patients whose sex is given, 56 were males, with a male/female ratio of 4:1. The age at onset of renal disease ranged from 2–68 years, with over two-thirds of the cases reported in children below the age of 15. This high incidence in children has been associated with seropositivity for the specific antigen in the mothers.[115,117] Blood pressure in the 12 patients whose levels are provided, most of whom were adults, was high. Urinalysis, where recorded, often revealed microscopic hematuria, pyuria, granular casts, and, in one case, red blood cell casts[107] (see Table 5.4).

Proteinuria, hypoalbuminemia, or nephrotic syndrome were present in all. Proteinuria ranged from 1–15.6 g/day. The serum albumin ranged from 1.2–3.4 g/100 ml. Blood urea nitrogen (BUN) and creatinine levels were within the normal range in most patients or only modestly increased, ranging from 7–38 mg/100 ml and 0.6–3.4 mg/100 ml, respectively, except in 1 patient whose BUN was 90 mg/100 ml and the creatinine 25 mg/100 ml. The C_{Cr} measured in 15 patients ranged from 30–150 ml/min, except in 1 patient[107] (see Table 5.4), in whom it was 5 ml/min. All except 4 patients were HBsAg-positive. The serum complement levels were either normal or at the lower range of normal values. Cryoglobulinemia was found in some, not detected in others, and not searched for in most.

TABLE 5.5.   Renal Biopsy Findings in Patients with Hepatitis B Virus-associated Nephropathy

Ref.	Year	No. of Patients	Diagnosis	IgG	IgA	IgM	HBsAg	HB?Ag	HBcAg	Complement	Electron Microscopy
93	1971	1	MGN	+	−	−	+	NR	NR	+	Focal mesangial sclerosis and hypercellularity
100	1973	1	MPGN	+	NR	NR	+	NR	NR	+	Endothelial and epithelial cell proliferation, no deposits
101	1974	3	MGN	+	+	+	+	NR	NR	+	Mesangial cell proliferation
			ISN + FSGN	−	±	+	+	NR	NR	+	
			MPGN	+	±	+	+	NR	NR	+	
106	1974	1	MGN	+	+	+	+	NR	NR	+	
107	1974	1	MGN	+	+	+	+	NR	NR	+	
102	1975	1	MesangPGN	+	+	+	+	NR	NR	+	Subendothelial deposits
103	1975	2	MGN	+	NR	+	+	NR	NR	+	
			MGN	+	NR	NR	+	NR	NR	+	
115	1975	5	MGN	+	NR	NR	NR	NR	NR	+	
		2	MPGN	NR	NR	NR	NR	NR	NR	NR	
		1	MesangPGN	NR	NR	NR	NR	NR	NR	NR	
		1	DPGN	+	NR	NR	NR	NR	NR	+	
108	1975	1	MGN	+	NR	NR	NR	NR	NR	+	
104	1975	1	MGN	+	±	+	+	NR	NR	+	
109	1975	1	MGN	+	+	+	+	NR	NR	+	Subendothelial deposits
110	1976	1	MesangPGN	+	−	−	+	NR	NR	+	
111	1977	1	MGN	+	−	NR	+	NR	NR	+	
112	1977	1	MGN	+	−	+	+	NR	NR	+	Subendothelial deposits
113	1978	1	MGN	+	±	+	+	NR	NR	NR	
117	1978	11	MGN	+(9/11)	+(2/11)	+(1/11)	−	NR	NR	+(7/11)	
118	1979	15	MGN	+(15/15)	+(2/15)	+(14/14)	−7, NR 8	NR	NR	+(11/15)	
97	1979	2	MGN	+	+	±	−	+	NR		
122	1980	21	MGN	+	+	+	−	NR	+(14/21)	+	
		1	MPGN								
		2	MesangPGN								
125	1982	1	MGN	+	NR	+	−	NR	NR	+	Epimembranous deposits
126	1985	2	MGN	+	±	+	NR	NR	NR	−	
133	1985	13	MGN	+(13/13)	+(1/13)	+(6/13)	−(8/8)	+(7/7)	−(4/4)	+(12/13)	

MGN = membranous nephropathy, FSGN = focal sclerosing glomerulosclerosis, DPGN = diffuse proliferative glomerulonephritis, MPGN = membranoproliferative glomeruloproliferative glomerulonephritis, MesangPGN = mesangioproliferative glomerulonephritis, ISN = interstitial nephritis, HBsAg = hepatitis B surface antigen, NR = not recorded.

Overt renal failure appears to be uncommon (see Table 5.4). Progression to end-stage renal disease and consequent death due to uremia, kidney transplantation, or maintenance hemodialysis[99,101,104,118,119] have been reported. In one report of 15 children, 7 had total remission and 4 had partial remission (0.2–0.8 g/day proteinuria) within a few months; 3 had persistent massive proteinuria; and 1 showed progressive deterioration of renal function, necessitating dialytic therapy.[118]

In adults the renal lesions, although less common than in children, appear to be progressive with persistent proteinuria and renal insufficiency.[93,99,104,106,119,126] Contrary to children, remission of nephrotic syndrome or proteinuria is not common in adults, renal failure is progressive in one-third of cases, and renal replacement therapy becomes necessary in 10% of patients with persistent antigenemia and massive proteinuria.[119] As a rule, recovery of the renal lesion occurs after spontaneous clearance of HBsAg from the serum.[119,135,143]

In the few patients in whom therapy with steroids or immunosuppression was attempted, treatment did not seem effective.[93,101,118] In fact, in the first case report of membranous glomerulonephritis attributed to HBV, the patient developed nephrotic syndrome while on steroid treatment for liver disease.[93] In the setting of chronic active hepatitis, which affects most adults who develop renal lesions, steroids may exert a deleterious effect on markers of viral replication,[136] and their use should be undertaken cautiously. Treatment with interferon of chronic carriers of HBsAg with associated membranous glomerulonephritis has been shown to result in changes of viral markers and remission of massive proteinuria, which was complete in some but only temporary or partial in others.[119,126–128] These results are obviously preliminary and inconclusive, but efforts at reducing viral markers may ultimately prove to be the best therapy. Thus, although not always effective, interferon therapy should be considered in patients with massive proteinuria and progressive disease.[129] Renal transplantation in chronic but asymptomatic carriers of HBsAg has been reported to have a high risk of progressive, sometimes fatal, liver disease in some[130,131] but not all[132] patients.

On renal biopsy (see Table 5.5), the predominant lesion, present in over 85% of patients, is classic membranous glomerulonephritis, characterized by basement membrane thickening; methenamine-silver stain shows epimembranous spikes, and electronmicroscopy shows subepithelial electron-dense deposits with a fairly monotonous regularity. Mild mesangial hypercellularity and matricial increase, as seen by light microscopy and confirmed by electron microscopy, are noted in some reports.

Crescentic glomerulonephritis has been described in 2 asymptomatic carriers of HBsAg, both presenting with nephrotic syndrome and acute renal failure.[137] HBeAg was demonstrated in the serum and glomerular tufts of both patients; neither had anti-GBM or ANCA antibodies. The initial kidney biopsy of 1 patient revealed membranous glomerulonephropathy, but crescentic glomerulonephritis was found 20 months later when he presented with renal failure. Renal failure progressed despite α-interferon treatment but responded to pulse methylprednisolone followed by three plasma exchanges. The development of crescentic glomerulonephritis probably reflects the severity of glomerular involvement with consequent disruption of glomerular capillaries and bleeding into Bowman's capsule, which accounts for the crescentic reaction in all such cases of rapidly progressive glomerulonephritis.[138,139]

Other histologic patterns of glomerular lesions reported with HBV are membranoproliferative glomerulonephritis, mesangioproliferative glomerulonephritis, proliferative glomerulonephritis, and focal sclerosing glomerulonephritis.[99,101,102,108,110,115,122,140] It is important to view these lesions in context. Thus, one patient with focal sclerosing glomerulonephritis, in whom tubulointerstitial nephritis was also present,[101] was a drug addict who had bladder neck contracture and a history of chronic urinary tract infection. Since both urinary reflux and drug addiction may result in nephropathy independently of HBV infection,[141,142] the finding of HBsAg in this patient may have been coincidental and another consequence of drug addiction rather than the cause of focal sclerosing glomerulonephritis, which has been associated more specifically with drug addiction and urinary reflux.[141,142] Thus, some of the reported lesions may well have been due to another etiology, with HBsAg an incidental finding.

Supporting evidence has been presented from careful electron microscopic study of the biopsy specimen of 98 children with HBs antigenemia first documented at the clinical onset of glomerulopathy.[143] Only 77 of the children had a uniform type of glomerulopathy characteristic of HBV-associated membranous glomerulonephropathy with abundant subepithelial electron-dense deposits. In addition, several had mesangial and subendothelial electron-dense deposits with a mild mesangial proliferative reaction but without the peripheral interposition and split basement membrane characteristic of membranoproliferative glomerulonephritis. Thus, in some cases classified as mesangioproliferative or membranoproliferative glomerulonephritis by light microscopy, careful scrutiny by electron microscopy may reveal principally the classic extramembranous deposits of membranous glomerulopathy. In such cases, when proliferative changes are seen, they are mild and not consistent with the classification of mesangioproliferative or membranoproliferative glomerulonephritis. In cases with lesions typical of membranoproliferative glomerulonephritis, the presence of HBsAg may be an epiphenomenon reflecting the endemic areas from where the reports emanated.[143]

On immunofluorescent examination, most cases reveal a full house of immunoglobulins—IgG, IgA, and IgM—together with early components of complement—C_1q and C_4—in a coarse, granular, beaded pattern along the glomerular basement membrane and mesangial areas. The more consistent and intense staining is that of IgG, with a slightly less intense staining of complement. IgM and IgA deposits have been either absent or detected only in trace amounts.

Immunofluorescence for HBsAg has been positive in the majority, but not all, of the cases (see Table 5.5). Where present, the distribution and pattern has been similar to that of IgG and complement. This may reflect the preeminent role of HBsAg as the most common circulating antigen; however, HBsAg has often been the only antigen searched for in serum as well as deposits. In reports in which renal tissue was negative for HBsAg, further examination has revealed the presence of either HBeAg[97] or HBcAg in deposits.[122,123] It seems, therefore, that any of the antigenic components of the HBV may be involved in the pathogenesis of glomerular lesions.[99]

The localization of HBV antigens in a granular pattern along the glomerular basement membrane in association with immunoglobulins, together with the demonstration of cryoprecipitable complexes of the different antigens and their antibodies from the serum of some patients,[95,97,122] may be construed as evidence in support of HBV infection as a primary cause of immune complex glomerulonephritis. Evidence implicating an immune complex pathogenesis was first provided from studies on an 8-year-old boy with fulminant viral hepatitis; the eluate from his kidneys was shown to contain antibody directed against HBsAg,[110] with the level of antibody activity to HBsAg 37 times higher in the eluate than in the serum. Subsequently, it was shown that the glomerular lesions can be reproduced experimentally by inoculation of baboons with human HBsAg.[144] Simultaneous serologic studies revealed a declining HBsAg titer 2 weeks after inoculation paralleling a rise in anti-HBs

antibodies. Renal changes shortly after inoculation consisted primarily of minor mesangial alterations. Repeat biopsy several months later showed more advanced lesions with capillary loop sclerosis and basement membrane thickening, like lesions in patients with chronic active hepatitis.

Thus, the primary renal lesions are those of an immune complex-mediated membranous nephropathy. The immunopathologic features of membranous nephropathy bear a striking resemblance to those observed with chronic bovine serum albumin-immune complexes in rabbits with a maintained, low-level antibody response to daily injections of small doses of antigen.[145,146] In view of the antigenic nature of the HBV and the chronic persistence of its antigens in some cases; together with persistent circulating immune complexes, it is not surprising that glomerular lesions have been observed. Why the glomerular lesions are not more frequent reflects a number of other factors that govern the effect on various organs, including quantity and size of the complexes as well as genetically determined differences in individual host responsiveness.[147]

Experimental studies in rats indicate that complexes with a molecular mass of 1,000,000 daltons or less precipitate in the glomerular basement membrane and subepithelial spaces to induce typical membranous glomerulonephropathy. Larger particles are cleared by the reticuloendothelial system, whereas smaller particles are unable to activate the mediator systems of immune-mediated injury.[146] The 20-nm spherical HBsAg particles, the most commonly demonstrated antigen, have a molecular mass of 3,000,000 daltons even without binding to antibody. Any immune complex containing molecular fragments of HBsAg of small size, but with the same immunoreactivity, may be responsible for the lesions. HBeAg, with a molecular mass of not more than 300,000 daltons even when bound to IgG, is of a size capable of inducing membranous nephropathy.

Independent of considerations of the size of particles necessary to initiate the glomerular lesions, spherical particles containing central cores of electron-dense material that were consistent with the ultrastructure of the HBV have been noted in renal biopsy specimens.[101] Electron microscopic examination at high magnification has been reported to reveal spherical particles containing central cores of electron-dense material, consistent with the ultrastructure of the HBV, within the subepithelial deposits of patients with membranous nephropathy.[101,148] In addition, HBV-DNA has been isolated from renal tissue extracts[149–151] and localized to the kidney by in-situ hybridization.[149,152] In a longitudinal study of patients with HBV-associated membranous nephropathy, in-situ hybridization demonstrated HBV-DNA in the glomeruli and tubules in 7 of 8 patients (87.5%) biopsied within 6 months after onset of disease, whereas it was detectable only in the tubular epithelium in 3 of 14 specimens (21%) obtained later than 6 months.[152] In 2 of the patients with massive proteinuria who progressed to end-stage renal disease, HBV-DNA remained detectable in the tubular epithelia, whereas it was no longer detectable in patients with mild or no proteinuria. Thus, the presence of HBV-DNA appears to show a direct correlation with the course of the disease, duration of proteinuria, and progression to renal failure. The glomeruli in which HBV-DNA was detected were also positive for HBeAg-AB immune complexes and IgG. There is increasing evidence that of the various antigenic components, HBeAg may have a more important pathogenetic role in coexistent membranous nephropathy.[119,152–154]

The exact incidence of HBV-associated glomerulonephritis is not known. Several reports, three from Poland[105,122,123] and one from Hungary,[116] suggest that the kidney tissue examined at autopsy or by biopsy from patients with glomerulonephritis and immunofluorescent evidence of an immune complex lesion but no liver pathology, is positive for HBsAg in as many as 16.8–56.2% of cases. This suggests that HBV might be involved in the pathogenesis of an exceptionally high percentage of cases of immune complex glomerulonephritis. Even though such results are intriguing, they must be viewed with caution. Certainly they do not reflect the experience in Japan,[115] France,[118] and North America.[120,121] The differences are likely due to the higher prevalence rate of hepatitis B viral infection in the general population of endemic areas.

Viewed from another perspective, HBs-antigenemia appears to be found in endemic areas for the virus in a higher proportion of patients with heterogeneous forms of glomerulonephritic lesions than in healthy people without evidence of kidney disease.[114–118,155,156] The renal lesions in such patients appears to span nearly the whole spectrum of renal pathology, although antigenemia seems to be more common in patients

with the characteristic lesions of membranous glomerulonephropathy (Table 5.6), which are more specific for viral infection.[143]

Polyarteritis nodosa also develops in association with HBV infection.[98] The renal lesions are classically indicative of arteritis with typical fibrinoid necrosis and perivascular infiltration. Angiographic studies usually reveal the typical aneurysmal dilatation. In some patients, fluorescent antibody studies have revealed variable deposition of HBsAg, IgG, IgM, and complement in a nodular pattern along the elastic membrane of the damaged vessels.

The incidence of circulating immune complexes is high early in the course of acute viral hepatitis. Modest degrees of reduction in GFR and abnormalities of urine sediment have been observed in patients with acute viral hepatitis.[157–159] The urinary sediment abnormalities—hematuria, proteinuria, and cylindruria—are seen early in the course of clinical liver disease and usually resolve within days or weeks.[157] The reduction in GFR and proteinuria (300–700 mg/day) may persist for months.[158,159] In a percutaneous biopsy study of 20 patients with acute viral hepatitis, glomerular changes noted in 10 patients included glomerular swelling and focal hypercellularity that appeared to consist primarily of epithelial cell hyperplasia and hypertrophy. In 3 patients, focal thickening of the basement membrane was found. The lesions were still present at 3 months but had resolved completely at 1 year.[159] Focal glomerular basement membrane thickening, mesangial electron-dense deposits on electron microscopy, and deposits of IgG and complement in a granular pattern along the glomerular basement membrane and mesangium on immunofluorescent staining also have been noted in cases of acute viral hepatitis.[123,158]

It seems, therefore, that renal glomerular changes in HBV infection are predominantly related to an immune-mediated process.[99,160] Two alternatives may account for the development of renal lesions: (1) direct deposition of antigenic fragments of the virion in the glomerular capillary wall, as suggested by demonstrations of HBsAg in urine, with the renal injury mediated subsequently through in situ immune complex formation, or (2) circulating immune complexes formed by the combination of one of the viral antigens with its antibody and trapped in the glomerular capillary wall that initiate a local

TABLE 5.6.   Hepatitis B Surface Antigen in Patients with Glomerular Abnormality

Reference	Year	Renal Diagnosis	No. Examined	No. Positive	Percent Positive
124	1973	Miscellaneous	182	37	20.3
114	1974	Membranoproliferative glomerulonephritis	57	5	8.7
		Diffuse proliferative glomerulonephritis	13	2	15.4
		Membranous glomerulopathy	32	3	9.4
		IgA nephropathy	59	2	3.4
		Focal sclerosing glomerulosclerosis	56	0	0
		Miscellaneous	50	5	10
		Control	3,152	19	0.54
105	1974	Chronic glomerulonephritis	32	16	50
115	1975	Chronic glomerulonephritis	105	8	7.8
155	1977	Nephrotic syndrome	21	3	14.2
117	1978	Membranous glomerulopathy	10	10	100
		Miscellaneous	152	7	4.6
		Control			2
118	1979	Membranous glomerulopathy	33	15	45.4
		Miscellaneous	170	3	1.76
		Nonglomerular kidney disease	100	4	4
116	1979	Immune complex glomerulonephritis + nephrotic syndrome	196	32	16.3
		Miscellaneous	80	4	5
		Control	18,799	186	0.99
156	1983	Miscellaneous	63	14	22.2
		Membranous glomerulopathy	14	14	100

inflammatory reaction. This may result in varying degrees of renal involvement, ranging from mild, reversible lesions to more severe, progressive lesions. The severity of renal involvement more likely depends on the duration of the antigenemia, variations in host responsiveness, and age of the patient. The long-term prognosis of renal lesions in patients with persistent antigenemia is unknown. The primary lesion that develops is membranous glomerulonephropathy, which is characteristically a slowly progressive disease with an indolent course accentuated by remissions and relapses. Long-term follow-up of cases of HBV-associated glomerulonephropathy should provide data on survival.

The relationship of the renal lesions to the clinical activity of liver disease is variable. All combinations have been described with (1) either hepatic or renal involvement as the initial presenting clinical illness, (2) renal involvement superimposed on chronic active hepatitis, or (3) renal and hepatic involvement occurring at the same time.[93,100–135] In some patients, the development of renal abnormalities coincides with the onset of acute hepatitis[118]; in others, the onset ranges from 1–20 years after acute hepatitis[112];

and in yet others, evidence of hepatic involvement remains either absent or subclinical.[118]

Human Immunodeficiency Virus Infection

In the rather brief period since the acquired immune deficiency syndrome (AIDS) was first identified in 1981, it has emerged as the most recent and relentlessly spreading epidemic disease confronting the human race. The number of identified cases of AIDS in the United States has increased exponentially. As of October 1993, the Centers for Disease Control and Prevention had received reports of 334,344 cases of AIDS. Worldwide, it is estimated that as many as 10 million people have been infected with the AIDS virus.[161] AIDS has become the fifth leading cause of death in people younger than 40 years. These alarming figures emphasize the emerging importance of the potential renal problems associated with AIDS.

As the protean manifestations of infection with HIV have come to be recognized, hepatic and renal abnormalities have emerged as rather common complications. The principal manifestations of renal involvement are reduced GFR, a high incidence of proteinuria, and various glomerular lesions, most notably focal and segmental glomerulosclerosis. The characteristic clinicopathologic renal disease that results from infection with the human immunodeficiency virus (HIV) has been termed HIV-associated nephritis (HIVAN).[162–165] The limited life expectancy of AIDS patients and their rapid demise from the multitude of infectious complications preclude full appreciation of the impact of renal changes.[166] Suffice it to say that the presence of renal failure has been identified as a marker of poor prognosis.[167] However, more than half of those who develop the renal lesions considered characteristic of HIV infection are otherwise asymptomatic carriers of the virus with no evidence of AIDS,[162] and their outcome depends on the infectious complications of the disease itself rather than the presence of kidney disease.[162–165]

The glomerular abnormalities in HIV-infected patients have been studied in kidney tissue obtained by percutaneous biopsy and at autopsy.[162–170] The lesions have been more common in tissue obtained at biopsy simply because the procedure has been performed only when abnormalities of renal function were present. On biopsied specimens the principal lesions are of focal and segmental glomerulosclerosis, with varying degrees of tubular atrophy, tubular dilatation, focal interstitial fibrosis, and infiltration with mononuclear cells.[163,168,170] Immunofluorescent study has shown granular deposits of IgM and C_3. The more predominant lesions noted at autopsy and in some of the biopsied specimens have been hypercellularity and moderate expansion of the mesangial matrix, which on immunofluorescent microscopy revealed mesangial deposits of IgG, IgM, and C_3, without glomerular sclerosis but with interstitial changes.[167–172]

Proteinuria is the most common abnormality noted on urinalysis. It is present in 35–40% of patients with AIDS encountered in major medical centers, and in 9–10% the proteinuria is in the nephrotic range.[162,167–172] The presence of modest proteinuria does not seem to correlate well with the glomerular lesions; in one series, about half the patients with normal glomeruli had quantitative proteinuria.[169] However, proteinuria in the nephrotic range is exceptional in the absence of focal and segmental glomerular sclerosis.[170,171] In patients with significant proteinuria, GFR is generally reduced, and their course involves rapid deterioration of renal function, eventuating in terminal renal failure in a few months.[166,168] The course of patients with mesangial hypercellularity appears to be relatively more indolent; such patients usually succumb to the ravages of AIDS before the onset of end-stage kidney disease.[169,170] Reversible acute renal failure and a variety of fluid and electrolyte disturbances may also occur during episodes of complicated superimposed infections or secondary to drug therapy with potentially nephrotoxic agents.[162,171]

A number of coexisting conditions may predispose HIV-infected patients to glomerular injury. The renal lesions and course of renal deterioration are quite similar to those described in intravenous substance abusers.[173] Some 35–45% of patients with AIDS are intravenous drug abusers, and seropositivity for HIV is high among intravenous drug abusers. In a study of 56 drug abusers with no evidence of renal disease, 41% were seropositive for HIV-III, 18% for HIV-II, and 9% for HIV-1.[174] In addition, as many as one-third of drug abusers have decreased helper cells and an inverted helper/suppressor T cell ratio—an abnormality that is characteristic of AIDS.[175] In fact, renal lesions are significantly more common in patients with AIDS who are intravenous drug users than in those who are homosexual.[162,170]

A second coexisting feature of interest is the fact that the lymphoproliferative disorders that develop in patients with AIDS have also been associated with glomerular abnormalities.[176] In fact, glomerular lesions were considered to be more common in patients with Kaposi's sarcoma in one report on AIDS[169] but not in others.[167,168]

A third coexistent predisposing feature is the susceptibility of AIDS patients to infectious organisms that have been incriminated as a cause of glomerular lesions, such as cytomegalovirus, streptococci, staphylococci, *Candida* sp., and salmonella.[177] Finally, increased levels of circulating immune complexes have been detected in patients with AIDS by some investigators[178,179] but not by others.[180]

In fact, the immunopathogenic mechanisms underlying infection with HIV are quite complex with varying stages of viral replication and viremia through the course of the disease,[181] during which direct viral infection of the renal glomerular and epithelial cells occurs.[182] Altered systemic or local antigen load, immune activation, and secretion of cytokines may well set the stage for renal disease. Certainly chronic exposure to the multitude of infective antigens to which

HIV-infected patients are exposed, in a setting of altered immune responsiveness, may contribute further to the development of renal lesions.[162]

Schistosomiasis

Hepatic involvement may develop with *Schistosoma mansoni* and less commonly with *S. japonicum* and *S. haematobium*. In the liver, a granulomatous eosinophilic reaction to the eggs results in periportal and septal fibrosis, intrahepatic portal vein destruction, and focal inflammatory infiltration with mononuclear cells; ultimately, the result is presinusoidal portal hypertension. The presenting features are those of portal hypertension; hepatic function is normal except for an increase in serum alkaline phosphatase.[183]

The glomerular lesions, which usually develop in individuals chronically and severely afflicted by schistosomiasis, consist of mesangial hypercellularity and hypertrophy with focal segmental or diffuse sclerosis. On immunofluorescent study, granular deposits of IgG, IgM, and complement are observed in the mesangial area and along the capillary walls. Electron microscopy reveals electron-lucent deposits within the thickened basement membrane and electron-dense deposits in the subendothelial and mesangial areas.[184–186]

A specific schistosomal antigen and its antibody have been identified in the serum of infected individuals.[187] A lesion similar to that seen in humans has been shown to develop in experimentally infected primates[188] and mice.[189] The schistosomal adult worm antigen has been identified in the glomeruli of experimentally infected mice[189] and by immunofluorescence in the mesangial area of human kidney tissue obtained at surgery or transcutaneous biopsy.[186,190]

Renal function is variable, ranging from normal to that of end-stage kidney disease.[185,186,191] Proteinuria is often present; nephrotic syndrome is a common presentation in patients with renal involvement. Glomerular changes may be present even in the absence of any clinical manifestation of renal disease.[188]

Malaria

A mild form of liver injury is a frequent accompaniment of malaria. Hepatomegaly occurs in about one-half of cases during the acute phase. Modest alterations in liver function usually return to normal following recovery from the acute episode. Jaundice, if present, is usually minimal and reflects hemolysis rather than hepatic injury. The hepatic phase may be prolonged, resulting in the clinical relapses encountered with *Plasmodium vivax* and *P. malariae* infections. *P. falciparum* is not associated with persistent hepatic infection but might result in massive hemolysis, centrilobular necrosis due to hypoxemia, and acute renal failure due to tubular necrosis.[177,183]

A definite relationship of *P. malariae* and *P. falciparum* to glomerular disease has been established.[192,193] In *P. malariae*, the degree of glomerular changes is variable and is related to some extent to duration and severity of disease.[192] In its mild form the changes are primarily limited to the mesangial area; in the more advanced form there is diffuse involvement of the glomerular capillary wall. The primary lesion is a thickening of the mesangium and glomerular basement membrane, which on silver staining reveal a duplication of argyrophilic material.[194] Cellular proliferation is unusual. Subendothelial deposits of membranelike material of variable density, as seen by electron microscopy, account for the basement membrane thickening. Minute lacunae scattered irregularly throughout the basement membrane have been considered to be a pathognomonic finding with this lesion, which has been termed quartan malarial nephropathy.[194]

The detection of elevated levels of antimalarial antibodies in the serum of patients with renal involvement[192,195] and the demonstration of coarse granular deposits of IgG, IgM, and complement in the kidney biopsies, which decrease with remission of the disease,[194,196] implicate an immune complex pathogenesis for the glomerular changes. Microscopic hematuria and proteinuria are characteristically present; massive proteinuria and nephrotic syndrome are the presenting picture in most patients. The prognosis of renal disease in quartan malaria tends to correlate with the degree of glomerular involvement. In patients who have extensive and generalized involvement and present with massive proteinuria, the lesion is progressive and renal insufficiency develops, whereas with mild focal involvement, remission and long-term survival are the rule.[197]

In *P. falciparum* malaria, the glomerular changes are characterized by hypercellularity, irregular thickening of the basement membrane, and polymorphonuclear leukocytic infiltration. Electron microscopy reveals electron-dense deposits in the subendothelial and paramesangial areas. Immunofluorescent studies reveal granular deposits of IgG, IgM, IgA, and complement in the mesangial region and along the glomerular basement membrane.[193,198] Malarial antigen has been demonstrated by fluorescent antibody technique and eluates of immunoglobulin malarial antibody activity, providing evidence for an immune complex-mediated mechanism. The urine abnormalities in falciparum nephritis range from microhematuria and proteinuria to massive proteinuria and nephrotic syndrome.[193,198] The prognosis of renal disease associated with *P. falciparum* is better than that of quartan malaria; abnormalities in renal function and urine sediment usually return to normal within 4–6 weeks after antimalarial therapy.[193]

Infectious Mononucleosis

A mild anicteric hepatitis almost always accompanies infections with Epstein-Barr virus. The hepatic lesion is characterized by areas of focal necrosis, portal tract lymphocytic inflammation, and infiltration of the sinusoids by atypical lymphocytes. Elevation of the serum transaminase levels is usual. In most patients the serum bilirubin level is less than 3 mg/100 ml, unless hemolysis supervenes. Splenomegaly, present in one-half of cases, reflects the lymphoid hyperplasia rather than portal hypertension. Hepatomegaly is rare and mild.[183]

Abnormalities in urine sediment, gross hematuria, nephrotic syndrome, and progressive renal failure have been described.[199–202] The most consistent findings in the kidneys are an aggregation of mononuclear cells in the interstitium and foci of tubular damage.[199,202] Mild glomerular changes, characterized by focal mesangial hypercellularity, also occur.[199,200,203] Electron microscopy and immunofluorescent studies have failed to provide convincing evidence for an immune complex mechanism for minor glomerular changes.

Other Infectious Diseases

Glomerular alterations have been reported in a number of other infectious diseases that affect the liver. Most of these are rare and usually mild and reversible.[177]

Infection with *Legionella pneumophila* (Legionnaires' disease) is frequently associated with hepatic involvement. The majority of patients have one or more abnormal liver function tests.

Mild elevations in serum transaminase, bilirubin, and alkaline phosphatase are detectable in 90% of patients. Abnormalities related to the kidneys range from proteinuria and hematuria to overt renal failure.[204–206] Hyaline and granular casts are seen, and red blood cells casts have been described.[205] Renal failure appears to be related to shock, rhabdomyolysis, and myoglobinuria.[205] The morphologic changes are those of acute tubulointerstitial nephritis.[206] In one of the rare cases in which renal changes were examined carefully, there were focal areas of glomerular epithelial detachment, marked endothelial swelling, and moderate increase in the mesangial matrix.[206] Immunofluorescent and electron microscopic studies failed to reveal evidence for immunoglobulin or complement deposits.

SYSTEMIC DISEASES

Amyloidosis

Although the liver is frequently involved in systemic amyloidosis, the clinical features of hepatic involvement and abnormalities of liver function tests are usually mild or absent.[207] Hepatomegaly occurs in one-half of cases and splenomegaly in one-third. Hepatic insufficiency is rare but may occur in some patients who present with jaundice, ascites, and edema.[208,209] Coexistent renal involvement should always be considered in patients with proteinuria.

Renal involvement is the most common systemic manifestation of amyloidosis.[210,211] The sites of early amyloid deposition in the kidneys are the mesangial area and capillary wall of the glomerulus and around the interstitial fibroblasts and blood vessels. The deposits vary from minimal and focal segmental deposits to diffuse and generalized replacement of the normal architecture by amyloid. The deposits, which are homogenous in appearance on light microscopy, may mimic diabetic glomerulosclerosis or membranous glomerulopathy and require proper staining or electron microscopic examination for identification.[212,213] Although the glomeruli are the most frequently involved, the tubules are not spared and tubular function impairment may dominate the clinical picture.[214] Cases of amyloidlike deposits, due to light chain deposits, which do not stain with Congo red but on electron microscopy reveal fibrillar structures, have been reported with kidney and hepatic involvement.[215]

Proteinuria is the most frequent finding associated with renal involvement; nephrotic syndrome ultimately develops in about two-thirds of cases. As a rule, the course of renal involvement is progressive; renal failure is the major cause of death,[210,211] although occasional remissions have been reported.[214]

Hemochromatosis

Hemochromatosis, a genetic disorder due to enhanced intestinal iron absorption and impaired regulation of reticuloendothelial iron metabolism, results in excessive deposition of iron in the liver and other body sites. The accumulation of hepatic iron is accompanied by portal fibrosis, which often progresses to cirrhosis and portal hypertension.[183]

Although renal disease is not part of the primary process, the development of diabetes mellitus in 80% of patients results in the expected glomerular changes. The classic changes of diabetic glomerular nodular and diffuse glomerulosclerosis have been reported within 4 years of the development of insulin requirement for the control of diabetes in patients with hemochromatosis.[216,217]

Sickle-cell Disease

The liver is often involved in sickle-cell disease. Hepatomegaly is present in over one-half of patients with sickle-cell anemia, and abnormalities of liver function (hyperbilirubinemia, elevated transaminase) are common and become worse during abdominal crises.

Various renal functional and structural abnormalities have been associated with sickle-cell disease.[218–220] Even in young patients with no evidence of clinical renal disease, the glomeruli are significantly enlarged and the capillary loops are congested and typically filled with sickled red blood cells. Such changes are particularly prominent in the juxtamedullary glomeruli.[221] Some degree of hypercellularity, particularly in the mesangial areas, is also an early sign. The mesangial changes have been attributed to iron-protein complexes accumulating in the mesangium.[222] Electron microscopy shows splitting of the basement membrane and confirms the mesangial hypercellularity.

Hematuria, which is the most common abnormality in patients with sickle-cell disease, is often nonglomerular, originating from the congested vessels of the pelvic mucosa. On the other hand, the proteinuria, which develops in 30–40% of patients, is of glomerular origin. Nephrotic syndrome develops in some and progresses to end-stage renal disease in a few. Glomerulosclerosis, interstitial fibrosis, tubular atrophy, and hemosiderin deposits are prominent features in all such cases.[223,224] In addition, immunoglobulins (IgG, IgM), complement components (C_1q and C_3), and renal tubular epithelial antigen have been demonstrated in a granular pattern along the glomerular basement membrane.[223,224] Cryoprecipitable complexes of renal tubular epithelial antigen-antibody have been detected in the circulation of patients with glomerular lesions and proteinuria. IgM and IgG eluted from the glomeruli have been shown to fix the proximal tubules of normal human kidney by direct immunofluorescence. This localization could be abolished by absorption of the eluate with renal tubular epithelial antigen.[223,224] Thus, the evidence for an immune deposit nephritis associated with sickle-cell anemia is fairly conclusive. A similar glomerular lesion mediated by identical immunopathogenic mechanisms can also occur in heterozygotes with sickle-cell trait.[225]

Collagen Diseases

Despite the fact that multisystem involvement is common in collagen diseases, hepatic involvement is not common. The liver is sometimes affected by drug-induced hepatotoxicity secondary to anti-inflammatory and immunosuppressive agents used in treatment. Occasionally, a subclinical form of collagen disease may be unmasked during the work-up of patients with chronic liver disease. Only rarely is liver involvement severe enough to warrant clinical attention.[183] On the other hand, glomerular changes are common and usually a dominant part of the clinical presentation.

Toxemia

The cardinal features of toxemia are hypertension, proteinuria, and edema; the extent of each varies considerably. The kidney is the main organ affected in this otherwise generalized disease with protean manifestations. Hepatic involvement, as part of the generalized vascular disorder, occurs in about one-half of cases of toxemia of pregnancy. The degree of hepatic involvement correlates with the severity of the toxemic state and is usually undetectable if the toxemia is clinically mild; however, it is present in varying degrees of severity in two-thirds of patients with eclampsia.[226,227]

Generalized glomerular changes constitute the most constant and probably most important pathologic feature of toxemia of pregnancy.[226,228–230] The glomeruli appear enlarged, swollen, and ischemic. There is marked swelling of the endothelial cells, which appear foamy and fill most of the capillary lumen; hence, the term glomerular capillary endotheliosis is used to describe the renal lesion.[230] The endothelial cells are separated from the basement membrane by a space filled with amorphous proteinaceous material that is flocculent in appearance with a fibrillar component composed at least partly of fibrin, as demonstrated by immunofluorescence studies.[228] The mesangial areas are swollen, and mesangial cell hyperplasia may be so extreme that it contributes to the capillary lumen narrowing caused by the endothelial cell swelling.

The degree of reduction in GFR and renal blood flow varies, depending on the severity of renal involvement. Abnormalities in urine sediment with hematuria, pyuria, and cylindruria are almost invariably present. Red blood cell casts have been reported. The amount of proteinuria varies with the extent of glomerular changes, ranging from modest increases detected on 24-hour protein quantitation to massive proteinuria well within the nephrotic range. All of these morphologic and functional changes, which are most prominent in the intermediate puerperium, are reversible once pregnancy is terminated.[231] By the second week, the glomerular lesions are largely resolved, although some changes may persist for months or even years.[232,233]

Acute Fatty Liver of Pregnancy

This rare but well-described hepatic disorder of unknown etiology occurs in the last trimester of pregnancy, usually, but not exclusively, in association with toxemia.[234] The typical presenting features are nausea, vomiting, abdominal pain and jaundice. Hemorrhagic complications are common. Renal failure may be a dominant feature; when present, it contributes significantly to the rather high mortality rate.[226,235,236] Improvement begins within 2–3 days of delivery with

gradual resolution of liver dysfunction and renal failure.

The classic glomerular changes of toxemia of pregnancy are present in women who present with toxemia. In other cases, the glomeruli reveal a mild diffuse global hypercellularity and variable degrees of irregular thickening of the basement membrane. The most frequent and uniform renal lesion is the accumulation of fat within the cells of the proximal tubules.[235–237]

Congenital Diseases

Congenital diseases of the kidney may be associated with various types of visceral involvement, including involvement of the liver. Most notable among these is polycystic kidney disease, but associated hepatic involvement has also been reported in juvenile nephrophthisis, medullary cystic disease, and cystic dysplastic kidneys.[238–241] Renal involvement in congenital diseases of the liver has also been reported.[242–245]

The renal lesions in such cases are primarily tubulointerstitial, and the glomeruli are rarely involved except for glomerulosclerosis, which is present in the eventual end-stage kidney disease that develops in most patients.

REFERENCES

1. Flint A: Clinical report on hydroperitoneum based on an analysis of forty-six cases. Am J Med Sci 1863; 4S:306–339.
2. Baldus WP, Summerskill WHJ: Liver-kidney interrelationships. In Schiff L (ed): Diseases of the Liver. Philadelphia: J.B. Lippincott Co., 1975;445–465.
3. Lichtman SS, Sohval AR: Clinical disorders associated with hepatic and renal manifestations, with especial reference to the so-called "hepatorenal syndrome." Am J Dig Dis 1937–1938;4:26–32.
4. Baxter JH, Ashworth CT: Renal lesions in portal cirrhosis. Arch Pathol 1946;41:476–488.
5. Fiessinger N, Varay A: Le rein des cirrhotiques. Presse Med 1938;46:1361–1362.
6. Kimmelstiel P, Wilson C: Intercapillary lesions in the glomeruli of the kidney. Am J Pathol 1936;12:83–98.
7. Horn RC, Smetana H: Intercapillary glomerulosclerosis. Am J Pathol 1942;18:93–100.
8. Raphael SS, Lynch MJG: Kimmelstiel-Wilson glomerulonephropathy. Its occurrence in diseases other than diabetes mellitus. Arch Pathol 1958;65:420–431.
9. Patek AJ, Seegal D, Bevans M: The coexistence of cirrhosis of the liver and glomerulonephritis. Report of 14 cases. Am J Med Sci 1951;221:77–85.
10. Fisher ER, Hellstron HR: The membranous and proliferative glomerulonephritis of hepatic cirrhosis. Am J Clin Pathol 1959;32:48–55.

11. Crowson CN, More RH: Glomerulotubular nephrosis correlated with hepatic lesions. II. Incidence and morphology of associated kidney and liver lesions in human autopsy material. Arch Pathol 1955;60:73–84.

12. Bloodworth JMB, Sommers SC: "Cirrhotic glomerulosclerosis": A renal lesion associated with hepatic cirrhosis. Lab Invest 1959;8:962–978.

13. Sakaguchi H, Dachs S, Grishman E, et al: Hepatic glomerulosclerosis. An electron microscopic study of renal biopsies of liver disease. Lab Invest 1965;14:533–545.

14. Guillan RA, Zelman S, Alonso DR: Hepatic glomerulosclerosis (an analysis of 60 cases). Am J Gastroenterol 1968;49:499–502.

15. Fisher ER, Perez-Stable E: Cirrhotic (hepatic) lobular glomerulonephritis. Correlation of ultrastructural and clinical features. Am J Pathol 1968;52:869–890.

16. Nochy D, Callard P, Bellon B, et al: Association of overt glomerulonephritis and liver disease: A study of 34 patients. Clin Nephrol 1976;6:422–427.

17. Manigand G, Paillas J, Morel-Maroger L, et al: Cirrhose du foie et nephropathie glomerulaire: a propos de trois observations de cirrhose hepatique latente, revelee par une nephropathie glomerulaire. Ann Med Intern 1969;120:323–334.

18. Manigand G, Morel-Maroger L, Simon J, Deparis M: Lesions renales glomerulaires et cirrhose du foie. Note preliminnaire sur les lesions histologique du rein au cours des cirrhoses hepatiques, d'apres 20 prelevements biopsiques. Rev Eur Etud Clin Biol 1970;15:989–996.

19. Callard P, Druet P, Feldmann G, et al: Glomerular immunoglobulin deposits in cirrhosis [Abstract]. Digestion 1974;10:309.

20. Callard P, Feldmann G, Prandi D, et al: Immune complex type glomerulonephritis in cirrhosis of the liver. Am J Pathol 1975;80:329–340.

21. Berger J, Yaneva H, Nabarra B: Glomerular changes in patients with cirrhosis of the liver. Adv Nephrol 1978;7:3–14.

22. Hovig T, Blomhoff JP, Holme R, et al: Plasma lipoprotein alterations and morphologic changes with lipid deposition in the kidney of patients with hepatorenal syndrome. Lab Invest 1978;38:540–549.

23. Woodroofe AJ, Gormly AA, McKenzie PE, et al: Immunologic studies in IgA nephropathy. Kidney Int 1980;18:366–374.

24. Suga T, Endoh M, Miura M, et al: Hepatic glomerulosclerosis with IgA deposition—report of three cases. Tokai J Exp Clin Med 1978;8:540–549.

25. Montoliu J, Darnell A, Grau JM, et al: Renal involvement in a syndrome of vasculitis complicating HbsAg negative cirrhosis of the liver. Proc Eur Dial Transplant Assoc 1984;21:677–682.

26. Singhal PC, Scharschmidt LA: Membranous nephropathy associated with primary biliary cirrhosis and bullous pemphigoid. Ann Allergy 1985;5:484–485.

27. Montoliu J, Darnell A, Torras A, Revert L: Glomerular disease in cirrhosis of the liver: Low frequency of IgA deposits. Am J Nephrol 1986;6:199–205.

28. Praga M, Costa JR, Shandas GJ, et al: Acute renal failure in cirrhosis associated with macroscopic hematuria of glomerular origin. Arch Intern Med 1987;147:173–174.

29. Fukuda Y: Renal glomerular changes associated with liver cirrhosis. Acta Pathol Jpn 1982;32:561–574.

30. Endo Y, Matsushita H, Nozawa Y, et al: Glomerulonephritis associated with liver cirrhosis. Acta Pathol Jpn 1983;33:333–346.

31. Liebowitz HR: Primary kidney disease in patients with cirrhosis of the liver. NY State J Med 1965;65:535–541.

32. Crawford DHG, Endre ZH, Axelsen RA, et al: Universal occurrence of glomerular abnormalities in patients receiving liver transplants. Am J Kidney Dis 1992;19:339–344.

33. Milner LS, Houser MT, Kolbeck PC, et al: Glomerular injury in end-stage liver disease—role of circulating IgG and IgM immune complexes. Pediatr Nephrol 1993;7:6–10.

34. Marriott JB, Oliveira DB: Antimitochondrial autoantibodies in antiglomerular basement membrane disease. Clin Exp Immunol 1993;93:259–264.

35. Bissuel F, Bizollon T, Dijoud F, et al: Pulmonary hemorrhage and glomerulonephritis in primary biliary cirrhosis. Hepatology 1992;16:1357–1361.

36. Kourilsky O, Leroy C, Peltier AP: Complement and liver cell function in 53 patients with liver disease. Am J Med 1973;55:783–790.

37. Andre F, Andre C: Cirrhotic glomerulonephritis and secretory immunoglobulin A. Lancet 1976;1:97.

38. Druet P, Letonturier P, Content A, Mandet C: Cryoglobulinemia in human renal diseases. A study of seventy-six cases. Clin Exp Immunol 1973;15:483–496.

39. Newell GC: Cirrhotic glomerulonephritis: Incidence, morphology, clinical features, and pathogenesis. Am J Kidney Dis 1987;9:183–190.

40. Nakamura M: IgA nephropathy associated with portal hypertension in liver cirrhosis. Intern Med 1994;33:488–490.

41. Coppo R, Basolo B, Rollins C, et al: Mediterranean diet and primary IgA nephropathy. Clin Nephrol 1986;26:72–82.

42. Amore A, Coppo R, Roccatelo D, et al: Experimental IgA nephropathy secondary to hepatocellular injury induced dietary deficiencies and heavy alcohol intake. Lab Invest 1993;6:714–723.

43. Smith SM, Yu GSM, Tsukamoto H: IgA nephropathy in alcohol abuse. Lab Invest 1990;62:179–184.

44. Smith SM, Tsukamoto H: Time dependency of IgA nephropathy induction in alcohol ingestion. Alcohol Clin Exp Res 1992;16:471–474.

45. Kater L, Jobsis AC, Baart EH, et al: Alcoholic hepatic disease: Specificity of IgA deposits in liver disease. Am J Clin Pathol 1979;71:51–57.

46. Sakaguchi H, Dachs S, Mautner W, et al: Renal glomerular lesions after administration of carbon tetrachloride and ethionine. Lab Invest 1964;13:1418–1426.

47. Scivittaro V, Amore A, Emancipator SN: Animal models as a means to study IgA nephropathy. Contrib Nephrol 1993;104:65–78.

48. Gyorgy P, Ehrich WE, Langer BW: Renal changes in dietary hepatic injury in rats. Proc Soc Exp Biol Med 1966;123:764–767.

49. Gormly AA, Smith PS, Seymour AE, et al: IgA glomerular deposits in experimental cirrhosis. Am J Pathol 1981;104:50–54.

50. Woodrooffe AJ, Gormly AA, Clarkson AR, et al: Experimental cirrhosis and deposition of glomerular IgA immune complexes. Contrib Nephrol 1984;40: 51–54.

51. Gallo GR, Emancipator SN, Lamm ME: Experimental cholestasis and deposition of glomerular IgA immune complexes. Contrib Nephrol 1984;40:55–61.

52. Schifferli JA, Taylor RP: Physiological and pathological aspects of circulating immune complexes. Kidney Int 1989;35:993–1003.

53. Laan-Klamer SM, Atmosierodjo-Briggs JE, Harms G, et al: A histochemical study about the involvement of rat liver cells in the uptake of heterologous immune complexes from the circulation. Histochemistry 1985; 82:477–482.

54. Sinniah R: Heterogeneous IgA glomerulopathy in liver cirrhosis. Histopathology 1984;18:947–962.

55. Sancho J, Gonzalez E, Egido J: Handling of IgA immune aggregates by liver cells. Contrib Nephrol 40:93–98, 1984.

56. Nakamura M: IgA nephropathy associated with portal hypertension in liver cirrhosis. Intern Med 1994; 33:488–489.

57. Ghabra N, Piraino R, Greenberg A, Banner B: Resolution of cirrhotic glomerulonephritis following successful liver transplantation. Clin Nephrol 1991;35:6–9.

58. Fleming SJ, Axelsen RA, Lynch SL, et al: Persistent glomerular abnormalities following orthotopic liver transplantation. Nephron 1991;58:486.

59. Distant DA, Gonwa TA: The kidney in liver transplantation. J Am Soc Nephrol 1993;4:129–136.

60. Keane WF, Mulcahy WS, Kasiske BL, et al: Hyperlipidemia and progressive renal disease. Kidney Int 1991;39(Suppl 31):S41–S48.

61. Salomon M, Sagaguchi H, Churg J, et al: Renal lesions in hepatic disease: A study based on kidney biopsies. Arch Intern Med 1965;115:704–709.

62. Sagaguchi H: Hepatic glomerulosclerosis—light microscopic study of autopsy cases. Acta Pathol Jpn 1968;18:407–415.

63. Nocy D, Druet P, Bariety J: IgA nephropathy in chronic liver disease. Contrib Nephrol 1984;40:268–275.

64. Schwartz DT: The relation of cirrhosis of the liver to renal hypertension. A review of 638 autopsied cases. Ann Intern Med 1967;66:862–869.

65. Arroyo V, Girès P: Arteriolar vasodilation and the pathogenesis of the hyperdynamic circulation and renal sodium and water retention in cirrhosis. Gastroenterology 1992;102:1077–1079.

66. Reeves G, Lowenstein LM, Sommers SC: The macula densa and juxtaglomerular body of cirrhosis. Ann Intern Med 1963;112:708–715.

67. Villamediana LM, Velo M, Olivera A, et al: Glomerular binding and contractile response to angiotensin II in rats with chronic experimental cirrhosis of the liver. Clin Sci 1991;80:143–147.

68. Laube H, Norris HT, Robbins SL: The nephromegaly of chronic alcoholics with liver disease. Arch Pathol 1967;84:290–294.

69. Tsushima Y, Tomino Y, Wang LN, et al: Immunofluorescent analysis of extracellular matrix (ECM) components in glomeruli of hepatic glomerulosclerosis. Nippon Jinzo Gakkai Shi 1993;35:949–955.

70. Wehner H, Andler D: Uber die intercapillare glomerulosklerose bei lebercirrhose. Virchows Arch [A] 1973; 360:265–272.

71. Wong F, Massie D, Colman J, Dudley F: Glomerular hyperfiltration in patients with well compensated alcoholic cirrhosis. Gastroenterology 1993;104:884–889.

72. Wong F, Massie D, Hsu P, Dudley F: Renal response to a saline load in well compensated alcoholic cirrhosis. Hepatology 1994;20:873–881.

73. De Santo NG, Anastasio P, Loguercio C, et al: Glucagon-independent renal hyperaemia and hyperfiltration after an oral protein load in Child A liver cirrhosis. Eur J Clin Invest 1992;22:31–37.

74. Wong F, Massie D, Hsu P, Dudley F: Indomethacin-induced renal dysfunction in patients with well-compensated cirrhosis. Gastroenterology 1993;104:869–876.

75. Arroyo V, Girès P: Arteriolar vasodilation and the pathogenesis of the hyperdynamic circulation and renal sodium and water retention in cirrhosis. Gastroenterology 1992;192:1077.

76. Fogo A, Ichikawa I: Growth of glomerular and interstitial cells: Evidence for a pathogenic linkage between glomerular hypertrophy and sclerosis. Am J Kidney Dis 1991;17:666–669.

77. Klahr S, Schreiner G, Ichikawa I: The progression of renal disease. N Engl J Med 1988;318:1657–1666.

78. Brenner BM, Meyer TW, Hostetter TH: Dietary intake and the progressive nature of kidney disease: The role of hemodynamically mediated glomerular injury in the pathogenesis of progressive glomerular sclerosis in aging, renal ablation and intrinsic renal disease. N Engl J Med 1982;307:652–659.

79. Sacerdoti D, Bologneisi M, Merkel C, et al: Renal vasoconstriction in cirrhosis evaluated by duplex Doppler ultrasonography. Hepatology 1993;17:219–224.

80. Monasterolo L, Peiretti A, Elias MM: Rat renal functions during the first days post-bile duct ligation. Renal Fail 1993;15:461–467.

81. Böhle A, Gise HV, Mackensen-Hahn S, Stark-Jacob B: The obliteration of the post-glomerular capillaries and its influence upon the function of both glomeruli and tubule. Klin Wochenschr 1981;59:1043–1051.

82. Jones WT, Rao DRG, Braunstein H: The renal glomerulus in cirrhosis of the liver. Am J Pathol 1961; 39:393–404.

83. Bearn AG, Kunkel HG, Slater RG: The problem of chronic liver disease in young women. Am J Med 1956;21:3–15.

84. Mistilis SP, Blackburn CRB: Active chronic hepatitis. Am J Med 48:484–495, 1970.

85. Silva H, Hall EW, Hill KR, et al: Renal involvement in active "juvenile" cirrhosis. J Clin Pathol 1965;18: 157–163.

86. Page AR, Good RA, Pollara B: Long-term results of therapy in patients with chronic liver disease associated with hypergammaglobulinemia. Am J Med 1969;47:765–774.

87. Benner EJ, Gourley RT, Cooper RA, Benson JA: Chronic active hepatitis with lupus nephritis. Ann Intern Med 1968;68:405–413.

88. Bridi GS, Falcon PW, Brackett NC, et al: Glomerulonephritis and renal tubular acidosis in a case of chronic active hepatitis with hyperimmunoglobulinemia. Am J Med 1972;52:267–278.

89. Bartholomew LG, Hagedorn AB, Cain JC, Baggenstoss AH: Hepatitis and cirrhosis in women with positive clot tests for lupus erythematosus. N Engl J Med 1958;259:947–956.

90. Mistilis SP, Skyring AP, Blackburn CRB: Natural history of active chronic hepatitis. I. Clinical features, course, diagnostic criteria, morbidity, mortality and survival. Aust Ann Med 1968;17:214–223.

91. Svec KH, Blair JD, Kaplan MH: Immunopathologic studies of systemic lupus erythematosus (SLE). 1. Tissue bound immunoglobulins in relation to serum antinuclear immunoglobulins in systemic lupus and in chronic liver disease with LE cell factor. J Clin Invest 1967;46:558–568.

92. Whittingham S, MacKay IR, Irwin J: Autoimmune hepatitis. Immunofluorescence reactions with cytoplasm of smooth muscle and renal glomerular cells. Lancet 1966;1:1333–1135.

93. Combes G, Stastny P, Shorey J, et al: Glomerulonephritis with deposition of Australian antigen-antibody complexes in glomerular basement membrane. Lancet 1971;2:234–237.

94. Lai FM, Lai KN, Lee JCK, Hom BL: Hepatitis B virus-related glomerulonephropathy in patients with systemic lupus erythematosus. Am J Clin Pathol 1987;88: 412–420.

95. McIntosh RM, Koss MN, Gocke DJ: The nature and incidence of cryoproteins in hepatitis B (H B, Ag) positive patients. Q J Med 1976;23–38.

96. Arnold W, Buschenfelde M: Immune complexes of Hb-Ag/anti-HB, in nuclei of HB-Ag positive chronic liver disease [letter]. N Engl J Med 1977;296:818.

97. Takekoshi Y, Tanaka M, Miyakawa Y, et al: Free "small" and IgG-associated "large" hepatitis Be antigen in the serum and glomerular capillary walls of two patients with membranous glomerulonephritis. N Engl J Med 1979;300:814–819.

98. Gocke DJ: Extrahepatic manifestations of viral hepatitis. Am J Med Sci 1975;270:49–52.

99. Johnson RJ, Couser WG: Hepatitis B and renal disease: Clinical, immunopathogenetic and therapeutic considerations. Kidney Int 1990;37:663–676.

100. Myers BD, Griffel B, Naveh D, et al: Membranoproliferative glomerulonephritis associated with persistent viral hepatitis. Am J Clin Pathol 1973;60:222–228.

101. Knieser MR, Jenis EH, Lowenthal DT, et al: Pathogenesis of renal disease associated with viral hepatitis. Arch Pathol 1974;97:193–200.

102. Stratta P, Camussi G, Ragni R, Vercellone A: Hepatitis-B antigenaemia associated with active chronic hepatitis and mesangioproliferative glomerulonephritis [letter]. Lancet 1975;2:179.

103. Blaker F, Hellwege HH, Kramer U, Thoenes W: Perimembranose glomerulonephritis bei chronischer hepatitis mit persistierendem hepatitis-B-antigen. Dtsch Med Wochenschr 1975;100:790–794.

104. Nagy J, Par A, Bajtai G, et al: Membranous glomerulonephritis induced by HB (Australia) antigen-antibody complexes. Acta Morphol Acad Sci Hung 1976;24:129–138.

105. Brzosko WJ, Krawczynski K, Nazarewicz T, et al: Glomerulonephritis associated with hepatitis-B surface antigen immune complexes in children. Lancet 1974; 2:478–482.

106. Ainsworth SK, Brackett NC, Hennigar GR, Givens LB: Glomerulonephritis with deposition of Australia antigen-antibody complexes in the glomerular basement membrane [Abstract]. Lab Invest 1974;30:369.

107. Kohler PF, Cronin RE, Hammond WS, et al: Chronic membranous glomerulonephritis caused by hepatitis B antigen-antibody immune complexes. Ann Intern Med 1974;81:448–451.

108. Baglin A, Domart M, Cassan P, et al: Syndrome nephrotique chez un toxicomane. Role possible du virus de l'hepatite B [Abstract]. Nouv Presse Med 1975;4:1051.

109. Moriyama M, Fukuda Y, Ishizaki M, et al: Membranous glomerulonephritis associated with active liver cirrhosis both involved by HB-antigen. Acta Pathol Jpn 1970;26:237–250.

110. Ozawa T, Levisohn P, Orsini E, McIntosh RM: Acute immune complex disease associated with hepatitis. Arch Pathol Lab Med 1976;100:484–486.

111. Cogan MG, Graber ML, Connor DG: Chronic active hepatitis and membranous glomerulonephritis. Am J Gastroenterol 1977;68:386–391.

112. Hirschel BJ, Benusiglio LN, Favre H, et al: Glomerulonephritis associated with hepatitis B. Report of a case and review of the literature. Clin Nephrol 1977;8:404–409.

113. Clinicopathological Conference: Two children with kidney disease. Br Med J 1978;2:867–872.

114. Lagrue G, Etivant MF, Sulvestre R, Hirbec G: Antigene Australie (Ag-HB) et glomerulonephrites. Nouv Presse Med 1974;3:1870–1872.

115. Guardia J, Pedreira JD, Martinez-Vasquez JM, et al: Glomerulonephrites chroniques avec antigene Hb. Nouv Presse Med 1975;4:2923–2925.

116. Nagy J, Bajtai G, Brasch H, et al: The role of hepatitis B surface antigen in the pathogenesis of glomerulopathies. Clin Nephrol 1979;12:109–116.

117. Takekoshi Y, Tanaka M, Shida N, et al: Strong association between membranous nephropathy and hepatitis B surface antigenaemia in Japanese children. Lancet 1978;2:1065–1068.

118. Kleinknecht C, Levy M, Peix A, et al: Membranous glomerulonephritis and hepatitis B surface antigen in children. J Pediatr 1979;95:946–952.

119. Lai KN, Li PKT, Liu SI, et al: Membranous nephropathy related to hepatitis B virus in adults. N Engl J Med 1991;324:1457–1463.

120. Venkataseshan VS, Lieberman K, Kim DU, et al: Hepatitis-B-associated glomerulonephritis: Pathology, pathogenesis and clinical course. Medicine 1990;69:200–216.

121. Southwest Pediatric Nephrology Study Group: Hepatitis B surface antigenemia in North American children with membranous glomerulopathy. J Pediatr 1985;106: 571–578.

122. Slusarczyk J, Michalak T, Nazarewicz T, et al: Membranous glomerulopathy associated with hepatitis B core antigen immune complexes in children. Am J Pathol 1980;98:29–43.

123. Morzyka M, Slusarczyk J: Kidney glomerular pathology in various forms of acute and chronic hepatitis. Arch Pathol Lab Med 1979;103:38–41.

124. Vox GH, Grobbelaar G, Milner LV: A possible relationship between persistent hepatitis B antigenaemia and renal disease in Southern African Bantu. S Afr Med J 1973;47:911–912.

125. Goldstein DA, Sherman D, Rakela J, Koss M: Nephrotic syndrome in a patient with liver disease. Am J Nephrol 1982;2:40–45.

126. Garcia G, Scullard G, Smith C, et al: Preliminary observation of hepatitis B-associated membranous glomerulonephritis treated with leukocyte interferon. Hepatology 1985;5:317–320.

127. Wong SN, Yu EC, Lok AS, et al: Interferon treatment for hepatitis B-associated membranous glomerulonephritis in two Chinese children. Pediatr Nephrol 1992;6:417–420.

128. Lisker-Melman M, Webb D, Di Bisceglie AD, et al: Glomerulonephritis caused by chronic hepatitis B virus infection: Treatment with recombinant human alpha-interferon. Ann Intern Med 1989;111:479–483.

129. Gilboa N, Neigut D: Interferon treatment of hepatitis B-associated membranous glomerulonephritis and nephrotic syndrome. Pediatr Nephrol 1993;7:328–329.

130. Pol S, Debure A, Degott C, et al: Chronic hepatitis in kidney allograft. Lancet 1990;335:878–880.

131. Parfrey PS, Forbes RDC, Hutchinson TA, et al: The impact of renal transplantation on the course of hepatitis liver disease. Transplantation 1985;39:610–615.

132. Agarwal SK, Dash SC, Tiwari SC, et al: Clinicopathologic course of hepatitis B infection in surface antigen carriers following living-related renal transplantation. Am J Kidney Dis 1994;24:78–82.

133. Yoshikawa N, Ito H, Yamada Y, Hashimoto H, et al: Membranous glomerulonephritis associated with hepatitis B antigen in children. A comparison with idiopathic membranous glomerulonephritis. Clin Nephrol 1985;23:28–34.

134. Masugi Y, Ishizaki M, Fukuda Y, et al: Immunopathologic studies of renal glomerular change in liver cirrhosis with special reference to its pathogenesis. Acta Pathol Jpn 1979;29:571–583.

135. Knecht GL, Chisari FV: Reversibility of HBV-induced glomerulonephritis and chronic active hepatitis after spontaneous clearance of serum HB-Ag. Gastroenterology 1978;78:1152–1156.

136. Scullard GH, Smith CL, Merrigan TC, et al: Effects of immunosuppressive therapy on viral markers in chronic active hepatitis B. Gastroenterology 1981;81:987–991.

137. Lai FM, Li PK, Sven MW, et al: Crescentic glomerulonephritis related to hepatitis B virus. Mod Pathol 1992;5:262–267.

138. Min KW, Gyorkey F, Gyorkey P, et al: The morphogenesis of glomerular crescents in rapidly progressive glomerulonephritis. Kidney Int 1974;5:47–56.

139. Bonsib SM: Glomerular basement membrane necrosis and crescent organization. Kidney Int 1988;33:966–974.

140. Tadokoro M: The clinicopathological studies of hepatitis B virus nephropathy. Nippon Jinzo Gakkai Shi 1991;33:257–266.

141. Senekjian HO, Stinebaugh BJ, Mattioli CA, Suki WN: Irreversible renal failure following vesicoureteral reflux. JAMA 1979;241:160–162.

142. Eknoyan G, Gyorkey F, Dichoso C, et al: Renal involvement in drug abuse. Arch Intern Med 1973;132:801–806.

143. Wrzolkowa T, Zurowska A, Uszycka-Karcz M, Picken M: Hepatitis B virus-associated glomerulonephritis: Electron microscopic studies in 98 children. Am J Kidney Dis 1991;18:306–312.

144. Gyorkey F, Hollinger FB, Eknoyan G, et al: Immune-complex glomerulonephritis, intranuclear particles in hepatocytes and in vivo clearance rates in subhuman primates inoculated with HB,Ag-containing plasma. Exp Mol Pathol 1975;22:350–365.

145. Uanue ER, Dixon FJ: Experimental glomerulonephritis: Immunological events and pathogenetic mechanisms. Adv Immunol 1967;6:1–90.

146. Germuth FG, Rodriguez E: The Immunopathology of the Renal Glomerulus. Boston: Little, Brown & Co., 1973.

147. Wiggins RC, Cochrane CG: Immunecomplexes-mediated biologic effects. N Engl J Med 1980;304:518–520.

148. Lin CY: Hepatitis B virus associated membranous nephropathy: Clinical features, immunologic profiles and outcomes. Nephron 1990;55:37–44.

149. Blum HE, Stowring L, Figus A: Detection of hepatitis B virus DNA in hepatocytes, bile duct epithelium and vascular elements by in situ hybridization. Proc Natl Acad Sci USA 1983;80:6685–6688.

150. Nowoslawaki A, Krawczynski K, Brzosko WJ: Tissue localization of Australia antigen immune complexes in acute and chronic hepatitis and liver cirrhosis. Am J Pathol 1972;68:31–56.

151. Halpern MS, England JM, Deery DT: Viral nucleic acid synthesis and antigen accumulation in pancreas and kidney of Pekin ducks infected with duct hepatitis B virus. Proc Natl Acad Sci USA 1983;80:4865–4869.

152. Lin CY: Hepatitis B virus deoxyribonucleic acid in kidney cells probably leading to viral pathogenesis among hepatitis B virus associated membranous nephropathy patients. Nephron 1993;63:58–64.

153. Hirose H, Udo K, Kojima M: Deposition of hepatitis B e antigen in membranous glomerulonephritis—identification by F(ab')$_2$ fragments of monoclonal antibody. Kidney Int 1984;26:338–341.

154. Ito H, Hattori S, Matusda I: Hepatitis B e antigen-mediated membranous glomerulonephritis. Lab Invest 1981;44:214–220.

155. Powell KC, Meadows R, Anders R, et al: The nephrotic syndrome in Papua New Guinea. Aetiological, pathological and immunological findings. Aust NZ J Med 1977;7:243–252.

156. Hsu HC, Lin GH, Chang MH, Chen CH: Association of hepatitis B surface (HBS) antigenemia and membranous nephropathy in Taiwan. Clin Nephrol 1983;20:121–129.

157. Farquhar JD: Renal studies in acute infections—(epidemic) hepatitis. Am J Med Sci 1949;218:291–297.

158. Eknoyan G, Gyorkey F, Dichoso C, et al: Renal morphological and immunological changes associated with acute viral hepatitis. Kidney Int 1972;1:413–419.

159. Conrad ME, Schwartz FD, Young AA: Infectious hepatitis, a generalized disease. A study of renal, gastrointestinal and hematologic abnormalities. Am J Med 1964;37:789–801.

160. Levy M, Kleinknecht C: Membranous glomerulonephritis and hepatitis B virus infection. Nephron 1980;26:259–265.

161. Institute of Medicine, National Academy of Sciences: Confronting AIDS. Directions of Public Health, Health Care and Research. Washington, DC: National Academy Press, 1986.

162. Bourgoignie JJ: Renal complications of human immunodeficiency virus type I. Kidney Int 1990;37:1571–1584.

163. D'Agati V, Suh J, Carbone L, et al: Pathology of HIV-associated nephropathy: A detailed morphologic and comparative study. Kidney Int 1989;35:1358–1370.

164. Glassock RJ, Cohen AH, Danovitch G, Parsa KP: Human immunodeficiency virus (HIV) infection and the kidney. Ann Intern Med 1990;112:35–49.

165. Seney FD, Burns DK, Silva FG: Acquired immunodeficiency syndrome and the kidney. Am J Kidney Dis 1990;16:1–13.

166. Rao TKS, Friedman EA, Nicastri A: The types of renal disease in the acquired immunodeficiency syndrome. N Engl J Med 1987;316:1062–1068.

167. Gardenswartz MH, Lerner CW, Seligson GR, et al: Renal disease in patients with AIDS: A clinicopathologic study. Clin Nephrol 1984;21:197–204.

168. Rao TKS, Filippone EJ, Nicastri AD, et al: Associated focal and segmental glomerulosclerosis in the acquired immunodeficiency syndrome. N Engl J Med 1984;310:669–673.

169. Pardo V, Aldana M, Colton RM, et al: Glomerular lesions in the acquired immunodeficiency syndrome. Ann Intern Med 1984;101:429–434.

170. Pardo V, Meneses R, Ossa L, et al: AIDS-related glomerulopathy: Occurrence in specific risk groups. Kidney Int 1987;31:1167–1173.

171. Humphreys MH, Schoenfeld PY: Renal complications in patients with the acquired immune deficiency syndrome (AIDS). Am J Nephrol 1987;7:1–7.

172. Luke DR, Sarnoski TP, Dennis S: Incidence of microalbuminuria in ambulatory patients with acquired immunodeficiency syndrome. Clin Nephrol 1992;38:69–74.

173. Eknoyan G, Gyorkey F, Dichoso C, Gyorkey P: Nephropathy in patients with drug addiction. Evolution of pathological and clinical features. Virchows Arch [A] 1975;365:1–13.

174. Robert-Guroff M, Weiss SH, Girou JA, et al: Prevalence of antibodies to HTLV-I, II and III in intravenous drug abusers from an AIDS endemic region. JAMA 1986;255:3133–3137.

175. Layon J, Idris A, Warzynski M, et al: Altered T-lymphocyte subsets in hospitalized intravenous drug abusers. Arch Intern Med 1984;144:1376–1380.

176. Dabbs DJ, Striker LM, Mignon F, Striker G: Glomerular lesions in lymphomas and leukemias. Am J Med 1986;80:63–70.

177. Eknoyan G, Dillman RO: Renal complications in infectious diseases. Med Clin North Am 1978;52:979–1003.

178. Siegal FP, Lopez C, Hammer GS, et al: Severe acquired immunodeficiency in male homosexuals manifested by chronic perianal ulcerative herpes simplex lesions. N Engl J Med 1981;305:1439–1441.

179. Pitchenick AE, Fischl MT, Dickinson GM, et al: Opportunistic infections and Kaposi's sarcoma among Haitians: Evidence of a new acquired immunodeficiency state. Ann Intern Med 1983;98:277–284.

180. Ammann AJ, Abrams D, Conant M, et al: Acquired immune deficiency in homosexual men: Immunologic profiles. Clin Immunol Immunopathol 1983;27:315–325.

181. Fanci AS: Multifactorial nature of human immunodeficiency virus disease: Implications of therapy. Science 1993;262:1011–1018.

182. Cohen AH, Sun NCJ, Shapshak P, Imagawa DT: Demonstration of human immunodeficiency virus in renal epithelium in HIV-associated nephropathy. Hum Pathol 1989;2:125–128.

183. Koff RS, Liver Disease in Primary Care Medicine. New York: Appleton Century-Crofts, 1980.

184. Sabbour MS, El-Said W, Abou-Gabal I: A clinical and pathological study of schistosomal nephritis. Bull WHO 1972;47:549–557.

185. Silva LC, Brito T, Camargo ME, et al: Kidney biopsy in the hepatosplenic form of infection with schistosoma mansoni in man. Bull WHO 1970;42:907–910.

186. Falcao HA, Gould DB: Immune complex nephropathy in schistosomiasis. Ann Intern Med 1975;83:148–154.

187. Madawar MA, Vollar A: Circulating soluble antigens and antibody in schistomiasis. Br Med J 1975;1:435–436.

188. Brito T, Gunji J, Camargo ME, et al: Glomerular lesions in experimental infections of schistosoma mansoni in Cebus apella monkeys. Bull WHO 1971;45:419–422.

189. Natali PG, Cioli D: Immune complex nephritis in schistosoma infected mice. Eur J Immunol 1976;6:359–364.

190. Higashi GL, Abdel-Salam E, Soliman M, et al: Immunofluorescent analysis of renal biopsies in uncomplicated Schistosoma haematobium infection in children. J Trop Med Hyg 1984;87:123–129.

191. Queiroz PF, Brito E, Martinelli R, Rocha H: Nephrotic syndrome in patients with Schistosoma mansoni infection. Am J Rop Med Hyg 1973;22:622–628.

192. Hendrickse RG: The quartan malarial nephrotic syndrome. Adv Nephrol 1976;6:229–247.

193. Bhamarapravati N, Boonpucknavig S, Boonpucknavig V, Yaemboonruang C: Glomerular changes in acute Plasmodium falciparum infection. Arch Pathol 1973;96:289–293.

194. White RHR: Quartan malarial nephrotic syndrome. Nephron 1973;11:147–162.

195. Ward PA, Kibukamusoke JW: Evidence for soluble immune complexes in the pathogenesis of the glomerulonephritis of quartan malaria. Lancet 1969;1:283–285.

196. Hendrickse RG, Glasgow EF, Adeniyi A, et al: Quartan malarial nephrotic syndrome. Lancet 1972;1:1143–1148.

197. Wing AJ, Hutt MS, Kibukamusoke JW: Progression and remission in the nephrotic syndrome associated with quartan malaria in Uganda. Q J Med 1972;41:273–289.

198. Berger M, Birch LM, Conte NF: The nephrotic syndrome secondary to acute glomerulonephritis during falciparum malaria. Ann Intern Med 1967;67:1163–1171.

199. Woodroffe AJ, Row PG, Meadows R, Lawrence JR: Nephritis in infectious mononucleosis. Q J Med 1974;43:451–460.

200. Wallace M, Leet G, Rothwell R: Immune complex-mediated glomerulonephritis with infectious mononucleosis. Aust NZ J Med 1974;4:192–195.

201. Tennant FS: The glomerulonephritis of infectious mononucleosis. Tex Rep Biol Med 1968;26:603–612.

202. Lee S, Kjellstrand CM: Renal disease in infectious mononucleosis. Clin Nephrol 1978;9:236–240.

203. Lowery TA, Rutsky EA, Hartley MW, Andreoli TE: Renal failure in infectious mononucleosis. South Med J 1976;69:1212–1215.

204. Tsai TF, Finn DR, Plikaytis BD, et al: Legionnaires' disease: Clinical features of the epidemic in Philadelphia. Arch Intern Med 1979;90:509–517.

205. Posner MR, Caudill MA, Brass R, Ellis E: Legionnaires' disease associated with rhabdomyolysis and myoglobinuria. Arch Intern Med 1980;140:848–850.

206. Oredugba O, Mazumbar DC, Smoller MB, et al: Acute renal failure in legionnaires' disease: Report of a case. Clin Nephrol 1980;13:142–145.

207. Levine RA: Amyloid disease of the liver. Correlation of clinical, functional and morphological features in forty-seven patients. Am J Med 1962;33:349–357.

208. Wollaeger EE: Primary systemic amyloidosis with symptoms and signs of liver disease: Diagnosis by liver biopsy; report of a case. Med Clin North Am 1950;34:1113–1118.

209. Rubinow A, Koff RS, Cohen AS: Severe intrahepatic cholestasis in primary amyloidosis. A report of four cases and a review of the literature. Am J Med 1978;64:937–946.

210. Lindeman RD, Scheer RL, Raisz LG: Renal amyloidosis. Ann Intern Med 1961;54:883–898.

211. Brandt K, Cathcart ES, Cohen AS: A clinical analysis of the course and prognosis of forty two patients with amyloidosis. Am J Med 1968;44:955–969.

212. Jao W, Pirani C: Renal amyloidosis: Electron microscopic observations. Acta Pathol Microbiol Scand [A] 1972;233:217–227.

213. Triger DR, Joeckes AM: Renal amyloidosis. A fourteen-year follow-up. Q J Med 1973;42:15–40.

214. Lowensten J, Gallo G: Remission of the nephrotic syndrome in renal amyloidosis. N Engl J Med 1970;282:128–132.

215. Ozawa K, Yamabe H, Fukushik K, et al: Case report of amyloidosis-like glomerulopathy with hepatic involvement. Nephron 1991;58:347–350.

216. Becher D, Miller M: Presence of diabetic glomerulosclerosis in patients with hemochromatosis. N Engl J Med 1960;263:367–373.

217. Ireland JT, Patnaik BK, Duncan LPJ: Glomerular ultrastructure in secondary diabetics and normal subjects. Diabetes 1967;16:628–635.

218. Vaamonde C, Oster JR, Strauss J: The kidney in sickle cell disease. In Suki WN, Eknoyan G (eds): The Kidney in Systemic Diseases, 2nd ed. New York: John Wiley & Sons, 1981;159–195.

219. Buckalew VM, Someren A: Renal manifestations of sickle cell disease. Arch Intern Med 1974;133:660–669.

220. Powars DR, Elliott-Mills DD, Chan L: Chronic renal failure in sickle cell disease: Risk factors, clinical course, and mortality. Ann Intern Med 1991;115:614–620.

221. Elfenbein IB, Patchefsky A, Schwartz W, Weinstein AG: Pathology of the glomerulus in sickle cell anemia with and without nephrotic syndrome. Am J Pathol 1974;77:357–374.

222. McCoy RC: Ultrastructural alterations in the kidney of patients with sickle cell disease and the nephrotic syndrome. Lab Invest 1969;21:85–95.

223. Pardo V, Strauss J, Kramer H, et al: Nephropathy associated with sickle cell anemia: An autologous immune complex nephritis. II. Clinicopathologic study of seven patients. Am J Med 1975;59:650–659.

224. Strauss J, Pardo V, Koss MN, et al: Nephropathy associated with sickle cell anemia. An autologous immune complex nephritis. 1. Studies on nature of glomerular-bound antibody and antigen identification in a patient with sickle cell disease and immune deposit glomerulonephritis. Am J Med 1975;58:382–387.

225. Ozawa T, Mass MF, Guggenheim S, et al: Autologous immune complex nephritis associated with sickle cell trait: Diagnosis of the haemoglobinopathy after renal structural and immunological studies. Br Med J 1976;1:369–371.

226. Burrow GN, Ferris TF: Medical Complication of Pregnancy. Philadelphia: W.B. Saunders, 1975;53–104, 351–374.

227. McKay DG: Clinical significance of the pathology of toxemia of pregnancy. Circulation 1964;30(Suppl 2):66–75.

228. Fisher ER, Pardo V, Paul R, Hayashi TT: Ultrastructural studies in hypertension. IV. Toxemia in pregnancy. Am J Pathol 1969;55:109–130.

229. Vassalli P, Morris RH, McCluskey RT: The pathogenic role of fibrin deposition in the glomerular lesions of toxemia of pregnancy. J Exp Med 1963;118:467–478.

230. Spargo B, McCartney CP, Winemiller R: Glomerular capillary endotheliosis in toxemia of pregnancy. Arch Pathol 1959;68:593–599.

231. Fiaschi E, Maccarato R: The histopathology of the kidney in toxaemia. Serial renal biopsies during pregnancy, puerperium and several years post-partum. Virchows Arch Pathol Anat Physiol Klin Med 1968;345:299–309.

232. Mautner W, Churg J, Grishman E, Dachs S: Preeclamptic nephropathy: An electron microscopic study. Lab Invest 1962;11:518–529.

233. Pirani CL, Pollack VE, Lannigan R, Folli G: The renal glomerular lesions of pre-eclampsia: Electron microscopic studies. Am J Obstet Gynecol 1963;87:1047–1070.

234. Vasiliauskas E, Rosenthal P: Is acute fatty liver of pregnancy a metabolic defect? Am J Gastroenterology 1994;89:1908–1910.

235. Morrin PAF, Handa SP, Valberg LS, et al: Acute renal failure in association with fatty liver of pregnancy. Recovery after fourteen days of complete anuria. Am J Med 1967;42:844–851.

236. Hatfield AK, Stein JH, Greenberger NJ, et al: Idiopathic acute fatty liver of pregnancy: Death from extrahepatic manifestations. Am J Dig Dis 1972;17:167–178.

237. Slater DN, Hague WM: Renal morphological changes in idiopathic acute fatty liver of pregnancy. Histopathology 1984;8:567–581.

238. Milutinovic J, Fialkow PF, Rudd TG, et al: Liver cysts in patients with autosomal dominant polycystic kidney disease. Am J Med 1980;68:741–744.

239. Witzleben CL, Sharp AR: Nephronophthisis-congenital hepatic fibrosis: An additional hepatorenal disorder. Hum Pathol 1982;13:728–733.

240. Kudo M, Tamura K, Fuse Y: Cystic dysplastic kidneys associated with Dandy-Walker malformation and congenital hepatic fibrosis. Report of two cases. Am J Clin Pathol 1985;84:459–463.

241. Harris HW, Carpenter TO, Shanley P, et al: Progressive tubulointerstitial renal disease in infancy with associated hepatic abnormalities. Am J Med 1986;81:169–176.

242. Popovic-Rolovic M, Kostic M, Sindjic M, Jovanovic O: Progressive tubulointerstitial nephritis and chronic cholestatic liver disease. Pediatr Nephrol 1993;7:396–400.

243. Chang Y, Twiss JL, Haronpian DS, et al: Inherited syndrome of infantile olivoponto cerebellar atrophy, micronodular cirrhosis and renal tubular microcysts: Review of the literature and a report of an additional case. Acta Neuropathol 1993;86:399–404.

244. Iitaka K, Sakai T: Renal tubular ectasia with congenital hepatic fibrosis. Pediatr Nephrol 1992;6:403–404.

245. Davis ID, Burke B, Freese D, et al: The pathologic spectrum of the nephropathy associated with alpha 1-antitrypsin deficiency. Hum Pathol 1992;23:57–62.

Chapter 6

THE SIGNIFICANCE OF HEPATITIS C VIRUS INFECTION IN THE CARE OF PATIENTS WITH RENAL DISEASE

DAVID ROTH, M.D.

Biology of Hepatitis C Virus
Epidemiology and Clinical Presentation
Diagnostic Testing for HCV Infection
  Immunodiagnosis
  Viral RNA Detection
  Clinical Applications
HCV Infection in Patients with End-Stage Renal Disease

Detection of Anti-HCV Antibody
Correlates of HCV Infection in the Dialysis Setting
Nosocomial Transmission of HCV
Treatment of HCV-infected Dialysis Patients
Transplantation
HCV in Clinical Nephrology
  Glomerulonephritis
  Essential Mixed Cryoglobulinemia

In recent years, hepatitis C virus (HCV) has loomed importantly as the primary cause of non-A, non-B hepatitis and a clinical problem of growing significance. This applies not only to the population at large, but specifically to patients with end-stage renal disease (ESRD) who undergo dialysis and immunosuppressed allograft recipients. Indeed, the magnitude of the problem is reflected by the fact that HCV, which was barely mentioned in previous editions of this book, now merits a comprehensive chapter.

BIOLOGY OF HEPATITIS C VIRUS

HCV has been identified as the causative agent for 80–90% of what had previously been referred to as non-A, non-B hepatitis.[1,2] The virus was first identified following successful cloning of the viral RNA genome from the pooled sera of chimpanzees experimentally infected with non-A, non-B hepatitis. Most of what is currently known about HCV comes from the study of genetically engineered proteins derived from the cloned sequences. Difficulty in propagating the virus in cell culture or positively visualizing the virion by electron microscopy has limited the study of its biology and pathogenesis.

HCV is a linear, single-stranded RNA virus with a genome comprising approximately 9,400 nucleotides.[3] The sequence contains a long open-reading frame capable of encoding a large viral polypeptide of ~3000 amino acids (Fig. 6.1). The 5'-untranslated region represents the most highly conserved section of the genome among varying worldwide hepatitis C viral isolates (> 97%). Therefore, this region of the genome provides the most sensitive primers for HCV RNA detection by polymerase chain reaction (vide infra).

The RNA sequence of HCV is similar to that of several other RNA viruses, including members of the pestivirus (e.g., bovine diarrhea virus) and flavivirus (e.g., yellow fever virus) families. The organization of the HCV genome is most similar to that of the flaviviruses: the carboxyterminus encodes nonstructural proteins that are required in viral replication and the aminoterminus encodes the structural proteins (envelope and capsid).

Replication of the HCV genome proceeds by a direct RNA-to-RNA mechanism, although the specifics of HCV RNA replication remain unknown. Because HCV is a positive-strand RNA virus, the presence of antigenomic or negative strand RNA has been considered a marker of active HCV replication. Quantitative analysis has demonstrated that the liver contains significantly more negative strand RNA than the serum, confirming the hepatocyte as the primary site of HCV replication. However, recent reports of viral

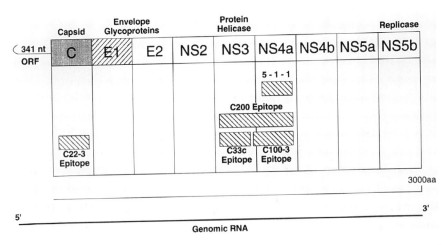

FIGURE 6.1. The organization of the hepatitis C viral genome. C = nucleocaspid gene, E1–E2 = envelope genes, NS2–NS5 = nonstructural genes involved in viral replication. The various epitopes correspond to antigenic regions of the genome that are determined serologically.

replication in T-lymphocytes suggest the possibility of alternative sites for viral replication. Further clarification of these issues will require the development of cell-culture systems for HCV.

EPIDEMIOLOGY AND CLINICAL PRESENTATION

The prevalence of HCV infection varies considerably worldwide. In the United States, seroprevalence of HCV in healthy blood donors has been reported to be ~0.5–1.2 %,[4] whereas considerably higher figures have been reported from Japan. The prevalence of HCV infection in specific at-risk populations, including health care workers (3–4%), multiply transfused and/or chronic hemodialysis patients (25%), and patients with a history of intravenous drug abuse (75%), is considerably greater than in the blood-donor pool.

The incubation period for a typical HCV infection is approximately 6–15 weeks following exposure. Nonspecific symptoms of liver injury appear first, to be followed by a rise in serum transaminases and bilirubin.

HCV infection progresses to chronic hepatitis in approximately 50–60% of cases.[5] Roughly 20% of patients with chronic HCV infection develop cirrhosis over the ensuing 5–15 years. During the period of chronic infection, liver transaminases typically follow a highly fluctuating course, with periods of hypertransaminasemia alternating with intervals of completely normal liver function tests (Fig. 6.2). This appears to be particularly true among immunosuppressed renal allograft recipients[6] and chronic hemodialysis patients,[7,8] in whom active HCV infection has been demonstrated in the setting of persistently normal transaminases.

In addition to the inherent risk of progressive liver disease, patients with chronic HCV infection are at increased risk for HCV-associated complications. An increased incidence of hepatocellular carcinoma (HCC) has been noted in patients with cirrhosis secondary to HCV infection.[9] The increased prevalence of both hepatitis B and hepatitis C infection in Japan enabled investigators to recognize an independent risk for HCC accompanying infection with either virus and a synergistic increase in the risk of neoplasia with coinfection. Extrahepatic syndromes linked to HCV infection include essential cryoglobulinemia and several histologic types of glomerulonephritis (vide infra).

DIAGNOSTIC TESTING FOR HCV INFECTION

Immunodiagnosis

The molecular characterization and cloning of HCV led to the production of large quantities of viral protein from recombinant organisms. When purified, the recombinant polypeptide can be used to produce a capture assay for reactive antibody that indicates exposure to HCV. The first generation anti-HCV immunoassay (ELISA I; Ortho Diagnostics) was licensed in May, 1990

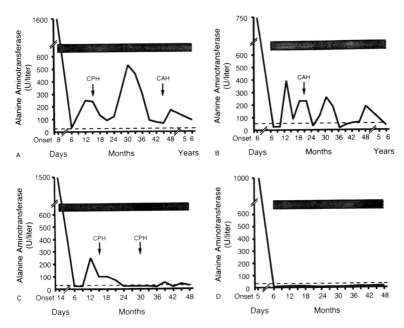

FIGURE 6.2. Representative patterns of alanine aminotransferase activity in patients with community-acquired HCV infection. The *dashed lines* show the upper limit of normal for alanine aminotransferase. The *arrows* indicate liver biopsies, CPH (a finding of chronic persistent hepatitis), and CAH (a finding of chronic active hepatitis). The *bars* indicate periods of positivity for anti-HCV on second-generation immunoassays. *A,* The course of chronic hepatitis C in a patient whose alanine aminotransferase level was abnormal on every determination throughout follow-up. *B,* Chronic hepatitis C in a patient whose alanine aminotransferase level was intermittently normal. *C,* Chronic hepatitis C in a patient with a prolonged period (up to 1 year) of normal alanine aminotransferase levels. *D,* Patient with biochemical resolution of hepatitis C as indicated by persistently normal alanine aminotransferase levels, but in whom HCV RNA was detected in serum samples up to 45 months after the onset of illness. (From Alter MJ, et al: The natural history of community-acquired hepatitis C in the United States. N Engl J Med 1992;327:1899–1905, with permission.)

and incorporated the C-100-3 polypeptide expressed in yeast (Table 6.1). The C-100-3 epitope corresponds with almost all of the NS4 protein of the HCV genome (see Fig. 6.1). Antibody to this protein develops in nearly all cases of post-transfusion non-A, non-B hepatitis.[1–3] A second-generation immunoassay (ELISA II; Ortho Diagnostics) is now commercially licensed and has replaced the ELISA I. The ELISA II detects antibodies to proteins derived from three distinct regions of the HCV genome. The c-200 recombinant antigen is an expression product of the NS3/NS4 region (see Fig. 6.1) and is derived from the region of the genome that encodes both the c33c and c100-3 recombinant antigens. The c22-3 recombinant antigen is a product of the putative nucleocapsid region of the HCV genome.

The recently licensed four-antigen recombinant immunoblot assay (RIBA) differs from the ELISA test by using a nitrocellulose strip-based methodology that is capable of detecting antibodies to

the recombinant HCV antigens 5-1-1, C100-3, c33c, and c22-3. During incubation of each strip with serum, anti-HCV antibodies react to the corresponding antigen. Results are reported as reactive (reactivity with at least two antigen bands), indeterminate (reactivity with a single antigen band), or nonreactive (no reactive bands).

Viral RNA Detection

The application of polymerase chain reaction (PCR) techniques to amplify reverse transcribed cDNA provided an opportunity to develop a highly sensitive assay for viral RNA. The ability to detect small numbers of viral RNA molecules in the blood or tissue specimens by PCR represents an extremely sensitive assay for HCV infection.[11] Several studies have demonstrated conclusively that primers specific for the 5'-untranslated region of the HCV genome are preferred, because this region is highly conserved among most worldwide

TABLE 6.1. Currently Available Assays for the Diagnosis of HCV Infection

Test System	Detecting	Comments
Anti-HCV antibody assay		
EIA-I*	Anti-c-100-3	Many false positives and negatives; 15–20-week interval after inoculation until seroconversion.
EIA-II*	Anti-c-100-3, c200, c33c, c22-3	Greater sensitivity and earlier diagnosis (12–14 wks) than EIA-I.
RIBA*	Anti-5-1-1, c100-3, c33c, c22-3	Improved specificity vs. ELISA assays; early diagnosis (similar to EIA-II).
Polymerase chain reaction		Only assay confirming active viral replication; allows earliest diagnosis of primary HCV infection (1–2 wks after inoculation).
5'-NCR primers	HCV RNA	
NS3-4 primers	HCV RNA	Less sensitivity with NS3-4 primers

EIA = enzyme-linked immunoassay (ELISA); RIBA = recombinant immunoblot assay.
* Commercially licensed.

HCV isolates studied to date.[3] Polymerase chain reaction tests using primers from the NS3-4 region have been shown to be considerably less sensitive than assays incorporating primers from the 5'-untranslated section of the genome.[12]

Clinical Applications

By 1986 most blood banks had incorporated alanine aminotransferase (ALT) and anti-HBC screening to identify blood donors at high risk for non-A, non-B hepatitis. The subsequent licensing of the first generation anti-HCV assay in 1990 and the earlier use of surrogate marker testing are credited with reducing the incidence of HCV infection over the ensuing years.[13] Currently, three assays are licensed for commercial anti-HCV testing. The first-generation ELISA (EIA-I) was extremely successful in predicting whether coded sera contained the agent responsible for post-transfusion non-A, non-B hepatitis, but many situations gave rise to false-positive and false-negative results. Patients with hypergammaglobulinemia and autoimmune chronic active hepatitis often tested positive by EIA-I in the absence of HCV infection.[14,15] False-negative tests have been seen in immunosuppressed individuals, patients with chronic renal failure, and patients with acquired immunodeficiency syndrome (AIDS). The second-generation ELISA (EIA-II) provides increased sensitivity and earlier detection of anti-HCV antibody compared with EIA-I.[1,16,17] EIA-II testing shortens the window of seroconversion from approximately 18 to 14 weeks following exposure.[16] The recombinant immunoblot assay (RIBA) increased the specificity of anti-HCV testing while maintaining the excellent sensitivity of the EIA-II.[14,18] In a series reported by

McHutchison et al.,[17] all RIBA-reactive samples were also positive by EIA-II testing. However, there appears to be a slight reduction in specificity with the EIA-II, especially in patients at low risk for HCV infection.

Validation of the RIBA was provided by Esteban and coworkers.[19] All RIBA-reactive patients had abnormal liver biopsies, although the severity of the histologic changes varied widely. Fully 69% of the RIBA-positive patients had either chronic active hepatitis (CAH) or cirrhosis. Of note, 35% of the patients with CAH had persistently normal transaminases, emphasizing the importance of liver biopsy for proper diagnosis and the low sensitivity of liver enzymes to ongoing infection. McGuinness and colleagues[12] screened 157 blood donors with anti-HCV assays and used PCR testing as a confirmatory test. Ninety percent of the patients who were RIBA-reactive with abnormal liver function tests had detectable HCV RNA by PCR. This figure dropped to 54% in RIBA-positive patients with normal liver enzymes. None of the ELISA-positive, RIBA-negative patients were PCR-positive, confirming the superior specificity of the RIBA.

HCV INFECTION IN PATIENTS WITH END-STAGE RENAL DISEASE

Detection of Anti-HCV Antibody

Hemodialysis. After the licensing of the EIA-I in May 1990, two papers documented a significant anti-HCV seropositivity among hemodialysis patients[20,21] (Table 6.2). Jeffers and coworkers[20] screened 90 patients in an urban dialysis unit and found a 12% prevalence of anti-HCV antibodies. HCV-positive patients had been more

TABLE 6.2. Evidence of HCV Infection in Hemodialysis Patients

Author	Ref.	EIA-I	EIA-II	HCV RNA	HCV Correlates
Zeldis (1990, U.S.)	21	16% (16/102)	—	—	BT, IVDA
Jeffers (1990, U.S.)	20	12% (11/90)	25% (16/63)	—	BT, IVDA
Hardy (1992, U.S.)	37	30% (26/87)	36% (31/87)	—	HD duration
Mondelli (1992, Italy)	24	31% (85/277)	55% (151/277)	—	BT, HD duration
Mazzotta (1992, Italy)	26	12% (9/74)	20% (15/74)	—	HD duration
Oguchi (1992, Japan)	22	17% (104/607)	44% (74/167)	—	BT, HD duration
Knudsen (1993, Denmark)	33	—	8% (28/340)	—	BT, HD duration
Chauveau (1993, France)	25	31% (36/115)	47% (52/110)	83% (42/52)	BT, HD duration
Dussol (1993, France)	31	—	29% (43/145)	52% (21/40)	BT, HD duration
Pol (1993, France)	7	—	—	85% (52/61)	BT, HD duration
Chan (1993, Hong Kong)	8	12% (6/51)	22% (6/51)	73% (8/11)	HD duration
Kuhns (1993, U.S.)	32	—	—	75% (12/16)	BT, IVDA

BT = blood transfusions, HD = hemodialysis, IVDA = intravenous drug abuse.

heavily transfused than the seronegative group and had a greater percentage of intravenous drug abusers. Similar results were reported in the same year by Zeldis and coworkers,[21] who identified antibodies in 16% of chronic hemodialysis patients.

Numerous subsequent reports have confirmed these initial findings.[8,22–24] Most centers detect anti-HCV antibody in 10–40% of hemodialysis patients. Recently published studies using EIA-II have demonstrated an almost two-fold increase in the prevalence of anti-HCV compared with EIA-I[8,22,24–26] (see Table 6.2). Clearly, earlier reports that relied on EIA-I underestimated the true prevalence of anti-HCV among hemodialysis patients.

Continuous Ambulatory Peritoneal Dialysis. Several groups have demonstrated a considerably lower prevalence of anti-HCV antibodies among patients on continuous ambulatory peritoneal dialysis (CAPD) compared with patients maintained on chronic hemodialysis.[27–30] Chan et al.[27] found that 5 of 278 (1.8%) CAPD patients were anti-HCV–positive vs. 10 of 61 (16%) hemodialysis patients (p < 0.001). As expected, the marked difference in the prevalence of anti-HCV antibodies was related to a significantly greater transfusion history in the hemodialysis patients. Besso et al.[28] reported 0% anti-HCV prevalence among 24 CAPD patients, whereas Huang and coworkers[29] detected anti-HCV antibodies in 15% of their CAPD patients. Of note, this figure dropped to 5.9% when patients with a prior history of hemodialysis were excluded.

The marked difference in the prevalence of anti-HCV antibodies among CAPD vs. hemodialysis patients undoubtedly relates to the number of blood transfusions. However, such findings also may indicate a greater HCV exposure in the dialysis setting through nosocomial transmission. This possibility is discussed in the next section.

HCV RNA Detection. The demonstration of circulating HCV RNA is considered indisputable evidence of active viral replication and potential infectivity. Several recently published studies have used the PCR to determine the prevalence of viremia among anti-HCV–positive (EIA-II) dialysis patients[7,8,31,32] (see Table 6.2). Pol et al.[7] detected HCV RNA in 52 of 61 (85%) EIA-II–positive patients. Similar results have been reported by Chan and coworkers[8] and Kuhns et al.;[32] both groups detected HCV RNA in greater than 70% of their EIA-II–positive patients. The consensus among several studies is that more than 75% of anti-HCV–seropositive dialysis patients are viremic (see Table 6.2). The implications of this finding for infection control in the dialysis unit and for treatment are considered in subsequent sections.

Correlates OF HCV Infection in the Dialysis Setting

Blood Transfusions. Numerous studies have reported a direct association between the number of blood transfusions and the prevalence of anti-HCV antibodies among hemodialysis patients.[20,23–25,31,33,34] Knudsen et al.[33] noted a statistically significant difference in the number of blood transfusions between anti-HCV–positive and indeterminate patients compared with anti-HCV–negative patients (30 vs. 13 transfusions, p < 0.01). Similarly, Muller and coworkers[23] demonstrated a direct correlation between the prevalence of anti-HCV antibodies and number of blood transfusions (1–10, 40%; >10, 76%;

r = 0.97; p < 0.001). A recent study of 145 French hemodialysis patients by Dussol et al.[31] supported these findings in that the number of blood transfusions was predictive of anti-HCV positivity in a multivariate analysis. In contrast, several other groups have failed to identify a significant association between number of transfusions and risk of anti-HCV positivity.[35,36] Fujiyama et al.[35] stratified patients by length of time on dialysis and found that patients with 0–2 years of dialysis had a 7.5% anti-HCV seropositivity compared with 58% among patients with more than 12 years of dialysis. An equal number of patients had been transfused in both groups (46% and 51%, respectively).

The results of a multicenter, prospective study sponsored by the Centers for Disease Control and Prevention was recently reported by Niu et al.[36] The study followed 499 patients from 11 chronic hemodialysis centers in different geographic regions of the United States to determine the prevalence and incidence of antibody to HCV and to evaluate the risk factors for HCV infection. Anti-HCV antibodies were detected in 52 of 499 (10%) patients at baseline. Logistic regression analysis revealed that anti-HCV positivity was not associated with a history of blood transfusions, whereas length of time on dialysis and use of injection drugs were significant variables. Intuitively, the increased exposure accompanying a greater number of blood transfusions would be expected to be associated with a greater incidence of anti-HCV positivity, especially among patients transfused prior to the availability of sensitive anti-HCV assays. Nonetheless, the risk of HCV infection appears to increase as duration of dialysis increases, independently of the number of blood transfusions, suggesting that intradialytic transmission may occur.

Duration of Dialysis. The association between duration of dialysis and increased prevalence of anti-HCV positivity has been confirmed in numerous studies.[22,25,31,33,36–38] Hardy et al.[37] screened 87 chronic dialysis patients and detected 31 (36%) anti-HCV–positive samples with RIBA. Logistic regression was used to model the probability of a positive RIBA result. A stepwise variable selection indicated that only time on dialysis was a significant predictor of a positive RIBA result.[37] In the multicenter study by Niu and coworkers,[36] a history of injecting drugs and length of time on dialysis (≥ 3 years) were the only variables associated with anti-HCV positivity

in a logistic regression analysis. Patients who had been transfused prior to 1986 and had ≥ 3 years on dialysis had an anti-HCV–positive rate of 20% compared with 3.7% among patients with the same transfusion history but < 3 years on dialysis (odds ratio, 6.5; p < 0.05).

Similar findings were noted in patients not transfused prior to 1986: patients with ≥ 3 years on dialysis had an anti-HCV prevalence rate of 15% vs. 4.6% among patients with < 3 years on dialysis (odds ratio, 3.6; p < 0.05). Thus, when adjusted for transfusion history, length of time on dialysis was a significant predictor of anti-HCV positivity.[36] If the length of time on dialysis is an independent predictor of anti-HCV status apart from the predictable and confounding influence of blood transfusions, then nosocomial transmission of HCV in the dialysis setting must be considered as a plausible explanation. Further discussion of the implications of such findings is presented in the section addressing special precautions and recommendations for infection control.

HCV Infection among Dialysis Staff. Past experience with hepatitis B virus (HBV) infection in dialysis units pointed out the risks of patient-to-patient as well as patient-to-staff transmission. The reported incidence of non-A, non-B hepatitis among hemodialysis staff has decreased from 0.5% in 1983 to 0.1% in 1990.[39] More accurate data are now available from studies that used ELISA assays to determine anti-HCV seroprevalence among dialysis staff.[22,24,27–29,36,37,40–42] Several of these studies reported a 0% prevalence of anti-HCV among dialysis personnel.[37,40–42] On the other hand, two reports from Italy reported anti-HCV antibody in 6.7% and 5.5% of staff members.[24,28] In the U.S. study of 11 chronic dialysis units,[36] 2 of 142 (1%) staff members were found to be anti-HCV–seropositive at baseline evaluation. There were no seroconversions over an 18-month observation period. Also of interest is the study of Oguchi et al.,[22] in which 3 of 150 (2%) staff members were determined to be anti-HCV–positive. In all 3 cases a history of needlestick accident was present, although 69% of all staff had reported a history of needlestick accidents. This suggests that the accidental transmission of HCV infection to staff members is unlikely. In contrast, 25 (17%) of the staff members were positive for anti-HBc, suggesting that HBV may be transmitted more easily than HCV. In any event, the prevalence of anti-HCV antibodies among dialysis staff is low and comparable to that found in other health care worker populations.[43,44] However, the reported seroprevalence among dialysis staff still exceeds similarly tested blood donors.

Serum Transaminases as a Marker of HCV Infection. From 1986 until the licensing of the EIA-I in 1990, abnormal alanine aminotransferase (ALT) activity and anti-HBc were used as surrogate markers for non-A, non-B, hepatitis.[45] Although the application of surrogate marker testing is credited with reducing the incidence of posttransfusion non-A, non-B hepatitis,[13] the sensitivity of transaminase elevations to detect hepatic dysfunction in the chronic hemodialysis population has been suspect.[46]. In fact, several recent studies have clearly demonstrated the unacceptably poor sensitivity of hypertransaminasemia to detect HCV infection in patients with ESRD.[7,8,3,47,48] In a recent study by Pol et al.,[7] only 16 of 52 (31%) HCV-infected patients with HCV RNA in the circulation had abnormal liver function tests. Furthermore, only 4 of 15 (26%) viremic patients with biopsy-proven chronic hepatitis had elevated liver enzymes. Similar findings were noted by Chan and coworkers,[8] who found only 33% of anti-HCV–positive hemodialysis patients to be hypertransaminasemic. In fact, of 10 anti-HCV–positive patients with normal liver enzymes, 8 (80%) were HCV-RNA–positive. Together such findings clearly demonstrate the low sensitivity of serum transaminases to detect ongoing HCV replication in patients on chronic hemodialysis and emphasize the need for more accurate and specific tests to diagnose HCV infection.

Concurrent HBV and HCV Infection. Studies of HBV and HCV interaction in co-infected patients have suggested that HCV may suppress or terminate the HBsAg carrier state.[49] Of interest, Kuhns et al.[32] detected HBV DNA by PCR in 2 coinfected dialysis patients, both of whom were HBsAg-negative. Thus, concurrent infection with HBV and HCV may complicate the diagnosis of chronic liver disease in patients with ESRD. Testing for viral nucleic acid may be necessary to determine adequately the status of hepatitis B and C virus infection in such patients.

Nosocomial Transmission of HCV

As discussed in the preceding section, length of time on dialysis has been demonstrated to be an independent predictor of HCV infection in hemodialysis patients.[23,24,36–38,50] Yamaguchi et al.[38] screened 1423 hemodialysis patients and found anti-HCV positivity in 64 of 349 (18%) who had not been transfused. Moreover, 25 of 57 (44%) patients who had been on dialysis for more than 10 years but had not been transfused were anti-HCV–positive. Muller[23] detected anti-HCV antibodies in 123 of 315 (39%) patients, of whom 33 (27%) had not been transfused and had no other identifiable risk factors for HCV. These results agree with those of Niu et al.,[36] who found no identifiable HCV risk factors in 19% of anti-HCV–positive patients, and Vandelli and coworkers,[50] who were unable to document a possible parenteral exposure to HCV in 10 of 19 (53%) newly diagnosed HCV-positive patients. Such findings raise two important issues regarding transmission of HCV in the dialysis setting: (1) What is the incidence of anti-HCV seroconversion among dialysis patients? (2) If nosocomial transmission of HCV occurs in dialysis units, should there be changes in the official policy and procedures governing infection control?

Several studies performed prior to the availability of anti-HCV testing documented outbreaks of non-A, non-B hepatitis in hemodialysis patients and implicated blood transfusions, person-to-person transmission, and contaminated environmental surfaces .[51,52] Niu et al.[42] recently reported an outbreak in a dialysis unit and correlated their findings with anti-HCV antibody testing. Of 56 potentially susceptible patients in a single dialysis unit, 11 (20%) seroconverted to anti-HCV positivity between January 1987 and March 1989; a cluster of cases occurred in the second half of 1987. No associations were found for dialysis on a particular schedule, incident of dialysis complication or excessive bleeding, exposure to a bleeding event from an anti-HCV–positive patient during dialysis, dialysis adjacent to an anti-HCV–positive patient, contact with a nurse who also cared for an anti-HCV–positive patient, or use of multidose medications. Routine equipment maintenance records documented a problem with sporadic overload of transducer protectors, which resulted in reflux of patient blood across the transducers between 1985 and 1989. Furthermore, inadequate infection control measures (lack of glove use and poor handwashing) was reported during the exposure period. Neither a common source nor direct person-to-person transmission could be documented. The authors concluded that strict adherence to longstanding infection control strategies were sufficient to control the spread of HCV in the dialysis setting.

This opinion has been questioned by several recently published studies. Jadoul et al.[53] examined the incidence of anti-HCV seroconversion among 401 patients dialyzed in 15 different units between May 1991 and November 1992. At baseline, 13.5% of patients were anti-HCV–positive by EIA-II testing. During the three consecutive 6-month periods of the study, EIA-II results became positive in 3 of 305 (1%), 4 of 314 (1.3%) and 1 of 313 (0.3%) patients, respectively, for an average yearly incidence of 1.7%. Three of the 8 seroconversions occurred in patients who had not been transfused. Three of the 8 patients who seroconverted were from the same unit, and all 3 had been dialyzed adjacent to an anti-HCV–positive patient. Sexual partners of these patients tested anti-HCV–negative, and there was no history of intravenous drug use.

Together such findings suggest nosocomial transmission of HCV, although the authors did not feel that isolation of the HCV-infected patient was warranted because of the absence of transmission in 10 of 13 units dialyzing HCV-positive patients. Further data supporting the concept of nosocomial HCV transmission come from a recent report by Garcia-Valdecasas et al.[54] Patients in three Spanish dialysis unit were screened over a 36-month period. During the first 12 months the incidence of HCV seroconversion was 1.35/100 patient months. However, among the cohort of patients sharing a machine with a HCV-positive patient, the figure rose to 2.87/100 patient months; the figure was only 0.49/100 patient months among the cohort not dialyzed on the same machine as an HCV-positive patient. During the ensuing 24 months, two of the units isolated HCV-positive patients on dedicated machines. The incidence of HCV seroconversion in these units declined from 1.59/100 to 0.26/100 patient months vs. 0.63/100 in the unit in which strict enforcement of universal precautions was the only change.

Although compelling data point to nosocomial transmission of HCV within the dialysis setting, the Centers for Disease Control has not yet altered official recommendations for control of non-A, non-B hepatitis in patients undergoing maintenance hemodialysis[55] (Table 6.3). Policy changes await the results of prospective longitudinal studies using PCR detection of HCV RNA to diagnose active infection and recent seroconversion.

Treatment of HCV-infected Dialysis Patients

Limited information is available concerning the treatment of the HCV-infected dialysis patient. Preliminary data have been reported by Koenig and coworkers[56] on the use of interferon α-2b (IFN α-2b) in the chronic dialysis patient with HCV infection. The authors administered IFN α-2b, 5×10^6 units thrice weekly, to 37 HCV-infected dialysis patients for 4 months. Twenty three of 37 completed the 4 months of therapy and 15 of 23 (65%) no longer had detectable HCV RNA in the serum. Seven of the 15 responders (47%) relapsed within 2 months of discontinuing IFN. Thus, only 8 of 37 (21%) patients initially treated with IFN had a successful response to therapy. More extensive and prolonged studies of the safety and efficacy of IFN α-2b or other antiviral therapies are needed before definitive recommendations can be made regarding the treatment of the HCV-infected dialysis patient.

If antiviral therapy is considered, a firm diagnosis of active HCV infection should be made by PCR testing for HCV RNA. Although greater than 75% of EIA-II–positive dialysis patients are viremic, antiviral therapy with interferon α-2b is not without risks and side effects; thus the initiation of treatment based solely on a positive ELISA assay is not sufficient. Although a recent study by Pol et al.[7] determined that 14 of 15 PCR-positive dialysis patients had histologic evidence of chronic hepatitis, data from Caramelo and coworkers[47] suggested that circulating viral RNA was not necessarily predictive of severe liver disease in the uremic patient. Thus, considering the limited data and the lack of consensus, a liver biopsy should be obtained prior to beginning interferon therapy.

TRANSPLANTATION

The success of renal transplantation as a therapy for end-stage renal disease has focused attention on factors affecting long-term patient and graft survival. Although the spectrum of liver disease following renal transplantation is varied,[57-60] chronic liver disease contributes substantially to late posttransplant morbidity. The screening of large numbers of kidney recipients demonstrated that HCV was the causative agent for most cases of what had previously been referred to as posttransplant non-A, non-B hepatitis.[61,62] Considering

TABLE 6.3.   Centers for Disease Control Recommendations for the Control of Non-A, Non-B Hepatitis and Hepatitis C in the Dialysis Center

1. Patients who are positive for anti-HCV or in whom non-A, non-B hepatitis has been diagnosed do not have to be isolated separately on dedicated machines. In addition, they can participate in dialyzer reuse programs.

2. Infection control strategies should emphasize basic barrier precaution, commonly referred to as universal precautions.

3. Patients should be monitored monthly for elevations in alanine aminotransferase and aspartate aminotransferase. Elevations in liver enzymes currently are more sensitive indicators of acute HCV infection than is anti-HCV.

4. Routine screening of patients or staff for anti-HCV is not necessary for purposes of infection control. Dialysis centers may wish to conduct serologic surveys of their patient populations to determine the prevalence of the virus in their center and, in the case of patients or staff with a diagnosis of non-A, non-B hepatitis, to determine medical management. In addition, if liver enzyme screening indicates the occurrence of an epidemic of non-A, non-B hepatitis in the dialysis setting, anti-HCV screening on serum samples collected during and subsequent to outbreaks may be of value. However, since anti-HCV in an individual cannot distinguish between chronic infection or infection that has resolved, its usefulness for infection control in the dialysis center setting is limited.

that 10–30% of hemodialysis patients in the United States are anti-HCV–positive,[20,21] pretransplant evaluation and contribution of HCV infection to long-term patient outcome are important issues.

Transmission.   Previous studies of asymptomatic blood donors have detected an anti-C100 seroprevalence of 0.5–1.2%. Using the anti-C100 ELISA, Pereira and colleagues[63] reported that 1.8% of the cadaver organ donors in their series were anti-HCV positive. Using the same assay, we screened 484 donor serum samples and identified 89 positive specimens (18%), of which 33 (6.8%) were RIBA-reactive.[64] An obvious explanation for the discrepancy between these results is not readily available, although it may simply reflect significant differences in the geographic prevalence of HCV infection. In fact, data from a collaborative nationwide survey involving several organ procurement organizations have demonstrated a wide range of anti-HCV positivity.[65] The observed higher prevalence of anti-HCV antibodies among cadaver organ donors compared with the general community may reflect lifestyle and socioeconomic factors that are more prevalent among people who become organ donors.

The transmission of HCV by solid-organ transplantation has been unequivocally demonstrated.[64,66] However, there remain notable discrepancies in the reported incidence of transmission among centers. Pereira and coworkers[66] detected HCV RNA in 7 of 26 (27%) organ recipients preoperatively and 23 of 24 (96%) during follow-up after transplantation from a HCV-carrier donor. They concluded that the likelihood of transmission of HCV with solid organ transplantation was high. Although such data are compelling and undoubtedly represent true viral transmission in a certain number of cases, several

questions remain unanswered. The authors did not specify whether the patients received blood products in the perioperative period. This point is especially relevant, because a number of the transplants were performed prior to the commercial licensing of the anti-C100 ELISA assay. Furthermore, the inclusion of several liver recipients is not relevant to the question because of inevitable transmission of a hepatotropic virus such as HCV. Finally, an analysis of historic, stored serum samples for HCV RNA generates many false-negative results. Thus any assessment of the extent of pretransplant viremia that relies on stored samples for comparison with freshly obtained posttransplant samples is likely to exaggerate the extent of seroconversion.

In our study, liver histology was available from 24 RIBA-positive organ donors. Chronic active or chronic persistent hepatitis was detected in 18 of 24 (75%) specimens, confirming that the majority of seropositive organ donors harbor active disease. Nevertheless, among the 27 kidney and heart recipients in whom the donor had either CAH or CPH on biopsy (with HCV RNA in 13 of 15), only 9 (33%) developed posttransplant liver dysfunction. Moreover, among 20 recipients of a kidney from a HCV-RNA–positive donor, only 6 (30%) developed biochemical evidence of liver disease. The remaining 14 patients maintained normal liver chemistries with a mean follow-up of 27±8 months. Such results contrast with those of Pereira et al.,[63] which report a high prevalence of liver disease in recipients of an organ from a HCV-carrier donor. Finally, we found no differences in 5-year patient and graft survival, regardless of the donor's serologic status.

A possible explanation for the discrepancy in reported HCV transmission involves differences

TABLE 6.4. HCV Infection in Renal Allograft Recipients

Author	Ref.	EIA-I No. Pos./No. Tested (%)	EIA-II No. Pos./No. Tested (%)	HCV-RNA No. Pos./No. EIA Pos. (%)
Roth (1991. US.)	68	179/596 (30)	—	—
Ponz (1991, Spain)	69	32/67 (48)	—	—
Baur (1991, Germany)	70	27/272 (10)	—	—
Klauser (1992, Austria)	71	43/324 (13)	—	—
Huang (1992, China)	74	59/120 (49)	—	—
Morales (1992, Spain)	61	66/200 (33)	—	—
Pol (1992, France)	62	20/127 (24)	—	—
Stemple (1993, U.S.)	72	76/716 (11)	—	—
Chan (1993, Hong Kong)	73	—	19/185 (10)*	18/19 (95)
Roth (1994, U.S.)	6	—	109/641 (17)	39/53 (74)

* Recombinant immunoblot assay.

in organ preservation. The New England Organ Bank uses slush preservation, whereas we have always used pulsatile perfusion. Preliminary studies from our center have demonstrated a greater than 99% reduction in the viral load in the kidney and detectable HCV RNA in the perfusate after several hours of pulsatile perfusion.[67] Conceivably, the reported differences in HCV transmission may be partly explainable on this basis, although other issues, including differing strain virulence patterns and recipient disease susceptibility associated with specific HLA specificities, require further study.

Seroprevalence of Anti-HCV Antibodies

Several investigators have reported the results of surveillance studies for anti-HCV antibodies among kidney recipients (Table 6.4). Using a second-generation anti-HCV assay, 17% of serum samples collected from patients transplanted at our center were anti-HCV–positive.[68] This figure is consistent with reports from other centers, in which 10-49% of transplant patients were anti-HCV–positive.[6,61,62,64,69–73] Such findings are not unexpected considering the high prevalence of anti-HCV antibodies among hemodialysis patients.[8,22,24–26]

Detection of HCV RNA.

In our series, HCV RNA was detected in the serum of 39 of 53 (74%) patients who were RIBA-positive when transplanted. This is consistent with a recent report by Chan et al.,[73] in which 95% of anti-HCV–positive patients were viremic (see Table 6.4). Also of note was the finding that 20 of 39 (52%) PCR-positive patients maintained normal transaminases throughout posttransplant follow-up. Ponz and colleagues detected liver disease in two-thirds of the anti-HCV carriers

transplanted at their center[69] Thus, 33–51% of the anti-HCV–positive transplant recipients in both reports maintained normal liver function tests, emphasizing the low sensitivity of liver transaminases to detect active viral replication. The same finding was noted previously in hemodialysis patients.[47] We recommend that every transplant patient with documented HCV infection and abnormal transaminases have a liver biopsy to characterize morphologically the extent of disease. This approach is supported by recent data from Rao et al., which demonstrate histologic progression to cirrhosis in serial biopsies obtained from transplant patients with chronic active hepatitis.[75] Until data are available describing the liver histology and clinical course in HCV-infected transplant patients with normal transaminases, recommendations on the timing and/or usefulness of a liver biopsy in this cohort cannot be made.

Quantitative PCR analysis of fresh serum from the 39 HCV-RNA–positive patients in our series demonstrated a wide range of viral copy number ($0.013\text{-}88 \times 10^6$/ml). Moreover, there was no correlation between HCV copy number and biochemical liver function abnormalities. This finding must be confirmed in a larger number of patients.

The rapid expansion of investigation in this field has led to the observation that HCV represents a variable group of agents, and multiple HCV strains have subsequently been identified worldwide.[3] We detected HCV strains HCV-1, BK, Hutch, and HCV-M among our patients (Table 6.5), one of which (BK) was originally reported from Japan.[76] Of interest, two patients were coinfected with two different strains of HCV. It is important to study the clinical consequence of infection with multiple HCV strains. In our relatively small series, we were unable to

TABLE 6.5. Quantitative Polymerase Chain Reaction and HCV Strain Identification*

	Posttransplant Liver Function		
	Normal (n = 32)	Abnormal (n = 34)	p Value
HCV RNA (copies/ml × 10⁶)	8.2 ± 13.8	6.9 ± 10.2	NS
Strain			
BK (n = 14)			
Hutch (n = 15)			
HCV-1 (n = 6)			
HCV-M (n = 4)			
HCV-1/BK (n = 1)			
HCV-1/Hutch (n = 1)			

Each value denotes the mean ± SD. Numbers in parentheses represent the number of patients in each group.
* Strain identification by restriction fragment length polymorphism of PCR product with confirmation by direct sequencing.
  Strain identification in patients with very low titers was not possible.

detect any clinical patterns that suggest differences in strain virulence. Nevertheless, the possibility that different HCV agents cause varying clinical outcomes requires investigation, especially in the immunosuppressed transplant recipient. An association between liver cirrhosis and hepatocellular carcinoma has been reported in HCV-infected Japanese patients,[77] and a recent report of hepatocellular carcinoma in a Japanese renal allograft recipient[78] suggests that increased surveillance for cirrhosis and/or early carcinoma is warranted for the HCV-infected transplant recipient. This may be especially true for patients infected with Southeast Asian strains of HCV.

Coinfection with HBV and HCV

Huang and colleagues[74] screened 120 Chinese renal transplant recipients and found 49.2% to be anti-HCV–positive, approximately one-half of whom were also HBsAg-positive. Among the entire 120 patients, 34% developed chronic hepatitis, although this figure rose to 50% (14 of 28) in coinfected patients. Furthermore, 21% of the dual-infected patients were found to have cirrhosis compared with none of the patients in the HCV-positive and HBV-negative groups. The authors concluded that coinfection with HCV and HBV can lead to a particularly aggressive form of liver disease in renal allograft recipients.

HCV-infected Kidney Recipients

We found RIBA positivity to be an independent predictor of posttransplant liver disease.[6] Chan et al.[79] reported similar results, although 75% of their anti-HCV–positive patients developed liver dysfunction compared with only 34% of our RIBA-positive cohort. We also observed a relationship between the dosage of antilymphocytic globulin (ALG) administered for induction therapy and the likelihood that the RIBA-positive patient would develop posttransplant liver disease. Antilymphocyte preparations predispose to viral reactivation; thus our findings are not surprising and emphasize the need to use such products with caution in RIBA-positive transplant recipients.

Patients who were seropositive for anti-HCV antibodies were more heavily transfused and were more likely to experience serious infectious events and acute rejection episodes (Table 6.6). Prior studies have suggested that transplant recipients with active viral replication (e.g., cytomegalovirus [CMV]) are further immunosuppressed as a consequence of interaction between viral infection and the host's immune responsiveness.[80,81] Further study, however, is required to elucidate properly the mechanisms whereby HCV infection may interfere with the host's immune surveillance.

Seemingly at odds with these findings was the nearly two-fold increase in acute rejection among the anti-HCV–positive patients. This finding contrasts with the results of Ponz et al.,[69] who reported no difference in rejection rates between anti-HCV–positive and –negative patients. Although an explanation is not readily apparent, several possibilities exist. It is likely that the amount of immunosuppression was markedly reduced following a serious infection, thus permitting an alloimmune response against the graft. In fact, 10 of 24 (41%) RIBA-positive patients with infection experienced at least 1 rejection episode. Alternatively, HCV infection may initiate a process that results in upregulation of MHC class II antigen expression in the allograft. Kidney recipients with active CMV infection have been described who either concomitantly or shortly thereafter developed acute rejection.[82]

TABLE 6.6.   Univariate Analysis According to Perioperative Anti-HCV Serostatus

Variable	Anti-HCV		p Value
	Positive (n = 109)	Negative (n = 200)	
Age (years)	47 ± 11.3	42.9 ± 12.5	NS
Gender (male/female)	66/43	115/85	NS
Follow-up (months)	65.7 ± 28.9	81.3 ± 30.3	< 0.001
Blood (no. of units)[a]	9.5± 13.4	6.9 ± 5.7	< 0.001
Preoperative liver function tests[b]	3/109 (2.7)	1/200 (0.5)	NS
Antilymphoblast globulin (mg)[c]	6983 ± 6169	6451 ± 5750	NS
Infections[d]	24.109 (22)	26/200 (13)	0.03
Rejections	40/109 (37)	41/200 (20)	0.002
Abnormal liver function test[e]	37/109 (34)	38/200 (19)	0.00

Each value denotes mean ± SD. Numbers in parentheses are percentages. Anti-HCV detected by recombinant immunoblast assay.
[a] Preoperative blood transfusions.
[b] Abnormal pretransplant liver function tests.
[c] Total antilymphoblast globulin administered as induction therapy.
[d] Requiring hospitalization and antimicrobial therapy.
[e] Chronically abnormal liver function tests after transplant.

In view of such risks, the anti-HCV–positive kidney recipient should be closely monitored for infection and allograft dysfunction. Furthermore, in light of the data linking ALG dosage with posttransplant liver dysfunction, the use of antilymphocyte preparations in the HCV-infected patient with allograft rejection becomes problematic. If possible, antilymphocyte products should not be used as first-line therapy to treat rejection in HCV-infected patients.

Transplant Evaluation of Anti-HCV–seropositive Patients

Although the anti-HCV–positive patient may be at increased risk for infection, rejection, and posttransplant liver disease, no difference has yet been demonstrated in patient and graft survival. For this reason, HCV infection should not be considered a contraindication to renal transplantation. However, it is advisable that the evaluation of the anti-HCV–positive transplant candidate should include PCR testing, if available, and liver biopsy to stage histologically the patient's disease. Staging is recommended regardless of the transaminase levels. Furthermore, careful studies of the safety and efficacy of antiviral therapy (ie. interferon) in patients with end-stage renal disease are needed to determine whether a course of antiviral treatment should precede transplantation. Patients with minimal changes or chronic persistent hepatitis are clearly suitable for transplant; however, sufficient data are not yet available to determine whether the HCV-infected patient with advanced chronic active hepatitis or early cirrhosis should be transplanted or remain on dialysis.

HCV IN CLINICAL NEPHROLOGY

Glomerulonephritis

Several histologic forms of immune complex-mediated glomerulonephritis have been linked to hepatitis B virus infection. It is not surprising, therefore, that infection with HCV has been recently associated with the development of membranoproliferative (MPGN) and membranous glomerulonephritis (MGN).

Rollino and coworkers[83] were the first to associate HCV infection with an immune-complex type of glomerulonephritis. They screened 27 patients with MGN and found 1 who was anti-HCV seropositive. The patient entered remission following steroid plus chlorambucil therapy. MGN was also diagnosed in 2 bone marrow recipients 9 and 18 months after transplantation [84] Both recipients were PCR-positive in both the serum and renal tissue.

Johnson et al.[85] described 8 patients with immune-complex glomerulonephritis of the membranoproliferative pattern associated with active HCV infection. In all 8 patients HCV RNA was detected in the serum, along with elevated serum aminotransferase and hypocomplementemia. Five of 8 had circulating cryoglobulins, and 3 of 4 biopsies studied with electron microscopy showed organized, finely fibrillar, cylindric or immunotactoidlike structures compatible with cryoglobulins. Four patients were treated with interferon α-2b for 2–12 months. All became HCV RNA-negative, and in 3 of 4 urinary protein excretion decreased to the normal range. The membranoproliferative pattern of GN has also been reported by two other investigators in association with

TABLE 6.7. Association of HCV with Essential Mixed Cryoglobulinemia

Ref.	Type of Mixed Cryos	RNA No. Pos./ No. Tested (%)	Serum HCV Antibodies EIA* No. Pos./No. Tested (%)	Serum HCV Antibodies RIBA† No. Pos./No. Tested (%)	Serum HCV RNA No. Pos./ No. Tested (%)	Cryoprecipitate HCV-Ab No. Pos./ No. Tested (%)	Cryoprecipitate HCV RNA No. Pos./ No. Tested (%)
89	Type II	4/4 (100)‡	8/19 (42)	8/19 (42)	16/19 (84)	1/4 (25)‡	4/4 (100)
90	Type II		50/51 (98)	33/50 (66)‡	13/16 (81)	21/51 (41)§	
91	Type II		21/30 (70)	21/30 (70)			
92	Type II and III		13/26 (50)	11/26 (42)			
93	Type II and III		129/161 (80)	88/100 (88)‡			
93	Secondary		44/66 (70)				
94	Type II and III		28/52 (54)			7/28 (25)‡	
95	Type II		13/15 (87)	13/15 (87)	5/7 (7)		
	TOTAL	4/4 (100)	306/417 (73)	202/292 (69)	34/42 (81)	29/83 (35)	4/4 (100)

* Second-generation enzyme immunoassay.
† Recombinant immunoblot assay.
‡ All patients were anti-HCV–positive.
§ Prevalence of anti-HCV increased to 94% after removal of IgM RF from cryoprecipitate.

HCV infection.[86,87] Of interest is a recent case report in which heavy proteinuria developed 3 months after liver transplantation in an HCV-infected patient.[87] Renal biopsy demonstrated changes compatible with MPGN. It is interesting to speculate why the nephropathy manifest itself early after transplant; the HCV infection had been present for a considerable time before transplant. Conceivably, the balance of antigen-antibody complexes was altered by the effect of immunosuppression on the circulating viral load.

Such cases illustrate several important clinical points. Patients with chronic liver disease and evidence of HCV infection who have abnormal urinalysis findings may have immune-complex glomerulonephritis. Such patients should be tested for cryoglobulins, rheumatoid factor, and serum complement concentrations as part of their evaluation. Renal biopsy should be obtained to confirm the diagnosis and to assist in the decision to use interferon α-2b.

Essential Mixed Cryoglobulinemia

The clinical syndrome of essential mixed cryoglobulinemia (EMC) is characterized by weakness, arthralgia, and purpura; some patients also have an immune-complex glomerular lesion referred to as cryoglobulinemic glomerulonephritis[88] Whereas 60–75% of mixed cryoglobulinemias are associated with infectious or lymphoprolifer-

ative disorders, hepatobiliary disease, connective tissue disease, or immunologically mediated glomerular disease, the remaining 30% have no underlying or associated disorder.

Efforts to identify a single antigen that is bound to polyclonal IgG and then binds, along with the polyclonal IgG, to a polyclonal or monoclonal IgM have been unsuccessful. Some investigators have suggested an association between hepatitis B virus infection and EMC, but such findings have not been consistently confirmed in subsequent studies.

Recently, several groups of investigators have detected a high prevalence of anti-HCV antibodies among patients with EMC[89–94] (Table 6.7). Moreover, several groups[89,90,95] have detected HCV RNA in anti-HCV–seronegative patients, confirming a significant incidence of false-negative serologic testing for anti-HCV antibodies among patients with EMC. Whereas 69% of patients with EMC were anti-HCV–reactive to sensitive second-generation assays, 81% were HCV RNA-positive by polymerase chain reaction (see Table 6.7)

In the study of Agnello and coworkers,[89] quantitative assays of HCV RNA (Table 6.8) demonstrated that greater than 99% of the HCV RNA in serum was cryoprecipitated. Furthermore, additional testing confirmed that the cryoprecipitation of HCV RNA from the serum was selective and specifically dependent on the type II cryoglobulins in HCV-infected serum.

TABLE 6.8.   Quantitative Studies of HCV RNA in Serum Samples and Cryoglobulins
from Patients with Type II Cryoglobulinemia

| Cryocrit (%) | HCV RNA | | | Relative HCV RNA Concentration in Cryoprecipitate* | Decrease in Serum HCV RNA after Cryoprecipitation (%) |
	Serum	Supernatant after Cryoprecipitate	Cryoprecipitate		
4	22 ng/ml	0.015 ng/ml	15 ng/ml	1000	> 99
8	50 pg/ml	0.030 pg/ml	30 pg/ml	1000	> 99
4	7 pg/ml	0.006 ng/ml	NT	NT	> 99
1	700 pg/ml	0.080 pg/ml	NT	NT	> 99

* Values were calculated with use of the following equation: cryoprecipitate HCV RNA concentration/supernatant HCV RNA concentration. NT = not tested.
Adapted from Agnello V, et al: N Engl J Med 1992;327:1490–1495.

A definitive role for HCV-immune complexes in the generation of the pathologic abnormalities of EMC awaits demonstration of HCV antigens in characteristic renal and vascular lesions. Although the data available thus far suggest a strong association of HCV infection with EMC, conclusive studies must still be conducted.

If HCV is involved in the pathogenesis of EMC, antiviral therapy may have a role in the treatment of patients with cryoglobulinemia. Several reports[89,96,97] have demonstrated that treatment with interferon results in marked clinical improvement. Most of these reports, however, are anecdotal and must be confirmed in larger series.

REFERENCES

1. Aach RD, Stevens CE, Hollinger FB, et al: Hepatitis C virus infection in post-transfusion hepatitis: An analysis with first and second-generation assays. N Engl J Med 1991;325:1325–1329.

2. Alter HJ, Purcell RH, Shih SW, et al: Detection of antibody to hepatitis C virus in prospectively followed transfusion recipients with acute and chronic non-A, non-B hepatitis. N Engl J Med 1989;321:1494–1500.

3. Houghton M, Weiner A, Han J, et al: Molecular biology of the hepatitis C viruses: Implications for diagnosis, development and control of viral disease. Hepatology 1991;14:381–388.

4. Esteban JI, Gonzalez A, Hernandez JM, et al: Evaluation of antibodies to hepatitis C virus in a study of transfusion associated hepatitis. N Engl J Med 1990;323:1107–1112.

5. Alter MJ, Margolis HS, Krawczynski K, et al: The natural history of community-acquired hepatitis C in the United States. N Engl J Med 1992;327:1899–1905.

6. Roth D, Zucker K, Cirocco R, et al: The impact of hepatitis C virus infection on renal allograft recipients. Kidney Int 1994;45:238–244.

7. Pol S, Romeo R, Zins B, et al: Hepatitis C virus RNA in anti-HCV positive hemodialysis patients: Significance and therapeutic implications. Kidney Int 1993;44:1097–1100.

8. Chan TM, Lok ASF, Cheng IKP, Chan R: Prevalence of hepatitis C virus infection in hemodialysis patients: A longitudinal study comparing the results of RNA and antibody assays. Hepatology 1993;17:5–8.

9. Tsukarma H, Hiyama T, Tanalsa S, et al: Risk factors for hepatocellular carcinoma among patients with chronic liver disease. N Engl J Med 1993;328:1797–1801.

10. Kuo G, Choo Q-L, Alter HJ, et al: An assay for circulating antibodies to a major etiologic virus of human non-A, non-B hepatitis. Science 1989;244:362–364.

11. Garson JA, Tedder RS, Briggs M, et al: Detection of hepatitis C viral sequences in blood donations by "nested" polymerase chain reaction and prediction of infectivity. Lancet 1990;335:1419–1422.

12. McGuinness PH, Bishop GA, Lien A, et al: Detection of serum hepatitis C virus RNA in HCV antibody-seropositive volunteer blood donors. Hepatology 1993;18:485–490.

13. Donahue JG, Munoz A, Ness PM, et al: The declining risk of post-transfusion hepatitis C virus infection. N Engl J Med 1992;327:369–373.

14. Alberti A, Chemello L, Cavaletto D, et al: Antibody to hepatitis C virus and liver disease in volunteer blood donors. Ann Intern Med 1991;114:1010–1012.

15. McFarlane IG, Smith HM, Johnson PJ, et al: Hepatitis C virus antibodies in chronic active hepatitis: Pathogenetic factor or false-positive result? Lancet 1990;335:754–757.

16. Farci P, London WT, Wong DC, et al: The natural history of infection with hepatitis C virus in chimpanzees: Comparison of serologic responses measured with first and second generation assays and relationship to HCV viremia. J Infect Dis 1992;165:1006–1011.

17. McHutchison JG, Person JL, Govindarajan S, et al: Improved detection of hepatitis C virus antibodies in high-risk populations. Hepatology 1992;15:19–25.

18. VanderPoel CL, Cuypers HTM, Reesink HW, et al: Confirmation of hepatitis C virus infection by new four-antigen recombinant immunoblot assay. Lancet 1991;337:317–319.

19. Esteban JI, Lòpez-Talavera JC, Genesca J, et al: High rate of infectivity and liver disease in blood donors with antibodies to hepatitis C virus. Ann Intern Med 1991;115:443–449.

20. Jeffers LJ, Perez GO, de Medina MD, et al: Hepatitis C infection in two urban hemodialysis units. Kidney Int 1990;38:320–322.

21. Zeldis JB, Depner TA, Kuramoto IK, et al: The prevalence of hepatitis C virus antibodies among hemodialysis patients. Ann Intern Med 1990;112:958–960.

22. Oguchi H, Miyasalra M, Tokunoga S, et al: Hepatitis virus infection (HBV and HCV) in eleven Japanese hemodialysis units. Clin Nephrol 1992;38:36–43.

23. Muller GY, Zabaleta ME, Arminio A, et al: Risk factors for dialysis-associated hepatitis C in Venezuela. Kidney Int 1992;41:1055–1058.

24. Mondelli MU, Cristina G, Piazza V, et al: High prevalence of antibodies to hepatitis C virus in hemodialysis units using a second generation assay. Nephron 1992;61:350–351.

25. Chauveau P, Courouce AM, Lemarec N, et al: Antibodies to hepatitis C virus by second generation test in hemodialysed patients. Kidney Int 1993;43:5149– 5152.

26. Mazzotta L, Landucci G, Pfanner L, et al: Comparison between first and second generation tests to determine the frequency of anti-HCV antibodies in uremic patients in replacement dialytic therapy. Nephron 1992;61:354–355.

27. Chan TM, Lok ASF, Cheng IKP: Hepatitis C infection among dialysis patients: A comparison between patients on maintenance hemodialysis and continuous ambulatory peritoneal dialysis. Nephrol Dial Transplant 1991;6:944–947.

28. Besso L, Rovere A, Peano G, et al: Prevalence of HCV antibodies in a uremic population undergoing maintenance dialysis therapy and in the staff members of the dialysis unit. Nephron 1992;61:304–306.

29. Huang C-C, Wu M-S, Lin D-Y, Liaw Y-F: The prevalence of hepatitis C virus antibodies in patients treated with continuous ambulatory peritoneal dialysis. Perit Dial Int 1992;12:31–33.

30. Ng Y-Y, Lee S-D, Wu S-C, et al: The need for second generation anti-hepatitis C virus testing in uremic patients on continuous ambulatory peritoneal dialysis. Perit Dial Int 1993;13:132–135.

31. Dussol B, Chicheportiche C, Cantaloube J-F, et al: Detection of hepatitis C infection by polymerase chain reaction among hemodialysis patients. Am J Kidney Dis 1993;22:547-580.

32. Kuhns M, de Medina M, McNamara A, et al: Detection of hepatitis C virus RNA in hemodialysis patients. J Am Soc Nephrol 1994;4:1491–1497.

33. Knudsen F, Wantzin P, Rasmussen K, et al: Hepatitis C in dialysis patients: Relationship to blood transfusions, dialysis and liver disease. Kidney Int 1993;43:1353– 1356.

34. Jonas MM, Zilleruelo GE, Larue SI, et al: Hepatitis C infection in a pediatric dialysis population. Pediatrics 1992;89:707–709.

35. Fujiyama S, Kawano S, Sato S, et al: Prevalence of hepatitis C virus antibodies in hemodialysis patients and dialysis staff. Hepato-Gastroenterology 1992;39:161–165.

36. Niu MT, Coleman PJ, Alter MJ: Multicenter study of hepatitis C virus infection in chronic hemodialysis patients and hemodialysis center staff members. Am J Kidney Dis 1993;22:568–573.

37. Hardy NM, Sandroni S, Danielson S, Wilson WJ: Antibody to hepatitis C virus increases with time on hemodialysis. Clin Nephrol 1992;38:44–48.

38. Yamaguchi K, Nishumura Y, Fukuoka N, et al: Hepatitis C virus antibodies in hemodialysis patients. Lancet 1990; 335:1409–1410.

39. Tokars JI, Alter MJ, Favero MS, et al: National surveillance of hemodialysis associated diseases in the United States, 1990. ASAIO J 1993;39:71–80.

40. Cantu P, Magnano S, Masini M, et al: Prevalence of antibodies against hepatitis C virus in a dialysis unit. Nephron 1992;61:337–338.

41. Lin H-H, Huang C-C, Sheen I-S, et al: Prevalence of antibodies to hepatitis C virus in the hemodialysis unit. Am J Nephrol 1991;11:192–194.

42. Niu MT, Alter MJ, Kristensen C, Margolis HS: Outbreak of hemodialysis-associated non-A, non-B hepatitis and correlation with antibody to hepatitis C virus. Am J Kidney Dis 1992;19:345–352.

43. Abb J: Prevalence of hepatitis C virus antibodies in hospital personnel. Zentralbl Bakteriol 1991;274:543–547.

44. Hofman H, Kunz C: Low risk of health care workers for infection with hepatitis C virus. Infection 1990;18:286– 288.

45. Koziol DE, Holland PV, Alling DW, et al: Antibody to hepatitis B core antigen as a paradoxical marker for non-A, non-B hepatitis agents in donated blood. Ann Intern Med 1986;104:488–495.

46. Wolf PL, Williams D, Coplon N, Coulson A: Low aspartate transaminase activity in serum of patients undergoing chronic hemodialysis. Clin Chem 1972;18:567–568.

47. Caramelo C, Ortiz A, Aquilera B, et al: Liver disease patterns in hemodialysis patients with antibodies to hepatitis C virus. Am J Kidney Dis 1993;22:822–828.

48. Oliva JA, Maymo RM, Carrio J, et al: Late seroconversion of C virus markers in hemodialysis patients. Kidney Int 1993;43:S153–S156.

49. Sheen IS, Liaw Y, Chuc, Pao C: Role of hepatitis C virus infection in spontaneous hepatitis B surface antigen clearance during chronic hepatitis B virus infection. J Infect Dis. 1992;165:831–834.

50. Vandelli L, Medici G, Savazzi AM, et al: Behavior of antibody profile against hepatitis C virus in patients on maintenance hemodialysis. Nephron 1992;61:260–262.

51. Gitnick G, Weiss S, Overby LR, et al: Non-A, non-B hepatitis: A prospective study of a hemodialysis outbreak with evaluation of a serologic marker in patients and staff. Hepatology 1983;3:625–630.

52. Marchesi D, Arici C, Poletti E, et al: Outbreak of non-A, non-B hepatitis in hemodialysis patients: A retrospective analysis. Nephrol Dial Transplant 1988;3:795–799.

53. Jadoul M, Cornu C, Strihou C, and the UCL Collaborative Group: Incidence and risk factors for hepatitis C seroconversion in hemodialysis. A prospective study. Kidney Int 1993;44:1322–1326.

54. Garcia-Valdecasas J, Bernal MC, Cerezo S, et al: Strategies to reduce the transmission of HCV infection in hemodialysis units. J Am Soc Nephrol 1993;4:347A

55. Favero MS, Alter MJ, Bland LA: Dialysis-associated infections and their control. In Bennett JV, Brachman P (eds): Hospital Infections, 3rd ed. Boston: Little, Brown, 1992;375–403.

56. Koenig P, Umlarift F, Lhotta K, et al: Treatment of hemodialysis patients suffering from chronic HCV-infection with interferon alpha. J Am Soc Nephrol 1993;4:361A.

57. Parfrey PS, Farge D, Forbe C, et al: Chronic hepatitis in end-stage renal disease: Comparison of HBsAg-negative and HBsAg-positive patients. Kidney Int 1985;28:959– 967.

58. Weir MR, Kirkman RL, Strom TB, Tilney NL: Liver disease in recipients of long-functioning renal allografts. Kidney Int 1985;28:839–844.

59. Boyce NW, Holdsworth SR, Hooke D, et al: Non hepatitis B-associated liver disease in a renal transplant population. Am J Kidney Dis 1988;11:307–312.

60. LaQuaglia MP, Tolkoff-Rubin NE, Dienstag JL, et al: Impact of hepatitis on renal transplantation. Transplantation 1981;32:504–507.

61. Morales M, Campo C, Castellano G, et al: Clinical implications of the presence of antibodies to hepatitis C after renal transplantation. Transplant Proc 1992;24: 78–80.

62. Pol S, Legendre C, Saltiel C, et al: Hepatitis C virus in kidney recipients: Epidemiology and impact on renal transplantation. J Hepatol 1992;15:202–206.

63. Pereira BJG, Milford EL, Kirkman RL, Levey AS: Transmission of hepatitis C virus by organ transplantation. N Engl J Med 1991;325:454–460.

64. Roth D, Fernandez JA, Babischkin S, et al: Detection of hepatitis C virus infection among cadaver organ donors: Evidence for low transmission of disease. Ann Int Med 1992;117:470–475.

65. Pereira BJG, Wright TL, Schmid CH, et al: Screening and confirmatory testing of cadaver organ donors for hepatitis C virus infection: A U.S. national collaborative study. Kidney Int 1994;46:886–892.

66. Pereira BJG, Milford EL, Kirkman RL, et al: Prevalence of hepatitis C virus RNA in organ donors positive for hepatitis C antibody and in the recipients of their organs. N Engl J Med 1992;327:910–915.

67. Zucker K, Cirocco R, Roth D, et al: Depletion of hepatitis C virus from procured kidneys using pulsatile perfusion preservation. Transplantation 1994;57:832–840.

68. Roth D, Fernandez JA, Burke GW, et al: Detection of antibody to hepatitis C virus in renal transplant recipients. Transplantation 1991;51:396–400.

69. Ponz E, Campistol JM, Bruguera M, et al: Hepatitis C virus infection among kidney transplant recipients. Kidney Int 1991;40:748–751.

70. Baur P, Daniel V, Pomer S, et al: Hepatitis C virus antibodies in patients after kidney transplantation. Ann Hematol 1991;62:68–73.

71. Klauser R, Franz O, Traindl O, et al: Hepatitis C antibody in renal transplant patients. Transplant Proc 1992; 24:286–288.

72. Stempel CA, Lake J, Kuo G, Vincenti F: Hepatitis C—its prevalence in end-stage renal failure patients and clinical course after kidney transplantation. Transplantation 1993; 55:273–276.

73. Chan T-M, Lok AS, Cheng KP, Chan RT: A prospective study of hepatitis C infection among renal transplant recipients. Gastroenterology 1993;104:862–868.

74. Huang C-C, Liaw Y-F, Lai M-K, et al: The clinical outcome of hepatitis C virus antibody-positive renal allograft recipients. Transplantation 1992;53:763–765.

75. Rao KV, Anderson WR, Kasiske BL, Dahl DC. Value of liver biopsy in the evaluation and management of chronic liver disease in renal transplant recipients. Am J Med 1993;94:241–250.

76. Takamizawa A, Mori C, Fuke I, et al: Structure and organization of the hepatitis C virus genome isolated from human carriers. J Virol 1991;65:1105–1113.

77. Nishioka K, Watanabe J, Furuta S, et al: A high prevalence of antibody to hepatitis C virus in patients with hepatocellular carcinoma in Japan. Cancer 1991;67:429–433.

78. Arita S, Asano T, Suzuki T, et al: Clinical study of hepatitis disorders in renal transplant recipients with special reference to hepatitis C. Transplant Proc 1992;24:1538–1540.

79. Chan TM, Lok ASF, Cheng IKP: Hepatitis C in renal transplant recipients. Transplantation 1991;52:810–813.

80. Linnemann CC, Kaufman CA, First MR, et al: Cellular immune response to cytomegalovirus infection after renal transplantation. Infect Immun 1978;22:176–180.

81. Rytel MW, Aguilar-Torres FG, Balay J, Heim LR: Assessment of the status of cell mediated immunity in cytomegalovirus infected renal allograft recipients. Cell Immunol 1978;37:31–40.

82. Pouteil-Noble C, Ecochard R, Landrivon G, et al: Cytomegalovirus infection—An etiological factor for rejection? Transplantation 1993;55:851-857.

83. Rollino C, Roccatello D, Giachino O, et al: Hepatitis C virus infection and membranous glomerulonephritis. Nephron 1991;59:319–320.

84. Davda R, Peterson J, Weiner R, et al: Membranous glomerulonephritis in association with hepatitis C virus infection. Am J Kidney Dis 1993;22:452–455.

85. Johnson RJ, Gretch DR, Yamabe H, et al: Membranoproliferative glomerulonephritis associated with hepatitis C virus infection. N Engl J Med 1993;328:465–470.

86. Cottiero R, Westrick E, Weinberg M: Membranoproliferative glomerulonephritis type I associated with chronic hepatitis C virus infection. J Am Soc Nephrol 1992;3:309A.

87. Burstein DM, Rodby RA: Membranoproliferative glomerulonephritits associated with hepatitis C virus infection. J Am Soc Nephrol 1993;4:1288–1293.

88. D'Amico G, Colasanti G, Ferrario F, Sinico RA: Renal involvement in essential mixed cryoglobulinemia. Kidney Int 1989;35:1004–1014.

89. Agnello V, Chung RT, Kaplan LM: A role for hepatitis C virus infection in type II cryoglobulinemia. N Engl J Med 1992;327:1490–1495.

90. Misiani R, Bellavita P, Fenili D, et al: Hepatitis C virus infection in patients with essential mixed cryoglobulinemia. Ann Intern Med 1992;117:573–577.

91. Disdier P, Harlé J-R, Weiller P-J: Cryoglobulinemia and hepatitis C infection. Lancet 1991;338:1151–1152.

92. Dammacco F, Sansonno D: Antibodies to hepatitis C virus in essential mixed cryoglobulinemia. Clin Exp Immunol 1992;87:352–356.

93. Galli M, Monti G, Monteverde A, et al: Hepatitis C virus and mixed cryoglobulinemias. Lancet 1992;1:989.

94. Ferri C, Greco F, Longobardo G, et al: Antibodies to hepatitis C virus in patients with mixed cryoglobulinemia. Arthritis Rheum 1991;34:1606–1610.

95. Pechére-Bertschi A, Perrin L, de Saussure P, et al: Hepatitis C: A possible etiology for cryoglobulinemia type II. Clin Exp Immunol 1992;89:419–422.

96. Bonomo L, Casato M, Afeltra A, Caccavo D: Treatment of idiopathic mixed cryoglobulinemia with alpha interferon. Am J Med 1987, 83:726–730.

97. Durand JM, Kaplanski G, Lefevre P, et al: Effect of interferon-α 2b on cryoglobulinemia related to hepatitis C virus infection. J Infect Dis 1992;165:778-779.

VENOOCCLUSIVE DISEASE OF THE LIVER FOLLOWING BONE MARROW TRANSPLANTATION

ROBERT SACKSTEIN, M.D., Ph.D.
NELSON J. CHAO, M.D.

Pathology
Incidence and Diagnosis
   Noninvasive Diagnostic Studies
   Clinical Grading of Severity
Predisposing Clinical Factors
   Pretransplant Factors
   Transplantation Factors

Pathophysiology
Clinical Course and Treatment
   Recent Therapeutic Options
Prophylaxis
Summary

Hepatic venoocclusive disease (VOD) is a clinical disorder characterized by concomitant hepatic and renal insufficiency; it is becoming an increasingly common complication of the high dose chemo/radiotherapy myeloablative regimens used in preparation for bone marrow transplantation (BMT). The first histopathologic characterization of VOD was in 1954 when Bras, Jelliffe, and Stuart reported on an obliterative process in hepatic veins in Jamaican children with cirrhosis.[1,2] The pathologic changes consisted of subendothelial intimal thickening with fibrous occlusion of the lumen in small and medium branches of the hepatic vein and associated centrilobular congestion with necrosis of pericentral hepatocytes. Clinically, the children presented with fluid retention, tender hepatomegaly, ascites, and progression to encephalopathy if sinusoidal obstruction was severe. The authors pointed to an association with consumption of Jamaican bush teas, now known to be the etiologic factor because they contain hepatotoxic pyrrolizidine (senezio) alkaloids.

Since these initial descriptions, VOD has been reported following hepatic radiation,[3,4] with the use of single agent chemotherapy at standard doses (usually after prolonged administration),[5–7] following renal transplant and azathioprine therapy,[8] and commonly following BMT[9–15] (Table 7.1). Although there are no accurate statistics about the incidence of VOD worldwide, the ingestion of toxic alkaloids is the most common cause of VOD in developing countries (especially India, Egypt, and the Caribbean), whereas in the U.S. and Europe VOD is encountered mostly as a complication of BMT.[8] This discussion focuses on VOD following BMT since this hepatic condition is responsible for most cases of acute hepatic and renal failure in the immediate posttransplant period.

PATHOLOGY

The histologic hallmark of VOD is thickening and obliteration of the central veins of the hepatic lobules and of small and medium-sized (< 300-μm diameter) intrahepatic veins (Fig. 7.1). VOD must be distinguished from hepatic vein thrombosis of the Budd-Chiari syndrome, which although it may present in a clinically similar manner, differs from VOD in that the disease process occurs in the major hepatic veins and the inferior vena cava. Furthermore, the conspicuous absence of platelet deposits in VOD following BMT distinguishes it from Budd-Chiari syndrome.

The acute lesion of VOD consists of narrowing of the venule lumina by subendothelial deposits of cellular debris, coagulated protein, reticulum, and macrophages, with associated sinusoidal congestion and damage to surrounding

TABLE 7.1. Causes of Hepatic Venoocclusive Disease*

Ingestion of pyrrolizidine alkaloids

Alkylating agents (especially busulfan and cyclophospha-mide)

Antimetabolites (especially cytosine arabinoside and 6-thioguanine; azathioprine after renal transplantation)

Ionizing radiation (alone or in combination with cyclophos-phamide)

* See text for references.

hepatocytes in zone 3 of the acinus. Such histologic changes may be scattered throughout the liver and, therefore, may be missed in liver biopsy. As venular and sinusoidal occlusion progresses, first by noncollagenous material and infiltrating foam cells and later by deposition of collagen, increasing sinusoidal congestion leads to ischemic necrosis of hepatocytes and intra-hepatic hypertension with hemorrhaging. The end-result of this process is dense nonportal, centrilobular cirrhosis. The severity of clinical VOD correlates with the extent of fibrosis and hepatocyte necrosis, not the distribution or degree of venular obstruction.[16]

INCIDENCE AND DIAGNOSIS

Venoocclusive disease is predominantly a clinical diagnosis without a clearly defined gold standard; consequently, the prevalence and incidence of VOD following BMT differ markedly among centers. Early estimates of incidence were 10–20%, but recent data suggest that as many as 50% or more of patients undergoing BMT develop VOD; liver dysfunction contributes to death in approximately 25% of such patients.[17] Reported differences in incidence rates among institutions are likely related to patient selection criteria, conditioning regimens, and changes in patient management over time. Although some variation in diagnostic criteria among institutions may explain differences in patient outcomes,[18] the diagnosis of VOD is generally based on the presence of two of the following three clinical criteria: tender hepatomegaly, sudden weight gain (generally identified by an increase greater than 2% of baseline, although some use a 5% increase as the threshold[15]), and hyperbilirubinemia (total serum bilirubin > 34 umol/L (2 mg/dl)). In strictest terms, the diagnosis depends on development of these signs in the absence of other possible explanations,

such as graft vs. host disease (GVHD), sepsis, congestive heart failure, hepatitis, or fungal liver disease, although each of these conditions may occur concomitantly with VOD. Timing constitutes a critical element in establishing the diagnosis. VOD commonly develops within 20 days following transplant, whereas liver injury due to GVHD usually is not manifested until later.

A change in liver size or tenderness is usually the first sign of VOD and occurs within 1 week following cytoreductive therapy and as early as 1 day after transplantation. Unexplained weight gain with salt and water retention also occurs as an early sign, usually within 1 week after transplantation. Sodium retention and weight gain may be related to the development of intrasinusoidal hypertension secondary to hepatic blood flow obstruction (see chapters 1 and 8). Fluid retention, as evidenced by peripheral edema, pleural effusion, or ascites, is usually demonstrated within 2 weeks after transplantation. When it occurs, renal failure (which mimics the hepatorenal syndrome; see below) may be manifested as early as 1–2 weeks after transplantation. In fact, renal sodium retention typically precedes the development of jaundice, which is usually a later sign.[14] The level of hyperbilirubinemia is variable; however, patients who are destined to have severe and often fatal VOD tend to have persistently higher peak levels of bilirubin.[17] Elevated liver function tests, specifically aspartate aminotransferase (AST) and alanine aminotransferase (ALT), may be observed, and alkaline phosphatase also may be elevated.

Clinically, the differential diagnosis of liver disease in posttransplant patients typically ranges from VOD to viral hepatitis (typically cytomegalovirus) or to GVHD in allogenic recipients. Only a small subset of VOD cases reported in the literature are diagnosed histologically. Because VOD occurs after ablation of the patient's bone marrow with concomitant thrombocytopenia, liver biopsy has not been routinely performed. Moreover, the morbidity associated with invasive procedures is compounded by the onset of coagulopathy accompanying liver disease. Nonetheless, transvenous biopsy performed by experienced physicians has been useful for the proper diagnosis and potential treatment of such patients when hepatic toxicity occurs.[19,20] The transvenous liver biopsy done through either the jugular or the femoral vein has provided adequate tissue specimens in approximately 80–90% of

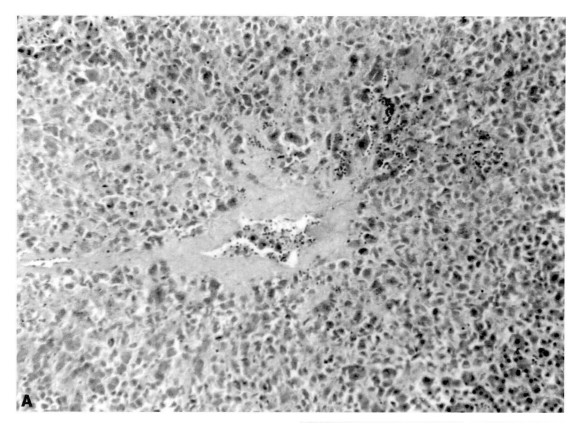

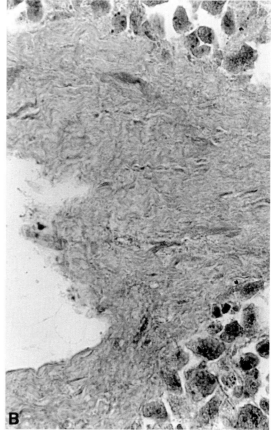

FIGURE 7.1. *A*, Venoocclusive disease of the liver in a bone marrow transplant patient, early stage. Note thickening of the wall of the centrilobular vein with early luminal narrowing (H & E, 25 × magnification). *B*, Same patient as A, high magnification (250 × magnification). Note extensive collagen fibrosis. (Figures courtesy of Dr. Ramon Sandin, H. Lee Moffitt Cancer Center.)

patients. Moreover, a transvenous approach allows the measurement of the hepatic wedge pressure. A gradient ≥ 10 mmHg between the wedged hepatic and free hepatic venous pressures has greater than an 80% positive predictive value for the histologic diagnosis of VOD.[19] The transvenous hepatic pressure measurements and biopsies should be performed only by experienced physicians, because such procedures are difficult to perform safely in light of posttransplant thrombocytopenia. Severe bleeding requiring surgical intervention or perforation through the capsule of the liver has occurred.

Even when liver tissue can be obtained, the diagnosis of VOD may still be confusing. The distribution of lesions in the liver may be patchy, and imposition of strict histologic standards for VOD is limited by the type of specimens collected, which often are very small fragments. Compounding this problem are differences in staining as well as interphysician variation in interpretation of histologic specimens. The most complete description of the histology of VOD has been reported by investigators in Seattle, who reviewed 355 cases of liver toxicity following BMT; 76 of these cases involved postmortem evaluation of tissue.[21] Correlation between clinical and histologic features of VOD revealed that histologic damage to structures in zone 3 of the liver occurred in 41 of 43 patients with clinical hepatic dysfunction; however, only 30 of the 43 had occlusion in the hepatic venules. Moreover, neither the percentage of venules with occlusion nor the degree of occlusion correlated with the clinical severity of VOD.

Noninvasive Diagnostic Studies

Doppler studies and ultrasound of the liver have been used in the diagnosis of VOD. Standard evaluation by ultrasound will rule out the presence of infiltrative liver disease or biliary dilatation and examines the presence and amount of ascites and the extent of hepatomegaly. Moreover, absence of visualization of the major hepatic veins by ultrasound is consistent with the diagnosis of VOD.[22–24] Doppler ultrasonography may reveal a slowing or reversal of the portal venous flow. One study has suggested that duplex sonography may provide a sensitive indicator of liver damage related to VOD through calculation of the hepatic artery resistive index (RI), defined as the difference between maximum and minimum systolic velocity divided by maximum systolic velocity. The RI was higher in patients with documented VOD than in normal volunteers or patients with GVHD.[25] However, a prospective controlled study is needed to determine the sensitivity and specificity of the changes observed by Doppler.

Liver-spleen scans and computed tomography (CT) with contrast are of limited utility in the diagnosis of VOD. Although these studies are most beneficial in the analysis of potential infiltrative liver disease, they may be useful in the setting of differentiating Budd-Chiari syndrome from VOD. The separate venous drainage of the caudate lobe into the inferior vena cava typically results in a normal appearance of the caudate lobe in Budd-Chiari syndrome, whereas such caudate sparing is not characteristic of VOD.

The diagnosis of VOD also may be corroborated by biochemical studies such as serum levels of aminopeptide of type III collagen. This peptide is released into the serum during the processing of precursor procollagen into type III collagen. Preliminary studies in children indicate that rising levels may predict the onset as well as the clinical course of VOD. Levels decreased in patients recovering from VOD, whereas they remained elevated in patients who died with progressive VOD.[26] At present, more information is needed about this approach to the diagnosis of VOD and, in particular, about its applicability in the diagnosis of VOD in adult patients.

Clinical Grading of Severity

To predict outcomes in patients with VOD, attempts have been made to categorize patients as having mild, moderate, or severe VOD based on the reversibility of liver dysfunction within 100 days after transplantation.[14,27] According to investigators at the Fred Hutchinson Cancer Center,[17] "mild" VOD requires no medication for fluid retention or for hepatic pain; "moderate" VOD requires sodium and fluid restriction and diuretics or pain medication; and "severe" VOD requires dialysis or is marked by liver dysfunction not reversible within 100 days or resulting in death.

Recently, a logistic regression model based on the degree of early weight gain and bilirubin levels at several intervals following BMT was developed to predict an unfavorable outcome for patients with VOD.[28] This approach was undertaken to assess whether early weight gain and bilirubin levels were indicative of severity of disease and whether the disease would be reversible. A comparison was made between patients who did not have VOD and patients with either severe or nonsevere VOD, and the regression model was used to generate coefficients for a probability equation allowing estimates that were highly specific but moderately sensitive. The authors propose that this approach may be useful to select patients in whom a potentially toxic intervention should be initiated (e.g., administration of tissue plasminogen activator) in an attempt to reverse progressing hepatic venular obstruction. However, despite the potential predictive value of this approach, the absence of clear benefit of interventional treatment at this time suggests that it may serve merely to offer insight into the need for prolonged supportive care (see discussion of clinical treatment below).

PREDISPOSING CLINICAL FACTORS

Because the criteria for the diagnosis of VOD have varied from institution to institution, the actual predisposing factors have not been uniformly corroborated from study to study. This is not surprising because of the many differences in choice of control patients, preparative regimens, patient selection criteria and whether analyses were performed in univariate or multivariate form, weighing certain risk factors more than others. In general, the clinical risk factors for developing VOD can be stratified into two categories: pretransplant factors and factors associated with transplantation.

Pretransplant Factors

Hepatitis. Probably the strongest risk factor identified in various studies is preexisting hepatitis. The association of VOD with baseline elevated AST, suggesting ongoing hepatitis, has been confirmed in large multivariate analyses from different institutions.[15,29,30] The risk of VOD may be proportionally increased relative to the degree of AST elevation. The basis for this association may be related to inflammatory hepatic injury with cytokine release induced, for example, by viral hepatitis. Such increased cytokines may result in increased tissue factor levels with enhancement of the thrombotic potential (see below). A second possibility is that the viral hepatitis may lead to increased levels of hepatic

transforming growth factor-beta (TGF-β),[31] with an associated increase in collagen synthesis (see below).

The observation that pretransplant hepatitis is uniformly associated with VOD is not without challenge. Other studies in which pretransplant viral hepatitis was endemic or present in all patients have not confirmed this association.[32,33] Explanations for the discrepancy may be related to differences in conditioning regimen or patient population. Still, a recent retrospective study using polymerase chain reaction rate to detect pretransplant presence of hepatitis C RNA has revealed a strong association between development of VOD and evidence of ongoing hepatitis C infection.[34]

Antimicrobial Therapy. Certain antimicrobial agents, particularly vancomycin and acyclovir, have been implicated, especially when given prior to transplantation. In multivariate analysis of 355 patients transplanted in Seattle, VOD was significantly associated with administration of acyclovir before transplantation and with administration of vancomycin during cytoreductive therapy.[17] A separate study found a threefold increase in the relative risk of hepatic toxicity in patients who receive broad-spectrum antibiotics for more than 26 days, with an increased risk if they received amphotericin B.[35] Moreover, vancomycin therapy correlated with persistent fever, which in itself is an additional risk factor for severe liver toxicity. The association of VOD and fever may be linked through infection, with resultant release of cytokines, such as interleukin-1 (IL-1) and tumor necrosis factor (TNF), that may have procoagulant effects (see below).

Refractory Disease. Refractory malignancy has been reported to be associated with a higher incidence of VOD.[15,36] However, a prospective analysis[37] has indicated that refractory disease in and of itself is not associated with a higher risk of VOD.

Gender. Two studies have suggested that female gender was associated with a higher risk, possibly related to the use of oral contraceptives during the preparative regimen and during transplantation.[30,35] However, gender risk has not been found to be statistically significant in univariate analysis in a recent large study.[17]

Hemostatic Factors. Since hemostatic factors are involved in VOD, one study has examined whether decreases in levels of naturally occurring anticoagulants could predict the occurrence of

VOD.[38] In a prospective analysis of 45 patients, protein C, protein S, and antithrombin III were measured prior to cytoreductive therapy and following BMT. In a multivariate analysis, protein C was the only independent variable that discriminated between VOD and non-VOD patients either prior to or after BMT. Patients with low protein C had a higher risk for developing VOD. A second study also found that protein C deficiency was present following autologous BMT and that antithrombin III levels were depressed.[39] Based on these studies and recent data suggesting that d-dimers may be useful in predicting deep venous thrombosis, a prospective study of d-dimers might be informative. Of interest, hemostatic activation of endothelial cells, as indicated by release of von Willebrand factor, does not appear to play a role in VOD.[40] Measured levels of von Willebrand factor antigen (vWF:ag) during the first 6 weeks after BMT did not correlate with development of VOD. However, levels of vWF:ag were higher in allograft patients, suggesting that endothelial activation may be more pronounced in this population.

Additional Factors.   Other factors that have been implicated in development of VOD include liver involvement with malignant disease, cytomegalovirus (CMV) serology, and age > 15 years.[29,41] The relative risk of second BMTs remain controversial; one report, however, has suggested an extremely high incidence of life-threatening VOD.[42] This observation has been corroborated in data from 114 recipients of a second bone marrow transplant.[43]

Transplantation Factors

Conditioning Regimen.   The type of conditioning regimen is probably the most important factor in the development of VOD. Unfortunately, many reports of VOD are anecdotal and do not provide a definitive answer to the specific identity of agents that induce VOD. The two most commonly used preparative regimens in BMT consist of fractionated total body irradiation/cyclophosphamide, and busulfan/cyclophosphamide. Both are associated with severe liver injury and VOD. In patients undergoing total body irradiation, the risk of VOD increases with a higher total dose of irradiation even with dose fractionation.[17,36] Moreover, dose rate may also be important. A low dose rate of 2 cGy/min has resulted in very low rates of VOD in two series.[44,45]

The chemotherapeutic agent most often implicated in development of VOD is busulfan,[46–48] an alkylating agent that is extremely effective in the conditioning regimen for allogenic bone marrow transplantation. Initially, there was confusion in the cause-effect relationship between busulfan and VOD. Early observations indicated that regimens in children based on adult doses of busulfan resulted in a very low incidence of hepatic VOD compared with the high incidence in adult patients. This difference is now understood as a consequence of the wide variability in the pharmacokinetics and distribution of busulfan associated with age. In young children the pharmacologic area under the curve (AUC) for busulfan is substantially lower than in adults. The volume of distribution, as well as clearance, appears to be as much as twice as high in children. Of note, there may be a three- to five-fold difference in busulfan levels among adult patients. Because of such data, efforts are now directed at using pharmacokinetic modeling for the AUC to determine the total dose of busulfan. Whether this approach will improve outcome by decreasing hepatic toxicity is not yet clear.

Source of Bone Marrow.   Several reports initially suggested that allogeneic BMT recipients have a higher incidence of VOD compared with autologous BMT recipients.[27,36] In the setting of allogeneic transplantation with mismatched or partially matched donors, the release of cytokines from alloreactive donor T cells may predispose or increase the likelihood for development of VOD. However, the many reports of VOD in patients receiving autologous BMT,[27,49] indicate that HLA incompatibilities are not prerequisite for VOD development.

Graft vs. Host Disease (GVHD).   VOD has been reported to occur more frequently in patients with GVHD,[50] although some studies have not confirmed this association.[15,17] The use of methotrexate for prophylaxis of GVHD in conjunction with the busulfan/cyclophosphamide regimen appears to be associated with a marked increase in the incidence of VOD: prophylaxis with a combination of methotrexate and cyclosporine was associated with a 70% incidence of VOD compared with the 18% incidence in historical controls on cyclosporine and methylprednisolone prophylaxis.[48]

It has been suggested that when T cell-depleted marrow is used, the incidence of VOD is reduced.[51] However, the decreased incidence of

VOD in T-cell depleted marrow recipients may be secondary to the elimination of methotrexate from the GVHD prophylaxis regimen. Although multivariate analyses have not identified an association between GVHD prophylactic regimens and increased risk for VOD disease,[17] there is no doubt that both methotrexate and cyclosporine are hepatotoxic and certainly can increase the severity, if not the incidence, of VOD.

Oral Mucositis. One study has correlated the development of oral mucositis with VOD.[52] The patients were treated with either busulfan and cyclophosphamide or fractionated total body irradiation and cyclophosphamide in preparation for BMT. Patients with oral mucositis were found to have 6.5 times higher likelihood of developing VOD. The sensitivity was 86% with a specificity of 73%, but the positive predictive value was only 35%. The authors suggest that both VOD and mucositis are toxic effects and that patients with hepatic abnormalities without oral mucositis are unlikely to have VOD if these preparatory regimens are used.

PATHOPHYSIOLOGY

Despite the clear association between preparative chemoradiotherapy regimens and VOD, there is little information about how such agents specifically cause VOD. In general, VOD develops in the setting of chemotherapeutic agents that undergo hepatic metabolism,[7] suggesting that the metabolic products may induce vascular injury in the beds at risk—the draining hepatic venous system. Ionizing radiation is thought to provoke VOD via direct microcirculatory damage manifested by endothelial edema and focal coagulation,[4] but it is not known whether edema precedes or results from fibrin deposition.

An understanding of the molecular pathogenesis of VOD associated with bone marrow transplantation has been hampered by the absence of a good animal model. Radiation-induced VOD has not been demonstrated in animals, although thrombotic occlusion of small hepatic vessels has been observed following radiation in dogs.[53] Of interest, in the primate model of VOD induced by injection of monocrotaline, the primary liver circulatory lesions are those of thrombotic occlusion, and platelet deposits are abundant.[54] In humans, available evidence suggests that platelets do not play a primary role in initiating the vascular occlusion of VOD as analyzed histologically

and by immunohistochemical analysis of platelet antigens.[55] Such studies, however, are hampered in that biopsy specimens in humans can be procured only after clinical identification of liver disease; thus, the timing of biopsies may miss the role of platelets in initiating VOD and emphasize instead the process of remodeling and replacement of platelet deposits by fibrin and collagen. Of note, although VOD is manifested during the period of thrombocytopenia after transplantation, its occurrence is associated with higher platelet transfusion requirements.[56] A prospective, randomized trial altering the threshold for platelet transfusions early in the posttransplant period may provide insight, albeit indirect, into the role of platelets in VOD.

As noted above, there is evidence that cytokines are increased after transplantation. The decrease in VOD observed in T-cell depleted transplants may be related to the decreased activation of T-cells and subsequent lower levels of cytokines such as IL-2. Data suggest that TNF-α levels are elevated prior to onset of VOD,[57] and it is known that this cytokine directly damages endothelial cells and acts as a procoagulant through effects on endothelial cells, platelets, and the common pathway of coagulation.[58] Cytokines known to regulate collagen deposition, such as transforming growth factor-β (TGF-β), have also been implicated in VOD. There is evidence that pretransplant levels of plasma TGF-β may predict which patients subsequently develop VOD.[59] TGF-β stimulates hepatocellular collagen synthesis and inhibits expression of collagenase; the net result is an increase in new and perhaps abnormally placed connective tissue.[60] The association between viral hepatitis and VOD may relate to levels of TGF-β; patients with viral hepatitis are known to have increased expression of TGF-β mRNA.[31]

In addition to effects on coagulation and collagen deposition, cytokines may promote the development of VOD through altering the endothelial, leukocyte, and platelet expression of membrane proteins that promote adhesive interactions.[61] Adhesion molecules of the integrin (e.g., LFA-1 and the VLA family), selectin (E-selectin and P-selectin) and immunoglobulin (e.g., ICAM-1) superfamilies have been identified in varying amounts on endothelial cells in various hepatic inflammatory conditions.[62–64] Alterations in expression of adhesion proteins most likely contributes to the cellular aggregation typically seen early in pathologic specimens of hepatic VOD. However, at present, the role of specific adhesion proteins in the pathogenesis of VOD is undefined.

CLINICAL COURSE AND TREATMENT

The course and outcome of VOD following BMT is complicated by development of other posttransplant conditions such as infection and GVHD. It is frequently difficult to decide whether a patient has died because of VOD or with VOD as a contributing factor. The major cause of death in the setting of hepatic failure due to VOD is the development of an hepato-renal-like syndrome with concomitant multi-organ failure; patients with severe VOD rarely die from progressive hepatic insufficiency alone. Data from Seattle indicate that full recovery from VOD is observed in approximately 70% of cases, usually by day 35, and that severe, irreversible VOD is correlated with onset of renal and cardiopulmonary failure within the first 20 days after transplantation.[17] At postmortem evaluation, the renal histology in such patients is usually normal, supporting the notion that renal failure is hemodynamic in nature, as in the hepatorenal syndrome.[65]

In addition to renal insufficiency, liver injury in VOD is associated with pulmonary complications (interstitial pneumonitis), possibly because of common regimen-related toxicity.[36,66] A recent report has suggested that increased lung uptake of [99]Tcm-sulfur colloid was a useful early indicator of development of VOD.[67] Pulmonary VOD, which is a rare complication, has also been reported in patients with both hepatic VOD and interstitial pneumonitis. However, an association between hepatic VOD and pulmonary VOD has not been confirmed.

Although VOD is the most common cause of renal failure in the immediate posttransplant period,[65] acute renal failure requiring dialysis occurs in only 20–25% of cases.[17,65] Renal insufficiency, defined by a doubling of the serum creatinine, occurs in greater than 50% of patients with VOD.[17] The development of renal insufficiency is associated with a doubling of mortality in the posttransplant period; death rates approach 90% in patients requiring dialysis.[65] The renal insufficiency of VOD is characterized by low urine sodium (typical values: $\leq$ 40 mEq/L; values in patients with renal failure: $\leq$ 20 mEq/L), despite aggressive treatment with diuretics.[65] Renal failure is associated with a serum blood urea nitrogen/serum creatinine ratio of $\geq$ 30. Approximately two-thirds of patients with acute renal failure following VOD are nonoliguric; volume overload is the major indication for dialysis.[65] In this regard, the renal failure accompanying hepatic dysfunction in VOD differs from the hepatorenal syndrome of end-stage liver disease, which is typified by oliguria. Although VOD underlies the development of renal failure, another clinical event, usually sepsis, is the final precipitant for renal failure requiring dialysis.[65]

The management of VOD is predominantly supportive (the reader is referred to chapter 3 for a greater discussion of management of renal failure in the hepatorenal syndrome). Primary measures are aimed at maintaining intravascular volume while decreasing third spacing, usually by infusing red cells, as well as albumin. Careful electrolyte balance and fluid management are of critical importance. Encephalopathy may develop and must be managed judiciously, especially in light of the potential of lactulose to precipitate volume depletion with further renal compromise secondary to the hemodynamically unstable, hepatorenal syndromelike state.

Recent Therapeutic Options

The rather dismal outcome of patients requiring hemodialysis for renal failure has precipitated evaluation of aggressive interventions to limit renal decompensation. Such approaches have included surgical relief with portacaval shunts to reduce hepatic pressures and decrease ascites.[68] In our experience, LeVeen peritoneovenous shunts have not been shown to be effective, but the more recent use of a transjugular intrahepatic portosystemic shunting (TIPS) catheter was found to be of benefit in 1 patient at our institution. The patient developed ascites, hyperbilirubinemia, and tender hepatomegaly. Because of a progressive rise in bilirubin and tense ascites, a TIPS catheter was placed, and within 72 hours the patient manifested a marked diuresis (up to 8 L/day) with rapid resolution of hyperbilirubinemia. Finally, although of limited practical application, orthotopic liver transplantation has been performed in some patients.[69]

The use of vasodilators in attenuating the hemodynamic changes in the liver and kidney in VOD have not yet gained investigative interest;

however, evidence suggests that continuous infusion of prostaglandin E₁ may be of benefit in the treatment of established VOD. This agent has both vasodilatory and antithrombotic effects that include activation of thrombolysis and inhibition of platelet activation. One trial[70] reported a striking improvement in all symptoms within 4–7 days of starting therapy, including decreases in both platelet transfusion requirements and total bilirubin.

Another thrombolytic agent of recent interest in the treatment of VOD is recombinant tissue plasminogen activator (TPA). TPA is a serum protease that locally activates the conversion of plasminogen to plasmin with subsequent clot lysis. TPA is frequently used in acute myocardial infarction, pulmonary emboli, and thrombolysis of arterial occlusions. Advantages of TPA over other thrombolytic agents include its short half-life and lack of side effects such as anaphylaxis, which is occasionally seen with streptokinase. The first reported case of successful treatment of severe VOD was a 45-year-old man who underwent autologous BMT for myeloma.[71] The patient received 50 mg of TPA for 3 hours/day for 4 days and had rapid resolution of liver dysfunction, as manifested by reversal of encephalopathy and ascites. A recent trial in 7 patients with severe clinical VOD used TPA at 10 mg/day for 2 days and continuous heparin infusion for 10 days. Four patients showed clinical improvement; 1 patient required discontinuation of heparin after 4 days because of severe bleeding.[72] Such preliminary data suggest that recombinant TPA may be relatively safe in severe VOD. Prospective trials are needed to assess this promising but risky treatment.

PROPHYLAXIS

Because of the poor outcome of established severe VOD, prophylaxis is of fundamental importance. Prophylaxis has focused primarily on strategies to prevent the formation of fibrin deposits. Initial clinical trials using heparin demonstrated variable results.[73–75] Early differences may have been related to patient selection or dose of heparin. The first evidence for a role of heparin in the prophylaxis of VOD was reported by Chan et al.[73] However, Bearman et al.[74] demonstrated that in their selected group of patients, heparin could be given only at low doses so that the partial thromboplastin time did not exceed 1.2 times

normal; otherwise, severe bleeding complications occurred. The authors concluded that 150 units/kg/day was a safe dose. More recently, a large prospective randomized study in 161 BMT recipients[75] demonstrated that continuous infusion of low-dose heparin (100 units/kg/day) resulted in a statistically significant decrease in the incidence of VOD. Seventy-seven of 80 patients received a full course of heparin from the onset of the conditioning regimen to 30 days following transplantation. Only 2.5% of the patients treated with heparin developed VOD compared with 14% of the patients in the control group. An uncontrolled trial from our institution suggests that this dose of heparin is safe and effective for the prevention of VOD. In the past 12 months since this prophylactic dose was instituted in all patients, only 1 case of severe VOD has occurred.

Another agent used for prophylaxis is prostaglandin E₁ (PGE₁). Clearly a major concern in use of PGE₁ is the development of a bleeding diathesis, especially in the setting of post-transplant thrombocytopenia. In one report from Seattle, 18 allogeneic BMT recipients at high risk for VOD were treated in a phase I/II trial.[76] Significant bleeding occurred in 9 patients, who were removed from the study on day 15. Toxicity included bullous skin lesions on edematous extremities as well as postural hypotension. Moreover, cyclosporine levels were higher in patients receiving PGE₁ than in matched historical controls, suggesting a possible drug interaction between PGE₁ and cyclosporine. The study concluded that severe VOD occurred more frequently in patients whose PGE₁ was stopped prior to day 15 than in patients who were able to complete the full course. Alternatively, it may be that PGE₁ was stopped in patients who developed severe VOD compared with patients with no or mild VOD, regardless of the protective effect. Another nonrandomized study of 109 consecutive patients suggested a marked decrease in incidence of VOD in the patients receiving PGE₁ compared with untreated controls.[41] The prophylactic PGE₁ dose was 500 mg/day for adults and 250 mg/day for children. In subset analyses, VOD developed in 62% of patients with prior known liver disease who did not receive PGE₁ compared with only 16% of patients who received PGE₁.

The synthetic bile salt ursodeoxycholic acid has also been utilized in prophylaxis of VOD.

This agent, commonly used in gallstone therapy, a nonhepatotoxic, relatively hydrophilic bile salt. The exact mechanism for the protective effect is unknown but may relate to increased clearance of native, hydrophobic toxic bile salts or to possible immunomodulatory properties.[77] When urso-deoxycholic acid was given prophylactically starting 1 day prior to the conditioning regimen, treated patients appeared to have a lower incidence and mortality rate from VOD then historical controls.[78] Prospective randomized trials are needed to confirm the efficacy of this agent in VOD prophylaxis.

Use of agents to block cytokine actions has attracted a significant amount of interest. Because TNF-α has been implicated as a potential etiologic agent in VOD, efforts have been directed at blocking its effects.[79] The most frequently used drug has been pentoxifylline, a synthetic methylxanthine that decreases production of TNF-α and also blocks its biologic effects. The initial pilot trial suggested that pentoxifylline was highly effective in decreasing the incidence of VOD.[79] Unfortunately, subsequent studies, including a randomized prospective study, failed to show a beneficial effect.[80,81]

SUMMARY

The expanding role of bone marrow transplantation in the treatment of malignancy—both hematologic and nonhematologic—has resulted in progressive increases in the incidence of VOD. Despite renewed scientific interest among marrow transplant specialists, hepatologists, and nephrologists, numerous fundamental questions about the pathophysiology of VOD remain to be answered. For example, the roles of vasoactive substances such as endothelin and nitric oxide have not been evaluated and are important subjects for future inquiry. The present state of knowledge dictates that the management of VOD be essentially supportive, with an emphasis on treating volume overload in the setting of acute renal failure. The current lack of effective treatment underscores the need (1) to identify further the specific risk factors so that they may be avoided and (2) to develop appropriate prophylactic measures. With a greater understanding of the pathophysiologic mechanisms underlying the development of VOD, novel approaches for prevention may evolve that will eliminate this life-threatening complication.

REFERENCES

1. Bras G, Jeliffe DB, Stuart KL: Veno-occlusive disease of the liver with nonportal type of cirrhosis occurring in Jamaica. Arch Pathol 1954;57:285–300.
2. McLean E: The toxic actions of pyrrolizidine (senecio) alkaloids. In Pharmacol Rev 1970;22:429–483.
3. Reed G, Cox AJ: The human liver after radiation injury: a form of veno-occlusive disease. Am J Pathol 1966; 48:597–612.
4. Fajardo L, Colby TV: Pathogenesis of veno-occlusive liver disease after irradiation. Arch Pathol Lab Med 1980;104:584–588.
5. Griner P, Elbadawi A, Packman CH: Veno-occlusive disease of the liver after chemotherapy: A report of two cases. Ann Intern Med 1976;85:578–582.
6. Gill RA, Onstad GR, Cardamone JM, et al: Hepatic veno-occlusive disease caused by 6-thioguanine. Ann Intern Med 1982;96:58–60.
7. Rollins B: Hepatic veno-occlusive disease. Am J Med 1986; 81:297–306.
8. Read AE, Wiesner RH, LaBrecque DR, et al: Hepatic veno-occlusive disease associated with renal transplantation and azathioprine therapy. Ann Intern Med 1986; 104:651–655.
9. Jacobs P, Miller JL, Uys CJ, Dietrich BE: Fatal veno-occlusive disease of the liver after chemotherapy, whole-body irradiation and bone marrow transplantation for refractory acute leukemia. South Afr Med J 1979;55:5–10.
10. Berk P, Popper H, Krueger GRF, et al: Veno-occlusive disease of the liver after allogeneic bone marrow transplantation: Possible association with graft-versus-host disease. Ann Intern Med 1979;90:158–164.
11. Beschorner W, Pino J, Boitnott JK, et al: Pathology of the liver with bone marrow transplantation: Effects of busulfan, carmustine, acute graft-versus-host disease, and cytomegalovirus infection. Am J Pathol 1980;99:369–385.
12. Wood W, Dehner LP, Nesbit ME, et al: Fatal veno-occlusive disease of the liver following high dose chemotherapy, irradiation and bone marrow transplantation. Am J Med 1980;68:285–290
13. Shulman H, McDonald GB, Matthews D, et al: An analysis of hepatic venocclusive disease and centrilobular hepatic degeneration following bone marrow transplantation. Gastroenterology 1980;79:1178–1191.
14. McDonald G, Sharma P, Matthews DE, et al: The clinical course of 53 patients with venocclusive disease of the liver after marrow transplantation. Transplantation 1985; 39:603–608.
15. Jones RJ, Beschorner WE, Lee SKS, et al: Venocclusive disease of the liver following bone marrow transplantation. Transplantation 1987;44:778–783.
16. Shulman HM, Hinterberger W: Hepatic veno-occlusive disease—liver toxicity syndrome after bone marrow transplantation. Bone Marrow Transplant 1992;10:197–214.
17. McDonald GB, Hinds MS, Fisher LD, et al: Veno-occlusive disease of the liver and multiorgan failure after bone marrow transplantation: A cohort study of 355 patients. Ann Intern Med 1993;118:255–267.
18. Blotstein MD, Paltiel OB, Thibault A, Rybka WB: A comparison of clinical criteria for the diagnosis of veno-occlusive disease of the liver after bone marrow transplantation. Bone Marrow Transplant 1992;10:439–443.

19. Shulman HM, McDonald GB: Utility of transvenous liver biopsy and hepatic venous pressure measurements in Seattle marrow transplant recipients. Exp Hematol 1990;18:699.

20. Carreras E, Granena A, Navasa M, et al: On the reliability of clinical criteria for the diagnosis of hepatic veno-occlusive disease. Ann of Hematol 1993;55:77–80.

21. Shulman HM, Hinds M, Schoch HG, McDonald GB: Liver toxicity after marrow transplantation: Correlation between coded autopsy histology and clinical features. Lab Invest 1992;66:586.

22. Kriegshauser JS, Charboneau JW, Letendre L: Hepatic venocclusive disease after bone marrow transplantation: Diagnosis with duplex sonography. Am J Radiol 1988;150:289–290.

23. Brown BP, Abu-Yousel M, Farner R, et al: Doppler sonography: A noninvasive method for evaluation of hepatic venocclusive disease. Am J Radiol 1990;154:721–724.

24. Dohmen K, Harada M, Ishibashi H, et al: Ultrasonographic studies on abdominal complications in patients receiving marrow-ablative chemotherapy and bone marrow or blood stem cell transplantation. J Clin Ultrasound 1991;19:321–333.

25. Herbetko J, Grigg AP, Buckley AR, Phillips GL: Venocclusive liver disease after bone marrow transplantation: Findings at duplex sonography. Am J Roentgenol 1992;158:1001–1005.

26. Eltumi M, Trivedi P, Hobbs J, et al: Monitoring of venoocclusive disease after bone marrow transplantation by serum aminopropeptide of type III procollagen. Lancet 1993;342:518–521.

27. Dulley FL, Kanfer EF, Appelbaum FR, et al: Venocclusive disease of the liver after chemoradiotherapy and autologous bone marrow transplantation. Transplantation 1987;43:870–873.

28. Bearman SI, Anderson LG, Mori M, et al: Venocclusive disease of the liver: Development of a model for predicting fatal outcome after marrow transplantation. J Clin Oncol 1993;11:1729–1736.

29. McDonald GB, Sharma P, Matthews DE, et al: Venocclusive disease of the liver after bone marrow transplantation: Diagnosis, incidence, and predisposing factors. Hepatology 1984;4:116–122.

30. Ganem G, Saint-Marc Girardin MF, Kuentz M, et al: Veno-occlusive disease of the liver after allogeneic bone marrow transplantation in man. Int J Radiat Oncol Biol Phys 1988;14:879–884.

31. Castilla A, Prieto J, Fausto N: Transforming of growth factors β1 and α in chronic liver disease. Effects of Interferon alfa therapy. N Engl J Med 1991;324:933–940.

32. Witherspoon RP, Storb R, Shulman HM, et al: Marrow transplantation in hepatitis-associated aplastic anemia. Am J Hematol 1984;17:269–278.

33. Lucarelli G, Galimberti M, Delfini C, et al: Marrow transplantation for thalassaemia following busulphan and cyclophosphamide. Lancet 1985;i:1355–1357.

34. Frickhofen N, Wiesneth M, Jainta C, et al: Hepatitis C virus infection is a risk factor for liver failure from venoocclusive disease after bone marrow transplantation. Blood 1994;83:1998–2004.

35. Nevill TJ, Barnett MJ, Klingemann H-G, et al: Regimen-related toxicity of a busulfan-cyclophosphamide conditioning regimen in 70 patients undergoing allogeneic bone marrow transplantation. J Clin Oncol 1991;9:1224–1232.

36. Bearman SI, Appelbaum FR, Buckner CD, et al: Regimen-related toxicity in patients undergoing bone marrow transplantation. J Clin Oncol 1988;6:1562–1568.

37. McDonald GB, Hinds M, Fisher L, Schoch HG: Liver toxicity following cytoreductive therapy for marrow transplantation: Risk factors, incidence, and outcome. Hepatology 1991;14:162A (459).

38. Faioni EM, Krachmainicoff A, Bearman SI, et al: Naturally occurring anticoagulants and bone marrow transplantation: Plasma protein C predicts the development of venocclusive disease of the liver. Blood 1993;81:3458–3462.

39. Gordon B, Haire W, Kessinger A, et al: High frequency of antithrombin 3 and protein C deficiency following autologous bone marrow transplantation for lymphoma. Bone Marrow Transplant 1991;8:497–502.

40. Collins PW, O'Driscoll GC, et al: von Willebrand factor as a marker of endothelial cell activation following BMT. Bone Marrow Transplant 1992;10:499–506.

41. Gluckman K, Jolivet I, Scrobohaci ML, et al: Use of prostaglandin E1 for prevention of liver veno-occlusive disease in leukaemic patients treated by allogeneic bone marrow transplantation. Br J Haematol 1990;74:277–281.

42. Radich J, Buckner CD, et al: Second allogeneic bone marrow transplants for patients relapsing after initial transplant with TBI-containing regimens. Blood 1991;78:241A.

43. Mrsic M, Horowitz MM, Atkinson K, et al: Second HLA-identical sibling transplants for leukemia recurrence. Bone Marrow Transplantation 1992;9:269–275.

44. Sloane JP, Farthing MJ, Powles RL: Histopathological changes in the liver after allogeneic bone marrow transplantation. J Clin Pathol 1980;33:344–350.

45. Locasciulli A, Bacigalupo A, Alberti A, et al: Predictability before transplant of hepatic complications following allogeneic bone marrow transplantation. Transplantation 1989;48:68–72.

46. Petersen FB, Buckner CD, Appelbaum FR, et al: Busulfan, cyclophosphamide and fractionated total body irradiation as a preparatory regimen for marrow transplantation in patients with advanced hematological malignancies: A phase I study. Bone Marrow Transplant 1989;4:617–623.

47. Morgan M, Dodds A, Atkinson K, et al: The toxicity of busulfan and cyclophosphamide as the preparative regimen for bone marrow transplantation. Br J Hematol 1991;77:529–534.

48. Essell JH, Thompson JM, Harman GS, et al: Marked increase in veno-occlusive disease of the liver associated with methotrexate use for graft-versus host disease prophylaxis in patients receiving busulfan/cyclophosphamide. Blood 1992;79:2784–2788.

49. Ayash LJ, Hunt M, Antman K, et al: Hepatic veno-occlusive disease in autologous bone marrow transplantation of solid tumors and lymphomas. J Clin Oncol 1990;8:1699–1706.

50. Berk PD, Popper H, Krueger GFR, et al: Veno-occlusive disease of the liver after allogeneic bone marrow transplantation. Ann Intern Med 1979;90:158–164.

51. Soiffer RJ, Dear K, Rabinowe S, et al: Hepatic dysfunction following T cell depleted allogeneic bone marrow transplantation. Transplantation 1991;52:1014–1019.

52. Wingard JR, Niehaus CS, Peterson DE, et al: Oral mucositis after bone marrow transplantation. A marker of treatment toxicity and predictor of hepatic veno-occlusive disease. Oral Surg Oral Med Oral Pathol 1991; 72:419–424.

53. Bicher HI, Dalrymple GV, Ashbrook D, et al: Effect of ionizing radiation on liver microcirculation and oxygenation. Adv Exp Med Biol 1976;75:497–503.

54. Allen JR, Carstens LA, Katagiri GJ: Hepatic veins of monkeys with veno-occlusive disease. Arch Pathol 1969; 87:279–289.

55. Shulman HM, Gown AM, Nugent DJ: Hepatic veno-occlusive disease after bone marrow transplantation: Immunohistochemical identification of the material within occluded central venules. Am J Pathol 1987;127: 549–558.

56. Rio B, Andreu G, Nicod A, et al: Thrombocytopenia in venoocclusive disease after bone marrow transplantation or chemotherapy. Blood 1986;67:1773–1776.

57. Holler E, Kolb HJ, Moller A, et al: Increased serum levels of tumor necrosis factor-α precede major complications of bone marrow transplantation. Blood 1990; 75:1011–1016.

58. van der Poll T, Büller HR, Cate H, et al: Activation of coagulation after administration of tumor necrosis factor to normal subjects. N Engl J Med 1990;322: 1622–627.

59. Anscher MS, Peters WP, Reisenbichler H, et al: Transforming growth factor-beta as a predictor of liver and lung fibrosis after autologous bone marrow transplantation for advanced breast cancer. N Engl J Med 1993; 328:1592–1598.

60. Andrus T, Bauer J, Gerok W: Effects of cytokines on the liver. Hepatology 1991;13:364–375.

61. Springer TA: Traffic signals for lymphocyte recirculation and leukocyte emigration: The multistep paradigm. Cell 1994;76:301–314.

62. Volpes R, Van Den Oord JJ, Desmet VJ: Immunohistochemical study of adhesion molecules in liver inflammation. Hepatology 1990;12:59–65.

63. Scoazec J-Y, Feldmann G: In situ immunophenotyping study of endothelial cells of the human hepatic sinusoid: Results and functional implications. Hepatology 1991; 14:789–797.

64. Volpes R, Van Den Oord JJ, Desmet VJ: Distribution of the VLA family of integrins in normal and pathological human liver tissue. Gastroenterology 1991;101:200–206.

65. Zager RA, O'Quigley J, Zager BK, et al: Acute renal failure following bone marrow transplantation: A retrospective study of 272 patients. Am J Kidney Dis 1989; 13:210–216.

66. Wingard JR, Mellits ED, Jones RD, et al: Association of hepatic veno-occlusive disease with interstitial pneumonitis in bone marrow transplant recipients. Bone Marrow Transplant 1989;4:685–689.

67. Jacobson AF, Teefey SA, Higano CA, Bianco JA: Increased lung uptake of 99Tcm-sulphur colloid as an early indicator of the development of hepatic veno-occlusive disease in bone marrow transplant patients. Nuc Med Comm 1993;14:706–711.

68. Murray JA, La Brecque DR, Gingrich RD, et al: Successful treatment of hepatic venocclusive disease in a bone marrow transplant patient with side-to-side portacaval shunt. Gastroenterology 1987;92:1073–1077.

69. Rapoport AP, Doyle HR, Starzl T, et al: Orthotopic liver transplantation for life-threatening veno-occlusive disease of the liver after allogenic bone marrow transplant. Bone Marrow Transplant 1991;8:421–424.

70. Ibrahim A, Pico JL, Maraninchi D, et al: Hepatic venoocclusive disease following bone marrow transplantation treated by prostaglandin E_1. Bone Marrow Transplant 1991;7(Suppl 2):53.

71. Baglin TP, Harper P, Marcus RE: Veno-occlusive disease of the liver complicating ABM-T successfully treated with recombinant tissue plasminogen activator (rt-PA). Bone Marrow Transplant 1990;5:439–441.

72. Bearman SI, Shuhart MC, Hinds MS, McDonald GB: Recombinant human tissue plasminogen activator for the treatment of established severe hepatic venoocclusive disease of the liver after bone marrow transplantation. Blood 1992;80:2458–2462.

73. Cahn JY, Flesch M, Plouvier E, et al: Venoocclusive disease of the liver and autologous bone marrow transplantation: Preventative role for heparin? Nouv Rev Fr Hematol 1985;27:27–28.

74. Bearman SI, Hind MS, Wolford JL, et al: A pilot study of continuous infusion heparin for the prevention of hepatic veno-occlusive disease after bone marrow transplantation. Bone Marrow Transplant 1990;5:407–411.

75. Attal M, Huguet F, Rubie H, et al: Prevention of hepatic venocclusive disease after bone marrow transplantation by continuous infusion of low-dose heparin: A prospective randomized trial. Blood 1992;79:1–7.

76. Bearman SI, Hinds MS, McDonald GB: Prostaglandin E_1 for the prevention of hepatic venocclusive disease: Results of a phase I study. Exp Hematol 1991;19:567–573.

77. Calmus Y, Gane P, Rouger P, Poupon R: Hepatic expression of class I and class II major histocompatibility complex molecules in primary biliary cirrhosis: Effect of ursodeoxycholic acid. Hepatology 1990;11:321–325.

78. Essell JH, Thompson JM, Harman GS, et al: Pilot trial of prophylactic ursodiol to decrease the incidence of venoocclusive disease of the liver in allogeneic bone marrow transplant patients. Bone Marrow Transplant 1992;10: 367–372.

79. Bianco JA, Appelbaum FR, Nemunitis J, et al: Phase I-II trial of pentoxifylline for the prevention of transplant related toxicities following allogeneic bone marrow transplantation. Blood 1991; 78:1205–1211.

80. Kahls P, Lechner K, Stockschlaeder M, et al: Pentoxyfylline did not prevent transplant-related toxicity in 31 consecutive allogeneic marrow transplant recipients. Blood 1992;80:2683–2686.

81. Clift RA, Bianco JA, Appelbaum FR, et al: A randomized controlled trial of pentoxifylline for the prevention of regimen-related toxicities in patients undergoing allogeneic marrow transplantation. Blood 1993;82:2025–2030.

Chapter 8

PATHOPHYSIOLOGY OF ASCITES FORMATION

MORTIMER LEVY, M.D., F.R.C.P.(C)

Source of Ascites
  Clinical Evidence for Hepatic Source
  Experimental Evidence for Hepatic Source
Factors Contributing to Formation of Ascites
  Hepatic Venous Outflow Block
  Hepatic Sinusoid
  Lymph Flow
  Reabsorption of Fluid from the Peritoneal Space
  Splanchnic Hemodynamics
  Myocardial Function
  Alterations in Hepatic Function: Decreased
    Albumin Synthesis
  Humoral Substances

Pathophysiology of Ascites Formation
  Vascular Overfilling Hypothesis
  Critical Function Threshold Theory
  Peripheral Arteriolar Dilatation Hypothesis
Clinical Studies
**Vascular Overfilling Becomes Vascular
  Underfilling**
Afferent Factors
Efferent Factors
Summary Statement

The term "ascites" is derived from the ancient Greek (denoting a distended bag or balloon) and, as used in current clinical practice, refers to a detectable collection of free fluid within the peritoneal space. It represents one of the most common features of advanced liver disease; in North America, it is most often encountered in association with alcoholic cirrhosis of the liver.

Although ascites may be present in association with numerous syndromes and diseases (Table 8.1), four basic disturbances lead to a significant collection of fluid within the peritoneal space: (1) increased pressure within the hepatic veins, hepatic sinusoids, or portal vein; (2) severe hypoalbuminemia; (3) altered permeability of the peritoneal membranes: and (4) overproduction of transudate, e.g., the ovary undergoing fertility hyperstimulation.[1] Because of the underlying scope of the text, this chapter considers the pathophysiology of ascites formation as it occurs in cirrhosis of the liver. Indeed, though cirrhosis remains the most common cause of ascites, other hepatic disturbances—e.g., severe acute hepatitis, metastatic involvement of the liver—also may cause this disturbance.

The parenchymal disturbances that eventually lead to a cirrhotic liver may occur over many years or even decades. It is therefore quite likely that a complex array of hormonal, neurohormonal, nutritional, hemodynamic and biochemical disturbances may contribute to the accumulation of ascites, and each is likely to vary in intensity throughout the extended period required for the full development of the cirrhotic liver. At any given time, therefore, a wide variety of derangements may influence the usual physiologic factors governing transcapillary (transsinusoidal) fluid exchange and renal handling of salt and water. Examination of the pathophysiology of ascites at a selected interval during what is invariably a long process yields at best only a snapshot view of the complete problem. This has been a major problem in understanding various aspects of the etiology of ascites, because most clinical observations have been made once ascites is present in great amount and at a time when hepatic integrity is markedly compromised.

Despite numerous factors mediating renal retention of sodium in advanced hepatic cirrhosis, it is clear that a set of hemodynamic perturbations preferentially directs fluid out of the hepatosplanchnic circulation and into the peritoneal space as ascites. Although such patients frequently

TABLE 8.1. Some Causes of Ascites

Right-sided heart failure

Obstruction of the supradiaphragmatic inferior vena cava or hepatic veins

Infiltrative disease of the liver (usually fatty) causing raised sinusoidal pressure (e.g., kwashiorkor)

Disturbed intrahepatic architecture (e.g., cirrhosis, metastatic disease)

Extrahepatic portal venous obstruction (especially if associated with hepatic disease)

Nephrotic syndrome or other causes of profound hypoalbuminemia

Tuberculous or malignant seeding of the peritoneal membrane

Hemodialysis associated ascites

Ovarian hyperstimulation syndrome

Myxedema

Pancreatic ascites (chronic pseudocysts)

Systemic lupus erythematosus

Chylous ascites

display edema of the lower extremities, the collection of fluid is usually due to secondary factors, such as increased venous pressure caused by tense ascites on the abdominal vena cava, rather than to a primary disturbance of fluid exchange within this vascular territory. Thus, a unique combination of factors contrives to localize fluid extravasation within the peritoneal compartment.

The volume of fluid found as ascites may be enormous; that is, it may often exceed 20 liters. Since this represents approximately 5–6 times the circulating plasma volume, progressive urinary sodium retention must occur to replenish the vascular space. Thus, some precise temporal relationship between ascites formation, alterations in the magnitude of the plasma volume, and urinary sodium retention must exist as an integral feature of the pathophysiology of ascites formation. Although localized disturbances in Starling forces may preferentially direct fluid into the capacious peritoneal cavity, only minimal amounts of ascites could collect if it were not for coexistent urinary sodium retention. Such retention permits large volumes of ascites to become sequestered until increments in peritoneal fluid pressure or other factors bring this process to an end.

The present chapter considers the factors contributing to the formation and pathophysiology of ascites. Such consideration, of necessity, involves discussion of disturbances in the renal excretion of sodium, neuroendocrine factors influencing such excretion, and temporal relationships among urinary sodium retention, alteration to the magnitude of the circulating plasma volume, and appearance of ascites.

SOURCE OF ASCITES

Ascitic fluid is derived from the vascular compartment subserving the hepatosplanchnic viscera. Considering the anatomy of the peritoneum and the abdominal viscera, ascitic fluid may be derived from the liver, intestinal capillaries, pancreas, or ovary. Realistically, ascites is invariably derived from the first two sources. In alcoholic cirrhosis, the evidence is rather impressive that the largest contribution to ascites is made by the liver rather than the intestinal viscera.[2–6] Although a great number of both experimental and clinical observations support this view, one could arrive at this conclusion on a priori grounds by knowing only two facts: (1) fluid leaves the vascular space only when the usual forces governing transcapillary exchange are disturbed, and (2) extrahepatic portal venous obstruction in both humans[6] and experimental animals[7] uncommonly leads to permanent ascites unless plasma albumin levels become depressed or liver function becomes compromised. Therefore, ascites will not accumulate to a significant degree in cirrhotic patients with portal hypertension unless circumstances favor transudation of fluid from the liver. Because the hepatic sinusoid is almost completely permeable to albumin,[8–10] this exchange vessel is not normally susceptible to variation in plasma colloid osmotic pressure, one of the major components in the Starling forces. Thus, only an increment in sinusoidal hydrostatic pressure predisposes to ascites formation, and the site of such a disturbance must be cephalad to presinusoidal resistances. In fact, in cirrhotic patients ascites usually does not develop without partial obstruction of hepatic venous outflow. Repeated alcoholic insult with frequent bouts of necrosis and inflammation produces scarring and disruption of the vascular and parenchymal architecture. Nodular regeneration eventually develops, and all of these factors increase postsinusoidal resistance, leading to partial hepatic venous outflow block (HVOB). Gradually, over the years, as the patient continues to abuse alcohol, the degree of HVOB increases, resulting eventually in progressive portal venous hypertension with all of its undesirable consequences. Because all of the splanchnic blood must leave this vascular territory through the hepatic veins, the progressive development of HVOB is obviously of great import; the hepatic veins carry approximately 25% of cardiac output back to the right heart.[7] Eventually, collateralization of venous blood flow and augmented lymphatic flow will obviate to some degree the imposed restrictions of HVOB. In simplistic terms, ascites accumulates only when the volume of blood entering the hepatosplanchnic vascular territory exceeds the combined volumes of blood leaving via the hepatic veins and fluid leaving via the large lymphatic channels.

If HVOB is the sine qua non for the advent of ascites, why is the hepatic sinusoid the preferential source of ascites rather than the splanchnic capillary? After all, blood supply to the liver is portal in nature; therefore, the classic response to venous obstruction (venous hypertension, collateral flow, and augmented lymph flow) should occur at two levels: (1) the sinusoid and (2) the splanchnic capillary. The reasons are to be found largely in the nature of the microvasculature in the liver as opposed to the visceral organs.

For teleologic reasons, one might predict that the intestinal microvasculature would autoregulate for capillary pressure rather than nutritional flow, since the intestines must reabsorb and secrete large volumes of fluid per day and absorb all body nutrients except oxygen.[11] Thus, edema of the intestinal wall would present a serious diffusional problem. Accordingly, most experimental studies have concluded that the formation of edema in the intestinal wall in the presence of venous hypertension occurs only with great difficulty.[11–15]

Wallentin[14] reported a study that examined the effect of prolonged elevation of venous outflow on capillary filtration in the intestine of cats. Although such a maneuver initially produced an augmentation in the flow of intestinal lymph, the filtration rate from the intestinal capillaries gradually declined; new isovolumetric states were obtained and edema of the intestinal wall prevented. The intestines were seen to be quite efficient in neutralizing changes in capillary hydrostatic pressure, presumably by permitting an increase in tissue pressure because of the increased volume of interstitial fluid.

Johnson[11] and Johnson and Hanson[12,13] have made similar observations in dogs. When venous pressure was increased in isolated loops of intestine, the increments in pressure were transmitted

back to the capillaries to the extent of only about 60%. This attenuation of the consequences of partial venous outflow block was thought to be due to precapillary vasoconstriction and postcapillary vasodilation, with the latter readjustment apparently playing a predominant role. Perhaps even more significant was the observation that as venous pressure continued to increase, the filtration coefficient across the capillary wall decreased. Such observations therefore support the view that it may be more difficult for edema to form in the intestinal wall because of both altered microvascular hemodynamics and increased tissue pressure.

More recently, Richardson et al[15] investigated permeability characteristics of colonic capillaries in dogs under conditions of venous hypertension. They observed that graded increments in venous outflow pressure resulted in a graded fall in blood flow because of a myogenic response to increased transmural pressure, as previously reported by Johnson[11] for the dog small intestine. Although lymph flow also increased, the ratio of lymph protein content to plasma protein content declined; therefore, the transcapillary oncotic gradient increased. Thus, Richardson et al.[15] concluded that as venous pressure rises, the colonic capillaries restrict the filtration of albumin and other macromolecules, thus permitting the transcapillary oncotic gradient to rise. The authors estimate that by this restriction the colonic capillaries tend to oppose further filtration from the capillaries that otherwise would occur because of the increased venous pressure. This is different from events occurring at the hepatic sinusoid, where in the presence of venous outflow obstruction, hepatic lymph protein increases rather than decreases.[16] If one assumes, according to the work of Johnson and Hanson,[11–13] that only 60% of the increased venous pressure is transmitted back to the capillary bed, the augmented transcapillary oncotic pressure buffers in excess of 50% of the imposed increment in hydrostatic pressure. Thus, for colonic capillaries, as for exchange vessels of the small intestine, a tendency to produce ascitic fluid in response to elevated portal venous pressure would be opposed by at least five separate forces: (1) a progressive fall in the filtration coefficient, (2) an increased lymph flow, (3) an increased transcapillary oncotic gradient, (4) an increment in tissue pressure, and (5) a decrease in arterial inflow. There is also evidence that, at least in the small intestine, as portal venous pressure rises, capillary derecruitment occurs, i.e., there is a fall in surface area of exchange vessels available for the extravasation of ascites.[13]

Another point to consider is the availability of splanchnic blood vessels for fluid formation. It is estimated that perhaps no more than 5% of total splanchnic blood flow is available for transperitoneal solute exchange.[17] If there is a similar restriction for fluid diffusion, the ease of ascites formation derived from the splanchnic capillary might be compromised and represent an additional explanation of why most ascites is apparently derived from the liver. It has been suggested that only capillaries situated near the reflection of mesentery over loops of bowel are involved in solute, and perhaps fluid, exchange.[18]

The behavior of the hepatic sinusoid is markedly different from that of the exchange vessels of the intestines. At least three mechanisms permit fluid to leave the exchange vessels of a given vascular territory: (1) blood flow may increase, thus raising hydrostatic pressure within the vessels; (2) there may be venous outflow block, also increasing hydrostatic pressure; and (3) there may be a marked fall in the plasma oncotic pressure. In the hepatic sinusoid, only increments in hydrostatic pressure caused by HVOB can direct fluid out of the vascular compartments. Lautt[19] has reviewed the unique characteristics of the hepatic microcirculation. In the liver, compared with other organs (e.g., skeletal muscle), the precapillary/postcapillary resistance ratio is very high: 50:1 vs. about 4:1 for muscle. As a result, capillary pressure within muscle is high, i.e., about 20 mmHg, and sinusoidal pressure is low, i.e. about 2 mmHg. Consequently, maximal vasodilation of the muscle lowers the resistance ratio to perhaps 1.5:1, thereby increasing capillary hydrostatic pressure significantly, perhaps by a factor of two. Under appropriate conditions, this alteration in local hemodynamics may produce a great deal of edema. In the liver, on the other hand, maximal vasodilation lowers the presinusoidal/postsinusoidal resistance ratio only to about 30:1, limiting the rise in intrasinusoidal pressure to perhaps 2 mmHg. Consequently, the tendency to increase the formation of hepatic lymph is minimal. Chapter 10 should be consulted for additional information on the role of the hepatic circulation in body fluid homeostasis.

The hepatic sinusoid is extremely permeable to protein; hepatic lymph protein is about 95% of simultaneously measured plasma protein.[16] Consequently, any reduction in plasma albumin results

in rapid equilibrium across the sinusoid, and the transsinusoidal oncotic gradient is virtually nonexistent. Under normal conditions, fluid exchange across the hepatic sinusoid is not much influenced by changing plasma levels of albumin. Consequently, the only available mechanism of influencing the formation of hepatic lymph is an increment in hydrostatic pressure caused by HVOB. In fact, partial obstruction to hepatic venous outflow is the most potent mechanism known for the production of ascites, and the formation of hepatic lymph is exquisitely sensitive to changes in hepatic venous outflow and, hence, sinusoidal pressure.

Liver blood volume is unusually large, accounting for about one-third of the volume of the liver, and together with the prehepatic splanchnic organs the hepatosplanchnic territory contains fully one-third of the total blood volume.[20] Although normally the hepatic component may serve as a mobile blood reservoir or as an effective blood buffer in times of fluid overload, this is less likely to occur in advanced cirrhosis. Hepatic microvascular sphincters are fibrosed and less compliant. Thus increments in portal inflow may have a far greater impact in raising intrahepatic sinusoidal pressure in diseased than in normal liver.[20]

Although hepatic blood volume and pressure may increase at various times during cirrhosis, the liver rarely becomes edematous.[7] The liver is protected by effective lymphatic filtration as sinusoidal pressures rise and by exudation across the liver surface into the capacious peritoneal cavity as regional capacity to remove lymph is exceeded.

In light of theoretical considerations suggesting that the nature of the respective exchange vessels predisposes the hepatic sinusoid to be the major site of ascites, what evidence indicates that this is really so?

Clinical Evidence for Hepatic Source of Ascites

If the splanchnic capillary were the major source of ascitic fluid, one might expect that in the presence of extrahepatic portal obstruction ascites would appear. For the most part, this does not happen.[6] Patients may develop portal hypertension to a degree equivalent to that found in alcoholic cirrhosis and experience its consequences (i.e., esophageal varices), but ascites usually appears only if liver damage or hypoalbuminemia supervenes.[6] Plasma volume is commonly expanded, as one could predict, because portal venous hypertension is associated with an increased holding capacity of the mesenteric venous system. Transient sodium retention must occur to restore the ratio of plasma volume to the new holding capacity of the vascular space if venous return and cardiac output are to be maintained. Some patients may develop ascites, but it is often transient.

In some diseases (e.g., schistosomiasis), the liver injury process is associated with augmented presinusoidal resistance to blood flow, and marked portal venous hypertension develops. Although varices and episodes of bleeding are a problem, ascites usually is not.[10,21] In clinical situations in which obstruction is postsinusoidal or extrahepatic, involving obstruction to hepatic venous outflow (e.g., severe congestive heart failure), ascites is usually quite prominent.

When portacaval fistulas are performed in patients with advanced cirrhosis and ascites, surgeons report that the operative field is constantly moist from effusion of fluid from the hepatic surface, whereas other exposed tissues tend to be dry.[22]

Experimental Evidence for Hepatic Source of Ascites

What laboratory evidence supports the view that the liver is the major source of ascitic fluid?

Several workers, including Freeman[23] and Mallet-Guy et al.,[2] have performed studies in which the liver was repositioned to a supradiaphragmatic position, following which the thoracic inferior vena cava was constricted. Ascitic fluid was formed only in the thoracic cavity. If cellophane bags were placed about the liver lobes, ascitic fluid would collect only in the bags.

With partial or even complete portal venous obstruction in dogs as well as other experimental animals, ascites does not form unless hypoproteinemia also develops. Even so, the ascitic fluid is scant and contains little protein.[21]

Gibson and Smith[24] produced cirrhosis in rats and noted that the weeping of fluid from the liver greatly exceeded that from the intestines. Moreover, as Morris[25] has shown, in response to acute supradiaphragmatic obstruction in dogs, lymph flow from the liver increases markedly, whereas flow from the intestinal lymphatics is much less.

At McGill University we have produced experimental cirrhosis in dogs that had a prior end-to-side portacaval fistula. Thus, although intrahepatic sinusoidal pressure was elevated, intrasplanchnic capillary pressure was normal. Yet ascites still developed within the usual period.[3] The construction of a side-to-side portacaval fistula (hence decompressing the liver) returns augmented thoracic duct lymph flow to normal in dogs with experimental HVOB, whereas an end-to-side fistula does little to reduce such flow.[26]

The marshaling of evidence that the liver is the major source of ascites dos not mean that such fluid is not derived from the intestines. Certainly, some surgeons report that the viscera are wet when the abdomen of a cirrhotic patient is entered surgically.[4] It is likely that ascitic fluid is derived from the splanchnic capillaries more in response to hypoalbuminemia than to portal hypertension. Several lines of evidence support this view. First, patients who develop nephrotic syndrome often have ascites as part of their clinical picture of anasarca. Because the hepatic sinusoid is so permeable to protein, the fall in albumin level is not apt to increase the formation of hepatic lymph. Since congestive heart failure or liver disease is not usually present, there is no driving force to derive ascites from the liver by restricting venous outflow. By exclusion, therefore, it must follow that the ascites is derived from the splanchnic capillaries. This physiololgic deduction is supported by experimental evidence. Morris[25] compared the effects of portal hypertension and saline infusions on hepatic and intestinal lymph flow in dogs. Although the production of HVOB produced a marked increment in hepatic lymph flow and little change in intestinal lymph flow, the rapid infusion of isotonic saline (thereby diluting plasma colloid osmotic pressure) produced rapid and marked changes in intestinal lymph flow but scarcely any change at all in hepatic lymph flow. Most available evidence, therefore, supports the view that, in all likelihood, most of the ascitic fluid is derived from the liver.

FACTORS CONTRIBUTING TO FORMATION OF ASCITES

Hepatic Venous Outflow Block

The peculiarities of the hepatic microcirculation ensure that only an elevated intrasinusoidal hydrostatic pressure, usually brought about by

HVOB, causes fluid to leave the sinusoid in significant amounts and to become hepatic lymph.

Numerous studies confirm the exquisite sensitivity of the rate of formation of hepatic lymph to alterations in hepatic venous outflow pressure.[26-34] Greenway and Lautt[26] reported a study of the effects of increasing hepatic venous pressure on the formation of hepatic lymph in anesthetized cats. The liver was inserted into a plethysmographic device, with the venous and arterial inflow remaining intact. A cannula was placed in the supradiaphragmatic vena cava, and the abdominal inferior vena cava was ligated below the level of the hepatic veins. By raising or lowering the outlet of the hepatic venous cannula, control over hepatic venous pressure could be maintained. After 20 minutes of augmented hepatic venous pressure, hepatic volume increased steadily for at least 4 hours. During this period hepatic blood volume was constant, and fluid with very high protein levels accumulated in the plethysmograph. With obstruction to the hepatic lymphatics the rate of fluid filtration out of the liver was directly proportional to the hepatic venous pressure. When hepatic volume pressure was restored to 0 mm Hg, the filtered fluid was not reabsorbed into the sinusoids. The authors concluded that transsinusoidal flux of fluid was exquisitely dependent on intrasinusoidal hydrostatic pressure and that virtually no protective mechanisms prevented filtration in the face of elevated hepatic venous pressure.

Brauer et al.[27] observed the effects of increased hepatic venous pressure in isolated perfused rat livers. In the face of HVOB, liver volume increased and a transudate similar to plasma in protein concentration appeared continuously on the hepatic surface. Such results contrast with reports about the intestines, in which an increment in venous pressure caused an increased filtration of fluid for no more than 5–8 minutes[12]; factors limiting accumulation of fluid are probably increased tissue pressure and decreased colloid osmotic pressure of the lymph.

An excellent physiologic study of transsinusoidal fluid dynamics in the canine liver during graded obstruction to hepatic venous outflow is pertinent.[30] A sequential, graded increase in hepatic venous pressure produced a stepwise increment in sinusoidal hydrostatic pressure and portal venous pressure. Sinusoidal pressure rose linearly with rising hepatic venous pressure, and, as other investigators have found, increments in

hepatic venous pressure are transmitted back to the sinusoids, undiminished in value. Fluid flux across the sinusoids accelerated quite rapidly; within 3 minutes of a new increment in pressure, lymph flow from the liver had increased and stabilized at a new steady-state level. This rapidity of response is almost certainly a reflection of the marked hydraulic conductance or extreme permeability of hepatic sinusoids.

The authors found that the formation of hepatic lymph was so dependent on increments in sinusoidal or intestinal pressure that lymph flow increased 63% for every millimeter of mercury elevation in interstitial pressure. At an interstitial pressure 4.13 times normal values, lymph flow was found to be 14 times that of control rates. As the authors point out, the physiologic significance of the exquisite sensitivity of lymph flow to changes in sinusoidal pressure is a "safety factor" against marked increments in hepatic interstitial pressure and the eventual formation of hepatic edema.

In the steady state, the amount of flow leaving the sinusoid ($J_v$sin) must be equivalent to Jvout, i.e., the amount of fluid leaving the liver either through the lymphatic channels or percolating across the capsular surface: $J_v\text{sin} = K_f(P_{sin} - P_{int})$ where K_f = sinusoidal filtration coefficient, P_{sin} = hydrostatic pressure within the sinusoid, and P_{int} = hydrostatic pressure within the hepatic interstitium. Assuming that the reflection coefficient for albumin is virtually zero (i.e., sinusoids are maximally permeable to albumin), these relationships mean that $P_{int} = P_{sin} - (J_v\text{out}/K_f)$. Thus, for a given increment in hydrostatic pressure within the sinusoid, a rise in hepatic pressure is minimized by an acceleration of lymph outflow, either into the thoracic duct or into the peritoneal space across the liver capsule.

Granger and Laine[29] pointed out that the liver reacts somewhat differently than most tissues, in which an increase in transcapillary flux of fluid and protein into the interstitium is more or less matched by lymphatic removal. Because the interstitium of the liver has a potential communication with the capacious peritoneal cavity, any retardation of lymph flow may result in the sequestration of fluid within the peritoneal space—a space of potentially enormous capacity (Fig. 8.1.)

The complete transmission of increments in hepatic venous pressure back to the hepatic sinusoids occurs in association with the assumption that the presinusoidal site is the major site of resistance to the flow of portal venous blood. The experimental techniques upon which this finding was based, however, may have been in error because of artifactual resistances from the measuring catheter. Recently however, studies in cats[35] and dogs[30] have demonstrated that presinusoidal portal resistance is low so that sinusoidal hydrostatic pressure approximates that of the portal vein. The pressure drop from portal vein to vena cava appears to occur primarily at a postsinusoidal site in a narrow band of intrahepatic vein. Nevertheless, augmented central venous pressure alters thoracic vena caval pressure and is quickly and completely transmitted to portal veins. Although the site of resistance may have changed conceptually and in reality, it is still an empiric fact that increments in hepatic venous pressure are responsible for increments in sinusoidal filtering pressure, which in turn are responsible for major increments in the formation of hepatic lymph.

Hepatic Sinusoid

The sinusoids are specialized capillaries within the hepatic parenchyma, designed to maximize the rate at which substances are presented to their walls and diffuse into the interstitium. They form an interconnected network of blood channels separated only by the thickness of a single sheet of parenchymal cells. Their perfusion is enormous, and because of their discontinuous lining, there is no effective barrier to exchange. When a marker such as carbon is injected into the circulation, it quickly appears in virtually every sinusoidal channel.[36,37]

Numerous investigators have determined that the hepatic sinusoid is so permeable that hepatic lymph protein content is about 95% of simultaneously measured plasma protein.[10,16,33] A consequence of this marked permeability is that the transsinusoidal oncotic gradient is virtually zero. Therefore, it matters little what happens to plasma albumin, because any change is quickly reflected in hepatic lymph. Consequently, a decline in serum albumin levels, and hence colloid osmotic pressure, is not instrumental in increasing amounts of hepatic lymph. Thus, in cirrhosis fluctuations in serum albumin concentration contribute to the sequestration of ascites at a site other than the hepatic sinusoid, i.e., the splanchnic capillary. Such a statement is correct only if we make two major assumptions: (1) intestinal capillaries do not become significantly more permeable to protein

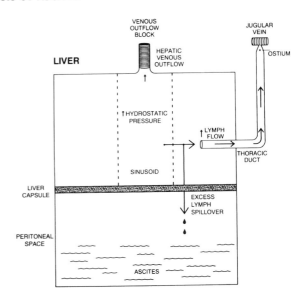

FIGURE 8.1. Partial obstruction to hepatic venous outflow produces raised intrahepatic sinusoidal pressure, which in turn is associated with augmented lymph production. Regional lymphatics carry hepatic lymph into the thoracic duct, where it is eventually returned to the venous compartment. Flow through the thoracic duct is limited because of the presence of an ostium. When lymph flow becomes excessive, it percolates across the hepatic capsule into the peritoneal cavity—a space of enormous potential capacity. Because of the availability of both efficient lymph removal and the peritoneal space as a reservoir in the presence of hepatic venous outflow block, diffusional integrity of the hepatic interstitium is maintained.

as cirrhosis progresses and as they become exposed to higher outflow pressures, and (2) the permeability characteristics of the hepatic sinusoids do not change during the cirrhotic process.

In fact, the second assumption is not true. Schaffner and Popper[38] have pointed out that in advanced cirrhosis a basement membranelike material is laid down about the sinusoids, converting them structurally into capillaries. Thus changes in serum albumin are expressed in changing fluid fluxes at the level of the hepatic sinusoid. Recent physiologic evidence supports this notion. Huet et al.[39] recently reported on multiple indicator dilution techniques carried out in cirrhotic patients. Labeled red blood cells (RBCs) and albumin were injected simultaneously into the portal vein or hepatic artery and outflow dilution patterns were secured from hepatic venous blood. In normal subjects, the space of distribution occupied by albumin exceeds that for RBCs by 60%. In other organs (e.g., the lungs) in which capillaries are not as permeable, the difference between the two markers is only 7%. In cirrhotic patients, the scatter was such that the volume of distribution for albumin ranged from approximately 7% to 60%. Thus, in cirrhotic patients a new diffusion barrier has appeared. Ultrastructural studies showed that in patients with marked liver disease (disturbed indocyanine green extractions) in which the ratio of distribution volumes for albumin and RBCs approximate unity, the microcirculation was characterized by a continuous capillary bed acting as a second barrier between vascular space and hepatocyte.

Early in the disease, therefore, the extreme permeability of the sinusoid does not permit hydraulic expression of a transsinusoidal oncotic gradient. Later in the disease, when liver function is more compromised, the appearance of a diffusion barrier may accelerate the formation of hepatic lymph as plasma albumin levels continue to decline. In fact, whereas in normal humans and dogs thoracic duct or hepatic lymph protein is about 90% that of simultaneously sampled plasma, in cirrhotic humans and dogs this percentage appears to be no longer correct. In patients with alcoholic cirrhosis, direct measurements indicate that in advanced disease, with abundant ascites, the hepatic lymph protein falls to about 50–55% of the plasma level.[8,10,33] In cirrhotic dogs, ascitic protein levels average one-third of plasma values, whereas in dogs with chronic constriction of the thoracic vena cava and ascites, the protein level in the transudate is about 75% of the plasma level. Hence, at some point in the cirrhotic process, depending on structural changes in the hepatic sinusoid, the low plasma albumin level undoubtedly facilitates formation of ascites.

Witte et al.[33] recently provided evidence that in cirrhotic humans longstanding portal venous hypertension does not stretch the pores of splanchnic capillaries and that augmented capillary permeability in the splanchnic bed does not facilitate formation of ascites. Hence, the first assumption appears to be correct.

In some species (e.g., dogs), interstitial hepatic pressure averages 5.8 mmHg, and intrasinusoidal hydrostatic pressure ranges between 5.8 and 7.0 mmHg.[30] Consequently, the transsinusoidal pressure gradient is virtually nonexistent. Because the oncotic gradient between the two sites is also virtually nonexistent, the factor regulating transsinusoidal fluid movement must be hydrostatic, and the protein movement into hepatic lymph must be largely convectional.

In cats, the situation is slightly different: at control hepatic venous pressures, the transsinusoidal oncotic gradient was found to be as high as 8.0 mmHg.[26,28] Moreover, the sinusoids appear to display some degree of selectivity to plasma proteins on the basis of molecular size. The sieving appeared to be consistent with an equivalent pore radius of 180–250 A. As venous pressure of the hepatic outflow increased, the plasma-lymph oncotic gradient tended to disappear as lymph protein concentration increased, and the sieving effect disappeared. Granger et al.[28] found that hepatic lymph flow was linear to increments in hepatic venous pressure and that when the flow rate was approximately 10 times that of the control, the equivalent pore radius of the sinusoid had risen to 1000 A. Since the molecular radius of albumin is approximately 40 A, it was comparatively free of sieving. In fact, Granger et al. calculated the lymph plasma ratio at control lymph flow rates to be about 0.9 for albumin.

Why does sieving disappear with increasing venous pressure? Granger et al.[28] considered a variety of explanations such as "stretched pore" effect; sieving of plasma proteins by the liver capsule; an interstitial matrix that alters diffusion patterns as tissue hydration changes; and contribution from the peribiliary capillary plexus, which also drains into the liver lymphatics. The peribiliary capillaries presumably have a continuous endothelium and exhibit conventional sieving characteristics to plasma proteins. Thus, the apparent protein selectivity of the hepatic sinusoid at normal outflow venous pressures in fact may be due to peribiliary capillaries as venous pressure increases and more and more hepatic lymph is formed; such selectivity would dilute the contribution from the peribiliary capillaries. Because the peribiliary capillaries contribute only 10% of hepatic lymph, such an explanation seems unlikely. Granger et al.[28] favor the likelihood that the hepatic interstitium is the rate-limiting barrier for the transport of proteins from blood and lymph.

Lymph Flow

As intrasinusoidal pressure climbs, the rate of formation of hepatic lymph dramatically increases. This fluid is returned to the vascular space via the regional hepatic lymphatics and thoracic duct. As long as the rate of return keeps up with the rate of formation, there should be no detrimental effect on hemodynamics or renal function, because the rate of combined portal and arterial inflow to the liver will be matched by hepatic venous outflow and lymphatic return. This statement, of course, assumes that the volume of an engorged lymphatic space should not be markedly increased. This volume has been measured in cirrhotic humans with ascites by Lieberman and Reynolds[40] using isotopic techniques and has been found to approximate 75 ml. Moreover, biopsy of the liver in patients with early alcoholic changes does not show edema, but rather fatty infiltration, hydropic degeneration, patchy hyaline necrosis, and early sclerotic and fibrotic changes.[20]

There is, however, an upper limit to the flow that can be carried by the thoracic duct and returned to the circulation. Presumably, this is due to fixed resistance at the thoracic duct ostium. In normal humans, such flows may be 800–1000 ml/day; in cirrhotic humans with ascites, flows of 8–10 L/day are not unusual, and values as high as 20 L/day have been recorded.[8] When the rate of formation of hepatic lymph exceeds the ability of the thoracic duct to return it to circulation, the hepatic lymph percolates into the peritoneal cavity. As Granger and Laine[29] have pointed out, the liver differs from most other organs, in which the transcapillary flux of fluid into the interstitial space is dynamically matched by its removal. In the liver, this simple arrangement does not hold because the hepatic interstitial space communicates directly with the potential space of the peritoneal compartment. Consequently, any tendency for hepatic interstitial pressure is stabilized by permitting fluid to pass through the hepatic capsule into the peritoneal space. In dogs, peritoneal compliance averages 10 ml/kg/mmHg.[29] Translated to a 70-kg human, this means that approximately 700 ml of fluid must accumulate within the peritoneal space to produce a 1-mmHg rise in intraabdominal pressure. Thus, the peritoneal cavity has great potential volume and acts as an important vent to the hepatic interstitium, as clearly demonstrated by experiments reported in rats that were made made cirrhotic with carbon tetrachloride.[41] Infusions of radioactive colloidal material into the portal vein are detected within minutes in the hepatic subcapsular region and traversing into the peritoneal space.

Although the markedly dilated lymphatic channels of experimental animals with cirrhosis of the liver as well as cirrhotic humans attest to the prominent role of this drainage route, there is perhaps no more dramatic demonstration of the role of the lymphatic channels in causing ascitic accumulation than the experiments reported by Farkouh,[42] Dumont and Mulholland,[43] and Zotti et al.[44] in chronic caval dogs. In this experimental model the supradiaphragmatic thoracic inferior vena cava is partially ligated. Because of obstruction to hepatic venous outflow, thoracic duct lymph flow markedly increases and large volumes of ascites form.[9] Because the thoracic duct was anastomosed into either the azygous venous system or esophagus, resistance to flow at the terminal end of the thoracic duct (provided by valves and narrowing) was alleviated. Thus ascites was either relieved or prevented from forming if the duct-vein shunt was performed prior to the caval constriction. Moreover, dogs with the shunt in place were quite capable of excreting an acute intravenous load of normal saline, whereas previously they had been avid salt retainers.[42]

A similar operation has been performed in cirrhotic humans with refractory ascites by anastomosing the thoracic duct to the subclavian[45] or jugular vein. Coodley and Matsumoto[45] also report a beneficial response with mobilization of the ascites. In dogs with experimental portal cirrhosis, Levy and Wexler[3] reported that in the earliest phase of cirrhosis, even before ascites is present, there is already a 300% increment in thoracic duct lymph flow. Dumont[46] presents an excellent review of the physiologic role of the thoracic duct with a fuller discussion on the flow capacity of the duct-venous junction.

Reabsorption of Fluid from the Peritoneal Space

Fluid, once in the peritoneal space, may be reabsorbed into the vascular space by one of two routes: (1) the diaphragmatic lymphatics, which then empty into the right thoracic duct,[47,48] or (2) the splanchnic capillaries. Ascites is not a static compartment, and exchange surely occurs between the vascular space and peritoneal compartment; yet such exchanges are limited. The lymphatic channels may already carry maximal amounts of lymph; the altered Starling forces within the splanchnic circulation make reabsorption of fluid difficult. Shear et al.[49] calculated that no more than 900 ml/day may be reabsorbed through the peritoneal membranes in patients with alcoholic cirrhosis of the liver.

Zink and Greenway[50] examined the factors influencing ascites reabsorption from the peritoneal space in anesthetized cats. They found that the major factor mediating reabsorption was intraperitoneal pressure. In fact, the rate of reabsorption was directly proportional to the intraperitoneal pressure, regardless of whether the ascitic fluid was free of protein or a full transudate. Fluid was reabsorbed with a protein content equivalent to that in peritoneal fluid. Presumably, the proteins are reabsorbed into the diaphragmatic lymphatics. The role of diaphragmatic lymphatics in the formation and reabsorption of ascites has been studied by Raybuck and associates[51] and by Lill et al.,[52] who produced almost total obliteration of peritoneal lymphatic drainage by abrading the peritoneal surface of the diaphragm and applying talcum power to the raw surface. Portal hypertension was produced by subtotal clipping of the portal vein. Portal hypertension alone or lymphatic obstruction alone did not contribute to increased ascites formation. The combination, however, produced modest accumulations of fluid of increased protein content. Thus, the subdiaphragmatic lymphatic plexus potentially plays an important role in the causation of ascites and undoubtedly has a major role in returning ascitic protein to the circulation.

What happens to diaphragmatic lymphatics in patients with chronic cirrhosis? The answer is not known with certainty, although hepatic capsular changes have been described by Tanikawa.[41] Certainly, in chronic caval dogs, marked changes have been described in capsular permeability. Waugh[53] demonstrated that after the disappearance of ascites, marked permeability changes occur in the capsule. In one dog studied 2.5 years after the initial caval ligation, ascites was no longer present despite an abdominal caval pressure $4\frac{1}{2}$ times greater than normal and an elevated portal venous pressure. To assess the permeability of the capsule, the liver was isolated in vitro and perfused with saline. No fluid escaped from the capsule, whereas saline transuded at a brisk rate from a similarly prepared normal liver. The capsule was observed to be quite fibrotic in chronic caval dogs.

Fibrotic changes also occur in the peritoneum of decompensated cirrhotics. Buhac and Jarmolych[54] studied postmortem samples of visceral peritoneum in 16 controls and 15 patients with terminal cirrhosis and ascites. The visceral peritoneum was at least 6 times thicker than normal and contained an increased number of blood vessels (which were quite dilated); lymphangiectasia was marked. The authors postulated that perhaps increased splanchnic blood flow contributes to cirrhotic ascites. Alternatively, the thickened peritoneal membrane may retard the transperitoneal movement of ascitic fluid into the vascular space. Thus, the accumulation and sequestration of ascitic fluid within the peritoneal compartment is a highly dynamic process with both formative and reabsorptive components. The studies of Raybuck et al.[51] demonstrate that interference with either component alone is not sufficient to result in the formation of ascites; interference with both components, however, is sufficient to produce detectable volumes of fluid within the peritoneal space.

Recently, Henriksen and colleagues[55–57] investigated the factors responsible for protein absorption from the ascitic compartment in humans with advanced cirrhosis of the liver. They found that filtration was the dominant transport mechanism of peritoneal protein exchange both in the influx and reabsorptive directions. Moreover, reabsorption into the vascular space appeared to be convective rather than diffusive. The usual pressure gradient from peritoneal cavity to right atrium is in accordance with convective transport. Such transport was thought to occur across the diaphragmatic lymphatics.

Splanchnic Hemodynamics

Alterations in splanchnic hemodynamics may influence the formation of ascites in several ways:

1. The increment in hepatic or splanchnic blood flow or both may be marked as the cirrhotic process advances. Because the microvasculature of the liver and intestines is faced with increasing hydrostatic pressure and decreasing plasma colloid osmotic pressure, an increased delivery of blood should result (assuming no change in the effective area of the exchange vessels) in augmented formation of lymph. When the flow of lymph becomes sufficiently exuberant, ascites forms—a manifestation of an expanded splanchnic lymph compartment. Because of progressive fibrotic changes within the cirrhotic liver, it is less able to buffer an increment in incoming portal blood flow, and augmented splanchnic inflow may well imply augmented hepatic sinusoidal

pressure, with a subsequent increased tendency to form lymphatic fluid.

2. The extensive development of portosystemic venous collaterals may influence urinary sodium excretion if splanchnic blood flow is markedly increased or the venovenous shunting of blood somehow (presumably by nervous reflex) directly influences the renal tubular handling of sodium. The second possibility has been investigated experimentally, and no evidence for such a phenomenon has been found.[3] One could not expect venovenous shunting to underfill the arterial circulation since portal blood has already passed through an extensive capillary bed. Although shunting of portal blood has been implicated in the renal retention of sodium by shunting humoral substances away from possible degradation by the liver, this mechanism does not seem likely. Patients with severe cirrhosis and refractory ascites often develop a marked natriuresis when treated with a portacaval shunt operation or a LeVeen peritoneovenous valve, despite the fact that intestinal blood continues to be shunted away from the liver[58-60] (see chapter 24). Dogs with experimental portal cirrhosis also exhibit a profound natriuresis after placement of a LeVeen valve.

3. The development of arteriovenous shunts within the splanchnic circulation may produce profound urinary sodium retention that aggravates the formation of ascites. The direct passage of arterial blood into the portal vein, for example, may profoundly raise portal venous pressure, which in turn may act as a potent stimulus to expand the splanchnic lymph compartment, of which the ascitic pool is but a subcompartment. Experimentally an aortoportal fistula in dogs is associated with marked edema of the bowel and formation of ascites.[61]

The question of splanchnic arterial inflow has received some consideration. On a priori grounds, one might anticipate that in the presence of portal hypertension, splanchnic and especially hepatic blood flow would be reduced. This is generally the case.[62] At best, it may be appropriate; after all, portal venous hypertension implies resistance to flow.

Some authors have argued that some degree of portal hypertension in human cirrhosis is due to fistulas between the hepatic artery and portal vein.[6,63] Certainly postmortem perfusion and corrosive casts have demonstrated a relative increment in hepatic artery mass,[62] and abnormal communications may be seen between the smaller

ramifications of the hepatic artery and portal vein.[6,62,64] The question arises, however, whether such channels are primary or secondary (i.e., a compensatory reaction to the inevitable reductions in portal venous inflow).

Lacroix and Leusen[65] reviewed the problem of hepatic hemodynamics in patients with alcoholic cirrhosis. Most studies show normal or reduced liver blood flow. As Reynolds[6] pointed out, most studies in cirrhotic humans have been performed with bromosulfophthalein; if liver extraction of this agent is poor, as it is in advanced liver disease, elevated values for blood flow will be artifactual.

Cohn and associates[66,67] studied the changes in hepatic and splanchnic blood flow in some detail. They used methods to measure blood flow that were independent of liver function, because in patients with disturbed liver function the classic extraction techniques become inaccurate. They injected a bolus of ^{131}I-serum albumin into the common hepatic artery while hepatic venous blood was continuously withdrawn. The resulting indicator dilution curve provided an accurate measurement of blood flow. In patients with chronic liver disease, the blood flow, although highly variable, was usually reduced.

Alterations in the mesenteric vessels are more complex and even more variable. Some patients with chronic alcoholic liver disease appear to have increased splanchnic inflow, whereas others appear to have reduced perfusion. These observations were based on the appearance and transit times of a radioactive marker through the splanchnic circulation following injections into the superior mesenteric artery.[67] Because HVOB produces portal hypertension by an obstruction to venous outflow, the splanchnic venous system is distended and engorged. An unchanged arterial inflow into such a system would result in a decreased transit time for the marker. However, many patients with cirrhosis and ascites have been found to have increased transit times, not only through the hepatic vasculature but also through the splanchnic vasculature. If the portal and mesenteric venous volume expands in the presence of portal venous hypertension, the rapid transit times must mean an augmented splanchnic blood flow, at least in some patients. It has been demonstrated previously that some patients with portal hypertension and splenomegaly may have augmented splenic flow rates.[62] Thus, it is possible that in some patients with advanced cirrhosis of the liver, particularly those with a hyperdynamic circulation, an increased flow of blood into a vascular territory where the venous resistance is already high may predispose to the formation of increased amounts of lymph and, hence, ascitic fluid.

Recently, Lebrec et al.[66] compared cirrhotic patients with portal hypertension and easily mobilized ascites with a group of cirrhotic patients with equivalent portal hypertension and refractory ascites. Total hepatic blood flow was comparable in both groups, as were postsinusoidal resistance and portal venous pressure. Significant differences were found in cardiac output (6.3 L/min in 8 patients with refractory ascites, 8.0 L/min in 25 patients with responsive ascites); the degree of portosystemic shunting (35% from superior mesenteric artery in patients with refractory ascites, 75% for responsive patients); and peripheral vascular resistance (1146 dyn/sec/cm^{-5} for refractory patients and 842 dyn/sec/cm^{-5} for responsive patients). Arterial blood pressure was comparable in both groups, as were liver function (as assessed by common methods) and serum albumin level.

Thus, a lower cardiac output and less portosystemic shunting characterized the group with refractory ascites. If less of the splanchnic arterial inflow were shunted off, there would be a greater tendency to increase portal venous pressure—a tendency that would be halted by the aggressive formation of ascites. Thus, venous pressure would be limited at the expense of expanding the ascitic compartment. The reduction in cardiac output in such patients would indicate underfilling of the arterial circuit (which explains the elevated peripheral vascular resistance) and provide an additional signal for urinary sodium retention. Although the causes for reduced shunting in cirrhotic patients with refractory ascites were not clear, Lebrec et al.[66] cite two reasons: (1) increased resistance to flow within the collateral vessels and (2) degree of HVOB. Although the differences were not significant for postsinusoidal resistance between the two groups, the value for refractory patients tended to be higher. For these two reasons, there is a greater tendency to form lymph. Because lymph flow is already maximal in cirrhotic patients with ascites, more ascites tends to form.

Experiments in dogs with an aortoportal vein fistula support the above observations.[61] When the portal vein is constricted, portal pressure remains low over the long term, in part because of collateral formation, increments in lymph flow and ascites do not result. When portal venous pressure is extremely elevated, as with direct connection to the aorta, portal pressure rises and ascites forms easily.

The variability of clinical data about splanchnic arterial inflow in cirrhotic humans is also found in animal models. We have found that although portal blood flow and hepatic arterial flow do not change in dogs with dimethylnitrosamine-induced portal cirrhosis, the volume of blood delivered to nonhepatic areas increased by 18.6% as dogs progressed to advanced cirrhosis.[68] This finding was associated with portal systemic venous shunting of 28% (normal: 5%).

In dogs with chronic biliary obstruction and cirrhosis, Bosch et al.[69] showed extensive portosystemic venous shunting of blood (49%) but a decrease in portal venous flow. Hepatic arterial flow did not change.

In the rat portal-hypertensive model, Vorobioff et al.[70] recently demonstrated that chronic portal hypertension (without liver disease) created by partially stenosing the portal vein is associated with a 50% decrease in splanchnic arteriolar resistance and a 56% increment in intestinal blood flow. Hepatic arterial flow doubled. Such hyperdynamic changes were associated with high-grade portosystemic venous shunting (96.2%), and total hepatic blood flow was actually decreased by 50%. Of interest was the observation that this model also mimicked the changes in systemic hemodynamics usually observed in advanced cirrhosis. Cardiac output significantly increased, and mean arterial blood pressure and peripheral vascular resistance decreased. The results appear to indicate that hyperdynamic splanchnic inflow rather than portal resistance is the major impetus for maintaining portal venous hypertension. As noted above, whether this factor is a major event in cirrhotic humans is unclear. Other factors that need to be explored are whether humoral substances (e.g., glucagon) or reduced resistance to circulating catecholamines plays a role in the putative splanchnic hyperemia of cirrhosis.

Nonetheless, a consensus is developing from both experimental and clinical studies[71–74] that a widespread decrease in peripheral arteriolar resistance is responsible for the hyperdynamic circulation often seen in advanced cirrhosis; in particular, splanchnic vasodilatation and an increment in splanchnic arterial inflow contribute significantly to portal hypertension. Even the kidney in well-compensated cirrhotic patients (without ascites) shows evidence of reduced microvascular flow resistance in one recent study.[74]

The recent awareness of the role of the nitric oxide system in controlling the circulation has prompted studies in experimental models of cirrhosis. Pizareta et al.[75] recently adduced evidence that in rats with experimental CCl_4 cirrhosis local formation of excessive NO may contribute to excessive splanchnic arterial inflow (and hence portal venous hypertension) as well as altered hemodynamics in other regional vascular beds.

In a recent thorough review, Benoit and Granger[76] conclude that although augmented splanchnic inflow may occur in cirrhotic patients, by far the most important component for the determination of increased portal venous pressure remains portal vascular resistance. HVOB probably remains the single most important determinant for the accumulation of ascites.

Myocardial Function

When cirrhotic patients become badly decompensated with large collections of ascites or develop functional renal failure, the performance of the left ventricle is often reduced. If advanced cirrhosis is associated with multiple arteriovenous fistulas, as many believe,[62] why cannot cardiac output increase sufficiently to maintain a normal arterial pressure in the face of a markedly reduced peripheral vascular resistance? Although there are several explanations, the reason appropriate to discussion of ascites formation relates to the actual function of the myocardium. Because cardiac output is often increased in cirrhotic patients, it is commonly assumed that the myocardium functions normally. However, Cohn and associates[66] demonstrated that this may not be true in alcoholic patients. If angiotensin is infused intravenously, peripheral vascular resistance is increased, and at this new level pulmonary wedge pressure tends to become quite elevated. Thus, although the left ventricle appears to function normally when the patient is relatively vasodilated, increasing the vascular resistance may precipitate heart failure. If heart failure is a common phenomenon when the afterload rises to normal values, it may be an added factor in the development of ascites.

Depression of myocardial function may also be a factor in the arterial hypotension so often observed in patients with advanced cirrhosis. Alcoholic cardiomyopathy, malnutrition, and various electrolyte abnormalities (Ca^{++}; Mg^{++}, PO_4, K^+) may interfere with ventricular performance and aggravate portal venous hypertension, in turn aggravating the tendencies to form ascites. Gould et al.[77] performed cardiac catheterization studies in cirrhotic patients with a presystolic gallop rhythm. Exercising increased left ventricular end-diastolic pressure in all 10 patients from an average of 6 to 19 mmHg. Pulmonary artery pressure also increased. Therefore, without the reduced afterload usually observed in patients with advanced cirrhosis and ascites, congestive heart failure and its subsequent consequences might easily be a major problem in the cirrhotic patient.

Alterations in Hepatic Function: Decreased Albumin Synthesis

The major changes that accompany progressive decline of liver function, at least as far as formation of ascites is concerned, are a decrease in the synthesis of albumin and a change in the way various humoral substances are metabolized.

The normal liver may synthesize 11–15 gm of albumin daily, but only 20–40% of that amount is synthesized in patients with advanced cirrhosis and hypoalbuminemia.[7] The serum levels may be further decreased as progressive urinary salt and water retention dilutes the colloid component of the extracellular fluid space, and a significant proportion of circulating albumin is sequestered within the ascitic fluid. What role does the declining level of serum albumin play in the formation of ascites? Theoretically, in the earlier stages of cirrhosis, declining levels of albumin should not contribute much to the formation of ascites, because the liver contributes the largest and perhaps the only source of fluid.[8] In addition to the experimental evidence, the protein content of thoracic duct lymph and ascitic fluid tends to be higher earlier in the course of ascites, signifying an hepatic source.[8] As time passes, the protein content tends to fall, in part because of dilution with protein-poor intestinal lymph and in part, perhaps, because of the phenomenon of sinusoidal capillarization, originally described by Schaffner and Popper.[38]

Although undoubtedly the advent of hypoalbuminemia, which complicates preexistent portal venous hypertension, predisposes to ascites

TABLE 8.2. Humoral Factors Thought to Contribute to Salt Retention in Cirrhotic Patients

Direct tubular effect
    Aldosterone; angiotensin II
    Catecholamines
    Estrogens
    Undetermined antinatriuretic agents (? from the liver)
    Resistance to atrial natriuretic peptide
    Reduced intrarenal secretion of urodilatin (?)

Mediated by renal ischemia or other vasoactive actions
    Angiotensin II
    Catecholamines
    Endothelin (?)
    Endotoxin (reabsorbed from the gastrointestinal tract)
    Deficient intrarenal kinins
    Deficient intrarenal vasodilator prostaglandins
    Increased thromboxane synthesis
    Vasoactive intestinal polypeptide (?)

formation, in certain clinical circumstances, such as severe congestive heart failure or Budd-Chiari syndrome, ascites develops in the absence of hypoalbuminemia. By the same token, hypoalbuminemia, if severe enough (as in severe nephrotic syndrome), predisposes to ascites formation in the absence of portal venous hypertension. It appears, therefore, that although hypoalbuminemia and intrahepatic hypertension may potentiate each other with regard to ascites formation, intrahepatic hypertension, at least in the earlier part of the disease, is predominant. As the cirrhotic process advances within the liver, progressive hypoalbuminemia probably becomes a more significant factor for the splanchnic contribution to ascites. Such observations aside, some workers have found correlations between the presence of ascites and hypoalbuminemia; others have not.[78] Moreover, intravenous infusions of hyperoncotic albumin usually no influence on ascites mobilization in cirrhotic patients, although plasma levels of albumin may rise.[79] Even if albumin is injected directly into the ascitic compartment, no increase in ascites formation takes place. Thus, despite the pivotal role of albumin in Starling's formulation of transcapillary fluid exchange, other forces clearly play a role in the determination of fluid formation; the level of albumin is no more than contributory.

Humoral Substances

Various hormones and humoral substances have been implicated in the pathophysiology of ascites formation. Rather than contributing to the mechanical sequestration of ascites within the peritoneal space, they are probably important in influencing or modulating renal tubular sodium handling (see chapters 12–18). Table 8.2 summarizes the more important humoral factors thought to contribute to urinary sodium retention in cirrhosis of the liver.

PATHOPHYSIOLOGY OF ASCITES FORMATION

The preceding section reviewed the mechanics of how ascites is formed and the factors contributing to its sequestration within the peritoneal space. As already indicated, if the only pathologic process in cirrhotic patients was derangement of Starling forces in the portal circulation, only minimal, clinically insignificant volumes of ascites would accumulate. It is the progressive replenishment of vascular space by retained salt and water that permits the continuous formation of ascites. Therefore, there must be some distinct temporal relationship between formation of ascites and onset of urinary sodium retention.

According to current textbooks, the relationship between ascites formation and urinary sodium retention should present no dilemma. The advent of portal venous hypertension and hypoalbuminemia increases the egress of fluid from hepatic sinusoids and splanchnic capillaries, leading to accumulation of ascites. This loss of fluid from the circulating plasma volume leads to a contraction of the vascular space, which in turn signals the renal tubule to retain salt and water. In such conventional terms, urinary sodium retention is secondary to formation of ascites and subsequent volume contraction, i.e., vascular underfilling.

Almost two decades ago Lieberman, Reynolds, and their colleagues[40,80,81] suggested on the basis of observations in patients with alcoholic cirrhosis of the liver that perhaps ascites forms because of vascular "overfilling." They noted that in alcoholic patients with cirrhosis and ascites (1) plasma volume was invariably expanded, (2) compensated patients who were given large doses of salt-retaining hormone began to sequester ascites, (3) paracentesis was not accompanied by reformation of ascites in a 4-hour period of observation, and (4) the nonsplanchnic plasma volume does not contract during formation of ascites. They suggested that advancing hepatic cirrhosis is associated with a salt-retaining signal to the renal tubule. As more and more salt and water are retained and plasma volume expands, the eventual encounter between abnormal Starling forces and an expanded plasma volume produces an accumulation of ascites. Thus, in their theory, ascites is secondary to urinary sodium retention, i.e., vascular overfilling.

Figure 8.2 summarizes the sequence of events in the hypotheses of underfilling and overfilling. In the traditional underfilling schema relating urinary sodium retention to ascites formation, the link between ascites accumulation and urinary sodium retention is contraction of the non-splanchnic component of the plasma volume. The overfilling hypothesis, as originally put forward,[80] included a component of urinary sodium retention required to replenish the blood that had become sequestered within the expanding mesenteric venous compartment, but the major component was thought to be a direct sodium-retaining signal to the renal tubule, nature unknown. The subsequent expansion of the plasma volume led to the formation of ascites because of the marked disturbance of Starling forces in the hepatoportal vascular territory. Once ascites began to form, plasma volume, whatever its previous value, must contract (Fig. 8.2), because widespread edema implies relative failure of the regional lymphatic vessels and fluid must leave the vascular compartment faster than it can reenter.

Thus, once ascites has formed, the pathophysiologic factors leading to urinary sodium retention are probably identical, no matter which theory is correct. An appropriate and complete description of the events relating sodium retention, magnitude of the plasma volume, and ascites formation, therefore, cannot be given in the presence of ascites; one must also study patients in the preascitic phase of the disease. In fact, this chapter argues that the causes of sodium retention in the presence of ascites are due largely to relative plasma volume contraction—i.e. ,vascular underfilling—and that these causes may be quite different than those in the preascitic phase of the disease. Table 8.3 summarizes some of these factors and when they are operative.

Most of the controversy in this area centers on the correct explanation of the factors that initiate urinary sodium retention in the preascitic phase of cirrhosis. There are at least three distinct theories: (1) vascular overfilling; (2) the hepatic functional threshold theory; and (3) vascular underfilling, caused in large part by peripheral arteriolar vasodilation.

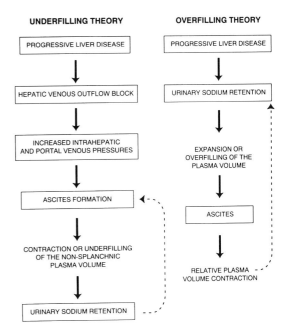

FIGURE 8.2. The temporal relationships among urinary sodium retention, changes in plasma volume, and ascites formation in both the underfilling and overfilling theories.

Vascular Overfilling Hypothesis*

The central tenet of the vascular overfilling hypothesis, as originally put forward by Leiberman, Reynolds, and colleagues, was that as chronic cirrhosis progresses, a sodium-retaining signal (nature unknown) to the renal tubule causes expansion of plasma volume. The encounter between the expanded plasma volume and the progressively abnormal Starling forces within the hepatoportal venous territory causes ascites to overflow. The original hypothesis has been refined by the present author in several ways as a result of studies in dogs with the experimental equivalent of human alcoholic cirrhosis. Initially, experiments were carried out in a canine model of portal cirrhosis, originally described by

---

* The author prefers the term "overfilling" to describe the theory that prior urinary sodium retention expands the plasma volume and that as an overexpanded circulating plasma volume is acted on by progressively disturbed Starling forces within the hepatoportal circuit, ascites forms. Some authors use the term "overflow hypothesis." However, because edema is always associated with the overflow of fluid from the vascular to the extravascular space, this term appears to be less helpful.

TABLE 8.3. Factors Causing Urinary Sodium Retention in Progressive Hepatic Cirrhosis

Operative through depletion of arterial blood volume
  Sequestration of blood in the portal venous system and
    portosystemic collaterals
  Formation of ascites
  Sequestration of blood in lower extremities
  Enlarged lymphatic dead space
  Hypoalbuminemia
  Bleeding from varices and other gastrointestinal sites
  Arteriolar dilatation
  Increasing capillary permeability to albumin associated
    with altered compliance of the interstitial space
  Reduction in ventricular preload (tense ascites)
  Reduced ventricular contractility
  Postural considerations
  Loss of muscle mass with corresponding depot of inter-
    stitial fluid available for vascular replenishment

Factors operative directly on renal tubule
  Increased efferent sympathetic nervous activity
  Low pressure intrahepatic baroreceptors with hepatorenal
    integration
  Decreased renal perfusion pressure
  Altered circadian rhythm for renal sodium handling
  Altered hepatic degradative and/or synthetic abilities
    influencing circulating humoral factors (e.g., estrogens
    or estrogenlike factors)
  Increased secretion of catecholamines, angiotensin,
    aldosterone, arginine vasopressin, endothelin
  Tubular insensitivity to atrial natriuretic peptide
  Alteration in intrarenal profile of autocoids (e.g., kinins,
    prostaglandins)

Madden et al.,[82] using dimethylnitrosamine as the initiating agent. Hepatic cirrhosis is produced over a 2-month period by sporadically feeding the hepatotoxin. The pathologic picture is exactly that of portal cirrhosis, and the dogs display clinical and biochemical features commonly found in patients with alcoholic cirrhosis (Table 8.4). The dogs usually remain in good health for a total of 4–5 months, after which they succumb to the cirrhotic process, usually by gastrointestinal bleeding. Later experiments were carried out in dogs with chronic biliary cirrhosis produced by chronic ligation of the common bile duct. Although the

TABLE 8.4. Features Observed in Dogs with Experimental Hepatic Cirrhosis

Jaundice
Disturbed liver function tests, including hypoalbuminemia
Muscle wasting
Ascites
Portal venous hypertension
Portasystemic venous collaterals
Hepatic encephalopathy
Gastrointestinal bleeding

histologic picture is that of biliary cirrhosis, a postsinusoidal obstructive process is also involved; the dogs exhibit the same symptoms and features as dogs with dimethylnitrosamine-induced cirrhosis. There are only two apparent differences: (1) the dogs may take 2–4 weeks longer to produce ascites, and (2) they appear to be more susceptible to anesthetic. Physiologically, however, they appear equivalent to the dogs with portal cirrhosis. Such approaches permit one to study various features of the cirrhotic dogs with great precision as they evolve from normal animals to animals with terminal illness. One may also date the onset of ascites with great precision. It is fairly easy to introduce experimental manipulations and to make predictions that can then be tested (Table 8.5).

If the dogs are fed a control diet with a fixed amount of sodium and housed in metabolic balance cages that facilitate the collection of urine, serial observations permit an estimate of the temporal relationships between formation of ascites and urinary retention of sodium. Figure 8.3 summarizes such data in a large group of experimental animals. During the control period of observation, the dogs were clearly in sodium balance. Sodium retention started some 15–16 days after the onset of cirrhosis, and ascites appeared about 10 days later. When plasma volume was measured 3 or 4 days after onset of sodium retention, there had been a significant increment compared with control values. Despite ongoing urinary sodium retention and plasma volume expansion, no ascites was detectable on careful abdominal examination. To ensure the validity of this important observation, 6 dogs were subjected to laparotomy when they were in positive sodium balance but had no detectable ascites. Visual inspection confirmed the absence of ascites. Additional sodium retention and plasma volume expansion were associated with formation of ascites about 10 days after onset of sodium retention.

Such data demonstrate clearly that sodium retention and plasma volume expansion preceded the formation of ascites. This relationship also was examined in another way. Five sodium-retaining dogs (balance studies) without ascites were placed on a high sodium diet (160 mEq/day). Within 2–3 days plasma volume had increased by 64 ml in association with marked ascites accumulation (2.0 ± 0.1 L). About 40% of the ascitic fluid was then removed by paracentesis, and the animals were returned to their cages for 24 hours

TABLE 8.5.   Predictions of Underfilling and Overfilling Theories

Feature	Traditional Underfilling Theory	Overfilling Theory
Urinary sodium retention	Secondary to ascites formation	Precedes ascites formation
Plasma volume expansion	None	Expansion that precedes ascites formation
Nonportal component of volume plasma	Contracted	Expanded
Ascites formation	Occurs concurrently with volume contraction	Occurs with volume expansion
Events following paracentesis	Ascites reforms	No reformation unless oral salt prescribed
Events following ascites mobilization with peritoneovenous valve	Urinary sodium excretion normal	Sodium excretion abnormal: retention with high salt intake
Urinary sodium excretion in face of end-to-side portacaval anastomosis (PCA)	Improvement in sodium excretion	Sodium retention remains
Urinary sodium excretion in face of side-to-side PCA	Urinary sodium excretion normal	Sodium excretion normal

without access to sodium. Twenty-four hours after paracentesis, plasma and ascitic volume, plasma albumin, and portal venous pressure remained unchanged. Following an increase in dietary sodium, plasma volume expanded by an additional 7% expansion ($p < 0.05$) with a marked increment in ascites within 2 days. Thus, despite the persistence of hemodynamic forces favoring the transudation of fluid out of the splanchnic capillaries, ascites did not reform until plasma volume was allowed to expand from its previous level. Such data are similar to those reported by Lieberman et al.[81] for patients with alcoholic cirrhosis. Thus, the first set of experimental data appeared to support the overfilling thesis for formation of ascites and firmly established that the appearance of ascites was preceded by urinary sodium retention. Similar results have been

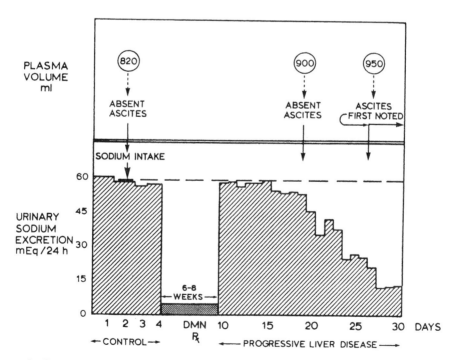

FIGURE 8.3.   Sodium balance in 8 dogs with experimental portal cirrhosis due to the oral administration of dimethylnitrosamine (DMN). The circled numbers are the values for plasma volume. Sodium intake was fixed at 60 mEq/day. Note that urinary sodium retention and plasma volume expansion precede the appearance of ascites. (From Levy M: Pathophysiology of ascites formation. In Epstein M (ed): The Kidney in Liver Disease, 3rd ed., 1988, with permission.)

reported in rats made cirrhotic with carbon tetrachloride and phenobarbital treatment by Lopez-Novoa et al.[83] Although ascites was not detected until the seventh week after initiation of treatment, positive sodium balance was observed from the fifth week onward. Moreover, in ascitic rats subjected to paracentesis and simultaneously placed on a very low sodium diet (35 µEq/day), there was no reformation of ascites for as many as 209 days of observation. Rats receiving greater salt intakes (600–1200 µEq/day) showed reformation of ascites within 2 days after paracentesis.

To establish that the antecedent sodium retention was not due entirely to volume contraction engendered by progressive engorgement of the mesenteric venous system and the spleen and extensive portosystemic collateral channels, similar balance studies were conducted on dogs with an end-to-side portacaval fistula (see below).

Status of Nonsplanchnic Plasma Volume

One of the predictions of both the underfilling and overfilling theories (see Table 8.5) relates to the status of the nonsplanchnic plasma volume during formation of ascites. In a series of experiments,

cirrhosis was induced in a group of dogs in whom a prior end-to-side portacaval fistula had been placed. This approach created a model in which cirrhosis and all of its biochemical and endocrine disturbances could be dissociated from portal venous hypertension and its hemodynamic consequences. Thus, any sodium retention would not be due to the need to replete an enlarged venous space, and if retention occurred prior to formation of ascites, the retained salt and water of necessity would expand all portions of the vascular space to an equivalent degree. This finding would imply that the nonsplanchnic portion of the circulation could not possibly be volume-contracted during ongoing formation of ascites. Thus, such an observation would support the overfilling theory, for the contraction of nonsplanchnic plasma volume could not stimulate the renal tubule to retain sodium. The results of this type of experiment in 5 cirrhotic dogs with a prior end-to-side portacaval fistula are shown in Figure 8.4. Several conclusions may be drawn:

1. The presence of portal venous hypertension and engorgement of the mesenteric venous compartment is not a sine qua non for urinary sodium

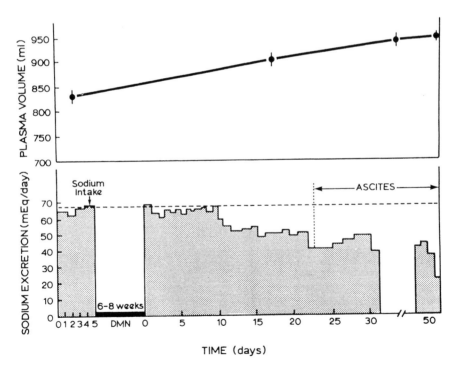

FIGURE 8.4.   Sodium balance in 5 cirrhotic dogs without portal hypertension because of prior construction of an end-to-side portacaval anastomosis. Note that urinary sodium retention and plasma volume expansion precede the appearance of ascites. DMN-dimethylnitrosamine. (From Levy M, Wexler MJ: Renal sodium retention and ascites formation in dogs with experimental cirrhosis but without portal hypertension or with increased splanchnic vascular capacity. J Lab Clin Med 1978;91:520–536, with permission.)

retention in cirrhotic dogs. That is not to say, however, that portal venous congestion cannot be a cause for urinary sodium retention, at least transiently. As the holding capacity of the mesenteric circulation increases with progressive portal venous hypertension, plasma volume must expand if venous return and cardiac output are to be maintained within physiologic limits. That transient urinary sodium retention must occur can be deduced from observations in patients with extrahepatic portal hypertension who clearly demonstrate expanded plasma volumes. This is similar to the situation encountered with "mineralocorticoid escape," in which the continuous administration of a high salt diet and large doses of intramuscular mineralocorticoid produce intense urinary sodium retention. After several days, however, progressive extracellular fluid (ECF) volume expansion causes a reduction in fractional tubular sodium reabsorption, and subjects return to sodium balance despite the continuing administration of a high salt diet and mineralocorticoid. The price of this return to balance is an expanded plasma volume, which dissipates only when the salt-retaining stimulus comes to an end.

2. In our canine model, the ascites is derived only from the hepatic parenchyma with no visceral contribution.

3. Because urinary sodium retention and plasma volume expansion occurred prior to the formation of ascites, contraction of the nonsplanchnic plasma volume could not have been a salt-retaining stimulus.

Moreover, because the retained salt and water would have expanded all portions of the vascular space to an equivalent degree and because Starling forces were not disturbed in the portal circulation, both splanchnic and nonsplanchnic portions of the vascular space would have become expanded. Indeed, this has been shown to be so by direct measurement.[3]

Our laboratory also measured splanchnic and nonsplanchnic plasma volumes directly in cirrhotic dogs with ascites that actively retained urinary sodium. We used dye dilution (Evans Blue T1824) with an exclusion technique in which measurements of plasma volume were made before and after exclusion of splanchnic volume from access to the dye by vascular constrictors. Such observations indicated that whereas total plasma volume increased by 161 ml on average, the nonsplanchnic or nonportal component also increased significantly—on average by 96 ml.

Our data represent the first direct observation that during formation of ascites and active urinary sodium retention, there is actual expansion—not contraction—of the nonportal or effective arterial blood volume.

Peripheral Vascular Resistance

Although the above experiments proved conclusively that actual contraction of the nonsplanchnic plasma volume was not necessary as a sodium-retaining stimulus prior to formation of ascites, it remained possible that underfilling of the arterial circulation occurred on the basis of reduced peripheral vascular resistance. Accordingly, a series of cirrhotic dogs were studied in sequential fashion as they passed from normality to a state of advanced disease for changes in cardiac output and peripheral vascular resistance as they related temporally to the onset of urinary sodium retention[85] (Fig. 8.5)

Changes in cardiac output and peripheral vascular resistance occurred only after sodium retention and plasma volume expansion had been noted. Thus, in this canine model of cirrhosis, the initiation of urinary sodium retention could be related neither to arithmetic contraction of the arterial blood volume nor to underfilling of this volume because of a reduction in cardiac output or peripheral vascular resistance. These data are discussed further in the section dealing with the peripheral arteriolar vasodilation theory.

Maintenance of Urinary Sodium Retention

The evidence produced in the canine cirrhotic model indicated that retention of urinary sodium begins prior to the formation of ascites, thus supporting the overfilling hypothesis. Another prediction of the overfilling hypothesis is that removal of the sequestered "third space" would not abolish the urinary sodium retention observed in cirrhotic dogs, i.e., the maintenance of sodium retention would depend not only on a large depot of edema but also on other factors.

With the advent of the LeVeen peritoneovenous valve,[58] it became possible to accomplish in dogs not only mobilization of ascites back into the vascular space but also prevention of its reformation. Five dogs with advanced cirrhosis were studied after they had developed large volumes of ascites and again after complete mobilization of ascites with a LeVeen shunt.[86]

Following placement of the shunt (which in reality serves as an iatrogenic thoracic duct), the

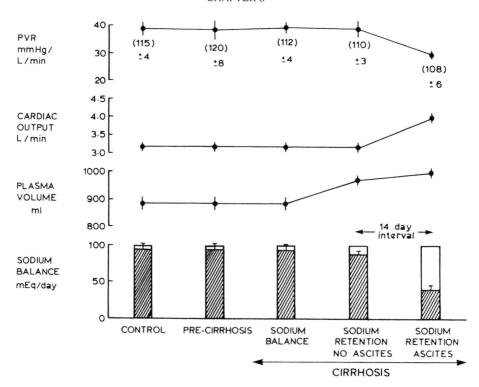

FIGURE 8.5. Temporal relationships among altered sodium balance, plasma volume, and systemic hemo-dynamics in 6 alert dogs with experimental portal cirrhosis. The height of the bars in the bottom panel refer to sodium intake; the shaded areas reflect 24-hr urinary excretion. Note that alterations in sodium balance and plasma volume expansion precede changes in cardiac output or peripheral vascular resistance (PVR). The numbers in parentheses at the top of the figure refer to arterial blood pressure. (From Levy M, Allotey JBK: Temporal relationship between urinary salt retention and altered systemic hemodynamics in dogs with experimental cirrhosis. J Lab Clin Med 1978;92:560–569, with permission.)

dogs displayed a marked diuresis and natriuresis; within 3 days volumes of ascites as large as 3.0 L were completely mobilized. Plasma volume increased, as did cardiac output, central venous pressure, and arterial blood pressure. Renal plasma flow and glomerular filtration rate (GFR) remained unchanged. Plasma renin and aldosterone levels fell to near-normal values. Despite such evidence of vascular fullness, the dogs still retained sodium, and when fed a high salt diet (120 mEq/day), they rapidly developed anasarca. Ascites did not reaccumulate despite marked urinary sodium retention and diffuse edema, presumably because of the functioning LeVeen valve. Such experimental results permit two important conclusions:

1. Despite expansion of the plasma volume, normal levels of plasma renin and aldosterone, augmented systemic hemodynamics, and normal renal perfusion, the dogs displayed urinary sodium retention in the absence of both a third space and volumetric contraction of the effective

blood volume. Thus, the maintenance of sodium retention in advanced cirrhosis depends on factors still operative when vascular fluid is no longer sequestered as ascites within the peritoneal cavity.

2. Ascites is in fact a manifestation of generalized edema. One could argue that because edema in the cirrhotic patient preferentially collects within the peritoneal space, it is a manifestation of localized disturbances of the Starling forces only within the portal venous system. Edema of the lower extremities is secondary to compression of the abdominal vena by tense ascites. However, by obviating the consequences of the disturbed Starling forces—i.e., by continuously removing the ascites—one could not abolish the sodium retention. Hence, the factors promoting tubular retention of sodium operate independently of the factors creating a localized edema state.

Various observations in the literature support the thesis that liver-damaged animals or patients may retain sodium in the absence of ascites. Levy and Wexler[3] demonstrated that urinary sodium retention may be quite marked in dogs with end-to-side portacaval fistula and hepatic atrophy. Davis and Ball[87] removed the ascites from chronic caval dogs and placed a tight plaster case about the abdomen so that fluid could not reform. Five of 8 dogs demonstrated marked sodium retention, whereas 3 returned to sodium balance. Orloff[5] studied 9 cirrhotic patients in whom ascites disappeared following a side-to-side portacaval fistula. Although all patients displayed a marked natriuresis in the immediate postoperative period, dietary sodium restriction was still necessary in follow-up visits (3–7 years), apparently to prevent edema formation. Further reports indicate that when patients with cirrhosis of the liver are subjected to portacaval shunt procedures, with marked reduction of portal venous pressure, the ascites may resolve but be replaced with peripheral edema. Thus, urinary sodium is being retained, but the retained salt and water are no longer preferentially directed into the peritoneal space. Instead, edema collects in the most dependent portions of the body.[88,89] Papper and Rosenbaum[90] demonstrated that oral administration of a salt load (225 mEq) to cirrhotic patients without ascites resulted in incomplete excretion compared with controls.

More recently, Ansley et al.[91] and Greig et al.[92] studied salt handling in cirrhotic patients who have received a LeVeen valve for treatment of refractory ascites. Ansley et al. demonstrated that 4 of 6 cirrhotic patients in whom ascites was completely mobilized, despite an average increment in GFR of 17 ml/min and a decrement in plasma aldosterone from 82 to 15 ng/100 ml (indicating vascular replenishment), were unable to increase sodium excretion spontaneously and required a potent diuretic to achieve natriuresis.

In the study by Greig et al., 11 patients who received a LeVeen shunt were examined up to 29 months postoperatively. All patients had patent shunts and no detectable ascites. On a diet of 20 mEq/day of sodium, mean excretion averaged 17.2 ± 5.3 mEq/day in 7 patients. Despite normal plasma levels of renin and aldosterone and a 100% increment in GFR (creatinine clearance) over preoperative values, 6 of 7 patients demonstrated marked sodium retention when challenged with 100 mEq/day of sodium. The mean 24-hour sodium excretion averaged 56.1 ± 16.5 mEq/day. The range of sodium excretion in the 7 patients

was 4–130 mEq/day. Thus, in cirrhotic humans as in cirrhotic dogs, the removal of ascites by continual peritoneovenous shunting is accompanied by vascular replenishment, reduction of markers of vascular fullness to normal levels (renin and aldosterone), and improvement in cardiac output and renal perfusion. Yet renal sodium handling remains abnormal. Such observations provide strong evidence that sodium retention in advanced cirrhosis is not dependent solely on a depot of ascites; that is, the maintenance of renal tubular sodium retention depends on factors other than vascular underfilling.

Factors Mediating Preascitic Sodium Retention

There is no doubt that plasma volume begins to expand early in the course of hepatic cirrhosis. The preascitic phase, therefore, must include a period of sodium retention, no matter how undetectable and subtle it may be. Probably the larger part of this sodium retention is directed toward the replenishment of a progressively expanding splanchnic venous bed and portosystemic collateral channels. If no other process intervened, however, the ratio of the enlarged plasma volume to the expanded splanchnic venous bed should be unchanged. The plasma volume should have increased only sufficiently to maintain venous return and cardiac output within physiologic limits as the holding capacity of the splanchnic venous territory increased. There should be no "extra" sodium retention. Yet at least three laboratories have provided evidence that the preascitic plasma volume expansion of cirrhosis is associated with suppression of plasma levels of renin and aldosterone.[93–95] If one accepts that renin and aldosterone are markers for fullness of the circulation, this finding is putative evidence that at least some component of first-phase or preascitic urinary sodium retention in cirrhosis is related to factors other than those that mediate ECF volume replenishment. That such an interpretation may be correct is shown by the fact that as ascites forms and the vascular volume contracts, these plasma markers begin to rise.[96]

Our laboratory has provided evidence from experiments performed in canine cirrhosis that some proportion of first-phase preascitic sodium retention is due to intrahepatic hypertension. Previous experiments[84,85] had shown that preascitic sodium retention observed in cirrhotic dogs occurs independently of changes in cardiac output or peripheral vascular resistance and portal hypertension. This finding suggested that some derivative of the cirrhotic liver may signal the renal tubule directly to augment sodium reabsorption; broadly speaking, such a signal may be due to a "sick" liver with compromised synthetic and degradative function or intrahepatic hypertension. To settle this question, we studied a series of cirrhotic dogs without intrahepatic or portal venous hypertension due to a side-to-side portacaval anastomosis.[97] The dogs were unable to form hepatic or splanchnic lymph and could not form ascites. Because the liver was severely cirrhotic, the absence of sodium retention implies that intrahepatic hypertension is a major cause of the component of first-phase sodium retention unrelated to requirements to replenish the effective blood volume. Eleven dogs on a diet of 35 mEq of sodium/day were followed for about 12 weeks and showed no evidence of either urinary sodium retention or plasma volume expansion (Fig. 8.6). When the dogs were fed a high salt diet (85 mEq/day) and given intramuscular injections of the mineralocorticoid desoxycorticosterone acetate (DOCA), they divided into two groups. Four dogs escaped the salt-retaining effects of DOCA, did not form ascites, and had

a natriuresis when the mineralocorticoid was stopped; they showed complete patency of the portacaval anastomosis and a gradient of only 1.6 cm H_2O. The other 7 dogs formed ascites in response to the intramuscular injections of DOCA, although they showed a natriuresis when the DOCA was stopped; the anastomosis was partially occluded with an elevated portal venous pressure and a gradient across the anastomosis of 7.0 cm H_2O. We interpreted such data to mean that a cirrhotic liver per se with markedly disturbed function does not signal the renal tubule to retain sodium. Intrahepatic hypertension must be present.

The statements by several groups[98–100] that low-pressure baroreceptors within the liver are capable of reacting to increased sinusoidal pressure are of interest. Kostreva et al.[98] recently demonstrated within the canine liver that activation of these baroreceptors also simultaneously increases reflex sympathetic efferent activity to the kidney and heart. Sympathetic activity to the heart was unassociated with tachycardia, suggesting some "special" effect. Given the role of the renal sympathetic nerves in mediating the tubular retention of sodium [101] and the possible role of the sympathetic nerves in modulating the

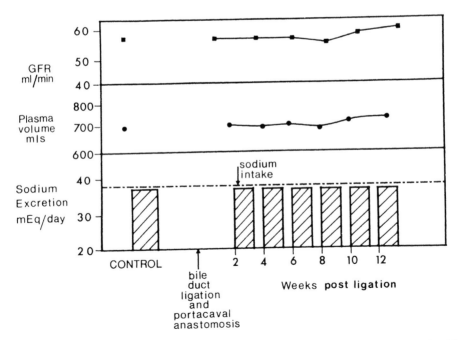

FIGURE 8.6. Sodium balance and plasma volume in cirrhotic dogs (chronic biliary ligation) with a side-to-side portacaval fistula that has normalized both intrahepatic and portal venous pressures. Ascites was absent; liver function was severely compromised in later stages of the disease process. (From Levy M, Wexler MJ: Salt and water balance in liver disease. Hosp Pract 1984;19:57–71; illustration by A Miller; with permission.)

release of the newly discovered atrial natriuretic factor,[102] it is possible that low-pressure intrahepatic baroreceptors act as an oscillating modulator of urinary sodium excretion through the renal nerves and release of atrial natriuretic factor. Because alterations in liver and portal pressure may occur physiologically with posture and respiration, Moreno and Burchell[103] made the tentative suggestion that variation in intrahepatic pressure may partly determine the magnitude of the plasma volume in cirrhotics.

Our laboratory recently adduced evidence that intrahepatic baroreceptors may indeed modulate urinary sodium excretion.[104] Dogs that were given low-grade thoracic caval constriction retained sodium for a period of about 6 days before returning to sodium balance without forming ascites. Complete hepatic denervation, with the same degree of thoracic caval constriction, reduced the salt-retaining period to 2–3 days, i.e. similar to the period observed for sham controls. Evidence from experiments in cirrhotic dogs also suggests that hepatic denervation may modulate urinary sodium retention in the preascitic state.[105]

That the earliest phases of cirrhosis include a component of urinary sodium retention not related strictly to defense of effective arterial blood volume has important implications. The earliest phase of edema must be associated with overfilling of the vascular compartment ,from which ascites overflows as Starling forces in the hepatoportal vascular territory become progressively disturbed. The formation of ascites that sequesters large volumes of fluid within the peritoneal space tends to empty the vascular compartment. This compartment becomes relatively underfilled, and sodium retention occurs in defense of plasma volume.

Several lines of evidence from clinical observations support the view that cirrhotic patients form ascites from an expanded plasma volume and that for the preascitic phase and at least some of the ascitic phase they are volume-replete. We have mentioned already the association between expanded plasma volumes and suppressed levels of plasma renin and aldosterone in cirrhotic patients who have not yet formed ascites. A review by Levy and Wexler[106] summarizes the remaining evidence. Briefly, the more important clinical observations supporting a biphasic relationship between the magnitude of the circulating plasma volume and the appearance of ascites are as follows:

1. Plasma volume expands in patients with obstruction of the portal vein even when ascites is absent and liver function remains uncompromised. This indicates that portal venous hypertension mandates an expanded splanchnic (and therefore total) plasma volume by virtue of augmenting the mesenteric venous holding capacity.

2. The excretion of salt and water is reduced in cirrhotic patients in whom humoral disturbances (increased plasma levels of renin, aldosterone, antidiuretic hormone, and catecholamines) indicate arterial hypovolemia. When such levels are normal, patients (generally without ascites) are normoexcretors of sodium and water.

3. Many patients with cirrhosis show uricosuria (an index of arterial hypovolemia), which reverses when the effective blood volume is reduced following infusion of a vasodilator.[107]

4. Evolution of the cirrhotic process is generally accompanied by progressive hypovolemia and azotemia, as the kidneys become underperfused because of a declining plasma volume and an increment in intrarenal vascular resistance.

The observation that plasma volume is expanded in cirrhotic patients before the appearance of ascites implies preascitic sodium retention. The appearance of ascites, which tends to empty the vascular compartment, also causes sodium retention, but in defense of the plasma volume. The evidence that ascites overflows from an expanded plasma volume seems overwhelming, particularly if one remembers that before edema (ascites) can accumulate, the protective or compensatory mechanisms tending to retard edema formation must be overwhelmed.

Critical Function Threshold Theory

Wensing, Branch and colleagues[108] popularized the notion that the onset of urinary sodium retention in experimental cirrhosis is related to a critical threshold of hepatic function. Although the overfilling theory presupposes that the cirrhotic liver is not merely a mechanical block within the portal circulation, the functional contribution to early sodium retention is thought to be based on sinusoidal hypertension and activation of low-pressure baroreceptors.

Wensing and colleagues[108,109] studied rats with experimental cirrhosis (phenobarbital and CCl_4 exposure) and in serial longitudinal studies found evidence of a critical threshold of liver function above which animals are in sodium balance, and below which animals excrete less urinary sodium than they consume in their daily diet. The sequential effect of positive sodium balance is eventually to produce ascites. In this schema, renal handling of sodium is directly related to a given degree of overall liver function, using the aminopyrine breath test (ABT) as the discriminating test. The surviving rats developed cirrhosis and gross ascites within 9–19 weeks after commencement of treatment. Treatment was terminated when ascites was detected. On average, the ABT remained normal for about 10 weeks and then linearly decreased throughout the balance of the study, although the rate of change among individual rats varied greatly. In the initial study, 13 of 15 rats eventually developed sodium retention (9–19 weeks) at a time when the ABT was markedly reduced. A subset of rats in which recovery was permitted developed a spontaneous sodium diuresis when the ABT recovered above a critical threshold (~40% of control function).

Two major criticisms must be directed at these studies:

1. Even in rats developing ascites, cessation of the CCl_4 dosing resulted in an apparent regression of the cirrhotic process and disappearance of ascites. This sequence of events does not parallel closely the clinical setting of alcoholic insult or even experiments in dogs with dimethylnitrosamine-induced cirrhosis in which withdrawal of the offending agent usually does not result in disappearance of ascites.

2. One has to assume that the ABT is correlated with general hepatic dysfunction or that the functioning hepatocyte mass is reduced. However, such provocative data support the idea that urinary sodium retention precedes the onset of ascites (1–2 weeks in experimental rats). Although the authors provide strong evidence that the onset of urinary sodium retention is linked to a critical threshold of liver function, which appears with an approximate 60% reduction of the ABT, it is unclear how this threshold is linked physiologically to the renal tubule. ABT dysfunction is a measure of mixed oxidase activity. It must not be implied, however, that such activity is responsible for the onset of sodium retention. Altered metabolic, synthetic, or degradative functions may be involved. Activation of hepatorenal reflexes (involving renal sympathetic efferents) also may be involved.

The investigators examined the possibility that the defect in hepatic mixed oxidase activity

expresses itself as a change in renal and/or systemic hemodynamics by studying 3 groups of rats: (1) controls, (2) cirrhotic rats with sodium retention and ABT results below the critical level, and (3) cirrhotic rats with sodium balance and the ABT data just above the critical threshold. The mean treatment period was similar for all three groups. Mean arterial blood pressure was about 125 mmHg in the control group, 105 mmHg in cirrhotic rats in sodium balance (p < 0.05), and 93 mmHg in the salt-retaining group. Thus, the advent of cirrhosis was associated with relative hypotension. However, no sequential measurements were made, and the authors' conclusion that hypotension and peripheral vasodilatation precede urinary sodium retention must remain speculative. Blood pressure measurements were obtained under anesthesia and after surgical stress, and it is possible that the results are due to increased susceptibility to anesthetic in cirrhotic rats compared with controls. Moreover, renin activity and renal renin production did not increase in cirrhotic rats and were not related to sodium retention. A striking feature of these studies is that whereas sodium excretion fell dramatically when the ABT declined slightly below threshold in cirrhotic rats, arterial blood pressure declined only slightly (about another 10% from cirrhotic rats in balance). Thus, it seems highly unlikely that hypotension, whatever its cause, could be responsible for the onset of urinary sodium retention.

The concept of a tight correlation between renal sodium retention and dysfunction of oxidative metabolism within the liver receives some support from clinical observations. Wood et al.[110] demonstrated that in compensated cirrhotic patients, the ability to excrete a sodium load in the urine over a 5-hour period is correlated with antipyrine elimination. Their results differed from the experimental data in rats in that the relationship was linear rather than representing a threshold. The ability to excrete the sodium load was also correlated with wedged hepatic venous pressure, i.e., with intrahepatic sinusoidal hypertension.

In simple terms, one would expect that the more advanced the cirrhotic process—which, after all, profoundly disturbs parenchymal architecture—the more severe the degree of hepatic dysfunction. To the extent that the altered parenchyma translates into perturbed physiologic functions, it is self-evident that as liver function worsens, one is more likely to see the consequences of advanced liver disease. Indeed, several investigators have shown a relationship between sodium retention and wedged hepatic venous or sinusoidal pressure.[90,111] In this author's view, the concept of a critical threshold rather than a linear and continuous relationship between some derivative of disturbed liver function and the onset of urinary sodium retention is not proved.

Peripheral Arteriolar Dilatation Hypothesis

The most recent attempt to explain the onset of urinary sodium retention in the preascitic phase of cirrhosis is the so-called peripheral arteriolar dilatation hypothesis (PADH), which was first presented in 1988 by Schrier and Epstein of the United States, Arroyo and Rodés of Spain, Bernardi of Italy, and Henrikson of Denmark.[112] An earlier version was formulated by Norris, Buell, and Kurtzman in 1987.[113] The kernel of the hypothesis as originally presented was that neither ascites accumulation with secondary hypovolemia nor primary renal sodium retention with plasma volume expansion and subsequent overflow ascites could be considered the initiating cause of salt and water retention in cirrhosis. Rather, the original hypothesis proposed that progressive peripheral arterial vasodilation initiated urinary sodium retention in the preascitic state. This hypothesis is based on the observation in both cirrhotic patients and animals with experimental hepatic cirrhosis that advanced liver disease is associated with an increment in cardiac output that is thought to be secondary to hyperdynamic circulation and a fall in systemic vascular resistance. The authors propose that peripheral vasodilatation increases the capacity of the arterial volume and decreases the effective filling pressure. The consequent decrease in fullness of the effective arterial blood volume (EABV) induces urinary sodium retention. This theory is borrowed from the "diversion" theory of Papper, an early and devoted hepatonephrologist, who suggested that despite the augmented cardiac output in patients with advanced cirrhosis, blood may be diverted from the kidney to nonrenal preferential areas (e.g., the viscera), thus leading to urinary sodium retention and reduced renal perfusion.[113a]

This tendency to underfilling is thought to induce compensatory responses such as mobilization of vasoconstrictor hormones (e.g., renin, aldosterone, catecholamines, vasopressin) and activation of the sympathetic autonomic system. The counterbalancing effects of these hormones, added to the tendency to refill the arterial compartment because of sodium retention, is thought to maintain arterial blood pressure in the early stages of the cirrhotic process. Thus, in the preascitic stages of the disease, plasma volume becomes expanded, cardiac output is thought to be eventually increased, and peripheral vascular resistance (PVR) is thought to be decreased. The predominant site of peripheral arteriolar dilatation is thought to be the splanchnic territory, although other sites (skin, muscle, lung) may participate. The cause of the splanchnic arteriolar dilatation is unknown, but it is thought to be related to the increment in portal venous pressure. The relative expansion of plasma volume is thought to return hormone levels to normal and to suppress the augmented sympathetic efferent activity. Repetitive decrements in PVR cause further volume expansion, leading eventually to ascites formation, permanent increment in vasoconstrictor hormones, and hyperkinetic circulation.

Schrier et al.[112] also used the hypothesis to explain the sequence of events in decompensated cirrhosis, when ascites forms and acute renal failure accompanies end-stage cirrhosis—i.e. the hepatorenal syndrome (Fig. 8.7). Schrier[114,115] also attempted to generalize the concept, extending it to explain sodium retention in other conditions such as congestive heart failure, arteriovenous fistulas, and pregnancy. The interested reader is urged to examine his review for more complete arguments concerning nonascitic edema.

What evidence supports and what evidence opposes the PADH?

Proponents of the PADH must be prepared to prove several suppositions. First, no other cause for preascitic urinary sodium retention is significant. It is difficult to see how a primary decrease in PVR can explain preascitic urinary sodium retention, when other factors are known to be present. It is self-evident that the progression of parenchymal disturbances within the cirrhotic liver is associated with progressive portal hypertension. As this variable worsens and blood is sequestered within the venous territory (as well as portosystemic collaterals), sodium is retained to restore the plasma volume–venous reservoir holding capacity ratio. Other causes for sodium retention are also present in the early phase. Indeed, denervating the liver in dogs with experimental hepatic cirrhosis eliminates the early

MAJOR TENETS OF THE PERIPHERAL
ARTERIAL VASODILATION HYPOTHESIS

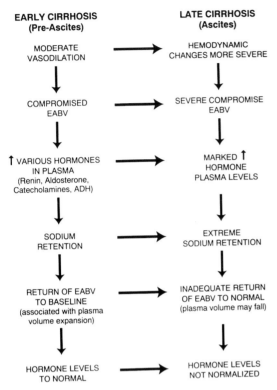

FIGURE 8.7. A schematic outline of how the peripheral arterial vasodilation theory purports to explain the sequence of events as they relate to the pathogenesis of urinary sodium retention, alteration in the magnitude of the EABV, renal function, and activation of various hormones in progressive liver cirrhosis.

component of sodium retention unrelated to portal venous sequestration in the preascitic state.[105] Unless the various early causes for urinary sodium retention can be separated experimentally, it is merely speculative to claim that peripheral arterial vasodilatation is the only or major cause of early urinary sodium retention in cirrhotic patients.

Second, proponents must show not only the existence of peripheral vasodilatation, but also a temporal relationship whereby a decline in peripheral vascular resistance precedes the onset of sodium retention in the preascitic phase. Two major difficulties are involved: (1) temporal studies have not supported a cause-and-effect relationship between depressed PVR and sodium retention, and (2) it is not always clear that hyperdynamic circulation (a supposed consequence of the PADH) is present in most cirrhotic patients.

Kowalski and Abelmann[116] were the first to examine systematically the nature of the hemodynamic changes in advanced alcoholic cirrhosis. They studied 22 hospitalized patients, of whom 19 had alcoholic cirrhosis (11 compensated, 8 decompensated); 17 of these 19 patients had vascular spiders. Cardiac output was measured by a dye-dilution technique. In only 7 of 22 patients was cardiac output elevated, and, except for one outlier, there was no apparent difference between compensated and decompensated patients. In addition, there was no consistent association between heart rate and cardiac output; heart size (as measured by x-ray techniques) was not increased; and there was no difference in blood pressure between the two groups. Thus, cardiac output was elevated in only one-third of cirrhotic patients.

Murray, Dawson and Sherlock[117] studied 24 patients with chronic portal cirrhosis. Of 17 patients in whom cardiac output was measured, 9 had normal values, 4 had only slightly elevated values, and 4 had markedly elevated levels, which accounted for the mean differences compared with 14 controls (3.68 ± 0.60 vs. 5.36 ± 1.98 L/min). Of interest, 6 patients with extensive extrahepatic portal venous obstruction and an extensive portosystemic collateral bed did not differ from controls. Thus , only half of the patients had elevated cardiac output. In a study reported by Kontos et al.,[118] only 10 of 16 cirrhotic patients had elevated cardiac output.

In series after series[119] only 30–70% of patients with cirrhosis have hyperdynamic circulations; the remainder are normal. Yet in patients with advanced liver disease an hyperkinetic state is supposedly fully developed. The suggestion has been made that the hyperkinetic state advances as the disease progresses, but even in advanced stages of disease, many patients may show no evidence of an hyperkinetic state. Mere hypotension is *not* sufficient evidence for such a state, because hypotension is often due to contraction of the EABV, active ascites formation, or gastrointestinal bleeding.

The notion that a progressive decline in PVR by itself may cause a hyperkinetic state is, of course, incorrect. Normal humans and animals receiving pharmacologic vasodilators undergo a reduction in vascular arterial capacitance with underfilling of the circulation[120] without an increment in cardiac output. The subsequent plasma volume expansion is ultimately responsible for the increase in cardiac output.

What evidence indicates that a decline in PVR precedes and is responsible for subsequent retention of urinary sodium? This issue has been assessed in various experimental models and in the clinical setting. Levy and Allotey[85] were the first to assess this variable in dogs with experimental portal cirrhosis. Appropriate indwelling catheters were inserted while the dogs were still normal, and serial measurements of arterial blood pressure, cardiac output, and PVR were made as the dogs became progressively cirrhotic over 8–12 weeks. The authors found that urinary sodium retention preceded the change in systemic hemodynamics, which occurred only when plasma volume had expanded and ascites was present. The study has been criticized on the basis that blood pressure tended to drift downward during the period of observation, and may have represented progressive vasodilatation. Although such observations have a certain inherent error, the changes were not statistically significant and were not large (blood pressure: 115 ± 4 mmHg during the control phase vs. 110 ± 3 mm Hg in the immediate preascitic phase). No change in cardiac output could be detected until ascites had supervened. Although the study may have technical problems, it is the only study to relate systemic hemodynamics to sodium excretion sequentially. More studies in this area are required.

Attempts also have been made to link the onset of preascitic urinary sodium retention to a prior perturbation in systemic hemodynamics in cirrhotic rats. Lopez et al.[71] studied temporal relationships in rats with CCl_4-induced cirrhosis that were spontaneously hypertensive (SHR). The study is flawed because of differences in renal perfusion–natriuresis relationships in hypertensive compared with nonhypertensive rats. Moreover, statistical analysis is faulty; paired t-tests were used to analyze multiple comparisons within one group. Sodium balance was normal for the first 7 weeks. During the eighth week, sodium retention correlated with a significant decline in systolic blood pressure. Only systolic rather than mean blood pressure was recorded by tail-cuff plethysmography, which is not the most accurate of measurements. During the eighth week the authors also noted the onset of urinary sodium retention. Of interest, no change in heart rate could be detected compared with control rats; cardiac output was left unmeasured. Although the authors admit that "it is impossible to ascertain whether the circulatory disturbances leading to the decrease in arterial pressure in cirrhotic SHR rats occurred before or simultaneously with the development of hypotension and sodium retention," they nonetheless conclude that their data support the PADH and are not consistent with the overfilling theory, despite the lack of significant evidence to determine the true temporal relationship between decline in blood pressure and onset of sodium retention. As we shall see, it is more likely that the reverse relationship is correct. Thus, the study showed an association between sodium retention and hypotension but not a pathophysiologic link. The investigators further cite patient and animal studies to support their point of view.[109,121–123] The clinical study[121] focused on hepatic hemodynamics and the renin-angiotensin-aldosterone (RAA) system in cirrhotic patients and found a direct correlation between plasma levels of RAA and wedged hepatic venous pressure, i.e., intrahepatic sinusoidal pressure. The data have nothing to say about the PADH; in fact, the data support the concept of vascular overfilling and the importance of low-pressure hepatic baroreceptors as the signal for primary sodium retention and the cause of ascites.

None of the cited animal studies support the PADH. Linas et al.[122] studied water excretion in cirrhotic rats and found that the nonosmotic release of arginine vasopressin (AVP) is responsible for defects in water excretion. Of interest, the rats (both Sprague-Dawley and Brattleboro cirrhotics) had marked elevation of plasma volume, whereas PVR an blood pressure were reduced but cardiac output remained normal. The two remaining citations are also irrelevant. The study by Wensing et al.[109] measured hemodynamics once only and correlates sodium excretion with aminopyrine clearance. The authors conclude that blood pressure falls and hemodynamics change as liver function declines but provide no sequential data. The study by Caramelo et al.,[123] also of CCl_4-induced cirrhotic rats, merely demonstrates altered systemic hemodynamics without attempting to perform sequential studies. The investigators showed altered capillary permeability following acute saline expansion in cirrhotic but not control rats. Of interest, despite the presence of a marked hyperkinetic circulation plasma levels of renin were not different in cirrhotic rats and controls.

In a study of sodium-retaining preascitic rats with CCl_4-induced cirrhosis, Fernandez-Munoz et al.[124] documented a hyperdynamic hypotensive state but did not correlate it with sodium retention. In a study of mice with chronic schistosomiasis and portal hypertension, Sarin et al.[125] documented a hyperdynamic circulatory state in the absence of cirrhosis but did not study the kinetics of sodium excretion.

Groszmann and colleagues at Yale have been particularly active in using the portal vein-ligated rat (PVL) to study the relationship among portal hypertension, change in PVR, and sodium excretion. Vorobioff et al.[70] ascertained that the PVL model produced an increment in portal inflow and cardiac output and a decline in PVR. These data, generally confirmed in other models of portal venous hypertension[126] and in clinical studies,[6] seem to suggest that the hyperkinetic state in cirrhosis is secondary to portal hypertension. Levy, Maher, and Wexler[127] also found that in dogs with chronic biliary cirrhosis, the prevention of portal hypertension with a side-to-side portacaval anastomosis also prevented alteration of systemic hemodynamics.

Albillos et al.[128] studied the temporal relationships between a decline in PVR and the onset of urinary sodium retention in rats. PVL rats were observed up to 4 days after onset of portal venous hypertension (hyperdynamic changes were well developed by this time). A decline in PVR and blood pressure was noted on the first day following the PVL. An increase in the ^{22}Na space was observed only on the second day. The authors concluded that sodium retention was secondary to the decline in PVR. The study, however, has several technical problems: analysis of multiple comparisons by inappropriate statistical techniques, no corresponding data for GFR or renal function, no urine collections to measure sodium excretion, and no measurements of plasma volume or hemodynamic parameters in rats different from those in which the exchangeable sodium space was measured.

The study has conceptual as well as technical problems. First, perturbations in peripheral vascular resistance occur on the first day after the experimental maneuver, with sodium retention on the following day—a situation markedly different from the clinical or even experimental progression of the cirrhotic process, in which such changes occur on a far more chronic basis. Second, because the constriction involves a vein returning some 25% of the cardiac output to the right heart, it is not surprising that blood pressure declines quickly following the PVL. Thus, the decline in arterial blood pressure may be due to blood sequestration rather than peripheral arteriolar vasodilatation.

Experiments in the PVL model that documented hyperdynamic circulation with an actual alteration in both splanchnic and peripheral arteriolar resistances were carried out 13 days after the PVL,[70] at an unspecified point,[129] or 10 days after the procedure.[130] Thus, although the studies have shown apparent sodium retention, it is likely due to venous congestion and hypotension rather than compromise of the EABV by widespread arteriolar dilatation. This conclusion is confirmed by the laboratory's techniques: when the evolution of the hyperkinetic state is studied in the PVL model,[131] the earliest point at which a true decrease in splanchnic venous resistance with increased portal venous inflow may be seen is the fourth day after PVL. Thus Albillos et al. documented urinary sodium retention secondary to an increment in portal venous holding capacity and not necessarily peripheral arteriolar dilatation. Such a conclusion has recently been reached by Moriura et al.[113a] in their study of acute portal hypertension in dogs. The authors demonstrated a reduction in cardiac output due to a reduction in venous return, which in turn was presumably due to pooling of blood in the portal venous circuit.

Using the same model, Colombato et al.[72] investigated temporal relationships among the hyperdynamic circulatory state, plasma volume expansion, and peripheral vasodilatation. Plasma volume was sequentially measured by ^{125}I-albumin dilution, cardiac output by a thermodilution technique, and arterial flows by Doppler flowmetry. A drawback of the study was that sets of animals were used in each successive day for up to 8 days after PVL. Although PVR, plasma volume, and cardiac output data were similar to those obtained by Albillos et al.[128] on the first day after PVL, evidence of vasodilatation on the first day was found only in the iliac artery; vasodilatation in the superior mesenteric artery (SMA) vascular bed was delayed until the fourth day after PVL, at which time plasma volume was maximally expanded. Even the data for the iliac artery are suspect, because there are no control values and PVL values are compared only with sham rats; furthermore, an increase in iliac flow cannot be detected until the fourth day. The decline in PVR on the first day is due entirely to the fall in blood pressure since CO remains normal.

Thus, there is no true change in peripheral vascular resistance probably until the fourth day. The authors conclude that plasma volume expansion is required for development of the full hyperkinetic state. When sodium is restricted in the diet, the hyperkinetic state seen in the PVL model is either attenuated or prevented.[132] This is not surprising, for expanded blood volume causes stress relaxation of the peripheral resistors and increases the holding capacity of the circulation.[133]

In an interesting study Ingles et al.[73] demonstrated that in conscious cirrhotic rats (CCl_4) without ascites an increase in both blood volume and total vascular capacity probably contributed to the hyperkinetic state.

Although animal data show eventual ECF volume expansion in PVL rats, early sodium retention is almost certainly due to the consequences of venous obstruction. Evidence that this model produces an hyperkinetic state is good, but it is clear that the hemodynamic perturbations are secondary to volume expansion, which may have many causes other than peripheral arteriolar vasodilation (e.g., sodium retention due to alteration in circulating humoral substances, increased intrahepatic pressures).

CLINICAL STUDIES

Numerous studies in patients with hepatic cirrhosis have also provided data about the possible pathophysiology of sodium retention in the preascitic state.

Epstein and colleagues[134] subjected cirrhotic patients to thermoindifferent water immersion. This technique is equivalent to infusing 2.0 L of isotonic saline within a 2-hour period and has the advantage of producing no change in plasma composition. This experimental maneuver is associated with significant natriuresis (see chapter 1). In cirrhotic patients with ascites who are subjected to this procedure, the natriuretic response tends to fall into one of three categories: about one-third of patients have a natriuretic response in the normal range; about one-third have a supranormal response, i.e., exaggerated natriuresis; and one-third have either no natriuretic response to immersion or a response that is markedly blunted.[134a,b]

Some investigators interpret such data as suggestive of central hypovolemia; the natriuresis subsequent to immersion occurs because the redistribution of plasma volume has refilled the central thoracic blood volume. Bichet and colleagues[135] produced evidence to support this view in their study of central hemodynamics during immersion for 5 hours. Cardiac output increased, as did right atrial pressure and wedged pulmonary capillary pressure. Following termination of immersion, all three parameters declined. Blood pressure did not change; immersion appeared to replenish or expand the central blood volume. The same investigators observed that water immersion produces water diuresis in appropriately loaded patients (20 ml/kg) and suppresses the circulating levels of AVP, thus providing additional evidence for central volume expansion.

Nicholls et al.[136] immersed in water cirrhotic patients initially described as normal excretors or nonexcretors after provision of a standard water load (20 ml/kg). Normal excretors eliminated more than 40% of the water in urine over a 4-hour period, whereas nonexcretors eliminated < 40%. Nonexcretors generally showed more ascites, hyponatremia and sodium retention than normal excretors. In response to water immersion, the patients showed a continuum of responses. Nonexcretors had higher plasma levels of AVP, renin, aldosterone, and norepinephrine that failed to suppress during immersion. Normal excretors displayed a greater natriuretic response as well as a tendency to normalize the elevated plasma hormone levels described above. Because the nonexcretors also tended to show an elevated intrarenal vascular resistance despite a CO similar to that of normal excretors, the investigators concluded that EABV was compromised to a greater degree in the nonexcretors with subsequent elevation of appropriate neurohumoral markers. They attributed this sequence of events to greater peripheral vasodilation earlier in the cirrhotic process and concluded that their findings supported the PADH.

Shapiro et al.[137] combined water immersion with norepinephrine infusions. They postulated that cirrhotic patients not responding to water immersion with natriuresis were already maximally vasodilated. Immersion further lowered blood pressure and prevented a response; if this effect could be countered with pressor infusion, such responders would become natriuretic after immersion. Although water immersion or norepinephrine infusion per se initiated a slight natriuresis, only the combination was effective in normalizing the natriuretic response. The authors concluded that decompensated cirrhotic patients retain sodium because of depleted EABV.

Attempts to correlate the natriuretic response of water immersion in cirrhotic patients with the clinical state have not been conclusive.[134] Although the issue has not been well studied, certain observations suggest that the degree of natriuretic response cannot be correlated with the degree of compensation, i.e., the presence or absence of ascites following thermoindifferent water immersion. Moreover, some investigators[134,138] have adduced evidence that the natriuretic response correlates with the degree to which neurohumoral markers are activated as a marker for depletion of EABV. Thus, decompensated cirrhotic patients not responding to water immersion with a significant natriuresis generally tend to have higher levels of plasma renin activity, aldosterone, AVP, and norepinephrine. But patients cannot always be so clearly demarcated. Thus, Skorecki, Blendis, and colleagues in Toronto[139] have observed that although cirrhotic patients with ascites divide approximately 50:50 into natriuretic responders and nonresponders following water immersion, plasma levels of atrial natriuretic peptide (a marker for fullness of EABV) were equivalent in each group, as was urinary excretion of cyclic guanosine monophosphate (cGMP), the second messenger for atrial natriuretic peptide (ANP).

In a study of water-loaded cirrhotic patients, Bichet, Van Putten, and Schrier[140] obtained evidence that plasma levels of norepinephrine, renin, aldosterone, and AVP were elevated in nonexcretors. Thus, nonexcretors had evidence of volume contraction. Although clinically detectable ascites was present in all 19 nonexcretors of the water load, it was also present in 2 of 7 patients with normal water excretion and no clear evidence of volume contraction. Moreover, all patients, whether normo- or nonexcretors, had evidence of hyperkinetic circulation and various degrees of ascites or peripheral edema or both before the study.

Such apparent discrepancies—in particular, the three types of natriuretic responses following water immersion reported by Epstein[134]—may best be explained in the following way. Preascitic urinary sodium retention causes plasma volume expansion. Because at least a portion of sodium retention is unrelated to defense of ECF volume, both splanchnic and nonsplanchnic portions of the circulation expand. EABV is also expanded.

As ascites begins to accumulate, the expanded plasma volume begins to contract. Because one cannot with precision stage the evolution of a progressive cirrhotic process and because most patients present in advanced stages of disease, it is obvious that a spectrum or continuum of patients will be examined. Patients with marked expansion of EABV (i.e., patients who are "overfilled") will have an exaggerated natriuresis, whereas patients who are approximately euvolemic will have a natriuretic response in the normal range and patients who are "underfilled" may well have an attenuated natriuretic response. If all patients were underfilled at the time of immersion, it is difficult to see how one could obtain exaggerated natriuretic responses. Although the above explanation is almost certainly an oversimplification, the results obtained from water immersion of cirrhotic patients do not unequivocally support the underfilling theory and may have alternative explanations.

Interesting clinical studies in cirrhotic patients have been reported recently by Rector and colleagues in Denver. Rector and Hossack[141] measured blood volumes, cardiac functions and dimensions, systemic hemodynamics, and various plasma hormones in cirrhotic patients with and without ascites. They found evidence for equivalent central filling in both groups and also found that atrial diameter was significantly larger in both groups than in controls, suggesting that central hypervolemia may develop even before ascites accumulates. They also found that the increments in CO and pulse rate and the usual decline in blood pressure and PVR were not correlated with urinary sodium excretion in ascitic patients. Although plasma volume was higher in patients with ascites than in patients without, portal pressure and therefore blood sequestration are likely to be more advanced in cirrhotic patients with ascites and so contribute to expanded plasma volume. The authors concluded that sodium retention in cirrhotics was unlikely to be triggered by central hypovolemia and suggested that it was due either to a primary stimulus (presumably from the liver) or from an arterial region of underfilling despite total volume expansion.

Additional studies by Rector et al.[142] have shown that cirrhotic patients with hyperdynamic circulation had an enlarged left ventricular diameter at both end-systole and end-diastole. No difference in CO, blood pressure, or PVR was found between ascitic and nonascitic patients. Because left ventricular volume is increased in end-systole, afterload cannot be diminished, and the increase in end-diastole indicates augmented vascular volume. The authors concluded that arterial underfilling is not the cause of an increased CO in cirrhotic patients and in a later study[143] concluded that arterial underfilling was not a cause for sodium retention in cirrhosis. This conclusion was reached by evaluating longitudinally a cohort of patients with liver cirrhosis. The authors made 40 multiple comparisons in 18 men with cirrhosis when ascites was either present, had appeared, or had disappeared. The premise was that if the PADH was correct, blood pressure and PVR might be expected to fall and plasma norepinephrine concentrations to rise in sequentially studied patients developing sodium retention; the opposite would be expected as sodium retention spontaneously resolves. In comprehensive studies these relationships were not found to hold up. Moreover, the authors note that in numerous series investigators have found no differences in blood pressure between cirrhotic patients with and without ascites. They concluded that no evidence supported the PADH.

Not all data are consistent with this viewpoint. Henriksen et al.[144] measured central blood volume in cirrhotics and found it to be reduced. Although such a finding is compatible with arteriolar vasodilation, other causes (e.g., sequestration of fluid within the peritoneal space) could be invoked, since the lowest values were found in patients with gross ascites.

Finally, Bernardi and colleagues[145,146] assessed hemodynamics and sodium retention in preascitic cirrhotic patients under varying postural conditions. They found no difference from controls after 2 hours of standing in either systemic hemodynamics or markers for fullness of EABV. CO rose, PVR fell, and ANP levels rose in cirrhotic patients only in the supine posture. The authors concluded that during upright posture cirrhotic patients compensate for an expanded portal venous tree and splanchnic dilatation by retaining sodium. During recumbency the excessive plasma volume produces hemodynamic changes. The authors view the increased CO and reduced PVR in recumbency as a physiologic adaptation. They argue that aldosterone-dependent sodium retention probably occurs in orthostasis in preascitic cirrhosis, but sodium balance is achieved in recumbency by suppression of aldosterone and increment in ANP.[146]

As a result of these studies and studies conducted by the Denver group, Bernardi[147] concluded that the major circulatory abnormalities in advanced cirrhosis—i.e., increased CO, decreased PVR, and decreased blood pressure—are caused by expanded blood volume rather than direct arteriolar vasodilatation. This author came to a similar conclusion based on studies[97,127] documenting that in cirrhotic dogs with a side-to-side portacaval anastomosis, in which hepatoportal hypertension is prevented despite a severely cirrhotic liver, plasma volume expansion and urinary sodium retention do not develop. In such a model, the usual perturbation to systemic hemodynamics does not develop. However, with provision of acute volume expansion or chronic expansion with a high salt diet and intramuscular mineralocorticoid,[146a] the increase in CO is highly significant. Bernardi concluded that the evidence was sufficiently strong to suggest that the initial hypothesis advanced by proponents of the PADH (of whom he was one) is in fact reversed.[147] It is probably incorrect to say that a primary reduction in PVR increases CO. Rather, volume expands, and preload increases; then CO increases and PVR declines as a compensatory response. The hyperdynamic circulation should be viewed as a physiologic adaptation to a primary hypervolemic condition. If arteriolar dilatation plays a major role in causing the retention of urinary sodium, with compensatory increments in vasoconstrictor hormones, it probably is important only in advanced ascitic stages of the cirrhotic process. Early, preascitic retention of urinary sodium probably has other, more significant causes, as outlined in the overfilling theory.

Several other recent observations cast doubt on the PADH, which tends to link both sodium retention and hyperkinetic circulation to prior peripheral vasodilatation. Henderson et al.[148] studied patients with orthotopic liver transplants for 2 years following the procedure. They found that elevated cardiac output and stroke volumes persisted at 2-year follow-up, even though liver function appeared to be normal. Kidney function was only mildly reduced, as judged by slightly elevated serum creatinine values (1.7 ± 0.4 mg/dl). No satisfactory explanation for this observation was given. It seems unlikely that the raised cardiac output can be explained on the basis of widespread decrement in peripheral vascular resistance.

Wong et al.[149] measured central blood volume in 24 cirrhotic patients (13 with ascites, 11 without) using radionuclide angiography. Mean blood pressure was similar in both groups and no different from control patients. Central blood volume was higher in cirrhotic patients than controls, but no difference was found between the two cirrhotic groups. Of interest, central blood volume could not be correlated to levels of aldosterone, plasma renin activity, or plasma ANP levels. End-systolic and end-diastolic volumes were similar between controls and cirrhotic patients despite an elevation of CO in the ascitic group and a fall in PVR. The authors concluded that there was a tendency to arterial underfilling despite the altered systemic hemodynamics of the ascitic group and that in the compensated nonascitic group the central volume expansion without evidence of peripheral vasodilation implied other mechanisms for the urinary sodium retention. These observations support the overfilling hypothesis rather than the PADH.

VASCULAR OVERFILLING BECOMES VASCULAR UNDERFILLING

The various hypotheses reviewed above speak to the urinary retention of sodium in the preascitic phase of a prolonged cirrhotic process. The overfilling hypothesis suggests that urinary sodium retention prior to the formation of ascites depends on two basic signals: the need to defend (1) plasma volume or (2) EABV. Sodium retention is due to factors such as increasing holding capacity in the portal venous system and progressive hypoalbuminemia. In addition, some degree of sodium retention is unrelated to the needs of EABV and results from activation of intrahepatic low pressure baroreceptors. This "extra" sodium retention expands the plasma volume, accounting for suppressed plasma renin and aldosterone levels in cirrhotic humans in the preascitic phase and for the observation that the nonportal or nonsplanchnic plasma volume is expanded during the active phase of ascites accumulation and urinary sodium retention. The observation that plasma volume expansion precedes ascites formation in dogs with an end-to-side portacaval anastomosis, in which plasma cannot be sequestered within an engorged venous system, also suggests that EABV is overfilled.

The PADH and the critical threshold hypothesis also could explain plasma volume expansion in the preascitic stage of cirrhosis. However, the evidence that either serves as the predominant cause of urinary sodium retention is weak. The experimental evidence for the overfilling hypothesis is far more compelling and is bolstered by clinical evidence.

Alcoholic patients with advanced cirrhosis and ascites often present with vascular depletion. On first consideration, this fact seems to militate against the overfilling hypothesis of ascites formation. Several points must be considered, however, before this hypothesis is dismissed. Strictly speaking, the overfilling hypothesis refers only to the temporal relationship between initiation of sodium retention and appearance of ascites. Once ascites is established in the presence of advanced liver disease, secondary phenomena may permit vascular underfilling and blunt the dependence of ascites formation on antecedent urinary sodium retention. Thus, inadequate salt intake, loss of fluids from the gastrointestinal tract in the form of vomitus or diarrhea, hemorrhage, diuretic abuse, and sequestration of blood and edema fluid in the lower extremities act to deplete the arterial blood volume. Replenishment from the large depot of ascites comes largely from fluid reabsorption into the splanchnic capillaries (regional lymphatics are already carrying maximal amounts of fluid). Splanchnic capillaries, however, exhibit altered Starling forces that do not favor reabsorption but rather efflux of fluid into the peritoneal space (portal venous hypertension and reduced colloid osmotic pressure). Indeed, Shear et al.[49] calculated that the maximal rate of transperitoneal transfer of ascites in such patients is approximately 900 ml/day. Consequently, any marked dissociation between vascular emptying and vascular filling or replenishment converts the patient into a volume-contracted model with reduction of effective arterial blood volume (Fig. 8.8). Even if ascitic fluid is reabsorbed into parietal rather than visceral capillaries supplying the peritoneum, the difficulty with which it is reabsorbed suggests constraints for reabsorption in this microvascular territory, perhaps due to hypoalbuminemia.

Therefore, an abundance of evidence suggests that traditional descriptions of ascites formation are oversimplified. A more complete and accurate description incorporates both overfilling and underfilling theories. Early in the cirrhotic process, preascitic sodium retention occurs for at least two distinct reasons. In part, sodium retention occurs in defense of ECF volume as progressive portal hypertension augments the holding

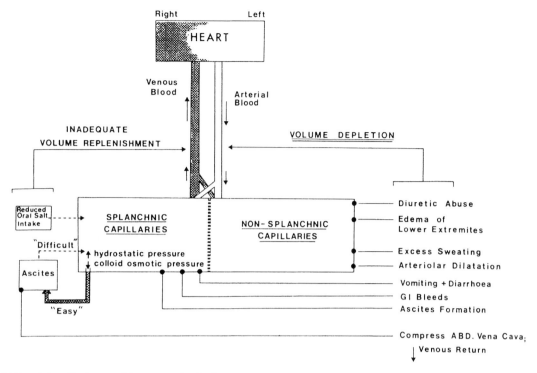

FIGURE 8.8. Patients with severe alcoholic cirrhosis of the liver may have many reasons for depleting the arterial blood volume. Repletion should come from the extensive depot of ascites, but reabsorption from the peritoneal space is difficult because of portal venous hypertension and a low plasma colloid osmotic pressure. Consequently, any marked discrepancy in such patients between factors mediating extracellular fluid volume depletion and replenishment of the vascular space may cause a hypovolemic "crisis." ABD = abdominal. (From Levy M: Pathophysiology of ascites formation. In Epstein M (ed): The Kidney in Liver Disease, 3rd ed. Baltimore: Williams & Wilkins, 1988, with permission.)

capacity of the splanchnic circulation and other events reduce peripheral vascular resistance. But sodium retention also occurs for reasons unconnected with defense of plasma or ECF volume; it is also due to signals emanating from the cirrhotic liver. Our laboratory has adduced evidence that intrahepatic hypertension may be the source for such a signal. This "extra" urinary sodium retention expands the plasma volume over and above what is strictly required to maintain normal systemic hemodynamics. Such expansion may suppress plasma levels of renin and aldosterone—two markers for fullness of the circulation. From such an overfilled vascular compartment, ascites will overflow when venous hypertension in the portal circuit is sufficiently disturbed. Once ascites collects in significant volume and peripheral vascular resistance falls (due to questionable arteriovenous shunts and arteriolar dilation), sodium retention occurs in defense of plasma volume, which begins to fall as ascites formation progresses. The vascular compartment becomes

relatively underfilled. Presumably at this point plasma levels of renin, aldosterone, catecholamines, and antidiuretic hormone begin to rise, and hyponatremia may supervene—all markers for arterial hypovolemia.

AFFERENT FACTORS

Although chapter 1 reviews in detail the factors influencing renal sodium handling in cirrhotic patients, with particular emphasis on both afferent and efferent events, a brief overview may be helpful at this point.

The bulk of evidence from experimental canine[3,84,86] and rat[83] models for portal cirrhosis supports the view that prior sodium retention is necessary before ascites accumulates in significant amounts within the peritoneal space. If this is so, what constitutes the nature of the afferent signal to the renal tubule? Experimental evidence from the canine model indicates that jaundice or hypoalbuminemia cannot be invoked.[86] Although aberrant humoral factors are most likely present, none has been implicated to date as a salt-retaining humoral substance. Levy[7] reviewed the 10 or so separate humoral factors thought to be released from the liver in different species and capable of influencing renal function. A strong possibility is that intrahepatic hypertension in some way sets in motion a train of events, mediated either by nervous or humoral pathways, that leads to augmented tubular reabsorption of sodium. Chronic caval dogs with intrahepatic hypertension but without compromised liver function also retain urinary sodium avidly in the presence of ascites, even when the ascitic depot has been completely mobilized with a LeVeen valve.[86] Caval dogs and cirrhotic dogs share intrahepatic hypertension: caval dogs because of mechanical obstruction and cirrhotic dogs because of disease. Because actual portal venous hypertension is relatively unimportant as a sodium-retaining stimulus,[3] it is tempting to speculate that in cirrhotic and caval dogs, hepatic venous or sinusoidal hypertension, or both represent the source of the sodium-retaining signal. Our laboratory has demonstrated that selective hepatic venous outflow block in dogs is a potent sodium-retaining stimulus in the absence of volume contraction or reduction of cardiac output.[150] Blendis and colleagues[151] and Orloff[5] have published similar data. Earlier data collected by Orloff[5] had suggested that normalizing intrahepatic pressures in dogs with selective hepatic venous occlusion may prevent urinary sodium retention. As reported above, results from our laboratory[97] support the view that intrahepatic hypertension may serve as a source for a sodium-retaining signal.

Preascitic first-phase sodium retention in cirrhosis has at least two components. One component is related to defense of effective blood volume and mediated by a tendency to volume contraction induced by augmented holding capacity of the splanchnic venous circulation and reduction in peripheral vascular resistance (due to arteriovenous fistulas and arteriolar dilation). The other component is unrelated to defense of the plasma volume or any requirements to replenish vascular volume. Data from our laboratory suggest that the activation of low-pressure intrahepatic baroreceptors by rising intrasinusoidal pressure plays an important role in mediating this component of urinary sodium retention. The possibility that salt-retaining humoral factors are also involved has not been completely ruled out.[152]

EFFERENT FACTORS

The sodium retention accompanying ascites formation is largely a tubular event. GFR may be depressed in patients with advanced cirrhosis (even though serum creatinine may be normal) and contribute to sodium retention; nevertheless, in the large majority of patients, urinary sodium retention is considered to be a tubular event. Moreover, some cirrhotic patients with ascites apparently demonstrate a supranormal GFR with markedly elevated renal perfusion.[153] Most radioactive xenon studies, however, particularly in decompensated cirrhotic patients, have demonstrated cortical hypoperfusion[154,154a,154b]; at least some of these studies have been criticized on technical grounds.[155] Moreover, improvement in renal perfusion following surgical shunt procedures to relieve portal venous hypertension or placement of a LeVeen valve is not necessarily associated with an improvement in urinary sodium excretion.[92]

The role of contracted effective blood volume as a cause for sodium retention in advanced liver disease is discussed in chapter 1, whereas the role of derangements of hormonal function (antidiuretic hormone, angiotensin-aldosterone system, and kinins) is considered in chapters 2 and 12–15.

A few comments about the role of estrogens are needed at this point. The liver normally plays a central role in estrogen metabolism by converting androgens to estrogens, interconverting weak and potent androgens, effecting estrogen conjugation, and excreting various sex steroids into the bile.[156] Changes in estrogen metabolism, therefore, may reasonably be expected with progressive deterioration of liver function and may contribute to renal sodium retention.

Increased estrogen levels are not known to alter renal hemodynamics, although available data are difficult to interpret.[157,158] Estrogens are thought to have a direct antinatriuretic effect on the renal tubule, possibly in the proximal tubule, and may have an effect on the liver, increasing production of renin substrate and thus circulating levels of angiotensin II.[157] Nevertheless, the evidence that estrogen-mediated hyperaldosteronism causes sodium retention is controversial. The bulk of evidence at the moment supports an extra-adrenal action for estrogens.[157,158]

The observation that estrogen-induced edema may occur without sustained effects on sodium and water balance suggests involvement of an extrarenal mechanism.[154] One possibility is estrogen-induced alterations in capillary permeability, which have been demonstrated in both humans and apes.[159]

SUMMARY STATEMENT

Progressive alcoholic cirrhosis of the liver is associated with severe disruption of the parenchymal and vascular architecture of the liver, leading eventually to hepatic venous outflow block. Severe fatty infiltration or central venous hyaline sclerosis with postsinusoidal obstruction may also lead to reduced venous outflow in the absence of true cirrhotic changes. The partial obstruction to hepatic venous outflow causes progressive increments in intrahepatic sinusoidal hydrostatic pressure and eventually leads to portal venous hypertension, although this latter phenomenon may be caused in part by the direct influx of hepatic arterial blood due to the appearance of direct arteriovenous communications. Recent evidence from various experimental models[70] suggests that portal hypertension per se is associated with splanchnic hyperemia. The transsinusoidal efflux of fluid within the liver is exquisitely dependent on changes in sinusoidal hydrostatic pressure. The extreme permeability characteristics of the vascular channel, as well as high presinusoidal resistance to flow in the arterial circuit, indicate that perturbations in venous outflow are virtually the sole mechanism whereby hydrostatic pressure within the hepatic sinusoid may become elevated and so cause augmented formation of hepatic lymph. The lymphatic "dead space" is minimized by virtue of efficient removal through regional lymphatics and the thoracic duct and by surface transudation into the peritoneal space. Fluid entering the lymphatics is returned to the venous circulation; fluid entering the peritoneal space is continuously removed by diaphragmatic lymphatics and reabsorption into splanchnic capillaries. As long as hepatic lymph is continuously returned to the venous circulation, there is, at this early stage, no significant effect on systemic hemodynamics or renal function, in particular, the tubular handling of sodium. At this stage, the splanchnic capillaries are probably not involved in forming large amounts of lymph.

As the disease advances, three major consequences of hepatic venous outflow block eventually appear:

1. The rate of formation of hepatic lymph exceeds the ability of the thoracic duct to return lymph to the venous circulation. At that point, transcapsular surface transudation becomes the major mechanism for keeping the hepatic interstitium relatively free of fluid and protein, and large volumes of ascites collect within the peritoneal space.

2. The development of severe portal venous hypertension has several consequences. The holding capacity of the entire mesenteric venous circulation (which holds about 75% of splanchnic blood) increases, necessitating some degree of urinary sodium retention, even if transient, to replenish vascular volume. The increase in intestinal capillary pressure, combined with a declining plasma colloid osmotic pressure, augments the formation of intestinal lymph, which eventually contributes to formation of ascites. A large depot of ascites may be considered, therefore, as an expanded subcompartment of hepatosplanchnic lymph.

3. Portal venous hypertension causes the formation of portacaval collateral channels. To the extent that splanchnic blood flow may increase or to the extent that arteriovenous communications develop, the facilitation of shunting arterial blood to the abdominal vena cava may serve as an additional salt-retaining stimulus.

As hepatic cirrhosis progresses, the permeability characteristics of the liver sinusoid appear to change, as it becomes less permeable to plasma protein. This alteration, together with the effect of declining plasma colloid osmotic pressure at the level of the intestinal capillary, facilitates the accumulation of ascites.

The tendency toward continuous sequestration of ascites within the peritoneal space is opposed by two forces: (1) the tendency toward fluid removal by diaphragmatic lymphatics and peritoneal capillaries and (2) the self-limiting force of increasing peritoneal pressure. The volume of peritoneal fluid increases until intraperitoneal pressure becomes sufficiently elevated to influence favorably fluid reabsorption by the peritoneal membrane. A new steady-state forms: all water and protein fluxes are increased, and ascites formation remains stable, but at the expense of a markedly distended abdomen. Although the accumulation of ascites increases pressure on the portal vein (in the supine position) by an amount equal to the depth of ascites, when the abdomen becomes stretched and the ascites tense, the

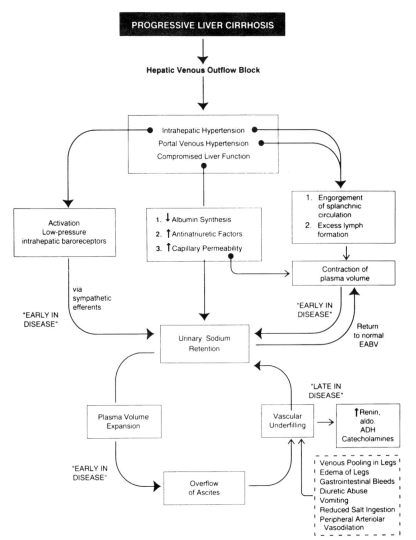

FIGURE 8.9. A summary of factors leading to urinary sodium retention and formation of ascites in progressive cirrhosis of the liver. Note that different salt-retaining signals may predominate in different phases of the disease and that "secondary" events late in the disease (e.g., venous pooling in the lower extremities, diuretic abuse, GI bleeding) may further contract the circulating plasma volume. Once ascites is present urinary sodium retention must defend the plasma volume, and numerous signals become operative upon the renal tubule. Preascitic causes of urinary sodium retention become subsumed by factors triggered by a contracted EABV.

pressure transmitted to the portal vein exceeds the pressure attributed to the layer of ascites. This may lead to severe consequences, such as reduction in venous return and cardiac output and trapping of venous blood in the lower extremities.

As the cirrhotic process disrupts the architectural features of the liver, it also compromises its synthetic and degradative functional properties. As the mechanical and hemodynamic consequences of hepatic venous outflow block set in motion a series of events leading to ascites formation, other disturbances within the liver (perhaps intrahepatic hypertension, altered synthesis of new humoral factors, decreased metabolism of antinatriuretic agents, decreased metabolism of antinatriuretic agents, or other disturbances?) independently signal the renal tubule to retain sodium. According to the vascular overfilling

hypothesis (strongly supported by animal experimental data), such sodium retention, which may occur in the absence of portal venous hypertension, causes plasma volume expansion, and the eventual encounter between the expanded plasma volume and the disturbed Starling forces initiates the formation of ascites and its collection within the peritoneal space. In this view, the accumulation of ascites is secondary to renal sodium retention and, at least initially, not its cause. The initiation of renal sodium retention, at least in canine and rat models of portal cirrhosis, appears to be independent of jaundice, hypoalbuminemia, hyperaldosteronism, decreases in peripheral vascular resistance, or contraction of the nonsplanchnic plasma volume. Thus, a reduction in the so-called effective arterial blood volume does not appear to be the sole initial signal for renal tubular sodium retention; also involved is a signal emanating from the cirrhotic liver.

As the formation of ascites becomes more extensive, involving the intestinal capillaries in addition to the liver; as venous blood is sequestered within the lower extremities; as the patient reduces salt intake (in part because of poor health and in part because of physicians' orders); as diuretics are administered to hasten urinary excretion of sodium; and as bleeding occurs from the gastrointestinal tract, the cirrhotic patient undergoes a tendency to empty or contract the arterial blood volume. The cirrhotic patient now displays vascular underfilling rather than overfilling, and a new set of physiologic disturbances occurs, including hyperaldosteronism, potassium wasting, increased circulating levels of angiotensin and catecholamines, and a tendency to reduced renal cortical perfusion. Replenishment of the contracted vascular space may become difficult because of dietary restriction of salt intake and because hemodynamic events within the splanchnic vascular and lymphatic circulations do not favor mobilization of the ascitic depot. The patient now displays all the features of volume contraction.

Newer evidence, both in human and experimental canine cirrhosis, has suggested that in advanced cirrhosis, even if (1) sequestration of ascites is prevented, (2) portal hypertension is alleviated, and (3) cardiac output, renal perfusion, and levels of plasma renin and aldosterone return to normal, cirrhotic humans and animals still exhibit marked urinary sodium retention. Thus, the maintenance of sodium retention also appears to be due, at least in part, to factors that have nothing to do with vascular underfilling. That is not to say, however, that a diminished effective blood volume plays no role in maintaining urinary sodium retention during advanced cirrhosis with ascites. The cirrhotic patient has ample opportunity to develop underfilling of the arterial blood volume, which in turn maintains a salt-retaining state (see Fig. 8.8). Epstein has reviewed evidence that a compromised effective arterial blood volume, rather than "nonvolume" factors, is the major cause for sodium retention in the cirrhotic patient with ascites (see chapter 1).

A schematic summary of the pathophysiology of ascites formation and factors leading to urinary sodium retention is displayed in Figure 8.9. Pathophysiology of ascites formation is far more complex than a simple disturbance in venous pressure and plasma albumin levels. It also involves derangements in endocrine, renal, cardiovascular, gastrointestinal, and metabolic physiology and encompasses structural alterations to the peritoneal membrane, hepatic capsule, and hepatic sinusoid. The interested reader who wishes a more complete discussion of the overfilling vs. underfilling theories for ascites formation is referred to additional sources.[160–162]

Acknowledgments. The research cited in this chapter was generously supported by grants from the Medical Research Council of Canada and the Kidney Foundation of Canada. Dr. Marvin J. Wexler, Department of Surgery, Royal Victoria Hospital, McGill University, Montreal, collaborated in many of the studies.

REFERENCES

1. Carr BR, Wilson JD: Disorders of the ovary and female reproductive tract. In Wilson JD, Braunwald E, Isselbacher K, et al (eds): Harrison's Principles of Internal Medicine, 12th ed. New York: McGraw Hill, 1991;1776–1795.
2. Mallet Guy P, Devic G, Feroldi J, Desfacques P: Etude experimentale des ascites: Stenoses veineuses post-hépatiques et transposition due foie dans le thorax. Lyon Chir 1954;49:153–165.
3. Levy M, Wexler MJ: Renal sodium retention and ascites formation in dogs with experimental cirrhosis but without portal hypertension or increased splanchnic vascular capacity. J Lab Clin Med 1978 91:520–53.
4. Hyatt RE, Smith JR: The mechanism of ascites: A physiologic appraisal. Am J Med 1954;16:434–448.
5. Orloff MJ: Pathogenesis and surgical treatment of intractable ascites associated with alcoholic cirrhosis. Ann NY Acad Sci 1970;170:213–238.
6. Reynolds TB: Portal hypertension. In Schiff L (ed): Diseases of the Liver, 4th ed. Philadelphia: J.B. Lippincott, 1975;330–367.
7. Levy M: The kidney in liver disease. In Brenner B, Stein JH (eds): Sodium and Water Homeostasis. New York: Churchill Livingstone, 1978;73–116.
8. Witte MH, Witte CL, Dumont AE: Progress in liver disease: Physiological factors involved in the causation of cirrhotic ascites. Gastroenterology 1971;61:742–750.
9. Witte MH: Ascitic, thy lymph runneth over. Gastroenterology 1979;76:1066–1068.
10. Witte CL, Witte MH, Dumont AE, et al: Lymph protein in hepatic cirrhosis and experimental hepatic and portal venous hypertension. Ann Surg 1968;168:567–577.
11. Johnson PC: Effect of venous pressure on mean capillary pressure and vascular resistance in the intestine. Circ Res 1965;16:294–300.
12. Johnson PC, Hanson KM: Capillary filtration in the small intestine of the dog. Circ Res 1966;19:766–773.
13. Johnson PC, Hanson KM: Relation between venous pressure and blood volume in the intestine. Am J Physiol 1963;204:31–34.

14. Wallentin I: Importance of tissue pressure for the fluid equilibrium between the vascular and interstitial compartments in the small intestine. Acta Physiol Scand 1966;689:304–315.

15. Richardson PDI, Granger DN, Mailman D, Kvietys PR: Permeability characteristics of colonic capillaries. Am J Physiol 1980;239(G):300–305.

16. Dumont AE, Witte CL, Witte MH: Protein content of liver lymph in patients with portal hypertension secondary to hepatic cirrhosis. Lymphology 1975;8: 111–113.

17. Nolph KD, Popovich RP, Ghods AJ, Twardowski Z: Determinants of low clearances of small solutes during peritoneal dialysis. Kidney Int 1978;8:111–113.

18. Nolph KD, Miller F, Rubin J, Popovich R: New directions in peritoneal dialysis concepts and applications. Kidney Int 1980;18(Suppl 10):S111–S116.

19. Lautt WW: Hepatic vasculature: A conceptual review. Gastroenterology 1977;73:1163–1169.

20. Lautt WW, Greenway CV: Hepatic circulation in homeostasis. In Epstein M (ed): The Kidney in Liver Disease, 3rd ed. Baltimore: Williams & Wilkins, 1988;244–264.

21. Sherlock S: Diseases of the Liver and Biliary System., 5th ed. Oxford: Blackwell Scientific Publications, 1975;455–444.

22. Markowitz JJ, Archibald J, Downie HG: Experimental Surgery, 5th ed. Baltimore: Williams & Wilkins 1964; 425–427.

23. Freeman S: Recent progress in the physiology and biochemistry of the liver. Med Clin North Am 1953;37: 109–126.

24. Gibson JB, Smith JC: The origin of ascites in experimental cirrhosis in the rat. Am J Pathol 1962;41: 535–547.

25. Morris B: The hepatic and intestinal contributions to the thoracic duct lymph. Q J Exp Physiol 1956;41: 318–325.

26. Greenway CV, Lautt WW: Effects of hepatic venous pressure on transsinusoidal fluid transfer in the liver of the anaesthetized cat. Circ Res 1970;26:697–703.

27. Brauer R, Holloway RJ, Leong GF: Changes in liver function and structure due to experimental passive congestion under controlled hepatic vein pressures. Am J Physiol 1957;197:681–695.

28. Granger DN, Miller T, Allen R, et al: Permselectivity of cat liver blood-lymph barrier to endogenous macromolecules. Gastroenterology 1979;77:103–109.

29. Granger HJ, Laine GA: Consecutive barriers to movement of water and solutes across the liver sinusoids. Physiologist 1980;23:83–85.

30. Laine GA, Hall JT, Laine SH, Granger HJ: Transsinusoidal fluid dynamics in canine liver during venous hypertension. Circ Res 1979;45:317–323.

31. Mitzner W: Hepatic outflow resistance, sinusoid pressure, and the vascular waterfall. Am J Physiol 1974; 227:513–519.

32. Lautt WW, Greenway CV: Hepatic venous compliance and the role of the liver as a blood reservoir. Am J Physiol 1976;231:292–295.

33. Witte MH, Witte CL, Dumont AE: Estimated net transcapillary water and protein flux in th liver and intestine of patients with portal hypertension from hepatic cirrhosis. Gastroenterology 1981;80:265–272.

34. Orloff MJ, Johansen KH: Treatment of Budd-Chiari syndrome by side-to-side portacaval shunt: Experimental and clinical results. Ann Surg 1978;188:494–512.

35. Lautt WW, Greenway CV, Legare DJ, Weisman M: Localization of intrahepatic portal vascular resistance. Am J Physiol 1986;251(G):375–381.

36. Krogh A: The Anatomy and Physiology of Capillaries [preprint]. New York: Hafner Publishing, 1959;63.

37. Goresky CA: The distribution of substances in a flow-limited organ. In Bergner PE (ed): The Liver in Compartments, Pools, and Spaces in Medical Physiology. Springfield, TN: US Atomic Energy Commission, 1967;423.

38. Schaffner FA, Popper H: Capitalization of hepatic sinusoids in man. Gastroenterology 1963;44:239–242.

39. Huet PM, Goresky CA, Lough JO: Cirrhosis of the liver: Functionally a 2-barrier system [abstract]. Presented at the 31st Annual Meeting of the American Association for the Study of Liver Disease. Chicago, 1980;25C.

40. Lieberman FL, Reynolds TB: Plasma volume in cirrhosis of the liver: Its relation to portal hypertension, ascites and renal function. J Clin Invest 1967;46:1297–1308.

41. Tanikawa J: Transperitoneal movement of radioactive colloidal gold in rats made cirrhotic with carbon tetrachloride. Jpn J Gastronenterol 1967;64:1209–1218.

42. Farkouh EF: Effects of internal drainage of thoracic duct on experimental ascites and salt excretion. M.S. Thesis. Department of Experimental Surgery, McGill University, Montreal, 1968.

43. Dumont AE, Mulholland JH: Effect of thoracic duct to esophagus shunt in dogs with vena caval obstruction. Am J Physiol 1963;204:289–292.

44. Zotti E, Lesage A, Bradham R, et al: Prevention and treatment of experimentally induced ascites in dogs by thoracic duct to vein shunt. Surgery 1966;60:28–34.

45. Coodley EL, Matsumoto T: Thoracic duct-subclavian vein anastomosis in management of cirrhotic ascites. Am J Med Sci 1980;279:163–168.

46. Dumont AE: The flow capacity of the thoracic duct venous junction. Am J Med Sci 1975;269–301.

47. Raybuck HE, Weatherford T, Allen L: Lymphatics in genesis of ascites in the rat. Am J Physiol 1960;198: 1207–1210.

48. Barrowman JA: Physiology of the Gastrointestinal Lymphatic System. Cambridge: Cambridge University Press, 1978;229–255.

49. Shear LS, Ching S, Gabuzda GJ: Compartmentalization of ascites and edema in patients with hepatic cirrhosis. N Engl J Med 1970;282:1391–1395.

50. Zink J, Greenway CV: Control of ascites absorption in anaesthetized cats. Gastroenterology 1977;73:1119–1124.

51. Raybuck HE, Allen L, Harms WS: Absorption of serum from the peritoneal cavity. Am J Physiol 1960;199: 1021–1024.

52. Lill SR, Parsons RH, Buhac I: Permeability of the diaphragm and fluid reabsorption from the peritoneal cavity in the rat. Gastroenterology 1979;76:997–1001.

53. Waugh WH: Local factors in the pathogenesis and course of experimental ascites. J Appl Physiol 1958; 13:493–500.

54. Buhac I, Jarmolych J: Histology of the intestinal peritoneum in patients with cirrhosis of the liver and ascites. Am J Dig Dis 1978;5:417–422.

55. Henriksen JH, Stage JG, Schlichting P, Winkler K: Intraperitoneal pressure, ascitic fluid and splanchnic vascular pressures and their role in prevention and formation of ascites. Scand J Clin Lab Invest 1980;40: 493–502.

56. Henriksen JH, Parving HH, Lassen NA, Winkler K: Filtration as the main transport mechanism of protein exchange between plasma and the peritoneal cavity in hepatic cirrhosis. Scand J Clin Lab Invest 1980;40: 503–513.

57. Henriksen JH: Variability of hydrostatic hepatic vein and ascitic fluid pressure and of plasma and ascitic fluid colloid osmotic pressure in patients with liver cirrhosis. Scand J Clin Lab Invest 1980;40:515–522.

58. Epstein M: The peritoneovenous shunt in the management of ascites and the hepatorenal syndrome. Gastroenterology 1982;82:790–799.

59. Fullen WD: Hepatorenal syndrome: Reversal by peritoneovenous shunt. Surgery 1977;82:337–340.

60. Blendis LM, Greig PD, Langer B, et al: The renal and hemodynamic effects of the peritoneovenous shunt for intractable hepatic ascites. Gastroenterology 1979;77: 250–256.

61. Witte CL, Chung YC, Witte MH, et al: Observations on the origin of ascites from experimental extrahepatic portal congestion. Ann Surg 1969;170:1002–1015.

62. Cohn JN: Renal hemodynamic alterations in liver disease. In Suki WW, Eknoyan G (eds): The Kidney in Systemic Disease. New York: John Wiley & Sons, 1976;223–234.

63. Groszmann RJ, Fravetz D, Parysow O: Intrahepatic arteriovenous shunting in cirrhosis of the liver. Gastroenterology 1977;73:201–204.

64. Cohn EM: Ascites: Pathogenesis and differential diagnosis. In Bockus HL (ed): Gastroenterology, 3rd ed, vol 4. Philadelphia: W.B. Saunders, 1976;48–56.

65. Lacroix E, Leusen I: La circulation hépatique et splanchnique. J Physiol (Paris) 1965;57:115–216.

66. Lebrec D, Kotclanski B, Cohn JN: Splanchnic hemodynamic factors in cirrhosis with refractory ascites. J Lab Clin Med 1979;93:301–309.

67. Kotelanski B, Groszmann R, Cohn JN: Circulation times in the splanchnic and hepatic beds in alcoholic liver disease. Gastroenterology 1972;63:102–111.

68. Levy M: Sodium retention and ascites formation in dogs with experimental portal cirrhosis. Am J Physiol 1977;233(F):572–585.

69. Bosch J, Enriques R, Groszmann RJ, et al: Chronic bile duct ligation in the dog: Hemodynamic characterization of a portal hypertension model. Hepatology 1983;3: 1002–1007.

70. Vorobioff J, Bredfeldt JE, Groszmann RJ: Hyperdynamic circulation in portal hypertensive rat model: A primary factor for maintenance of chronic portal hypertension. Am J Physiol 1983;244(G):52–57.

71. Lopez C, Jimenez W, Arroyo W, et al: Temporal relationship between the decrease in arterial pressure and sodium retention in conscious spontaneously hypertensive rats with carbon tetrachloride-induced cirrhosis. Hepatology 1991;13:585–589.

72. Columbato LA, Albillos A, Groszmann RJ: Temporal relationship of peripheral vasodilatation plasma volume expansion and the hyperdynamic circulatory state in portal-hypertensive rats. Hepatology 1992; 15:323–328.

73. Ingles AC, Hernandez I, Garcia-Estan J, et al: Increased total vascular capacity in conscious cirrhotic rats. Gastroenterology 1992;103:275–281.

74. Wong F, Massie D, Coluan J, Dudley F: Glomerular hyperfiltration in patients with well-compensated alcoholic cirrhosis. Gastroenterology 1993;104:884–889.

75. Pizcueta P, Piqué JM, Fernandez M, et al: Modulation of the hyperdynamic circulation of cirrhotic rats by nitric oxide inhibition. Gastroenterology 1992;103: 1909–1915.

76. Benoit JN, Granger DN: Splanchnic hemodynamics in chronic portal hypertension. Semin Liver Dis 1986; 6:287–298.

77. Gould L, Shariff M, Zahir M, Dilieto M: Cardiac hemodynamics in alcoholic patients with chronic liver disease and a presystolic gallop. J Clin Invest 1969; 48:860–864.

78. Summerskill WHJ, Baldus WP: Ascites. In Schiff L (eds): Diseases of the Liver, 4th ed. Philadelphia: J.B. Lippincott, 1975;424–444.

79. Patek AJ, Mankin H, Colcher H, et al: Effects of intravenous injection of concentrated human serum albumin upon blood plasma ascites and renal function in 3 patients with cirrhosis of the liver. J Clin Invest 1948; 27:135–144.

80. Lieberman FL, Ito S, Reynolds TB: Effective plasma volume in cirrhosis with ascites: Evidence that a decreased volume does not account for renal sodium retention, a spontaneous reduction in glomerular filtration rate (GFR), and a fall in GFR during drug-induced diuresis. J Clin Invest 1969;48:975–981.

81. Lieber man FL, Denison EK, Reynolds TB: The relationship of plasma volume, portal hypertension, ascites and renal sodium in cirrhosis: The "overflow" theory of ascites formation. Ann NY Acad Sci 1970;170:202–206.

82. Madden JW, Gertman PM, Peacock EE: Dimethylnitrosamine induced hepatic cirrhosis: A new canine model of an ancient human disease. Surgery 1970;68: 260–268.

83. Lopez-Novoa JM, Rengel MA, Hernando L: Dynamics of ascites formation in rats with experimental cirrhosis. Am J Physiol 1980;238(F):353–357.

84. Levy M: Sodium retention and ascites formation in dogs with experimental portal cirrhosis. Am J Physiol 1977;233(F):572–585.

85. Levy M, Allotey JBK: Temporal relationships between urinary salt retention and altered systemic hemodynamics in dogs with experimental cirrhosis. J Lab Clin Med 1978;92:560–569.

86. Levy M, Wexler MJ, McCaffrey C: Sodium retention in dogs with experimental cirrhosis following removal of ascites by continuous peritoneovenous shunting. J Lab Clin Med 1979;94:933–946.

87. Davis JO, Ball WC: Effects of a body cast on aldosterone and sodium excretion in dogs with experimental ascites. Am J Physiol 1958;192:538–542.

88. Bergstrund I, Ekman C, Kohler R: Inferior vena caval obstruction in hepatic cirrhosis. Acta Radiol 1964;2:1–8.

89. Davis JO, Holman JE, Carpenter CC, et al: An extra-adrenal factor essential for chronic renal retention in presence of increased sodium retaining hormone. Circ Res 1964;14:17–31.

90. Papper S, Rosenbaum JD: Abnormalities in the excretion of water and sodium in "compensated" cirrhosis of the liver. J Lab Clin Med 1952;40:523–530.

91. Ansley JD, Bethel RA, Bowen PA, Warren WD: Effect of peritoneovenous shunting with the LeVeen valve on ascites, renal function and coagulation in six patients with intractable ascites. Surgery 1978;83:181–187.

92. Greig PD, Blendis LM, Langer B, et al: Renal and hemodynamic effects of the peritoneovenous shunt. II. Long term effects. Gastroenterology 1981;80:119–125.

93. Bernardi M, Trevisani F, Santini R, et al: Aldosterone related blood volume expansion in cirrhosis before and during the early phase of ascites formation. Gut 1983;24:761–766.

94. Wilkinson SP, Williams R: Renin-angiotensin-aldosterone system in cirrhosis. Gut 1980;21:545–554.

95. Wernze H, Speck HJ, Muller G: Studies on the activity of the renin-angiotensin-aldosterone system in patients with cirrhosis of the liver. Klin Wochenschr 1978;56:389–397.

96. Bichet DG, Van Putten VJ, Schrier RW: Potential role of increased sympathetic activity in impaired sodium and water excretion in cirrhosis. N Engl J Med 1982;307:1552–1557.

97. Unikowsky B, Wexler MJ, Levy M: Dogs with experimental cirrhosis of the liver but without intrahepatic hypertension do not retain sodium or form ascites. J Clin Invest 1983;72:1594–1604.

98. Kostreva DR, Castaner A, Kampine JP: Reflex effects of hepatic baroreceptors on renal and cardiac sympathetic nerve activity. Am J Physiol 1980;238(R):390–394.

99. Andrews WHH, Palmer JF: Afferent nervous discharges from the canine liver. Q J Exp Physiol 1967;52:964–970.

100. Niijima A: Afferent discharges from venous pressoreceptors in liver. Am J Physiol 1977;232:76–81.

101. Dibona GV, Sawin LL: Role of the renal nerves in renal adaptation to dietary sodium restriction. Am J Physiol 183;245(F):322–328.

102. DeBold AG, Borenstein HB, Veress AT, et al: A rapid and potent natriuretic response to intravenous injection of atrial myocardial extract in rats. Life 1981;28:89–94.

103. Moreno AM, Burchell AR: Respiratory regulation of splanchnic and systemic venous return in normal subjects and in patients with hepatic cirrhosis. Surg Gynecol Obstet 1982;15:257–267.

104. Levy M, Wexler MJ: Sodium excretion in dogs with low grade caval constriction: Role of hepatic nerves. Am J Physiol 1987;253(F):672–678.

105. Levy M, Wexler MJ: Hepatic denervation alters first-phase urinary sodium excretion in dogs with cirrhosis. Am J Physiol 1987;253(F):664–671.

106. Levy M, Wexler MJ: Salt and water balance in liver disease. Hosp Pract 1984;19:57–71.

107. Decaux G: Uric acid and urea clearance in cirrhosis secondary to increased "effective vascular volume." Am J Med 1982;73:328–334.

108. Wensing G, Sabra R, Branch RA: The onset of sodium retention in experimental cirrhosis in rats is related to a critical threshold of liver function. Hepatology 1990;11:779–786.

109. Wensing G, Sabra R, Branch RA: Renal and systemic hemodynamics in experimental cirrhosis in rats: Relation to hepatic function. Hepatology 1990;12:13–19.

110. Wood LJ, Massie D, Mclean AJ, Dudley FJ: Renal sodium retention in cirrhosis: Tubular site and relation to hepatic dysfunction. Hepatology 1988;8:831–836.

111. Rocco VK, Ware AJ: Cirrhotic ascites. Ann Intern Med 1986;105:573–585.

112. Schrier RW, Arroyo V, Bernardi M, et al: Peripheral arterial vasodilation hypothesis: A proposal for the initiation of renal sodium and water retention in cirrhosis. Hepatology 1988;5:1151–1157.

113. Norris SM, Buell JC, Kurtzman NA: The pathophysiology of cirrhotic edema: A reexamination of the "underfilling" and "overflow" hypothesis. Semin Nephrol 1987;7:99–105.

113a. Papper S, Vaamonde CA: The kidney in liver disease. In Strauss MB, Welt LG (eds): Diseases of the Kidney, 2nd ed. Boston: Little, Brown, 1971;1139–1153.

114. Schrier RW: Pathogenesis of sodium and water retention in high-output and low-output cardiac failure, nephrotic syndrome cirrhosis and pregnancy. Part I. N Engl J Med 1988;319:1065–1072.

115. Schrier RW: Pathogenesis of sodium and water retention in high-output and low-output cardiac failure, nephrotic syndrome cirrhosis and pregnancy. Part II. N Engl J Med 1988;319:1127–1134.

116. Kowalski, Abelmann WH: The cardiac output at rest in Laennec's cirrhosis. J Clin Invest 1953;32:1025–1032.

117. Murray JF, Dawson AM, Sherlock S: Circulatory changes in chronic liver disease. Am J Med 1958;24:358–364.

118. Kontos HA, Shapiro W, Mauck HP, Patterson JL: General and regional circulatory alterations in cirrhosis of the liver. Am J Med 1964;37:526–534.

119. Lee SS, Bomzon A: The heart in liver disease. In Bomzon A, Blendis LM (eds): Cardiovascular Complications of Liver Disease. Boca Raton, FL: CRC Press, 1990;81–102.

120. Pagani M, Watner SF, Braunwald E: Hemodynamic effects of intravenous sodium nitroprusside in the conscious dog. Circulation 1978;57:144–157.

121. Bosch J, Arroyo V, Betriu A, et al: Hepatic hemodynamics and the renin-angiotensin-aldosterone system in cirrhosis. Gastroenterology 1980;78:92–99.

122. Linas SL, Anderson RJ, Guggenheim SJ, et al: Role of vasopressin in impaired water excretion in conscious rats with experimental cirrhosis. Kidney Int 1981;20:173–180.

123. Caramelo C, Fernandez-Munoz D, Santos JC, et al: Effect of volume expansion on hemodynamics, capillary permeability and renal function in conscious cirrhotic rats. Hepatology 1986;6:129–134.

124. Fernandez-Munoz D, Caramelo C, Santos JC, et al: Systemic and splanchnic hemodynamics in conscious rats with experimental cirrhosis without ascites. Am J Physiol 1985;249:G236–G 240.

125. Sarin S, Mosca P, Sabba C, Groszman RJ: Hyperdynamic circulation in a chronic murine schistosomiasis model of portal hypertension. Hepatology 1991;13:581–584.

126. Vorobioff J, Bredfeldt JE, Groszmann RJ: Increased blood flow through the portal system in cirrhotic rats. Gastroenterology 1984;87:1120–1126.

127. Levy M, Maher E, Wexler MJ: Euvolemic cirrhotic dogs in sodium balance maintain normal systemic hemodynamics. Can J Physiol Pharmacol 1988;66:80–83.

128. Albillos A, Colombato LA, Groszmann RJ: Vasodilatation and sodium retention in prehepatic portal hypertension. Gastroenterology 1992;102:931–935.

129. Groszmann RJ, Vorobioff J, Riley E: Measurement of splanchnic hemodynamics in portal-hypertensive rats: Application of γ-labeled microspheres. Am J Physiol 1982;242G:156–160.

130. Chojkier M, Groszman RJ: Measurement of portal systemic shunting in the rat by rising γ-labeled microspheres. Am J Physiol 1981;240:G321–375.

131. Sikuler E, Kravetz D, Groszmann RJ: Evolution of portal hypertension and mechanisms involved in its maintenance in a rat model. Am J Physiol 1985;248:G618–G625.

131a. Moriura S, Nimura S, Kato M, et al: Effects of acute portal hypertension by portal venous stenosis on systemic hemodynamics in dogs. Eur Surg Res 1990;22:113–119.

132. Genecin P, Polio J, Groszmann RJ: Na+ restriction blunts expansion of plasma volume and ameliorates hyperdynamic circulation in portal hypertension. Am J Physiol 1990;259:G298–G503.

133. Prather JW, Taylor AE, Guyton AC: Effect of blood volume, mean circulatory pressure and stress relaxation on cardiac output. Am J Physiol 1969;216:467–472.

134. Epstein M: Renal effects of head-out water immersion in humans: A 15-yr update. Physiol Rev 1992;72:563–621.

134a. Epstein M, Pins DS, Schneider N, Levinson R: Determinants of deranged sodium and water homeostasis in decompensated cirrhosis. J Lab Clin Med 1976;87:822–839.

134b. Epstein M, Levinson R, Sancho J, et al: Characterization of the renin-aldosterone system in decompensated cirrhosis. Circ Res 1877;41:818–829.

135. Bichet DG, Groves BM, Schrier RW: Mechanisms of improvements of water and sodium excretion by immersion in decompensated cirrhotic patients. Kidney Int 1983;24:788–794.

136. Nicholls KM, Shapiro MD, Groves BS, Schrier RW: Factors determining renal response to water immersion in nonexcretor cirrhotic patients. Kidney Int 1986;30:417–421.

137. Shapiro MD, Nicholls KM, Groves BM, et al: Interrelationship between cardiac output and vascular resistance as determinants of effective arterial blood volume in cirrhotic patients. Kidney Int 1985;28:266–211.

138. Warner LC, Leung WM, Campbell P, et al: Role of resistance to atrial natriuretic peptide in the pathogenesis of sodium retention in hepatic cirrhosis. In Brenner BM, Laragh JH (eds): Progress in Atrial Peptide Research, vol. 3. New York: Raven Press, 1989;185–204.

139. Skorecki KL, Leung WM, Campbell P, et al: Role of atrial natriuretic peptide in the natriuretic response to central volume expansion induced by head-out immersion in sodium-retaining cirrhotic subjects. Am J Med 1988;85:375–382.

140. Bichet DG, Van Putten VJ, Schrier RW: Potential role of increased sympathetic activity in impaired sodium and water excretion in cirrhosis. N Engl J Med 1982;307:1522–1557.

141. Rector WmG, Hossack KF: Pathogenesis of sodium retention complicating cirrhosis: Is there room for diminished "effective" arterial blood volume? Gastroenterology 1988;95:1658–1662.

142. Lewis FW, Adair O, Rector WG Jr: Arterial vasodilation is not the cause of increased cardiac input in cirrhosis. Gastroenterology 1992;102:1024–1029.

143. Rector WF, Robertson A, Lewis FW: Arterial underfilling does not cause sodium retention in cirrhosis. Am J Med 1993;95:286–295.

144. Henriksen JH, Bendsten F, Sorensen TIA, et al: Reduced central blood volume in cirrhosis. Gastroenterology 1989;97:1506–1513.

145. Bernardi M, DiMarco C, Trevisani F, et al: Hemodynamic status of preascitic cirrhosis: An evaluation under steady state conditions and after postural change. Hepatology 1992;16:341–346.

146. Bernardi M, DiMarco C, Trevisani F, et al: Renal sodium retention during upright posture in preascitic cirrhosis. GAstroenterology 1993;105:188–193.

146a. Levy M, Maher E: Unpublished observations.

147. Bernardi M: Hyperdynamic circulation in cirrhosis. Physiology or pathophysiology? [letter to the editor]. Gastroenterology 1993;104:1579–1580.

148. Henderson JM, Mackay GJ, Hooks M, et al: High cardiac output of advanced liver disease persists after orthotopic liver transplantation. Hepatology 1992;15:258–262.

149. Wong F, Liu P, Tobe S, et al: Central blood volume in cirrhosis: Measurement by radionuclide angiography [abstract]. Hepatology 1993;18:101A.

150. Levy M: Renal function in dogs with acute selective hepatic venous outflow block. Am J Physiol 1974;227:1074–1083.

151. Campbell V, Greig P, Cranford J, et al: Canine models of water and salt retention in acute portal hypertension: Assessment of hemodynamic stability [abstract]. Clin Res 1980;28:677.

152. Epstein M: The sodium retention of cirrhosis: A reappraisal. Hepatology 1986;6:312–315.

153. Vaamonde CA, Papper S (eds): Diseases of the Kidney, 3rd ed. Boston: Little, Brown, 1979;1289–1320.

154. Kew MC, Brunt PW, Varma RR, et al: Renal and intrarenal blood flow in cirrhosis of the liver. Lancet 1971;2:504–510.

154a. Epstein M, Berk DP, Hollenberg NK, et al: Renal failure in the patient with cirrhosis: The role of active vasoconstriction. Am J Med 1970;49:175–184.

154b. Epstein M, Schneider N, Befeler B: Relationships of systemic and intrarenal hemodynamics in cirrhosis. J Lab Clin Med 1977;89:1175–1187.

155. Hollenberg NK, Mangel R, Fung HY: Assessment of intrarenal perfusion with radioxenon: A critical review of analytical factors and their implications in man. Semin Nucl Med 1970;6:193–216.

156. Van Thiele DH, Lester R: Sex and alcohol. N Engl J Med 1974;291:251–253.

157. Christy NP, Shaver JC: Estrogens and kidney. Kidney Int 1974;6:366–376.

158. Katz AI, Lindheimer MD: Actions of hormones on the kidney. Annu Rev Physiol 1977;39:97–134.

159. Akroyd OE, Zuckerman S: Factors in sexual skin edema. J Physiol 1938;94:13–25.

160. Better OS, Shrier RW: Disturbed volume homeostasis in patients with cirrhosis of the liver. Kidney Int 1983; 23:303–311.

161. Rocco VK, Ware AJ: Cirrhotic ascites. Ann Intern Med 1986;105:573–585.

162. Rector WMG Jr: Sodium retention and ascites formation. In Rector WMG Jr (ed): Complications of Chronic Liver Disease. St. Louis: Mosby, 1992;68–84.

Chapter 9

HEPATIC CIRCULATION IN HOMEOSTASIS

W. WAYNE LAUTT, Ph.D.
CLIVE V. GREENWAY, M.D.

Overview
Microvasculature
Hepatic Blood Flow
  Hepatic Arterial Regulation
  Regulation of Portal Venous Pressure
  Active and Passive Effects on Hepatic Venous
    Resistance
  Calculation of Hepatic Vascular Resistance

Hepatic Blood Volume
  Hepatic Blood Volume in Liver Disease
Hepatic Fluid Exchange
  Fluid Exchange in Cirrhosis
Summary

The vascular bed of the liver is unique in virtually every aspect of its functions. The classical definitions of vascular functions are the resistance functions, determining total flow and distribution of flows; the capacitance (blood volume reservoir) functions; and the exchange functions, which rely primarily on diffusion of substances between the plasma and parenchymal cells. An additional important function of the vessels that offer resistance to portal blood flow and to blood flow exiting the liver is the regulation of intrahepatic and splanchnic venous pressures. Understanding of these vascular functions in the liver has recently advanced considerably. All have major implications for cardiovascular homeostasis and renal function, and all are altered in the diseased liver.

The splanchnic vascular bed accounts for 25% of cardiac output and includes all of the abdominal organs except the kidney. Whereas the renal role in cardiovascular homeostasis is long-term, the hepatic vascular roles are much more acutely associated with immediate buffering of disturbances both local (within the splanchnic system) and systemic. The liver operates in several ways to maintain total hepatic blood flow and cardiac venous return at a constant level despite various fluxes in flows of the many vascular beds that drain into the portal vein and thence to the liver. In addition to the direct vascular buffering roles played by the liver, the hepatic sensory system is unusually rich. Pressure, temperature, perhaps flow, chemical composition (sodium, potassium, long-chain fatty acids, and glucose), and osmotic and oncotic pressure of hepatic blood are sensed by afferent nerves for use in poorly understood ways.

This chapter provides a conceptual overview of the normal hepatic vascular bed, followed by discussion of alterations in the cirrhotic liver. The discussion of the diseased circulation will be as conceptual as possible; data are discussed only insofar as they allow interpretation or speculation with reference to known normal physiologic processes. Summarizing a review of alcoholic liver disease, Orrego et al.[1] confessed, "It is clear that we have not been able to transform most of the information available into knowledge." A recent major review of normal hepatic vasculature should be consulted for the detailed references on which most of the following discussion is based.[2]

OVERVIEW

The liver sits astride a massive river of portal venous blood that flows out of the highlands of the intestine (60%), stomach (20%), spleen (10%), and pancreas (10%), carrying blood of low oxygenation but rich in nutrients and ingested toxins. A major proportion (35–100%) of hepatic oxygen supply is derived from the hepatic artery, which supplies about 25% of total hepatic blood flow. Hepatic blood flow accounts for about 25% of cardiac output.

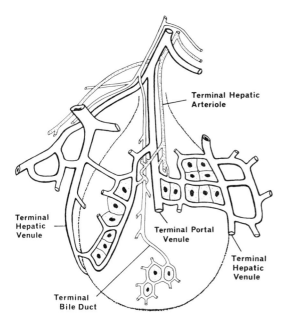

Terminal Hepatic
Arteriole

Terminal
Hepatic
Venule

Terminal Portal
Venule

Terminal
Hepatic
Venule

Terminal
Bile Duct

FIGURE 9.1. The acinus is the functional unit of the liver.[3] There are about 100,000 acini per human liver; each is about 2 mm in diameter. Acini cluster like grapes at the end of vascular stalks comprising the terminal branches of portal veins, hepatic arteries, and bile ducts. Blood flows into the center (zone 1) of the acinus and outward to drain into terminal venules at the periphery (zone 3). Zone 1 is well oxygenated and rich in nutrients, hormones, and toxins. Because flow in adjacent sinusoids is concurrent, zone 3 has the lowest oxygenation, and short-circuiting of substances across the vascular system does not occur nor do vasoactive substances in zone 3 diffuse back upstream to zone 1, where the hepatic arterial resistance vessels exist. Based on the acinar concept of Rappaport.[3]

Hepatic blood volume is unusually large, accounting for about 30% of liver volume and representing 12% of the total blood volume of the body. The prehepatic splanchnic organs contain another 21% of the blood volume of the body. Thus, the entire vascular bed, whose venous pressure is regulated by the liver, represents a large and mobile blood reservoir.

Portal venous pressure is 6–10 mmHg, which is not significantly higher than hepatic sinusoidal pressure. Virtually all of the pressure drop from the portal vein to the vena cava occurs across sphincterlike areas in the hepatic veins. Resistance sites in the presinusoidal portal venules and postsinusoidal hepatic veins respond to active and passive stimuli. The liver is the most vascular of any organ, with blood flowing on two sides of most

parenchymal cells, and net vascular resistance to flow is insignificant except at localized control points at the inlet and outlet.

MICROVASCULATURE

The portal vein and hepatic artery subdivide within the liver, and the terminal branches of each vessel travel in intimate contact to the center of each of the 100,000 hepatic functional units, the acini (Fig. 9.1). The acinus, a cluster of parenchymal cells about 2 mm in diameter, is supplied with portal and arterial blood that enters into the central zone (Rappaport's zone 1), where it is well mixed.[3]

Blood flows outward to the periphery of the acinus with concurrent flow in adjacent sinusoids. All exit points from terminal hepatic venules are at the periphery (zone 3) of the acinus; diffusion from zone 3 to zone 1 is not possible. This vascular arrangement allows the activity of the parenchymal cells to develop strong gradients from zone 1 to 3, including the ability to extract selected compounds with virtually 100% efficiency. Blood passing the full length of a sinusoid (220–480 μm) is sequentially distributed to approximately 20 hepatocytes.[4] There is substantial evidence that the microvascular environment of the hepatocyte regulates hepatocyte function. Heterogeneity of hepatic enzyme distribution across the acinus has been reviewed,[5–7] and the classification of chemically induced injury has been discussed relative to the acinus and its zones.[8]

The terminal portal venule and arteriole travel to the center of the acinus enclosed within a limiting plate of parenchymal cells. Within the conduit formed by the limiting plate is a fluid space, the space of Mall, and terminal bile ductules and lymph vessels taking fluids away from the acinus. Within this space, the hepatic arteriole breaks up into a network of arterioles that lies in contact with the portal venule and bile ductule. This region is discussed later in relation to blood flow regulation.

Blood flow distribution within the liver shows considerably more heterogeneity than early studies had suggested. Heterogeneity of flow is most obvious with the smallest areas of comparison. Individual sinusoids show episodic flow varying from swift passage of red blood cells to the opposite extreme of fully stagnant sinusoids. At the grossest level, flow distribution to individual entire lobes also shows some degree of dynamic heterogeneity which may be affected by the hydrostatic pressures induced by gravity, specific microvascular anatomic differences between the surface and deeper parts of the liver, and various active stimuli. The significant heterogeneity shown for local flow on immediately adjacent portions of the liver surface indicates that extreme caution is needed when using small areas of flow determination to reflect changes in the entire organ.[8a] The functional implications of the gross levels of heterogeneity are not clear. However, heterogeneity does not appear to be significantly increased in studies of large animals under in vivo conditions, even under conditions of low flow, norepinephrine (NE) infusion, sympathetic nerve stimulation, or raised venous pressure.[9–11] The surface few millimeters of the liver receive approximately 25% more arterial flow than deeper tissues. Portal flow distribution within liver lobes most often shows a pattern of highest flow to the top, tapering to lowest flow to the bottom (the dorsal side on animals placed on a surgical table). This degree of heterogeneity of perfusion appears to be controlled by dynamic and multiple interacting forces.[8a]

If portal blood flow in one area is reduced, arterial flow is elevated. Both blood supplies are well mixed in zone 1, and substances are equally well extracted if delivered via either the arterial or portal circuit.[12,13] Marked heterogeneity of tissue perfusion, however, is quite common in isolated liver preparations, and pharmacokinetic studies of such preparations must be interpreted with caution. For example, increasing hepatic extraction seen with increased blood flow may represent merely increased sinusoidal perfusion of sinusoids previously underperfused. In the normal liver it seems likely that one function of the hepatic arterial buffer response (see below) is to maintain homogeneity of liver perfusion. If local portal venous stasis occurs, the hepatic artery within that acinus should dilate to increase the higher pressure arterial input, thereby flushing the sinusoids and restoring sinusoidal blood flow.

The hepatocytes are arranged in a syncytium of plates of a single cell in thickness. The rich sinusoidal network forms multiple interconnecting lacunae that flood the plates of parenchymal cells on both sides. The sinusoidal endothelial cells were previously believed to contain large pores that offered no resistance to passage of plasma constituents. It has become clear recently that these large pores were artifacts of preparation, and it now appears that the sinusoidal cells contain fenestrae of 100–300 Å diameter.[14] The fenestrae are capable of sieving albumin.[14] Thus contact with parenchymal cells is highly likely to be altered for any compounds bound to albumin and lipoprotein by changes in fenestrae diameter. Morphologic studies suggest that the fenestrations are reduced in size by norepinephrine and serotonin[15] and increased by elevated venous pressure[14,16] and acute or chronic alcohol exposure.[17]

HEPATIC BLOOD FLOW

The portal vein supplies the majority of hepatic blood flow; however, the liver is unable to regulate portal blood flow. Intrahepatic vascular resistance may be elevated acutely to the extent that portal pressure rises to 2–3 times normal levels without altering portal flow. Portal flow undergoes wide variation depending on the activities of the organism. Because the liver cannot regulate portal flow, the only control of flow within the liver is via the hepatic artery.

Hepatic Arterial Regulation

Analogy, intuition, and indirect observation suggested that the hepatic artery was regulated by the metabolic activity of the liver cell mass. No direct data support this view, and several lines of evidence strongly indicate that this view is untenable.[18] Alteration of hepatic oxygen supply, attained by isovolemic hemodilution, led to reduced oxygen content in the inflow and outflow vessels with no dilation of the hepatic artery. Similarly, stimulation of hepatic enzymes with dinitrophenol or inhibition with SKF 525A (2-diethyl-aminoethyl 2,2-diphenylvalerate hydrochloride) did not lead to the expected vascular effects on the hepatic artery. If oxygen demand was increased, the liver simply extracted more oxygen from the blood to maintain oxygen uptake. Even in a situation such as chronic alcohol exposure, in which oxygen uptake is massively increased, the hepatic artery does not show vasodilation.[19]

Coincidental observation of increased liver metabolism and increased arterial flow is not proof of metabolic control over the hepatic artery. For example, these dual effects of bile salts have been clearly demonstrated to be separate and independent actions.[20] As discussed earlier, the unidirectional flow of the hepatic acinus precludes diffusion of compounds from the sinusoidal

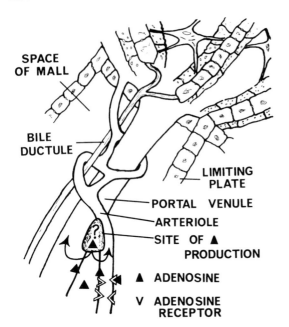

SPACE
OF MALL

BILE
DUCTULE

LIMITING
PLATE

PORTAL VENULE

ARTERIOLE

SITE OF ▲
PRODUCTION

▲ ADENOSINE

V ADENOSINE
RECEPTOR

FIGURE 9.2 Adenosine washout hypothesis. The area shown is the portal triad, which represents the vascular stalk leading into the center of each acinus. The terminal branches of the hepatic arteriole, portal venule, and bile ductule lie within an enclosed space delimited by a limiting plate of cells. The fluid surrounding these vessels and contained within the limiting plate comprises the space of Mall. The data are consistent with the hypothesis that adenosine is continuously secreted into the space of Mall (independent of general parenchymal cell oxygen supply or demand) and that the local concentration of adenosine determines the tone of the hepatic artery. The adenosine can be washed away into the portal vein and hepatic arterial flow. The hepatic arterial buffer response is accounted for, for example, by reduced portal blood flow washing away less adensoine and accumulated adenosine leading to dilation of the hepatic artery.[21] The mechanism of classic autoregulation is explained by the same hypothesis; for example, increased arterial blood flow and a subsequent washout of adenosine. The reduced adenosine concentration accounts for the resultant arterial constriction.[29] (From Lautt WW, et al: Adenosine as putative regulator of hepatic arterial flow (the buffer response). Am J Physiol 1985;248:H331–H338, with permission.)

blood to the hepatic arterial resistance vessels upstream; therefore, metabolites released by parenchymal cells cannot regulate the hepatic artery.

If the metabolic activity of the hepatic parenchymal cells does not directly control hepatic arterial flow, what does regulate arterial flow?

The hepatic artery is regulated by both intrinsic and extrinsic factors. The intrinsic regulation consists of two known mechanisms, both of which are explained by a final common pathway, adenosine concentration. This regulatory mechanism represents the first report of flow-dependent flow regulation. The first form of intrinsic regulation is the classic arterial autoregulation. As the arterial pressure rises, the hepatic artery responds by constricting, and this response previously was viewed as myogenic in origin. The second form of intrinsic regulation is the hepatic arterial buffer response (HABR).[21] If portal blood flow is reduced, the hepatic artery dilates; if portal flow increases, the hepatic artery constricts.

Hepatic Arterial Buffer Response. HABR has been referred to by different terms, such as the reciprocal flow or reciprocal hemodynamic relationship. Evidence indicates, however, that there is no reciprocity in the responses; that is, changes in the hepatic arterial perfusion do not alter portal vascular flow[22] or resistance.[23] Apparent changes in portal resistance in response to hepatic arterial flow changes[24] were due to incorrect methods of calculating resistance based on the assumption that intrahepatic resistance is presinusoidal rather than postsinusoidal (see below). Previous hypotheses have been evaluated,[21,22] and our current view is that both forms of intrinsic regulation can be accounted for by the adenosine washout hypothesis.[21]

This hypothesis (Fig. 9.2) states that adenosine is released, at a constant rate, into fluid in the space of Mall surrounding the hepatic arterial resistance vessels and portal venules. The space of Mall is contained within a limiting plate that separates it from other fluids. The concentration of adenosine is regulated by washout into the portal vein and hepatic artery. If portal blood flow is reduced, less adenosine is washed away from the space of Mall, and the elevation in adenosine levels leads to dilation of the hepatic artery with a subsequent increase in hepatic arterial flow. This flow-dependent regulation does not depend on the oxygen supply. Several criteria support the hypothesis that adenosine mediates the buffer response:

1. Adenosine produces dilation of the hepatic artery. Hepatic arterial conductance can be almost tripled by adenosine.[25]

2. In order for portal blood flow to wash away adenosine from the area of the arterial resistance vessels, portal blood must have access to the

hepatic arterial resistance vessels. Vasoactive compounds infused into the portal vein have one-half to one-third the effect of the same dose infused directly into the hepatic artery. This has been shown for a wide range of direct acting vasoactive substances including adenosine and bile salts.[2,24]

3. Dipyridamole, an adenosine uptake antagonist, potentiates dilation induced by exogenous adenosine effects as well as the magnitude of the hepatic arterial buffer response.[26]

4. Pharmacologic antagonists of adenosine also produce competitive blockade of the buffer response. Several adenosine antagonists have been used, but in our experience 8-phenyltheophylline has proved the most useful. This selective, competitive antagonist results in parallel inhibition of the arterial buffer response and the vasodilator effects of infused adenosine.[25] Complete dose-response curves of the antagonistic effect of 8-phenyltheophylline on the hepatic arterial buffer response indicate that this selective antagonist can eliminate the buffer response completely. It is a common observation with in vivo pharmacologic studies that endogenously released compounds are less effectively antagonized than exogenously mediated substances. This is also seen with the buffer response in that the dose of 8-phenyltheophylline required to block 50% of the maximal vasodilator effect of exogenous adenosine is 0.3 mg/kg ,whereas the ID_{50} dose for the buffer response is 1.3 mg/kg. This difference in ability to block exogenous vs. endogenous compounds must be taken into consideration in mechanistic studies. Buffer responses have also been demonstrated in the human liver, and the presence of an effective buffer response following liver transplantation has been suggested to be a valuable index of viability of the transplant.[27] The mechanism and putative roles of the hepatic arterial buffer response recently have been reviewed.[21,28]

Hepatic Arterial Autoregulation. The mechanism of autoregulation is similar to that for the buffer response in that adenosine can also be washed away from the space of Mall by arterial blood. When arterial blood pressure is increased, arterial blood flow is increased and leads to increased washout of adenosine and constriction of the hepatic artery. Although autoregulation is not powerful in the hepatic artery, it can be antagonized in a dose-related manner by administration of a selective, competitive antagonist of adenosine.[29]

Impact and Roles of Hepatic Arterial Regulation. Constancy of hepatic blood flow is important for at least two major homeostatic reasons:

1. Hepatic clearance of many compounds, including hormones such as aldosterone and corticosterone,[30,31] is blood flow-dependent. If a hormone level is to be rapidly adjustable by altered output from the endocrine gland, rapid turnover of the hormone must occur. It is important that the high catabolic rate be maintained as constant as possible so that the hormone levels can be accurately controlled by glandular output. If hepatic blood flow were not prevented from rapid, transient changes secondary to similar changes in the portal venous flow, endocrine homeostasis would be imperiled.

2. The effect of altered hepatic blood volume on cardiovascular status is related to the hepatic arterial buffer response and autoregulation. Hepatic blood volume is passively altered in response to changes in total hepatic blood flow (see below). By tending to maintain hepatic blood flow and hence portal and intrahepatic pressures at a constant value, transient alterations in hepatic blood volume and, therefore, in venous return are minimized.

The effect of the buffer response is seen in the dramatic differences noted for the effects of vasoactive compounds on the hepatic circulation, depending on the site of administration. Isoproterenol infused separately into the superior mesenteric artery or directly into the hepatic artery produces a dose-related vasodilation of each artery. Intravenous infusion of isoproterenol leads to dilation of the superior mesenteric artery; but despite equal dilator concentrations of isoproterenol reaching both arteries, the hepatic artery is seen to respond much less effectively. At low doses, the hepatic artery actually constricts. This constriction is due to the arterial buffer response to elevated portal flow, as proved by using a vascular clamp to hold the superior mesenteric arterial flow at control levels. When portal flow is not permitted to rise, the hepatic artery dilates to a similar extent as the superior mesenteric artery.[32,33] In many cases, the hepatic artery shows a response that is determined primarily by the HABR rather than by the pharmacologic agent in the lumen of the blood vessel. Because of the confounding effect of the buffer response on hepatic vascular responses and the interaction of the buffer response with systemic stimuli, studies purporting to show direct effects on the hepatic artery must ensure that portal venous flow remains constant during the test. An attempt to elevate hepatic arterial flow therapeutically by using an intravenous dilator may actually result in the opposite flow effect if the splanchnic arteries are dilated and portal flow increases. This probably explains why intravenous adenosine dilated all arteries other than the hepatic artery in dogs[34] and why intravenous vasopressin has been reported to dilate the hepatic artery.[35]

Although the mechanism whereby hepatic blood flow is regulated according to total blood flow is beneficial for the homeostatic status of the entire organism, the separation of metabolic demand from vascular supply may have negative consequences for the liver. In conditions such as uncorrected hyperthyroidism and chronic alcohol exposure, hepatic oxygen uptake may double,[36] possibly leading to hypoxia in the cells farthest downstream from the inflow vessels. In this pathologic state, the hepatic artery is not dilated despite the fact that the hepatocytes are hypoxic. This hypothesis recently has been supported by the observation that chronic alcohol exposure in rats led to elevated hepatic oxygen uptake with no elevation in hepatic arterial flow.[19] This suggests a possible therapeutic intervention in alcoholic liver disease by pharmacologic dilation of the hepatic artery to eliminate the hypoxic status. In most situations in which oxygen supply is potentially endangered, the liver is protected from hypoxia by the fact that increases in hepatic arterial flow compensate for reductions in portal blood flow, thus resulting in a disproportionate increase in oxygen delivery to the liver. Although total hepatic blood flow is reduced during hemorrhage, the increased proportion of blood flow accounted for by the hepatic artery significantly protects the liver from becoming hypoxic.[37] Mathie and Blumgart[38] have shown that even the 22% buffer capacity (hepatic artery compensates for 22% of change in portal flow) in anesthetized dogs results in normal levels of oxygen delivery to the liver. Studies done for other purposes, in which buffer capacities can be calculated, suggest buffer capacities in the range of 22–100% in cats, dogs and rats.[21,39–41]

In addition, within a wide physiologic range, reductions in oxygen delivery or elevations in hepatic metabolic rate can be dealt with adequately by increased oxygen extraction from the available blood supply. The liver was once believed to be an organ verging on hypoxia in the normal state; however, this belief clearly has been refuted.[18,42] The current view is that the liver receives considerably more oxygen than is normally required and that any changes in liver metabolism within a physiologic range result simply in alterations in hepatic oxygen extraction without the need for hepatic arterial dilation.

Major questions related to the HABR remain unanswered. Although the HABR is not regulated by oxygen requirement of the liver, it is not clear whether the buffer capacity shows an altered gain in the presence of a metabolically altered liver or whether such modulation of the response may result from altered constituents of the portal venous blood (e.g., altered oxygen or vasoactive compounds). It has not been proved (although all data are consistent with the hypothesis) that the release of adenosine is completely oxygen-independent or that it occurs at a constant rate. The precise site of this regulatory mechanism has not been localized, although the data are consistent with adenosine regulation in the space of Mall. The buffer capacity in conscious animals and in various physiologic states has not been quantified, and the biochemical pathway of adenosine production within the space of Mall is not known. The production of adenosine seems unlikely to derive from breakdown of adenine nucleotide or cyclic adenosine monophosphate, because both compounds are affected by the level of oxygen supply. The current speculation is that adenosine is likely to derive from demethylation of S-adenosylhomocysteine in a manner similar to that shown for the heart.[43]

Extrinsic Arterial Regulation. Extrinsic humoral regulation of the hepatic artery is less well understood,[2,24] and it appears that in several situations the HABR is able to confound extrinsic stimuli. The hepatic artery shows vasoactive responses to direct intraarterial or intraportal infusions of most vasoactive compounds in a manner not unlike other arteries. Several vasodilator peptides and hormones released from the splanchnic system into the portal blood have been shown to produce hepatic arterial dilation when given in pharmacologic amounts; however, no physiologic role as a regulator of hepatic arterial flow has yet been demonstrated for any of these compounds. The lack of constriction of the hepatic artery in the postprandial state,[44] despite an elevated portal venous flow, suggests the presence of some dilator agent that is able to counteract the HABR. Possible dilator candidates include bile salts, hypertonic solutions, gastrin, secretin, and glucagon.[2,24]

The hepatic artery is richly innervated by sympathetic nerves. Nerve-induced vasoconstriction is mediated by α-adrenergic receptors. In dogs the constriction is well maintained, whereas in cats the constriction "escapes" despite continued stimulation. The situation in humans is unknown. Effects and roles of hepatic nerves on vascular and metabolic parameters have been reviewed elsewhere.[45–48]

Hepatic Artery in Cirrhosis. The HABR is active in the diseased human liver until terminal stages are reached. As portacaval shunts form and divert blood flow away from the liver, the hepatic artery provides proportionately more of the hepatic blood flow. The ability of the hepatic artery to dilate in response to an acute obstruction of portal flow is the best prognostic indicator for outcome of surgical portacaval shunts.[49] Unfortunately, this relationship contains a "catch-22." The reason to perform the shunt is to depressurize the portal vein, yet if the HABR is functional, the arterial dilation minimizes the reduction of portal pressure induced by reduced portal flow.[50] Thus, patients in whom the hepatic artery does not dilate have the best improvement in portal pressure but the least likelihood of surviving surgery.

The hepatic artery serves to buffer acute changes in portal flow to hold total blood flow steady. Despite the fact that many patients have a hyperdynamic splanchnic inflow with elevated splenic blood flow,[51–53] variable proportions of this flow are diverted via shunts past the liver so that portal venous inflow to the liver is severely reduced. Large changes in portal flow clearly cannot be compensated adequately by the relatively much smaller arterial flow. Thus, the cirrhotic liver is usually severely underperfused.[54] Because total hepatic blood flow determines hepatic clearance rate for many nutrients and hormones (e.g., steroids[30]), many of the hormonal disturbances in cirrhotic patients may be attributed to reduced hepatic extraction secondary to reduced flow. Substances normally extracted from the portal blood undergo an added clearance impairment due to the portacaval shunts. In addition, if the exchange properties are altered and if the liver is hypoxic, other hormonal and metabolic changes are possible.

Regulation of Portal Venous Pressure

Whereas the liver cannot regulate portal flow, it does regulate portal and intrahepatic pressure. This pressure is important for regulation of fluid exchange and for determining splanchnic blood volume. Earlier views held that the portal venule provided significant vascular resistance and that the pressure drop from the portal vein to the central venous system was primarily across these presinusoidal sites. Our current view is that most of the resistance to portal blood flow occurs across the hepatic veins and, specifically, across a distinct sphincterlike zone. In the basal, normal liver, the portal and sinusoidal vascular resistance to blood flow is very low, and portal venous pressure usually equals sinusoidal pressure.

The hepatic venous sphincters constrict in response to NE, angiotensin, hepatic nerve stimulation (cats and dogs), and histamine (dogs). In addition, however, portal pressure rises above sinusoidal pressure in response to significant presinusoidal portal vascular resistance.[55,56] The hepatic venous resistance site is distensible and can dilate to the point that a very small pressure gradient exists between portal and central venous pressure. The distensibility of the resistance sites in the hepatic veins and portal venules is dramatically acted upon by the distending blood pressure within the vessels. Passive changes in resistance, secondary to changes in distending blood pressure, are in the same range as the resistance responses to active stimuli such as sympathetic nerve activation. A mathematical relationship between the distending pressure and resistance has been defined, and physiologic consequences of the distensibility also have been described. Discussion of these issues is prefaced by an outline of the basic observations and assumptions related to pre- and postsinusoidal venous resistance sites.

Hepatic Venous Sphincters. Wedged hepatic venous pressure has long been known to be similar to portal venous pressure.[57] It has been traditionally assumed that the blood pressure measured at the tip of the wedged pressure catheter does not report a true pressure typical of the blood vessel in which the catheter is wedged. It also has been assumed that the measured pressure represents some upstream pressure transmitted to the venous catheter via a static column of blood produced by occlusion of the outflow vessel. The pressure measured via the static column would represent the pressure at the first site of collateral vessels. Wanless et al.[58] assumed that the small portal venules represent the first collaterals; Groszmann and Atterbury[59] assumed that the collaterals are the sinusoids in the normal liver. We assumed that the collaterals exist throughout the liver, including the hepatic veins proximal to the hepatic venous sphincters. Each set of assumptions leads to somewhat different conclusions about the sites of regulation of portal and intrahepatic pressure and may have extreme significance for the concept of portal hypertension and the microcirculatory disruptions in cirrhosis.

A full discussion of these theories and their consequences is beyond the scope of this chapter, but the essential differences are based on what each theory assumes is measured by a catheter passed into a hepatic vein. In the basal state and in many cirrhotic livers, wedged hepatic venous pressure is virtually equal to portal venous pressure. If the wedged pressure measures portal pressure (i.e., no collaterals at all), then portal hypertension may be the result of raised resistance at any vascular segment distal to the portal vein. The pressure would be elevated if the hepatic veins, sinusoids, or portal veins were constricted. If, however, the first collaterals are represented by the sinusoids, the raised portal pressure must be due to vascular resistance distal to the sinusoids, i.e., postsinusoidal resistance; the common view is that this resistance, especially in diseased liver, is largely in the terminal sinusoids and terminal hepatic venules. Our assumption of collaterals even in the hepatic venules leads to the hypothesis that pressure measured by the wedged or unwedged catheter is a true representation of the pressure in functionally analogous, adjacent veins. The site of vascular resistance, therefore, is within quite large hepatic veins. Several lines of evidence support this hypothesis.

As the pressure catheter is advanced via the vena cava into the hepatic veins, pressure is similar to central venous pressure until the catheter tip passes through a narrow length of hepatic vein (Fig. 9.3). This region has the characteristics of a smooth muscle sphincter,[23,55,56,60] and morphologic studies support the existence of sphincter-like regions in large hepatic veins.[57] These sphincters are localized to third-order branches (ramuli, according to the nomenclature of Elias and Petty[61]) of the hepatic veins in cats[60] and in the terminal 1–2 cm of the lobar hepatic vein proper in dogs.[23] The sudden rise of pressure from central venous pressure (CVP) to portal venous pressure (PVP) as the catheter is advanced usually has been assumed to represent

wedging of the catheter,[62,63] and the pressure readings were assumed to be via a static column. Several factors indicate that this measurement is not a "wedged" pressure:

1. The catheter is not wedged and can be advanced at least an additional 1–2 cm beyond the sphincter, even in cats.[60]

2. We use catheters with sealed tips, and pressure is recorded via sideholes cut 3 and 7 mm from the tip. We assume that the ability to record a valid pressure beyond the sphincter but distal to the sealed catheter tip depends on the existence of collaterals between the veins proximal to the sphincters. The sphincters are contracted by neural (see Fig. 9.3) and pharmacologic stimuli, and the site of the sphincter is not altered by catheter size or state of contraction,[23,55,60] as would be expected if the "sphincter" in fact represented an artifact of wedging in the vein.

3. In dogs—an unusual species in that the hepatic sphincter is located in the terminal portion of the lobar hepatic vein—it is possible to position a catheter in the hepatic vein, proximal to the sphincter site, via an incision in the surface of the liver. By locating a small hepatic venous tributary and passing a catheter downstream into the hepatic vein, pressure similar to portal pressure can be demonstrated. Histamine-induced sphincter contraction led to equal and parallel elevations in portal venous pressure and in hepatic venous pressure proximal to the hepatic veins in a position in which it is impossible to be measuring a "wedged" pressure.[23]

Portal Venous Resistance. Vascular resistance proximal to the hepatic venous sphincters is normally very low. As the open-ended or closed-ended hepatic venous catheter is advanced into the hepatic veins and passes through the sphincter, the pressure measured proximal to the sphincter, referred to as lobar venous pressure (LVP), is insignificantly different from portal venous pressure (PVP). The gradient from portal-to-lobar venous pressure reflects the total vascular resistance between the recording catheters and includes the portal venules, sinusoids, and small hepatic venules. If this gradient is insignificant, as in the basal state, during passive volume collapse due to occlusion of hepatic blood inflow, during passive engorgement due to elevated CVP (in cats and dogs), and during histamine-induced hepatic sphincter contraction (in dogs),[23] then resistance proximal to the hepatic sphincters is also insignificant. This conclusion has been

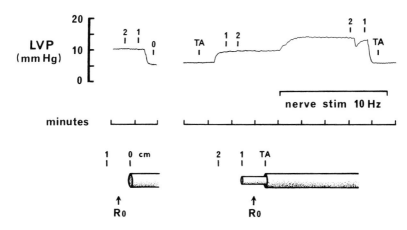

FIGURE 9.3. Demonstration of hepatic venous sphincters in dogs. A hepatic venous pressure profile was obtained by withdrawing a large catheter (PE 240, external diameter 2.42 mm) from a wedged position in the hepatic veins in 1-cm steps (*left panel*) until recorded pressure dropped to near central ventral pressure. The location of the resistance site (sphincter) is indicated by the large pressure drop (Ro). With the large catheter left in place (within 1 cm of Ro) and tied at the jugular vein, a small catheter (Pe 90, external diameter of .27 mm) was passed down the inside of the large catheter until the tips aligned (TA). Pressure was monitored via the small catheter, which was then advanced into the hepatic vein and seen to pass the Ro site within the first cm. At 2 cm proximal to Ro, the lobar venous pressure (LVP) was similar to that recorded with the large catheter. The hepatic nerves were then stimulated at 10 Hz, and the LVP rose in response. As the catheter is withdrawn in 1-cm steps, the major site of resistance (Ro) is still seen across the vascular segment that provided the resistance in the control state. This test demonstrates that the pressures measured as LVP do not depend significantly on the size of the catheter and that the Ro site can be consistently located relative to a constant point (the fixed catheter). Similar pressures and profiles are measured using small catheters with sealed tips and recording from side holes. (From Legarre DJ, Lautt WW: Hepatic venous resistance site in the dog: Localization and validation of intrahepatic pressure measurements. Can J Physiol Pharmacol 1987;65:352–359, with permission.)

extensively validated in dog[23] and cat[60] liver and is consistent with the data (but not the conclusions) of previous reports based on normal[2] and diseased animal and human livers.

Significant presinusoidal vascular resistance caused by pharmacologic agents and sympathetic nerves leads to a greater rise in PVP than LVP. Although it is clear that a significant gradient of portal-to-lobar venous pressure indicates significant vascular resistance proximal to the hepatic venous sphincters, the specific site of resistance could be any or all of the following: portal veins and venules, sinusoids, hepatic venules. We tentatively conclude that, in normal livers, the portal-to-lobar venous pressure gradient represents portal vascular resistance. This supposition is supported by the complex vascular responses[2,45,46] to stimulation of the hepatic nerves in cats:

1. Hepatic blood volume is rapidly decreased, and this response is well maintained throughout nerve stimulation.

2. Hepatic venous sphincters constrict and lead to a well-maintained rise in LVP.[55]

3. The hepatic artery constricts, but the flow reduction then undergoes an escape (in cats but not in dogs) despite continued nerve stimulation,

4. The portal-to-lobar venous pressure gradient initially develops but also undergoes vascular escape (in cats but not in dogs), even if the hepatic artery is occluded throughout the entire stimulation.[55]

It seems possible that the escape of the PVP-LVP gradient indicates that the resistance site is presinusoidal rather than sinusoidal. The calculated resistance based on blood flow measurements and the pressure gradients, PVP minus LVP and LVP minus CVP, respectively, indicate that the postsinusoidal resistance is well maintained for 5 minutes of constant nerve stimulation, whereas the putative presinusoidal resistance undergoes complete vascular escape similar to the presinusoidal arterial resistance. The fact that the postsinusoidal resistance (hepatic venous sphincters) and the volume responses are well maintained, even after escape of a significant portal-to-lobar venous gradient, suggests that the capacitance vessels, including sinusoids , do not contribute to the pressure gradient between the portal and lobar veins. Such arguments are the basis for interpreting the gradient from PVP to LVP (or wedged pressure) as representing portal vascular resistance, whereas the gradient LVP to vena caval pressure primarily represents hepatic venous sphincter resistance.

Active and Passive Effects on Hepatic Venous Resistance

Regulation of Venous Resistance. Both presinusoidal and postsinusoidal venous resistance sites within the liver are passively distensive. This distensibility accounts for the mechanism of passive autoregulation of PVP. According to this theory, portal blood flow can be increased over dramatic ranges with minor changes in PVP because of the passive distensibility of the resistance sites. The initial observations that led to the conclusion of significant passive distensibility of resistance sites[64] were followed by attempts to describe the quantitative relationship between distending blood pressure and venous resistance. The distending blood pressure is best estimated from the average of pressures upstream and downstream from the resistance sites.[65,66] Resistance changes inversely with the distending pressure cubed (Pd[3]) over physiologically relevant ranges of Pd.[66] The graphic relationship between resistance and 1/Pd[3] is linear and extrapolates through the zero ordinate, indicating that at infinite distending blood pressure vascular resistance approaches zero. The slope of the line is an index of contractility (IC), which does not change in response to changes in hepatic blood flow or CVP. The calculated resistance, however, changes dramatically in response to these influences. The measured resistance depends on the interactions between active contractile tone and passive distending forces. The use of the IC calculation allows differentiation between active and passive effects, because the IC is acutely affected only by changes in active vascular tone. The IC model has been validated[66] and used to describe active contractile responses of both presinusoidal and postsinusoidal resistance sites.

Use of the resistance calculation may grossly underestimate the active vascular response to stimuli such as norepinephrine infusions. This underestimation occurs when active vasoconstriction leads to increased intrahepatic and portal pressure; this increased pressure then produces passive distension of the resistance vessels to counteract in part the active response. In the absence of passive consequences secondary to altered distending pressure, the percentage change in resistance and the percentage change in IC should be similar. Stimulation of the hepatic nerves, for example, increased IC of the hepatic venous resistance site by 563%, whereas the calculated resistance increased by only 222%. The difference is explained by the fact that the Pd had also increased from 6.6 to 8.4 mmHg.

This differentiation may become extremely important in assessing the mechanism of action of drugs designed to treat portal hypertension. If, for example, a drug such as propranolol is administered, the effect is to decrease both portal blood flow and PVP. It has been assumed that the decrease in PVP is secondary to reduced flow through a constant hepatic or collateral resistance. The IC model indicates that a decrease in portal flow results in a decrease in PVP and that the decrease in Pd results in a passive recoil of the resistance vessels, thus minimizing the change in PVP.

Over the past several years considerable discussion has focused on the relative importance of elevated portal blood flow in cirrhotic patients with a hyperdynamic circulation vs. the importance of elevated intrahepatic resistance. The IC model allows calculation of the IC, which in turn allows clear calculation of the effect of changes in blood flow on the pressure. The relationship between pressure and flow in the portal vein is approximately linear over a wide range of blood flows; the relationship becomes steeper, indicative of a greater effect of flow on pressure, as the IC rises to pathologic levels. The relationship between hepatic blood flow and hepatic venous resistance and intrahepatic pressure (lobar venous pressure = LVP) is shown in Figure 9.4.

Physiologic Consequences of Venous Resistance Distensibility. As noted previously, venous distensibility provides the mechanism by which portal pressure is maintained within a narrow range in the face of dramatic changes in portal flow. A decrease in hepatic blood flow from 50 to 20 ml/min/kg results in a decrease of intrahepatic pressure by only 1.4 mmHg and portal pressure by 2.0 mmHg. In this instance, presinusoidal resistance increased by 226% and hepatic venous resistance by 57%.[68] Surprisingly, changes in IC values within physiologic limits do not notably alter the efficiency of the autoregulation between flow and pressure, as predicted by the IC model and as demonstrated by lack of significant change in the slope of the flow-pressure curve during infusion of NE, which raised portal venous IC from 40 to 80 and hepatic venous IC from 31 to 78 IC units .[68] Calculated IC values for the cirrhotic liver would be estimated to be in the range of 500 units, and the pressure-flow relationship becomes much steeper at this extreme level (see discussion of portacaval shunts).

PVP is well maintained within narrow limits, partially as a result of the venous distensibility, but several other factors are also involved. First, the majority of vascular resistance in the basal state is postsinusoidal, and most types of cirrhosis appear to have a primary elevation in resistance at the postsinusoidal site. Therefore, the total blood flow, as distinct from portal flow, is of primary consequence, because it is the mixed hepatic arterial and portal flow that must pass through the elevated resistance of the postsinusoidal vessels. Changes in portal blood flow activate the HABR, as previously discussed. Thus, a decrease in portal flow is partially compensated by an increase in arterial flow. The hepatic artery becomes fully constricted at high portal flows and fully dilated at low portal flows;[69] thus the hepatic artery buffers the portal flow changes so that total flow across the venous resistance tends to be maintained. This mechanism protects intrahepatic pressure. Such a role for the hepatic artery is consistent with the observation[70] that equal changes in portal and arterial flow produce equal changes in hepatic pressure, as reflected in volume changes.

It is important, however, not to overemphasize the role of the HABR and venous distensibility as the major means of regulating PVP. The effect of portal flow on PVP becomes less as the basal resistance becomes less, even if the resistance is not distensible. If there were no resistance, changes in flow would produce no changes in pressure. The resistance across the liver is extremely low, as reflected by a pressure gradient of approximately 3 mmHg in the basal state. Consider the differences in distensible vs. nondistensible venous resistance in a normal liver. With the normal baseline hepatic venous IC of 20 units, a venous pressure of 4 mmHg, and a portal pressure of 7 mmHg, the intrahepatic pressure would change only by 2.5 mmHg as blood flow was changed from 10 to 50 ml/kg/min. However, if the resistance site were not distensible and remained

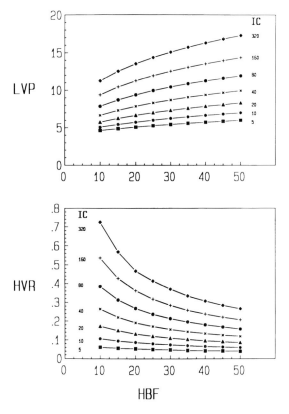

FIGURE 9.4. Predicted lobar venous pressure (LVP, mmHg) upstream from hepatic venous resistance sits and hepatic venous resistance (HVR, mm Hg·ml^{-1} min· kg) as total hepatic blood flow (HBF, ml·min^{-1}·kg^{-1}) is altered. The family of curves is obtained for a wide range of IC values predicted from computer-assisted estimates based on the previously derived equation (IC = R·Pd^3).[66] Downstream venous pressure is assumed constant at 4 mm Hg. Changing HBF produces effects on HVR secondary to altered Pd. (From Lautt WW, Legare DJ: Passive autoregulation of portal venous pressure: Distensible hepatic resistance. Am J Physiol 1992;263:G702–G708, with permission.)

constant over the entire flow range, the LVP still would change only by 4.6 mmHg. The distensible resistance becomes more crucial as a mechanism to autoregulate pressure as the basal resistance becomes more elevated. A final factor in considering the portal regulatory scheme is the effect of intrahepatic pressure changes on hepatic volume (see below). If portal flow rises and leads to elevated intrahepatic pressure, the hepatic volume expands and reduces venous return to the heart, which, in turn, leads to reduced cardiac output and splanchnic blood flow.[71] Thus, in the healthy liver, multiple mechanisms interact to regulate

PVP. How all of these various factors interrelate in the diseased liver is unclear. Furthermore, the interactions are made more complex by collateral portacaval shunts which are also distensible.

A second physiologic consequence of the distensible venous resistance in the liver is related to the ability of the liver to serve as a volume buffer to prevent large transient changes in CVP with the resultant large changes in cardiac output (described more fully in the section on hepatic blood volume).

Vascular Characteristics of the Portacaval Shunt Vessels. A model of portal vein stenosis in cats was recently used to develop complete portacaval shunting of the portal blood flow.[72] The shunt vessels were also demonstrated to be passively distensible, and the quantitative relationship between distending pressure and distensible resistance also followed the cubic relationship of the IC model, in which IC is a constant product of resistance and Pd[3]. Several recent reports also indicate that the shunt vessels are able to respond actively to a wide variety of pharmacologic agents.[73,74] As with intrahepatic resistance vessels, it may become crucial for evaluation of pharmacologic effects to differentiate between calculated resistance and calculated IC values. Drugs that affect portal flow may have an effect on resistance both actively through changes in tone of the shunt vessels and passively in response to the altered distending pressure. Passive effects do not influence the IC, which is altered acutely only by active contractile responses. In the cat model of portal stenosis, the calculated IC for the shunt vessels is in the range of 500 units, and the flow-pressure relationship is considerably steeper than in a normal liver.

Portal and Intrahepatic Pressure in Cirrhosis. Based on the preceding conclusions from experiments in normal animals, we are tempted to speculate on the pressures measured in the clinical setting. Following the above logic, if wedged hepatic venous pressure in the normal liver is a measure of LVP, the same may be true in the cirrhotic liver. Groszmann and Atterbury[59] assumed that wedged pressure measures sinusoidal pressure in the normal liver but that the sinusoidal collaterals are eliminated in the diseased liver; thus wedged pressure measures portal pressure. In our opinion, it is more likely that the elevation in wedged pressure is due to elevated vascular resistance in large hepatic veins, probably at the sphincters.

A key question is whether a catheter with a sealed tip, measuring pressure from sideholes, is also capable of measuring a pressure similar to portal pressure in the normal and diseased human liver. If this capability can be shown, it would suggest that marked venous collaterals exist and that the "wedged" pressure is synonymous with LVP and maintained by downstream hepatic venous resistance. Presence of a sphincter can be easily determined by slow withdrawal of the catheter to produce a hepatic venous pressure profile. If such a demonstration is done in both normal and diseased livers, the site of intrahepatic and PVP regulation may be confirmed to reside with the hepatic venous sphincters.

In most forms of cirrhosis, portal pressure, sinusoidal pressure ,and "wedged hepatic venous pressure" are similar. We speculative that the hepatic veins, and most probably the hepatic sphincters, are the site of increased resistance. Whereas the sphincters are distensible in the normal liver and, thus, lead to a pressure-flow curve that shows small portal pressure changes for quite large flow changes, the sphincters (or other resistance sites) in the diseased liver are less compliant and the pressure-flow curve is much steeper.[50] For this reason, flow changes that would not cause marked pressure effect in the normal liver, may greatly alter portal pressure in the diseased liver.

Others have suggested that the hepatocyte enlargement seen in cirrhosis is a major cause of portal hypertension by virtue of occlusion of sinusoids.[75] This theory appears unlikely. We have shown that hepatic blood volume in normal cat and dog livers can be reduced to extremely low levels without contribution of significant vascular resistance from the sinusoids or portal vessels (during nerve stimulation after resistance vessels have escaped and during well-maintained volume reduction in cats[55] and secondary to large reductions in hepatic inflow in cats and dogs[23,60]). The earlier view that fibrin and collagen depositions account for vascular resistance has been deemphasized by the demonstration that elevated intrahepatic pressure occurs prior to and in the absence of collagen deposition in the space of Disse.[75] Unfortunately, both studies rely on correlation of pathologic parameters with portal pressure. As with any serious disease state, multiple factors correlate with the severity of disease and, therefore, with each other. It appears unlikely that intrahepatic pressures measured with a needle puncture technique[76,77] would show pressures similar to portal pressure unless sinusoidal pressure was similar to portal pressure. If the sinusoids themselves were the site of resistance, some sort of graded pressure would be expected.

Recent studies have shown that both verapamil (a calcium channel blocker)[78] and intravenous clonidine (through reflex inhibition of hepatic sympathetic nerves)[79] reduce intrahepatic resistance to portal flow in the cirrhotic liver. These studies strongly suggest some pathophysiologic constriction of hepatic vein sphincter rather than resistance due to fibrosis.

We recently used a chronic bile duct ligation model in cats to produce hepatic fibrosis. Despite the grossly altered morphology and demonstration of fibrotic areas concentrated in the portal tracts, the initial increased resistance occurred at postsinusoidal sites (10 days), whereas additional presinusoidal resistance developed only after 21 days of occlusion. Thus, this study is also consistent with the hypothesis that sinusoidal and presinusoidal resistance is normally so low that even considerable additional obstruction due to fibrosis does not lead to an elevation of resistance that has consequences for the vascular resistance and pressure gradients.[79a]

Of interest, the bile duct-ligated livers showed a selective decrease in response to hepatic nerve stimulation but maintained normal responses to infused catecholamines. This study thus suggests a selective hepatic neuropathy. Studies described later in relation to hepatic blood volume responses support this conclusion.

Recently Shibayama and Nakata[80] reported that the major site of vascular resistance in cirrhotic rats was in the portal venules. This study, however, is incompatible with the observation that intraportally administered radioactive albumin appeared on the surface of livers in cirrhotic rats with the same time sequence as in rats with partial hepatic venous outflow, whereas in control rats little radioactivity exuded from the surface.[81] This study suggests that rats may be similar to all other species in showing elevated sinusoidal pressure in cirrhosis.

Calculation of Hepatic Vascular Resistance

Virtually all pharmacologic studies of portal vascular resistance have previously assumed that portal pressure is determined by presinusoidal

vascular resistance so that resistance was calculated as (PVP–CVP) divided by portal blood flow. Presinusoidal portal resistance, normally very low, is correctly calculated as (PVP–LVP) divided by portal venous flow. The major intrahepatic resistance to the portal blood, located at the hepatic venous sphincters, is calculated as (LVP–CVP) divided by *total* hepatic blood flow. This explains the erroneous conclusion that reduction of portal pressure after occlusion of the hepatic artery reduces portal venous resistance.[24] The hepatic artery occlusion reduces intrahepatic pressure because of the reduction of flow across the hepatic venous sphincter, and correctly calculated postsinusoidal resistance is unchanged. Hepatic arterial resistance is usually calculated using the pressure gradient from systemic arterial pressure to CVP; however, because sinusoidal pressure is insignificantly different from portal pressure, the correct gradient is arterial minus portal pressure. For strict accuracy the LVP is preferable to portal pressure, because the difference between PVP and LVP (sinusoidal) may be as much as 1–2 mmHg. The maximal error from using portal pressure, however, is trivial. The maximal error from using the incorrect flow to calculate venous resistance is not trivial.

Selection of the appropriate index to reflect hemodynamic responses requires consideration of fundamental and simple mathematical realities. Changes in arterial vascular tone in vivo result primarily in changes in blood flow, and such vascular responses are best assessed using vascular conductance rather than resistance, which is the inverse of conductance. Several quite dramatic examples illustrate the difference between the two indices,[82–84] but the most obvious example is demonstrated by calculation of the hemodynamic response to a massive vasoconstrictor stimulus that results in blood flow approaching zero. In this case, vascular conductance approaches zero, but resistance approaches infinity. Resistance calculations, therefore, are misleading and cannot be used for classic pharmacodynamic calculations.[85] The rule of thumb is that the physiologic parameter that undergoes the largest change in response to a change in vascular tone should be in the numerator of the equation. Therefore, in studies of arterial vascular beds using a constant flow perfusion system in which changes in vascular tone result in changes of perfusion pressure, arterial resistance is the appropriate calculation. Similarly, in the portal venous system, maximal physiologic changes in intrahepatic vascular tone result in changes in portal and intrahepatic pressure with no significant changes in flow. For this reason, the venous resistance calculation is appropriate, whereas venous conductance calculation is inappropriate.

The ability to differentiate active from passive changes in vascular tone requires calculations of the IC (IC = R·Pd^3). For the presinusoidal site, Pd is equal to the average of portal venous and intrahepatic pressure as estimated by either wedged hepatic venous pressure or LVP, as previously discussed. The appropriate blood flow for this calculation is portal venous. The IC calculation for the hepatic venous site uses a Pd calculated from the mean of intrahepatic pressure and CVP at the site of the hepatic veins entrance to the vena cava. In this case, the appropriate flow is the total of hepatic arterial and portal venous flow. Mathematical characteristics of the use of IC include the following:

1. In a simple circuit without a dual blood inflow, such as that seen with isolated preparations perfused only through the portal vein, the IC values of two resistance sites in series are additive.

2. If blood flow in the portal vein passes partially through the diseased liver and partially through the vascular shunts, the proportion of blood flow through the liver and shunts is maintained in the presence of reduced portal blood flow if the IC of both sites is not altered.

3. In a nondistensible vascular bed, a change in vascular tone results in equal percentage changes in resistance and IC. Significant differences in changes of the two parameters are attributed to the simultaneous changes in the distending pressure.

HEPATIC BLOOD VOLUME

To serve as a physiologic blood reservoir, an organ must contain blood that can be mobilized without major negative consequences to itself. The liver is a major blood reservoir; about 25–30% of its volume is accounted for by blood.[2] Of this blood volume, 50–60% can be expelled by stimulation of hepatic sympathetic nerves without impairment of liver function. The hepatic capacitance vessels contract in direct response to α_2-adrenergic and angiotensin agonists. Passive collapse due to reduced blood flow is dramatic in the liver. Factors affecting hepatic blood volume were recently reviewed.[2,71]

Capacitance, or total blood volume, consists of stressed and unstressed volume.[86–88] Stressed volume depends on the relationship between intrahepatic pressure (see previous discussion of LVP measurement) and hepatic compliance. Compliance, a measure of the distensibility of the vascular bed, is defined as the change in volume per unit of change in pressure (many studies incorrectly interchange capacitance and compliance). If the linear relationship between intrahepatic pressure and volume is extrapolated to zero pressure, the intercept is positive, that is, a theoretical volume remains in the liver at zero venous pressure. This extrapolated volume is the unstressed volume. These concepts have major physiologic importance. The unstressed volume accounts for about 40% of total hepatic volume[89] and is hemodynamically inactive in that relationships between pressure, flow, and volume would not be altered if it did not exist. Only the stressed volume plays a role in hemodynamic events.

Active venoconstriction occurs mainly, if not entirely, by changing the unstressed volume;[88] that is, compliance is not changed. The effect of norepinephrine on liver volume is to convert unstressed volume to stressed volume without altering compliance.[89] Active contraction of the capacitance vessels transfers blood from the inactive pool of unstressed volume to the active pool of stressed volume, which maintains venous pressure and venous return. In contrast, passive blood mobilization is secondary to reduced intrahepatic pressure, and the volume of blood is expelled according to the compliance of the vascular bed.

Although both active and passive regulation may occur, they operate via the two separate pools and have quite different consequences. Determining the extent of active and passive regulation requires determination of changes in stressed and unstressed volume, hepatic compliance, and intrahepatic pressures. Two examples, discussed elsewhere in more depth,[2] illustrate the complex interactions and the need for intrahepatic pressure measurements. The response to sympathetic nerves and norepinephrine involves reduced hepatic blood flow. The passive effect of reduced blood flow is to produce a linearly related decrease in intrahepatic pressure and hence in stressed volume. However, to conclude that a major component of the volume response to norepinephrine is secondary to the passive effects of flow reduction is not correct. When flow is reduced by mechanical reduction of hepatic inflow, intrahepatic pressure falls and passive reduction in hepatic blood volume occurs (stressed volume).

However, during sympathetic nerve stimulation, intrahepatic pressure rises because of constriction of the hepatic venous sphincters; thus the passive consequence of the intrahepatic pressure would be to expand rather than to decrease stressed volume.

During the response to hemorrhage, active mechanisms reduce liver volume by reducing unstressed volume; venous return, cardiac output, hepatic blood flow, and intrahepatic pressures are protected. If, however, all of the putative active regulators are removed (by adrenalectomy, hepatic denervation, nephrectomy, and hypophysectomy), the effect of removed blood is more profound; the reduced cardiac output leads to greater decreases of flow and pressures, and the effect on hepatic stressed volume is increased. The liver still compensates for about 21% of the hemorrhaged volume.[90] Thus, although the passive effect of reduced liver flow is large, without knowing the intrahepatic pressure one cannot assess the degree of volume change that is active (unstressed volume) or passive, secondary to recoil of the compliant hepatic vascular bed (stressed volume).

The integrity of the venous capacitance system is crucial to determination of the overall effect of vasoactive compounds on cardiac output and systemic blood pressure. If peripheral resistance is decreased and the capacitance vessels are simultaneously constricted (elevated cardiac preload), the cardiac output is markedly elevated but arterial pressure may remain unaltered. If arterial and venous dilation occur simultaneously, cardiac output may remain unaltered but arterial pressure declines dramatically. Simultaneous contraction of arterial resistance vessels and venous capacitance vessels leads to large elevations in systemic blood pressure with minimal effects on cardiac output, whereas contractions of arterial resistance vessels with inactive capacitance vessels results in reduced cardiac output. Such interrelationships have been discussed more fully in previous reviews,[2,88,91] and a computer model of the circulation is available (Greenway, by request).

Hepatic Blood Volume In Liver Disease

The capacitance functions of cirrhotic livers have not been examined. However, a recent study of active and passive responses of the hepatic capacitance vessels was carried out in a bile duct ligation model (2 weeks).[92] Despite considerable

morphologic disruption, including extensive biliary hyperplasia and fibrotic encroachment into the portal triad region, the compliance of the studied livers was not significantly altered. The passive response to a decrease in portal inflow produced the same reduction of liver volume expressed per mmHg change in portal pressure in diseased and control livers. It is anticipated that a cirrhotic liver with portal hypertension and much more severe fibrosis is unlikely to have a normal compliance. Such livers also had small elevations in postsinusoidal resistance at 10 days and an additional small resistance in the presinusoidal site at 21 days. Thus the portacaval pressure gradient rose from 1.5 to 5 mmHg.[93]

Whereas the normal liver compensated for approximately 20% of blood loss during hemorrhage, the diseased livers compensated only for approximately 11%.[92] The responses to intraportal and intraarterial norepinephrine infusions remained unchanged and were similar in both normal and diseased animals, regardless of the site of infusion. This similarity suggests that arterial and portal flows have equal access to the capacitance vessels. The response to sympathetic nerve stimulation, however, was decreased, suggesting a selective hepatic neuropathy induced by bile duct ligation. Whether hepatic neuropathy is a consistent feature of other forms of liver disease or a consequence of the notable disruption in the portal triad, through which the nerves pass to the liver parenchyma, is not clear. This study suggests that the response of hepatic blood volume to hemorrhage is mediated by passive compliant responses (stressed volume) to reduced portal pressure and active responses (unstressed volume) to nerve stimulation. Chronic bile duct ligation, however, produces selective hepatic neuropathy, resulting in loss of the active component and reduced ability to compensate for blood loss.

In a normal liver, acute congestion leads to loss of capacitance response to nerve stimulation.[94] If such a loss also occurs with chronic congestion, the impact on hemodynamic stability may be significant. It is predicted that hepatic compliance would be reduced as a result of the increased stiffness secondary to fibrosis; however, the proportion of the elevated hepatic volume in the cirrhotic liver that is accounted for by stressed and unstressed volume and the compliance of this tissue are clearly matters of speculation. Given the important role of the hepatic capacitance vessels in determining the overall cardiovascular response to antihypertensive agents and other cardiovascular drugs,[71,91] both questions are of some significance. In addition, severely cirrhotic patients are likely to die as a result of a hemorrhagic episode resulting from rupture of varices. The major organ that normally responds to hemorrhage may be incapable of adequate response in the severely diseased state. The normal liver expands or contracts to compensate for about 25% of an altered circulating blood volume. Rapid blood volume expansion (e.g., liquid consumption), therefore, may be expected to result in cardiovascular perturbations as a result of the less efficient volume-buffering capacity of the diseased liver.

Normally an acute change in portal flow is compensated by the HABR; thus total hepatic blood flow does not change to a great degree. If total flow does change, the distensible hepatic venous sphincters dilate or constrict and thus buffer changes in intrahepatic and portal pressure. If intrahepatic pressure does not change as a result of compensatory systems, passive changes in hepatic blood volume do not occur. In the diseased liver, the hepatic artery may not buffer flow as effectively; the hepatic sphincters may be fibrosed and, therefore, less compliant and unable to buffer the pressure changes secondary to changes in flow. Both factors may explain the observation that changes in portal flow have a much greater impact on intrahepatic and portal pressure in cirrhotic than in normal livers.[50] The effect of the altered pressure on what must be a stiffer, less compliant hepatic capacitance system is unknown.

HEPATIC FLUID EXCHANGE

The factors controlling movement of fluid across capillary walls were delineated by Starling and are described by the following equation:

$$F = CFC \left[(P_c - P_i) - r (OP_c - OP_i) \right]$$

where P_c and P_i are the hydrostatic pressure in the capillary and interstitial fluid, respectively; OP_c and OP_i are the colloid osmotic pressures in the capillary and interstitial fluid, respectively; r is the osmotic reflection coefficient for protein; F is the net fluid movement across the vascular walls; and CFC is the capillary filtration coefficient (the product of capillary permeability and surface area). The major physical force controlling net fluid exchange in the liver is sinusoidal hydrostatic pressure. Elevation of hepatic venous pressure results in partial transmission of this pressure to the sinusoid and produces a constant filtration rate that is maintained for at least 8 hours, provided that plasma volume is maintained.[95] The filtered fluid does not represent pooling in an interstitial fluid compartment, because it could be quantitatively collected from a plethysmograph in which the intact liver with ligated lymphatics was contained. The liver thus clearly lacks the protective mechanisms that limit filtration in the intestine and skeletal muscle.

The filtration rate across the liver during a stable (20–30-minute) elevation in hepatic venous pressure was 0.08 ml/min/mmHg increase in vena caval pressure per 100 gm of liver in cats and dogs.[88] Hepatic compliance is very high, and an elevation in hepatic venous pressure not only causes fluids to filter out of the vascular compartment but also results in blood pooling in the liver.

Hepatic lymphatics appear to arise in the space of Mall around the portal tract, forming extensive lymphatic plexuses that anastomose with other lymphatic plexuses on the surface of the liver beneath the capsule. It is presumed that the fluid exudate on the surface of the liver with elevated hepatic venous pressure has traversed this lymphatic network. The fluid of the space of Disse is not in direct contact with the space of Mall, which is contained within a limiting plate of parenchymal cells. Small porelike structures identified[57] in the limiting plate permit passage of fluid from the space of Disse to the space of Mall and thence to the hepatic lymphatics. Thus, compounds that are filtered into hepatic lymph from the sinusoidal space have two filtration barriers to pass, the sinusoidal fenestrae and the gaps in the limiting plate. It is not clear whether the gaps in the limiting plate are under physiologic regulation; however, the observation that hepatic nerve stimulation leads to dramatic increases in intrahepatic pressure but reduced fluid exudation across the surface of the liver[96] is highly suggestive of considerable physiologic control.

The liver does not become edematous as a result of increased fluid filtration. The lack of edema is indicated by lack of alteration of hepatic oxygen uptake[96] and by the observation that the filtered fluid can be collected quantitatively from a plethysmograph.[94] Protection of the liver against edema appears to be achieved by lymphatic drainage and, when formation of lymph exceeds the capacity of the major lymph trunks, by exudation of lymph from the surface of the liver. The fluid that pools in the peritoneal cavity does not appear to be reabsorbed by the liver; rather it is reabsorbed from the peritoneal cavity in a manner directly dependent on intraperitoneal pressure.[98]

Fluid Exchange In Cirrhosis

Schaffner and Popper[99] described the pathologic changes in cirrhotic livers as capillarization that involves the porous sinusoidal wall and gives it the appearance of the more impermeable capillaries of other organs. Collagen fibers and basement membranes appear in the space of Disse, and microvilli are lost from the sinusoidal pole of hepatocytes. However, the effect of lost villi facing the sinusoid may be offset by the observations that the hepatocytes tend to separate and that the widened interhepatocyte spaces have more microvilli.[100] As the disease progresses, the lymph that drains into the thoracic duct becomes more dilute. The protein content may be reduced by more effective seiving due to capillarization, or it may be that the liver contributes less lymph and the dilute lymph represents filtration from other splanchnic organs. The full implications of capillarization are unclear; in fact, it may be more of a morphologic than a functional phenomenon, since chronic exposure of livers to alcohol results in reduced numbers of fenestrae but increased fenestrae diameter.[101]

SUMMARY

The hepatic circulation is modified in all forms of liver disease. The hepatic arterial flow is regulated by an adenosine washout mechanism to maintain total hepatic blood flow at relatively constant levels. This hepatic arterial buffer response (e.g., dilation in response to reduced portal flow) also plays a role in regulation of intrahepatic and portal pressure and may be a major factor in determining the viability of diseased livers with portacaval shunts. Transplanted livers that fail to show an arterial dilation in response to transient occlusion of portal inflow have a poor prognosis. Portal venous flow is not directly controlled by the liver, and changes in hepatic vascular resistance lead only to changes in portal pressure. The normal liver has insignificant presinusoidal portal vascular resistance, and portal pressure is similar to sinusoidal pressure. Virtually all of the pressure drop from the portal vein

to the vena cava occurs across the sphincterlike regions of the hepatic veins that can be stimulated by sympathetic nerves and blood-borne constrictors. Active vasoconstriction may result in highly significant increases in presinusoidal resistance and significant pressure gradients between the portal vein and the intrahepatic sinusoidal pressure. A similar situation has been suggested in alcoholic cirrhosis, and most of the elevated vascular resistance may be localized to the hepatic veins, perhaps to the hepatic venous sphincters.

The hepatic presinusoidal (portal venous) and postsinusoidal (hepatic venous) resistance sites are passively distensible, and this distensibility accounts for passive autoregulation of portal blood pressure, as demonstrated by the trivial effect of large changes in portal flow on portal pressure. The dynamic interaction between distending blood pressure and distensible resistance is described adequately by the IC model, whereby resistance changes inversely as distending pressure cubed.

The biliary hyperplasia and portal triad fibrosis characteristic of bile duct-ligated models of liver disease before onset of true cirrhosis and portal hypertension do not alter the compliance of the capacitance vessels or the responses of capacitance vessels and venous resistance vessels to blood-borne catecholamines; however, capacitance and resistance responses to hepatic nerve stimulation are reduced, and the liver is unable to respond effectively to blood loss. Hepatic blood volume represents a large and rapidly mobilized blood reservoir that has a major effect on venous return and hence on cardiac output response to vasoactive agents as well as to postural adjustments and compensation for expanded or contracted total blood volume.

The impact of cirrhosis with portal hypertension on liver capacitance functions has not been evaluated, but it is anticipated to be significant because of reduced compliance. The ability to mobilize blood passively from the stressed volume of the liver secondary to reduced blood flow (and pressure) may become impaired. In addition, the sympathetic nerves may become ineffective in mobilizing unstressed volume in congested livers. Such factors may account, in part, for increased susceptibility of cirrhotic patients to hemorrhagic shock. Recent advances in knowledge of vascular control and roles in the normal liver provide the background by which abnormal functions may be studied and interpreted.

Acknowledgments.　　Much of the work described in this chapter was supported by grants from the Medical Research Council of Canada and the Manitoba Heart and Stroke Foundation. The manuscript was prepared by Karen Sanders. The intellectual and technical contributions of Dallas Legare to these studies is gratefully acknowledged.

REFERENCES

1. Orrego H, Israel Y, Blendis LM: Alcoholic liver disease: Information in search of knowledge? Hepatology 1981;1:267–283.
2. Greenway CV, Lautt WW: Hepatic circulation. In Schultz SG, Wood JD, Rauner BB (eds): Handbook of Physiology: The Gastrointestinal System I, vol. 1. New York: Oxford University Press, 1989;1519–1564.
3. Rappaport AM: Microvascular methods—the transilluminated liver. In Lautt WW (ed): Hepatic Circulation in Health and Disease. New York: Raven Press, 1981;1–12.
4. Gumucio JJ, Miller DL: Functional implications of liver cell heterogeneity. Gastroenterology 1981;80:393–403.
5. Gumucio DL: Functional and anatomic heterogeneity in the liver acinus: Impact on transport. Am J Physiol 1983;244:G578–G582.
6. Goresky CA, Groom AC: Microcirculatory events in the liver and spleen. In Handbook of Physiology: Cadiovascular System, vol. 4. Baltimore: Williams & Wilkins, 1984;689–780.
7. Thurman RG, Kauffman FC, Jungermann K: Regulation of Hepatic Metabolism. New York: Plenum Press, 1986.
8. Plaa GL: Toxicology of the liver. In Casarett LJ, Doull J (eds): Toxicology: The Basic Science of Poisons. New York: Macmillan, 1975;170–189.
8a. Lautt WW, Schafer J, Legare DJ: Hepatic blood flow distribution: Consideration of gravity, liver surface, and norepinephrine on regional heterogeneity. Can J Physiol Pharmacol 1993;71:128–135.
9. Greenway CV, Oshiro G: Intrahepatic distribution of portal and hepatic arterial blood flows in anaesthetized cats and dogs and the effects of portal occlusion, raised venous pressure and histamine. J Physiol (Lond) 1972;227:473–485.
10. Greenway CV, Oshiro G: Comparison of the effects of hepatic nerve stimulation on arterial flow, distribution of arterial and portal flows and blood content in the livers of anaesthetized cats and dogs. J Physiol (Lond) 1972;227:487–501.
11. Cousineau D, Goresky CA, Rose CP, Lee S: Reflex sympathetic effects on liver vascular space and liver perfusion in dogs. Am J Physiol 1985;248:H186–H192.
12. Mathie RT: Hepatic blood flow measurement with inert gas clearance. J Surg Res 1986;41:92–110.
13. Lautt WW, Legare DJ, Daniels TR: The comparative effect of administration of substances via the hepatic artery or portal vein on hepatic arterial resistance, liver blood volume, and hepatic extraction in cats. Hepatology 1984;4:927–932.
14. Granger DN, Miller T, Allen R, et al: Permselectivity of cat liver blood-lymph barrier to endogenous macromolecules. Gastroenterology 1979;77:103–109.
15. Wisse E, Van Dierendonck JH, De Zanger RB, et al: On the role of the liver endothelial filter in the transport of particulate fat (chylomicrons and their remnants) to parenchymal cells and the influence of certain hormones on the endothelial fenestrae. In Popper H, Bianchi L, Gudat F, Reutter W (eds): Communications of Liver Cells. England: MTP Press, 1980;195–200.
16. Fraser R, Bowler LM, Day WA, et al: High perfusion pressure damages the sieving ability of sinusoidal endothelium in rat livers. Br J Exp Pathol 1980;61:222–228.
17. Fraser R, Bowler LM, Day WA: Damage of rat liver sinusoidal endothelium by ethanol. Pathology 1980;12:371–376.
18. Lautt WW: Relationship between hepatic blood flow and overall metabolism: The hepatic arterial buffer response. Fed Proc 1983;42:1662–1666.
19. Bredfeldt JE, Riley EM, Groszmann RJ: Compensatory mechanism in response to an elevated hepatic oxygen consumption in chronic ethanol-fed rats. Am J Physiol 1985;248:G507–G511.
20. Lautt WW, Daniels TR: Differential effect of taurocholic acid on hepatic arterial resistance vessels and bile flow. Am J Physiol 1983;244:G366–G369.
21. Lautt WW: Mechanism and role of intrinsic regulation of hepatic arterial blood flow: The hepatic arterial buffer response. Am J Physiol 1985;249:G549–G556.
22. Lautt WW: Role and control of the hepatic artery. In Lautt WW (ed): Hepatic Circulation in Health and Disease. New York: Raven Press, 1981;203–220.
23. Legare DJ, Lautt WW: Hepatic venous resistance site in the dog: Localization and validation of intrahepatic pressure measurements. Can J Physiol Pharmacol 1987;65:352–359.
24. Richardson PD, Withrington PG: Liver blood flow 2. Effects of drugs and hormones on liver blood flow. Gastroenterology 1981;81:356–375.
25. Lautt WW, Legare DJ: The use of 8-phenyltheophylline as a competitive antagonist of adenosine and an inhibitor of the intrinsic regulatory mechanism of the hepatic artery. Can J Physiol Pharmacol 1985;63:717–722.
26. Lautt WW, Legare DJ, d'Almeida MS: Adenosine as putative regulator of hepatic arterial flow (the buffer response). Am J Physiol 1985;248:H331–H338.
27. Henderson JM, Gilmore GT, Mackay GJ, et al: Hemodynamics during liver transplantation: The interactions between cardiac output and portal venous and hepatic arterial flows. Hepatology 1992;16:715–718.
28. Lautt WW: Adenosine-mediated regulation of hepatic blood flow. In Phillis JW (ed): Adenosine and the Adenine Nucleotides as Regulators of Cellular Function. Orlando, FL: CRC Press, 1991;213–220.
29. Ezzat WR, Lautt WW: Hepatic arterial pressure-flow autoregulation is adensoine mediated. Am J Physiol 1987;252:H836–H845.
30. Messerli FH, Nowaczynski W, Honda M, et al: Effects of angiotensin II on steroid metabolism and hepatic blood flow in man. Circ Res 1977;40:204–207.
31. Lautt WW: The hepatic artery: subservient to hepatic metabolism or guardian of normal hepatic clearance rates of humoral substances. Gen Pharmacol 1977;8:73–78.

32. d'Almeida MS, McQuaker JE, D'Aleo L, Lautt WW: Competing effects of intravenously infused dilator agents and raised portal blood flow on hepatic arterial conductance. Proc West Pharmacol Soc 1988;31:113–115.

33. Lautt WW, d'Almeida MS, McQuaker JE, D'Aleo L: Impact of the hepatic arterial buffer response on splanchnic vascular responses to intravenous adenosine, isoproterenol and glucagon. Can J Physiol Pharmacol 1988;66:807–813.

34. Lagerkranser M, Irestedt L, Sollevi A, Andreen M: Control and splanchnic hemodynamics in the dog during controlled hypotension with adenosine. Anesthesiology 1984;60:547–552.

35. Greenway CV, Stark RD: Hepatic vascular bed. Physiol Rev 1971;51:23–65.

36. Israel Y, Orrego H: Hepatocyte demand and substrate supply as factors in the susceptibility to alcoholic injury: Pathogenesis and prevention. Clin Gastroent 1981;10:355–373.

37. Greenway CV, Lawson AE, Stark RD: The effect of haemorrhage on hepatic artery and portal vein flows in the anaesthetized cat. J Physiol (Lond) 1967;193:375–379.

38. Mathie RT, Blumgart LH: The hepatic haemodynamic response to acute portal venous blood flow reductions in the dog. Pflugers Arch 1983;399:223–227.

39. Fernandez-Munoz D, Caramelo C, Santos JC, et al: Systemic and splanchnic haemodynamic disturbances in conscious rats with experimental liver cirrhosis without ascites. Am J Physiol 1985;249:G316–G320.

40. Groszmann RJ, Blei AT, Kniaz JL, et al: Portal pressure reduction induced by partial mechanical obstruction of the superior mesenteric artery in the anesthetized dog. Gastroenterology 1978;75:187–192.

41. Hughes RL, Mathie RT, Fitch W, Campbell D: Liver blood flow and oxygen consumption during metabolic acidosis and alkalosis in the greyhound. Clin Sci 1980;60:355–361.

42. Bauereisen E, Lutz J: Blood circulation and oxygen uptake in liver. Z Gastroent 1975;13:70–76.

43. Lloyd HGE, Schrader J: The importance of the transmethylation pathway for adenosine metabolism in the heart. In Gerlach E, Becker BF (eds): Topics and Perspectives in Adenosine Research. Berlin: Springer-Verlag, 1987;199–208.

44. Chou CC: Splanchnic and overall cardiovascular hemodynamics during eating and digestion. Fed Proc 1983;42:1658–1661.

45. Lautt WW: Hepatic nerves—a review of their functions and effects. Can J Physiol Pharmacol 1980;58:105–123.

46. Lautt WW: Afferent and efferent neural roles in liver function. Prog Neurobiol 1983;21:323–348.

47. Gardemann A, Puschel GP, Jungermann K: Nervous control of liver metabolism and hemodynamics. Eur J Biochem 1992;207:399–411.

48. McCuskey RS: Intrahepatic distribution of nerves: A review. In Popper H, Bianchi L, Gudat F, Reutter W (eds): Communications of Liver Cells. England: MTP Press, 1980;115–120.

49. Burchell AR, Moreno AH, Panke WF, Nealon TF: Hepatic artery flow improvement after portocaval shunt: A single hemodynamic clinical correlate. Ann Surg 1976;184:289–300.

50. Zimmon DS, Kessler RE: Effect of portal venous blood flow diversion on portal pressure. J Clin Invest 1980;65:1388–1397.

51. Kontos HA, Shapiro W, Mauck HP, Patterson GL: General and regional circulatory alterations in cirrhosis of the liver. Am J Med 1964;37:526–535.

52. Kowalski HJ, Abelman WH: The cardiac output at rest in Laennec's cirrhosis. J Clin Invest 1953;32:1025–1033.

53. Lebrec D, Bataille C, Bercoff E, Valla D: Hemodynamic changes in patients with portal venous obstruction. Hepatology 1983;3:550–553.

54. Huet PM, Villenevue JP, Marleau D, Viallet A: Hepatic circulation: applicable human methodology. In Lautt WW (ed): Hepatic Circulation in Health and Disease. New York: Raven Press, 1981;57–74.

55. Lautt WW, Greenway CV, Legare DJ: Effect of hepatic nerves, norepinephrine, angiotensin, elevated central venous pressure on postsinusoidal resistance sites and intrahepatic pressures in cats. Microvasc Res 1987;33:50–61.

56. Lautt WW, Legare DJ: Effect of histamine, norepineprhine and nerves on vascular resistance and pressures in dog liver. Am J Physiol 1987;252:G472–G478.

57. Child CG: The Hepatic Circulation and Portal Hypertension. Philadelphia: W.B. Saunders, 1954.

58. Wanless IR, Medline A, Phillips MJ: Pathology of the hepatic vasculature including hepatic vascular tumors. In Lautt WW (ed): Hepatic Circulation in Health and Disease. New York: Raven Press, 1981;257–281.

59. Groszmann RJ, Atterbury CE: Clinical applications of the measurement of portal venous pressure. J Clin Gastroenterol 1980;2:379–386.

60. Lautt WW, Greenway CV, Legare DJ, Weisman H: Localization of intrahepatic portal vascular resistance. Am J Physiol 1986;14:G375–G381.

61. Elias H, Petty D: Gross anatomy of the blood vessels and ducts within the human liver. Am J Anat 1952;90:59–111.

62. Bohlen HG, Maass-Moreno R, Rothe CF: Hepatic venular pressures of rats, dogs, and rabbits. Am J Physiol 1991;261:G539–G547.

63. Maass-Moreno R, Rothe CF: Contribution of the large hepatic veins to postsinusoidal vascular resistance. Am J Physiol 1992;262:G14–G22,

64. Lautt WW, Legare DJ, Greenway CV: Effect of hepatic venous sphincter contraction on transmission of central venous pressure to lobar and portal pressure. Can J Physiol Pharmacol 1987:65:2235–2243.

65. Greenway CV, Lautt WW: Distensibility of hepatic venous resistance sites and consequences on portal pressure. Am J Physiol 1988;254:H452–H458.

66. Lautt WW, Greenway CV, Legare DJ: Index of contractility: Quantitative analysis of hepatic venous distensibility. Am J Physiol 1991;260:G325–G332.

67. Lautt WW, Legare DJ: Evaluation of hepatic venous resistance responses using index of contractility (IC). Am J Physiol 1992;262:G510–G516.

68. Lautt WW, Legare DJ: Passive autoregulation of portal venous pressure: Distensible hepatic resistance. Am J Physiol 1992;263:G702–G708.

69. Lautt WW, Legare DJ, Ezzat WR: Quantitation of the hepatic arterial buffer response to graded changes in portal blood flow. Gastroenterology 1990;98:1024–1028.

70. Bennett TD, Rothe CF: Hepatic capacitance responses to changes in flow and hepatic venous pressure in dogs. Am J Physiol 1981;240:H18–H28.

71. Greenway CV, Lautt WW: Blood volume, the venous system, preload, and cardiac output. Can J Physiol Pharmacol 1986;64(4):383–387.

72. Ingles A, Legare DJ, Lautt WW: Development of portacaval shunts in portal-stenotic cats. Can J Physiol Pharmacol 1993;71:671–674.

73. Groszmann RJ, Blei AT, Atterbury, CE: Portal hypertension. In Arias IM, Jakoby WB, Popper H, Schachter D, Shafritz DA (eds): The Liver: Biology and Pathobiology, 2nd ed. New York: Raven Press, 1988;1147–1159.

74. Koshy A, Sekiyama T, Hadengue A, et al: Effects of α1 and β-adrenergic antagonists and 5- hydroxytryptamine receptor antagonist on portal-systemic collateral vascular resistance in conscious rats with portal hypertension. J Gastroent Hepatol 1992;7:449–454.

75. Orrego H, Blendis LM, Crossley IR, et al: Correlation of intrahepatic pressure with collagen in the Disse space and hepatomegaly in humans and in the rat. Gastroenterology 1981;80:546–556.

76. Boyer TD, Triger DR, Horisawa M, et al: Direct transhepatic measurement of portal vein pressure using a thin needle. Gastroenterology 1977;72:584–589.

77. Orrego H, Amenabar E, Lara G, et al: Measurement of intrahepatic pressure as index of portal pressure. Am J Med Sci 1964;247:278–282.

78. Reichen J, Le M: Verapamil favorably influences hepatic microvascular exchange and function in rats with cirrhosis of the liver. J Clin Invest 1986;78:448–455.

79. Willet IR, Jennings G, Esler M, Dudley FJ: Sympathetic tone modulates portal venous pressure in alcoholic cirrhosis. Lancet 1986;2:939–943.

79a. Lautt WW, d'Almeida MS, unpublished data, 1993.

80. Shibayama Y, Nakata K: Localization of increased hepatic vascular resistance in liver cirrhosis. Hepatology 1985;5:643–648.

81. Tanikawa K: Ultrastructural Aspects of the Liver and its Disorders. New York: Igaku-Shoin, 1979;167.

82. Lautt WW: Resistance or conductance for expression of arterial vascular tone. Microvasc Res 1989;37:230–236.

83. d'Almeida MS, Lautt WW: The effect of glucagon on autoregulatory escape from hepatic arterial vasoconstriction in the cat. Proc West Pharmacol Soc 1989; 32:265–267.

84. d'Almeida MS, Lautt WW: Expression of vascular escape: Conductance or resistance. Am J Physiol 1992; 262:H1191–H1196.

85. Lautt WW, McQuaker JE: Methodological approach to pharmacodynami calculations of vascular responses in vivo. Proc West Pharmacol Soc 1989;32:227–230.

86. Rothe CF: Reflex control of veins and vascular capacitance. Physiol Rev 1983;63:1281–1342.

87. Rothe CF. Properties of veins. In Abramson DI, Dobrin PB (eds): Blood Vessels and Lymphatics in Organ Systems. Orlando, FL: Academic Press, 1984;85–96.

88. Greenway CV, Lautt WW: Effects of hepatic venous pressure on transsinusoidal fluid transfer in the liver of the anesthetized cat. Circ Res 1970;26:697–703.

89. Greenway CV, Seaman KL, Innes IR: Norepinephrine on venous compliance and unstressed volume in cat liver. Am J Physiol 1985;248:H468–H476.

90. Lautt WW, Brown LC, Durham JS: Active and passive control of hepatic blood volume responses to hemorrhage at normal and raised hepatic venous pressure in cats. Can J Physiol Pharmacol 1980;58:1049–1057.

91. Greenway CV: Mechanisms and quantitative assessment of drug effects on cardiac output using a new model of the circulation. Pharmacol Rev 1981;33:213–251.

92. Schafer J, d'Almeida MS, Weisman H, Lautt WW: Reduced hepatic blood volume responses to hemorrhage and nerve stimulation but normal compliance and norepinephrine effects in cats with chronic bile duct ligation. Hepatology 1993;18:969–977.

93. Greenway CV: Hepatic plethysmography. In Lautt WW (ed): Hepatic Circulation in Health and Disease. New York: Raven Press, 1981;41–54.

94. Greenway CV, Lautt WW: Effects of hepatic venous pressure on transsinusoidal fluid transfer in the liver of the anesthetized cat. Circ Res 1970;26:697–703.

95. Greenway CV: Hepatic fluid exchange. In Lautt W (ed): Hepatic Circulation in Health and Disease. New York: Raven Press, 1981;153–167.

96. Lautt WW: Effects of acute, passive hepatic congestion on blood flow and oxygen uptake in the intact liver of the cat. Circ Res 1977;41:787–790.

97. Zink J, Greenway CV: Intraperitoneal pressure in formation and reabsorption of ascites in cats. Am J Physiol 1977;2:H185–H190.

98. Schaffner F, Popper H: Capillarization of hepatic sinusoids in man. Gastroenterology 1963;44:239–242.

99. Phillips MJ, Steiner JW: Electron microscopy of liver cells in cirrhotic nodules. Am J Pathol 1965;46:985–1006.

100. Mak KM, Lieber CS: Alterations in endothelial fenestrations in liver sinusoids of baboons fed alcohol: A scanning electron microscopic study. Hepatology 1984; 4:386–391.

Chapter 10

HEMODYNAMICS, DISTRIBUTION OF BLOOD VOLUME, AND KINETICS OF VASOACTIVE SUBSTANCES IN CIRRHOSIS

JENS H. HENRIKSEN, M.D.
SØREN MØLLER, M.D.

Hemodynamics
  Assessment of Blood Flow
  Mean Transit Time (Circulation Time)
Blood Volume
  Central and Arterial Blood Volume
Vasoactive Substances
  Kinetics and Disposal of Vasoactive Substances
  Kinetics of Atrial Natriuretic Factor

Kinetics of Calcitonin Gene-related Peptide
Kinetics of Nitric Oxide
Kinetics of Catecholamines
Kinetics of Endothelin
Relationship between Hemodynamics, Distribution of Blood Volume, and Kinetics of Vasoactive Substances
Summary

Cirrhosis is associated with a spectrum of circulatory disturbances.[1–3] Besides increased portal-sinusoidal pressure and splanchnic blood flow, the systemic circulation displays characteristic alterations: (1) increases in cardiac output, heart rate, and plasma and blood volume and (2) decreases in renal blood flow, systemic vascular resistance, and arterial blood pressure.[4–6] Moreover, recent investigations show that circulation times are abnormal in patients with cirrhosis and portal hypertension.[7–10] As substantiated in chapter 9, systemic vasodilation plays a central role in the circulatory derangement in cirrhosis. In addition to opening up arteriovenous shunts, vasodilatation may be mediated by an alteration in the balance between vasodilators and vasoconstrictors. The activation of vasoconstrictor systems—the renin-angiotensin-aldosterone system (RAAS), the sympathetic nervous system (SNS), and vasopressin—is now well documented, in cirrhosis and is described in chapters 1, 12, and 19. But the case with vasodilators is different; several candidates have been proposed—vasoactive intestinal polypeptide, substance P, glucagon, atrial natriuretic factor (ANF), prostaglandins, kinins, endothelial-derived relaxing factor (EDRF or nitric oxide), enkephalins, endotoxins, and cytokines—but so far research has failed to turn up a specific substance.[11–23]

Vasodilatation may be mediated by substances that are either produced in excess or that escape degradation in the diseased liver. Many vasoconstrictors and vasodilators are abundantly extracted from tissue, and their overall clearance and disposal may depend on blood flow.[24] Changes in the circulation, therefore, may result in altered disposal and changes in the circulating levels of particular bioactive substances. The consequence is a complex interaction between hemodynamics and the modulators responsible for the altered circulation.

The genesis and perpetuation of fluid retention in cirrhosis remain unclarified.[25–29] The overflow theory of ascites formation suggests that fluid overflows into the peritoneal cavity as a result of circulatory overfilling.[30,31] Conversely, another theory posits circulatory underfilling as the central mechanism.[26,32,33] Whereas the finding of an increased plasma volume suggests overfilling,[30,31] the natriuretic effect in some patients of water immersion or implantation of a peritoneovenous shunt suggests central underfilling.[34,35] The size of the central vascular compartment in which volume receptors and baroreceptors are located is an important problem, not only for the pathogenesis of fluid retention, but also to understand whether the hyperdynamic circulation is mediated through an increased cardiac preload or

TABLE 10.1. Methods and Quantities in the Assessment of Blood Flow

Methods	Overall Flow Rate (ml/min)	Perfusion Coefficient (ml/min·100 gm)	Regional Tissue Flow (ml/min·100 gm)	Flow Velocity (mm/sec)	Capillary Flow	Arteriovenous Shunt Flow		Flow Distribution (%)	Flow Change (%)
Indicator (thermo) dilution	+				+	plus	+		
Fick's method	+				+	plus	+		
Venous occlusive plethysmography		+			+	plus	+		
^{133}Xe clearance (washout)			+		+			(+)*	+
Microspheres	(+)†		+		+		+	+	+
Laser Doppler				+	+				+
Pulsed Doppler	(+)‡			+					+

* If ^{133}Xe is supplied by artery.

† In animal experiments.

‡ Under the assumption that vascular cross-sectional area can be estimated with adequate precision.

a reduced afterload.[5,36–38] Moreover, a knowledge of the mechanisms behind the hemodynamic disturbances in cirrhosis may have important implications for therapy.[25,29,39]

This chapter outlines the basic elements of hemodynamics in cirrhosis, provides an updated review of recent investigations of circulatory alterations in different vascular areas and distribution of blood volume, and discusses newly discovered bioactive substances with potential effects on the circulation and their kinetics in relation to circulatory disturbances in cirrhosis.

HEMODYNAMICS

Cardiac output and heart rate are generally higher in patients with severe liver insufficiency than in patients with almost normal liver function.[3,6,40] Vasodilation has been described in several vascular areas, including lungs, splanchnic system, skin, and muscle. Before discussing the distribution of the increased cardiac output in cirrhosis, we should consider a few basic aspects of methodology.

Assessment of Blood Flow

Measurement of blood flow may assess only capillary perfusion (e.g., ^{133}xenon washout, laser Doppler), whereas other techniques give the sum of capillary perfusion and shunt flow (e.g., venous occlusion plethysmography, indicator dilution). Some techniques determine the perfusion coefficient, i.e., the flow rate per gram of tissue

(^{133}xenon washout, venous occlusion plethysmography), whereas others determine the overall flow rate (indicator dilution, Fick's principle) or the linear blood velocity (Doppler sonography). Although the microsphere technique may give the absolute flow in animal experiments, it gives only the relative flow in humans under noninvasive conditions. The diversity of flow measurements (Table 10.1) has led to confusion, and the method should be selected according to factors such as type of flow to be determined and presence of shunts.[41]

Although studies have demonstrated that the splanchnic inflow is increased[6,42] and the renal blood flow diminished,[6,43] the other organs and tissues that receive the increased cardiac output have yet to be established in humans.[6]

Blood flow in the skin is probably increased, particularly in the hands and fingers,[44] and intravital microscopy has demonstrated substantial dilatation of capillaries in the nail beds.[45] Spider nevi represent arteriolar dilatation, although recent investigations have failed to demonstrate a relation between the presence of spider nevi and cutaneous blood flow.[45]

Skeletal muscle blood flow seems to be increased in patients with cirrhosis,[46] although disturbances in the perfusion of skeletal muscle are insufficiently investigated, partly because of technical and methodologic difficulties. Because of wasting in patients with cirrhosis, an elevated perfusion coefficient (ml/min·100 gm) does not necessarily mean overall blood flow (ml/min) in skeletal muscle is increased because the muscle mass may be substantially reduced. Such problems have caused confusion; present knowledge of blood flow in skeletal muscle of cirrhotic patients is insufficient.

Some cirrhotic patients have a decrease in arterial oxygen saturation[47-49] because of disturbances in ventilation and perfusion and shunting through microscopic or larger arteriovenous fistulas in the lungs.[50,51] Portal-pulmonary collateral flow has also been described,[52] and patients with cirrhosis have reduced pulmonary vascular resistance.[50,51,53] Although some patients may exhibit organic lung disease, the majority have a reversible disorder, recently described as the hepatopulmonary syndrome.[54] This syndrome is characterized by low arterial oxygenation, pulmonary shunts and abnormal ventilation-perfusion ratios, low pulmonary vascular resistance, high perfusion, and reduced lung diffusion capacity.[54] The disturbances are reversible and disappear after liver transplantation.[50]

The cerebral blood flow is poorly investigated in patients with liver disease. It is decreased in patients with acute and chronic severe hepatic encephalopathy, although in some patients with coma it seems to be elevated, with cerebral edema as the outcome.[55,56]

Thus, the distribution of the increased cardiac output (Fig. 10.1) needs further investigation; at present it is not possible to give a complete picture of the distribution of abnormal blood flow.

Mean Transit Time (Circulation Time)

Kinetics deals with the relation of mass, volume, and concentration with time in the body. Circulation times and mean transit time ($\bar{t}$) have been extensively treated in the kinetic theory by various authors.[41,57-60] In brief, the mean transit time—i.e., the average time required for all elements of a given material to pass through a specified system—can be viewed as the volume of the compartment relative to the flow through the compartment (Fig. 10.2). This view is analogous to the clearance concept, which is the excretion rate relative to plasma concentration. For example, if cardiac output is 4 L/min and blood volume is 5 L, the mean overall circulation time is 1.25 minutes; therefore, the average time required for a red cell to pass the aortic valve twice is 1.25 minutes. If cardiac output is reduced to 2.5 L/min or increased to 15 L/min, the mean overall circulation time is 2 minutes or 20 seconds,

Cardiac Output

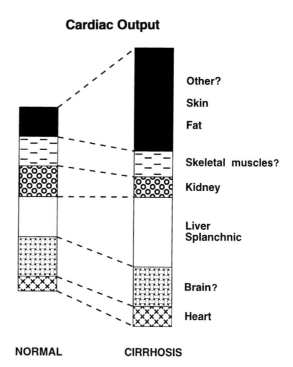

NORMAL   CIRRHOSIS

FIGURE 10.1. Regional distribution of cardiac output in normal subjects and cirrhotic patients. Note that increased cardiac output in cirrhosis mainly affects the splanchnic and peripheral perfusion, whereas the renal blood flow is decreased. Cerebral, subcutaneous, and skeletal muscle blood flow are poorly investigated in cirrhosis.

respectively. Conversely, if one determines the blood flow rate and mean circulation time as the mean transit time of an indicator substance, the volume can be derived from the fundamental kinetic equation: volume = flow rate × mean transit time (see Fig. 10.2).

The central circulation time is substantially reduced in patients with cirrhosis compared with age-matched controls[7-10] (Fig. 10.3). The overall circulation time (i.e., blood volume divided by cardiac output) is somewhat reduced in cirrhotic patients. In contrast, cirrhotic patients have a normal noncentral circulation time (overall circulation time minus central circulation time): that is, circulation time in the peripheral parts of the arterial tree, systemic capillary bed, and venous bed, including the splanchnic system, is normal. Segmental circulation times may be determined after bolus injection of gamma-emitting indicator into the central veins or right heart followed by external detection (residue detection) with a gamma camera.[9] The transit time of different

Basic Concept

Volume = Flow x Mean Transit Time

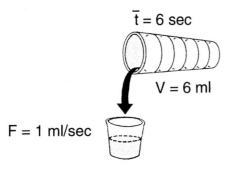

$$\bar{t} = 6 \text{ sec}$$

$$V = 6 \text{ ml}$$

$$F = 1 \text{ ml/sec}$$

Central and arterial blood volume

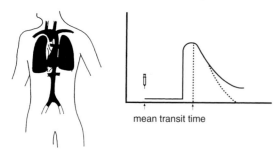

mean transit time

CBV = Cardiac output x Mean transit time

FIGURE 10.2 Principles of circulation times, regional blood volumes, and blood flow. *Upper panel* illustrates the fundamental kinetic relation between the mean transit (circulation) time ($\bar{t}$), volume (V), and flow (F). The mean transit time may be determined as the time-weighted area under the indicator curve. The central and arterial blood volume (CBV)—i.e., the blood volume in the cardiac cavities, lungs, and central arterial tree—is assess as the mean transit time multiplied by the cardiac output (*lower panel*).

segments of the central circulation may be estimated by a complicated mathematical process involving deconvolution. With this technique, Hartleb and Rudzki[9] found a substantial reduction in central circulation time and segmental circulation times in patients with decompensated cirrhosis.

The reduced circulation times in some of the vascular bed in cirrhosis reflect not only a hyperdynamic circulation with increased cardiac output but also an abnormal distribution in blood volume.[6,33,61,62] Thus, the combination of hyperdynamic perfusion and reduced vascular volume

highly accelerates the flow in that part of the vascular bed. In addition to increased overall blood and plasma volumes, an alteration in the balance of vasodilator and vasoconstrictor activity in resistance and capacitance vessels may contribute to the abnormal size of parts of the vascular bed.[63,64]

BLOOD VOLUME

Increased plasma and blood volume in patients with cirrhosis has been described by Tristani and Cohn[65] and Lieberman and Reynolds.[30] Increased volume was first ascribed to an increase in the splanchnic vascular bed as a result of portal congestion. However, decompression with surgical portacaval shunt decreased the plasma volume only from 64 to 55 ml/kg,[30] which was still significantly higher than in controls. Because the transvascular transport of plasma proteins is accelerated in patients with cirrhosis,[30,66,67] codetermination of some parts of the extravascular space by the conventional albumin dilution technique may involve a methodologic error. Moreover, the ratio between peripheral and whole-body hematocrit is somewhat decreased in cirrhotic patients[30,68]; hence calculation of the blood volume may give erroneous results unless the red cell volume is measured directly. e.g., by ^{51}Cr-labeled red cells.[68] It is now evident, however, that such reservations lead only to minor errors in determination of plasma and blood volume.[8,66,67] Plasma and blood volumes are increased in patients with cirrhosis, even in the compensated stage of the disease.[8,10,30,31,65–70] Nevertheless, increased overall plasma and blood volume does not exclude the possibility of an abnormal distribution of blood volume with hypovolemic and hypervolemic parts of the vascular bed. In fact, a number of findings suggest hypovolemia in some parts of the circulation: highly enhanced sympathetic nervous activity, activation of the RAAS, elevated circulating vasopressin, low arterial blood pressure, and reduced renal perfusion.[5]

Central and Arterial Blood Volume

The size of the central and arterial blood volume (CBV)—i.e., the blood volume in the heart cavities, lungs, and central arterial tree (up to points that are temporally equidistant from the heart to the aortic bifurcation)—was recently determined

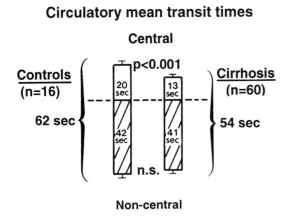

Circulatory mean transit times

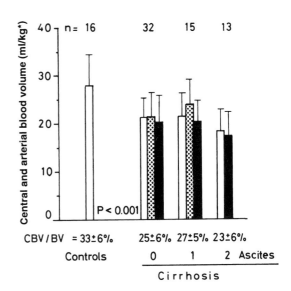

CBV/BV = 33±6%   25±6% 27±5% 23±6%

FIGURE 10.3. Circulatory mean transit times in normal subjects and cirrhotic patients. The central circulation time is significantly reduced in patients with cirrhosis compared with controls, whereas the noncentral circulation times are nearly equal. The overall circulation time, assessed as total blood volume divided by cardiac output, equals the sum of the central and noncentral circulation times and is slightly but significantly reduced in cirrhosis (54 vs. 62 sec, $p < 0.01$). Data from Henriksen et al.[7,8,10]

by Henriksen et al. as the cardiac output multiplied by mean transit time of the indicator[7,8,10] (see Fig. 10.2). This volume was substantially reduced in patients with cirrhosis (Fig. 10.4) with the lowest values in patients with tense ascites and reduced systemic vascular resistance.[8] The value was decreased also in patients without fluid retention. Particularly with early fluid retention, whether the patients are centrally over- or under-filled[35,71–73] is still disputed.

The term effective blood volume has been defined in various ways.[74] According to one definition, it is the nonhepatosplanchnic blood volume[30,75]; according to another, it is the part of the blood volume that affects volume receptors and baroreceptors (see chapters 1, 3, and 8). From an anatomic point of view the first definition is simpler and has been applied in animal studies, because it is possible experimentally to exclude the hepatosplanchnic parts of the circulation[75] and thereby to assess the size of effective blood volume. Determined thus, the effective blood volume proved to be increased in animals with experimental cirrhosis.[75] If one applies the second definition, the activity of essential neurohumoral systems may reveal whether volume receptors and baroreceptors are stimulated or suppressed.[5] Problems concerning the size of effective blood

ml/kg* Central and arterial blood volume

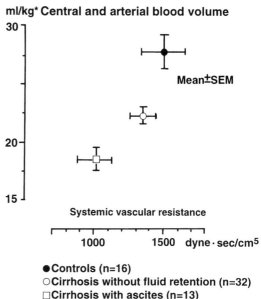

● Controls (n=16)
○ Cirrhosis without fluid retention (n=32)
□ Cirrhosis with ascites (n=13)

FIGURE 10.4. The central and arterial blood volume (CBV) expressed in ml/kg ideal body weight in normal subjects and cirrhotic patients with various amounts of ascites. Open box = no treatment, shaded box = spironolactone, solid box = spironolactone combined with loop agents. CBV/BV indicates percentage CBV of total blood volume (upper panel). Central and arterial blood volume in relation to systemic vascular resistance (lower panel). Data from Henriksen et al.[7,8,10]

volume have not been solved in humans because of inadequate tools for direct measurements. Because volume sensors are located in the heart and lungs and baroreceptors in the aortic arch and carotid sinus,[76–78] it seems appropriate to equate

Blood Volume

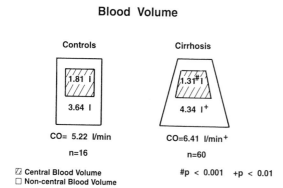

FIGURE 10.5. Reduced central and expanded noncentral blood volume in patients with cirrhosis compared with normal subjects. Data from Henriksen et al.[7,8,10]

Cirrhosis

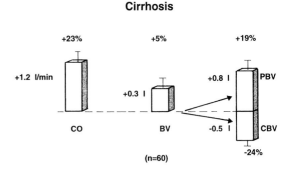

FIGURE 10.6. Average changes in cardiac output (CO), total blood volume (BV), noncentral blood volume (PBV), and central and arterial blood volume (CBV) in cirrhosis. Note that the percentual changes in PBV and CBV are almost identical to the change in CO. Data from Henriksen et al.[7,8,10]

central and arterial blood volume, as determined by the indicator technique, with the volume that produces signals of vascular filling to pertinent receptors. Determined thus, effective blood volume is reduced in patients with advanced cirrhosis and ascites.

Analysis of segmental circulation times and blood flow discloses an abnormal distribution in the blood volume of cirrhotic patients (Fig. 10.5) The noncentral blood volume is increased in almost exactly the same proportion as the cardiac output (Fig.10.6). However, the central and arterial blood volume is reduced despite an increase in overall blood volume. Why cirrhotic patients are unable to maintain a normal-sized central and arterial blood volume (effective blood volume) despite fluid retention thus remains an enigma.

Changes in body position produce major changes in circulation times and flow (Table 10.2). Head-up tilting reduced cardiac output substantially and prolonged the central circulation time, resulting in a further decrease in the central and arterial blood volume.[8,79] Conversely, head-down tilting produced a small increase in the central and arterial blood volume.[8] As expected, lower body negative pressure reduces central and arterial blood volume dramatically.[8]

In patients with cirrhosis, the central and arterial blood volume is negatively correlated to the size of portal venous pressure (Fig. 10.7). The central and arterial blood volume was directly correlated to the systemic vascular resistance (see Fig. 10.4), suggesting that the greater the vasodilatation, the greater the central hypovolemia.[7,8,10] Systemic vasodilation, portal congestion, and sequestration of fluid in the peritoneal cavity are

probably the main causes of the shift in blood volume from the central parts of the circulation, including the arterial tree, to the systemic veins and hepatosplanchnic bed, with activation of volume receptors and baroreceptors as the outcome.

VASOACTIVE SUBSTANCES

A large number of vasoactive substances have been identified.[11–24] Most can be classified as either vasodilators or vasoconstrictors. However, some have different actions in different vascular beds, and some may stimulate the release of other endogenous substances with an opposite effect. For instance, epinephrine is a vasoconstrictor in the kidney but may act as a dilator in heart and skeletal muscle.[80] Endothelin 1 (ET-1) is a powerful vasoconstrictor in the coronary circulation and kidney[81–83] but may release nitric oxide (NO), which blurs the response.[84] Vasoconstrictors and vasodilators are discussed in detail in chapters 17 and 18.

Kinetics and Disposal of Vasoactive Substances

The past decades have seen a substantial increase in the number of identified vasoactive substances, and refined analyses now allow reliable determination of the concentration of several such substances in plasma and tissue. Production, release, regulation, and function have attracted considerable interest. However, the degradation and disposal of vasoactive substances also must be considered, because the circulating level is

TABLE 10.2. Cardiac Output, Central Mean Circulation Time, and Central and Arterial Blood Volume in Patients with Cirrhosis

Body Position	Cardiac Output (L/min)	Central Mean Circulation Time (sec)	Central and Arterial Blood Volume (ml/kg)
Supine (n = 6)	6.9 ± 2.7*	13.7 ± 3.7	22.6 ± 7.8
60° head-up	4.8 ± 1.9	16.1 ± 4.0	18.5 ± 4.8
% change	−30.4%	+17.5%	−18.1%
p value	< 0.01	< 0.005	= 0.05
Supine (n = 4)	5.8 ± 2.1	14.5 ± 3.4	20.7 ± 4.3
15° head-down	7.0 ± 1.3	12.7 ± 1.3	22.4 ± 4.6
% change	+19.6%	−12.4%	+8.2%
p value	< 0.05	ns	< 0.05

* Mean ± SD.

From Henriksen JH, Bendtsen F, Sørensen TA, et al: Reduced central blood volume in cirrhosis. Gastroenterology 1989; 97:1506–1513, with permission.

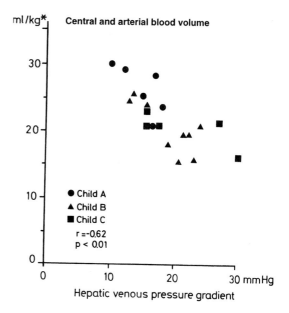

FIGURE 10.7. Relation between central and arterial blood volume and portal venous pressure, determined as hepatic venous pressure gradient. (Modified from Henriksen JH, Bendtsen F, Gerbes AL, et al: Estimated central blood volume in cirrhosis: Relationship to sympathetic nervous activity, beta-adrenergic blockade and atrial natriuretic factor. Hepatology 1992;16:1163–1170.)

governed by a balance between presence in and removal from the plasma.[24] Particularly in patients with reduced hepatic metabolic function, as in cirrhosis, an elevated circulating level may reflect a decreased rate of disposal. Before considering specific examples, a brief general description of whole-body and organ kinetics is useful.

Whole-body kinetics may be studied after a single injection or continuous infusion of a particular substance.[24] If the turnover is rapid, continuous infusion is appropriate because of problems with distribution and collection of samples after a single injection. Regardless of the technique, plasma samples must be collected at the proper location (e.g. systemic or pulmonary artery), especially when the substance has a high turnover rate or is degraded in lung or peripheral tissues.[41,85] Otherwise, the use of a peripheral venous sample leads to overestimation of the metabolic clearance rate.[86]

Organ kinetics may be assessed by the Fick technique, which uses catheterization of the artery and organ vein. This technique assumes the presence of mixed blood at the organ inlet as well as at the outlet.[41] Whereas this assumption is reasonably justified in the arterial system, organ veins, such as the hepatic vein, may not be well mixed, especially in diseases with unequal perfusion (e.g.cirrhosis). The arteriovenous extraction ratio (i.e., the fraction of a substance that is removed during one passage of plasma through the organ or tissues) is easily assessed, if disposal alone takes place in the organ.[41] But if both release and disposal take place in the same organ

(e.g., neurotransmitters), special techniques, often requiring the use of radiolabeled substances, are needed.[87]

Early animal experiments suggested the existence of a circulating vasodilator that might be produced by or escape degradation in the diseased liver.[88] Eligible candidates include the prostaglandins, but their action is documented only in the kidney[11,89,90] (see chapter 14). Substance P is markedly increased in the plasma from patients with hepatic coma[15] but normal in most patients with cirrhosis and well-preserved liver function.[16] Vasoactive intestinal polypeptide and methionine enkephalin have also been suggested but not proved.[14,18,91] According to experimental evidence, glucagon is implicated in the splanchnic and systemic vasodilatation of cirrhosis.[19,20] The circulating level of glucagon is related to portosystemic collateral flow in portal hypertension as well as to systemic hemodynamic changes.[17] Increased glucagon also may contribute to vasodilatation by reducing the vascular sensitivity to endogenous vasoconstrictors. This section deals more extensively with the kinetics of catecholamines, three newly discovered peptides—atrial natriuretic factor (ANF),[92] calcitonin gene-related peptide (CGRP), and NO, all of which are potent vasodilators[21,86,93,94]—and endothelin 1 (ET 1), a recently discovered vasoconstrictor.[81–83]

Kinetics of Atrial Natriuretic Factor

In addition to its natriuretic effect, atrial natriuretic factor (ANF) possesses vasodilatory properties, modifies the baroreflex, and inhibits the release of renin (see chapter 15). Low, normal, and high circulating levels of ANF have been described in patients with cirrhosis,[35,92,95–98] and it is still debated whether increased circulating ANF is due to decreased disposal in the diseased liver or increased cardiac release.[98–101]

ANF is abundantly extracted from organs and tissues.[7,100,102,103] It is highly extracted in the kidney and the hepatointestinal system, including the superior collateral drainage through the azygos vein.[7,100,102,103] Recently it was reported that the overall hepatointestinal clearance of ANF in cirrhosis is normal or even somewhat increased.[101] Thus, increased circulating levels of ANF seem to reflect increased release rather than decreased disposal. Because the extraction of ANF from peripheral tissue may be significant,[7,102,103] peripheral samples of venous plasma may underestimate the circulating level.

The mechanisms behind or mechanisms that mediate increased ANF in cirrhosis are unclear, and it is still debated whether ascites contributes to increased release by changing the transmural atrial pressure and spatial relations in the heart.[92] Unlike the elevated pressure in congestive heart failure, pressure in the right and left atria is almost normal in patients with cirrhosis[6,7,10,54] and correlates with ANF level only to a minor extent.[92,104] Increased ANF alone cannot explain the increased systemic vasodilatation in cirrhosis (see chapter 15).

Kinetics of Calcitonin Gene-related Peptide

Calcitonin gene-related peptide (alpha-CGRP), a potent vasodilator, was recently discovered in humans.[105,106] This 37-amino-acid neuropeptide has been localized to the central and peripheral nervous systems, including skeletal muscle, cardiovascular system, urogenital tract, and digestive tissues.[105,107–109] DNA studies have shown the existence of a second CGRP (beta-CGRP) gene in humans.[110] Beta-CGRP differs from alpha-CGRP only in three amino acids. However, the two types of CGRP bind to the same receptor.[111] On a molar basis CGRP seems to be the most potent vasodilator peptide described so far.[106] Recent studies have shown that CGRP colocalizes with substance P in both central and peripheral nerves.[93] Either singly or in combination with substance P and its stimulatory effect on acetylcholine synthesis, CGRP may contribute to systemic vasodilation in cirrhosis.

Determination of CGRP in plasma from artery and different organ veins showed no significant arteriovenous difference in patients with cirrhosis and controls.[113] The most likely explanation for this finding is the occurrence of both release and disposal in the same vascular area, as with other neurotransmitters and neuromodulators (e.g., NE, substance P). The circulating level of CGRP is directly related to the severity of disease as assessed from the Child scores.[13] Gupta et al.[114] recently confirmed the finding of highly increased circulating CGRP, especially in patients with ascites and hepatorenal syndrome. The relation to hemodynamics and volume distribution is discusses below.

Kinetics of Nitric Oxide

The existence of an endothelium-derived relaxing factor (EDRF) with potent vasodilating properties was first described in 1980.[115] The substance was later identified as nitric oxide (NO), which is synthesized from L-arginine in the vascular endothelium by NO synthase.[116] The production of NO is stimulated by mechanical factors, such as sheer stress and increase in blood flow and by endogenous vasodilators (e.g. bradykinin) and endotoxins. Liberated from endothelial cells, NO has a half-life of less than 30 seconds.[116] Recent studies have suggested that tumor-necrosis factor-α (TNF-α) also induces release of NO and that TNF-α may play a role in vasodilatation in patients with hypertension.[117] NO production can be inhibited by competitive inhibitors of NO synthase, such as N^Gmonomethyl-L-arginine (L-NMMA)[21,18]

In 1991 Vallance and Moncada proposed that NO is implicated in peripheral vasodilatation in cirrhotic patients.[119] To support this hypothesis, several studies have shown that blockade of NO formation significantly improves systemic hyperdynamic circulation, increases blood pressure, and decreases plasma volume and sodium retention.[21,118,120] In the splanchnic area, blockade of NO synthase leads to contraction of the splanchnic arterial vessels and decrease in the hepatosplanchnic blood flow.[121,122] However, a recent study of cirrhosis by Calver et al. showed increased blood flow in the forearm but no increased vasoconstriction after NO inhibition.[123] Thus, the importance of NO in the peripheral and splanchnic circulation in chronic liver disease is still under debate, and more studies are needed to define clearly its role[124] (see chapter 17).

Kinetics of Catecholamines

Several studies have shown increased circulating levels of norepinephrine (NE) in cirrhosis.[91,125–129] A central question was whether the increase is due only to reduced disposal or reflects increased spillover from postsynaptic sympathetic neurons as a result of enhanced sympathetic nervous activity. Studies in which tritium-labeled NE was infused and plasma was selectively sampled from different parts of the circulation make clear that reduced disposal is minor, if present, and that the increased circulating level of NE in cirrhosis reflects enhanced sympathetic nervous activity,[126,128,130–132] especially in the kidney, hepatointestinal system, heart, skeletal muscle,[128] and some areas of the skin.[130–134] Renal venous NE reflects renal sympathetic burst frequency,[135] and an inverse relation has been found between renal venous NE and renal blood flow, thus indicating that enhanced renal sympathetic nervous activity contributes significantly to reduced renal blood flow in cirrhosis.[126, 131,133]

Epinephrine is extracted from major organs and peripheral tissues. To assess the circulating level of epinephrine, it is therefore important to collect blood samples from the artery. Because NE is released and extracted in the same vascular area, the concentrations of NE in the artery and cubital veins are almost similar in normal subjects and patients with cirrhosis. Thus cubital venous samples more or less reflect the circulating level of endogenous NE but not of epinephrine. For kinetic study of NE, samples should be taken from the proper location (systemic artery, pulmonary artery) to quantify the unidirectional fluxes from catecholamine.[134] The relation to hemodynamics and volume distribution is considered below.

Kinetics of Endothelin

Besides acting as powerful vasoconstrictors, the sympathetic nervous system (SNS), the RAAS, and vasopressin have salt-water retaining effects on the kidney.[4,37,39,91] Overactivity in these systems is an important element in maintaining arterial blood pressure in cirrhosis (see chapters 2, 12, and 19). Within the last five years an increased level of a fourth vasoconstrictor, endothelin-1 (ET-1), has been described.[136–141] ET-1, a 21-amino-acid peptide, is derived from the larger preproendothelin. Three peptides, ET-1, endothelin-2, and endothelin-3, have now been identified. ET-1 is produced and released from endothelial cells, and receptors are found in myocardium, kidney, adrenal gland, intestine, spleen, lung, and liver.[142] Endothelin-3 is neurogenically derived. The origin of endothelin-2 is unknown, and at present it cannot be measured in plasma. ET-1 has potent vasoconstricting properties and is about five times as potent as angiotensin II on a molar basis.[142] ET-1 also induces liberation of NO, which may obscure some of its vasoconstrictive action.[21,118-119,134,142] Administration of ET-1 is followed by decreases in glomerular filtration rate, renal blood flow, urinary volume, and sodium excretion.[82,142,143] The cardiovascular effects of ET-1 are an increase in mean arterial blood pressure and systemic vascular resistance and a decrease in heart rate and cardiac output[142,144]; decrease in cardiac output probably is due to baroreceptor reflex.[145]

Lerman,[136] Uemasu et al.,[137] Uchihara et al.,[138] and Møller et al.[141] reported increased immunoreactivity of circulating ET-1. Veglio,[139] on the other hand, found decreased ET-1 in cirrhotic patients without renal failure, with and without ascites. The reason for this discrepancy is unknown, but probably it is due to the use of a less specific assay in Veglio's study.[139] Moore et al.[140] found highly increased levels of plasma ET-1 in cirrhotic patients with hepatorenal syndrome. Møller et al.[141] recently reported a positive correlation between serum concentration of creatinine and circulating level of ET-1 and a negative correlation between ET-1 and serum concentration of sodium in patients with cirrhosis. Similarly, a negative correlation was found between systolic and diastolic blood pressures on one hand and circulating ET-1 on the other. Such results implicate ET-1 in the hemodynamic and homeostatic disturbances in cirrhosis. Moreover, Møller et

Vasodilation in Cirrhosis

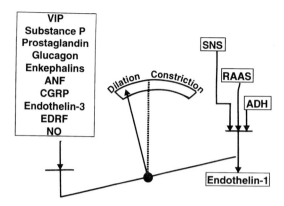

FIGURE 10.8. Balance between vasodilatory and vasoconstricting forces in cirrhosis. VIP = vasoactive intestinal peptide, ANF = atrial natriuretic factor, CGRP = calcitonin gene-related peptide, EDRF = endothelium-derived relaxing factor, NO = nitric oxide, SNS = sympathetic nervous system, RAAS = renin-angiotensin-aldosterone system, ADH = anitdiuretic hormone or vasopressin.

al.[141] found a positive relation between ET-1 and both Child score and portal venous pressure, suggesting a role for ET-1 in line of with that of the SNS, RAAS, and vasopressin.

The hepatic extraction of renin, vasoactive intestinal polypeptide, glucagon, ANF, NE, and epinephrine has been reported to be normal in patients with cirrhosis. Therefore, it must be concluded that, in the main, the increased circulating levels of various vasoactive substances are due to increased release rather than decreased disposal (see chapter 18).

RELATION AMONG HEMODYNAMICS, DISTRIBUTION OF BLOOD VOLUME AND KINETICS OF VASOACTIVE SUBSTANCES

Neurohumoral regulation is important for adjustment of the cardiovascular system and volume regulation. Fig. 10.8 summarizes the balance between vasoconstrictors and potential vasodilators in cirrhosis. That the vasoconstrictor systems (RAAS, SNS, and vasopressin) are highly activated in the decompensated stage of cirrhosis is well documented, but the vasodilator systems are far less elucidated and to some extent speculative. However, recent research has shown that circulating CGRP is inversely correlated with systemic vascular resistance in patients with cirrhosis

(Fig. 10.9).[146] This suggests a role for CGRP in systemic vasodilatation. Moreover, Møller et al.[146] recently reported a negative covariation between circulating CGRP and both central circulation time and size of central and arterial blood volume (Fig.10.9). This covariation further suggests that CGRP plays a role in the abnormal distribution of blood volume with central hypovolemia.

Central and arterial blood volume is directly correlated with systemic vascular resistance[135] (see Fig. 10.4), thus confirming that the greater the vasodilation, the greater the central hypovolemia.[7,8,10] The abnormal distribution of blood volume in cirrhosis therefore seems to be closely related not only to essential hemodynamic disturbances, such as portal hypertension and systemic vasodilation, but also to the concentration of CGRP.[113,114] But other bioactive substances, such as nitric oxide, may be involved,[21,118–119] and the mechanisms behind systemic vasodilatation and abnormal distribution of blood volume still constitute a major and largely unsolved question in cirrhosis.

In normal subjects, the SNS plays an important role in cardiovascular adaptation to upright position and physical exercise.[147] In the first case, the SNS response is mediated by activation of volume receptors and baroreceptors.[37] In the second case, SNA is enhanced through central activation.[147] Animal studies have also shown that increased portal and sinusoidal pressure leads to activation of sympathetic nerves to the heart and kidney, which are mediated by a non–volume-dependent hepatic baroreceptor[148,149] (see chapter 8). In patients with cirrhosis, all of the above mechanisms may contribute to sympathoadrenal overactivity, activation of the RAAS, and neuropituitary release of vasopressin. Thus, arterial blood pressure is decreased, and signs of reduced arterial blood volume suggest that baroreceptors are unloaded and thereby contribute to enhanced sympathetic nervous activity. Henriksen et al.[10] recently reported an inverse relation between size of central and arterial blood volume on one hand and arterial and renal venous levels of NE on the other. This finding suggests that central and arterial hypovolemia is a significant afferent stimulus to both renal and overall sympathetic overactivity. Accordingly, in patients with ascites, implantation of a peritoneovenous shunt, which expands the central blood volume and decompresses the splanchnic area, lowers the elevated plasma concentration

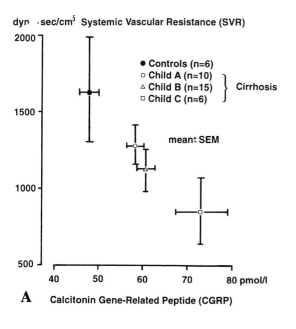

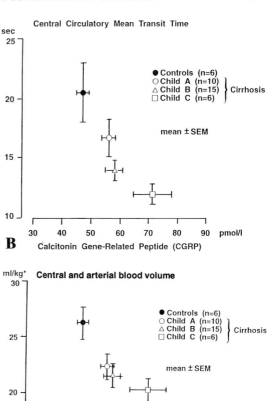

FIGURE 10.9. *A*, Inverse relation between the circulating level of calcitonin gene-related peptide (CGRP) and systemic vascular resistance in cirrhosis. *B*, Inverse relation between circulating CGRP and central circulation time. *C*, Inverse relation between central and arterial blood volume and circulating CGRP. (Data from Møller et al.[146])

of NE .[35,71] Several investigators have found a direct relation between portal pressure and circulating level of NE.[125–128,131,133] This finding, of course, may suggest that sympathetic overactivity is involved in the development of portal venous hypertension. Supporting this view is the concomitant reduction in portal pressure and plasma NE during treatment with clonidine, a centrally acting alpha-2-agonist with sympatholytic activity.[150,151] On the other hand, the finding is also in keeping with the existence of a non-volume-dependent hepatic baroreceptor. The inverse relation between clearance of indocyanine green (a measure of hepatic function and blood flow) and a direct relation between the Child-Pugh score and arterial levels of NE and epinephrine may suggest that hepatic dysfunction and metabolic derangement are also afferent mediators of enhanced sympathetic nervous activity in cirrhosis.[152]

In previous publications the values for systemic arterial blood pressure in cirrhosis were measured in patients resting supine and awake either by the cuff method or invasively through an arterial catheter.[2,6,7–10,18,30,33,35,38,48,50,69,71,126,130,152–156] The 24-hour arterial blood pressure and heart rate were not recorded. Recently, however, Møller et al.[157] reported the results of 24-hour determinations in cirrhotic patients. During the day, the systolic, diastolic, and mean arterial blood pressures were substantially reduced compared with age- and sex-matched controls, whereas at night the values were unexpectedly normal (Fig. 10.10). In contrast, the heart rate was significantly above normal both during the day and at night. Consequently, the drop from daytime to nighttime and the rise from nighttime to daytime showed lower values than those of controls. It is known from other diseases, such as uremia and different types of heart failure, that the circulation of patients classified as "nondippers" is abnormally regulated.[158–159] The fact that at night the patients had a combination of normal blood pressure and increased heart rate suggests abnor-

24-hour Measurements in Cirrhosis (n=35) and Controls (n=35)

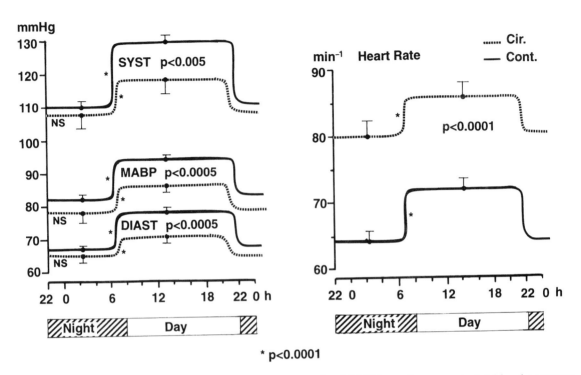

FIGURE 10.10. Variations in systolic (SYST), diastolic (DIAST), and mean arterial blood pressure (MABP) and heart rate during 24-hour ambulatory blood pressure measurements in normal subjects (*solid lines*) and cirrhotic patients (*dashed lines*). Note the differences in systemic blood pressure during daytime. At night no significant difference in blood pressure was recorded. Significant change from nighttime to daytime (p < 0.0001). (Data from Møller et al.[157])

mal regulation of the circulation also in cirrhosis. Rest in the supine position for a long time (as during sleep) would be expected to lessen the abnormal distribution of blood volume and to improve the ability to maintain a normal sleeping arterial blood pressure only at the cost of increased heart rate and cardiac output. The upright position during the day or shifting from the supine to the upright position may further aggravate central hypovolemia, and a normal arterial blood pressure cannot be maintained even when the heart rate and cardiac output are increased. The negative correlation of the arterial blood pressure with the Child score during the day and at night confirms that the hemodynamic derangement is related to the severity of liver disease.

SUMMARY

Recent investigations have shown that the central circulation time is substantially reduced with cirrhosis and inversely correlated with portal pressure. The noncentral circulation time is normal. Consequently, the increased blood volume is abnormally distributed with a reduced central and arterial blood volume and an augmented noncentral blood volume. Increasing evidence suggests that the decreased systemic and splanchnic vascular resistance is of primary pathogenic importance in the development of circulatory disturbance (hyperkinetic circulation, low arterial blood pressure, and low central and arterial blood volume) and neurohumoral abnormalities.

In addition to enhanced sympathetic nervous activity, activation of the renin-angiotensin-aldosterone system, and elevated levels of circulating vasopressin, ET-1 also has been implicated in hemodynamic regulation in cirrhosis. Various studies have substantiated increased circulating concentrations of ET-1 in cirrhosis. Significant relations to systemic hemodynamics and the

Child-Pugh score indicate that ET-1 has a role in hyperdynamic circulation and hepatorenal syndrome.

In addition, systemic vascular resistance is directly correlated with central and arterial blood volume, suggesting that the greater the vasodilatation, the greater the central hypovolemia. Although such findings point to the existence of one or more vasodilators, so far research has failed to turn up a specific substance. Various vasodilating agents, such as glucagon, substance P, enkephalins, prostaglandins, and atrial natriuretic factor, are candidates. But the results have been conflicting. Recent research has shown that circulating calcitonin gene-related peptide is inversely correlated with systemic vascular resistance in patients with cirrhosis. Several reports have focused on nitric oxide in cirrhosis and hepatorenal syndrome. In animal studies inhibition of nitric oxide production is associated with a significant increase in arterial blood pressure, glomerular filtration rate, and sodium excretion; future research may elucidate its role in liver disease.

In conclusion, patients with cirrhosis and portal hypertension are unable to maintain a normal-sized central and arterial blood volume (effective blood volume). Conversely, the non-central blood volume is expanded and may aggravate the increased splanchnic blood flow and portal hypertension. The systemic circulatory changes in general are related to the degree of portal hypertension and severity of liver failure and are more pronounced in patients with fluid retention than in those without. Systemic vasodilatation and portal hypertension with portosystemic collaterals are probably the main causes of the shift in blood volume from the arterial tree and central parts of the circulation to the hepatosplanchnic bed and systemic veins, with activation of volume receptors and baroreceptors as the outcome.

Acknowledgment. This work was supported by Kong Christian d. X's Fond, Fonden til Laegevidenskabens Fremme, and the John and Birthe Meyer Foundation. The authors with to express their gratitude to Flemming Bendtsen, MD, Niels Juel Christensen, MD, Alexander L. Gerbes, MD, Niels A. Lassen, MD, Helmer Ring-Larsen, MD, Thorkild I.A. Sørensen, MD, and Kjeld Winkler, MD, for excellent and fruitful collaboration throughout the last decade and to Ms. Bente Henriksen for her helpful assistance in preparing the manuscript.

REFERENCES

1. Kowalski HJ, Abelmann WH: The cardiac output at rest in Laennec's cirrhosis. J Clin Invest 1953;32:1025–1031.
2. Murray JF, Dawson AM, Sherlock S: Circulatory changes in chronic liver disease. Am J Med 1958; 24:358–367.
3. Sherlock S: Vasodilatation associated with hepatocellular disease: Relation to functional organ failure. Gut 1990;31:365–367
4. Ring-Larsen H: Hepatic nephropathy related to hemodynamics. Liver 1983;3:265–289
5. Schrier RW, Arroyo V, Bernardi M, et al: Peripheral arterial vasodilation hypothesis: A proposal for the initiation of renal sodium and water retention in cirrhosis. Hepatology 1988;8:1151–1157.
6. Bomzon A, Blendis LM (eds): Cardiovascular Complications of Liver Disease. Boca Raton, FL: CRC Press, 1990.
7. Henriksen JH, Schutten HJ, Bendtsen F, Warberg J: Circulating atrial natriuretic peptide (ANP) and central blood volume (CBV) in cirrhosis. Liver 1986;6:361–368.
8. Henriksen JH, Bendtsen F, Sørensen TIA, et al: Reduced central blood volume in cirrhosis. Gastroenterology 1989;97:1506–1513.
9. Hartleb M, Rudzki K: Segmental mean transit times of ^{99M}technetium with central vascular space in liver cirrhosis. Liver 1992;12:191–198.
10. Henriksen JH, Bendtsen F, Gerbes AL, et al: Estimated central blood volume in cirrhosis: Relationship to sympathetic nervous activity, beta adrenergic blockade and atrial natriuretic factor. Hepatology 1992;16:1163–1170.
11. Zipser RD, Radvan GM, Kronborg IJ, et al: Urinary thromboxane B_2 and prostaglandin E_2 in the hepatorenal syndrome: Evidence for increased vasoconstrictor and decreased vasodilator factors. Gastroenterology 1983;84:697–703.
12. Pérez-Ayuso RM, Arroyo V, Camps J, et al: Renal kallikrein excretion in cirrhotics with ascites: Relationship to renal hemodynamics. Hepatology 1984;4:247–252.
13. Calam J, Unwin RJ, Sing J, et al: Renal function during vasoactive intestinal peptide (VIP) infusions in normal man and patients with liver disease. Peptides 1984; 5:441–443.
14. Henriksen JH, Staun-Olesen P, Fahrenkrug J, Ring-Larsen H: Vasoactive intestinal polypeptide (VIP) in cirrhosis: Arteriovenous extraction in different vascular beds. Scand J Gastroenterol 1980;15:787–792.
15. Hörtnagel H, Singer EA, Lenz K: Substance P is markedly increased in plasma of patients with hepatic coma. Lancet 1984;i:480–483.
16. Henriksen JH, Schaffalitzky de Muckadell OB, Bülow JB: Does liver-intestine significantly degrade circulating endogenous substance P in man? Scand J Gastroenterol 1986;21:300–304.
17. Pizcueta PM, Bosch J: Role of endogenous vasoactive systems in the pathogenesis of circulatory abnormalities in cirrhosis. In Gentillini P, Arias IM, Arroyo V, Schrier RW (eds): Liver Diseases and Renal Complications. New York: Raven Press, 1990;247-253.

18. Thornton JR, Dean H, Losowsky MS: Is ascites caused by impaired hepatic inactivation of blood borne endogenous opioid peptides? Gut 1988;29:1167–1172.

19. Benoit JH, Zimmermann B, Premen AJ, et al: Role of glucagon in the splanchnic hyperemia of chronic portal hypertension. Am J Physiol 1986;251:G674–G677.

20. Kravetz D, Arderiu MT, Bosch J, et al: Hyperglucagonemia and hyperkinetic circulation following porta caval shunt in the rat. Am J Physiol 1987;252:G252–G261.

21. Claria J, Jiminéz W, Ros J, et al: Pathogenesis of arterial hypotension in cirrhotic rats with ascites: Role of endogenous nitric oxide Hepatology 1991;15:343–349.

22. Vinel JP, Denoyel P, Viossat I, et al: Atrial natriuretic peptide, plasma renin activity, systemic vascular resistance and cardiac output in patients with cirrhosis. J Gastroenterol Hepatol 1989;4:529–535.

23. Triger DR: Endotoxinemia in liver disease—time for appraisal? J Hepatol 1991;12:136–138.

24. Henriksen JH: Kinetics of whole-body and organ degradation. In Henriksen JH (ed): Degradation of Bioactive Substances: Physiology and Pathophysiology. Boca Raton, FL: CRC Press, 1991;3–32.

25. Rodes J (ed): Pathophysiology of ascites and functional renal failure. Barcelona: Salvat, 1987;1-58.

26. Henriksen JH, Ring-Larsen H: Ascites formation in liver cirrhosis: The how and the why. Dig Dis 1990;8: 152–162.

27. Wilkinson SP, Moore KP, Arroyo V: Pathogenesis of ascites and hepatorenal syndrome. Gut 1991;(Suppl): S12–S17.

28. Gerbes AL: Pathophysiology of ascites formation in cirrhosis of the liver. Hepato-Gastroenterology 1991; 38:360–364.

29. McCormick PA, McIntyre N: Pathogenesis and management of ascites in chronic liver disease. Br J Hosp Med 1992;47:738–744.

30. Lieberman FL, Reynolds TB: Plasma volume in cirrhosis of the liver. Its relations to portal hypertension, ascites, and renal failure. J Clin Invest 1967;47:1297–1308.

31. Lieberman FL, Denison EK, Reynolds TB: The relationship of plasma volume, portal hypertension, ascites, and renal sodium retention in cirrhosis. The overflow theory of ascites formation. Ann NY Acad Sci 1970;170:202–212.

32. Epstein FH: Underfilling versus overfilling in hepatic ascites. N Engl J Med 1982;307:1577–1578.

33. Skorecki KL, Brenner BM: Body fluid homeostasis in congestive heart failure and cirrhosis with ascites. Am J Med 1982;72:323–338.

34. Epstein M: Peritoneovenous shunt in the management of ascites and the hepatorenal syndrome. Gastroenterology 1982;82:790–799.

35. Campbell P, Skorecki K, Logan A, et al: Acute effects of peritoneovenous shunting on plasma atrial natriuretic peptide in cirrhotic patients with massive refractory ascites. Am J Med 1988;84:112–119.

36. Lewis FW, Adair O, Rector WC Jr: Arterial vasodilation is not the cause of increased cardiac output in cirrhosis. Gastroenterology 1992;102:1024–1029.

37. Henriksen JH: Systemic hemodynamic alterations in hepatic cirrhosis. Eur J Gastroenterol Hepatol 1991;3: 705–713.

38. Bernardi M, Di Marco, Trevisani F, et al: The hemodynamic status of pre-ascitic cirrhosis: An evaluation under steady-state conditions and after postural change. Hepatology 1992;16:341–346.

39. Henriksen JH, Ring-Larsen H: Renal effects of drugs used in the treatment of portal hypertension. 1993;18: 688–695.

40. Albano O, Groszmann RJ, Sabba C, Taylor KJW: Systemic and regional hemodynamics in liver disease. In Albano O, Groszmann RJ, Sabba C, Taylor KJW (eds): Proceedings of International Symposium of Systemic and Regional Hemodynamics in Liver Disease, Bari, June 3–5, 1990.

41. Lassen NA, Perl W: Tracer Kinetic Methods in Medical Physiology. New York: Raven, 1979.

42. Benoit JN, Granger DN: Splanchnic hemodynamics in chronic portal hypertension. Semin Liver Dis 1986;6: 287–298.

43. Epstein M, Berk DP, Hollenberg NK, et al: Renal failure in patients with cirrhosis. The role of active vasoconstriction. Am J Med 1970;49:175–185.

44. Martini GA: Uber fingernagelveranderungen bei lebercirrhosis als folge veranderter peripherer durchblutung. Klin Wochenschr 1956;34:25–31

45. Pirovno M, Linder R, Boss C, et al: Cutaneous spider naevi n liver cirrhosis: Capillary, Microscopical and hormonal investigations. Klin Wochenschr 1988;66: 298–302.

46. Lunzer M, Newman SP, Sherlock S: Skeletal muscle blood flow and neurovascular reactivity in liver disease. Gut 1973;14:354–359.

47. Rodman T, Sobel M, Close PH: Arterial oxygen unsaturation and the ventilation perfusion defect of Laennec's cirrhosis. N Engl J Med 1960;263:73–79.

48. Koshy A, Moreau R, Cerini R, et al: Effects of oxygen inhalation on tissue oxygenation in patients with cirrhosis: Evidence for an impaired arterial baroreflex control. J Hepatol 1989;9:240–245.

49. Hadengue A, Benhayoun MK, Lebrec D, Benhamou J-P: Pulmonary hypertension prevalence and relation to splanchnic hemodynamics. Gastroenterology 1991; 100:520–528.

50. Eriksson LS, Söderman C, Ericzon BG, et al: Normalization of ventilation-perfusion relationships after liver transplantation in patients with decompensated cirrhosis: Evidence for a hepatopulmonary syndrome. Hepatology 1990;12:1350–1357.

51. Hedenstierna G, Söderman C, Eriksson LS, Wahren J: Ventilation -perfusion inequality in patients with nonalcoholic liver cirrhosis. Eur Respir J 1991;4:711–717.

52. Calabresi P, Abelmann WH: Porto-caval and porto-pulmonary anastomoses in Laennec's cirrhosis and in heart failure. J Clin Invest 1957;36:1257–1265.

53. Rodriguez-Roisin R, Roca J, Agusti AG, et al:Gas exchange and pulmonary vascular reactivity in patients with liver cirrhosis. Am Rev Respir Dis 1987;135:1085–1092.

54. Söderman C: Central hemodynamics and ventilation-perfusion relationships in patients with liver cirrhosis. The hepatopulmonary syndrome. Stockholm: Repro Print AB, 1993;1–50.

55. Ware AJ, D'Agostino AN, Combers B: Cerebral oedema: A major complication of massive hepatic necrosis. Gastroenterology 1971;61:877–884.

56. Ede RJ, Gimson AES, Bihari D, Williams R: Controlled hyperventilation in the prevention of cerebral oedema in fulminant hepatic failure. J Hepatol 1986;2:43–51.

57. Bradley SE, Marks PA, Reynell PC, Meltzer J:The circulating splanchnic blood volume in dog and man. Trans Assoc Am Physicians 1953;66:294–299.

58. Chinard FP, Enns T, Nolan MF: Pulmonary extravascular water volumes form transit time and slope data. J Appl Physiol 1962;17:179–183.

59. Zierler KL: Circulation times and the theory of indicator-dilution methods for determining blood flow and volume. In Hamilton WF, Dow P (eds): Handbook of Physiology, vol. 1. Washington, 1962;585–644.

60. Kassissia I, Rose CP, Goresky CA, et al: Flow-limited tracer oxygen distribution in the isolated perfused rat liver. Effects of temperature and hematocrit. Hepatology 1992;16:763–775.

61. Winkler K, Bass L, Henriksen JH, et al: Heterogeneity of splanchnic vascular transit times in man. Clin Physiol 1983;3:537–544.

62. Better OS, Schrier RW: Disturbed volume homeostasis in patients with cirrhosis of the liver. Kidney Int 1983; 23:303–311.

63. Schrier RW, Howard RL: Unifying hypothesis of sodium and water regulation in health and disease. Hypertension 1991;18:164–168.

64. Groszmann RJ: Hyperdynamic state in chronic liver diseases. J Hepatol 1993;17:538–540.

65. Tristani FE, Cohn JN: Systemic and renal haemodynamics in oliguric hepatic failure: Effect of volume expansion. J Clin Invest 1967;46:1894–1906.

66. Henriksen JH, Parving H-H, Lassen NA, Winkler K: Filtration as main mechanism of increased protein extravasation in liver cirrhosis. Scand J Clin Lab Invest 1980;40:121–128.

67. Henriksen JH: Protein-kinetic and hemodynamic studies in patients with liver cirrhosis. Evidence of a lymph-imbalance theory of ascites formation. Clin Physiol 1981;1:565–578.

68. Larsen OA, Winkler K, Tygstrup N: 'Extra' plasma in the liver calculated from the hepatic hematocrit in patients with portocaval anastomosis. Clin Sci 1963;25: 357–360.

69. Bosch J, Arroyo V, Betriu A, et al: Hepatic hemodynamics and the renin-angiotensin-aldosterone system in cirrhosis. Gastroenterology 1980;78:92–99.

70. Gines P, Arroyo V: Paracentesis in the management of cirrhotic ascites. J Hepatol 1993;17:514–518.

71. Blendis LM, Sole MJ, Campbell P, et al: The effect of peritoneovenous shunting on catecholamine metabolism in patients with hepatic ascites. Hepatology 1987; 7:143–148.

72. Rector WG Jr, Hossack KF: Pathogenesis of sodium retention complicating cirrhosis: Is there room for diminished 'effective' arterial blood volume? Gastroenterology 1988;95:1658–1663.

73. Bernardi M, Trevisani F, Santini C, et al: Aldosterone related blood volume expansion in cirrhosis before and after early phase of ascites formation. Gut 1983;24: 761–766.

73a. Wong F, Liu P, Tobe S, et al: Central blood volume in cirrhosis. Measurement with radionuclide angiography. Hepatology 1994;19:312–321.

73b. Henriksen JH, Møller S, Bendtsen F, et al: Assessment of central blood volume in cirrhosis by radionuclide angiography. What does it really mean? Hepatology 1994;20:1652–1653.

74. Henriksen JH: 'Effective blood volume' in liver cirrhosis. In Gentillini P, Arias IM, Arroyo V, Schrier RW (eds): Liver Diseases and Renal Complications. New York: Raven Press, 1990;235–244.

75. Levy M: Sodium retention and ascites formation in dogs with experimental portal cirrhosis. Am J Physiol 1977;233:F572–F585.

76. Rowel LB, Detry J-MR, Blackman JR, Wyss C: Importance of the splanchnic vascular bed in human blood pressure regulation. J Appl Physiol 1972;32:213–220.

77. Sagawa K: Baroreflex control of systemic arterial pressure and vascular bed. In Shepard JT, Abboud FM (eds): Handbook of Physiology, Section 2: The Cardiovascular System, vol. III. Baltimore: Williams & Wilkins, 1983;453–496.

78. Thames MB: Neural control of renal function: Contribution of cardiopulmonary baroreceptors to the control of the kidney. Fed Proc 1977;37:1209–1213.

78a. Møller S, Søndergaard L, Møgelvang J, et al: Decreased right heart blood volume determined by magnetic resonance imaging: Evidence of central underfilling in cirrhosis. Hepatology 1995;22:472–478.

79. Henriksen JH, Bendtsen F, Sørensen TIA, et al: There is room for diminished central and arterial blood volume in cirrhosis. Hepatology 1991;13:1261.

80. Guyton AC (ed): Textbook of Medical Physiology, 8th ed. Philadelphia: W.B. Saunders, 1991;667–678.

81. Yanagisawa M, Kurihara H, Kimura S, et al: A novel potent vasoconstrictor peptide produced by vascular endothelial cells. Nature 1988;332:411–415.

82. Miller WL, Redfield MM, Burnett JC Jr: Integrated cardiac, renal, and endocrine actions of endothelin. J Clin Invest 1989;991–992.

83. Firth JD, Roberts FC, Raine EG Jr: Effect of endothelin on the function of the isolated perfused wording rat heart. Clin Sci 1990;7965:221–225.

84. Luscher TF: Endothelium-derived relaxing and contracting factors: Potential role in coronary artery disease. Eur Heart J 1989;10:847–857.

85. Henriksen JH, Christensen NJ, Ring-Larsen H: Pulmonary extraction of circulating noradrenaline in man. Eur J Clin Invest 1986;16:327–423.

86. Christensen NJ, Garlbo H, Gjerris A, et al: Whole-body and regional clearance of noradrenaline and adrenaline in man. Acta Physiol Scand Suppl 1984; 527:17–20.

87. Christensen NJ, Henriksen JH: Degradation of endogenous catecholamines. In JH Henriksen (ed): Degradation of Bioactive Substances: Physiology and Pathophysiology. Boca Rotan, FL: CRC Press, 1991; 289–305.

88. Shorr E: Hepatorenal vasotropic factors, experimental cirrhosis, liver injury. Transactions of the Sixth Conference, May 1–2, 1947. New York: Josiah Macy Foundation, 1947;33–39.

89. Arroyo V, Planas R, Gaya J, et al: Sympathetic nervous activity, renin-angiotensin system and renal excretion of prostaglandin E_2 in cirrhosis. Relation to functional renal failure and sodium and water excretion. Eur J Clin Invest 1983;13:271–278.

90. Epstein M, Lifschitz M: Renal eicosanoids as determinants of renal function in liver disease. Hepatology 1987;7:1359–1367.

91. Henriksen JH, Staun-Olsen P, Mogensen NB, Fahrenkrug J: Circulating endogenous vasoactive intestinal polypeptide (VIP) in patients with uraemia and liver cirrhosis. Eur J Clin Invest 1986;16:211–216.

92. Warner L. Skorecki K, Blendis LM, Epstein M: Atrial natriuretic factor and liver disease. Hepatology 1993; 17:500–513.

93. McEwan J, Larkin S, Davies G, et al: Calcitonin gene-related peptide: A potent dilator of human epicardial coronary arteries. Circulation 1986;74:1243–1247.

94. Bunker CB, Reavley C, O'Shaugnessy DJ, Dowd PM: Calcitonin gene-related peptide in treatment of severe peripheral vascular insufficiency in Raynaud's phenomenon. Lancet 1993;342:80–82.

95. Gerbes AL, Arendt RM, Paumgartner G: Atrial natriuretic factor: Possible implications in liver disease. J Hepatol 1987;5:123–132.

96. Bonkovsky H, Hartle DK, Mellen BG, et al: Plasma concentrations of immunoreactive atrial natriuretic peptide in hospitalized cirrhotic and non-cirrhotic patients: Evidence for a role of deficient atrial natriuretic peptide in pathogenesis of cirrhotic ascites. Am J Gastroenterol 1988;83:531–535.

97. Salerno F, Badalamenti S, Moser P, et al: Atrial natriuretic factor in cirrhotic patients with tense ascites. Gastroenterology 1990;98:1063–1070.

98. Hollister AS, Rodeheffer RJ, White FJ, et al: Clearance of atrial natriuretic factor by lung, liver, and kidney in human subjects and the dog. J Clin Invest 1989;83:623–628.

99. Moreau R, Pussard E, Brenard R, et al: Clearance of atrial natriuretic peptide in patients with cirrhosis. Role of liver failure. J Hepatol 1991;13:351–357.

100. Henriksen JH, Bendtsen F, Schütten HJ, Warberg J: Hepatic intestinal disposal of endogenous human alpha atrial natriuretic factor 99-126 in patients with cirrhosis. Am J Gastroenterol 1990;85:1155–1159.

101. Henriksen JH, Bendtsen F, Gerbes AL: Azygos and hepatic extraction of atrial natriuretic factor (ANF) in patients with cirrhosis. No evidence of reduced disposal. J Hepatol 1993;17:419–420.

102. Crozier IG, Nicholls MG, Ikram H, et al: Atrial natriuretic peptide in humans. Production and clearance by various tissues. Hypertension 1986;8:11–15.

103. Schütten HJ, Henriksen JH, Warberg J: Organ extraction of atrial natriuretic peptide (ANP) in man. Significance of sampling site. Clin Phys 1987;7:125–132.

104. Bendtsen F, Gerbes AL, Henriksen JH: Disposal of atrial natriuretic factor (ANF 99-126) in patients with cirrhosis: Effect of beta-adrenergic blockade. Scand J Clin Lab Invest 1993;53:549–554.

105. Morris HR, Panico M, Etienne T, et al: Isolation and characterization of human calcitonin gene-related peptide. Nature 1984;308:746–748.

106. Tipping JR: CGRP: A novel neuropeptide from the calcitonin gene is the most potent vasodilator know. J Hypertension 1986;4(Suppl 5):S102–S105.

107. Rosenfeld MG, Mermod JJ, Amara SG, et al: Production of a novel neuropeptide encoded by the calcitonin gene via tissue specific RNA processing. Nature 1983;304:129–135.

108. Tschopp FA, Henke H, Petermann JB, et al: Calcitonin gene-related peptide and its binding sites in the human central nervous system and pituitary. Proc Natl Acad Sci USA 1985;82:248–252.

109. Cysteic Y, Hayashi N, Kasahara A, et al: Calcitonin gene-related peptide in the hepatic and splanchnic vascular systems of the rat. Hepatology 1986;6:676–681.

110. Steenbergh PH, Hoppener JW, Zandberg J, et al: A second human calcitonin/CGRP gene. FEBS Lett 1985;183:403–407.

111. Foord SM, Craig RK: Isolation and characterization of a human calcitonin gene-related peptide receptor. Eur J Biochem 1987;170:373–379.

112. McEwan JR, Bentamin N, Larkin S, et al: Vasodilation by calcitonin gene-related peptide and by substance P. A comparison of their effects on resistance and capacitance vessels of human forearms. Circulation 1988; 77:1072–1080.

113. Bendtsen F, Schifter S, Henriksen JH: Increased circulating calcitonin gene-related peptide (CGRP). J Hepatol 1991;12:118–123.

114. Gupta S, Morgan TR, Gordan GS: Calcitonin gene-related peptide in hepatorenal syndrome. J Clin Gastroenterol 1992;14:122–126.

115. Furchgott RF, Zawadski JV: The obligatory role of endothelial cells in the relaxation of arterial smooth muscle by acetylcholine. Nature 1980; 288:373–376.

116. Whittle BJR, Moncada S: Nitric oxide—The elusive mediation of the hyperdynamic circulation of cirrhosis. Hepatology 1992;16:1089–1092.

117. Khoruts A, Stahnke L, McClain CJ, et al: Circulation tumor necrosis factor, interleukin-I and interleukin-6 concentrations in chronic alcoholic patients. Hepatology 1991;13:267–276.

118. Pizueta P, Pique JM, Fernandez M, et al: Modulation of the hyperdynamic circulation of cirrhotic rats by nitric oxide inhibition. Gastroenterology 1992;103:1909–1915.

119. Vallance P, Moncada S: Hyperdynamic circulation in cirrhosis: A role for nitric oxide. Lancet 1991;337: 776–78.

120. Lee F-Y, Colombato LA, Albillos A, Groszmann RJ: N-nitro-L-argine administration corrects peripheral vasodilatation and systemic capillary hypotension and ameliorates plasma volume expansion and sodium retention in portal hypertensive rats. Hepatology 1993; 17:84–90.

121. Wu YP, Burns RC, Sitzmann JG: Effects of nitric oxide and cyclooxygenase inhibition on splanchnic hemodynamics in portal hypertension. Hepatology 1993; 18:1416–1421.

122. Sieber CC, Lopez-Talavera JC, Groszman RJ: Role of nitric oxide in the vitro splanchnic vascular hyporeactivity in ascitic cirrhotic rats. Gastroenterology 1993; 104:1750–1754.

123. Calver A, Harris A, Maxwell JD, Vallance P: Effect of local inhibition of nitric oxide synthesis of forearm blood now and dorsal hand vein size in patients with alcoholic cirrhosis. Clin Sci 1994;86:203–208.

124. Sogni P, Moreau R, Ohsuga M, et al: Evidence for normal nitric oxide mediated vasodilator tone in conscious rats with cirrhosis. Hepatology 1992;16:980–983.

124a. Bomzon A, Blendis LM: The nitric oxide hypothesis and the hyperdynamic circulation in cirrhosis. Hepatology 1994;20:1343–1350.

124b. Groszmann RJ: Hyperdynamic circulation of liver disease 40 years later: Pathophysiology and clinical consequences. Hepatology 1994;20:1359–1363.

125. Henriksen JH, Christensen NJ, Ring-Larsen H: Noradrenaline and adrenalone concentrations in various vascular beds in patients with cirrhosis. Relation to hemodynamics. Clin Physiol 1981;1:293–304.

126. Henriksen JH, Ring-Larsen H, Kanstrup I-L, Christensen JJ: Splanchnic and renal elimination and release of catecholamines in cirrhosis. Evidence of enhanced sympathetic nervous activity in patients with decompensated cirrhosis. Gut 1984;25:1034–1043.

127. Bichet DG, van Putten VJ, Schrier RW: Potential role of increased sympathetic activity in impaired sodium and water excretion in cirrhosis. N Engl J Med 1982; 307:1552–1557.

128. Floras J, Legault L, Morali G, et al: Increased sympathetic outflow in cirrhosis and ascites: Direct evidence from intraneural recordings Ann Intern Med 1991; 114:373–380.

129. Bernardi M, Trevisani F, Santini C, et al: Plasma norepinephrine, weak neurotransmitters, and renin activity during active tilting in liver cirrhosis: Relationship with cardiovascular homeostasis and renal function. Hepatology 1983;3:56–64.

130. Nicholls KM, Shapiro MD, Van Putten VJ, et al: Elevated plasma norepinephrine concentrations in decompensated cirrhosis. Association with increased secretion rates, normal clearance rates, and suppressibility by control blood volume expansion. Circ Res 1985;56:457–461.

131. Willet I, Esler M, Burke F, et al: Total and renal sympathetic nervous system activity in alcoholic cirrhosis. J Hepatol 1985;1:639–648.

132. Henriksen JH, Christensen NJ, Ring-Larsen H: Continuous infusion of tracer norepinephrine may miscalculate unidirectional nerve uptake of norepinephrine in man. Circ Res 1989;65:388–395.

133. Ring-Larsen H, Hesse B, Henriksen JH, Christensen NJ: Sympathetic nervous activity and renal systemic hemodynamics in cirrhosis—plasma norepinephrine concentration, hepatic extraction, and renal release. Hepatology 1982;2:304–310.

134. Christensen NJ, Henriksen JH: Degradation of endogenous catecholamines. In Henriksen JH (ed): Degradation of Bioactive Substances: Physiology and Pathophysiology. Boca Raton, FL: CRC Press, 1991;289–305.

135. Kopp U, Bradley T, Hjemdahl P: Renal venous outflow and urinary excretion of norepinephrine, epinephrine and dopamine during graded renal nerve stimulation. Am J Physiol 1983;244:E52–E60.

136. Lerman A, Click RL, Narr BJ, et al: Elevation of plasma endothelin associated with systemic hypertension in humans following orthotopic liver transplantation. Transplantation 1991;51:646–650.

137. Uemasu J, Matsumoto H, Kawasaki H: Increased plasma endothelin levels in patients with liver cirrhosis. Nephron 1992;60:380.

138. Uchihara M, Izumi N, Sato C, Marumo F: Clinical significance of elevated plasma endothelin concentration in patients with cirrhosis. Hepatology, 1992;16:95–99.

139. Veglio F, Pinna G, Melchio R, et al: Plasma endothelin levels in cirrhotic subjects. J Hepatol 1992;15:85–87.

140. Moore K, Wendon J, Frazer M, et al: Plasma endothelin immunoreactivity in liver disease and the hepatorenal syndrome. N Engl J Med 1992;327:174–178.

141. Møller S, Emmeluth C, Henriksen JH: Elevated circulating plasma endothelin-1 concentrations in cirrhosis. J Hepatol 1993;19:285–290.

141a. Gerbes AL, Møller S, Gülberg V, Henriksen JH: Endothelin-1 and -3 plasma concentrations in patients with cirrhosis: Role of splanchnic and renal passage and liver function. Hepatology 1995;21:735–739.

141b. Saló J, Francitorra A, Follo A, et al: Increased plasma endothelin in cirrhosis. Relationship with systemic endotoxemia and response to change in effective blood volume. J Hepatol 1995;22:389–398.

141c. Møller S, Gülberg V, Henriksen JH, Gerbes AL: Endothelin-1 and -3 in cirrhosis. Relations to systemic and central hemodynamics. J Hepatol 1995;23:135–144.

142. Masaki T, Yanagisawa M: Physiology and pharmacology of endothelins. Med Res Rev 1992;12:391–421.

143. Simonson MS, Dunn MJ: Endothelin peptides and the kidney. Annu Rev Physiol 1993;55:249–265.

144. Goetz KL, Wang BC, Madwed JB, et al: Cardiovascular, renal, and endocrine responses to intravenous endothelin in conscious dogs. Am J Physiol 1988;255: R1064–R1068.

145. Van Den Buuse M, Itoh S: Central effects of endothelin on baroreflex of spontaneously hypertensive rats. J Hypertension 1993;11:379–387.

146. Møller S, Bendtsen F, Schifter S, Henriksen JH: Increased circulating calcitonin gene-related peptide in cirrhosis: A marker of systemic vasodilatation and central hypovolaemia. J Hepatol 1995;23(Suppl 1):113.

147. Galbo H: Hormonal and Metabolic Adaption to Exercise. Stuttgart: Thieme Verlag, 1983.

148. Kostreva DR, Castaner A, Kampine JP: Reflex effect of hepatic baroreceptors on renal and cardiac sympathetic nerve activity. Am J Physiol 1980;238:R390–R394.

149. Lang F, Tschernko E, Shulze E, et al: Hepatorenal reflex regulating kidney function. Hepatology 1991; 14:590–594.

150. Moreau R, Lee SS, Hadenque A, et al: Hemodynamic effect of a clonidine-induced decrease in sympathetic tone in patients with cirrhosis. Hepatology 1987;7: 149–154.

151. Albillos A, Banares R, Barrios C, et al: Oral administration of clonidine in patients with alcoholic cirrhosis. Hemodynamic and liver function effects. Gastroenterology 1992;102:248–254.

152. Bendtsen F: Oesophageal varices prior to bleeding. Diagnosis and physiological and therapeutic effect of propanolol in cirrhosis. Dan Med Bull 1993;40:306–316.

153. Fernandez-Seara J, Prieto J, Quiroga J, et al: Systemic and regional hemodynamics in patients with liver cirrhosis and ascites with and without functional renal failure. Gastroenterology 1989;97:1304–1312.

154. Llach J, Gines P, Arroyo V. et al: Prognostic value of arterial pressure endogenous vasoactive systems, and renal function in cirrhosis with ascites. Gastroenterology 1988;94:482–487.

155. Moreau R, Hadengue A, Soupison T, et al: Abnormal pressor response to vasopressin in patients with cirrhosis: Evidence for impaired buffering mechanisms. Hepatology 1990;12:7–12.

156. MacGilchrist AJ, Sumner D, Reid JL: Impaired pressor reactivity in cirrhosis: Evidence for a peripheral vascular defect. Hepatology 1991;13:689–694.

157. Møller S, Wiinberg N, Henriksen JH: Non-invasive 24-hour ambulatory arterial blood pressure monitoring in cirrhosis. Hepatology 1995;22:88–95.

158. O'Brien E, Sheriden J, O'Malley K: Dippers and non-dippers. Lancet 1988;2:397.

159. Verdecchia P, Schillaci G, Porcellati C: Dippers versus non-dippers. J Hypertension 1991;9:42–44.

Chapter 11

LOW-PRESSURE BARORECEPTORS II— NEW PERSPECTIVES

The Phrenic Nerve as a Visceral Reflex Pathway

DAVID R. KOSTREVA, Ph.D.

Hepatic Phrenic Afferents
Low-pressure Baroreceptors
Parenchymal Mechanoreceptors
Clinical Significance
Inferior Vena Cava Mechanoreceptors with Phrenic Afferents

Pericardial Mechanoreceptors with Phrenic Afferents
Clinical Significance
Neural Integration of the Low-pressure Baroreceptor Reflexes
Summary

This chapter addresses the latest concepts concerning low-pressure baroreceptors based on findings since the previous edition of this book.

It is well known that the liver receives its afferent and efferent innervation from the vagal and sympathetic nerves.[1-7] However, in 1940 Alexander[1] concluded from indirect experimental evidence that the phrenic nerve may also innervate the liver. He conducted experiments in cats in which he sectioned the vagal innervation of the liver and removed the celiac ganglion. Two weeks after surgery, histologic studies were conducted on the livers to determine whether any innervation remained. Alexander observed some myelinated fibers still intact in the denervated livers and concluded that they were "undoubtedly afferent phrenic nerve components." Until our recent publication,[8] Alexander's study was the only evidence in the literature to suggest that the phrenic nerve innervates the liver.

Our initial findings demonstrating that the phrenic nerve in fact innervates the liver were discovered purely through serendipity. While training a pediatric anesthesiologist how to do nerve recordings in animal studies, I decided to use the phrenic nerve for recording efferent activity. Near the end of one of the experiments we recorded afferent nerve activity from the cut central end of the phrenic nerve. While probing the diaphragm to verify that we could indeed record afferent nerve activity from diaphragmatic mechanoreceptors, we probed the pericardium, where to our surprise we found an abundance of mechanoreceptors. We then probed the central tendon of the diaphragm, which by all accounts in the literature is devoid of mechanoreceptors. In spite of these accounts we were able to record mechanoreceptor responses. However, after opening the abdominal cavity and probing the abdominal surface of the central tendon, we could not elicit mechanoreceptor responses. While probing the liver parenchyma and hepatic veins, however, we found an abundance of mechanoreceptor afferent nerve activity coursing through the phrenic nerve originations in the liver and hepatic veins.

We embarked on three full-scale studies in anesthetized dogs to characterize both hepatic and pericardial mechanoreceptors with phrenic afferents and to investigate their reflex roles. The purpose of the hepatic mechanoreceptor study was to determine whether phrenic afferent nerve activity could be recorded during stimulation of mechanosensitive receptors in the liver parenchyma, gallbladder, hepatic veins, and inferior vena cava. The dogs were prepared surgically to yield an unimpeded view of the thoracic phrenic nerve as well as the right side of the liver and inferior vena cava. The right phrenic nerve was isolated near the first rib in some animals, whereas in others the right C5 branch of the phrenic nerve was used for recording afferent nerve activity. While recording phrenic afferent nerve activity,

Hepatic Mechanoreceptors with Phrenic Afferents

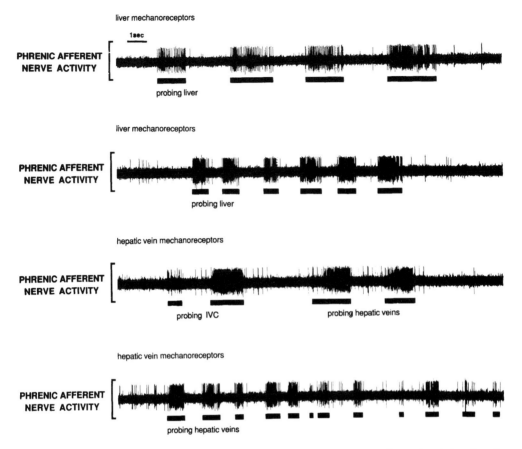

FIGURE 11.1. Raw unprocessed phrenic efferent nerve activity recorded from the right phrenic nerve originating from hepatic parenchymal (*top two panels*), hepatic vein (*bottom two panels*), and inferior vena caval mechanoreceptors (*second panel from bottom*). The horizontal bars indictae the period of mechanical stimulation.

the gallbladder, hepatic veins, inferior vena cava, diaphragm, and parenchyma of the quadrate, right medial, and right lateral lobes of the liver were mechanically probed with a cotton-tipped swab soaked in mineral oil. Pressure was applied to each area for several seconds while changes in phrenic nerve activity were recorded (Fig. 11.1).

HEPATIC PHRENIC AFFERENTS

Low-pressure Baroreceptors

Our study demonstrated for the first time the existence of mechanoreceptors in the hepatic vein, hepatic parenchyma, and inferior vena cava.[8] Gentle mechanical probing of the two most anterior hepatic veins arising from the right medial lobe elicited distinct increases in phrenic

afferent nerve activity (see Fig. 11.1). These mechanoreceptors appeared to be slowly adapting in nature, because they maintained excitability throughout the duration of mechanical probing. The hepatic vein mechanoreceptors were found at points as distal as the junction of the hepatic veins with the inferior vena cava.

The hepatic vein receptors were tested for sensitivity to increases in inferior vena caval pressure by occlusion of the inferior vena cava rostral to the diaphragm and to increases and decreases in systemic arterial pressure. Changes in arterial pressure were produced with a pressurized hemorrhage bottle connected to both femoral arteries via catheters. Changes in hepatic venous pressure produced by vena caval occlusion did not elicit changes in afferent nerve activity. Increases in arterial pressure also had no effect.

Parenchymal Mechanoreceptors

Mechanoreceptors were also demonstrated in the liver parenchyma of the right medial lobe distinctly separate from the visible hepatic veins. Probing or pinching the liver parenchyma was an adequate stimulus to activate mechanoreceptors with phrenic afferents (see Fig. 11.1). Changes in phrenic afferent nerve activity from liver parenchymal mechanoreceptors were found only in the right medial lobe. The mechanoreceptors were not responsive to changes in venous or arterial pressure. In addition, probing the gallbladder or increasing the pressure within the gallbladder with a catheter and warm saline had no effect on phrenic afferent nerve activity in any of the animals.

Clinical Significance

Clinical observations suggest that referred pain from a diseased gallbladder may be felt in the right shoulder, possibly via the phrenic nerve. Our study in dogs[8] does not support this specific premise; probing or manipulation of pressure within the gallbladder produced no change in phrenic afferent nerve activity. However, pain information from the liver parenchyma may use the phrenic afferent pathway. In gallbladder disease, the source of pain referred to the right shoulder is perhaps not the gallbladder but rather the surrounding liver parenchyma.

The phrenic afferent innervation of the hepatic veins may have a sensory role in the regulation of intrahepatic and/or portal venous blood pressure, which is known to be controlled by the smooth muscle sphincters in the hepatic veins. Legare and Lautt[9] demonstrated that in dogs the primary site of hepatic venous resistance is localized to a narrow sphincterlike region approximately 0.5 cm in length within 1–2 cm of the junction of the vena cava and hepatic veins. They showed that 62% of the pressure drop from the portal vein to the inferior vena cava in the basal state occurred over this 0.5-cm segment of hepatic vein. The investigators noted "that these resistance sites provide virtually all of the vascular resistance that is responsible for the drop in portal venous pressure as the blood passes through the liver." In addition, they stated that "in the dog, the portal venous pressure in the basal state is virtually determined by vascular resistance within the hepatic veins." The same resistance site was identified by Walker et al.,[10] Yeager et al.,[11] Arey,[12] Arey and Simonds,[13] and Brissaud and Sabourin.[14]

Our findings demonstrate that the same region of the hepatic veins is also richly innervated by phrenic afferent neurons connected to mechanoreceptors in the walls of the hepatic veins. The mechanoreceptors described above may well play a sensory role in the regulation of intrahepatic and/or portal venous blood pressure, which is controlled by the smooth muscle sphincters in the hepatic veins.

Because light touch also elicited marked increases in hepatic afferent nerve activity, lung inflation exerting pressure on the diaphragm and liver may be an adequate physiologic stimulus for some of the hepatic phrenic afferents. Furthermore, when the abdominal accessory muscles of respiration contract, intraabdominal pressure increases and may increase pressure on the liver and hepatic veins, moving them against the central tendon. Such pressure may be an important physiologic stimulus for hepatic vein receptors. The interaction of the central tendon with the lungs during inspiration may provide a normal physiologic breath-to-breath stimulation of hepatic receptors with phrenic afferents.

INFERIOR VENA CAVA MECHANORECEPTORS WITH PHRENIC AFFERENTS

Mechanosensitive areas with phrenic afferents were also found in the inferior vena cava. The mechanoreceptor areas were distributed along a band of muscle that wraps around the inferior vena cava adjacent and rostral to the diaphragm. This muscle band appears to be derived from the diaphragm as an extension along the inferior vena cava. The mechanoreceptors responded briskly to mechanical stimulation and remained sensitive throughout the stimulation period (see Fig. 11.1).

PERICARDIAL MECHANORECEPTORS WITH PHRENIC AFFERENTS

The phrenic nerve and its function have intrigued physiologists since 1863, when Luschka[15] first suggested that the phrenic nerve innervates the diaphragm with both motor and sensory fibers. In 1891 Ferguson[16] conducted the first anatomic studies verifying the fact that the phrenic nerve contains sensory fibers. He subjected cats to a C3–C6 dorsal root ganglionectomy, which produced a degeneration of phrenic afferents, and demonstrated that 30% of the phrenic nerve is

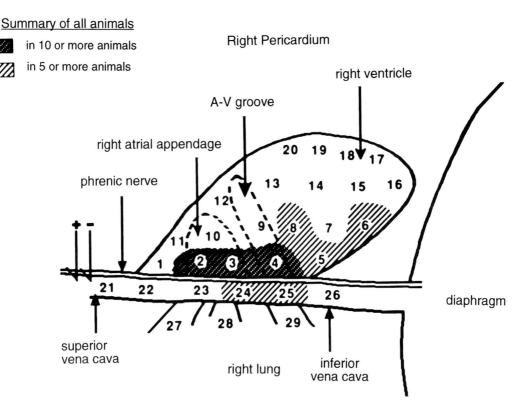

FIGURE 11.2.   Regions of the right pericardium that were studied systematically. The *dark shaded areas* indicate mechanoreceptor activity recorded in 10 or more of 18 animals. The *light shaded areas* indicate mechanoreceptor activity recorded in at least 5 but less than 10 of the 18 animals. The + and – indicate the position of the recording electrodes.

composed of afferent nerve fibers. In 1962 an identical study conducted by Landau et al.[17] in dogs demonstrated that 40–50% of the phrenic nerve was afferent. In 1961 Ruckebusch[18] presented the first direct evidence that phrenic afferents innervate pericardial mechanoreceptors in cats. Since the work of Ruckebusch, the phrenic afferent innervation of the pericardium remained unstudied until we initiated studies in dogs.[19]

The objectives of the pericardial study were to determine (1) whether receptors with phrenic afferents can be found in both right and left sides of the pericardium in dogs; (2) the kinds of stimuli that activate the receptors; (3) the anatomic distribution of the mechanoreceptors by constructing a pericardial surface map; and (4) which of the three pericardial layers contain the pericardial receptors with phrenic afferents.

The study was conducted in anesthetized dogs in which the left and right phrenic nerves were isolated near the first rib for recording of phrenic afferent nerve activity. Maps were constructed so that 20 distinct regions of the left and right

pericardium could be consistently identified and probed for mechanoreceptor location (Fig. 11.2). Areas of the right pericardium with mechanoreceptors that elicit the greatest increases in phrenic afferent nerve activity overlay the right atrial appendage (Fig. 11.2 and Fig. 11.3) and the adjacent inferior vena cava (see Fig. 11.2). The areas of the left pericardium eliciting the greatest increases in phrenic afferent nerve activity were the most inferior regions overlying the atrioventricular groove and the left lateral surface located between the atrioventricular groove within 2 cm of the apex.

The layers of the pericardium (fibrous, parietal, and visceral or epicardial) were also studied to determine which layer contained the mechanoreceptors. In all animals, mechanoreceptors were found only in the fibrous or outer layer of the pericardium. The majority of the mechanoreceptors with phrenic afferents were located in a 1–2-cm band of the fibrous pericardium paralleling the phrenic nerve on both the left and right sides (see Fig. 11.2). In addition, the right side

Pericardial Mechanoreceptors   RC5

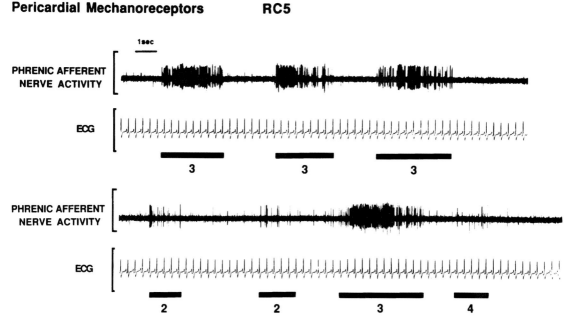

FIGURE 11.3.   Raw unprocessed phrenic afferent nerve activity recorded from the right C5 branch (RC5) of the phrenic nerve originating from the pericardial mechanoreceptors in areas 2, 3, and 4 (see Fig. 11.2). The horizontal bars indicate the period of mechanical stimulation.

appears to have a greater density of pericardial mechanoreceptors than the left side.

Clinical Significance

The physiologic role of the pericardial phrenic afferents are not understood. A potential role may be related to central transmission of pain sensation from the pericardium to the brain. In 1932 Capps[20] published clinical observations about pain arising from the pleura, pericardium, and peritoneum and portrayed the phrenic nerve as conveying sensory innervation from the fibrous pericardium. Other evidence, such as that provided by Fisch,[21] strongly suggests that pericardial afferents may be responsible for angina that cannot be attributed to coronary arterial disease.

In addition, pericardial receptors with phrenic afferents may have a respiratory reflex function, because phrenic afferents are known to project to the medullary respiratory centers,[22,23] including the Botzinger complex.[24] This theory seems entirely reasonable, because the phrenic nerves are the primary motor nerves for the diaphragm. The potential for reflex integration of phrenic neural information arising from pericardial afferents, diaphragm afferents, and hepatic afferents is now obvious; respiration may be a common

physiologic denominator for the reflex function of such phrenic afferents.

A Reflex Role for Phrenic Afferents on Respiratory Drive

The potential for visceral-phrenic neural integration led us to investigate whether hepatic, diaphragm, or pericardial phrenic afferents influence the drive to respiration. In a study in anesthetized dogs with elevated pCO_2 (35–50 torr), the author's own phrenic efferent nerve activity was used to drive ventilation with a solenoid-controlled ventilator. Altered drive to respiration was measured in response to selected regional stimulation of phrenic nerve afferents using a constant current stimulator. Stimulation of afferents from the phrenic nerve cut just above the diaphragm had no effect on respiratory drive (Fig. 11.4, bottom panel). Therefore, neither hepatic nor diaphragm phrenic afferents seem capable of increasing respiratory drive. However, when the phrenic nerve was electrically stimulated above the level of the heart, which included phrenic afferents arising from the pericardium, a marked increase in respiratory drive was demonstrated by an increase in both frequency and amplitude of left phrenic efferent nerve activity (see Fig. 11.4,

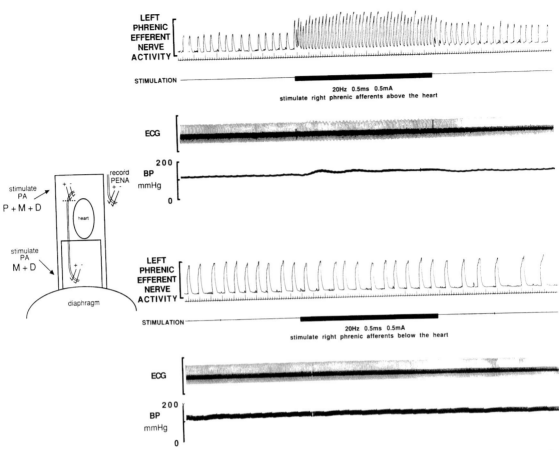

FIGURE 11.4. Reflex effects of electric stimulation of phrenic afferents *below* (M + D) and *above* (P + M + D) the heart. The *top two panels* depict the responses to stimulation of all phrenic afferents, including the pericardial afferents that increase the amplitude and frequency of the left phrenic efferent nerve activity. ECG = electrocardiogram; BP = systemic blood pressure. The *bottom two panels* depict the responses to stimulation of the hepatic and diaphragm phrenic afferents. (M + D) = mediastinal plus diaphragm plus liver; (P + M + D) = pericardial plus mediastinal plus diaphragm plus liver.

top panel). Thus one of the physiologic roles for the pericardial mechanoreceptors with phrenic afferents may be to increase respiratory rate and tidal volume. Of interest, in patients with pulmonary embolism, respiratory rate and tidal volume increase concomitantly with an increase in right heart and venous pressures. Elevated right-heart pressures may stimulate the pericardial mechanoreceptors with phrenic afferents, thereby eliciting a reflex alteration of respiration.

NEURAL INTEGRATION OF THE LOW-PRESSURE BARORECEPTOR REFLEXES

As new sites for low-pressure baroreceptors are discovered (Table 11.1), the potential for reflex integration and interaction among various sites

also increases. Figure 11.5 depicts both afferent and efferent limbs of potential low-pressure baroreceptor reflexes with vagal, sympathetic, and phrenic neural pathways. The vagal and phrenic afferent information is integrated in the brain, whereas sympathetic afferent information may be integrated at the level of the sympathetic ganglia, spinal cord, or brain. A likely example of a spinal cord or perhaps a sympathetic chain/ganglia reflex was described by Herman and Kostreva,[25] who demonstrated that renal sympathetic afferents reciprocally influence neural activity traveling to the heart and thereby alter cardiac function, which in turn increases cardiac metabolism.

There is also evidence for a hierarchy of low-pressure baroreceptor reflexes. While studying hepatic afferents,[26] we demonstrated that in dogs occlusion of the inferior vena cava at the level of

TABLE 11.1. Low-pressure Baroreceptors

Atria	Hepatic veins
Right ventricle	Spleen
Pericardium	Mesenteric bed
Pulmonary artery, veins	Kidney
Vena cava	Hind limb veins
Liver	

TABLE 11.2. Pathologic Activation of Low-pressure Baroreceptors

Congestive heart failure	Kidney disease
Cardiac tamponade	Cushing's disease
Pulmonary artery stenosis	Hypoproteinemia
Valvular disease	Lymphatic obstruction
Rheumatic	Positive pressure ventilation
Congenital anomaly	Pulmonary embolism
Pulmonary vascular disease	Anesthesia
Liver disease—cirrhosis	

the diaphragm produced a marked increase in venous pressure in the liver and mesenteric and renal beds, which reflexly increased cardiopulmonary and renal sympathetic efferent nerve activity. After hepatic denervation, sympathetic efferent nerve activity decreased rather than increased. Similar inhibition was produced by occlusion of a single renal vein. This study suggests a hierarchy of low-pressure baroreceptor reflexes. When the hepatic receptors are stimulated, their reflex response overrides that elicited by the kidneys. How or whether other low-pressure baroreceptor reflexes are involved in this hierarchy remains unknown. However, such interactions may be important in various disease states in which one or more reflexes may become either under- or overemphasized by nerve damage or pathologic alteration of the mechanoreceptors.

Such findings suggest another exciting frontier of reflexogenic control systems that may be highly important in maintaining normal physiology. Alteration of low-pressure baroreceptor reflexogenic control systems also may play a role in the genesis and progress of various disease states (Table 11.2).

Congestive heart failure, for example, is characterized by a marked increase in central venous pressure that probably activates the majority of low-pressure baroreceptors. Even positive pressure ventilation during anesthesia is known to produce oscillations in central venous pressure that may cause periodic stimulation of various low-pressure baroreceptors.

Inactivation of low-pressure baroreceptors also may have important pathophysiologic consequences. Some of the pathologic conditions that could cause neural inactivation of low-pressure baroreceptor reflexes are found in Table 11.3. For example, diabetic neuropathy targets the autonomic innervation of the kidney, heart, and other organs, thereby blunting or completely eliminating normal neural reflex pathways that may be vital to the function of these and other organs. Neuropathic diseases affecting either the peripheral or central nervous systems may alter the functional pathways mediating low-pressure baroreceptor reflexes. For example, in Guillain-Barré

Neural Reflex Pathways for Low-Pressure Baroreceptors

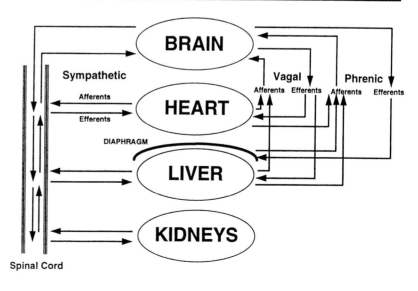

FIGURE 11.5. Sympathetic, vagal, and phrenic neural reflex pathways for low-pressure baroreceptors originating in the heart, liver, and kidneys. Also depicted are the diaphragm afferents and efferents via the phrenic nerve.

TABLE 11.3. Pathologic Inactivation of
Low-pressure Baroreceptors

Spinal cord injury	Neuropathies
Diabetic neuropathy	Cardiac surgery
Stroke	Organ transplantation
Shy-Drager syndrome	Kidney
Multiple sclerosis	Liver
Guillain-Barré syndrome	Heart

syndrome baroreceptor deafferentation may produce tachycardia, hypertension and sympathetic hyperactivity.[27] The precise effects of Guillain-Barré syndrome on low-pressure baroreceptor reflexes remain unknown.

In addition to neuropathic diseases that denervate various organ systems, heart, liver, and kidney transplantation as well as kidney and spleen removal certainly may result in denervation and elimination of some low-pressure baroreceptors systems. However, such surgical procedures provide the clinical investigator with new avenues for human studies that will help to determine the normal and pathologic roles and relative importance of low-pressure baroreceptor reflex mechanisms in man.

SUMMARY

In conclusion, some new low-pressure baroreceptors and mechanoreceptors were described as having a unique afferent neural pathway, namely, the phrenic nerve. The list of low-pressure baroreceptors presented in the previous edition of this book has now been extended to include mechanoreceptors with phrenic afferents found in the liver, hepatic veins, inferior vena cava, and pericardium. Although the reflex role of the hepatic and vena cava phrenic afferents remains unknown, the pericardial phrenic afferents may be involved in altering respiratory drive.

REFERENCES

1. Alexander WF: The innervation of the biliary system. J Comp Neurol 1940;72:357–370.
2. Friedman MI: Hepatic nerve function. In Arias IM, Propper H, Schachter D, Shafritz DA (eds): The Liver: Biology and Pathobiology. New York: Raven, 1982;663–673.
3. Friedman MI: Hepatic nerve function. In Arias IM, Jakoby WB, Propper H, Schachter D, Shafritz DA (eds): The Liver: Biology and Pathobiology, 2nd ed. New York: Raven, 1988;949–959.
4. Lautt WW: Hepatic nerves: A review of their function in liver function. Can J Physiol Pharmacol 1980;58:105–123.
5. Lautt WW: Afferent and efferent neural roles in liver function. Prog Neurobiol 1983;21:323–348.
6. Richardson PDI, Withrington PG: Liver blood flow. I. Intrinsic and nervous control of liver blood flow [abstract]. Gastroenterology 1981;81:159.
7. Ungvary G, Donath T: On the monoaminergic innervation of the liver. Acta Anat 1969;72:446–459.
8. Kostreva DR, Pontus SP: Hepatic vein, hepatic parenchymal, and inferior vena caval mechanoreceptors with phrenic afferents. Am J Physiol 1993;265:G15–G20.
9. Legare DJ, Lautt WW: Hepatic venous resistance site in the dog: Localization and validation of intrahepatic pressure measurements. Can J Physiol Pharmacol 1987;65:352–359.
10. Walker WF, MacDonald JS, Pickard C: Hepatic vein sphincter mechanism in the dog. Br J Surg 1960;48:218–220.
11. Yeager VL, Anderson DJ, Taylor JJ: Smooth muscle in the hepatic artery, portal vein and hepatic vein within the liver of the raccoon and guinea pig. Experientia Basel 1985;41:262–265.
12. Arey LB: Throttling veins in the livers of certain mammals. Anat Rec 1941;81:21–33.
13. Arey LB, Simonds JP: The relation of the smooth muscle in the hepatic veins to shock phenomena. Anat Rec 1920;17–18:219.
14. Brissaud E, Sabourin C: Sur la constitution lobulaire du foie et les voies de la circulation sanguine intra-hepatique. CR Seances Soc Biol 1888;40:757–762.
15. Luschka H: Die Anatomie des Menschens, vol. 12. Tubingen: Lauupp and Siebeck, 1863;215.
16. Ferguson J: The phrenic nerve. Brain 1891;14:282–283.
17. Landau BR, Akert K, Roberts TS: Studies on the innervation of the diaphragm. J Comp Neurol 1962;119:1–10.
18. Ruckebusch Y: Influx afferents d'origine pericardique dans les nerfs phreniques. CR Soc Biol Paris 1961;155:524–527.
19. Kostreva DR, Pontus SP: Pericardial mechanoreceptors with phrenic afferents. Am J Physiol 1993;264:H1836–H1846.
20. Capps J: An Experimental and Clinical Study of Pain in the Pleura, Pericardium and Peritoneum. New York: Macmillan, 1932.
21. Fisch S: On the origin of cardiac pain. A new hypothesis. Arch Intern Med 1980;140:754–755.
22. Macron JM, Marlot D: Effects of stimulation of phrenic afferent fibers on medullary respiratory neurons in cats. Neurosci Lett 1986;63:231–236.
23. Speck D, Revelette: Excitation of dorsal and ventral respiratory group neurons by Phrenic nerve afferents. J Appl Physiol 1987;62:946–951.
24. Speck D: Botzinger complex region role in phrenic-to-phrenic inhibitory reflex of cat. J Appl Physiol 1989;67:1364–1370.
25. Herman NL, Kostreva DR: Alterations in cardiac [14C]deoxyglucose uptake induced by two renal afferent stimuli. Am J Physiol 1986;251:R867–R877.
26. Kostreva DR, Castaner A, Kampine JP: Reflex effects of hepatic baroreceptors on renal and cardiac sympathetic nerve activity. Am J Physiol 1980;238:R390–R394.
27. Fagius J, Wallin BG: Microneurographic evidence of excessive sympathetic outflow in the Guillain-Barré syndrome. Brain 1983;106:589–600.

Chapter 12

RENIN-ANGIOTENSIN SYSTEM IN LIVER DISEASE

MURRAY EPSTEIN, M.D., F.A.C.P.

Physiology of the Renin-Angiotensin System
  Components of the Renin-Angiotensin System
  Control of Renin Secretion
  Vasoactive Interrelationships
  Measurement of Components of the Renin-
    Angiotensin System
**Alterations of the Renin-Angiotensin System in
  Liver Disease**
  Plasma Renin Activity
  Sequential Studies in a Single Patient During
    Prolonged Observation
  Angiotensin II
  Renin Substrate

Angiotensin-Converting Enzyme (Kininase II)
Plasma Angiotensinase Activity
Mechanisms of Increased Renin-Angiotensin Levels
  Decreased Hepatic Extraction by the Liver
  Increased Renin Secretion
Responsiveness of the Renin-Angiotensin System
**Renin-Angiotensin System as a Determinant of
  Renal Hemodynamics**
Prognosis and the Renin-Angiotensin System
Renin-Angiotensin System in Renal Failure
**Pharmacologic Blockade of the Renin-Angiotensin
  System**
Summary

Almost 100 years ago, Tigerstedt and Berg-man[1] identified a pressor substance in saline extracts of the kidney, which they named "renin." Their discovery attracted little attention until 1934, when Goldblatt and associates[2] reported that an increase in renin secretion and hypertension resulted from the induction of renal ischemia in dogs. During the subsequent half-century, studies of this hormone have assumed enormous importance in investigations of the pathogenesis of many disease states, including the role of the kidney in the regulation of fluid and electrolyte balance in cirrhosis.

This chapter provides an overview of the alterations of the renin-angiotensin system in liver disease. As such, it constitutes a framework within which other chapters will consider specific problems, including (1) the effects of renin inhibition and (2) the mechanisms contributing to hyperreninemia (see chapter 3). Because the renin-angiotensin system is complex and because the appropriateness of measuring any particular component varies with the clinical circumstances and the needed information, this review begins with a consideration of normal physiology.

PHYSIOLOGY OF THE RENIN-ANGIOTENSIN SYSTEM

The physiology of the renin-angiotensin system has been discussed recently in several excellent and extensive reviews,[3–9] and is described here only briefly. A simplified outline of the renin-angiotensin-aldosterone system is depicted in Figure 12.1. The enzyme renin is synthesized and stored by cells at the vascular pole of the renal glomerulus. Both the afferent and efferent arterioles are anatomically and functionally associated with a group of specialized cells at the origin of the distal tubule that form the macula densa. The entire structure is referred to as the juxtaglomerular apparatus. This site is the center of a feedback loop that regulates blood pressure and intravascular volume by modulating the rate of renin secretion. In response to an appropriate signal, renin is released into both renal venous blood and renal lymph. The substrate for renin, angiotensinogen, is an α-globulin synthesized by the liver. Renin reacts in the plasma with angiotensinogen to split off a largely inactive decapeptide, angiotensin I. As it courses through the circulation, the two end amino acids, histidyl and leucine, are removed by

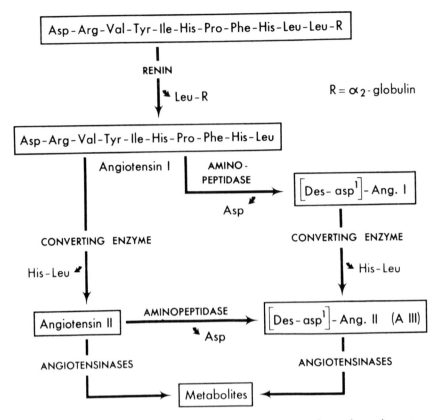

FIGURE 12.1.   An overview of the components of the renin-angiotensin system.

a converting enzyme to form the 8-amino acid polypeptide angiotensin II, which is largely responsible for the several physiologic and pathophysiologic effects of the renin-angiotensin system. Recent reports have suggested that angiotensin II is further hydrolyzed to form the heptapeptide angiotensin III, which has a less potent pressor effect than angiotensin II but plays a role in stimulating adrenal aldosterone secretion. Even smaller peptide products of angiotensin (6 amino acids or less) are not presently believed to have important physiologic roles.

Components of the Renin-Angiotensin System

Renin Substrate

Renin substrate, or angiotensinogen, is the protein substrate from which renin enzymatically cleaves angiotensin I. The available evidence indicates that angiotensinogen in the circulation is produced by the liver. The concentration of angiotensinogen in plasma can be altered by a number of hormones and manipulations. Thus, the administration of adrenocortical steroids, estrogens, and

angiotensin II as well as nephrectomy increases circulating angiotensinogen levels. Under most physiologic circumstances, however, glucocorticoids and angiotensin II are probably the most important physiologic regulators.

Renin

Renin is a specific protease that releases angiotensin I from renin substrate. Recent studies indicate that larger forms of renin, or prorenin, may be synthesized and stored in the kidney as well as in other organs and that these forms of renin may be activated by alterations in pH, temperature, and proteolytic enzymes.[10] The number and variety of structures of either prorenin or big renin remain unsettled.

In humans, active and inactive forms of renin are present in kidney and plasma. The inactive form can be converted to an active form by exposure to acid (pH 3.0) or proteolytic enzymes or by incubation in the cold. The relative amounts of the inactive and active forms appear to vary under different circumstances and in different disease states. The relationship between the active and inactive forms remains unsettled, and until in vivo conversion is demonstrated, the clinical significance of inactive renin remains to be established. Confusion may arise, however, when interpreting data about renin levels in the literature because different in vitro assays of renin may measure only the active form or both the active and inactive forms of renin (see below).

Angiotensin I-Converting Enzyme

Angiotensin l-converting enzyme (ACE) exists in large concentrations in the lung. It was long thought to be present solely in lung; however, the available evidence indicates that ACE is present in the kidney, in other organs, and possibly in peripheral plasma. ACE has recently assumed greater clinical significance as a result of the availability of drugs that are relatively specific ACE inhibitors. Included among these is a nonpeptide originally isolated from the venom of the snake *Bothrops jararaca*. Subsequently, an orally active ACE inhibitor (referred to as SQ 14225) has become available. Currently many ACE inhibitors are available for clinical use.[11] The application of such ACE inhibitors to studies aimed at elucidating the pathophysiologic role of the renin-angiotensin-aldosterone system is reviewed in detail elsewhere[12] in this chapter.

Angiotensin

Angiotensin I, the primary product of renin's action on angiotensinogen, is relatively inactive physiologically. In turn, it is converted by converting enzyme to the 8-amino acid chain referred to as angiotensin II. Angiotensin II is one of the most potent vasoconstrictor agents on a molar basis. In addition, angiotensin II is a potent stimulator of aldosterone production by the adrenal cortex. Finally, angiotensin II may have a direct effect on sodium transport in the kidney. Angiotensin II is further degraded by a series of enzymes collectively referred to as angioteninases. One of the several products of degradation of angiotensin II is the 7-amino acid peptide angiotensin III. Although angiotensin III is potent at stimulating aldosterone production by the adrenal cortex, it is relatively ineffective as a vasoconstricting agent, with the possible exception of the renal vasculature.

Control of Renin Secretion

Several lines of evidence indicate that at least nine factors control the release of renin from the juxtaglomerular cells:

1. Baroreceptor mechanism
2. Macula densa
3. Stimulation of renal sympathetic nerves
4. Circulating angiotensin II levels
5. Prostaglandins
6. Plasma potassium concentration
7. Atrial natriuretic factor
8. Other hormonal and electrolyte factors
9. Physiologic factors

Baroreceptor Mechanism

Many observations provide evidence for an intrarenal vascular receptor in the control of renin release. Over 35 years ago, Tobian and coworkers[13] postulated the presence of a baroreceptor, or stretch receptor, that modulates the control of renin release. According to this hypothesis, the juxtaglomerular apparatus—in specific, the juxtaglomerular cells—may act as stretch receptors. An increase in mean arterial pressure and cellular stretch would result in an inhibition of renin release; conversely, a diminution in juxtaglomerular cell tension would enhance renin release.

Subsequently, using the nonfiltering dog kidney model, Blaine and Davis[14] provided convincing evidence for an intrarenal vascular receptor in the control of renin release. They were able to investigate vascular factors independent of changes at the macula densa, alterations related to renal nerves or adrenal catecholamines, and other potential influences on renin release. Striking increases were demonstrable in renin synthesis and release following reduction in renal blood flow because of either hemorrhage or aortic constriction. This occurred in the absence of changes in glomerular filtration rate or other exogenous influences.

Although such studies support a role for an autonomous intrarenal vascular receptor as a potential control mechanism for renin release, the specific nature of the receptor is still poorly understood. Whether the receptor responds to changes in systemic or renal perfusion pressure, stretch, changes in intravascular pressure or transmural pressure within the arteriolar wall of the juxtaglomerular apparatus, or changes in arteriolar wall tension is not known. Current data suggest that activation of a renal vascular receptor, regardless of the state of renal arteriolar vasomotion, results in renin release. This mechanism probably accounts for the release of renin whenever renal arterial pressure is lowered, either as part of generalized systemic hypotension (e.g., hemorrhage, diuretic-induced plasma volume depletion) or in localized renal hypotension (e.g., partial clamping of the renal artery). It has been suggested that this system is little involved with blood pressure control under normal circumstances but assumes an important role when circulatory homeostasis is markedly diminished or stressed.

Evidence has accrued from recent studies in humans that changes in central blood volume modulate renin release[15] (see chapter 1). Egan et al.[16] suggested that changes in cardiopulmonary mechanoreceptor stimulation mediate changes in plasma renin activity (PRA) through a neurohormonal reflex. Furthermore, they concluded that unloading both low-pressure baroreceptors and arterial baroreceptors induced the largest increases in PRA, suggesting an interaction between the two types of receptors.

Role of the Macula Densa

Current concepts indicate that manipulations that augment the distal delivery of sodium and chloride, under conditions in which they may be transported at the level of the macula densa, may affect renin release. Initially, Vander[17] proposed that a decrease in the load of sodium delivered to the macula densa portion of the distal tubule stimulates renin release. On the other hand, Thurau[18] presented evidence for a direct relationship between alterations in tubular fluid milieu, the macula densa, and renin synthesis and release. The interrelationship between tubular function and glomerular function, with alterations effected by activation of the renin-angiotensin system as perceived by a stimulus at the macula densa, has been termed the "tubuloglomerular feedback" mechanism. According to this hypothesis, alterations in tubular function, probably involving the distal portion of the proximal tubule and the loop of Henle, result in changes in tubular fluid composition within the macula densa segment of the distal nephron. The exact nature of the alterations in tubular fluid composition that are sensed at the macula densa remain the subject of speculation. At first, sodium, as a function of concentration or load, was suggested as the stimulus perceived by the macula densa. Subsequent studies, however, have suggested that alterations in chloride, the accompanying anion, may constitute the signal perceived by the macula densa.

Considerable evidence suggests that there is a macula densa system for the physiologic control

of renin release, but little is known about the relative importance of this receptor in the physiologic or pathophysiologic control of renin-angiotensin system activity. Recent studies suggest that the macula densa receptor control of renin release may be of greater importance at lower perfusion pressures.

Sympathetic Nervous System

Stimulation of renal sympathetic nerves or infusion of catecholamines stimulates renin release. Increased sympathetic activity may be responsible for the increase in PRA with exercise and stress and may play a role in the response to upright posture and hemorrhage. Such stimulation is thought to be mediated by β-receptor activity. (see chapter 19.)

Circulating Angiotensin II

As renin is released from the juxtaglomerular cells into the renal arterial blood, some angiotensin is formed and, in turn, is converted to the active angiotensin II within the kidney. This intrarenal angiotensin II exerts a direct feedback suppression of the release of renin that is unrelated to its vasoconstrictive activity. This suppression of renin release can be blocked by nonpressor analogs of angiotensin that, in and of themselves, stimulate renin release.

Prostaglandins

Increased prostaglandin activity results in enhanced renin release. This subject is considered in greater detail below in the section about vasoactive interrelationships (see also chapter 14).

Plasma Potassium Concentration

Increased plasma potassium inhibits renin secretion. Since the infusion of potassium did not affect renin secretion in a nonfiltering kidney model, the mechanism by which potassium acts presumably involves an inhibition of tubular sodium reabsorption so that more sodium is delivered to the macula densa.

Atrial Natriuretic Factor

Infusion of atrial natriuretic factor (ANF) induces a prompt and marked inhibition of renin secretion in dogs despite a concurrent fall in arterial pressure.[19] A reduction in PRA during ANF infusion has also been observed in normal humans.[19] The mechanisms whereby ANF reduces PRA have not been fully defined, but renal

TABLE 12.1. Factors Influencing Circulating Renin and Angiotensin

Sodium balance
Potassium balance
Posture and activity
Circadian rhythm
Menstrual cycle (higher in the luteal phase)
Drugs that influence renin release

Stimulate Renin Release	*Suppress Renin Release*
Benzothiadiazine-type diuretics (thiazides)	Licorice
Spironolactone	Carbenoxolone
Amiloride	Methyldopa
Diazoxide	Clonidine
Antibiotics (gentamicin, viomycin, capreomycin)	β-Receptor blocking agents
β-Agonists	Prazosin
Caffeine	Prostaglandin inhibitors (indomethacin, ibuprofen, aspirin)
Chlorpromazine	Vasopressin
Glucagon	Somatostatin
Estrogen	

hemodynamic alterations are likely to be involved. Furthermore, the ANF-induced increase in glomerular filtration rate (GFR), by increasing the filtered load of solute, may lead to increased sodium chloride delivery to the macula densa, thus inducing PRA suppression. A direct inhibitory effect of ANF on renin release is also possible (see chapter 15).

Other Hormonal and Electrolyte Factors

Additional hormonal and electrolyte factors are also involved in the control of renin release. The sodium ion may suppress renin independently of its participation in body fluid volume homeostasis. Furthermore, vasopressin in physiologic doses inhibits renin release.[20]

Physiologic Factors

Aside from the influence of various hormones and ions, renin levels may change in response to other factors. As shown in Table 12.1, such factors include age, race, posture, sodium intake, time of day, and menstrual cycle. PRA declines with increasing age both in normotensive and hypertensive people. This may reflect simply a progressive decrease in the functional mass of juxtaglomerular cells; thus, care should be taken to use populations of similar age in establishing normal levels. Race also affects renin levels. Blacks have lower PRA levels whether they are normotensive or hypertensive.

The profound effects of posture on the renin-angiotensin axis are extremely important. Standing is associated with a sharp rise in peripheral blood PRA and angiotensin II levels within 5 minutes, with a peak in 90–120 minutes; the levels remain high thereafter. The effects of posture on PRA may be mediated through changes in stimulation of baroreceptors, as noted previously.

Sodium balance is a major determinant of renin-angiotensin activity. Sodium deprivation leads to an increase in PRA; high dietary sodium intake depresses PRA. Potassium also modulates renin release. Potassium loading exerts an inhibiting effect on the renin-angiotensin system; potassium depletion increases plasma renin. The relative importance of potassium in the regulation of the renin-angiotensin system remains to be established; some investigators suggest that it is relatively minor and readily overwhelmed by the effects of changes in sodium balance. There is a distinct circadian rhythm of PRA independent of activity and posture, with the highest levels occurring during the early morning.

Various medications have been shown to exert important effects on renin release. Diuretic agents and vasodilators stimulate renin release; methyldopa, clonidine, and ß-receptor blocking agents tend to suppress renin.

Vasoactive Interrelationships

The influence of the renin-angiotensin axis on systemic blood pressure, volume homeostasis, and renal function cannot be considered in isolation because of the interdependence of the renin-angiotensin system and other vasoactive phenomena. As emphasized in a previous review,[21] interaction between the renin-angiotensin system and other vasoactive systems (i.e., bradykinin,

TABLE 12.2. Measurement of the Three Components of the Renin-Angiotensin System

Component to Be Measured	Methodology
Renin substrate	Amount of angiotensin generated by the addition of excessive renin
Renin activity	Amount of angiotensin generated by the system, without additions
Renin concentration	Amount of angiotensin generated when the amount of renin substrate is fixed

prostaglandins) is complex. This suggests that cautious interpretation of early results is warranted.

Of these vasoactive phenomena, the interrelationships between the renin-angiotensin system and prostaglandins have received much attention. Increased renin-angiotensin system activity results in increased prostaglandin synthesis and release; conversely, increased prostaglandin activity results in enhanced renin release. Furthermore, the administration of prostaglandin synthetase inhibitors, which greatly diminish circulating prostaglandins, results in a decrease in renin-angiotensin system activity. Such results suggest a positive feedback between synthesis and release of prostaglandin and activity of the renin-angiotensin system. The physiology of renal prostaglandins and their interrelationship with the renin-angiotensin system are considered in chapter 14.

The interaction between the renin-angiotensin axis and prostaglandin activity may be directly or indirectly modulated by other vasoactive systems. Catecholamines and sympathetic nervous system activity influence renin and prostaglandin release, resulting in the possibility of a complex series of interactions. Prostaglandin synthesis and release are enhanced by renal nerve stimulation and norepinephrine, factors that also increase renin-angiotensin system activity. Furthermore, a feedback interdependence of prostaglandins with catecholamines modulates adrenergic tone; prostaglandins of the E type inhibit catecholamine release from adrenergic nerve endings and prostaglandins of the F type facilitate adrenergic/catecholamine effects.

An interdependence between the renin-angiotensin system and the kallikrein-kinin system may be inferred from the previous discussion on the similarity of ACE and kininase II. This interdependence goes beyond the sharing of a common enzyme. As an example, Flamenbaum and co-workers[22] demonstrated a direct effect of bradykinin on renin synthesis and release. In addition, the infusion of bradykinin resulted in an increased secretory rate for prostaglandins of both the E type and F type. The physiology of the kallikrein-kinin system and its interrelationship

with both the renin-angiotensin system and renal prostaglandins are considered in greater detail in chapter 14.

Measurement of Components of the Renin-Angiotensin System

Because renin cannot yet be measured directly, evaluation of the activity of the renin-angiotensin system under both normal and pathologic conditions usually entails measurement of other components of the system. Although techniques to measure concentrations of circulating angiotensin I and angiotensin II are available, the procedures are technically tedious and tricky. Since the values correlate well with those obtained by the more easily and widely performed assays of renin activity, neither circulating angiotensin I nor angiotensin II is commonly measured in clinical practice.

Table 12.2 summarizes the principles underlying the measurement of the diverse components of the renin-angiotensin system. The most commonly used measurement is PRA. The usual procedure for assay of PRA is the measurement of the amount of angiotensin I generated by incubation of the patient's substrate and enzyme. The amount of angiotensin generated in the reaction between renin and angiotensinogen under defined conditions (temperature, pH, substrate concentration, and incubation time) is determined by radioimmunoassay. Despite extensive experience, a number of technical problems have not been worked out, and disagreements about the best procedure persists. Even after the American Association of Clinical Chemists published its "Selected Method,"[23] numerous valid objections have persisted. Methods that do not add substrate in excess measure *plasma renin activity*. When exogenous substrate is added in excess so that the amount of angiotensin produced reflects the effects on the actual amounts of renin present rather than any limitation imposed by changes in substrate availability, the results are expressed as *plasma renin concentration* (PRC). Under most situations, the relative alterations in PRC are reflected in PRA and the latter test is sufficient. Because PRA reflects angiotensin formation as occurring in the circulation with existing substrate concentrations, it is thought by some to constitute a better index of angiotensin formation in vivo. *Renin substrate concentration* also may be measured by incubating known amounts of plasma with added excess of human renin; the total amount of angiotensin formed then reflects the concentration of substrate under defined conditions.

As noted earlier, confusion may arise because different in vitro assays of plasma renin may measure only the active form or both active and inactive forms together. Assays of PRC, widely used in England and Australia, measure both since they activate the inactive form by using a pH below 4.0. It has been suggested that such assays should be viewed as measuring "total" renin. The radioimmunoassays for PRA, based on the technique of Haber et al.,[24] are widely used in the United States. They keep the pH above 4.0 and therefore measure only the active form. At least one instance has been reported wherein the use of a PRC assay measuring both active and inactive forms produced results different from those found by the use of a PRA assay measuring only the active form. However, with the method of Haber et al., plasma must be rapidly frozen to obviate the problem of cryoactivation, which occurs in chilled plasma specimens.

Although the availability of commercially prepackaged kits suggests that this determination is within the capability of most radioisotope laboratories, considerable care must be exercised in its performance, which presents methodologic pitfalls of greater complexity than many other commonly used radioimmunoassays. Furthermore, even accurately performed renin measurements can be interpreted only if samples are obtained under clinically defined circumstances; random, single determinations are often meaningless.

ALTERATIONS OF THE RENIN-ANGIOTENSIN SYSTEM IN LIVER DISEASE

Plasma Renin Activity

Numerous investigators have undertaken studies to document the activity of the renin-angiotensin system in patients with liver disease, most commonly by measuring PRA but also by reporting on the histologic appearance of the juxtaglomerular apparatus, PRC levels, and circulating concentrations of angiotensin II. The conditions of study have varied with regard to factors known to alter the activity of the renin-angiotensin system (age of patients, body posture, and time of day for venous sampling, dietary sodium intake, and drug treatment); consequently, comparisons of results between studies are not always possible.

Over 35 years ago, Reeves and colleagues[25] conducted an autopsy study in 45 patients with cirrhosis and ascites and reported that whereas the total renal juxtaglomerular cell counts were similar to those in noncirrhotic controls, type II and III juxtaglomerular cells (i.e., moderately granulated) were more numerous in cirrhotic patients. The investigators interpreted this finding as suggesting that the rate of renal renin secretion was increased in the interval prior to the patients' demise.

Thirty five years ago Hartroft and Hartroft[26] demonstrated that the juxtaglomerular index is higher in patients with cirrhosis and ascites than in normal subjects. In 1967 Ayers[27] reported that the PRA of such patients is markedly higher and the renin substrate concentration lower than in control subjects. Subsequent studies by many investigators have established that many patients with advanced liver disease manifest perturbations of several components of the renin-angiotensin system, including plasma renin activity and renin substrate.[28–38] Nevertheless, disagreement centers on the frequency with which PRA stimulation occurs in cirrhosis.

A brief review of some of the salient features of studies in which renin-angiotensin activity has been determined points out the bases for such controversy. Table 12.3 is not meant to constitute an exhaustive summary of all relevant articles; rather, it highlights important features from several of the more frequently cited articles in which renin-angiotensin activity has been measured. Many studies have determined PRA (or PRC, or both) without commenting on concomitant changes of many of the factors that influence circulating renin and angiotensin concentrations. Although some investigators have rigorously controlled sodium intake, others have either failed to control this important determinant of renin or have utilized varying sodium intakes without attempting to segregate plasma renin levels according to sodium intake.

Although potassium is thought to exert an important effect on the renin-aldosterone system,

TABLE 12.3.   Representative Studies of Plasma Renin Activity in Patients with Liver Disease

Authors (Reference)	Patient Population	Number of Patients	PRA (ng/ml/hr)* in Study Population	PRA (ng/ml/hr)* Normal Values
Schroeder et al. 1970 (28)	Cirrhosis with ascites	17	12.6 × 10⁻⁴ U/ml (10 of 17 were elevated)	0–3.5 × 10⁻⁴ U/ml
	Cirrhosis, ascites, and renal failure	7	174 × 10⁻⁴ U/ml	
Barnardo et al. 1970 (29)	Cirrhosis without ascites	3	33 ± 42 (SD) ng/L/min	< 22.9 ng/L/min
	Cirrhosis with ascites	30		
Kondo et al. 1974 (30)	Cirrhosis without ascites	17	2.3 ± 0.9 (SD)	1.5± 0.6 (SD)
	Cirrhosis with ascites	10	4.0 ± 3.0 (SD)	
	Chronic hepatitis	17	1.8 ± 0.7 (SD)	
Rosoff et al. 1975 (31)	Cirrhosis with ascites	8	Supine 6.0 ± 2.4 (SE) Erect 8.4 ± 3.1 (SE)	2.2 ± 0.5 (SE) 5.9 ± 0.4 (SE)
Epstein et al. 1977 (32)	Cirrhosis without ascites	2	9.4 ± 1.6	3.4–13.9 (±2 SD)
	Cirrhosis with ascites	14		
Wernze et al. 1978 (34)	Cirrhosis with ascites (untreated)	23	2.2 ± 1.7 (SD)	2.1 ± 1.0 (SD)
	Cirrhosis without ascites	12	1.4 ± 0.8 (SD)	(0.4–4.2 is range)
Arroyo et al. 1979 (35)	Cirrhosis with ascites	68	0.12–18.1 is range	1.1 ± 0.5 (SD)
Wilkinson et al. 1979 (36)	Cirrhosis and CAH			1.82 ± 0.57 (SD) nmol/L/hr
	Without ascites	15	Mean = 0.91 nmol/L/hr	(0.92–2.96 is range)
	Increasing ascites	35	Mean = 3.99 nmol/L/hr	
	With renal failure	17	Mean = 9.50 nmol/L/hr	
Chonko et al. 1977 (33)	Cirrhosis with ascites	6	8.4 ± 2.3	
		5	< 1	< 1
Mitch et al. 1979 (37)	Cirrhosis with ascites	14	4.0 ± 1.0 (range: 0.4–17.4)	0.3 ± 0.1 (SE)
	Cirrhosis without ascites	10	4.6 ± 2.1 (range: 0.1–18.9)	
Hata et al. 1979 (38)	Cirrhosis without ascites	7	1.7 ± 0.4 (SE)	0.3–3.0 is range
	Cirrhosis with ascites	8	3.7 ± 0.8 (SE)	
Bernardi et al. 1983 (41)	Cirrhosis without ascites	16	0.53 ± 0.32 (SD)	1.37 ± 0.39 (SD)
	Cirrhosis with ascites	21	2.68 ± 1.61 (SD)	
Sellars et al. 1985 (40)	Cirrhosis with ascites/edema and in sodium balance	16	Supine 1.9 pmol/L/min Erect 4.4 pmol/L/min	Supine 3.4 pmol/L/min Erect 6.8 pmol/L/min
	Cirrhosis with ascites/edema and sodium retention	13	Supine 29.7 pmol/L/min Erect 50.7 pmol/L/min	
Bernardi et al. 1986 (42)	Cirrhosis with ascites	9	2.3 ± 0.3 (SEM)	1.1 ± 0.3 (SEM)
	Cirrhosis without ascites	7	0.5 ± 0.2 (SEM)	

PRA = plasma renin activity, CAH = chronic active hepatitis.

* All values reported as ng/ml/hr unless otherwise indicated; all values are PRA except in the study of Schroeder et al., who used plasma renin concentration.   *Table continued on opposite page.*

only 7 of the 17 reviewed studies attempted to control potassium intake, and only 7 studies reported on the concomitant serum potassium concentrations. Finally, in light of the presence of a distinct circadian rhythm for PRA, independent of physical activity and posture, it is noteworthy that one-third of the studies did not specify the time at which blood was obtained for PRA determinations.

Despite these caveats regarding interpretation, it is apparent that renin levels are frequently elevated in patients with advanced liver disease. Furthermore, the degree of augmentation of the renin-angiotensin system may correlate with clinical status. Brown et al.[39] were among the first to propose a correlation between ascites and the degree of PRA elevation. In 1964 they used a bioassay technique to determine PRA levels in 18 cirrhotic patients. They were able to correlate elevated PRA levels with the extent of compensation, reporting that PRA levels were in the normal range in compensated cirrhotic patients (without ascites) and elevated in decompensated cirrhotic patients (with unequivocal ascites). In contrast, Kondo et al.[30] reported that PRA levels were

TABLE 12.3.   Representative Studies of Plasma Renin Activity in Patients with Liver Disease (*cont.*)

Assay	Sodium Intake (mEq/day)	Potassium Intake (mEq/day)	Serum Potassium	Posture	Time of Day	Medications
RIA	12	Not specified	Not specified	Supine	Not specified	None
	12	Not specified	Not specified	Supine	Not specified	None
Bioassay	135 in 16 patients	90	Not specified	Supine	Not specified	None
	22 in 9 patients	90	Not specified	Supine	Not specified	None
Bioassay	Not Na restricted	Not specified	Not specified	Supine	Morning	None
	Not Na restricted	Not specified	Not specified	Supine	Morning	None
	Not Na restricted	Not specified	Not specified	Supine	Morning	None
RIA	80	Not specified	> 3.4	Supine	Not specified	None
	80	Not specified	> 3.4	Erect	Not specified	None
RIA	10	100	Not specified	Seated	8 a.m.	None
RIA	120–150	70–90	3.8 ± 0.5 (SD)	Supine	7:30–9:30 a.m.	None
			4.3 ± 0.3 (SD)			
RIA	40	Not specified	Not specified	Supine	Not specified	None
RIA	40–50	Not specified	Not specified	Supine	Morning	None
RIA	300	Not specified	Not specified	Supine	Morning	None
RIA	Not Na restricted	Not specified	3.8 ± 0.1	Supine	Morning	None
RIA	Not specified	Not specified	Not specified	Supine	Not specified	None
RIA	40	80	4.22 ± 0.70	Not specified	10 a.m.	None
			4.16 ± 0.50			
RIA	Not specified	Not specified	4.1 ± 0.5	Supine	9–11 a.m.	None
				Erect		
			3.9 ± 0.4	Supine		
RIA	40	90	4.4 ± 0.1	Erect	Mean of	None
			4.2 ± 0.2	Supine	24-hr period	

RIA = radioimmunoassay.

increased significantly in cirrhotic patients with or without ascites compared with normal controls.

Wilkinson et al.[36] reported that PRA was either normal or reduced in patients without ascites. Patients with accumulating ascites manifested extremely variable PRA levels; that is, it was reduced in 5 of 35 patients, normal in 16, and increased in the remaining 14 patients. Mean PRA for the group with ascites exceeded that in patients without ascites.

Hata et al.[38] reported that the mean PRA in cirrhotic patients with ascites was significantly higher than that in patients without ascites. Of their 8 patients with ascites, 5 manifested elevated PRA levels; whereas 3 had PRA levels within the normal range.

Subsequent reports from other investigators as well as observations from the author's laboratory are at variance with the above findings. For example, the report of Mitch et al.[37] questions the segregation of hyperreninemia to ascitic patients. The availability in their report of individual PRA values in a large group of normal controls as well as cirrhotic patients with or without ascites permits the reader to examine the frequency of PRA elevation in patients with and without ascites. Mean PRA in their patients with ascites (4.0 ± 1.2 ng/ml hr) did not differ from the mean PRA in the 9 patients without ascites (4.6 ± 2.1). Although not stated, compensated patients appeared as likely to manifest PRA elevations as ascitic patients.

Wernze et al.[34] characterized the diverse components of the renin-angiotensin axis in a group of 77 patients with cirrhosis of the liver. In addition to categorizing the patients according to presence or absence of ascites, they also divided patients with respect to diuretic administration. The investigators demonstrated that untreated cirrhotic patients with ascites manifested PRA and PRC levels that did not differ from those of controls. Cirrhotic patients without ascites (group IV) also had PRA and PRC levels within the normal range. The investigators concluded that activation of the renin-angiotensin axis was unlikely in cirrhotic patients with ascites in the absence of diuretic administration.

This conclusion contrasts with a report by Sellars et al.,[40] who examined two groups of patients with ascites and/or edema and a group of normal controls. The patients in one group were in sodium balance, whereas patients in the other group were retaining sodium. Both groups were on unrestricted sodium intake and had not used diuretics for at least 4 weeks. In the sodium-retaining group, PRA was strikingly increased compared with the group in sodium balance or the control group, although some patients manifested normal values. Sellars et al. concluded, therefore, that the stimulation of the renin-angiotensin system in cirrhotic patients may occur without diuretic treatment.

In two subsequent studies, Bernardi et al.[41,42] reported that PRA was significantly higher in patients with cirrhosis and ascites than in cirrhotic patients without ascites. In one of the studies,[41] however, 50% of the patients with ascites had PRA values within the normal range, and in the other study[42] 3 of 9 patients had normal levels of PRA values.

Although D'Arienzo et al.[43] and Burmeister et al.[44] reported elevated PRA levels in a group of cirrhotic patients, their data are difficult to interpret. The patients had recently received spironolactone[43,44]; thus, the elevated values may have been attributable in part to the effects of the drug.

We reexamined this question and have been unable to confirm the putative high frequency with which PRA stimulation has been reported in advanced liver disease.[32] PRA levels were determined under rigorously controlled experimental conditions in a group of 28 cirrhotic patients. Liver disease was associated with excessive alcohol intake in all 28 patients, and all were negative for hepatitis B surface antigen by radioimmunoassay. None had clinical findings that suggested underlying or antecedent cardiac or renal disease. Significant vascular, parenchymal, or neoplastic renal disease was excluded by history, physical examination, and laboratory tests and, in some subjects, by intravenous pyelography. No patient received diuretics during the 10 days prior to study. Twenty-three patients were studied during decompensation, arbitrarily defined by the presence of unequivocal ascites or edema.

All subjects were housed during the entire study in an environmentally controlled metabolic ward at a constant temperature. Each consumed a daily diet containing 10 mEq of sodium, 100 mEq of potassium, and 800–1000 ml of water. The composition of the diet remained unchanged throughout the study, and 24-hour urine collections were made daily for determination of sodium, potassium, and creatinine. After a mean of 5 days on the constant diet, at which time the urinary sodium was less than 10 mEq/24 hr and weight had remained stable, each patient underwent a determination of PRA. On the morning of study, plasma was obtained twice for PRA determinations during the seated posture at 8 and 8:30 a.m. PRA was determined by the radioimmunoassay technique of Haber et al..[24] The results of the two determinations for each patient were averaged. The results were compared with those of a large group of normal controls studied under identical conditions.[45,46]

We observed that 18 of the 28 cirrhotic patients manifested basal plasma renin levels that were within the normal range for seated normal subjects (Fig. 12.2). Of the remaining 10 patients, 4 manifested suppressed PRA levels and 6 had distinctly elevated PRA levels. The increases in PRA varied independently of the degree of ascites.[32]

Sequential Studies in a Single Patient During Prolonged Observation

Additional support for the concept that the degree of hyperreninemia varies independently of the clinical status of the patient is derived from observations in patient McD. We followed

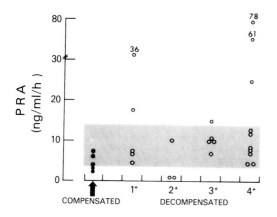

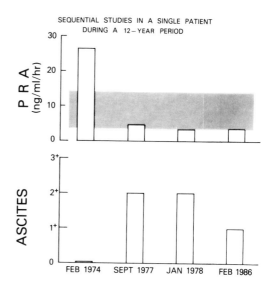

FIGURE 12.2. An assessment of the relationship between plasma renin activity (PRA) levels and degree of ascites accumulation in 28 cirrhotic patients. *Closed circles* correspond to compensated (absence of ascites and edema) patients. The *open circles* correspond to patients with varying degrees of ascites, edema, or both. The *shaded area* subtends the mean ± 2 SD for 14 normal subjects studied under identical conditions of sodium and potassium intake, posture, and time of day. As can be seen, relatively few patients manifested increments in PRA despite advanced liver disease and ascites accumulation.

FIGURE 12.3. The relationship between plasma renin activity (PRA) and ascites accumulation in patient McD during sequential studies over a 12-year period. The *shaded area* subtends the mean ± SD for 14 normal subjects studied under identical conditions of sodium and potassium intake, posture, and time of day. During the initial study period at a time when the patient manifested neither edema nor ascites, his PRA level was greatly elevated (26.2 ng/ml/hr). During the subsequent two studies at 43 and 47 months, there was a striking dissociation between ascites, which had reaccumulated, and PRA levels, which had decreased markedly. During restudy 8 years later ascites had diminished despite similar PRA values.

prospectively the PRA levels of patient McD for a prolonged time during which his clinical course waxed and waned, with periods of transition from decompensation to compensation to decompensation. Figure 12.3 depicts the results during four study periods when the patient's clinical status changed markedly. During the initial study period (February 1974), at a time when the patient manifested neither edema nor ascites, his PRA level was greatly elevated (26.2 ng/ml/hr). During the subsequent three studies at 43, 47, and 144 months, there was a striking dissociation between ascites, which had reaccumulated, and PRA levels, which had decreased markedly. These observations are consistent with the formulation that PRA varies independently of clinical status.

Angiotensin II

In view of the documentation that plasma renin substrate (PRS) levels may be depressed in cirrhosis (see below), it is appropriate to inquire to what extent angiotensin II levels are elevated in cirrhotic patients and to what extent they constitute appropriate indices for assessing the activity of the renin-angiotensin system. Although the number of studies that have determined

angiotensin II levels in liver disease are relatively few compared with the wealth of studies that have measured PRA and PRC, the available data suggest that angiotensin II levels parallel PRA and PRC in cirrhosis (Table 12.4). Thus, Saruta et al.[47] assessed simultaneously PRA and angiotensin II levels in a large group of patients with cirrhosis. Angiotensin II was determined by radioimmunoassay using a modification of the method of Gould et al.[48] As reported elsewhere, both of these components of the renin-angiotensin system were elevated in cirrhotic patients. Furthermore, despite decrements in PRS levels, the excellent correlation between PRA and angiotensin II suggested that PRA constitutes a useful index of renin-angiotensin activity in cirrhosis.

Similarly, Wernze et al.[34] demonstrated a good correlation between PRA (as well as PRC) and angiotensin II in a large group of patients with cirrhosis of the liver. They interpreted their data

TABLE 12.4.   Studies of Plasma Angiotensin II in Patients with Liver Disease

Authors (Reference)	Patient Population	No. of Patients	Angiotensin II (pg/ml)	
			Study Population	Normal Range
Kondo et al. (30)	Cirrhosis without ascites	17	200 ± 128 (SD)	124 ± 69 (SD)
	Cirrhosis with ascites	10	285 ± 156 (SD)	
	Chronic hepatitis	17	163 ± 106 (SD)	
Wernze et al. (34)	Cirrhosis with ascites (untreated)	23	14.1 ± 9.0 (SD)	13.7 ± 6.9 (SD)
	Cirrhosis without ascites	12	9.9 ± 4.8 (SD)	

RIA = radioimmunoassay.

as indicating that, despite suppression of renin substrate levels, PRA is an appropriate index of renin secretion.

Renin Substrate

Over 50 years ago, Haynes and Dexter[49] were the first to report low levels of renin substrate in the plasma of patients with liver disease. Subsequent reports have amply confirmed these early observations. Even though defective hepatic production was considered the most likely cause of depressed PRS concentrations, increased utilization secondary to elevated renin levels was also considered as a factor.

Aside from affecting the reaction of renin with substrate to form angiotensin, PRS deficiency may mediate the renal failure of liver disease. Specifically, Berkowitz and associates[50,51] postulated that renin substrate depletion per se may be the principal etiologic factor responsible for the hemodynamic abnormalities that accompany the hepatorenal syndrome (HRS). According to this formulation, the reduction in renin substrate results in reduced angiotensin levels; therefore, the normal inhibitory feedback mechanism is impaired and renin secretion persists. The investigators infused substrate in the form of fresh-frozen plasma to patients with HRS and demonstrated a significant transient improvement in renal function as assessed by an increase in urine volume and creatinine clearance (C_{Cr}). Of interest, the amelioration and subsequent deterioration of renal function coincided with the rise and fall in renin substrate concentrations. Similarly, sequential observations following hepatic transplantation have disclosed that a rise in renin substrate may precede transient improvements in renal function.

In contrast, Horisawa and Reynolds[52] treated 10 patients with liver disease and HRS with exchange transfusions. One patient recovered from renal failure, but 8 died after exchange transfusion with no appreciable improvement in renal function. Because renin substrate levels increased after exchange transfusions in 6 of the patients, the investigators interpreted their findings as militating against the "renin substrate theory."

Angiotensin-converting Enzyme (Kininase II)

ACE was first reported to be slightly elevated in liver cirrhosis by Andersen.[53] However, only 5 patients were investigated, and a bioassay technique was used to assess ACE activity. Schwiesfurth and Wernze[54] determined serum ACE activity in 81 patients with liver disease: 18 patients with acute viral hepatitis and 63 patients with cirrhosis of the liver. ACE was assayed fluorometrically using the synthetic substrate benzyloxycarbonyl-phenylalanylhistidyl-leucine. The investigators noted that serum ACE activity was elevated in all groups of patients with liver disease compared with controls. Patients with ascites manifested the greatest increase in ACE activity.

The significance of these findings is difficult to ascertain. First, the functional significance of circulating ACE remains speculative. The vascular bed of the lung has enormous amounts of ACE compared with plasma, and most circulating angiotensin I is converted to angiotensin II in the pulmonary vascular bed. If indeed ACE is elevated in liver disease and if such elevations reflect an increase of ACE in the vascular bed, it is not inconceivable that this would facilitate the conversion of angiotensin I to angiotensin II. Thus, one should be able to observe an increase in the ratio of angiotensin II to angiotensin I. Clearly, additional studies are warranted to explore these questions.

Plasma Angiotensinase Activity

Biron et al.[55] reported that plasma angiotensinase activity was significantly increased in

TABLE 12.4. Studies of Plasma Angiotensin II in Patients with Liver Disease (cont.)

Assay	Sodium Intake (mEq/day)	Potassium Intake (mEq/day)	Serum Potassium	Posture	Time of Day	Medications
RIA	Not Na restricted	Not specified	Not specified	Supine	Morning	None
	Not Na restricted	Not specified	Not specified	Supine	Morning	None
	Not Na restricted	Not specified	Not specified	Supine	Morning	None
RIA	120–150	70–90	3.8 ± 0.5 (SD)	Supine	7:30–9:30	None
			4.3 ± 0.3 (SD)	Supine	a.m.	

patients with cirrhosis. The investigators demonstrated a correlation between the degree of hepatic impairment (as assessed by the magnitude of hyperbilirubinemia and bromosulfophthalein retention) and the elevation of angiotensinase activity. Kokubu and associates[56] confirmed these results, demonstrating increased angiotensinase activity in the plasma of patients with diverse hepatic diseases including cirrhosis, acute infectious hepatitis, and obstructive jaundice.

The interpretation of the above findings is difficult. First, there is no general agreement about how one should measure angiotensinase activity. Second, the disappearance of angiotensin II is more rapid in regional circulation than in vitro.[57] Such findings imply that a significant portion of angiotensinase activity may be localized to the vascular endothelium and that limited information about the activity of angiotensinases is obtained by measuring its activity in peripheral venous blood. Finally, although the concept of an accelerated or delayed metabolism of angiotensin II is of interest, the functional significance of such a possibility remains to be established.

MECHANISMS OF INCREASED RENIN-ANGIOTENSIN LEVELS

Plasma renin levels depend on both the rate of production of renin by the kidney and the rate of hepatic renin inactivation. As indicated below, both mechanisms probably contribute to the elevated plasma renin levels of cirrhosis.

Decreased Hepatic Extraction

Several lines of evidence suggest that renin is inactivated in large part by the liver.[58–65] Extraction of renin by the canine liver has been reported to approximate about 20–25%, and the mean extraction in patients with normal liver function is 26%.[56] Wernze et al.[65] reported that the hepatic

clearance of renin is reduced in both compensated (68% of normal) and decompensated (43% of normal) cirrhotic patients compared with hypertensive control subjects with normal liver function. In addition, Barnardo et al.[59] demonstrated that PRA was significantly higher in blood from the hepatic vein than in blood drawn simultaneously from the brachial artery of cirrhotic patients and that the portal venous PRA also exceeded peripheral PRA levels. The authors suggested that cirrhotic patients have a splanchnic source of reninlike activity. In addition to hepatic inactivation of renin, excretion of renin in the bile may also contribute to the clearance of renin from plasma,[64] and this excretory route is thought to be altered in advanced cirrhosis. Together such studies suggest that the elevated peripheral PRA levels of cirrhosis are attributable, in part, to a diminished hepatic clearance rate of renin.

Although a diminished hepatic extraction of renin clearly contributes to the elevated renin levels in liver disease, evidence indicates that this is not the major determinant of hyperreninemia. Mitch et al.[37] assessed plasma renin levels and the hepatic extraction of renin in 24 patients with alcoholic liver disease. The results were compared with those from a group of normal subjects undergoing evaluation as prospective kidney transplant donors. As anticipated, PRA levels were markedly increased and hepatic renin extraction was decreased in the patients with liver disease. However, there was a marked discrepancy between PRA elevation (13.5-fold) and the decrease in hepatic renin extraction (only 2.4-fold compared with controls), suggesting that hepatic renin extraction is not the primary determinant of PRA augmentation in patients with liver disease. Bosch et al.[66] also provided evidence that the prepotent determinant of increased PRA is increased renin secretion by the kidney.

Although angiotensin II is inactivated in the liver as well as other tissues,[67–70] a decrease in hepatic clearance of angiotensin II per se probably does not influence plasma angiotensin II levels. Because the clearance rate of angiotensin II by tissues other than the liver is unaltered in cirrhotic patients, an impaired hepatic clearance of angiotensin II would not markedly influence plasma angiotensin II levels.

Increased Renin Secretion

There are at least two explanations for increased renin secretion in cirrhosis: (1) renal hypoperfusion may be the primary event with a resultant activation of the renin-angiotensin axis or (2) activation of the renin-angiotensin system may constitute the primary event.

In an attempt to assess whether the increased renin secretion of cirrhosis is secondary to the renal hypoperfusion or whether the hyperreninemia is primary with secondary renal vasoconstriction, Barnardo et al.[29] altered one of the variables (renal perfusion) and determined the effect on PRA. The infusion of dopamine in subpressor doses resulted in an increase in paraaminohippurate clearance in all 13 subjects (mean increase of 58%). In 10 instances, augmentation in renal perfusion was associated with a decrease in PRA. Thus, the investigators suggested that the increased PRA is probably secondary to the renal hypoperfusion rather than its cause. Unfortunately, the possibility that dopamine may directly affect renin release renders the interpretation of these studies difficult.

The conclusion of Barnardo et al. was not supported by the findings of Arroyo et al.,[35] who examined the relationship between renin activity (as assessed by PRC as well as PRA) and both renal plasma flow and GFR. In a large group of cirrhotic patients with ascites but without azotemia, renin levels failed to correlate with either GFR or renal plasma flow. Additional studies in 12 patients in whom the renal vein was catheterized disclosed that the renin secretion rate also failed to correlate with either renal plasma flow or GFR. The authors interpreted their data as indicating that alterations in total renal perfusion are not major determinants of renin secretion in nonazotemic cirrhotic patients with ascites.[35]

Evidence from our laboratory supports the role of diminished effective volume as a major determinant of increased renin release in advanced liver disease.[32] Studies in cirrhotic patients demonstrate that head-out water immersion results in a striking suppression of PRA. The demonstration that this manipulation, which merely altered the distribution of plasma volume without increasing total plasma volume[15] (see chapter 1), suppressed PRA lends strong support to the formulation that diminished effective volume is a major determinant of the augmented PRA levels encountered in many patients with cirrhosis. Regardless of the mechanism(s), the activation of the renin-angiotensin system has profound implications for renal function.

In addition to assessing the role of alterations in central blood volume in mediating the augmented secretion of renin in cirrhosis, the present study may afford additional insights into the humoral regulators of renin secretion, such as catecholamines, the potassium ion, angiotensin II, atrial natriuretic factor, and antidiuretic hormone.[4,19,71]

Potassium may constitute a determinant of renin release with potassium depletion increasing PRA (see above). To the extent that patients with advanced liver disease are frequently potassium-depleted and hypokalemic,[72] it was of interest to assess whether depressed serum potassium levels might constitute determinants of PRA augmentation. As seen in Figure 12.4, the PRA levels failed to correlate inversely with hypokalemia (not significant; r = 0.234). The lack of correlation between serum potassium levels and PRA agrees with the findings of Wernze et al.[34] and Mitch et al.[37]

Renin release may vary inversely with plasma sodium concentration.[73,74] Brown and associates[73] demonstrated an inverse correlation between plasma sodium concentration and renin release and suggested that the sodium ion may constitute a determinant of renin release. This formulation has attained additional support from the studies of Tuck et al.[74] We therefore examined the relationship of serum sodium concentration and PRA levels in 28 cirrhotic patients and observed an inverse correlation (r = -0.392; p < 0.05). The current demonstration of this relationship agrees with the findings of Wernze et al.,[34] who reported that both PRA and PRC were inversely related to plasma sodium levels.

Although such findings are consistent with the concept that the serum sodium concentration is a determinant of renin release, an alternative explanation is possible. Because hyponatremia is thought to constitute an index of the severity of impaired renal diluting ability, the inverse correlation between hyponatremia and PRA may merely indicate that the more advanced the liver disease (and the attendant maldistribution of circulating blood volume), the greater the activation of the renin-angiotensin system.

As noted earlier, increased activity of the renal sympathetic nerves is thought to account for increased renin release under certain conditions. The role of increased adrenergic activity in mediating the hyperreninemia of advanced liver disease is unsettled. On the one hand, Wilkinson et al.[75] reported that clinically β-effective adrenergic blockade induced by propranolol or practolol resulted in a profound (81%) suppression of PRA in 11 cirrhotic patients. In contrast, Shohat et al.[76] reported that oral propranolol failed to suppress PRA in a group of patients with cirrhosis and ascites. Additional studies are necessary to clarify this point.

Epstein et al.[77] examined the effects of head-out water immersion on plasma norepinephrine (NE) in cirrhotic patients. The mean levels of NE before immersion with the patients in the seated posture was elevated 3-fold compared with normal subjects under identical conditions. Seven of the 16 patients manifested levels within the normal range, whereas the remaining 9 manifested elevated values. Immersion did not significantly alter NE in the cirrhotic patients, but PRA was markedly suppressed. During immersion, there was a striking dissociation between PRA and the corresponding plasma NE levels. These observations suggest that the increased levels of NE in cirrhotic patients may not contribute to the increase in PRA.

The possibility that changes in basal ANF levels constitute determinants of PRA responsiveness should be considered. In a series of studies, we examined simultaneous plasma ANF and PRA levels in a group of 11 cirrhotic patients.[78–80] There was a marked dissociation between plasma ANF levels, which were within the normal range, and PRA levels, which tended to be elevated. Furthermore, there was a striking dissociation between the changes in ANF and PRA during immersion. These observations suggest that the stimulation of the renin-angiotensin system in cirrhosis is probably not attributable to diminished ANF levels. Additional studies are necessary to clarify this point.

RESPONSIVENESS OF THE RENIN-ANGIOTENSIN SYSTEM

Despite extensive study, the responsiveness of the renin-angiotensin-aldosterone system in

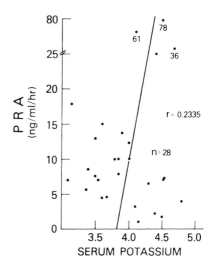

FIGURE 12.4. Relationship between plasma renin activity (PRA) and serum potassium levels in 28 cirrhotic patients studied under rigorously controlled conditions of sodium and potassium intake, posture, and time of day. PRA levels failed to correlate inversely with hypokalemia (not significant; r = 0.324).

cirrhosis to stimulatory or suppressive manipulations remains unsettled. Moreover, despite a few previous investigations of the responsiveness of the renin-angiotensin-aldosterone axis to volume alterations in cirrhosis,[31,33,76,81] significant differences in experimental design render comparisons difficult. Chonko et al.[33] studied 11 patients with Laënnec's cirrhosis following chronic sodium loading with a 300-mEq sodium/day diet. They reported that the initially elevated PRA levels were not suppressed in 6 of 11 patients (group A) despite a 6.1 ± 0.8 kg weight gain. The 6 patients also failed to suppress plasma aldosterone (PA).

Rosoff et al.[31] studied the PRA and PA response to volume and postural stimuli in a group of patients with cirrhosis and refractory ascites and reported that although patients manifested greater than normal elevations of PRA and PA in response to assumption of the upright posture, PRA and PA were not enhanced further by volume manipulations. Thus, dietary sodium restriction failed to increase further either PRA or PA levels. Moreover, the induction of an 11.4-kg weight loss in 2 patients following the administration of furosemide and triamterene resulted in either no change or a decrease in PA concentrations.[31] Similarly, Saruta et al.[82] observed a blunted response of PA to the stimulatory maneuver of dietary sodium restriction plus upright posture.

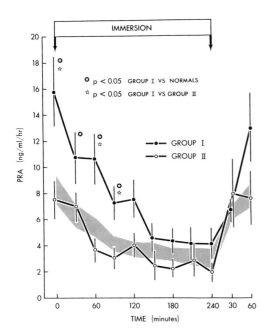

FIGURE 12.5. Effect of water immersion on plasma renin activity (PRA) in 16 cirrhotic patients in balance on a 10-mEq sodium diet. *Shaded area* represents the mean ± SE for 9 normal controls undergoing immersion while receiving an identical diet.[46] The immersion-induced suppression of PRA in group II patients paralleled that of normal controls undergoing an identical study. (Reprinted by permission of the American Heart Association, Inc., from Epstein M, et al: Characterization of the renin-aldosterone system in decompensated cirrhosis. Circ Res 1977;41:823.)

Although other investigators have studied the responsiveness of the renin-angiotensin-aldosterone axis to acute volume expansion using infusions of exogenous volume expanders, the results conflict. Wong et al.[81] infused saline (0.9% at 500 ml/hr for 4 hr) in a group of decompensated cirrhotic patients following equilibration on a 10-mEq sodium diet. They reported a suppression of both PRA and PA. Similarly, they observed that albumin (50 gm infused over 2 hr) suppressed PRA and PA. Similarly, Shohat et al.[76] assessed the response to acute saline loading and reported a suppression of PRA and PA at 60 minutes, with a further suppression at 150 minutes after infusion.

In an attempt to investigate this problem further, we assessed renin-aldosterone responsiveness using the model of water immersion. It was noted earlier that water immersion obviates this hazard because it is associated with a decrease in total plasma volume and body weight rather than with the increase that attends saline infusion.[15,83] Furthermore, in contrast to saline infusion, the "volume stimulus" induced by immersion occurs without concomitant changes in plasma composition, including serum sodium and potassium concentrations, which might alter PRA and PA.[84,85]

Sixteen patients with alcoholic chronic liver disease were studied. After a mean of 5 days on the constant diet, at which time the urinary sodium was less than 10 mEq/24 hr and weight was stable, each patient underwent a control (Control) study, followed 2 or 3 days later by water immersion to the level of the neck (Immersion). During both the control and immersion studies, venous blood (4 ml) was collected at 30-minute intervals for PRA and PA determinations.

Examination of the individual natriuretic responses of the 16 patients during immersion disclosed a continuum of markedly different responses. Eight patients had no or a barely discernible natriuretic response during immersion and were classified arbitrarily as group I. In contrast, the remaining 8 patients manifested a profound natriuresis that equalled or exceeded the 37 ± 8 (SE) μEq/min (peak value) documented in normal subjects during identical study conditions who ingested an identical diet of 10 mEq sodium, 100 mEq potassium.[46] These 8 patients were designated group II.

The effects of 4 hours of immersion on PRA are shown in Figures 12.5 and 12.6. When the alterations of PRA are considered separately for group I and group II, an interesting pattern emerges. Since the preimmersion values of group I patients were 2-fold greater than those of group II patients, the PRA response to immersion is depicted both in terms of absolute changes (Fig. 12.5) and as percentage change from the preimmersion hour (Fig. 12.6). Figure 12.5 shows that the basal PRA levels prior to immersion in group II patients were appropriate for sodium-depleted subjects and did not differ from mean PRA levels for normal seated subjects in balance on an identical sodium and potassium diet (p > 0.4).[46] Immersion resulted in a significant suppression of PRA within 60 minutes of study (p < 0.01). By 240 minutes, mean PRA was suppressed to 22 ± 5% of prestudy values (Fig. 12.6), not different from the findings in normal seated subjects.[46] In contrast, group I patients manifested basal PRA levels prior to immersion that were 2-fold greater than the comparable values in group II patients and sodium-depleted normal subjects (Fig.12.5).

Despite these differences in basal PRA, mean PRA was suppressed in group I patients to 31 ± 8% of prestudy values, not different from the 78 ± 5% suppression manifested by group II patients during immersion (p > 0.2) (Fig. 12.6).

The results of the study demonstrate that the renin-aldosterone system is highly responsive to a standardized volume stimulus. Thus, group II patients who manifested an appropriate natriuresis in response to immersion were able to suppress both PRA and PA in a manner analogous to that of normal subjects studied under identical experimental conditions. It is of even greater interest that even the group I patients, whose PRA and PA levels were markedly higher than those of group II patients, were still able to suppress PRA and PA to nadir levels that were comparable with those of both normal subjects and group II patients. Cessation of immersion in both group I and group II patients was associated with a prompt recovery in PRA and PA to the prestudy levels.

The ability of group I patients to suppress PRA and PA to the same extent as group II patients merits comment. Chonko et al.[33] observed that their group A cirrhotic patients (who failed to suppress PRA and PA) had significantly higher PRA and PA levels on day 1 than did their group B patients (appropriate suppression of PRA and PA). It is not readily apparent why cirrhotic patients with the most marked degree of activation of the renin-aldosterone system manifested differing patterns of responsiveness in the study of Chonko et al.[33] and in our study.

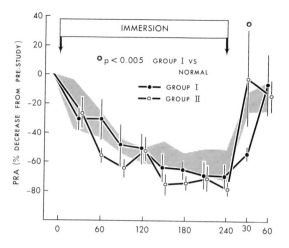

FIGURE 12.6. Comparison of the effects of immersion on plasma renin activity (PRA) in group I and group II cirrhotic patients and in normal controls in balance on an identical 10-mEq Na diet. Data are expressed in terms of percentage change from the preimmersion hour. *Shaded area* represents the mean ± SE for controls. Group I patients manifested a 69 ± 8 suppression of PRA, not different from the 78 ± 12% suppression manifested by group II patients (p > 0.2). Neither cirrhotic group differed from normal controls (p > 0.2).

RENIN-ANGIOTENSIN SYSTEM AS A DETERMINANT OF RENAL HEMODYNAMICS

Activation of the renin-angiotensin system exerts profound effects on renal hemodynamics and function. Angiotensin II induces an increase in renal vascular resistance, with a parallel reduction in renal plasma flow.[86] Glomerular filtration rate, however, tends to fall much less than renal plasma flow, and consequently filtration fraction increases.[86,87] The hemodynamic effects of angiotensin II have been attributed to preferential vasoconstriction of efferent arterioles, so that afferent arterioles are less affected.[88–90] Such alterations promote an increase in the glomerular capillary hydrostatic pressure and consequently an increase in the mean transcapillary ultrafiltration pressure, which tends to offset the angiotensin II induced decrease in renal plasma flow and serves to maintain GFR by increasing the filtration fraction.[90] Angiotensin II also stimulates mesangial cell contraction, thereby lowering the glomerular capillary ultrafiltration coefficient (Kf).[90,91] Because of its effects on glomerular hemodynamics, angiotensin II plays a critical role in the autoregulation of GFR—the maintenance of GFR at near constant values despite wide fluctuations in renal perfusion pressure.[88,92]

PROGNOSIS AND THE RENIN-ANGIOTENSIN SYSTEM

Long-term survival in patients with cirrhosis and ascites has been related statistically to a number of variables, including arterial pressure, plasma norepinephrine, urinary sodium excretion, and the combination of hyponatremia and impaired renal function. It has also been suggested that plasma levels of renin are of prognostic value.

A recent study by the Barcelona group investigated the incidence, predictive factors, and prognosis of the hepatorenal syndrome in cirrhosis

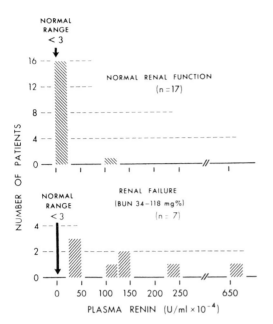

FIGURE 12.7. Relationship between renal function and plasma renin levels in 24 patients with cirrhosis and ascites. The range for normal subjects $(0-3.5 \times 10^{-4}$ Goldblattt U/ml) on dietary sodium restriction is depicted by the *stippled area* to the left of the *lower panel*. Seventeen patients had normal renal function *(upper panel)*, whereas 7 patients had azotemia with blood urea nitrogen levels ranging from 34 to 188 mg/dl *(lower panel)*. In contrast to the normal or modestly elevated plasma renin levels in cirrhotic patients with normal glomerular filtration rates, most patients with azotemia manifested profound elevations in plasma renin levels, greatly exceeding the values of the nonazotemic group. (Based on data from Schroeder ET, et al:[28] Plasma renin level in hepatic cirrhosis: Relation to functional renal failure. Am J Med 49:186–191, 1970.)

with ascites.[93] After following 234 nonazotemic cirrhotic patients with ascites for a median of 17 months (range: 0.2–123 months), they suggested that PRA elevation may constitute merely a nonspecific marker for the florid systemic hemodynamic alterations that complicate the course of such patients. Ginès et al.[93] demonstrated that patients with a more contracted effective arterial blood volume, as indicated not only by higher PRA levels but also by lower mean arterial pressure, higher plasma norepinephrine concentration, and more intense renal sodium and water retention, had a higher risk of developing hepatorenal syndrome during extended follow-up. Ginès et al.[93] proposed that such findings are consistent with the peripheral arterial vasodilation

hypothesis i.e., that HRS constitutes an extreme expression of arterial vascular underfilling (see chapter 1).

RENIN-ANGIOTENSIN SYSTEM IN RENAL FAILURE

Although the alterations of the renin-angiotensin system are prominent in advanced liver disease in general, they are particularly pronounced in patients with decompensated cirrhosis and azotemia.

Barnardo et al.[29] examined the relationship between renal function and PRA in a large group of patients with cirrhosis and varying degrees of renal functional impairment. PRA correlated with C_{Cr} and effective renal plasma flow. Although mean PRA was 17.0 ± 17.5 ng/L/min in patients with a C_{Cr} greater than 79 ml/min, it was higher (30.7 ± 34.4) in patients with C_{Cr} ranging from 50 to 79 ml/min. Patients with the most profound degree of renal functional impairment (C_{Cr} of < 50 ml/min) manifested the most profound elevation of PRA (108 ± 44 ng/L/min). Wilkinson et al.[36] noted that cirrhotic patients with renal failure secondary to both the HRS and acute tubular necrosis had PRA levels that greatly exceeded those manifested by cirrhotic patients with increasing ascites but without azotemia. Perhaps the most carefully documented study assessing the relationship of the renin-angiotensin system to renal function is that of Schroeder et al.[28] The investigators examined the relationship between renal function and plasma renin levels (determined as PRC) and observed that cirrhotic patients with impaired renal function manifested the most profound elevations in plasma renin levels (Fig. 12.7). Of the 24 patients with cirrhosis and ascites, 17 had normal renal function, whereas 7 had azotemia with blood urea nitrogen levels ranging from 34 to 118 mg/dl. Whereas cirrhotic patients with normal GFR had normal or modestly elevated plasma renin levels, most patients with azotemia manifested profound elevations in plasma renin levels greatly exceeding the values of the nonazotemic group.

In light of compelling studies demonstrating that the blood vessels of the human kidney are exquisitely sensitive to small increments in circulating angiotensin II, the augmented levels of renin documented in patients with HRS may contribute to the pathogenesis of the HRS. Figure 12.8 is an attempt to summarize the mechanisms

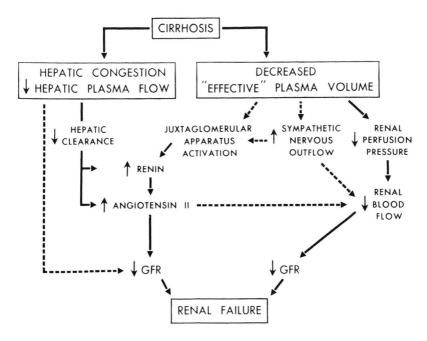

FIGURE 12.8. Probable mechanisms whereby the renin-angiotensin system and the sympathetic nervous system interact to produce renal failure. Both a diminished effective volume and impaired hepatic clearance of renin-angiotensin result in a marked enhancement of circulating plasma renin activity with a resultant decrease in glomerular filtration rate (GFR). An increase in sympathetic nervous system activity (attributable to decreased effective volume) decreases GFR both by diminishing renal perfusion and by activating the renin-angiotensin system.

whereby an increased rate of secretion of renin by the kidney, in concert with decreased hepatic inactivation of renin, contributes to the elevated plasma renin levels of cirrhosis. The figure demonstrates further how activation of the renin-angiotensin system interacts with neural and hemodynamic events to produce renal failure.

The delineation of the etiologic role of the renin-angiotensin system in mediating the renal functional impairment of cirrhosis and the application of angiotensin antagonists in such studies are considered in the next section.

PHARMACOLOGIC BLOCKADE OF THE RENIN-ANGIOTENSIN SYSTEM

The demonstration that the renin-angiotensin-aldosterone system is activated in patients with decompensated cirrhosis as well as patients with HRS has stimulated investigations of the possible efficacy of ACE inhibitors in this setting.[94–100] Earlier studies by Pariente et. al.[94] and Daskalopoulos et al.[95] suggested that captopril may induce adverse effects in patients with decompensated cirrhosis. The investigators observed a decrease in GFR, a decrease in sodium excretion, and development of hypotension as side effects of captopril administered as a single dose of 25–150 mg to patients with cirrhosis of the liver.[94,95] Wood et al.[97] reported that captopril therapy at a dose of 6.25 or 12.5 mg every 8 hours produced a significant fall in MAP and was associated with side effects such as postural hypotension, reduced GFR and increasing encephalopathy.

Brunkhorst and coworkers[98] investigated the effects of captopril (6.25 mg 4 times/day) in cirrhotic patients with ascites. An increase in sodium excretion in 12 of 13 patients with diuretic resistance was observed. Doses of diuretics varied from very low to very high.

Gentilini et al.[99] recently investigated the effects of a low dose of captopril (12.5 mg) on renal hemodynamics and function in 38 patients with cirrhosis of the liver and in a group of controls. In a randomized, double-blind, placebo-controlled, crossover trial, they studied the effects of captopril on renal plasma flow, glomerular filtration rate (measured by radioisotopic techniques), and sodium excretion. They used a lower dose of captopril than most previous investigators in an attempt to obviate the confounding effects of decreases in arterial pressure. Patients with ascites, portal hypertension, sodium retention, and low arterial pressure were included, although none had advanced liver disease. The investigators demonstrated that in healthy subjects, captopril induced a significant 18% increase in renal plasma flow, whereas glomerular filtration rate was unchanged. In contrast, glomerular filtration rate decreased significantly in cirrhotic patients with (from 108 ± 7 to 78 ± 9 ml/min) and without ascites (from 102 ± 4 to 88 ± 3 ml/min), whereas renal plasma flow did not change. Urinary sodium excretion also significantly decreased in ascitic patients (from 44 ± 4 to 31 ± 4 μmol/min). Because renal plasma flow did not change in response to captopril, the investigators interpreted the results as indicating efferent vasodilation, thus suggesting that activation of the renal renin-angiotensin system acts to maintain glomerular filtration rate through efferent vasoconstriction. The reduction in glomerular filtration rate was associated with an acute decrease in sodium excretion in patients with ascites, probably as a result of reduction in filtered sodium load, because renal perfusion pressure and fractional sodium excretion did not change.

In contrast to the above observations, Van Vliet et al.[100] recently reported that low-dose captopril (<12.5 mg) induced a natriuretic response in patients who had previously manifested a blunted natriuretic response to furosemide and spironolactone therapy. They investigated the efficacy of a low dose of captopril in 8 patients with massive ascites resistant to therapy of salt and fluid restriction and increasing doses of spironolactone and furosemide. Mean duration of diuretic use was 73 days (range: 7–240 days). After at least 3 days of observation on 80 mg furosemide and 100 mg spironolactone, captopril was added. Consequently, 4 of 8 patients responded to captopril with a natriuresis and diuresis. Of interest, the mean dosage of captopril in the responders was equal to that in the nonresponders. The investigators concluded that the addition of low-dose captopril to relatively low doses of diuretics has the potential to reverse a blunted natriuresis in cirrhotic patients without induction of hepatic encephalopathy, renal impairment, or electrolyte disturbances. The reasons for discrepant findings in renal sodium handling are not readily apparent.

SUMMARY

Many patients with advanced liver disease manifest alterations of several components of the renin-angiotensin system; plasma renin activity is augmented, whereas renin substrate concentration is depressed. A review of the available studies indicates that the precise magnitude of such alterations is difficult to discern, because many of the variables that affect the renin-angiotensin system were not controlled or recorded.

Although marked perturbations occur in many patients with liver disease, it is important to emphasize the great variability in the frequency with which such alterations occur, the magnitude of the abnormalities, and the response within the same patient over time. Renin-angiotensin stimulation has been postulated to correlate with the degree of compensation as well as with renal perfusion; however, the associations are not clearcut. Finally, although most earlier investigations have suggested that pharmacologic blockade with ACE inhibitors confers no benefit, recent isolated studies using low doses of ACE inhibitors have suggested that not all results are negative. Clearly, additional studies using a low dosage of either an ACE inhibitor or possibly an angiotensin II receptor antagonist are warranted.

REFERENCES

1. Tigerstedt R, Bergman PG: Niere und Kreislauf. Skandinavisches Archiv für Physiologie 1898;8:223–271.
2. Goldblatt H, Lynch J, Hanzal RF, Summerville WW: Studies on experimental hypertension. I. The production of persistent elevation of systolic blood pressure by means of renal ischemia. J Exp Med 1934;59:347–379.
3. Haber E: The role of renin in normal and pathological cardiovascular homeostasis. Circulation 1976;54:849–861.
4. Davis JO, Freeman RH: Mechanisms regulating renin release. Physiol Rev 1976;56:1–56.
5. Peach MJ: Renin-angiotensin system: Biochemistry and mechanism of action. Physiol Rev 1977;57:313–370.
6. Reid IA, Morris BJ, Ganong WF: The renin-angiotensin system. Ann Rev Physiol 1978;40:377–410.
7. Sealey JE, Laragh JH: The renin-angiotensin-aldosterone system for normal regulation of blood pressure and sodium and potassium homeostasis. In Laragh JH, Brenner BM (eds): Hypertension: Pathophysiology, Diagnosis and Management. New York: Raven Press, 1990;1287–1317.
8. Navar LG, Rosivall L: Contribution of the renin-angiotensin system to the control of intrarenal hemodynamics. Kidney Int 1984;25:857–868.
9. Navar LG, Saccomani G, Mitchell KD: Synergistic intrarenal actions of angiotensin on tubular reabsorption and renal hemodynamics. Am J Hypertens 1991;4:90–96.

10. Sealey JE, Atlas SA, Laragh JH: Prorenin and other large molecular weight forms of renin. Endocr Rev 1980;1:365–391.

11. Opie L: Angiotensin Converting Enzyme Inhibitors. Scientific Basis for Clinical Use. New York: Wiley-Liss, 1992.

12. Hollenberg NK: Renin, angiotensin, and the kidney: Assessment by pharmacological interruption of the renin-angiotensin system. In Epstein M (ed): The Kidney in Liver Disease, 3rd ed. Baltimore: Williams & Wilkins, 1988;374-389.

13. Tobian L, Tomboulian A, Janecek J: The effect of high perfusion pressures on the granulation of juxtaglomerular cells in an isolated kidney. J Clin Invest. 1959;38:605–610.

14. Blaine EH, Davis JO: Evidence for a renal vascular mechanism in renin release: New observations with graded stimulation by aortic constriction. Circ Res 1971;28 (Suppl II):118–126.

15. Epstein M: Renal effects of head-out water immersion in humans: A 15-year update. Physiol Rev 1992;72:563–621.

16. Egan B, Fitzpatrick MA, Julius S: The heart and the regulation of renin. Circulation 1987;(1 Pt 2):I130–I133.

17. Vander AJ: Control of renin release. Physiol Rev 1967;47:359–382.

18. Thurau K: Influence of sodium concentration at macula densa cells on tubular sodium load. Ann NY Acad Sci 1966;139:388–399.

19. Atlas SA, Laragh JH: Physiological actions of atrial natriuretic factor. In Mulrow PJ, Schrier R (eds): Atrial hormones and other natriuretic factors. Bethesda, MD: American Physiological Society, 1987;53–76.

20. Hesse B, Nielsen I: Suppression of plasma renin activity by intravenous infusion of antidiuretic hormone in man. Clin Sci Mol Med 1977;52:357–360.

21. Flamenbaum W, Schmitt GW: The role of prostaglandins in the pathophysiology of renal failure associated with liver disease. In Epstein M (ed): The Kidney in Liver Disease. New York: Elsevier/North-Holland, 1978;285-298.

22. Flamenbaum W, Gagnon J, Ramwell P: Bradykinin-induced renal hemodynamic alterations: Renin and prostaglandin relationships. Am J Physiol 1979;237:F433–F440.

23. Lash B, Fleischer N: Radioimmunoassay of angiotensin I, for estimation of plasma renin activity. Clin Chem 1974;20:620–623.

24. Haber E, Koerner T, Page LB, et al: Application of a radioimmunoassay for angiotensin I to the physiologic measurements of plasma renin activity in normal human subjects. J Clin Endocrinol Metab 1969;29:1349–1355.

25. Reeves G, Lowenstein LM, Sommers SC: The macula densa and juxtaglomerular body in cirrhosis. Arch Int Med 1963;12:708–715.

26. Hartroft WS, Hartroft PM: New approaches in the study of cardiovascular disease: Aldosterone, renin, hypertension and juxtaglomerular cells. Fed Proc 1961;20:845–854.

27. Ayers CR: Plasma renin activity and renin-substrate concentration in patients with liver disease. Circ Res 1967;20:594–598.

28. Schroeder ET, Eich RH, Smulyan H, et al: Plasma renin level in hepatic cirrhosis: Relation to functional renal failure. Am J Med 1970;49:186–191.

29. Barnardo DE, Summerskill WHJ, Strong CG, Baldus WP: Renal function, renin activity and endogenous vasoactive substances in cirrhosis. Am J Dig Dis 1970;15:419–425.

30. Kondo K, Nakamura R, Saito I, et al: Renin, angiotensin II and juxtaglomerular apparatus in liver cirrhosis. Jpn Circ J 1974;38:913–921.

31. Rosoff L Jr, Zia P, Reynolds T, Horton R: Studies of renin and aldosterone in cirrhotic patients with ascites. Gastroenterology 1975;69:698–705.

32. Epstein M, Levinson R, Sancho J, et al: Characterization of the renin- aldosterone system in decompensated cirrhosis. Circ Res 1977;41:818–829.

33. Chonko AM, Bay WH, Stein JH, Ferris TF: The role of renin and aldosterone in the salt retention of edema. Am J Med 1977;63:881–889.

34. Wernze H, Spech HJ, Muller G: Studies on the activity of the renin-angiotensin-aldosterone system (RAAS) in patients with cirrhosis of the liver. Klin Wochenschr 1978;56:389–397.

35. Arroyo V, Bosch J, Mauri M, et al: Renin, aldosterone and renal haemodynamics in cirrhosis with ascites. Eur J Clin Invest 1979;9:69–73.

36. Wilkinson SP, Smith IK, Williams R: Changes in plasma renin activity in cirrhosis: A reappraisal based on studies in 67 patients and "low renin" cirrhosis. Hypertension 1979;1:125–129.

37. Mitch WE, Whelton PK, Cooke CR, et al: Plasma levels and hepatic extraction of renin and aldosterone in alcoholic liver disease. Am J Med 1979;66:804–810.

38. Hata T, Ogihara R, Mikami H, et al: Blood pressure response to (1-sarcosine, 8-isoleucine) angiotensin II in patients with liver cirrhosis and ascites. Jpn Circ J 1979;43:37–41.

39. Brown JJ, Davies DL, Lever AF, Robertson JIS: Variations in plasma renin concentration in several physiological and pathological states. Can Med Assoc J 1964;90:201–206.

40. Sellars L, Shore AC, Mott V, Wilkinson R: The renin-angiotensin-aldosterone system in decompensated cirrhosis: Its activity in relation to sodium balance. Q J Med (New Ser) 1985;56:485–496.

41. Bernardi M, Trevisani F, Santini C, et al: Aldosterone related blood volume expansion in cirrhosis before and during the early phase of ascites formation. Gut 1983;24:761–766.

42. Bernardi M, Palma De R, Trevisani F, et al: Chronobiological study of factors affecting plasma aldosterone concentration in cirrhosis. Gastroenterology 1986;91:683–691.

43. D'Arienzo A, Ambrogio G, Siervi Di P, et al: A randomized comparison of metoclopramide and domperidone on plasma aldosterone concentration and on spironolactone-induced diuresis in ascitic cirrhotic patients. Hepatology 1985;5:854–857.

44. Burmeister P, Schölmerich J, Diener W, Gerok W: Renin, aldosterone and arginine vasopressin in patients with liver cirrhosis: The influence of ascites retransfusion. Eur J Clin Invest 1986;16:117–123.

45. Epstein M, Re R, Preston S, Haber E: Comparison of the suppressive effects of water immersion and saline administration on renin-aldosterone in normal man. J Clin Endocrinol Metab. 1979;49:358–363.

46. Epstein M, Pins DS, Sancho J, Haber E: Suppression of plasma renin and plasma aldosterone during water immersion in normal man. J Clin Endocrinol Metab. 1975;41:618–625.

47. Saruta T, Kondo K, Saito I, Nakamura R: Characterization of the components of the renin-angiotensin system in cirrhosis of the liver. In Epstein M (ed): The Kidney in Liver Disease. New York: Elsevier/North-Holland, 1978;207–223.

48. Gould AB, Skeggs LT, Kahn JR: Measurement of renin and substrate concentrations in human serum. Lab Invest 1966;15:1802–1813.

49. Haynes FW, Dexter L: The renal humoral pressor mechanism in man. IV. The hypertensinogen content of plasma of normal patients and patients with various diseases. J Clin Invest 1945;23:78–81.

50. Berkowitz HD: Renin substrate in the hepatorenal syndrome. In Epstein M (ed): The Kidney in Liver Disease. New York: Elsevier/North Holland, 1978;251–270.

51. Berkowitz HD, Calvin C, Miller LD: Significance of altered renin substrate in the hepatorenal syndrome. Surg Forum 1972;23:342–343.

52. Horisawa M, Reynolds TB: Exchange transfusion in hepatorenal syndrome with liver disease. Arch Intern Med 1976;136:1135–1137.

53. Andersen JB: Converting enzyme activity in liver disease. Acta Pathol Microbiol Scand 1967;71:1–7.

54. Schweisfurth H, Wernze H: Changes of serum angiotensin I converting enzyme in patients with viral hepatitis and liver cirrhosis. Acta Hepatogastroenterol 1979;26:207–210.

55. Biron P, Baldus WP, Summerskill WHJ: Plasma angiotensinase activity in cirrhosis. Proc Soc Exp Biol Med 1964;116:1074–1077.

56. Kokubu T, Ueda E, Fujimoto S, et al: Plasma angiotensinase activity in liver disease. Clin Chim Acta 1965;12:484–488.

57. Vane JR: The release and fate of vaso-active hormones in the circulation. Br J Pharmacol 1969;35:209–242.

58. Wernze H, Fujii J: Hepatische Inaktivierung und Pressorische Wirkung von Angiotensin. Z Gesamte Exp Med 1966;140:128–135.

59. Barnardo DE, Strong CG, Baldus WP: Failure of the cirrhotic liver to inactivate renin: Evidence for a splanchnic source of renin-like activity. J Lab Clin Med 1969;74:495–506.

60. Leary WPP, Ledingham JGG: Renal and hepatic inactivation of angiotensin in rats: Influence of sodium balance and renal artery compression. Clin Sci Mol Med 1970;38:573–582.

61. Schneider EG, Davis JO, Baumber JS, Johnson JA: The hepatic metabolism of renin and aldosterone. A review with new observations on the hepatic clearance of renin. Circ Res 1970;27(Suppl 1):175–183.

62. Christlieb AR, Couch NP, Amsterdam EA, et al: Renin extraction by the human liver. Proc Soc Exp Biol Med 1968;128:821–823.

63. Heacox R, Harvey AM, Vander AJ: Hepatic inactivation of renin. Circ Res 1967;21:149–152.

64. Horky K, Rojo-Ortega JM, Rodríguez J, Genest J: Renin uptake and excretion by liver in the rat. Am J Physiol 1970;219:387–390.

65. Wernze H, Seki A, Schneider KW, Jesse R: Hepatische Extraktion und Clearance von Renin bei Lebercirrhosen. Klin Wochenschr 1972;50:302–310.

66. Bosch J, Arroyo V, Betriu A, Mas A, et al: Hepatic hemodynamics and the renin-angiotensin-aldosterone system in cirrhosis. Gastroenterology 1980;78:92–99.

67. Johnson DC, Ryan JW: Degradation of angiotensin II by a carboxypeptidase of rabbit liver. Biochim Biophys Acta 1968;160:196–203.

68. Kokubu T, Fujimori S, Hiwad K, et al: Inactivation of angiotensin II in liver. Jpn Circ J 1967;31:879–883.

69. Leary WP, Ledingham JG: Inactivation of angiotensin II analogues by isolated perfused rat liver and kidney. Nature 1970;227:178–179.

70. Biron P, Meyer P: Hepatic extraction of angiotensin after carbon tetrachloride intoxication. Rev Can Biol 1968;27:277–279.

71. Oparil S, Haber E: The renin-angiotensin system. N Engl J Med 1974;291:389–401.

72. Pérez GO, Oster JR: Altered potassium metabolism in liver disease. In Epstein M (ed): The Kidney in Liver Disease, 2nd ed. New York: Elsevier Biomedical, 1983; 183–201.

73. Brown JJ, Davies DL, Lever AF, Robertson JIS: Plasma renin concentration in human hypertension. I. Relationship between renin, sodium and potassium. BMJ 1965; 2:144–148.

74. Tuck ML, Dluhy RG, Williams GH: A specific role for saline or the sodium ion in the regulation of renin and aldosterone secretion. J Clin Invest 1974;53:988–995.

75. Wilkinson SP, Bernardi M, Smith IK, et al: Effect of β-adrenergic blocking drugs on the renin-aldosterone system, sodium excretion, and renal haemodynamics in cirrhosis with ascites. Gastroenterology 1977;73:659–663.

76. Shohat J, Iaina A, Serban I, et al: The effect of propranolol on renal sodium handling in patients with cirrhosis. Biomedicine 1979;31:128–131.

77. Epstein M, Larios O, Johnson G: Effects of water immersion on plasma catecholamines in decompensated cirrhosis. Miner Electrolyte Metab 1985;11:25–34.

78. Epstein M, Preston R, Aceto R, et al: Dissociation of plasma irANF and renal sodium handling in cirrhotic humans undergoing water immersion [abstract]. Kidney Int 1987;31:269.

79. Epstein M, Loutzenhiser R, Friedland E, et al: Increases in circulating atrial natriuretic factor during immersion-induced central hypervolemia in normal humans. J Hypertension. 4(Suppl 2):S93–S99, 1986.

80. Epstein M, Loutzenhiser R, Friedland E, et al: Relationship of increased plasma ANF and renal sodium handling during immersion-induced central hypervolemia in normal humans. J Clin Invest 1987;79:738–745.

81. Wong PY, Carroll RE, Lipinski TL, Capone RR: Studies on the renin-angiotensin-aldosterone system in patients with cirrhosis and ascites: Effect of saline and albumin infusion. Gastroenterology 1979;77:1171–1176.

82. Saruta T, Saito I, Nakamura R, Oka M: Regulation of aldosterone in cirrhosis of the liver. In Epstein M (ed): The Kidney in Liver Disease. New York: Elsevier/North-Holland, 1978;271–282.

83. Epstein M: Cardiovascular and renal effects of head-out water immersion. Application of the model in the assessment of volume homeostasis. Circ Res 1976;39: 619–628.

84. McCaa RE, Bower JD, McCaa CS: Relative influence of acute sodium and volume depletion on aldosterone secretion in nephrectomized man. Circ Res 1973;33: 555–562.

85. Himathongkam T, Dluhy RG, Williams GH: Potassium-aldosterone-renin interrelationships. J Clin Endocrinol Metab 1975;41:153–159.

86. Navar LG, Langford HG: Effects of angiotensin in the renal circulation. In Page IH, Bumpus FN (eds): Angiotensin: Handbook of Experimental Pharmacology, vol. 37. Berlin: Springer-Verlag, 1974;455–474.

87. Fagard RH, Cowley AW, Navar LG, et al: Renal response to slight elevations of renal arterial plasma angiotensin II concentration in dogs. Clin Exp Pharmacol Physiol 1986;3:531–538.

88. Meyers BD, Deen WM, Brenner BM: Effects of norepinephrine and angiotensin II on the determinants of glomerular ultrafiltration and proximal tubule fluid reabsorption in the rat. Circ Res 1975;37:101–110.

89. Hall JE, Guyton AC, Jackson TE, et al: Control of glomerular filtration rate by renin-angiotensin system. Am J Physiol 1977;233:F366–F372.

90. Ballermann BJ, Zeidel ML, Gunning ME, Brenner BM: Vasoactive peptides and the kidney. In Brenner BM, Rector FC Jr. (eds): The Kidney, 4th ed. Philadelphia: W.B. Saunders 1991;510-583.

91. Ausiello DA, Kreisberg J, Roy C, Karnovsky MJ: Contraction of cultured rat glomerular cells of apparent mesangial origin after stimulation with angiotensin II and arginine vasopressin. J Clin Invest 1980;65:754–760.

92. Gagnon JA, Keller HI, Kokotis W, Schrier RW: Analysis of role of renin-angiotensin system in autoregulation of glomerular filtration. Am J Physiol 1970;219:491–496.

93. Ginès A, Escorsell A, Ginès P, et al: Incidence, predictive factors, and prognosis of the hepatorenal syndrome in cirrhosis with ascites. Gastroentorology 1993;105: 229–236.

94. Pariente EA, Bataille C, Bercoff E, Lebrec D: Acute effects of captopril on systemic and renal haemodynamics and on renal function in cirrhotic patients with ascites. Gastroenterology 1985;88:1255–1259.

95. Daskalopoulos G, Pinzani M, Murray N, et al: Effects of captopril on renal function in patients with cirrhosis and ascites. J Hepatol 1987;4:330–336.

96. Stanek B, Renner F, Sedimayer A, Stilberbauer K: Effect of captopril on renin and blood pressure in cirrhosis. Eur J Clin Pharmacol 1987;33:249–254.

97. Wood LJ, Goergen S, Stockigt JR, et al: Adverse effects of captopril in treatment of resistant ascites, a state of functional bilateral renal artery stenosis. Lancet 1985; ii:1008–1009.

98. Brunkhorst R, Wrenger E, Kuhn K, et al: Effekte einer captopril therapie auf die natrium-und wasserausscheidung bei patienten mit leberzirrhose und aszites. Klin Wochenschr 1989;67:774–783.

99. Gentilini P, Romanelli RG, La Villa G, et al: Effects of low-dose captopril on renal hemodynamics and function in patients with cirrhosis of the liver. Gastroenterology 1993;104:588–594.

100. Van Vliet AA, Hackeng WH, Donker AJM, Meuwissen SGM: Efficacy of low-dose captopril in addition to furosemide and spironolactone in patients with decompensated liver disease during blunted diuresis. J Hepatol 1992;15:40–47.

Chapter 13

ALDOSTERONE IN LIVER DISEASE

MURRAY EPSTEIN, M.D., F.A.C.P.

Physiology of Aldosterone
   Normal Control of Aldosterone Release
   Physiologic Responses to Aldosterone
   Role of the Liver in Aldosterone Metabolism
Alterations of Aldosterone in Liver Disease
   Frequency of Hyperaldosteronism and Correlation
      with Clinical Status
   Sequential Studies in a Single Patient during a
      48-Month Period

Control of Aldosterone Secretion in Liver Disease
   Aldosterone Responsiveness
Effects of Aldosteronism on the Kidney
   Sodium
   Potassium
   Acid-Base
Summary

Aldosterone is prominent among the hormones demonstrated to modulate renal tubular function. Since its isolation and characterization in 1953,[1] the mechanism(s) regulating the secretion of this steroid hormone has been the subject of extensive investigation. Studies during the past three decades have disclosed that aldosterone secretion is perturbed in patients with liver disease and that such derangements may constitute important determinants of fluid and electrolyte abnormalities in patients with advanced liver disease.

In light of its relatively early discovery and characterization,[1,2] it is not altogether surprising to note that the majority of publications dealing with renal hormones in liver disease have focused on perturbations in aldosterone. As a result, aldosterone has achieved a prominence with regard to the pathogenesis of sodium retention and edema formation that appears to exceed its true role. In this chapter we review briefly the control mechanisms governing aldosterone release in normal physiology in order to provide a framework for considering the derangement of aldosterone control in liver disease and its relative contribution to sodium retention.

PHYSIOLOGY OF ALDOSTERONE

Normal Control of Aldosterone Release

Aldosterone is the hormone secreted by the *zona glomerulosa* of the adrenal cortex. It accounts for less than 0.25% of the total adrenal steroid output and circulates in very low concentrations (approximately 10^{-9} to 10^{-10} M). By virtue of its ability to stimulate active transepithelial sodium transport at physiologic concentrations, aldosterone is classified as a mineralocorticoid. In contrast to the feedback relationship between adrenocorticotropic hormone (ACTH) and cortisol, the regulation of aldosterone secretion is much more complex and the subject of continuing controversy. Extensive evidence indicates that the secretion of aldosterone is maintained primarily by four factors: (1) the renin-angiotensin axis, (2) potassium, (3) ACTH, and (4) sodium. A role for ANF in modulating aldosterone has recently been delineated.

Renin-Angiotensin System

An abundance of evidence indicates that the renin-angiotensin system plays a major role in bringing about the increase in aldosterone secretion produced by diverse stimuli, including sodium deficiency, hemorrhage, upright posture, and the redistribution of circulating volume by manipulations such as constriction of the inferior vena cava and head-out water immersion. Most studies in humans suggest that aldosterone is linked with the renin-angiotensin system in a negative feedback loop[3] (Fig. 13.1). Thus, changes in volume and/or sodium are monitored by the juxtaglomerular apparatus, eventuating in alterations in renin release. As detailed in chapter 12 of this volume, renin acts through a series of steps to produce an-

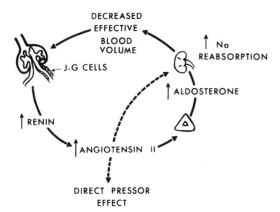

FIGURE 13.1. An overview of the components and physiology of the renin-angiotensin-aldosterone system. The schematic demonstrates how aldosterone is linked with the renin-angiotensin system in a feedback loop. At the time of a diminution in effective blood volume, activation of the renin-angiotensin-aldosterone system results in the conservation of sodium by acting at the level of the distal tubule to promote sodium reabsorption (and thereby extracellular fluid volume). Thus, by augmenting effective blood volume, aldosterone closes the negative feedback loop.

giotensin II, which stimulated the glomerulosa cells of the adrenal cortex to secrete aldosterone. By acting at the level of the distal tubule to promote sodium reabsorption, aldosterone can augment effective blood volume, thereby closing the negative feedback loop (Fig. 13.1).

Potassium

Potassium is a potent stimulus of aldosterone secretion.[3-6] Studies utilizing the infusion of potassium, either systemically or directly into the adrenal arterial supply, as well as in vitro studies with beef adrenal slices, support a direct role for the potassium ion in the regulation of aldosterone secretion. Studies in normal humans have indicated that oral potassium loading on varied dietary sodium intakes increases aldosterone excretion and/or secretion.[5,6] It has been demonstrated that the effect of potassium on aldosterone excretion is independent of reciprocal changes in intravascular volume as well as the status of the renin-angiotensin system. The importance of this control mechanism is underscored by the demonstration of a dominance of the potassium ion in the control of aldosterone secretion in primary aldosteronism[3] and in anephric patients.[7]

Adrenocorticotropic Hormone (ACTH)

While ACTH is the most potent aldosterone agonist, several lines of evidence suggest that it is only of minor importance in regulating aldosterone secretion in normal subjects.[8] As an example, subjects who have isolated ACTH deficiency (i.e., patients on long-term steroid therapy) manifest qualitatively normal aldosterone responses to sodium restriction and acute stimulatory maneuvers. Thus, although aldosterone may be under the physiologic control of ACTH under certain conditions, ACTH appears to be of lesser importance than either potassium or the renin-angiotensin system in the overall control of aldosterone secretion.

Atrial Natriuretic Factor

In the intact dog and normal humans, atrial natriuretic factor (ANF) induces a reduction in plasma aldosterone concentration in association with a fall in plasma renin activity.[9] Thus, the aldosterone-suppressing effect could be in part secondary to the presumed concurrent fall in plasma angiotensin II. There is evidence, however, that ANF can directly inhibit aldosterone production in vivo, since its effects on renin and aldosterone can be dissociated in certain circumstances.[9] In patients with congestive heart failure, ANF infusion causes a major decrease in plasma aldosterone concentration despite the fact that its ability to inhibit renin secretion is severely blunted.

Plasma Sodium Concentration

While there is general agreement that the renin-angiotensin system is the principal mediator of the increased aldosterone secretion that occurs in response to sodium deficiency, there is also evidence that a decrease in plasma sodium concentration per se may directly stimulate the secretion of aldosterone. Experimental manipulations that reduce the sodium concentration of the blood perfusing the adrenal have been reported to increase the rate of aldosterone secretion without consistent effects on corticosterone or cortisol secretion. Conversely, local increases in adrenal arterial plasma sodium concentration (from 7 to 15 mEq/L) decreased aldosterone secretion in sodium-deficient sheep by approximately 25%.[10] In summary, although alterations in plasma sodium concentration may modulate aldosterone release, the relatively large changes in sodium concentration required to produce such effects render it unlikely that plasma sodium concentration per se normally constitutes an important factor in the control of aldosterone secretion.

Physiologic Responses to Aldosterone

Aldosterone exerts a number of effects on renal tubular function that are relevant to an understanding of those derangements in the fluid and electrolyte homeostasis that complicate advanced liver disease. It therefore seems appropriate to review briefly the effects of aldosterone on sodium, potassium, and acid excretion in normal physiology.

Sodium

The administration of aldosterone to a normal subject causes a decrease in sodium excretion and moderate gain of weight incident to expansion of extracellular volume. There is no change in glomerular filtration rate (GFR). Blood pressure may or may not rise modestly. If the normal subject is ingesting a normal diet, the decrease in sodium excretion persists until a total of approximately 300–500 mmol of sodium are retained, at which point "escape" occurs; i.e., the weight gain ceases and sodium excretion returns to control levels, despite continued administration of the hormone. This phenomenon—loss of the sodium-retaining effect of aldosterone despite its continued administration—is called "mineralocorticoid escape." The term was introduced by Relman and Schwartz[11] to describe the regulatory mechanisms that override the hormonal effects of mineralocorticoid on the renal tubule.

The rapidity with which "escape" supervenes depends on how quickly the excess sodium is accumulated, which in turn is determined by the magnitude of sodium intake and the dose of mineralocorticoid administered.[12,13] Thus, subjects ingesting large quantities of sodium who rapidly gain weight will undergo escape within a few days. In contrast, those whose sodium intake is low accumulate salt and water at a slower pace, and a week or more may pass by before escape occurs. Indeed, neither weight gain nor escape will occur if sodium is totally restricted.

The phenomenon of mineralocorticoid escape has stimulated a great deal of study. It has been demonstrated that escape occurs in dogs despite reductions of renal blood flow and GFR. Other studies have shown that escape is independent of systemic arterial pressure and dilution of plasma proteins or angiotensin, and is not preventable by adrenalectomy. Furthermore, it could not be associated with changes of renal venous pressure, the presence of renal nerves, or the renin-angiotensin system. It has been proposed that the extracellular volume expansion produced by administration of mineralocorticoid and sodium stimulates the production or release of a natriuretic factor into the circulation during mineralocorticoid escape. Such a natriuretic factor would thus mediate mineralocorticoid escape. (For a detailed discussion of the status of natriuretic hormones, see chapter 16.)

In contrast to the situation in normal humans, a number of disease states are characterized by the relentless accumulation of sodium in response to mineralocorticoid excess (either administered or endogenous) with edema formation. Prominent among the latter clinical states is advanced liver disease.[14,15]

The nephron sites of enhanced sodium reabsorption subsequent to aldosterone action and those responsible for "escape" may not be the same. Although it is certain that mineralocorticoids enhance sodium reabsorption in the cortical collecting tubule,[13] whether they have a direct effect on other tubule segments remains controversial.[4]

Potassium

The exogenous administration of mineralocorticoid to a normal subject on a normal diet (i.e., an adequate sodium intake and a potassium intake of about 100 mEq/day) results almost immediately in an increase in potassium excretion. In contrast to renal sodium handling in which a new steady state is attained after a few days, potassium excretion is unrelenting and the kaliuresis persists until severe potassium deficiency results. If sodium intake is severely restricted, however, potassium loss will be lessened markedly or obviated altogether (see reference 15a for a discussion of role of hyperaldosteronism in altered potassium metabolism).

Acid Excretion

Several lines of evidence indicate that mineralocorticoid hormones play a prominent role in acid-base balance. The administration of mineralocorticoids promotes hydrogen ion secretion by the distal nephron with resultant increased urinary acid excretion. If allowed to persist, metabolic alkalosis ensues. Initially, the urine becomes acidic with increased titratable levels of acid and ammonium ion. As metabolic alkalosis develops, the urine again becomes alkaline, with hydrogen ion excretion equal to production (For a detailed discussion of acid-base abnormalities in liver disease, see chapter 4.)

Role of the Liver in Aldosterone Metabolism

The degradation of aldosterone occurs principally in the liver.[16] The metabolic clearance rate of aldosterone is dependent upon hepatic blood flow; the plasma circulating through the liver is cleared of its content of non-protein-bound aldosterone in a single pass through this organ. Tait et al.[17] reported that the liver is responsible for approximately 85% of the metabolic clearance rate (MCR) of aldosterone. Lommer et al.[18] demonstrated that under normal conditions, the hepatic extraction of aldosterone (which reflects biochemical transformation and biliary extraction) varies between 95% and 98%. Furthermore, these authors noted that the renal extraction of aldosterone (which reflects metabolism and excretion) varies between 14% and 27% of arterial plasma aldosterone (PA). Finally, Lommer et al.[18] suggested that the hepatic clearance rate of aldosterone correlated well with hepatic plasma flow.

In cirrhotic patients, hepatic plasma flow and hepatic clearance of aldosterone are markedly diminished. In these patients, the degree of reduction in the hepatic clearance rate of aldosterone appears to be related to the degree of impairment of hepatic function.[16]

Coppage et al.[19] studied the disappearance rate of $7\text{-}^3H\text{-}d\text{-}$aldosterone from plasma in normal subjects and in cirrhotic patients. In normal subjects, the half-time ($t_{1/2}$) of circulating aldosterone ranged from 26 to 39 minutes, with a mean $t_{1/2}$ of 34 minutes. In contrast, cirrhotic patients manifested values for $t_{1/2}$ ranging from 43 to 81 minutes (mean of 63 minutes), which were prolonged markedly compared with those of normal subjects.

It thus follows that in chronic liver disease, whether due to cirrhosis or to venous congestion, hepatic blood flow is impaired and the clearance of aldosterone from plasma is correspondingly reduced. In the following sections the prevalence and magnitude of hyperaldosteronism in liver disease and the primary mechanisms mediating such changes are examined.

ALTERATIONS OF ALDOSTERONE IN LIVER DISEASE

Following the isolation and characterization of aldosterone, the importance of the liver in its metabolism became readily apparent. As early as 1962, Ayers et al.[20] demonstrated that the disappearance of tritiated aldosterone from the plasma was delayed in dogs with passively congested livers. Following hepatectomy, the disappearance of aldosterone from the circulation was further delayed. These observations led to a number of investigations of the metabolism of aldosterone in liver disease.

In 1951, Bongiovanni and Eisenmenger[21] reported increased quantities of a sodium-retaining substance with the characteristics of aldosterone in the urine of patients with cirrhosis. Subsequently, many investigators confirmed the presence of hyperaldosteronism in liver disease by demonstrating elevated aldosterone excretory or secretory rates.[19,22–29]

Although these early studies documented a profound degree of secondary hyperaldosteronism in patients with cirrhosis and ascites, they were based on urinary excretory and secretory rates calculated from analyses of the urinary metabolite. Since the excretory pattern of aldosterone metabolites is altered in the presence of hepatic or renal impairment,[16,30] the interpretation of these studies is difficult. Subsequent studies attempted to circumvent these questions by delineating aldosterone stimulation in cirrhosis by determining PA levels. Thus, Kliman and Peterson[31] developed an improved double isotope dilution derivative method for determining PA levels with greater specificity than was previously possible. Using this method, Peterson studied a small number of patients with cirrhosis and ascites and observed the occurrence of elevated PA levels.[32] More recently, the widespread availability of a radioimmunoassay method for measuring PA has facilitated the characterization of PA in a large group of patients with advanced liver disease. In the following section, we examine the results of these studies and the inferences drawn from them.

Frequency of Hyperaldosteronism and Correlation with Clinical Status

It is widely accepted that aldosterone levels are frequently elevated in patients with advanced liver disease. Furthermore, it has been postulated that the presence of hyperaldosteronism correlates with the presence of ascites, or edema, or both. Nevertheless, disagreement centers on the frequency with which PA stimulation occurs in cirrhosis. A brief review of some of the salient features of studies in which aldosterone has been determined points up bases for such controversy. Table 13.1 is not an exhaustive summary of all relevant articles on this subject; rather, it highlights prominent features from several of the more frequently cited articles in which PA has been determined.[33–44] Many investigators have measured PA without commenting on concomitant changes of many of the factors that influence aldosterone release. While some investigators have rigorously controlled sodium intake, others either have failed to control this important determinant of aldosterone metabolism or have used varying sodium intakes without attempting to segregate PA levels according to sodium intake.

Although potassium is thought to exert an important effect on aldosterone release, not all of the reviewed studies attempted to control potassium intake. While a few investigators have reported on the concomitant serum potassium concentrations, none has correlated individual PA levels with the corresponding serum potassium concentrations. Finally, in light of the presence of a distinct circadian rhythm in PA, independent of activity and posture, it is noteworthy that some studies did not specify the time in which blood was obtained for PA determinations.

Rosoff et al.[33] measured basal PA levels in eight cirrhotic patients with moderately tense ascites while on an 80-mEq sodium intake. They reported markedly elevated baseline aldosterone levels in all eight patients; the PA levels were 4–6-fold greater than those found in normal subjects under similar study conditions.

Saruta et al.[16] determined PA levels in 28 cirrhotic patients. At the time of study, the subjects were ingesting a diet containing 130–170 mEq of sodium and 90–110 mEq of potassium. Mean PA in the 11 cirrhotic patients without ascites was 67 ± 27 (SD) pg/ml, not different from the values in control subjects 73 ± 22 pg/ml. In contrast, mean PA in the cirrhotic patients with ascites was 144 ± 65 pg/ml, 2-fold greater than in both the compensated (e.g., no ascites) cirrhotic patients and the normal controls. Of the patients with ascites, approximately one-half had elevated PA levels.

Wernze et al.[36] characterized PA levels in a group of 77 patients with cirrhosis of the liver. In addition to categorizing the patients according to the presence or absence of ascites, the patients were further divided with respect to diuretic administration. These investigators reported that mean PA in untreated cirrhotic patients with ascites (his Group I) was 128 ± 58 pg/ml (SD), a value that did not differ from mean PA in untreated cirrhotic patients without ascites (Group IV) (102 ± 68) (SD). These investigators concluded that in the absence of diuretic administration, hyperaldosteronism was unlikely to occur in the cirrhotic patients with ascites.

Mitch et al.[38] provided additional information regarding the relationship of clinical status and hyperaldosteronism. The availability in their report of individual PA values in a large group of normal controls as well as cirrhotic patients with or without ascites permits the reader to examine the frequency of PA elevation in patients with and without ascites. Mean PA in their patients with ascites (138 ± 22 pg/ml) did not differ from the mean PA of 124 ± 36 pg/ml in patients without ascites. When one calculates the normal range for PA utilizing the individual PA values for their 12 normal controls, it is apparent that the majority of cirrhotic patients with ascites manifested PA levels within the normal range (mean + 2 SD = < 164 pg/ml).

In contrast to these findings, Sellars et al.[39] suggested that PA levels correlated with clinical status. They observed an increase in plasma aldosterone in ascitic patients who were retaining sodium as compared with patients in sodium balance.

In three recent studies, Bernardi et al.[40–42] observed that PA was significantly elevated in patients with cirrhosis and ascites compared with cirrhotic patients without ascites and a normal control group. It should be noted, however, that in one of the studies,[40] 50% of the cirrhotic patients with ascites manifested plasma aldosterone levels within the normal range. In the two other studies, 10 of 23[41] patients and 3 of 9[42] patients with cirrhosis and ascites had normal plasma aldosterone values.

Although Burmeister et al.[43] also demonstrated that cirrhotic patients with ascites manifested elevated PA levels, their study was confounded by diuretic administration (including spironolactone) in seven of the patients. Madsen et al.[44] studied nine cirrhotic patients without edema or ascites and observed that PA was not elevated.

TABLE 13.1.   Plasma Aldosterone in Liver Disease*

Authors (Reference)	Patient Population	No.	Plasma Aldosterone (pg/ml)	
			Study Population	Normal Range
Rosoff et al. 1975 (33)	Cirrhosis with ascites	8	1190 ± 340 (SE) (Supine) 1870 ± 540 (SE) (Erect)	50 ± 10 (SD) 100 – 200
Epstein et al. 1977 (34)	Cirrhosis without ascites	2	423 ± 62	135 ± 599 (2 SD)
	Cirrhosis with ascites	14		
Wernze et al. 1978 (36)	Cirrhosis with ascites (untreated)	23	128 ± 58 (SD)	115 ± 35 (SD)
	Cirrhosis without ascites	12	102 ± 68 (SD)	115 ± 35 (SD)
Arroyo et al. 1979 (37)	Cirrhosis with ascites	68	48 – 2780 (range)	105 ± 31 (SD)
Mitch et al. 1979 (38)	Cirrhosis without ascites	10	132 ± 19 (SE)	81 ± 12 (SE)
	Cirrhosis with ascites	14		
Chonko et al. 1977 (35)	Cirrhosis with ascites	11	177 ± 22 (6 patients) < 60 (5 patients)	< 63 ± 6 < 63 ± 6
Bernardi et al. 1983 (40)	Cirrhosis without ascites	16	58 ± 39 (SD)	99 ± 32 (SD)
	Cirrhosis with ascites	21	138 ± 105 (SD)	
Sellars et al. 1985 (39)	Cirrhosis with ascites/edema and in sodium balance	16	Supine 70 Erect 126 (pmol/L)	Supine 80 Erect 182
	Cirrhosis with ascites/edema and sodium retention	13	Supine 337 (pmol/L) Erect 432 (pmol/L)	
Bernardi et al. 1985 (41)	Cirrhosis with ascites	23	258 (range 42–637)	< 150
Madsen et al. 1986 (44)	Cirrhosis without edema or ascites	9	172 (range 56–289)	133 (range 42–256)
Bernardi et al. 1986 (42)	Cirrhosis with ascites	9	267 ± 55 (SEM)	60 ± 4 (SEM)
	Cirrhosis without ascites	7	54 ± 11 (SEM)	

RIA, radioimmunoassay.

*All values for plasma aldosterone (except when otherwise indicated) are expressed as pg/ml to facilitate comparison between studies.

We have recently reexamined this question and have been unable to confirm the putative high frequency with which PA stimulation has been reported to occur in advanced liver disease. Plasma aldosterone levels were determined under rigorously controlled experimental conditions in a group of 28 cirrhotic patients. Liver disease was associated with excessive alcohol intake in all 28 patients, and all were negative for hepatitis B surface antigen by radioimmunoassay (RIA). None had clinical findings that suggested underlying or antecedent cardiac or renal disease. Significant vascular, parenchymal, or neoplastic renal disease were excluded by history, physical examination, laboratory tests, and, in some subjects, intravenous pyelography. No patient received diuretics during the 10 days prior to study. Twenty-three patients were studied during decompensation, arbitrarily defined by the presence of unequivocal ascites, or edema, or both.

All subjects were housed during the entire study in an environmentally controlled metabolic ward at a constant temperature. Each consumed a daily diet containing 10 mEq sodium, 100 mEq potassium, and 800–1000 ml of water. The composition of the diet remained unchanged throughout the study. Twenty-four hour urine collections were made daily for determination of sodium, potassium, and creatinine. After a mean of 5 days on the constant diet, at which time the urinary sodium was less than 10 mEq/24 hours and the weight remained stable, each subject underwent a determination of PA. On the morning of study, plasma was obtained twice for PA determinations during the seated posture, at 8 AM and 8:30 AM. Plasma aldosterone was measured by an RIA technique, which allowed the direct assay of aldosterone in plasma extracts without the necessity of prior fractionation.[45] This RIA utilized a new antibody with a very high affinity constant (10^{-11} m/L), so that 50% displacement was obtained with only 8 pg aldosterone.[45] With this approach, aldosterone could be assayed utilizing only 0.1 ml plasma. The coefficient of variation for interassay determinations was 10.2%. The values of the two determinations for each patient were averaged. The results were compared with those of a large

TABLE 13.1.　Plasma Aldosterone in Liver Disease (*Cont.*)

Assay	Sodium Intake (mEq/day)	Potassium Intake (mEq/day)	Serum Potassium	Posture	Time of Day	Medications
RIA	80	Not specified	> 3.4	Supine	Not specified	None
	80	Not specified	> 3.4	Erect	Not specified	None
RIA	10	100	Not specified	Seated	8 AM	None
RIA	120–150	70–90	3.8 ± 0.5 (SD)	Supine	7:30–9:30 AM	None
RIA	120–150	70–90	4.3 ± 0.3 (SD)	Supine	7:30–9:30 AM	None
RIA	40	Not specified	Not specified	Supine	Not specified	None
RIA	Unrestricted	Not specified	Not specified	Supine	Morning	None
RIA	300	Not specified	Not specified	Supine	Morning	None
RIA	300	Not specified	Not specified	Supine	Morning	None
RIA	40	80	4.2 ± 0.7	Not specified	10 AM	None
			4.2 ± 0.5			
RIA	Not specified	Not specified	4.1 ± 0.5	Supine Erect	9–11 AM	None
			3.9 ± 0.4	Supine Erect		
RIA	40	80	Not specified	Not specified	10 AM	None
RIA	Not specified	Not specified	Not specified	Supine	9 AM	Not specified
RIA	40	90	4.4 ± 0.1	Supine	Mean of 24 h period	None
			4.2 ± 0.2			

group of normal subjects studied under identical conditions.[46,47]

The results are depicted in Figure 13.2. We observed that 21 of the 28 cirrhotic patients manifested basal PA levels within the normal range for seated normal subjects. Of the remaining seven patients, three manifested suppressed PA levels while four had distinctly elevated PA levels. The

increases in PA varied independently of the degree of ascites.

Serum potassium levels were determined simultaneously and ranged from 3.1 to 4.8 mEq/L, with a mean of 3.9 ± 0.1 mEq/L. Plasma aldosterone levels did not correlate with the corresponding serum potassium levels ($r = -0.155$, ns).

FIGURE 13.2.　An assessment of the relationship between plasma aldosterone (PA) levels and degree of ascites accumulation in 28 cirrhotic patients. *Closed circles* indicate compensated (absence of ascites and edema) patients. *Open circles* indicate patients with varying degrees of ascites and/or edema. The shaded area subtends the mean ± 2 SD for 14 normal subjects studied under identical conditions of sodium and potassium intake, posture, and time of day. As can be seen, relatively few patients manifested increments in PA despite advanced liver disease and ascites accumulation.

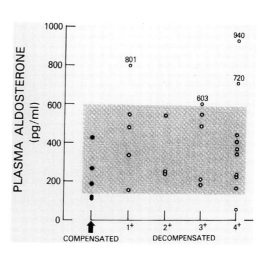

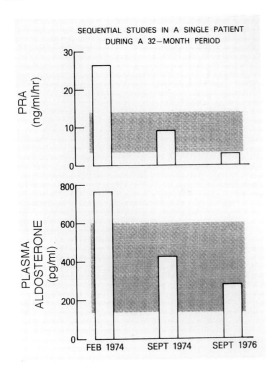

SEQUENTIAL STUDIES IN A SINGLE PATIENT
DURING A 32-MONTH PERIOD

FIGURE 13.3. Alterations in plasma renin activity (PRA) and plasma aldosterone (PA) in patient McD during sequential studies over a 32-month period. The *shaded area* subtends the mean ± 2 SD for 14 normal subjects studied under identical conditions of sodium and potassium intake, posture, and time of day. During all three study periods, the patient manifested neither edema nor ascites. These observations demonstrate the occurrence of marked variability in PRA and PA levels despite an unaltered clinical status with regard to the presence of ascites and edema accumulation.

Sequential Studies in a Single Patient During A 48-Month Period

Additional support for the concept that the degree of hyperaldosteronism may vary independently of the clinical status of the patient is derived from observations in patient McD. We were fortunate to have the opportunity to follow prospectively the plasma renin activity (PRA) and PA levels of this patient over a 48-month period, during which his clinical course waxed and waned with periods of transition from decompensation to compensation to decompensation. Sequential determinations of PA were obtained following discontinuation of all medications under identical conditions of diet and posture. For ease of presentation, the relationship of PRA and PA to clinical status is depicted in separate

figures (Figs. 13.3 and 13.4). Figure 13.3 depicts the results during three occasions when the patient manifested neither edema or ascites. During the initial study in February 1974, both the PRA (26.2 ng/ml/hour) and PA (765 pg/ml) levels were elevated. On subsequent retesting, both levels decreased markedly. At the time of the final study in September 1976, his PA had decreased by 64%, to 276 pg/ml. These observations demonstrate the occurrence of marked variability in PA levels despite an unaltered clinical status.

Figure 13.4 depicts the relationship between ascites accumulation and PA levels during a 48-month period. During the initial study in February 1974, at a time when the patient did not manifest either edema or ascites, his PA level was markedly elevated (765 pg/ml). Forty-five months later, at a time when ascites had reappeared (2+), his PA level had declined to 482 pg/ml. During his final study in 1978, PA had decreased further to 205 pg/ml. During all three periods, serum potassium concentration was unaltered. The demonstration of a dissociation between ascites accumulation and PA levels lends further credence to the formulation that PA varies independently of clinical status.

In summary, it is apparent that PA levels are frequently augmented in patients with advanced liver disease, albeit to a lesser extent than suggested previously. Furthermore, while elevated PA levels have been postulated to correlate with the degree of compensation, such an association is not clear cut. While elevated PA levels are encountered more frequently in patients with ascites than in nonascitic patients, most patients with ascites do not manifest increased PA concentrations.

Control of Aldosterone Secretion in Liver Disease

Although it is quite clear that the secretion of aldosterone is augmented in advanced liver disease, the relative contributions of diverse factors to aldosterone hypersecretion are not fully established. Included among such factors are the renin-angiotensin system, the serum concentrations of potassium and sodium, ANF, and ACTH.[3-10]

Renin-Angiotensin System

The most important determinant of aldosterone secretion in cirrhosis is the renin-angiotensin system. Many studies in both normal humans and normal experimental animals have supported the postulate that alterations of aldosterone secretion in response to volume changes are mediated primarily by alterations of the renin-angiotensin system.[3,46,48] In contrast to the above studies, much controversy centers on the role of the renin-angiotensin system as a determinant of PA in cirrhosis. Saruta et al.[16] have assessed the relationship between PRA and PA in a large group of cirrhotic patients and observed that PA varied independently of PRA. On the other hand, Chonko et al.,[35] Epstein et al.,[34] Wernze et al.,[36] Arroyo et al,[37] Mitch et al.,[38] and Bosch et al.[49] have all demonstrated a close correlation between PRA and PA in patients with cirrhosis.

In contrast to the above static determinations of PRA and PA in liver disease, we elected to assess kinetically the relationship of the renin-angiotensin system and aldosterone to immersion-induced central volume expansion (see pp. 9–10). These studies demonstrated a parallelism between the suppression of PRA and PA in response to immersion, supporting the formulation that the stimulation of aldosterone secretion in cirrhosis is mediated to a great extent by the renin-angiotensin system.

Perhaps the most compelling evidence in support of the importance of the renin-angiotensin system in the regulation of aldosterone is derived from studies utilizing angiotensin antagonists. Despite problems inherent in the application of such agents in the setting of decompensated liver disease (see chapter 12), a number of investigators have carried out limited studies utilizing such inhibitors in the setting of advanced liver disease. Schroeder et al.[50] administered a specific antagonist of angiotensin II (saralasin or P-113) and demonstrated that blockade induced by this agent effectively lowered elevated PA levels in four of five salt-deprived patients.

Arroyo et al.[51] assessed the effect of angiotensin II blockade induced by the administration of the competitive antagonist saralasin (P-113) on several variables including PA in three patients with functional renal failure (i.e., hepatorenal syndrome). The infusion of saralasin at a low dose (0.4 µg/kg/min) resulted in a decrease in PA in all patients, although the decrement was relatively modest in two of three patients. Cessation of the infusion was associated with a return of PA to control levels in all three instances.

Finally, Anderson et al.[52] assessed the acute effects of saralasin on plasma aldosterone in five

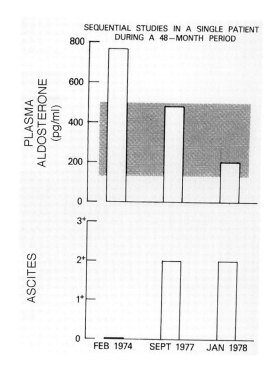

FIGURE 13.4. The relationship between plasma aldosterone (PA) and ascites accumulation in patient McD during sequential studies over a 48-month period. The *shaded area* subtends the mean ± 2 SD for 14 normal subjects studied under identical conditions of sodium and potassium intake, posture, and time of day. During the initial period, at a time when the patient manifested neither edema nor ascites, his PA level was markedly elevated (765 pg/ml). During the subsequent two studies at 45 and 48 months, there was a striking dissociation between ascites which had reaccumulated and PA levels which had decreased markedly.

cirrhotic patients with and two patients without ascites while ingesting both a 10-mEq sodium and 200-mEq sodium diet. Saralasin induced significant decrements in PA levels in all patient groups (see also 52a).

In contrast to the above studies, Wilkinson et a.[53] reported a dissociation between the suppressive effects of propranolol or practolol on PRA and aldosterone excretion. They demonstrated that clinically effective β-adrenergic blockade resulted in an 81% suppression of PRA, while the effect on aldosterone excretion (AER) was variable (with AER increasing in 5 of 11 patients) (Fig. 13.5). These investigators suggested that factors other than the renin-angiotensin system are responsible for the control of aldosterone secretion in many cirrhotic patients. It should be noted, however, that a subsequent study that assessed the effects of β-adrenergic blockade in cirrhosis failed to confirm the findings of Wilkinson et al. Thus, Shohat et al.[54] reported that oral propranolol administration failed to suppress PRA, or plasma, or urinary aldosterone in a group of patients with cirrhosis and ascites.

In the few instances in which such a correlation between PRA and aldosterone was not demonstrated, additional considerations may account for this discrepancy. In this regard, the findings of Saruta et al.[16] are of interest. As noted earlier, these workers examined the relationship between PRA and PA in a group of 28 cirrhotic patients and failed to discern a correlation between these two variables. Although earlier studies from their laboratory disclosed that PRA correlated closely

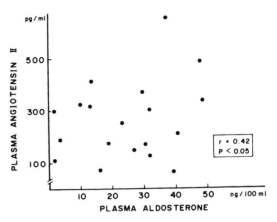

FIGURE 13.6. An examination of the relationship between plasma angiotensin II and plasma aldosterone (PA) in 19 patients with cirrhosis of the liver. There was a significant correlation between angiotensin II and PA. (Reprinted by permission from Saruta et al: Regulation of aldosterone in cirrhosis of the liver. In Epstein M (ed): The Kidney in Liver Disease. New York: Elsevier/North Holland, 1978, pp 271–282.)

with plasma angiotensin II levels in patients with cirrhosis,[16] they postulated that in some instances, angiotensin generation may be influenced by the depletion of renin substrate. The latter investigators therefore assessed the relationship between PA and plasma angiotensin II levels (rather than PRA) in 19 patients with cirrhosis of the liver. As shown in Figure 13.6, there was a significant correlation between PA and angiotensin II ($r = 0.42$; $P < 0.05$), in contrast to the lack of correlation between PRA and PA.

Another possible explanation for a dissociation between PRA and PA in liver disease is the possible contribution of angiotensin III. As noted elsewhere (chapter 12), it has been proposed that, in addition to angiotensin II, the heptapeptide analogue of angiotensin II (i.e., angiotensin III) participates in the control of aldosterone.[55] Since it is conceivable that angiotensin III may be increased in patients with nonhypertensive secondary aldosteronism, such as hepatic cirrhosis, there is a possibility that the augmented aldosterone secretion of cirrhosis may be mediated in part by angiotensin III.

Finally, it is conceivable that the relative clearance of renin and aldosterone by the liver may account, in part, for the lack of correlation between PRA and PA in some patients with liver disease. As noted above, the hepatic clearance rate

ALDOSTERONE EXCRETION

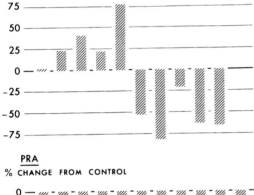

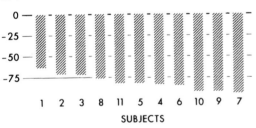

FIGURE 13.5. Relationship of plasma renin activity (PRA) to aldosterone excretion following β-adrenergic blockade induced by propranolol and practolol. Effective β-adrenergic blockade induced marked decrements in PRA in all 11 patients ranging from 64% to 92%. In contrast, the effect on aldosterone excretion was variable with only 5 of 11 patients manifesting a decrease in aldosterone excretion. (Adapted from data of Wilkinson SP et al: Effect of β-adrenergic blocking drugs on the renin-aldosterone system, sodium excretion, and renal haemodynamics in cirrhosis and ascites. Gastroenterology 1977;73:659–663.)

of renin (70 ml/min) is significantly less than that of aldosterone (500 ml/min). Whether such differences in hepatic clearance rate of these two hormones may influence the relationship between PRA and PA in liver disease remains to be established.

Potassium

As discussed in a previous edition of this book[15a] potassium is a potent stimulus of aldosterone secretion. Indeed, it has been proposed that potassium ion is the prepotent mediator of aldosterone secretion in anephric patients and patients with primary aldosteronism. Despite its importance in such conditions, the frequent occurrence of hypokalemia in patients with decompensated cirrhosis and elevated aldosterone levels suggests that potassium does not constitute a major determinant of aldosterone release in cirrhosis.

Plasma Sodium Concentration

Several lines of evidence indicate that a decrease in plasma sodium concentration per se may directly stimulate the secretion of aldosterone. Since hyponatremia is a frequent occurrence in patients with cirrhosis and ascites, and since many observers have noted an inverse relationship between PA and serum sodium concentration in this setting, it has been suggested that hyponatremia per se may contribute to aldosterone release. While this is an attractive speculation, such a possibility seems unlikely. The degree of hyponatremia necessary to affect aldosterone release is relatively large (vide supra), a condition that obtains in only a minority of patents with cirrhosis and ascites. Rather, an alternative explanation is possible. Since the hyponatremia is thought to constitute an index of the severity of impaired renal diluting ability, the inverse correlation between hyponatremia and PA may merely indicate that the more advanced the liver disease (and the attendant maldistribution of circulating blood volume), the greater the activation of the renin-angiotensin-aldosterone system.

Adrenocorticotropic Hormone (ACTH)

While ACTH under certain conditions may stimulate aldosterone secretion, the observation that the majority of cirrhotic patients have normal plasma cortisol levels[16] militates against the importance of ACTH in contributing to the increased aldosterone levels in cirrhosis.

Atrial Natriuretic Factor

Theoretical considerations suggest that a decrease of plasma ANF in cirrhotic patients with ascites may constitute a mechanism whereby plasma aldosterone is elevated. A review of the available data indicates that such a formulation is unlikely. First, the majority of available studies have indicated that ANF levels are normal or elevated (rather than depressed) in patients with decompensated cirrhosis and hyperaldosteronism. Furthermore, studies which have dynamically assessed ANF and PA simultaneously in response to a volume expansive maneuver, i.e., head-out water immersion, have failed to demonstrate a statistically significant inverse correlation. (Epstein et al., unpublished observations, 1988). Additional studies will be required to delineate the relationship of plasma aldosterone and ANF in response to volume expansive maneuvers in cirrhotic patients.

Aldosterone Responsiveness

As noted in chapter 12, the responsiveness of the renin-angiotensin-aldosterone system in liver disease has been a subject of considerable attention. As detailed previously,[34] we have applied the water immersion model to an assessment of aldosterone responsiveness in 16 patients with decompensated cirrhosis.

Examination of the individual natriuretic responses of the 16 subjects during immersion disclosed a continuum of markedly different responses. Eight subjects had no or a barely discernible natriuretic response during immersion and were classified arbitrarily as Group I. In contrast, the remaining eight subjects manifested a profound natriuresis that equaled or exceeded the 37 ± 8 (SE) μEq/min (peak value) documented in normal subjects during identical study conditions and ingesting an identical 10-mEq sodium, 100-mEq potassium diet46 (see also Fig. 1.3 in chapter 1). The latter eight subjects were designated Group II.

The effects of immersion on PA are shown in Figures 13.7 and 13.8. Eleven of the patients had basal PA levels within the normal range for normal seated subjects in balance on an identical sodium and potassium diet (mean ± 2 SD, 135–599 pg/ml). Of the remaining five patients, one had a low basal PA level of 132 pg/ml, while four patients had distinctly elevated PA levels (612–975 pg/ml). When divided according to their natriuretic responses, all four patients with elevated PA levels were in Group I.

Figures 13.7 and 13.8 depict the alterations in PA for Group I and Group II patients. Since the basal PA levels prior to immersion in Group I patients were almost 2-fold greater than the comparable values in Group II patients ($P < 0.05$), the PA response to immersion is presented both in terms of absolute changes (Fig. 13.7) and as percentage change from the preimmersion hour (Fig. 13.8). Despite these differences in basal PA, the magnitude of the immersion-induced suppression of PA of the two groups was similar; by 240 minutes, the 57 ± 6% suppression of PA manifested by Group I patents was not different from the 60 ± 4% suppression of Group II patients ($P > 0.5$) (Fig. 13.8). Similarly, the extent of recovery 1 hour after cessation of immersion was similar in the two groups (to 94 ± 9% of preimmersion values for Group I patients versus 90 ± 15% for Group II patients, $P > 0.5$).

EFFECTS OF HYPERALDOSTERONISM ON THE KIDNEY

As noted above, aldosterone exerts a number of effects on renal function that contribute wholly or partly to the fluid and electrolyte abnormalities of liver disease. While these effects are considered in greater detail elsewhere in this volume (pp. 12–14), their possible contribution to the renal functional abnormalities of liver disease is considered briefly here.

Sodium

With the demonstration that cirrhosis is frequently associated with increased levels of aldosterone, it has been tempting to attribute the sodium retention of liver disease to the encountered hyperaldosteronism. Thus, a traditional viewpoint emerged that aldosterone is the major determinant of the sodium retention.[56,57] As elaborated elsewhere in this book (pp. 12–14) and in several recent editorials,[58,59] many lines of evidence have challenged this formulation. Many investigators have reported a striking dissociation between elevated PA levels on the one hand and increasing sodium excretion on the other.[33,34] Additional studies utilizing the model of head-out water immersion have assessed in a kinetic manner the responses of PA and renal sodium excretion to acute central volume expansion.[34] Collectively, these studies demonstrated a dissociation between the suppression of circulating aldosterone and the absence of the natriuresis in many subjects. The total evidence presently available, therefore, appears to favor the postulate that the hyperaldosteronism of cirrhosis is a permissive factor in many patients, and that the predominant component of the abnormal renal sodium handling is often a diminished distal delivery of filtrate.

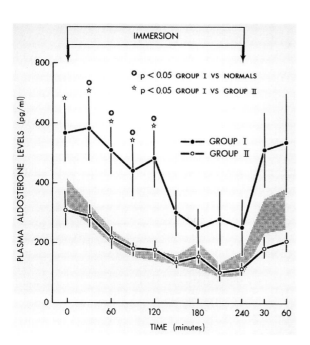

FIGURE 13.7. Effect of water immersion on plasma aldosterone (PA) in 16 cirrhotic patients in balance on a 10-mEq sodium diet. *Shaded area* represents the mean ± SE for nine normal control subjects undergoing immersion while receiving an identical diet.[46] The immersion-induced suppression of PA in Group II patients paralleled that of normal controls undergoing an identical study. Although prestudy PA levels in Group I patients were 2-fold greater than those of both Group II patients and normal subjects, PA was suppressed markedly during immersion, attaining levels not different from Group II or normal subjects. (Reprinted by permission of the American Heart Association, Inc. from Epstein M et al: Characterization of the renin-aldosterone system in decompensated cirrhosis. Circ Res 1977;41:825.)

Potassium

It is well established that the administration of aldosterone increases potassium excretion. The magnitude of the potassium losses, however, are dependent on the sodium intake of the subject and on the quantity of sodium reaching the distal nephron. In the context of the frequent occurrence of hyperaldosteronism in patients with advanced liver disease, it has been tempting to attribute the pathogenesis of potassium depletion to the effects of aldosterone excess. Whether potassium depletion, indeed, occurs as frequently as claimed and whether aldosterone excess contributes importantly to its genesis is considered in detail elsewhere.[15a]

Acid-Base

By virtue of its ability to promote distal hydrogen ion secretion and hypokalemia, aldosterone contributes importantly to acid-base homeostasis. In the context of the prevalence of hyperaldosteronism in patients with advanced liver disease, it is probable that aldosterone excess contributes to the pathogenesis of the metabolic alkalosis frequently manifested by such patients following diuretic administration. The mechanisms by which aldosterone participates in the pathogenesis of such changes and their importance in the acid-base derangements of liver disease are considered in a critical review elsewhere in this book (see chapter 4).

SUMMARY

It is apparent that many patients with advanced liver disease manifest alterations of aldosterone metabolism characterized by diminished hepatic clearance and increased plasma levels of aldosterone. A review of the available studies indicates that the precise magnitude of such alterations is difficult to discern, since many of the variables that affect aldosterone release were not controlled (or not recorded). Despite such failings, it is apparent that PA levels are frequently augmented in patients with advanced liver disease, albeit to a lesser extent than suggested previously.

Although marked perturbations occur in many patients with liver disease, it is important to emphasize that there is great variability with regard to the frequency with which such alterations occur, the magnitude of the abnormalities,

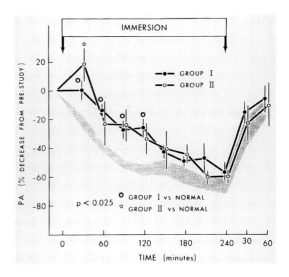

FIGURE 13.8. Comparison of the effects of immersion on plasma aldosterone (PA) in Group I and Group II cirrhotic patients and in normal control subjects in balance on an identical 10-mEq sodium diet. Data are expressed in terms of percentage change from the preimmersion hour. *Shaded area* represents the mean ± SE for control subjects. Group I patients manifested a 57 ± 6% suppression of PA, not different from the 60 ± 11% suppression manifested by Group II patients ($P > 0.5$). Neither group of cirrhotic patients was different from normal control subjects ($P > 0.4$).

and intrapatient variability over time. Elevated PA levels have been postulated to correlate with the degree of compensation, but such an association is not clear cut. While elevated PA levels are encountered more frequently in patients with ascites than in nonascitic patients, most patients with ascites do not manifest increased PA concentrations. Other chapters will consider specific aspects wherein aldosterone excess contributes to sodium retention (chapter 1) and acid-base derangements (chapter 4).

REFERENCES

1. Simpson SA, Tait JF, Wettstein A, Neher R, von Euw J, Reichstein T: Isolierung eines neuen kristallisierten Hormons aus Nebennieren mit besonders hoher Wirksamkeit au den Mineralstoffwechsel. Experientia 1953;9:333–335.
2. Simpson SA, Tait JF: Recent progress in methods of isolation, chemistry, and physiology of aldosterone. Recent Prog Horm Res 1955;11:183–220.
3. Reid IA, Ganong WF: Control of aldosterone secretion. In Genest J, Koiw E, Kuchel O (eds): Hypertension. New York: McGraw Hill, 1977;265–292.

4. Knochel JP, White MG: The role of aldosterone in renal physiology. Arch Intern Med 1973;131:876–884.

5. Gann DS, Delea CS, Gill JR Jr, Thomas JP, Bartter FC: Control of aldosterone secretion by change of body potassium in normal man. Am J Physiol 1964;207:104–108.

6. Himathongkam T, Dluhy RG, Williams GH: Potassium-aldosterone-renin interrelationships. J Clin Endocrinol Metab 1975;41:153–159.

7. Bayard F, Cooke CR, Tiller DJ, Beitins IZ, Kowarski A, Walker WB, Migeon CJ: The regulation of aldosterone secretion in anephric man. J Clin Invest 1971;50:1585–1595.

8. Ganong WF, Alpert LC, Lee TC: ACTH and the regulation of adrenocortical secretion. N Engl J Med 1974; 290:1006–1011.

9. Atlas SA, Laragh JH: Physiological actions of atrial natriuretic factor. In Mulrow PJ, Schrier R (eds): Atrial Hormones and Other Natriuretic Factors. Bethesda, MD: American Physiological Society, 1987;53–76.

10. Blair-West JR, Coghlan JP, Denton DA, Goding JR, Wintour M, Wright RD: The direct effects of increased sodium concentration in adrenal arterial blood on corticosteroid secretion in sodium deficient sheep. Aust J Exp Biol Med Sci 1966;44:455–474.

11. Relman AS, Schwartz WB: Effect of DOCA on electrolyte balance in normal man and its relation to sodium chloride intake. Yale J Biol Med 1952;24:540–588.

12. Ross EJ: Effects on the kidney. In Ross EJ (ed): Aldosterone and Aldosteronism. London: Lloyd-Luke Ltd., 1975;74–92.

13. Knox FG, Burnett JC Jr: Mechanism of mineralocorticoid escape. In Lichardus B, Schrier RW, Ponec J (eds): Hormonal Regulation of Sodium Excretion. Amsterdam: Biomedical Press, 1980;19–31.

14. Denison EK, Lieberman FL, Reynolds TB: 9-a-Fluorohydrocortisone induced ascites in alcoholic liver disease. Gastroenterology 1971;61:496–503.

15. Wilkinson SP, Smith IK, Moodie H, Poston L, Williams R: Studies on mineralocorticoid "escape" in cirrhosis. Clin Sci 1979;56:401–406.

15a. Perez GO, Oster JR: Altered potassium metabolism in liver disease. In Epstein M (ed): The Kidney in Liver Disease, 2nd ed. New York: Elsevier Biomedical, 1983; 183–201.

16. Saruta T, Saito I, Nakamura R, Oka M: Regulation of aldosterone in cirrhosis of the liver. In Epstein M (ed): The Kidney in Liver Disease, New York: Elsevier/North Holland, 1978;271–282.

17. Tait JF, Bougas J, Little B, Tait SAS, Flood C: Splanchnic extraction and clearance of aldosterone in subjects with minimal and marked cardiac dysfunction. J Clin Endocrinol 1965;25:219–228.

18. Lommer D, Dusterdieck G, Jahnecke J, Vecsei P, Wolff HP: Sekretion, Plasmakonzentration, Verteilung, Stoffwechsel und Ausscheidung von Aldosteron bei Gesunden und Kranken. Klin Wochenschr 1968;46:741–751.

19. Coppage WS Jr, Island DP, Cooner AE, Liddle GW: The metabolism of aldosterone in normal subjects and in patients with hepatic cirrhosis. J Clin Invest 1962;41: 1672–1680.

20. Ayers CR, Davis JO, Lieberman F, Carpenter CCJ, Berman M: The effects of chronic hepatic venous congestion on the metabolism of d,l-aldosterone and d-aldosterone. J Clin Invest 1962;41:884–895.

21. Bongiovanni AM, Eisenmenger WJ: Adrenal cortical metabolism in chronic liver disease. J Clin Endocrinol 1951;11:152–173.

22. Axelrad BJ, Cates JE, Johnson BB, Luetscher JA Jr: Aldosterone in urine of normal man and of patients with oedema. Br Med J 1955;1:196–199.

23. Dyrenfurth I, Stacey CH, Beck JC, Venning EH: Aldosterone excretion in patients with cirrhosis of the liver. Metabolism 1957;6:544–555.

24. Summerskill WHJ, Crabbe J: Effect of amphenone therapy on urinary excretion of aldosterone and sodium in hepatic cirrhosis and ascites. Lancet 1957;2:1091–1095.

25. Wolff HP, Koczorek KhR, Buchborn E: Aldosterone and antidiuretic hormone (Adiuretin) in liver disease. Acta Endocrinol 1958;27:45–58.

26. Hurter R, Nabarro JDN: Aldosterone metabolism in liver disease. Acta Endocrinol 1960;33:168–174.

27. Peterson RE: Adrenocortical steroid metabolism and adrenal cortical function in liver disease. J Clin Invest 1960;39:320–331.

28. Cope CL, Nicolis G, Fraser G: Measurement of aldosterone secretion rate in man by the use of a metabolite. Clin Sci 1961;21:367–380.

29. Vecsei P, Dusterdieck G, Jahnecke J, Lommer D, Wolff HPD: Secretion and turnover of aldosterone in various pathological states. Clin Sci 1969;36:241–256.

30. Ross EJ: Biosynthesis and metabolism. In Ross EJ (ed): Aldosterone and Aldosteronism. London: Lloyd-Luke Ltd, 1975;10–52.

31. Kliman B, Peterson RE: Double isotope derivative assay of aldosterone in biological extracts. J Biol Chem 1960; 235:1639–1643.

32. Peterson RE: The miscible pool and turnover rate of adrenocortical steroids in man. Recent Prog Horm Res 1958;6:231–261.

33. Rosoff L Jr, Zia P, Reynolds T, Horton RL: Studies of renin and aldosterone in cirrhotic patients with ascites. Gastroenterology 1975;69:698–705.

34. Epstein M, Levinson R, Sancho J, Haber E, Re R: Characterization of the renin-aldosterone system in decompensated cirrhosis. Circ Res 1977;41:818–829.

35. Chonko AM, Bay WH, Stein JH, Ferris TF: The role of renin and aldosterone in the salt retention of edema. Am J Med 1977;63:881–889.

36. Wernze H, Spech HJ, Muller G: Studies on the activity of the renin-angiotensin-aldosterone system (RAAS) in patients with cirrhosis of the liver. Klin Wochenschr 1978;56:389–397.

37. Arroyo V, Bosch J, Mauri M, Viver J, Mas A, Rivera F, Rodes J: Renin, aldosterone and renal haemodynamics in cirrhosis with ascites. Eur J Clin Invest 1979;9:69–73.

38. Mitch WE, Whelton PK, Cooke CR, Walker WG, Maddrey WC: Plasma levels and hepatic extraction of renin and aldosterone in alcoholic liver disease. Am J Med 1979;66:804–810.

39. Sellars L, Shore AC, Mott V, Wilkinson R: The renin-angiotensin-aldosterone system in decompensated cirrhosis: Its activity in relation to sodium balance. QJ Med 1985;56:485–496.

40. Bernardi M, Trevisani F, Santini C, De Palma R, Gasbarrini G: Aldosterone related blood volume expansion in cirrhosis before and during the early phase of ascites formation. Gut 1983;24:761–766.

41. Bernardi M, Servadei D, Trevisani F, Rusticali AG, Gasbarrini G: Importance of plasma aldosterone concentration on the natriuretic effect of spironolactone in patients with liver cirrhosis and ascites. Digestion 1985;31:189–193.

42. Bernardi M, De Palma R, Trevisani F, Santini C, Capani F, Baraldini M, Gasbarrini G: Chronobiological study of factors affecting plasma aldosterone concentration in cirrhosis. Gastroenterology 1986;91:683–691.

43. Burmeister P, Schölmerich J, Diener W, Gerok W: Renin, aldosterone and arginine vasopressin in patients with liver cirrhosis: The influence of ascites retransfusion. Eur J Clin Invest 1986;16:117–123.

44. Madsen M, Pedersen EB, Danielsen H, Jensen LS, Sørenson SS: Impaired renal water excretion in early hepatic cirrhosis. Lack of relationship between renal water excretion and plasma levels of arginine vasopressin, angiotensin II, and aldosterone after water loading. Scand J Gastroenterol 1986;21:749–755.

45. Sancho J, Haber E: A direct microassay for aldosterone in plasma extracts. J Clin Endocrinol Metab 1978;47:391–396.

46. Epstein M, Pins DS, Sancho J, Haber E: Suppression of plasma renin and plasma aldosterone during water immersion in normal man. J Clin Endocrinol Metab 1975;41:618–685.

47. Epstein M, Re R, Preston S, Haber E, Re R: Comparison of the suppressive effects of water immersion and saline administration on renin-aldosterone in normal man. J Clin Endocrinol Metab 1979;49:358–363.

48. Epstein M, Haber E, Re R: A kinetic assessment of aldosterone responsiveness in secondary hyperaldosteronism and in anephric man. In James VHT, Serio M, Giusti G, Martini L (eds): The Endocrine Function of the Human Adrenal Cortex. London: Academic Press, 1978;493–508.

49. Bosch J, Arroyo V, Betriu A, Mas A, Carrilho F, Rivera F, Navarro-Lopez F, Rodes J: Hepatic hemodynamics and the renin-angiotensin-aldosterone system in cirrhosis. Gastroenterology 1980;78:92–99.

50. Schroeder ET, Anderson GH, Goldman SH, Streeten DHP: Effect of blockade of angiotensin II on blood pressure, renin and aldosterone in cirrhosis. Kidney Int 1976;9:511–519.

51. Arroyo V, Bosch J, Rivera F, Rodes J: The renin angiotensin system in cirrhosis: Its relation to functional renal failure. In Bartoli E, Chiandussi L (eds): Hepato-Renal Syndrome. Padova: Piccin Medical Books, 1979;202–221.

52. Anderson GH Jr, Anderson T, Streeten DHP, Schroeder ET: Acute effects of saralasin on plasma aldosterone in different pathophysiological conditions. J Clin Endocrinol Metab 1980;50:529–536.

52a. Saruta T, Eguchi T, Saito I: Angiotensin antagonists in liver disease. In Epstein M (ed): The Kidney in Liver Disease, 2nd ed. New York: Elsevier Biomedical, 1983;441–450.

53. Wilkinson SP, Bernardi M, Smith IK, Jowett TP, Slater JDH, Williams R: Effect of β-adrenergic blocking drugs on the renin-aldosterone system, sodium excretion, and renal haemodynamics in cirrhosis with ascites. Gastroenterology 1977;73:659–663.

54. Shohat J, Iaina A, Serban I, Theodor E, Eliahou HE: The effect of propranolol on renal sodium handling in patients with cirrhosis. Biomedicine 1979;31:128–131.

55. Peach MJ, Sarstedt CA, Vaughan ED: Changes in cardiovascular adrenal cortical responses to angiotensin III induced by sodium deprivation in the rat. Circ Res 1976;38(Suppl 2):117–121.

56. Vesin P: Water, electrolyte, and acid-base disorders in liver disease. In Maxwell MH, Kleeman CR (eds): Clinical Disorders of Fluid and Electrolyte Metabolism, 2nd ed. New York: McGraw-Hill, 1972;873–895.

57. Wilkinson SP, Smith ILK, Williams R: Sodium retention, the renin-angiotensin aldosterone system, and the intrarenal distribution of plasma flow in cirrhosis with unimpaired renal function. In Epstein M (ed): The Kidney in Liver Disease, 1st ed. New York: Elsevier/North Holland, 1978;55–66.

58. Epstein M: Renal sodium handling in cirrhosis: A reappraisal. Nephron 23:211–217, 1979.

59. Epstein M: Determinants of abnormal renal sodium handling in cirrhosis: A reappraisal. Scan J Clin Lab Invest 1980;40:689–694.

Chapter 14

LIPID-DERIVED AUTACOIDS AND RENAL FUNCTION IN LIVER CIRRHOSIS

GIACOMO LAFFI, M.D.
GIORGIO LA VILLA, M.D.
MASSIMO PINZANI, M.D.
PAOLO GENTILINI, M.D.

Prostaglandins and Thromboxanes
  Biochemical and Physiologic Aspects
  Renal Prostaglandins in Cirrhosis
  Thromboxane A$_2$ and Renal Function in Cirrhosis
  Renal Prostaglandins in Hepatorenal Syndrome
  Altered Systemic Production and Metabolism of
    Prostacyclin
  Administration of Prostaglandins

Leukotrienes
  Biochemical and Physiologic Aspects
  Leukotrienes and the Hepatorenal Syndrome
Platelet-Activating Factor
  Biochemical and Physiologic Aspects
  Platelet-activating Factor in Cirrhosis
**Cytochrome P-450 Metabolites of Arachidonic
  Acid**

Eicosanoids are a family of locally active substances (autacoids) that originate from arachidonic acid (AA) or another essential fatty acid with 20 carbon atoms. Prostaglandins (PGs), leukotrienes (LTs), and the other compounds of the eicosanoid family have been detected in almost every tissue or body fluid and are thought to be involved in the regulation of a broad spectrum of functions in response to different stimuli. Over the past three decades, the renal eicosanoid system has been a major area of research. The available methodologic approaches have yielded much information about the biologic significance of AA metabolites in the regulation of renal function. More recently, the introduction of new technologies, including cloning and gene sequence analysis of the major enzymes involved in AA metabolism, has provided important new information.

This chapter deals with the renal AA metabolism in cirrhosis, focusing mainly on the products of PG endoperoxide synthase (PES, formerly known as cyclooxygenase complex), which have been studied more extensively in this setting.

PROSTAGLANDINS AND THROMBOXANES

Biochemical and Physiologic Aspects

Biosynthesis of Prostaglandins

Arachidonic acid, a polyunsaturated fatty acid with 20 carbon atoms and 4 double bonds (C20:4ω6), is the most important eicosanoid precursor (Fig. 14.1). The synthetic pathway of AA involves desaturation of the dietary precursor linoleic acid (C18:2ω6) to gamma linolenic acid (C18:3ω6), which is elongated to dihomo-gamma linolenic acid (C20:3ω6) and further desaturated to AA. These reactions occur in the liver, and the rate-limiting step of AA biosynthesis is desaturation of linoleic acid by delta-6-desaturase.

Arachidonic acid is esterified into cellular membrane phospholipids, mainly in position 2 of membrane phospholipids, in the phosphatidyl-inositol fraction. Phosphatidyl-choline and phosphatidyl-ethanolamine are esterified to AA to a lesser extent. The latter two phospholipids, however, occur in the membrane in greater amounts than phosphatidyl-inositol and may represent an

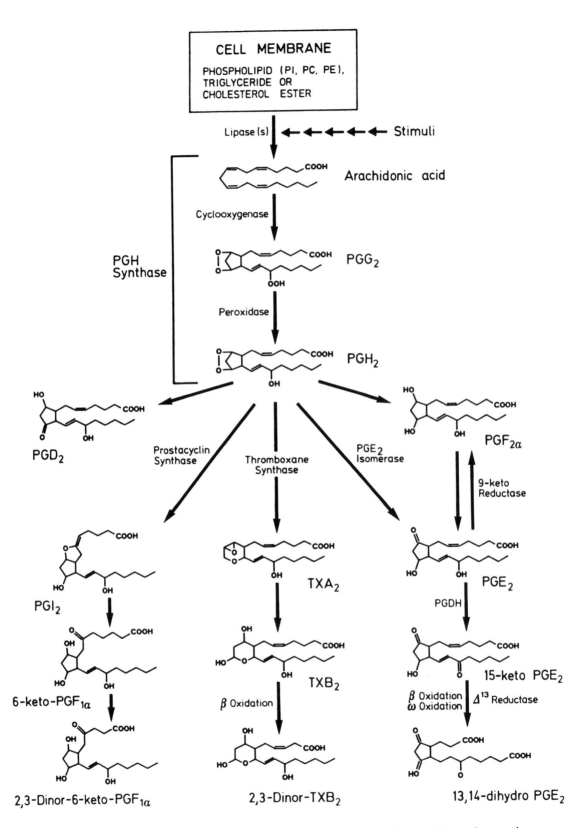

FIGURE 14.1   Arachidonic acid metabolism via the prostaglandin endoperoxide synthase pathway.

important source of AA. The amounts of free AA are negligible in nonstimulated cells. Therefore, the release of AA from cellular stores is the key factor for the synthesis of biologically active derivatives in response to physical and chemical stimuli.

Three possible pathways have been recognized. The first involves sequential degradation of phosphatidyl-inositol via a sequence of reactions beginning with phospholipase C and followed by di- and monoglyceride lipase.[1,2] The second involves conversion of phosphatidyl-ethanolamine or phosphatidyl-choline to phosphatidic acid by phospholipase D, followed by formation of diglyceride and monoglyceride.[1-3] The third and most important pathway begins with the activation of a phospholipase A_2 (PLA_2), which directly acts on a phospholipid that, depending on the specific PLA_2 involved, may be 1,2-diacyl- or 1-O-alkyl-2-acyl-phosphatidyl-inositol, phosphatidyl-ethanolamine, or phosphatidyl-choline.[3-5] Several hormones and autacoids activate PLA_2 via a G-protein dependent activation of cellular phospholipases. Phospholipase C catalyzes the breakdown of phosphatidyl-inositol to inositol triphosphate (IP3), thus triggering an increase in the concentration of cytosolic free calcium, which in turn is responsible for the calmodulin-dependent activation of PLA_2. Physical and nonspecific stimuli may activate PLA_2 directly via calcium influx.[6] In some instances, cells synthesize prostanoids using AA mobilized in the neighboring cells[7] and/or contained in circulating lipids.[8]

The next step in PG biosynthesis is the conversion of AA into the PG endoperoxide PGH_2, the first compound of the dienoic series, through activity of PES (see Fig. 14.1). The same enzyme, when acting on dihomo-gamma linolenic acid or eicosapentaenoic acid, induces the formation of PGs of the monoenoic (PG_1) or trienoic (PG_3) series, respectively.[9] Two PES isoenzymes have been recognized, PES-1 and PES-2.[7] The first isoenzyme is widely present in most cellular types of virtually all mammalian tissue, whereas PES-2 occurs only in prostate, brain, testis, and lung, being practically undetectable in the kidney and other major organs.[3] PES has two catalytic activities. The first is the cyclooxygenase activity, in which AA is cyclisated and oxygenated to form PGG_2. This compound is converted to PGH_2 by peroxidase activity. These reactions occur at different, although neighboring, catalytic

sites. In fact, treatment of PES-1 with aspirin, indomethacin, or fatty acid analogs, blocks cyclooxygenase without affecting peroxidase activity.[10,11] Cyclic endoperoxides are highly unstable, having a half-life of about 5 minutes; in some circumstances, however, they may exert biologic activity by binding to receptors for thromboxane A_2 (TXA_2).

After its synthesis, PGH_2 is immediately converted to one of the major biologically active prostanoids—PGD_2, PGE_2, $PGF_{2\alpha}$, PGI_2, and TXA_2. Conversion involves specific isomerases (synthases) or reductases and is rather cell-specific, with differentiated cells producing appreciable amounts of only one of the major PGs. Hence, freeing of AA within platelets results in the synthesis of TXA_2, whereas in endothelial cell freeing of AA predominantly yields PGI_2. PGH_2 is converted to PGD_2 and PGE_2 by simple isomerization (nonoxidative rearrangement). These reactions are mediated by PGD and PGE synthase, respectively. $PGF_{2\alpha}$ is formed through reduction of PGH_2, a reaction probably catalyzed by a $PGF_{2\alpha}$ synthase that is dependent on reduced nicotinamide adenine dinucleotide phosphate (NADPH)[12]. Finally, PGH_2 may be converted to PGI_2 by prostacyclin synthase or to TXA_2 by thromboxane synthase.

Sources and Nephronal Distribution of PES Products

Prostaglandins are autacoids and by definition exert biologic actions on renal cells when they are released in the discrete anatomic microenvironment along the nephron. Release of PGs may occur either from cellular constituents of the renal tissue (autocrine/paracrine actions) or from infiltrating cells such as neutrophils and platelets during inflammatory reactions. Several methodologic approaches have been used to assess the sources and nephronal distribution of renal prostanoids. In general, these studies have yielded consistent results. However, differences in the relative generation rates and distribution, likely due to interspecies variations, have been often reported.[13] Most of the information summarized here derives from (1) immunohystochemical studies mapping the location of PES with fluorescent-tagged antibodies[14]; (2) evaluation of PG synthesis by microdissected tubular segments or isolated glomeruli[15,16]; and (3) cell culture studies using glomerular epithelial cells,[17] mesangial cells,[18,19] medullary collecting tubular cells,[20] and medullary interstitial cells.[21]

Prostaglandin endoperoxide synthase activity is present in arterial and arteriolar endothelial cells, including glomerular afferent and efferent arterioles.[22] The predominant metabolite produced at these sites is PGI_2.[22] In isolated whole glomeruli from humans and pigs, the predominant metabolite appears to be PGI_2[23, 24] rather than PGE_2, as seen in rats and rabbits. At this level and in most species, $PGF_{2\alpha}$ is produced in consistent amounts together with PGI_2 and PGE_2, whereas virtually no TXA_2 is produced.[15] Analysis of individual glomerular cell subpopulations has provided insight into the intraglomerular generation of prostanoids. Human mesangial cells in culture are capable of generating PGE_2, and, to a lesser extent, $PGF_{2\alpha}$ and PGI_2. In addition, they show, both in culture and in whole tissue, positive staining for PES and prostacyclin synthase.[24]

Mesangial cells have also been proposed as a potential source for the intraglomerular release of PG, particularly in response to specific stimuli such as immune complexes and endotoxins.[25,26] The profile of PES products generated by glomerular epithelial cells appears to be similar to that of mesangial cells, although some reports indicate a predominance of PGI_2.[27] The profile of PG generation by glomerular endothelial cells is not yet fully elucidated. However, preliminary reports indicate a predominant production of vasodilatory PES derivatives, particularly PGI_2. Studies using either microdissection techniques or tubular cell cultures have indicated that PGE_2 represents the predominant metabolite generated in the tubule (80–90% of the measured PGs); variations among the other products are insignificant.[28,29] Synthesis of PGs is very low in the proximal and distal convoluted tubules. Greater synthetic capacity has been found in the thin limb of Henle's loop, medullary thick ascending limb, and the medullary, and cortical collecting tubules.[27,28] PGE_2 is also the major PES metabolite generated in medullary interstitial cells.[30]

Stimuli for the Renal Generation of PES Products

Several hormonal, chemical, or physical stimuli may cause the generation and local release of PGs in different segment of the nephron. Angiotensin II (AII)-mediated PG release is the best characterized with respect to physiologic importance and cellular mechanisms. In vivo studies performed in anesthetized dogs have demonstrated that infusion of AII increased the secretion of PGs in both renal venous effluent and urine.[31,32] In addition, in humans intravenous administration of AII results in increased synthesis and urinary excretion of PGE_2. In cultured renal cells, particularly mesangial and medullary interstitial cells, activation of AII receptors is coupled to a phospholipase C-dependent increase in intracellular Ca^{2+} concentration, which in turn results in AA release from membrane phosphoinositol lipids.[27,33]

The intrarenal synthesis of PGs is also markedly increased in response to catecholamines as well as afferent renal nerve activity. Intravenous administration of norepinephrine to healthy subjects results in increased renal excretion of PGE_2 and 6-keto-$PGF_{1\alpha}$, the nonenzymatic derivative of PGI_2.[34] This effect appears to result from α-adrenergic stimulation, since blockade of α-adrenergic receptors abolishes or attenuates the release of PGs. The effects of other catecholamines, such as dopamine or isoproterenol, appears to be much less evident.[35,36]

Kinins have been shown to increase PG synthesis by isolated renal tissue and renal cells in culture. Indeed, some of the glomerular as well as tubular actions of kinins have been attributed to the secondary increase in PGs.[37–39] Moreover, several lines of evidence suggest that arginine vasopressin (AVP) and AVP analogs stimulate PG synthesis in whole kidney, isolated renal tissue, and cultured kidney cells. However, this effect appears to be relevant at the collecting tubule level. Indeed, most studies have indicated that AVP increases PGE_2 synthesis in collecting ducts.[40,41]

Hormonal stimulation of PG synthesis assumes a key role in some pathophysiologic conditions. In general, the renal cortical and medullary synthesis and release of PGE_2 and PGI_2 subserves a compensatory action in maintaining the integrity of renal function under stress.

In addition to hormonal stimuli, chemical and physical stimuli have been shown to elicit renal synthesis and release of PGs, including platelet activating factor (PAF), endotoxins, reactive oxygen species, ischemia or hypoxia, and alterations in membrane fluidity.[42–48]

Finally, PGs are synthesized and released following the administration of diuretics such as furosemide,[49] ethacrynic acid,[50] and bumetanide.[51] In all cases, the acute increments of PG excretion are short-lived and the effects on sodium excretion and the release of renin outlast the enhancement of PG excretion.

Renal Metabolism and Urinary Excretion of PES Products

All PES products have a limited half-life. In general the half-life of PGs is 3–5 minutes, whereas that of TXA_2 is about 30 seconds. PGs undergo both enzymatic and nonenzymatic pathways, whereas the elimination of TXA_2 is exclusively nonenzymatic. Spontaneous hydrolysis of PGI_2 and TXA_2 generates 6-keto-$PGF_{1\alpha}$ and TXB_2, respectively (see Fig. 14. 1). These stable hydrolysis products are usually measured, and their rates of formation are considered representative of those of the parent molecules. PGE_2 and $PGF_{2\alpha}$ are enzymatically degraded, initially by 15-PG dehydrogenase and subsequently by 13,14-keto-reductase, to form 13,14-dihydro-15-keto derivatives of the parent molecules.[52,53] Further metabolism of these compounds by omega oxidation leads to the formation of dinor derivatives. The end products of all these degradative reactions possess minimal biologic activity.

The conversion of PGE_2 into $PGF_{2\alpha}$, which involves the NADPH-dependent 9-ketoreductase reaction, represents a physiologically relevant transformation of PES products within the kidney. This enzymatic activity, particularly enriched in suspension from the thick ascending limb of Henle's loop, may contribute significantly to urinary $PGF_{2\alpha}$ excretion.

Renal PGs that escape local degradation are secreted into the renal venous and lymphatic circulation[54] or excreted into urine. Because filtered PGs are degraded in the proximal tubule, it is unlikely that changes in PG concentration in the renal artery influence urinary excretion. Indeed, tritiated PGE_2 infused in humans is recovered only in small amounts (less than 0.1%) in the urine,[55] and in animals stimulation of PGE_2 synthesis from one kidney does not influence PGE_2 excretion by the other kidney.[56]

Prostaglandins reach the lumen of the nephron by both active secretion and passive entry. Active secretion uses the organic acid secretory pathway and is inhibited by probenecid and related compounds.[57,58] Although urinary PGs represent only a small amount of PGs synthesized in the kidney, measurement of urinary PGs or their metabolites provides a reliable estimation of basal as well as stimulated PG synthesis under most circumstances. In addition, renal PG excretion provides an integrated estimate of renal PG production, whereas the necessarily episodic sampling of renal venous plasma limits the measurements to a single or few time points.

Urinary PGE_2 excretion is an acceptably reliable index of renal PGE_2 synthesis. In fact, maneuvers that either increase or decrease renal PGE_2 synthesis are followed by parallel changes in urinary PGE_2 excretion, indicating that urinary PGE_2 excretion reflects intrarenal production, provided that no contamination by seminal fluid (rich in PGE_2) occurs. Renal excretion of the stable metabolites 6-keto-$PGF_{1\alpha}$ and TXB_2 are believed to reflect renal production of their parent compounds, PGI_2 and TXA_2, respectively. Drugs that selectively spare renal PES (such as low-dose aspirin) do not affect the urinary excretion of 6-keto $PGF_{1\alpha}$ or TXB_2, thus showing that urinary excretion is independent of extrarenal synthesis.[59] However, considerable amounts of 6-keto-$PGF_{1\alpha}$ and TXB_2 infused in the renal artery (32% and 13%, respectively) are recovered unmetabolized in the urine.[55] Hence, an increased systemic production of these compounds (e.g., in thromboembolic diseases) may be associated with higher urinary excretion rates.[60]

Measurements of urinary PGs give no information about their nephronal source. Furthermore, urinary PGs result predominantly from medullary synthesis, as confirmed by the observation that selective chemical destruction of rat renal papilla decreases urinary PG excretion by 75%. Therefore, it is possible that evaluation of urinary PGs fails to show changes in PG production by the cortical vasculature and glomeruli.[61]

Receptors and Intracellular Signals for PES Metabolites

Prostaglandin receptors are present at all of the diverse sites of action of PGs, including the vasculature, glomeruli, medullary thick limb, collecting tubules, and medullary interstitial cells. The number of distinct receptors that mediate PG actions explains the diversity of effects of prostanoids within the kidney. In general, PG receptors are named for the natural PG for which they have the greatest affinity. The PGE_2 receptor is presently the best characterized both biochemically and functionally. Particularly relevant for renal physiology is the existence of two classes of PGE_2 receptors (EP): EP_1, which has a similar affinity for $PGF_{2\alpha}$ and is linked to the activation of phospholipase C, and EP$_2$, which is linked to the activation of adenylate cyclase. As with all other PG receptors, these two classes of PGE$_2$ receptors are coupled to the above effector mechanisms through G proteins.[62] Specific receptors for PGI$_2$ (IP, linked to adenylate cyclase), PGF$_{2\alpha}$ (FP, linked to phospholipase C), and TXA$_2$ (TP, linked to phospholipase C) have been characterized more recently.

As a generalization, vasorelaxant PGs (PGE$_2$ and PGI$_2$) produce an increase in the intracellular levels of cyclic adenosine monophosphate (cAMP) through activation of adenylate cyclase, whereas vasoconstrictor eicosanoids have negligible effects on adenylate cyclase but stimulate phospholipase C to initiate contractile and mitogenic effects. In addition, TXA$_2$ is able to activate PLA$_2$, thus stimulating the release of AA. The increase in intracellular cAMP antagonizes glomerular and mesangial contraction induced by various agonists, including TXA$_2$ and angiotensin II. Activation of phospholipase C induced by TXA$_2$ and endoperoxide analogs (acting as stable mimetics of TXA$_2$) leads to a rapid increase in cytosolic calcium because of the effects of IP3 to mobilize calcium from intracellular stores.[61] Such observations, made by using stable analogs of PGE$_2$ and TXA$_2$, have been confirmed with selective receptor antagonists. Although receptor antagonists for PGF$_{2\alpha}$ are not currently available, the calcium and inositol phosphate responses induced by PGF$_{2\alpha}$ (at least in cultured mesangial cells) are quite similar to those induced by TXA$_2$.

Both PGE$_2$ receptors (EP1 and EP2) have been described in glomerular mesangial cells. The EP2 receptor, linked to adenylate cyclase, is the most represented. When the stimulatory effect on adenylate cyclase is blocked, unopposed activation of phospholipase C by PGE$_2$ results in cell contraction.[63] Because mesangial cells play a key role in the regulation of glomerular hemodynamics, the presence of both receptors may lead to a correct balance of the effects of PGE$_2$ at this level. Within the tubular epithelium, the major sites of action of PGs are in the ascending limb of Henle's loop and in the cortical and medullary collecting tubule. At this level, PGE$_2$ is the best-studied eicosanoid with regard to signaling and physiologic actions. At least two classes of PGE$_2$ receptors have been described in the collecting tubule and in the thick ascending limb of the loop of Henle.[64] Low concentrations of PGE$_2$ inhibit

AVP-stimulated water reabsorption by the collecting tubule and sodium chloride reabsorption by the thick ascending limb. These effects are due to the activation of a receptor linked to an inhibitory guanosine triphosphate (GTP)-binding protein (G$_i$) that leads to a reduction of intracellular levels of cAMP.[64] However, at higher concentrations, PGE$_2$ can activate a receptor that is linked to a stimulatory GTP-binding protein (G$_s$) and increases cAMP, thus enhancing water and sodium reabsorption.

Biologic Actions of PES Products in the Kidney

In agreement with their general physiologic role, the main function of renal PES products is to mediate or modulate the action of other hormones and autacoids involved in the regulation of renal vascular tone, mesangial and glomerular functions, and handling of salt and water. Indeed, inhibition of PES activity, in the absence of exogenous administration or endogenous release of hormones such as AII or AVP, has limited effects on renal function.[65,66] On the other hand, in certain pathophysiologic conditions, the increased local release of PES products may be directed either to compensate for the excess of hormonal vasoconstrictors (as in the case of vasodilatory PES products) or to mediate vasoconstriction during obstructive injury (as in the case of TXA$_2$).

Effects on Smooth Muscle and Mesangial Cell Function. A clearcut division of PES products into smooth-muscle relaxant (PGE$_2$ and PGI$_2$) and constrictor agents (TXA$_2$ and PGF$_{2\alpha}$) is supported by a large body of experimental evidence. These concepts also apply to the renal vasculature. The release of vasodilator PGs (PGE$_2$ and PGI$_2$) by smooth muscle and mesangial cells in response to renal vasoconstrictors such as AII, AVP, norepinephrine, PAF, and serotonin has relevant consequences for the preservation of renal perfusion and glomerular filtration in conditions characterized by an enhanced systemic or local release of these agents. In addition to modulating the actions of vasoconstrictors, endogenous PGs also mediate the actions of some vasodilator agents; for example, PGI$_2$ mediates the vasorelaxant actions of dopamine, magnesium, epidermal growth factor, and the renal vasodilatory response to a protein meal.

Effects on Renin Release. Renin release is regulated by different mechanisms, the most important of which are β–adrenergic control, renal baroreceptor mechanisms, and macula densa regulation. In vitro studies have clarified the role of PGs in the regulation of renin release. Kidney cortical slices stimulated with PGI_2 or PGE_2 show enhanced renin release.[67,68] The role of PGs is most apparent in the macula densa-regulated release of renin. In particular, stimulation of renin secretion by the macula densa mechanism, which depends on the extent of sodium chloride delivery to and reabsorption by the distal convoluted tubule, is inhibited by blocking PES activity.

Effects on Renal Blood Flow and Glomerular Filtration Rate. Despite the prominent vasodilatory actions of many PES products on the renal circulation, there is little evidence that basal renal eicosanoid synthesis plays a role in regulating either renal blood flow (RBF) or glomerular filtration rate (GFR). Accordingly, inhibition of renal PG synthesis up to 75% of normal does not alter RBF or GFR in dogs,[69,70] rats,[71,72] or humans.[71,73] However, in every condition characterized by an increased vasoconstrictor action of AII and catecholamines, inhibition of PES activity may lead to significant reduction of RBF. PGs are also not critical for renal autoregulation of RBF and GFR; PES inhibitors do not interfere with autoregulatory adjustments of renal vascular resistance following variations of renal perfusion pressure.[74–76]

Effects on Tubule Transport. PES products have important effects on salt and water transport through direct actions on the tubular epithelium. These functional effects are thought to be independent of any hemodynamic changes induced by PES products. The effects of PGs on sodium reabsorption in the proximal tubule seem negligible or minor.[77] In the medullary thick ascending limb of Henle's loop, both PGE_2 and PGI_2 inhibit sodium influx.[78,79] These compounds exert similar effects in the cortical and medullary collecting tubules. The inhibitory effect of PGE_2 on sodium reabsorption is probably due to the activation of a GTP-binding protein with consequent decrease of agonist-stimulated cAMP.[80,81] The effects of PGs on sodium reabsorption do not seem to be critical in every species, and studies using PES inhibitors have yielded conflicting results. The administration of indomethacin and aspirin in humans generally reduces urinary sodium excretion, and chronic administration of nonsteroidal antiinflammatory drugs (NSAIDs) results in edema in 5–10% of subjects.[82–84] However, these drugs inhibit PG synthesis also in the central nervous system and in the cardiovascular and endocrine systems, thus making difficult a precise interpretation of in vivo observations.[61]

Hormonally regulated water transport across the collecting duct appears to be a major process under the influence of PGs. Administration of intrarenal infusions of PGs causes a water diuresis and attenuates the hydroosmotic effects of AVP. Conversely, NSAIDs enhance the concentrating effects of AVP. Several in vivo studies[71,84,85] have suggested that PGs regulate both basal and AVP-stimulated water reabsorption. This effect appears related to the suppression of cAMP generation induced by AVP. In addition, studies of microdissected rabbit cortical collecting duct cells have shown that the inhibitory effect of PGE_2 can be reversed by pretreatment with pertussis toxin, suggesting the involvement of a pertussis toxin-sensitive G_i.

As already mentioned, there is abundant evidence that AVP and its analogs stimulate renal PG synthesis. Stimulation of the pressor AVP receptor V_1 acutely increases PG production by activating PLA_2. This effect is not elicited by acute stimulation of the V_2 (antidiuretic) receptor, whereas it is induced by chronic stimulation. Such observations are compatible with the hypothesis that AVP action is autoregulated by AVP-induced PGE_2 synthesis.

Renal Prostaglandins in Cirrhosis

Evidence of the major role of renal PGs in the regulation of renal hemodynamics and function in cirrhosis with ascites was first obtained by Boyer et al.,[86] who demonstrated that the administration of indomethacin to cirrhotic patients with ascites was followed by a reduction of effective renal plasma flow (RPF) and GFR and an increase in serum creatinine concentration. In another study, Zipser et al.[87] provided further evidence for the contention that cirrhotic patients with ascites have a PG-dependent renal function. In fact, the urinary excretion of immunoassayable PGE_2 was higher in 5 cirrhotic women with ascites than in 12 normal women, indicating an activation of the renal PG system. On the other hand, inhibition of the renal PG system with NSAIDs had deleterious effects on renal function of patients with cirrhosis.

Following such investigations, a large series of studies was performed to define the role of the renal PG system in different groups of cirrhotic

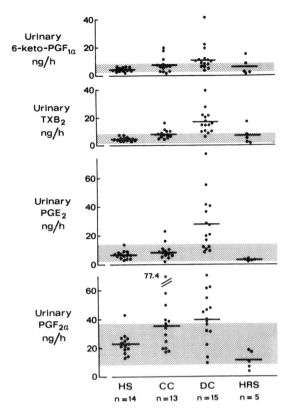

FIGURE 14.2. Urinary excretion rates of 6-keto-PGF$_{1\alpha}$, TXB$_2$, PGE$_2$, and PGF$_{2\alpha}$ in healthy subjects (HS), 13 patients with compensated cirrhosis (CC), 15 patients with decompensated cirrhosis (DC), and 5 patients with hepatorenal syndrome (HRS). *Stippled areas* indicate the normal range (mean ± SD). (From Laffi G, La Villa G, Pinzani M, et al: Altered renal and platelet arachidonic acid metabolism in cirrhosis. Gastroenterology 1986;90:274–282, with permission.)

patients, with and without ascites, and in animals with experimental cirrhosis. The following sections describe the results of these studies.

Measurements of Renal PES Derivatives

Compensated Cirrhosis. Cirrhotic patients without ascites excrete into urine greater amounts of PGE$_2$, PGF$_{2\alpha}$, 6-keto-PGF$_{1\alpha}$, and TXB$_2$ than healthy subjects,[88–93] indicating increased renal production of all major renal AA metabolites. In general, the excretion rates of AA metabolites in patients with compensated cirrhosis were comparable to rates observed in patients with ascites. In addition, analysis by gas chromatography/mass spectrometry (GC/MS) indicates that 6-keto-PGF$_{1\alpha}$ and TXB$_2$ are excreted into urine in greater amounts by patients with compensated

liver diseases than by healthy subjects.[94] As discussed below, patients with compensated liver disease also show an increased urinary excretion of 2,3-dinor derivatives of PGI$_2$ and TXA$_2$, which are indexes of the systemic production of the parent compounds.[94]

Studies based on the administration of NSAIDs confirmed that the integrity of the renal PG system contributes to the maintenance of renal function in patients with compensated cirrhosis. In fact, administration of NSAIDs to such patients usually induces a reversible impairment of renal function, as indicated by a decrease in RPF, GFR, urine flow rate, and urinary sodium excretion.[91,95]

Cirrhosis with Ascites. In cirrhotic patients with ascites but without renal failure, the urinary excretion of vasodilating PGE$_2$ and 6-keto-PGF$_{1\alpha}$ and vasoconstricting PGF$_{2\alpha}$ and TXB$_2$, as assessed by radioimmunoassay (RIA), is significantly higher than in healthy subjects[88–95] (Fig. 14.2). Such patients usually have high plasma renin activity (PRA) and high plasma concentrations of aldosterone, norepinephrine, and AVP, which are thought to be due to reduction of effective plasma volume.[96] The activation of these systems accounts for much of the increased renal PG synthesis, which in turn antagonizes the vasoconstricting effects of AII, norepinephrine, and AVP, thus contributing to the maintenance of renal hemodynamics and function. In fact, despite the striking activation of these systems, RPF and GFR are usually comparable to those of healthy subjects.

Inhibition of the renal PG synthesis removes the vasodilatory modulus and exaggerates the effects of constrictor agents. In fact, as discussed in greater detail below, administration of NSAIDs is accompanied by renal vasoconstriction, reduction of GFR, and, in some instances, transient acute renal failure similar to that of the hepatorenal syndrome (HRS). Within 24–48 hours after withdrawal of NSAIDs, renal function recovers completely, indicating that renal failure is related strictly to inhibition of renal PGs. Finally, HRS occurs in the setting of marked reduction in PGE$_2$ excretion together with an impressive increase in PRA and plasma norepinephrine levels (see below). Such data clearly indicate that renal function in cirrhosis depends on the integrity of the renal PG system.[97] In this respect, cirrhosis is comparable to other clinical conditions, such as renal ischemia, extracellular volume depletion, anesthesia, surgery, reduced cardiac output, and renal disease.[98] Common element to most of these

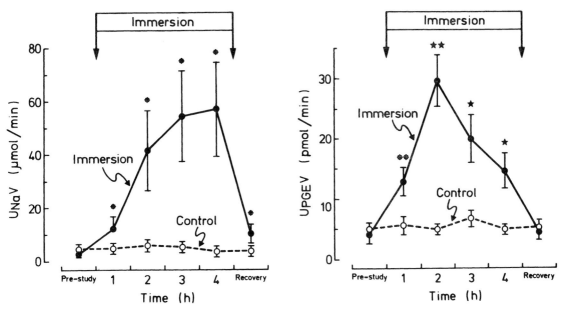

FIGURE 14.3. Effects of water immersion on the urinary excretion rats of sodium (*left panel*) and PGE$_2$ (*right panel*) in 13 cirrhotic patients (11 with ascites). * = p < 0.05. ** = p < 0.01; star = p < 0.005, 2 stars = p < 0.001. (From Epstein M, Lifschitz M, Ramachandran M, Rappaport K: Characterization of prostaglandin E responsiveness to decompensated cirrhosis: Implications for renal sodium handling. Clin Sci 1982;63: 555–563, with permission.)

conditions is reduction in effective circulating plasma volume, associated with activation of vasoconstricting systems, such as the RAA and sympathetic nervous systems, and nonosmotic secretion of AVP.[98]

Prostaglandins and Renal Sodium Handling in Cirrhosis

The role of renal PGs in the regulation of sodium excretion in cirrhosis is not yet completely defined. To explore the relationship between renal sodium handling and urinary PGE$_2$ excretion, Epstein et al.[99] submitted 13 cirrhotic patients (11 with unequivocal ascites) to head-out water immersion, a maneuver that redistributes blood volume, induces central hypervolemia, and enhances urinary PGE$_2$ excretion in healthy subjects (Fig. 14.3). Compared with the control phase, water immersion induced an 8-fold increase in mean urinary PGE$_2$ excretion, which was 3-fold higher than that observed in normal subjects under identical conditions. Water immersion also induced a wide continuum of natriuretic responses, characterized by either a sluggish or barely discernible natriuresis or appropriate or even exaggerated natriuresis. Of interest, a significant, direct relationship was observed between

urinary PGE$_2$ excretion and cumulative sodium excretion during immersion (r = 0.61, p < 0.05), suggesting that renal PGE$_2$ may be involved in the regulation of sodium excretion in cirrhosis.

A role for renal PGs in the regulation of renal sodium handling was also suggested by Lianos et al.,[100] who infused AII into 15 cirrhotic patients with ascites, at rates sufficient to increase systolic blood pressure by approximately 10–15 mmHg. AII infusion induced a variable natriuretic response in 7 patients, ranging from 9–2200% of the baseline value, whereas in the remaining 8 patients sodium excretion decreased by 18–88%. The natriuretic response was accompanied by an increase in PGE$_2$ excretion, which, however, decreased in patients in whom AII induced a reduction of sodium excretion. The latter patients tended to have higher baseline PGE$_2$ excretion rates. They also were more sensitive to the effects of PES inhibition and less sensitive to the pressor effects of AII. After partial inhibition of renal PG synthesis with indomethacin, natriuretic responses to AII were attenuated or reversed, and antinatriuretic responses accentuated. These results were interpreted as indicating that the sodium excretion pattern induced by an exogenous AII challenge in cirrhotic patients with ascites depends on the renal PG system and as supporting the hypothesis that renal PGs have a major role in regulating renal function in such patients.

A recent study by Wong et al.[95] in patients without ascites helped to clarify the mechanism involved in the regulation of renal sodium handling by PGE_2. Indomethacin caused a reduction in sodium excretion due to both a decrease in GFR (and thus in filtered sodium load) and an increase in tubular reabsorption, as indicated by the reduction of fractional sodium excretion. The lithium clearance technique indicated that the main site of increased sodium reabsorption was the proximal tubule.

Other studies, however, failed to show any relationship between urinary PGE_2 excretion and renal sodium handling. Rector[101] measured urinary PGE_2 in three groups of cirrhotic patients: (1) with negative sodium balance and no ascites; (2) with ascites and good responses to diuretics; and (3) with diuretic-resistant ascites. No differences were observed in the urinary excretion of PGE_2 among the three groups in baseline conditions. Moreover, intravenous furosemide was followed by similar changes in urinary PGE_2 excretion in both diuretic-responsive and diuretic-resistant patients.

Prostaglandins and Water Metabolism

Perez-Ayuso et al.[102] evaluated the ability to excrete water load in 27 patients with cirrhosis and ascites and in 10 healthy subjects. Plasma AVP levels and urinary excretion of PGE_2 were also evaluated. Cirrhotic patients with negative free water clearance in baseline conditions were also unable to dilute their urine further and to reduce plasma AVP after the water load, whereas in patients with positive free water clearance in basal condition the water load was followed by further dilution of urine and reduction in plasma AVP levels. However, plasma AVP levels after water load in the latter group were significantly higher than levels in healthy subjects. In other words, patients with positive free water clearance were able to dilute their urine despite higher than normal AVP levels. Urinary PGE_2 excretion significantly increased in such patients after water load, whereas it was unchanged in patients unable to dilute their urine. These results suggest that in patients with cirrhosis maintenance of water excretion despite high levels of AVP depends on renal synthesis of PGE_2, which counteracts the water-retaining effect of AVP. On the other hand, a reduced renal synthesis of PGE_2 may impair water excretion in cirrhotic patients with negative free water clearance.

The importance of renal PGs in modulating free water clearance was further outlined in other studies. Administration of demeclocycline (900 mg/day) caused a significant increase in free water clearance and serum sodium concentration in 7 of 9 patients with hyponatremia.[103] Demeclocycline was also associated with an increase in urinary PGE_2 excretion, suggesting that its beneficial effects were due, at least in part, to the stimulation of renal PGE_2 synthesis. Boyer et al.[86] observed that administration of indomethacin impaired free water clearance only in patients showing a greater than 15% decrease in RPF. This study, however, did not clarify whether the reduction in free water clearance was due to impairment of renal hemodynamics or to suppression of the antagonizing effect of PGE_2 on the tubular action of endogenous AVP.

Data by Perez-Ayuso et al.[102] provided further insights into the intrinsic mechanisms by which PGE_2 modulates renal water handling in cirrhosis. The administration of an intravenous bolus of lysine acetylsalicylate (450 mg, equivalent to 250 mg of acetylsalicylic acid) together with water load to 12 patients with cirrhosis and ascites led to impairment of renal hemodynamics in 50% of patients, whereas urinary PGE_2 excretion and free water clearance decreased in all patients. In 6 patients, therefore, the impairment in free water clearance induced by lysine acetylsalicylate was independent of changes in renal hemodynamics (Fig. 14.4). Because plasma AVP was unchanged in the patients studied, such results support the hypothesis that renal PGs modulate renal water handling by antagonizing the tubular action of endogenous AVP.

Experimental Models of Liver Diseases

Zambraski and Dunn[104] assessed urinary PG excretion in dogs with chronic bile duct ligation (CBDL), an experimental model of liver disease resembling secondary biliary cirrhosis. The authors observed increases of approximately 100%, 80%, and 500% in the urinary excretion of PGE_2, $PGF_{2\alpha}$, and 6-keto-$PGF_{1\alpha}$, respectively. Of interest, PG excretion was similar in both ascitic and nonascitic animals, indicating that renal PG system was activated in both groups. The administration of indomethacin reduced PG excretion in both sham operated and CBDL dogs, but only

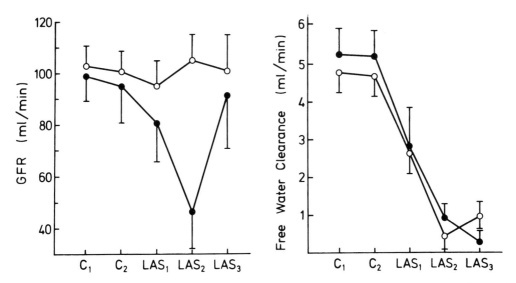

FIGURE 14.4. Glomerular filtration rate (*left panel*) and free water clearance (*right panel*) before and after the intravenous administration of 450 mg of lysine acetylsalicylate in 12 patients with cirrhosis and ascites. Patients are divided into two groups according to whether GFR decreased (*solid circles*) or did not decrease (*open circles*) after administration of the drug. Data are given as the mean ± SEM. C_1, C_2, LAS_1, LAS_2, and LAS_3 represent five 30-minute clearance periods before (C) and after (LAS) drug administration. (From Arroyo V, et al: Pathophysiology of ascites and functional renal failure in cirrhosis. J Hepatol 1988;6:239–257, with permission.)

the CBDL dogs experienced an increase in renal vascular resistance and a decrease in RPF and GFR. Such changes were of the same extent in ascitic and nonascitic animals. In CBDL dogs, mean arterial pressure, which was approximately 25% lower than in sham operated animals at baseline, significantly increased after indomethacin.

The critical role of PGs in maintaining renal function in CBDL dogs was confirmed in a study by Levy et al.,[105] who observed a marked decrease of RPF and GFR after indomethacin. When the development of portal hypertension was prevented by performing an end-to-side portacaval anastomosis at the time of bile duct ligation, indomethacin had no effects on renal perfusion independent of ascites. In contrast, prevention of ascites formation by LeVeen shunting did not modify the deleterious effects of indomethacin on RPF and GFR. Finally, administration of saralasin or captopril prevented the decline in RPF and GFR after indomethacin. The authors suggested that portal hypertension is an important factor mediating PG dependency of renal function in cirrhosis and that the mediation may be via nervous reflexes, which in turn may induce an activation of the RAA system.

The importance of the RAA system as a major stimulus for renal PG synthesis was outlined by

another experiment[106] in rats with CCl_4-induced cirrhosis, which showed a close chronologic relationship between urinary aldosterone excretion, sodium retention and the urinary excretion of 6-keto-$PGF_{1\alpha}$ and TXA_2. However, at difference with what occurs in human cirrhosis, in this study the urinary excretion of PGE_2 and $PGF_{2\alpha}$ was significantly lower in cirrhotic than in control animals.

Inhibition of PES Activity and Renal Function in Cirrhosis

NSAIDs are widely used to investigate the role of the renal PG system in regulating renal function and sodium and water excretion in humans and experimental animals, in both healthy and disease states, including cirrhosis. However, systemic administration of NSAIDs inhibits PG synthesis at both renal and extrarenal sites, including the central nervous system and the cardiovascular and endocrine systems. This may lead to changes in release of neurohypophyseal hormones, cardiac output and vascular resistance, and PRA and plasma concentrations of aldosterone and catecholamines, all of which may influence renal function.[61] Attribution of the effects of NSAIDs to the inhibition of PG synthesis within the kidney, therefore, may be misleading. On the other hand, recognition that NSAIDs may impair renal function in cirrhotic patients has major clinical importance because of their broad use.

As previously mentioned, inhibition of renal PG synthesis with NSAIDs induces no appreciable decline in renal hemodynamics or sodium and water excretion under ordinary circumstances, indicating that renal function does not depend on the integrity of the renal PG system. However, when effective blood volume is decreased and vasoconstrictor hormones are activated to maintain cardiovascular homeostasis (as in cirrhosis of the liver), renal function indeed depends on the integrity of renal PG synthesis and is therefore more susceptible to the effect of NSAIDs.

As indicated above, the first evidence of the deleterious effects of NSAIDs on renal function in cirrhotic patients with ascites was provided in 1979 by Boyer et al.[86] and Zipser et al.[87] Boyer et al. observed a 23% reduction in RPF, a 19% decrease in GFR ,and a 29% increase in serum creatinine following the administration of 50 mg of indomethacin every 6 hours for 1 day. Resting blood pressure and pulse rate slightly fell after indomethacin. Zipser et al.[87] observed that the reduction in creatinine clearance and the increase in serum creatinine induced by NSAIDs paralleled the decrease in urinary excretion of PGE_2. NSAIDs also reduced PRA and PAC, confirming that renal PGs stimulate renin release. Finally, NSAIDs increased the pressor effect of exogenous AII.

The impairment in renal hemodynamics following NSAID administration is extremely variable in patients with cirrhosis. In susceptible patients, as little as 25 or 50 mg of indomethacin reduced GFR by 90%, causing anuric renal failure. In all cases, renal impairment is reversible, lasting as long as the NSAIDs are administered. Within 24–48 hours after cessation of NSAIDs, renal perfusion returns to baseline levels, suggesting that renal impairment results from functional rather than anatomic changes.[86,87,107]

Several factors, including the degree of liver failure and the presence of sodium retention and ascites, may affect the renal response to NSAIDs, which is strictly related to the derangement of systemic and renal hemodynamics. Liver failure may affect the disposition of NSAIDs, thus representing an additional factor that interferes with drug activity. Most NSAIDs are tightly bound to albumin and have a small volume of distribution.

Because cirrhotic patients frequently have reduced serum albumin levels, the concentration of unbound drug may increase, as in case of azapropazone. Pharmacokinetic studies on naproxen, azapropazone, and sulindac indicate that clearance is reduced in patients with cirrhosis due to liver failure, leading to prolonged half life and increased nephrotoxicity.[108]

Several lines of evidence indicate that patients with ascites and avid sodium retention (and therefore with more pronounced reduction in effective plasma volume and more marked activation of vasoconstricting systems) show greater susceptibility to renal failure after NSAID administration.[86,87,109] In the study by Boyer et al.,[86] 12 of 15 patients with ascites but only 1 of 5 patients without ascites developed a decrease in RPF after indomethacin, and only ascitic patients submitted to low-sodium diet also showed a reduction of GFR. Furthermore, the decrease in RPF correlated inversely with 24-hour urinary sodium excretion. Zipser's group[87,109] clearly showed that the adverse effects of NSAIDs on RPF and GFR were especially marked in patients with sodium excretion lower than 1 mmol/day (Fig. 14.5). Susceptible patients also had greater PRA and plasma aldosterone concentration, together with higher urinary excretion of PGE_2, TXB_2, and 6-keto-$PGF_{1\alpha}$.[109] Kawasaki et al.[110] observed that survival was lower in patients with a greater than 15% decrease in GFR after indomethacin. Such patients had lower prothrombin times and albumin levels and greater prevalence of ascites, confirming that patients with more severe liver disease and ascites are more susceptible to the effect of NSAIDs.

The administration of diuretics and severe restriction of sodium intake may enhance the nephrotoxic effect of NSAIDs. Indeed, both procedures may favor a further reduction in effective plasma volume, thus activating the RAA and sympathetic nervous systems and secretion of AVP. Planas et al.[111] suggested that intravenous furosemide, which increases renal PG synthesis, may protect patients with cirrhosis and ascites from renal failure after acute administration of NSAIDs. Other studies, however, did not support this contention. In the study by Daskalopoulos et al.,[112] indomethacin reduced creatinine clearance from 99 ± 18 to 45 ± 10 ml/min in 9 patients with cirrhosis and ascites. After intravenous furosemide (80 mg), indomethacin still reduced GFR from 103 ± 28 to 59 ± 14 ml/min.

The deleterious effects of NSAIDs, although usually less severe, also have been observed in patients with compensated cirrhosis. Uemura et al. [91] administered indomethacin to 7 patients without ascites and 9 with ascites. Both groups developed a 35–40% decrement in RPF. In the ascitic group, this phenomenon was associated with a reduction in GFR and an increase in serum creatinine. Sodium excretion decreased in both compensated (from 99 ± 56 to 62 ± 43 mmol/day, mean $\pm$ SD) and decompensated (from 102 ± 28 to 59 ± 28 mmol/day) cirrhotic patients, but the difference was significant only in the ascitic group. PRA, AII, and aldosterone concentrations tended to decrease in both groups after indomethacin administration. In a more recent study, Wong et al.[95] administered a single oral dose of indomethacin to compensated patients with alcoholic cirrhosis. The drug induced 34% and 33% decreases in GFR and RPF, respectively, together with a concomitant 32% increase in renal vascular resistance. Urinary flow rate and sodium excretion also significantly decreased by 27 and 43%, respectively, whereas urine osmolality increased. All of these effects disappeared between 3 and 4 hours after drug administration. An interesting observation from this study is that the absolute and percentage decrease in GFR was greater in patients with the highest baseline values, suggesting that renal PGs may be important in the pathogenesis of the glomerular hyperfiltration sometimes observed in such patients. These data are consistent with the hypothesis that alterations of systemic and renal hemodynamics and renal function also occur in patients with compensated cirrhosis, as suggested by the peripheral vasodilation hypothesis of ascites formation.[96] Indeed, studies from our laboratory show that in cirrhotic patients with and without ascites GFR is reduced after converting enzyme inhibition with captopril at a dose (12.5 mg) that does not affect arterial pressure.[113]

NSAIDs have different intrinsic capacities to inhibit PES activity. Indomethacin has the greatest inhibiting potency among the NSAIDs; 1–4 doses of 50 mg each per day reduces GFR in almost all patients with cirrhosis and ascites.[86,87,107] Ibuprofen, naproxen, and aspirin are somewhat less potent inhibitors of renal PG synthesis. Indeed, the increase in sodium excretion after intravenous furosemide, which also depends on the integrity of the renal PG system, was reduced by 80% with indomethacin (100 mg), 50% with naproxen

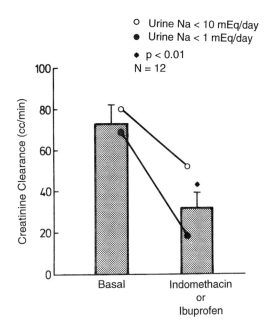

FIGURE 14.5. Effects of indomethacin or ibuprofen on creatinine clearance. Drug administration for 24 hours reduced creatinine clearance in all patients. The 7 patients with basal urine sodium less than 1 mEq/day had lower basal clearance and greater fall with drug administration than did the 5 subjects who excreted 1–10 mEq sodium/day. *Bars* represent mean $\pm$ SEM. (From Zipser RD, Hoefs JC, Speckart JF, et al: Prostaglandins: Modulators of renal function and pressor resistance in chronic liver disease. J Clin Endocrinol 1979;48:895–900, with permission.)

(500 mg), and 18% with oral acetylsalicylate (1800 mg)[114]

Sulindac (sulindac sulfoxide) was suggested to be qualitatively different from other NSAIDs because of its selective sparing of renal PES activity. Ciabattoni et al.[115] reported that sulindac did not reduce renal PG excretion in healthy women and patients with Bartter's syndrome, nor did it affect RPF, GFR, and urinary PG excretion in patients with chronic glomerulonephritis, who are susceptible to the nephrotoxic effects of ibuprofen. The sparing effect of sulindac on renal PG synthesis was related to its metabolic pathway.[108] Sulindac is a prodrug, lacking significant inhibitory activity for PES. After administration, sulindac sulfoxide is reduced, mainly in the liver, to sulindac sulfide, which inhibits PES and thus PG synthesis. Sulindac sulfide can be reoxidized to sulindac sulfoxide, which is eliminated either directly or as the further oxygenation product, sulindac sulfone. Unlike other NSAIDs, the active metabolite of sulindac does not appear in the urine after sulindac sulfoxide administration, whereas urinary excretion of sulindac sulfoxide and sulfone is significant. Therefore, it was suggested that sulindac does not impair renal PG synthesis because of the remarkable capacity of the kidney to inactivate sulindac sulfide and probably because the active metabolite is strongly bound to plasma proteins, thus escaping glomerular filtration.[115] However, further studies[116] in healthy subjects showed that sulindac blunts the increase in urinary PGE_2 excretion after administration of furosemide. In patients with underlying rheumatologic disease and mild reduction of renal function, an 11-day course with sulindac induced a significant reduction of urinary PGE_2 excretion together with a significant decrease in RPF and an increase in serum creatinine.[117]

Different studies addressed the effects of sulindac on the renal PG system and renal hemodynamics in animals with experimental cirrhosis and cirrhotic patients. Sulindac sulfide (5 mg/kg) was administered intravenously to 4 CBDL and 4 sham-operated dogs.[118] Both groups showed a 60–90% reduction in PGE_2, $PGF_{2\alpha}$, and 6-keto-$PGF_{1\alpha}$ excretion rates. In CBDL animals, the reduced urinary excretion of PGs was associated with a reduction in RPF, GFR, and urine volume, and greater amounts of sulindac sulfide were recovered in urine. Such findings indicate that the kidney, at least in CBDL animals, has a limited capacity to oxidize the sulfide to the sulfoxide form. Administration of sulindac sulfoxide to CBDL animals was followed by a substantial reduction in urinary PG excretion rates, GFR, and RBF. Furthermore, detectable levels of sulindac sulfide were found only in CBDL animals.

Daskalopoulos et al.[112] compared the effects of indomethacin and sulindac on baseline and furosemide-stimulated GFR, urine volume and urinary excretion of sodium and PGE_2. Unlike indomethacin, sulindac modified none of these parameters in baseline conditions. However, the drug was effective in reducing, although to a lesser extent than indomethacin, furosemide-stimulated diuresis (38% vs. 55%), natriuresis (52% vs. 67%; Fig. 14.6), and urinary PGE_2 excretion (74% vs. 81%). In a further study,[109] a 5-day course of sulindac (400 mg/day) significantly reduced the urinary excretion of PGE_2, TXB_2 and, to a lesser extent, 6-keto $PGF_{1\alpha}$, in 10 cirrhotic patients with ascites, but it did not impair renal hemodynamics (Fig. 14.7). Plasma levels of

sulindac sulfide were two-fold higher in cirrhotic patients (12 μmol/L) than in controls (5 μmol/L). Quintero et al.[119] reported that a 3-day course of sulindac (400 mg/day) in patients with cirrhosis and ascites reduced urinary excretion of PGE_2 by 84% and GFR by 40%. Of interest, plasma levels of sulindac sulfide were four-fold higher in cirrhotic patients than in controls (27 vs. 7 μmol/L). Such data indicate that, in the presence of liver failure, conversion of inactive prodrug (sulindac sulfoxide) to the active metabolite (sulindac sulfide) is delayed and that the active metabolite, once formed, has a very low biliary clearance that leads to cumulative higher plasma levels than in controls.[109] In cirrhotic patients, therefore, conventional doses of sulindac cause an evident reduction in urinary PG excretion. When high levels of active sulfide accumulate, a reduction in renal hemodynamics may also occur. Alterations of sulindac pharmacokinetics were also reported by Juhl et al.[120] in patients with alcoholic cirrhosis, who showed impaired conversion of sulfoxide to sulfide, delayed plasma peak concentration of active drug, and four-fold higher plasma levels of sulfide than healthy subjects. Available evidence, therefore, does not support the hypothesis that sulindac spares renal PG synthesis and renal function in cirrhosis.

Nonacetylated salicylates have a reduced ability to inhibit platelet, gastric, and possibly renal PES activity, although apparently retaining similar antiinflammatory activity. One study[121] compared the renal effects of oral indomethacin (50 mg) and diflunisal (1500 mg) in 9 patients with alcoholic cirrhosis and ascites in baseline conditions and after 80 mg of furosemide. Indomethacin reduced baseline GFR (from 91 ± 11 to 76 ± 11 ml/min) and blunted furosemide-stimulated diuresis and natriuresis. Diflunisal appreciably affected none of these parameters. The adverse effects of indomethacin on renal function were associated with a remarkably greater decrease in urinary PGE_2 excretion (50% vs. 10%), whereas both drugs caused a similar marked reduction of serum thromboxane levels (94% and 80%, respectively). Zambraski et al.[122] evaluated the effect of intravenous salicylic acid on renal function and urinary PG excretion in control and CBDL miniature swine. Salicylic acid did not significantly alter RPF or GFR in either normal or CBDL animals and caused a significant increase in diuresis and natriuresis in both groups. Surprisingly, urinary PGE_2 excretion decreased after salicylic acid in

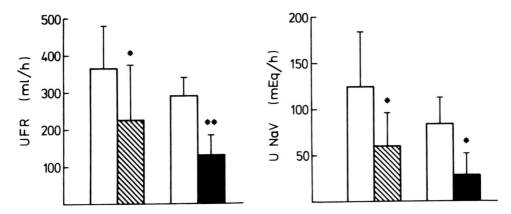

FIGURE 14.6. Effects of acute administration of sulindac or indomethacin on furosemide-induced changes in urine flow rate (UFR, *left panel*) and sodium excretion (UNaV, *right panel*) in patient with cirrhosis and ascites. Open bars = furosemide, dashed bars = furosemide + sulindac, solid bars = furosemide + indomethacin; * = p < 0.05, ** = p < 0.01 vs. furosemide alone. (From Daskalopoulos G, Kronborg I, Katkow W, et al: Sulindac and indomethacin suppress the diuretic action of furosemide in patients with cirrhosis and ascites: Evidence that sulindac affects renal prostaglandins. Am J Kidney Dis 1985;6:217–221, with permission.)

both groups. The mechanisms responsible for the diuretic and natriuretic effects of salicylate were not evaluated, nor was the drug investigated in human cirrhosis.

Recently, attention has focused on another NSAID, imidazole 2-hydroxybenzoate. In vitro and in vivo studies indicate that this drug does not affect synthesis of renal PGs but selectively inhibits synthesis of TXA_2.[123] The renal effects of imidazole 2-hydroxybenzoate were recently evaluated in cirrhotic patients with and without ascites in double-blind, cross-over studies.[124,125] Imidazole 2-hydroxybenzoate did not affect renal function or inhibit renal PG production in basal conditions, nor did it affect furosemide-stimulated diuresis and natriuresis in patients with ascites; however, serum TXB_2 levels were reduced. Further studies are needed to assess the effects of imidazole 2-hydroxybenzoate in patients with ascites, in comparison with NSAIDs known to impair renal function, and to ascertain its safety in patients with cirrhosis.[126]

Renal Prostaglandins and Diuretics

The intravenous administration of furosemide to healthy subjects enhances urinary PG excretion.[127] Studies on the effects of NSAIDs on furosemide-induced diuresis and natriuresis in healthy subjects yielded conflicting results. In fact, NSAIDs induced a 30% reduction of the natriuretic response in some studies, whereas in others no significant effect was observed.[59] Therefore, the

integrity of the renal PG system does not seem to determine effectiveness of furosemide in inducing diuresis and natriuresis in healthy subjects.[59]

In contrast, PGs are important for the effectiveness of loop diuretics in conditions of reduced effective blood volume, such as cirrhosis. Intravenous administration of furosemide to cirrhotic patients is followed by a variable increase in urinary PGE_2 excretion.[112] Although there is no clear relationship between the urinary excretion of PGs and the extent of furosemide-induced natriuresis,[101,128] studies with NSAIDs clearly indicate that diuretic effectiveness depends on an intact renal PG system. In fact, the administration of NSAIDs to cirrhotic patients invariably blunts the natriuretic and diuretic effect of furosemide[111,112,114] (see Fig. 14.6). As previously mentioned, the extent of the inhibition is related to the inhibitory potency of the drug on PES. The effects of intravenous acetylsalicylic acid on renal hemodynamics and the diuretic and natriuretic response to furosemide were investigated by Planas et al.[111] in 6 patients with cirrhosis and ascites. The effects of intravenous furosemide on GFR, RPF, urine volume, and sodium excretion were evaluated before and after the administration of lysine acetylsalicylate, which caused a marked reduction of furosemide-induced natriuresis and diuresis but did not significantly affect either GFR or RPF. Such results indicate that PGs are involved in the modulation of furosemide-induced diuresis and natriuresis

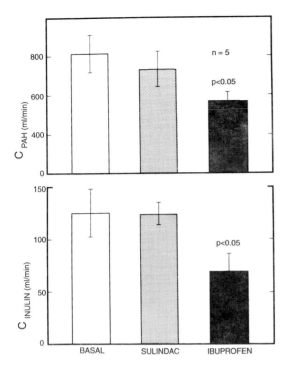

FIGURE 14.7. Effects of sulindac and ibuprofen on renal plasma flow (PAH clearance, *top*) and glomerular filtration rate (inulin clearance, *bottom*) in 5 patients with cirrhosis and ascites who developed a decrease in renal clearance during treatment with ibuprofen. (From Laffi G, Daskalopoulos G, Kronborg I, et al: Effects of sulindac and ibuprofen in patients with cirrhosis and ascites: An explanation for the renal-sparing effect of sulindac. Gastroenterology 1986;90:182–187, with permission.)

through a predominantly tubular effect. This view is supported by other studies showing that both sulindac[112] and acetylsalicylic acid[114] reduce natriuresis and diuresis in absence of significant changes in GFR. Prostaglandins are also involved in the natriuretic response to spironolactone,[114] which is markedly reduced by indomethacin (82%), naproxen (52%), and aspirin (33%).

Recent evidence favors a role for PGI_2 as a mediator of the diuretic and natriuretic effects of diuretics in cirrhosis. In one study,[129] the increase in urinary sodium excretion induced by spironolactone was strictly and significantly related to the urinary excretion of 6-keto-$PGF_{1\alpha}$, which significantly increased, whereas urinary PGE_2 and TXB_2 did not change. PGI_2 also may be involved in modulating the effects of diuretics on renal hemodynamics. Quiroga et al.[130] administered intravenous furosemide to 21 nonazotemic cirrhotic patients with ascites. In 15 (group A), furosemide induced an increase in GFR, whereas in the remaining 6 (group B) GFR decreased. Changes in GFR correlated with urinary excretion of 6-keto-$PGF_{1\alpha}$, which also increased in group A and decreased in group B. In contrast, urinary PGE_2 excretion increased to a similar extent in both groups. Furosemide-induced diuresis and natriuresis were also more evident in group A than in group B.

Thromboxane A_2 and Renal Function in Cirrhosis

Thromboxane A_2 is a potent vasoconstrictor that influences the tone of afferent and efferent arterioles as well as mesangial cell contraction, thereby affecting both RBF and GFR.[131] Moreover, TXA_2 may modify glomerular permeability to proteins and is a positive modulator of the antidiuretic effect of AVP.[132,133] Despite little evidence for a role of TXA_2 in the regulation of renal function in healthy subjects,[65] several reports indicate that it may be involved in the pathogenesis of certain renal diseases, such as renal allograft rejection,[134] relapsing minimal change nephrotic syndrome,[135] and systemic lupus erythematosus.[136]

Several groups showed that the urinary excretion of TXB_2, as measured by RIA, is increased in cirrhotic patients with ascites.[68,89,90,92] More recently, GC/MS analysis of TXB_2 and 2,3-dinor-TXB_2, indexes of renal and systemic production of TXA_2, respectively, has shown that urinary excretion of both compounds is higher in patients with ascites than in healthy subjects.[94] The augmented urinary excretion of TXB_2, at least in patients with ascites, seems to be related mainly to an increased renal synthesis of TXA_2: administration of low-dose aspirin caused a 90% decrease in serum TXB_2 levels during whole blood clotting, an index of platelet TXA_2 synthesis, without affecting urinary TXB_2 excretion[88] (Fig. 14.8).

The role of the increased renal TXA_2 production in determining the impairment of renal function in patients with cirrhosis and ascites is still unclear. We evaluated the effects of OKY 046, a TX-synthase inhibitor, in healthy subjects and cirrhotic patients with ascites in baseline conditions and after furosemide.[137,138] Selective TX-synthase inhibition resulted in a significant reduction of urinary TXB_2 excretion, ranging between 50% and 60% of control values in both groups, without appreciable change in PGE_2 and 6-keto-$PGF_{1\alpha}$ excretion (Fig. 14.9). This phenomenon

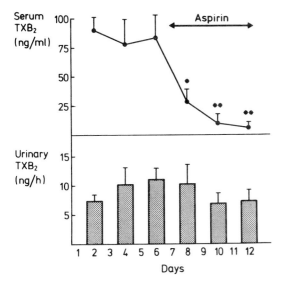

FIGURE 14.8. Effects of low-dose aspirin (0.45 mg/kg/day for 6 days) on platelet TXA_2 generation during whole blood clotting (as expressed by serum TXB_2 concentration) and urinary TXB2 excretion in 4 patients with compensated cirrhosis. * = $p < 0.05$, ** = $p < 0.02$ vs. baseline levels. (From Laffi G, La Villa G, Pinzani M, et al: Altered renal and platelet arachidonic acid metabolism in cirrhosis. Gastroenterology 1986;90;274–282, with permission.)

was associated with a significant increase in free water clearance after furosemide in both cirrhotics and controls (Fig. 14.10) and with an increment in furosemide-induced natriuresis in cirrhotic patients. Such data suggest that renal TXA_2 is involved in the regulation of water handling in healthy subjects and cirrhotic patients. An additional study, performed by administering ONO-3708, a TXA_2 antagonist, added further evidence to this contention.[139] A 4-hour infusion of ONO-3708 (3 µg/kg/min) was effective in blocking TXA_2 receptors; bleeding time increased two-fold, and platelet aggregation induced by U-46619, a TXA_2 analog, was blunted in all patients. ONO-3708 induced a significant increase in urine flow rate and free water clearance, together with a significant, although slight, increase in RPF. Available data do not allow definitive determination of whether TXA_2 influences water metabolism through a prevalent effect on renal hemodynamic or a positive modulation of AVP-dependent water reabsorption in the collecting duct. Nevertheless, the lack of correlations between changes in RPF and free water clearance during ONO administration suggests that the latter hypothesis is more likely.

Renal Prostaglandins in Hepatorenal Syndrome

Hepatorenal syndrome (HRS) is defined as unexplained, progressive renal failure in patients with liver disease but no known cause of renal failure. The main pathogenetic feature of HRS is reduced renal perfusion with preferential renal cortical ischemia.[140]

The marked alterations in renal hemodynamics may be related to both extreme activation of vasoconstricting and sodium-retaining factors (which in turn is the consequence of the striking reduction in effective plasma volume) and reduced production of vasoactive substances such as PGs, which help to maintain renal hemodynamics (see Fig. 14.2). Patients with acute alcoholic hepatitis who develop HRS were found to have very low urinary PGE_2 excretion compared

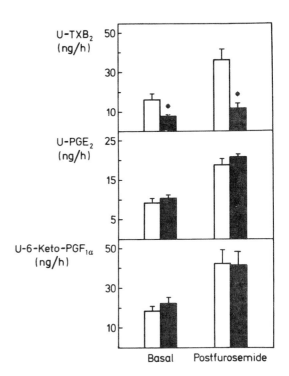

FIGURE 14.9. Basal and postfurosemide urinary (U) excretion of TXB_2, PGE_2, and 6-keto-$PGF_{1\alpha}$ before (day 1, *open bars*) and after (day 2, *solid bars*) oral administration of OKY 046, a TX-synthase inhibitor, in 8 cirrhotic patients with ascites (mean ± SEM). * = $p < 0.005$ vs. day 1. (From Pinzani M, Laffi G, Meacci E, et al: Intrarenal thromboxane A_2 generation reduces the furosemide-induced sodium and water diuresis in cirrhosis with ascites. Gastroenterology 1988;95:1081–1087, with permission.)

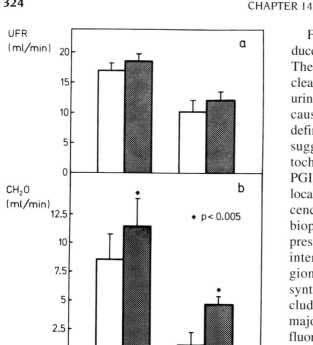

FIGURE 14.10. Furosemide-induced changes in urine flow rate (UFR, *panel a*) and free water clearance (CH_2O, *panel b*) in 8 healthy subjects (HS) and 8 cirrhotic patients with ascites (C) before (day 1, *open bars*) and after (day 2, *dotted bars*) oral administration of OKY 046, a TX-synthase inhibitor (mean ± SEM). (From Pinzani M, Laffi G, Meacci E, et al: Intrarenal thromboxane A_2 generation reduces the furosemide-induced sodium and water diuresis in cirrhosis with ascites. Gastroenterology 1988;95:1081–1087, with permission.)

with patients with acute renal failure and healthy subjects with reduced water intake and similar urinary flow rates.[141] Urinary excretion of the vasoconstrictor TXB_2 was increased in the same patients. In 3 patients who survived, progressive improvement of renal function was associated with a progressive decrease in urinary TXB_2 excretion. Such results led to the suggestion that an imbalance between vasoconstrictor and vasodilator AA metabolites, reflected by the increased ratio of TXB_2 to PGE_2, may be a relevant factor in the pathogenesis of HRS.[141] However, administration of dazoxiben, a TX-synthase inhibitor, failed to have any beneficial effect on renal function in patients with HRS,[142] despite an approximately 50% reduction in urinary TXB_2 excretion. It is possible, however, that greater availability of PG endoperoxides, due to inhibition of TXA_2 synthase, would mimic the renal effects of TXA_2.

Further studies confirmed the finding of reduced PGE_2 excretion in patients with HRS.[88,89,92] The pattern of 6-keto-PGF_{1\alpha}, however, is less clear; in fact, reduced, normal, or even increased urinary excretion has been observed.[88,89,94,143] The causes of reduced renal PGE_2 synthesis are not definitively assessed. A possible explanation was suggested by data obtained in an immunohistochemical study on renal medullary PGH and PGI_2 synthase expression.[24] Both enzymes were localized and semiquantitated by immunofluorescence in postmortem renal tissues obtained by biopsy or nephrectomy. PGI_2 synthase was expressed in peritubular capillaries, adjacent renal interstitial cells, and glomerular mesangial regions. Immunofluorescent staining for PGI_2 synthase was marked in all kidney samples, including those from 3 patients with HRS. The major site of PGH synthase-positive immunofluorescence was located in epithelial cells of the collecting tubule. A less intense staining was observed in cells of the thin ascending limb of the loop of Henle. No evidence for PGH staining was observed in patients with HRS, suggesting that reduced enzymatic activity in renal cells may contribute to impaired PGE_2 synthesis.

A study by Moore et al.[94] added further information about the role of altered systemic and renal production of TXB_2 and 6-keto-PGF_{1\alpha} in patients with HRS. The authors evaluated the renal and systemic synthesis of TXA_2 and PGI_2 by measuring the urinary excretion of TXB_2, 6-keto-PGF_{1\alpha}, and their 2,3-dinor-derivatives in patients with different degree of liver dysfunction and patients with HRS. The urinary excretion rate of all metabolites was markedly elevated during the early stages of HRS and decreased in parallel with creatinine clearance, suggesting that the excretion of these prostanoids depends on renal function. Both patients with severe liver failure but without renal failure and patients with HRS showed the highest urinary excretion of prostanoids of renal (TXB_2 and 6-keto-PGF_{1\alpha}) and extrarenal origin (2,3-dinor-6-oxo-PGF_{1\alpha} and 2,3-dinor-TXB_2) compared with healthy subjects and cirrhotic patients with and without ascites. After correction for creatinine clearance, there was a strong correlation between prostanoid excretion and serum bilirubin in patients with liver disease. Such results indicate that production of both PGI_2 and TXB_2 is increased in patients with severe liver disease, regardless of the presence of renal failure.

The above data confirm that cirrhotic patients with HRS have reduced renal production of vasodilating PGE_2, which may be involved in the pathogenesis of HRS. The relevance of the increased renal and extrarenal TXA_2 synthesis in the pathogenesis of HRS, if any, remains to be established. Available data also indicate that systemic synthesis of PGI_2 is increased in such patients. The pathophysiologic relevance of this observation is discussed below.

Altered Systemic Production and Metabolism of Prostacyclin

Patients with cirrhosis of the liver exhibit a characteristic circulatory disturbance, with high cardiac output and low vascular resistance.[96] In addition, they show reduced sensitivity to pressor hormones such as AII and norepinephrine, plasma levels of which are usually elevated in decompensated cirrhosis.[144]

Augmented synthesis and/or reduced catabolism of vasodilating substance(s) was proposed as a possible cause of the circulatory derangement of cirrhotic patients. The potential role of PGs in modulating vascular reactivity in cirrhotic patients was outlined by Zipser et al.,[87] who showed that indomethacin or ibuprofen, when administered to patients with cirrhosis and ascites, normalized the pressor response to AII.

In another study, the administration of indomethacin to cirrhotic patients with ascites induced a significant increase in peripheral vascular resistance and reduction of cardiac output, liver blood flow, and portal pressure.[145] The authors suggested that endogenous PGs may play a role in increased cardiac output and diminished vascular resistance. In addition, by promoting splanchnic vasodilation, PGs may contribute to increased portal pressure.

Increased systemic synthesis of PGI_2 may be involved in the alterations of systemic hemodynamics in cirrhotic patients. Guarner et al.[143] evaluated the urinary excretion rate of 2,3-dinor-6-keto-$PGF_{1\alpha}$, the major urinary metabolite of systemically produced PGI_2, in cirrhotic patients with and without ascites and in a group of patients with HRS. The urinary excretion rate of 2,3-dinor-6-keto-$PGF_{1\alpha}$ was significantly higher in all groups of patients, including those with HRS. Because patients with the highest urinary excretion of 2,3-dinor-6-keto-$PGF_{1\alpha}$ (> 230 pg/mg creatinine) had significantly lower blood pressure

and higher PRA and PAC, it was hypothesized that systemic PGI_2 production may contribute to alterations in systemic hemodynamics in patients with liver cirrhosis.[143] As reported above, the results the study by Guarner et al.[143] of urinary 2,3-dinor-6-keto-$PGF_{1\alpha}$ were confirmed by Moore et al.[94] with GC/MS.

Different hypotheses have been formulated to explain the increased systemic PGI_2 synthesis in cirrhosis. Hamilton et al.[146] studied rats with portal hypertension induced by partial ligation of the portal vein. After 1 week, the portal veins of the diseased rats released greater amounts of PGI_2 than portal veins of control rats. Moreover, a close correlation was observed between portal pressure and PGI-like activity, suggesting that the increased PGI_2 production may be an adaptive response to the increased pressure in portal endothelium. On the other hand, Guarner et al.[147] suggested that increased urinary excretion of 2,3-dinor-6-keto-$PGF_{1\alpha}$ was not related to portal hypertension but to substances released by intestinal bacteria that bypass the liver. In fact, the urinary excretion of 2,3-dinor-6-keto-$PGF_{1\alpha}$ was even higher in patients whose portal pressure had been reduced by portacaval shunting, whereas intestinal decontamination with nonabsorbable antibiotics resulted in significant reduction of urinary excretion.

Studies by Goerig et al.[148] lend further support to the contention that such factors are products of intestinal bacteria, such as endotoxin. The authors observed increased activity of PG synthases in different tissues after portacaval shunt in rats. Similar changes in synthase activity was also observed after intravenous infusion of endotoxin, suggesting that endotoxemia secondary to portacaval shunt may be the factor stimulating systemic production of PG.

The increased systemic synthesis of PGI_2 may have other implications in patients with advanced liver disease, who have complex alterations of coagulation, including reduced platelet number and function. In a recent study we observed that patients with reduced platelet aggregation also had high platelet levels of cAMP, the second messenger of PGI_2.[149] Increased endothelial production of PGI_2 may therefore be involved in both altered hemodynamics and reduced platelet function in cirrhotic patients.

On the other hand, the augmented urinary excretion of 2,3-dinor-6-keto-$PGF_{1\alpha}$ in cirrhotic patients may not be due to increased systemic production of PGI_2. Portosystemic shunting may lead to decreased hepatic metabolism of PGI_2, with reduced formation of omega-carboxy- and 15-keto-13,14-dihydro-derivatives of PGI_2, so that increased amounts are eliminated as 2,3,-dinor-6-keto-$PGF_{1\alpha}$.[150] Indeed, 10–16 ng/kg^{-1}/min^{-1} of PGI_2 are needed to induce vasodilation in healthy volunteers. Because the fractional excretion of PGI_2 as 2,3-dinor-6-keto-$PGF_{1\alpha}$ is 6.8%, the amount of endogenous PGI_2 required to cause systemic vasodilatation would result in a urinary excretion rate of 2,3-dinor-6-keto-$PGF_{1\alpha}$ between 3000 and 4500 ng/hr, which is 100-fold greater than that observed in decompensated liver disease (4–53 ng/hr).[19] Systemically produced PGI_2, therefore, does not seem to play a major role in mediating vasodilation in cirrhosis.[94]

Administration of Prostaglandins

Reduced renal synthesis of PGE_2 in the setting of marked activation of the RAA and sympathetic nervous systems and AVP hypersecretion is considered an important factor in the pathogenesis of HRS.[151,152] Therefore, several authors tried to restore intrarenal PG availability by oral or parenteral administration of exogenous PGs. This approach, however, suffers several limitations. PGs are local hormones and, following their intracellular synthesis, act on the parent or neighboring cells in an autocrine or paracrine fashion. Therefore, it is unlikely that administration of exogenous PGs restores impaired PG synthesis at cellular levels in different districts of the kidney. Exogenously administered PG may be rapidly degraded during passage through the pulmonary circulation, where 95% of infused PGE_2 is usually inactivated. Moreover, exogenous PGs may result in altered systemic hemodynamics and hypotension, that blunt their renal effects.

In 1972, Fichman et al.[153] infused PGA_1 into 6 cirrhotic patients with ascites and severe renal failure. Only 2 had a mild improvement in GFR, urine flow rate, and sodium excretion. Arieff and Chidsey[154] administered PGA_1 intravenously to 20 patients with cirrhosis and ascites. PGA_1 was effective in increasing RPF and GFR only in patients with relatively preserved renal function. Boyer et al.[86] infused PGA_1 (0.3 µg/kg/ min) into 13 cirrhotics patients with normal renal function. The infusion was effective in increasing RPF mainly in the group defined as nonresponders to indomethacin. When indomethacin was administered before PGA_1 infusion, RPF and GFR increased in both responders and nonresponders, although the effect was greater in responders. Zussman et al.[155] failed to reverse HRS with intrarenal administration of PGE_1. More recently, Gines et al.[156] confirmed that intravenous PGE_2 (0.5 µg/min for 1 hr, followed by 1 µg/min for another hour) does not improve GFR, free water clearance, or sodium excretion in cirrhotic patients with functional renal failure.

Fevery et al.[157] described reversal of HRS in 4 patients receiving the oral PGE_2 analog misoprostol (0.4 mg 4 times/day). During treatment there was a remarkable increase in urine flow rate, reduction in serum creatinine, and normalization of hyponatremia. Urinary sodium excretion increased from 0.4-3 to 15–40 mmol/24 hr in 2 patients and to 3–5 mmol/24 hr in the other 2 patients. Three patients, however, received albumin or other plasma expanders before and during misoprostol treatment. The possibility, therefore, that plasma expansion may account, at least partially, for the favorable effects on renal function cannot be ruled out. Indeed, these results were not confirmed by Gines et al.,[158] who administered misoprostol (0.2 mg every 6 hours for 4 days) to cirrhotic patients with functional renal failure without observing appreciable changes in GFR, sodium excretion, free water clearance, or natriuretic response to intravenous furosemide. Considering these results, administration of exogenous prostaglandins seems to have no substantial role in ameliorating renal function in patients with functional renal failure.

Exogenous PGs were also administered in an attempt to prevent the deleterious effect of NSAIDs on renal function in cirrhotic patients. In a double-blind, cross-over study, 10 patients with cirrhosis and ascites received indomethacin together with either misoprostol or placebo.[158] Misoprostol was somewhat effective in preventing the indomethacin-induced fall in sodium excretion at 4 hours, but urinary sodium fell to the levels observed in control groups after 8 hours. Indomethacin reduced the 4-hour creatinine clearance by 49% and misoprostol plus indomethacin by 34%. In another study, oral misoprostol prevented the deleterious effects of indomethacin on renal hemodynamics in a series of cirrhotic patients without ascites.[159]

Dietary Manipulations

Under normal conditions the liver has a central role in regulating the synthesis and metabolism of lipids. Advanced liver diseases are therefore associated with severe alterations of total and esterified plasma cholesterol, apolipoproteins, phospholipids and constitutive fatty acids of phospholipids, cholesterol esters, and plasma membranes.[160,161] A key factor in lipid metabolism is lecithin-cholesterol acyltransferase (LCAT), an enzyme synthesized in the liver and secreted into the circulation. LCAT catalyzes the transfer of a long chain fatty acyl group from the 2-position of lecithin to the 3-β-hydroxyl group of cholesterol, forming cholesterol esters and lysolecithin. Reduced activity of LCAT results in profound alterations in the composition of lipoproteins, including accumulation of cholesterol and lecithin. The molar ratios of cholesterol to phospholipid and lecithin to sphingomyelin are therefore increased. Cholesterol and phospholipid molecules on the surface of lipoproteins tend to exchange and equilibrate with their counterparts in lipoproteins of different density classes and also with molecules in cell plasma membranes. Therefore, alteration in lipid composition of the lipoprotein surface, as in advanced liver diseases, results in corresponding changes in the lipid composition of cell membranes.[160] Profound alterations of fatty acid composition in plasma phospholipids and plasma membranes have also been reported.[160,161] Monosaturated fatty acids are increased, whereas polyunsaturated fatty acids are significantly decreased, particularly AA.[161,162] The reasons for the deficiency in plasma AA are unclear. AA is a minor component of the diet and in humans derives almost completely from dietary linoleic acid. The ratio of linoleic to AA in patients with liver disease is elevated, indicating impaired conversion of linoleic to AA by the liver.[163] It has been suggested that the liver is a major source of AA for other organs and tissues, exporting it in the phospholipids of lipoproteins. Thus a decreased hepatic conversion of linoleic to AA probably explains much of the AA deficiency in severe chronic liver disease; reduced dietary content and impaired absorption of linoleic acid may also be contributory factors.

Reduced AA content has been observed in circulating cells such as platelets[162] and erythrocytes[164] from cirrhotic patients and also in brush border membranes from kidney epithelial cells of rats with biliary obstruction[165]; when the renal content in AA falls below a critical level, substrate deficiency may limit PG synthesis.

On the other hand, PG synthesis may also be reduced by profound alterations of plasma membranes in cirrhotic patients. Imai et al.[166] analyzed the lipid composition of highly purified renal cortical brush border membranes obtained from BDL rats. The cholesterol/phospholipid ratio was significantly increased 3 days after bile duct ligation and remained elevated after 15 days. Such alterations, together with reduced content of polyunsaturated fatty acids, modify the physicochemical characteristics of plasma membranes, leading to decreased fluidity and therefore impairing both receptor-agonist interaction and consequent signal-transduction mechanisms. Under such conditions, mobilization of AA and consequent PG synthesis in response to different stimuli may be reduced.[160,166]

Administration of precursors of AA may be beneficial, because they may either restore the AA content of plasma membranes or correct the altered ratio between polyunsaturated and monosaturated fatty acids. Epstein et al.[167] administered an 8-hour infusion of a 10% emulsion of safflower oil containing about 77% linoleic acid to 6 healthy subjects, in a dose of 1.5 gm/kg body weight. This treatment induced a profound increase in immunoassayable 6-keto-PGF$_{1\alpha}$, whereas the increase in PGE$_2$ was less noticeable. Rimola et al.[168] evaluated the effect of acute intravenous infusion of 10% Intralipid (an emulsion of soya bean oil containing more than 50% of linoleic acid) on urinary PG excretion and renal function in 7 patients with cirrhosis and HRS. The infusion induced an increase in serum linoleic acid but did not affect serum AA, urinary excretion of PGE$_2$, TXB$_2$, and 6-keto-PGF$_{1\alpha}$, or renal function. Such results, however, do not definitively rule out a role for dietary manipulation in liver diseases. In fact, more prolonged administration of linoleic acid may be effective in ameliorating the defect. Moreover, because defective hepatic delta-6-desaturase activity may preclude the conversion of linoleic to linolenic acid, the administration of other precursors, such as linolenic or AA, may be more effective.

LEUKOTRIENES

Biochemical and Physiologic Aspects

Leukotrienes (LTs) B$_4$, D$_4$, and E$_4$ are biologically active AA derivatives via the 5-lipooxygenase pathway.[169,170] Synthesis of LTs first requires

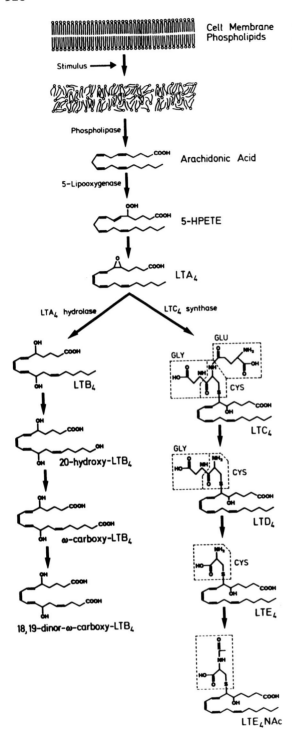

FIGURE 14.11. Arachidonic acid metabolism via the lipooxygenase pathway.

5-lipooxygenase (Fig. 14.11). The same enzyme catalyzes the conversion of 5-HPETE to the labile 5,6-epoxide LTA_4. This compound may be further metabolized in two pathways:

1. LTA_4 is converted to LTB_4 by LTA_4 hydrolase. Unlike 5-lipooxygenase, which is selectively distributed within myeloid cells, LTA_4 hydrolase has a wider distribution. LTB_4 therefore is produced by at least three routes: (1) enzymatic conversion of LTA_4 in the same cell in which LTA_4 is produced by 5-lipooxygenase activity; (2) enzymatic conversion of LTA_4 in another cell after export from the cell of origin (transcellular metabolism); and (3) nonenzymatic hydrolysis of LTA_4 to the inactive 6-trans-LTB_4 and 12-epi-LTB_4 stereoisomers after release in the extracellular space.

2. LTA_4 is converted to LTC_4 by conjugation with reduced glutathione at carbon atom 6; this reaction is catalyzed by LTC_4 synthase, a microsomal enzyme of the glutathione-S-transferase family. LTC_4 synthase is also widely distributed in tissues; thus transcellular metabolism is probably a major pathway of LTC_4 production.

Peptidolytic metabolism of LTC_4 yields the other active compounds of the LT family: (1) LTD_4, obtained through removal of glutamic acid by β-glutamyl transpeptidase activity, and (2) LTE_4, which derives from cleavage of LTD_4 with the release of glycine, a reaction catalyzed by several dipeptidases. LTC_4, D_4, and E_4 represent the biologically active constituents of the so-called slow-reacting substance of anaphylaxis.

Unlike PGs, which are widely produced in the body, LTs are synthesized by a limited number of cell types, which express the enzyme activities for the 5-lipooxygenase pathway. These cell types mainly include circulating leukocytes and fixed cells of the macrophage system.[170] Isolated glomeruli and mesangial cells have been reported to produce small amounts of 5-HETE, LTB_4, LTC_4, and LTE_4. Of course, intrarenal LT production may also occur, at least in pathophysiologic conditions, by invading polymorphonuclear cells and monocyte/macrophages. Furthermore, renal tissue contains LTA_4 hydrolase and therefore may generate LTB_4 from LTA_4 produced locally by invading leukocytes.

Circulating LTs have a short half-life (30–60 seconds) in most species. The liver and the kidney are the main organs responsible for rapid clearance of LTs. Hepatobiliary elimination predominates over renal excretion in all species

the release of free AA from cell membranes, usually by action of phospholipase A_2. Free AA is thus converted to 5S-hydroperoxy-6,8-trans-11,14-cis-eicosatetraenoic acid (5-HPETE) by investigated so far; however, the relative contribution of renal excretion is greater in primates than in rats. One hour after intravenous administration of labeled LTC_4 in rats, about 80% of the radioactivity is recovered from bile and only 1.5% from urine. In the monkey *Macaca fascicularis*, about 40% of administered ^3H-LTC_4 is recovered as metabolites in bile and about 20% in urine within 5 hours. Following hepatic uptake, LTs undergo partial metabolism and are excreted in the bile. Enterohepatic circulation of these compound has been reported, but this phenomenon is of minor importance, at least in physiologic conditions.

Impairment of hepatic uptake and biliary elimination of LTs results in an increase in plasma levels and renal excretion, as observed in a mutant strain of rats with a hereditary defect of hepatobiliary elimination of conjugated bilirubin, dibromosulfonphthalein, and ouabain. More importantly, hepatobiliary elimination of LTs is reduced in intra-and extrahepatic cholestasis and in rats receiving endotoxin, which also stimulates LT release.[169]

The biologic actions of LTs are mediated by distinct receptors. The signal transduction pathway for both LTB_4 and LTD_4 receptors is modulated by guanine nucleotide-binding proteins (G-proteins) and involves phospholipase C, a transient increase in intracellular calcium, and activation of protein kinase C. LTs are released in response to several different stimuli; therefore, abnormal synthesis of LTs has been suggested to have a role in allergic and inflammatory diseases. LTB_4 is a potent chemotactic agent for polymorphonuclear leukocytes, eosinophils, and monocytes. At higher concentrations, it stimulates aggregation and promotes degranulation and generation of superoxide anion. This compound also has an immunoregulatory effect on T cells. The cysteinyl LTs (relative potencies: $LTD_4 > LTC_4 > LTE_4 >$ N-acetyl-LTE_4) contract respiratory, vascular, and intestinal smooth muscles and may increase vascular permeability. In particular, LTC_4 and LTD_4 are powerful bronchoconstrictors, acting principally on smooth muscle in peripheral airways. In humans, LTC_4 and LTD_4 cause hypotension, perhaps due in part to decrease in intravascular volume and cardiac contractility secondary to LT-induced reduction in coronary blood flow.

In the kidney, LTC_4 and LTD_4 have a marked vasoconstricting effect, especially on efferent arterioles, and depress RPF, GFR, and the ultrafiltration coefficient (K_f). Depression of K_f is due mainly to the receptor-mediated contraction of mesangial cells. LTs also elicit mitogenic responses in mesangial and glomerular epithelial cells of rats and humans. Little evidence suggests that LTs may be involved in the regulation of epithelial cell transport processes, thus influencing sodium and water excretion.

Experimental data suggest that LTD_4 synthesis and release by polymorphonuclear and other infiltrating cells may be involved in the reduction of GFR and K_f in the early phases of nephrotoxic serum nephritis, whereas LTB_4 may contribute to the amplification of functional and histologic damage through its chemoattractant and activating effects on inflammatory cells.

The short half-life of circulating LTs, together with the possibility of artifactual LT production during blood sampling, precludes reliable measurement under most circumstances. Determination of levels in bile, when available, and urine is therefore the method of choice to assess the systemic production of LTs in physiologic and pathophysiologic conditions.

Leukotrienes and the Hepatorenal Syndrome

Two studies have investigated the urinary excretion of LTs in patients with cirrhosis and HRS. Huber et al.[171] found that patients with HRS had higher urinary excretion rates of LTE_4, the major metabolite of LTC_4 and D_4, than healthy subjects, patients with noncirrhotic renal failure, and cirrhotic patients without HRS. Cirrhotic patients without HRS had a slight increase in LTE_4 excretion compared with healthy subjects. Furthermore, N-acetyl-LTE_4 was detected only in the urine of patients with HRS. Similar results were obtained by Moore et al.,[172] who found that urinary LTE_4 excretion, corrected for creatinine clearance, was remarkably higher in patients with HRS than in healthy subjects and patients with compensated and decompensated cirrhosis, severe liver dysfunction and chronic renal failure. The investigators also evaluated the endogenous metabolism of LTs by infusing ^3H-LTC_4 into 2 healthy subjects and 1 patient with HRS; they observed that renal clearance of LTE_4 was reduced in HRS. This observation, together with increased urinary excretion of LTE_4, was interpreted as suggesting increased LT production in HRS. The pathogenetic relevance of such observations remains unclear.

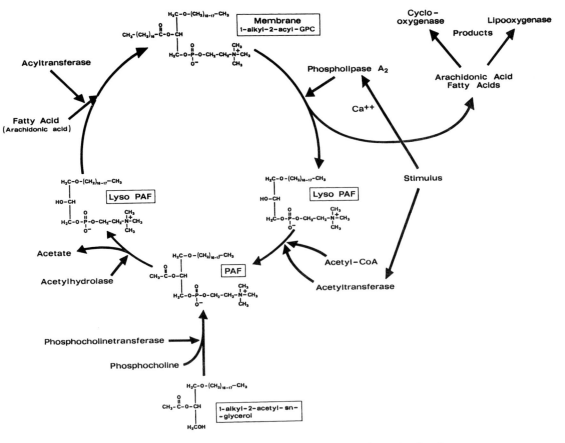

FIGURE 14.12.   Synthesis and metabolism of platelet activating factor.

PLATELET ACTIVATING FACTOR

Biochemical and Physiologic Aspects

Platelet-activating factor (PAF) has the basic structure 1-O-alkyl-2-acetyl-sn-glycero-3-phosphocholine.[9,73] The alkyl group in position 1 varies in length from 12 to 18 carbon atoms. In human polymorphonuclear cells, PAF consists predominantly of a mixture of the 16- and 18-carbon ethers. Like PGs, PAF is not stored in cells but synthesized only upon activation. This synthetic route is known as the remodeling pathway (Fig. 14.12). The first step is activation of phospholipase A_2, which catalyzes the hydrolysis of the sn-2 fatty acyl residue from alkyl choline phosphoglycerides to yield an intermediate compound, 1-O-alkyl-sn-glycero-3-phosphocholine (lyso-PAF), and a free fatty acid, usually AA. Several cell types producing PAF in response to appropriate stimuli also synthesize AA derivatives under the same circumstances. In the next step lyso-PAF is converted to PAF by the addition of acetate, a reaction catalyzed by the enzyme acetyl-coenzyme A:lyso-PAF acetyl-transferase. A second route to PAF, the de novo pathway, involves the synthesis of 1-O-alkyl-2-acetyl-sn-glycerol, which is then converted to PAF by CDP-choline:1-alkyl-2-acetyl-sn-glycerol choline-phosphotransferase. This pathway is analogous to phosphatidylcholine synthesis, but the enzymes are specific for the appropriate precursors. The remodeling pathway does not require de novo protein synthesis, and the rapidity of its onset indicates direct enzyme activation, which may involve a phosphorylation step. It has been suggested that the de novo pathway serves to produce a small amount of PAF constitutively in the kidney, which has a tonic effect on blood pressure and other physiologic responses.

Many cell types are able to synthesize PAF, including platelets, neutrophils, monocytes, mast cells, and vascular endothelial cells. Some cells, such as platelets and neutrophils, not only produce PAF but also are targets for PAF activation. PAF was originally described as a soluble factor in blood; thus it is evident that in some instances

PAF is released in the bloodstream. However, PAF synthesized by endothelial cells is not secreted. We recently found that stimulated polymorphonuclear cells obtained from healthy subjects and cirrhotic patients secrete less than 5% of synthesized PAF, whereas more than 90% remains within the cells.[174] Such findings have led to the suggestion that PAF may sometimes act as an intracellular messenger. According to another hypothesis, PAF acts on the surface of the cells as an intercellular messenger. Such a role has been described in endothelial cells and neutrophils. In endothelial cells, a substantial fraction of PAF is located on the surface and mediates the adhesion of circulating cells, such as neutrophils, on the endothelium.[9,173] PAF is degraded to the inactive lyso-PAF by a PAF acetylhydrolase that is highly specific for phospholipids with short acyl chains at the sn-2-position; this enzyme is present in plasma and various cells and tissues. Lyso-PAF is then converted to a 1-O-alkyl-2-acyl-glycerophosphocholine by an acyltransferase.

Platelet-activating factor regulates both physiologic events and pathologic responses, particularly in inflammation and allergy.[9,173] In fact, it is a potent aggregating agent and chemotactic factor for polymorphonuclear cells, monocytes, and macrophages. It stimulates the release of LTs and lysosomal enzymes and the generation of superoxide anion in polymorphonuclear cells. In addition to activation of circulating cells, PAF has a wide range of effects on the cardiovascular system[9] and kidney.[175] The infusion of PAF into animals induces hypotension through various factors ,such as decrease in cardiac output, reduction of resistance in some vascular beds, and decrement in circulating blood volume secondary to peripheral pooling and marked extravasation. Unilateral infusion of PAF into the renal artery of anesthetized dogs causes a dose-dependent decrease in RPF and an even more marked decline in GFR, urinary flow rate, and sodium excretion. The effects of PAF on renal function are potentiated by indomethacin.[175]

Platelet-activating Factor in Cirrhosis

Few studies have investigated the behavior of PAF in cirrhosis. Caramelo et al.[176] measured acetylhydrolase activity and PAF levels in blood and ascitic fluid from cirrhotic patients. The highest levels of circulating PAF were found in decompensated cirrhotic patients, whereas compensated patients showed values intermediate between those of patients with decompensated cirrhosis and controls. PAF levels in ascitic fluid were similar to levels in blood. Values of acetylhydrolase in serum were similar in all groups. The authors suggested that the high plasma levels of PAF were due to enhanced production rather than decreased catabolism. They also speculated that the high levels of PAF may be of pathogenetic relevance in the derangement of systemic and renal hemodynamics in cirrhotic patients.

Measurement of circulating levels of PAF has limited value, because PAF is an autacoid and therefore exerts its actions in autocrine and paracrine manners. Moreover, as reported above, PAF is thought to act as intracellular and/or intercellular messenger; therefore, only a minimal amount is secreted outside the cell. Results obtained by administration of selective PAF antagonists to animals with experimental cirrhosis gave more consistent evidence of the potential role of PAF in cirrhosis. Villamediana et al.[177] showed that rats with carbon tetrachloride-induced cirrhosis developed hyperdynamic circulation, with enhanced cardiac output, decreased mean arterial pressure and peripheral vascular resistance, and increased vascular permeability. The cirrhotic rats also had higher levels of circulating PAF than controls. Of greater interest, intravenous injection of BN 52021, a PAF antagonist, induced a decrease in cardiac output and an increase in peripheral vascular resistance. Arterial pressure increased slightly but not significantly. In another study, Kleber et al.[178] infused PAF into cirrhotic rats and observed an increase in heart rate and a decrease in arterial pressure, cardiac index, and RPF, whereas total peripheral resistance was unchanged. PAF had no significant effect on portal tributary blood flow. The authors also observed that two different PAF antagonists prevented the reduction in RPF induced by endotoxins.

In combination, such data suggest that an abnormal PAF synthesis may be involved in the derangement of systemic and renal hemodynamics in cirrhotic patients.

CYTOCHROME P-450 METABOLITES OF ARACHIDONIC ACID

A cytochrome P-450–dependent monooxygenase system identified in mammalian kidney catalyzes the enzymatic transformation of AA via (1) allylic oxidation, which leads to formation of

12- or 15-HETE; (2) olefin epoxidation, which leads to formation of 5,6-, 8,9-, 11,12-, and 14,15-epoxides (the epoxyeicosatrienoic acids [EETs]); and and omega or omega^{-1} oxidation, which leads to formation of 20-HETE and 19-HETE, respectively.[131,179] EETs can be hydrated to their corresponding vicinal diols, the dihydroxy-eicosatetraenoic acids (DHTs). This pathway for AA metabolism has been demonstrated in renal cortical and medullary tissue of several species, and P-450 AA derivatives have been found in human urine. Like PES derivatives, these compounds are believed to modulate cellular activity, and their effects are usually confined to the local environment of the cell of origin. To date, a role for renal cytochrome P-450 derivatives of AA has been postulated in the control of salt and water transport, in the regulation of Na-K-ATPase activity, and in the pathogenesis of hypertension.[179]

Cytochrome P-450–dependent metabolism of arachidonic acid was investigated by incubating isolated microsomes from the renal cortex and medulla of rats with experimental cirrhosis (both with and without ascites) and control rats, with ^{14}C-AA.[180] The conversion of labeled AA to cytochrome P-450–dependent metabolites was significantly reduced in the cortex and outer medulla of cirrhotic rats. HPLC separation of metabolites showed that this phenomenon was due mainly to reduced synthesis of a substance comigrating with 11,12-epoxieicosatrienoic acid. More recently, Muredach et al.[181] found increased urinary excretion of 5,6-epoxy-eicosatrienoic acid in a group of patients with cirrhosis and ascites. The pathophysiologic implications of these finding are still unknown.

Acknowledgments. Much of the authors' research reported in this chapter was supported by grants from the Italian Liver Foundation and the Italian Ministero per l'Università e la Ricerca Scientifica e Tecnologica.

REFERENCES

1. Balsinde J, Diez E, Mollinedo F: Arachidonic acid release from diacyl-glycerol in human neutrophils. J Biol Chem 1991;266:15638–15643.
2. Gronich JH, Bonventre JV, Nemenoff RA: Purification of a high-molecular-mass form of phospholipase A$_2$ from rat kidney activated at physiological calcium concentrations. Biochem J 1990;271:37–43.
3. Smith WL: Prostanoid biosynthesis and mechanisms of action. Am J Physiol 1992;263:F181–F191.
4. Morrison AR: Biochemistry and pharmacology of renal arachidonic acid metabolism. Am J Med 1986;80 (Suppl 1A):3–11.
5. Dennis EA, Rhee SG, Billah MM, Hannun YA: Role of phospholipases in generating lipid second messengers in signal transduction. FASEB J 1991;5:2068–2077.
6. Schlondorff D, Perez J, Satriano JA: Differential stimulation of PGE$_2$ synthesis in mesangial cells by angiotensin and A23187. Am J Physiol 1982;248:C119–C126.
7. Smith WL, Marnett LJ, DeWitt DL: Prostaglandin and thromboxane biosynthesis. Pharmacol Ther 1991;49:153–179.
8. Habenicht AJR, Salbach P, Goerig M, et al: The LDL receptor pathway delivers arachidonic acid for eicosanoid formation in cells stimulated by platelet derived growth factor. Nature (London) 1990;345:634–636.
9. Campbell WB: Lipid-derived autacoids: Eicosanoids and platelet-activating factor. In Goodman Gilman A, Rall TW, Nies AS, Taylor P (eds): The Pharmacological Basis of Therapeutics, 8th ed. New York: Pergamon Press, 1990;600–617.
10. Marshall PJ, Kulmacz RJ: Prostaglandin H synthase: Distinct binding sites for cyclooxygenase and peroxidase substrates. Arch Biochem Biophys 1988;266:162–170.
11. Mizuno K, Yamamoto S, Lands WEM: Effects of nonsteroidal anti-inflammatory drugs on fatty acid cyclooxygenase and prostaglandin hydroperoxidase activity. Prostaglandins 1982;23:743–757.
12. Kuchinke W, Barski O, Watanabe K, Hayaishi O: A lung type prostaglandin F synthase is expressed in bovine liver: cDNA sequence and expression in E. Coli. Biochem Biophys Res Commun 1992;183:1238–1246.
13. Bonvalet JP, Pradelles P, Farman N: Segmental synthesis and actions of prostaglandins (PGs) along the nephron. Am J Physiol 1987; 253:F377–F387.
14. Smith WL, Bell TG: Immunohistochemical localization of the prostaglandin-forming cyclooxygenase in renal cortex. Am J Physiol 1978;235:F451–457.
15. Farman N, Pradelles P, Bonvalet JP: Determination of prostaglandin E$_2$ synthesis along rabbit nephron by enzyme immunoassay. Am J Physiol 1986;251:F238–F244.
16. Farman N, Pradelles P, Bonvalet JP: PGE$_2$, PGF$_{2\alpha}$, 6-keto-PGF$_{1\alpha}$, and TXB$_2$ synthesis along the rabbit nephron. Am J Physiol 1987;252:F53–F59.
17. Pfeilschifter J: Cross-talk between transmembrane signalling systems: A prerequisite for the delicate regulation of glomerular haemodynamics by mesangial cells. Eur J Clin Invest 1989;19:347–361.
18. Ardaillou N, Hagege J, Nivez MP, et al: Vasoconstrictor-evoked prostaglandin synthesis in cultured human mesangial cells. Am J Physiol 1985;248:F240–F246.
19. Scharschmidt LA, Simonson MS, Dunn MJ: Glomerular prostaglandins, angiotensin II, and nonsteroidal antiinflammatory drugs. Am J Med 1986;81(Suppl 2B):30–42.
20. Grenier FC, Rollins TE, Smith WL: Kinin-induced prostaglandin synthesis by renal papillary collecting tubule cells in culture. Am J Physiol 1981;241:F94– F104.
21. Dunn MJ, Staley RS, Harrison M: Characterization of prostaglandins production in tissue culture of rat renal medullary cells. Prostaglandins 1976;12:37–49.
22. Terragno NA, Terragno A, Early JA, et al: Endogenous prostaglandin synthesis inhibitor in the renal cortex. Effects on production of prostacycline by renal blood vessels. Clin Sci 1978;55(Suppl):199–202.

23. Stahl RA, Paravicini M, Schollmeyer P: Angiotensin II stimulation of prostaglandin E_2 and 6-keto-$F_{1\alpha}$ formation by isolated human glomeruli. Kidney Int 1984;26:30–34.

24. Govindarajan S, Nast CC, Smith WL, et al: Immuno-histochemical distribution of renal prostaglandin endoperoxide synthetase and prostacyclin synthetase: Diminished endoperoxide synthetase in the hepatorenal syndrome. Hepatology 1987;7:654–659.

25. Schriener GF, Kiely JM, Cotran RS, Unanue ER: Characterization of resident glomerular cells expressing Ia determinants and manifesting restricted interactions with lymphocytes. J Clin Invest 1981;68:920–931.

26. Badr KF, DeBoer DK, Takahashi K, et al: Glomerular responses to platelet activating factor in the rat: Role of thromboxane A_2. Am J Physiol 1989;256:F35–F43.

27. Schlondorff D, Ardaillou R. Prostaglandins and other arachidonic acid metabolites in the kidney. Kidney Int 1986;29:108–119.

28. Farman N, Pradelles P, Bonvalet JP: PGE_2, $PGF_{2\alpha}$, 6-keto-$PGF_{1\alpha}$, and TxB_2 synthesis along the rabbit nephron. Am J Physiol 1987;252:F53-F59.

29. Schlondorff D, Satriano JA, Schwartz GJ: Synthesis of prostaglandin E_2 in different segments of isolated collecting tubules from adult and neonatal rabbits. Am J Physiol 1985;248:F134–F144.

30. Maridonneau-Parini I, Fradin A, Touqui L, Russo-Marie F: Effect of intracellular oxygen-free radicals on the formation of lipid-derived mediators in rat renomedullary interstitial cells. Biochem Pharmacol 1985; 34:4137–4143.

31. Hill TWK, Moncada S: The renal haemodynamic and excretory actions of prostacyclin and 6-oxo-PGF_1 in anesthetized dogs. Prostaglandins 1979;17:87–98.

32. Aiken JW, Vane JR: Intrarenal prostaglandin release attenuates the renal vasoconstrictor activity of angiotensin. J Pharmacol Exp Ther 1973;184:678–687.

33. Ardaillou N, Nivez MP, Striker G, Ardaillou R: Prostaglandin synthesis by human glomerular cells in culture. Prostaglandins 1983;26:773–784.

34. Nakamura KT, Page WV, Sato T, et al: Ontogeny of isoproterenol-stimulated renin secretion from sheeps renal cortical slices. Am J Physiol 1989;256:F1258–1263.

35. Cooper CL, Malik KU: Prostaglandin synthesis and renal vasoconstriction elicited by adrenergic stimuli are linked to activation of alpha-1 adrenergic receptors in the isolated rat kidney. J Pharmacol Exp Ther 1984; 233:24–31.

36. Needleman P, Kauffman AH, Douglas JR Jr, et al: Specific stimulation and inhibition of renal prostaglandin release by angiotensin analogs. Am J Physiol 1973;224:1415–1419.

37. Blasingham MC, Nasjletti A: Contribution of renal prostaglandins to the natriuretic action of bradykinin in the dog. Am J Physiol 1979;237:F182–187.

38. Colina-Chourio J, McGiff JC, Miller MR, Nasjletti A: Possible influence of intrarenal generation of kinins on prostaglandin release from the rabbit perfused kidney. Br J Pharmacol 1976;58:165–172.

39. Cooper CL, Schaffer JE, Malik KU: Mechanism of action of angiotensin II and bradykinin on prostaglandin synthesis and vascular tone in the isolated rat kidney. Effect of Ca^{++} antagonists and calmodulin inhibitors. Circ Res 1985;56:97–108.

40. Bell C, Mya MKK: Release by vasopressin of E-type prostaglandins from the rat kidney. Clin Sci Mol Med 1977;52:103–106.

41. Cooper CL, Malik KU: Mechanism of actions of vasopressin on prostaglandin synthesis and vascular function in the isolated rat kidney: Effect of calcium antagonist and calmodulin inhibitors. J Pharmacol Exp Ther 1984;229:139–147.

42. Margolis BL, Bonventre JV, Kremer SG, et al: Epidermal growth factor is synergistic with phorbol esters and vasopressin in stimulating arachidonate release and prostaglandin production in renal glomerular mesangial cells. Biochem J 1988;249:587–592.

43. Lefkowith JB, Schreiner G: Essential fatty acid deficiency depletes rat glomeruli of resident macrophages and inhibits angiotensin II-induced eicosanoid synthesis. J Clin Invest 1987;80:947–956.

44. Badr KF, Kelley VE, Rennke HG, Brenner BM: Roles for thromboxane A_2 and leukotrienes in endotoxin-induced acute renal failure. Kidney Int 1986;30:474-480.

45. Adler S, Sthal RA, Baker PJ, et al: Biphasic effect of oxygen radicals on prostaglandin production by rat mesangial cells. Am J Physiol 1987;252:F743–F749.

46. Basci A, Wallin JD, Shah SV: Effect of stimulated neutrophils on cyclic nucleotide content in isolated rat glomeruli. Am J Physiol 1987;252:F429–F436.

47. Roszinski S, Jelkmann W: Effect of PO_2 on prostaglandin E_2 production in renal cell cultures. Respir Physiol 1987;70:131–141.

48. Jackson RM, Chandler DB, Fulmer JD: Production of arachidonic acid metabolites by endothelial cells in hyperoxia. J Appl Physiol 1986;61:584–591.

49. Williamson HE, Bourland WA, Marchand GR: Inhibition of furosemide induced increase in renal blood flow by indomethacin. Proc Soc Exp Biol Med 1975; 8:164–167.

50. Williamson HE, Bourland WA, Marchand GR: Inhibition of ethacrynic acid induced renal flow by indomethacin. Prostaglandins 1974;8:297–301.

51. Olsen VB, Ahnfelt-Ronne I: Bumetanide induced increase of renal blood-flow in conscious dogs and its melitien to renal hormones. Acta Pharmacol Toxicol 1976;38:219–228.

52. Hoult JR, Moore PK: Pathways of prostaglandin F_2 metabolism in mammalian kidneys. Br J Pharmacol 1977;61:615–626.

53. Katzen DR, Pong SS, Levine L: Distribution of prostaglandin E 9-keto reductase and $NADP^+$ dependent 15-hydroxyprostaglandin dehydrogenase in the renal cortex and medulla of various species. Res Commun Chem Pathol Pharmacol 1975;12:781–787.

54. Sejersted OM, Vikse A, Eide I, Kiil F: Renal venous and urinary PGE_2 output during intrarenal arachidonic acid infusion in dogs. Acta Physiol Scand 1984;121:249–259.

55. Zipser RD, Martin K: Urinary excretion of arterial prostaglandins and thromboxanes in man. Am J Physiol 1982;242:E171–E177.

56. Frolich JA, Wilson TW, Sweetman BJ, et al: Urinary prostaglandins: Identification and origin. J Clin Invest 1975;55:763–770.

57. Bito LZ, Baroody RA: Comparison of renal prostaglandin and p-aminohippuric acid transport processes. Am J Physiol 1978;237:F20–F24.

58. Irish JM III: Secretion of prostaglandin E$_2$ by rabbit proximal tubules. Am J Physiol 1979;237:F268–F273.

59. Patrono C, Dunn MJ: The clinical significance of inhibition of renal prostaglandin synthesis. Kidney Int 1987;32:1–12.

60. Zipser RD, Lifschitz MD: Prostaglandins and related compounds. In Epstein M (ed): The Kidney in Liver Disease. Baltimore: Williams & Wilkins, 1988;393–416.

61. Menè P, Dunn MJ: Vascular, glomerular, and tubular effects of angiotensin II, kinins, and prostaglandins. In Seldin DW, Giebisch G (eds): The Kidney: Physiology and Pathophysiology, 2nd ed. New York: Raven Press, 1992;1205–1248.

62. Halushka PV, Mais DE, Mayeux PR, Morinelli PA: Thromboxane, prostaglandin and leukotriene receptors. Annu Rev Pharmacol Toxicol 1989;29:213–219.

63. Troyer DA, Gonzalez OF, Douglas JG, Kreisberg JI: Phorbol ester inhibits arginine vasopressin activation of phospholipase C and promotes contraction of, and prostaglandin production by, cultured mesangial cells. Biochem J 1988;251:907–912.

64. Smith WL, Sonnemburg WK, Allen ML, et al: The biosynthesis and actions of prostaglandins in the renal collecting tubule and thick ascending limb. In Dunn MJ, Patrono C, Cinotti GA (eds): Renal Eicosanoids. New York: Plenum Press, 1989;131–147.

65. Zipser RD: Effects of selective inhibition of thromboxane synthesis on renal function in humans. Am J Physiol 1985;248:F753.

66. Munger K, Baylis C: Sex differences in renal hemodynamics in rats. Am J Physiol 1988;254:F223.

67. Data JL, Gerber JG, Crump WJ, et al: The prostaglandin system: A role in baroreceptor control of renin release. Circ Res 1978;42:454.

68. Franco-Saenz R, Suzuki S, Tan SY, Murlow PJ: Prostaglandin stimulation of renin release: Independence of β-adrenergic receptor activity and mechanism of action. Endocrinology 1980;106:1400.

69. Altsheler P, Klahr S, Rosenbaum R, Slatopolsky E: Effects of inhibitors of prostaglandin synthesis on renal sodium excretion in normal dogs and dogs with decreased renal mass. Am J Physiol 1978;235:F338–F344.

70. DeForrest JM, Davis JO, Freeman RH, et al: Effects of indomethacin and meclofenamate on renin release and renal hemodynamic function during chronic sodium depletion in conscious dogs. Circ Res 1980;47:99–107.

71. Berl T, Raz A, Wald H, et al: Prostaglandin synthesis inhibition and the action of vasopressin: Studies in man and rat. Am J Physiol 1977;232:F529–F537.

72. Conrad KP, Colpoys MC: Evidence against the hypothesis that prostaglandins are the vasodepressor agents of pregnancy. Serial studies in chronically instrumented, conscious rats. J Clin Invest 1986;77:236–245.

73. De Witt DL, Smith WL: Primary structure of prostaglandin G/H synthase from sheep vesicular gland determined from the complementary DNA sequence. Proc Natl Acad Sci USA 1988;85:1412–1416.

74. Anderson RJ, Taher MS, Cronin RE, et al: Effect of β-adrenergic blockade and inhibitors of angiotensin II and prostaglandins on renal autoregulation. Am J Physiol 1975;229:731–736.

75. Finn W, Arendshorst WJ: Effect of prostaglandin synthetase inhibitors on renal blood flow in the rat. Am J Physiol 1976;231:1541–1545.

76. Carlson DE, Schramm LP: Humoral and mechanical factors modulating neural input to renal vasculature. Am J Physiol 1978;235:R64–R75.

77. Dominguez JH, Pitts TO, Brown T, et al: Prostaglandin E$_2$ and parathyroid hormone: Comparison of their actions on the rabbit proximal tubule. Kidney Int 1984; 26:404.

78. Ingelfinger JR, Pratt RE, Dzau VJ: Regulation of extrarenal renin during ontogeny. Endocrinology 1988;122: 782–786.

79. Stokes JB: Effect of prostaglandin E$_2$ on chloride transport across the rabbit thick ascending limbs of Henle. Selective inhibition of the medullary portion. J Clin Invest 1979;64:495–502.

80. Culpepper RM, Andreoli TE: Interactions among prostaglandin E$_2$, antidiuretic hormone, and cyclic adenosine monophosphate in modulating Cl absorption in single mouse medullary thick ascending limbs of Henle. J Clin Invest 1983;71:1588–1601.

81. Culpepper RM, Andreoli TE: PGE$_2$, forskolin, and cholera toxin interactions in modulating NaCl transport in mouse mTALH. Am J Physiol 1984;247:F784–792.

82. Donker AJM, Arisz L, Brentjens JRH, et al: The effect of indomethacin on kidney function and plasma renin activity in man. Nephron 1976;17:288–296.

83. Gullner HG, Gill JR Jr, Bartter FC, Dusing R: The role of the prostaglandin system in the regulation of renal function in normal women. Am J Med 1980;69:718–724.

84. Haylor J: Prostaglandin synthesis and renal function in man. J Physiol 1980;298:383–396.

85. Henrich WL, Berl T, McDonald KM, et al: Angiotensin II, renal nerves, and prostaglandins in renal hemodynamics during hemorrhage. Am J Physiol 1978;235: F46–F51.

86. Boyer TD, Zia P, Reynolds TB: Effects of indomethacin and prostaglandin A$_1$ on renal function and plasma renin activity in alcoholic liver disease. Gastroenterology 1979;77:215–222.

87. Zipser RD, Hoefs JC, Speckart JF, et al:. Prostaglandins: Modulators of renal function and pressor resistance in chronic liver disease. J Clin Endocrinol Metab 1979;48:895–900.

88. Laffi G, La Villa G, Pinzani M, et al: Altered renal and platelet arachidonic acid metabolism in cirrhosis. Gastroenterology 1986;90:274–282.

89. Rimola A, Gines P, Arroyo V, et al: Urinary excretion of 6-keto-PGF$_{1\alpha}$, thromboxane B$_2$, and prostaglandin E$_2$ in cirrhosis with ascites: Relationship to functional renal failure (hepatorenal syndrome). J Hepatol 1986; 3:111–117.

90. Guarner C, Colina I, Guarner F, et al: Renal prostaglandins in cirrhosis of the liver. Clin Sci 1986;70:477–484.

91. Uemura M, Tsujii T, Fukui H, et al: Urinary prostaglandins and renal function in chronic liver diseases. Scand J Gastroenterol 1986;21:75–81.

92. Parelon G, Mirouze D, Michel F, et al: Prostaglandines urinaires dans le syndrome hepatorenal du cirrhotique: Role du thromboxane A$_2$ et d'un desequilibre dus acides gras polyinsatures precurseurs. Gastroenterol Clin Biol 1985;9:290–297.

93. Arroyo V, Planas R, Gaya J, et al: Sympathetic nervous activity, renin-angiotensin system and renal excretion of prostaglandin E_2 in cirrhosis. Relationship to functional renal failure and sodium and water excretion. Eur J Clin Invest 1983;13:271–278

94. Moore K, Ward PS, Taylor GW, Williams R: Systemic and renal production of thromboxane A_2 and prostacyclin in decompensated liver disease and hepatorenal syndrome. Gastroenterology 1991;100:1069–1077.

95. Wong F, Massie D, Hsu P, Dudley F: Indomethacin-induced renal dysfunction in patients with well-compensated cirrhosis. Gastroenterology 1993;104:869–876.

96. Schrier RW, Arroyo V, Bernardi M, et al: Peripheral arterial vasodilation hypothesis: A proposal for the initiation of renal sodium and water retention in cirrhosis. Hepatology 1988;8:1151–1157.

97. Zipser RD: Role of renal prostaglandins and the effects of nonsteroidal anti-inflammatory drugs in patients with liver disease. Am J Med 1986;81(Suppl 2B): 95–103.

98. Dunn MJ: Renal prostaglandins. In Dunn MJ (ed): Renal endocrinology. Baltimore, Williams & Wilkins 1973;1–74.

99. Epstein M, Lifschitz M, Ramachandran M, Rappaport K: Characterization of prostaglandin E responsiveness in decompensated cirrhosis: Implications for renal sodium handling. Clin Sci 1982;63:553–563.

100. Lianos EA, Alavi N, Tobin M, et al: Angiotensin-induced sodium excretion in cirrhosis. Role of renal prostaglandins. Kidney Int 1982;21:70–77.

101. Rector WG: Urinary prostaglandin E_2, sodium retention, and diuretic responsiveness in patients with chronic liver disease. Am J Gastroenterol 1987;82:347–351.

102. Perez-Ayuso RM, Arroyo V, Camps J, et al: Evidence that renal prostaglandins are involved in renal water metabolism in cirrhosis. Kidney Int 1984;26:72–80.

103. Perez-Ayuso RM, Arroyo V, Camps J, et al: Effects of demeclocycline on renal function and urinary prostaglandin E_2 and kallikrein in hyponatremic cirrhosis. Nephron 1984;36:30–37.

104. Zambraski EJ, Dunn MJ: Importance of renal prostaglandins in control of renal function after chronic ligation of the common bile duct in dogs. J Lab Clin Med 1984;103:549–559.

105. Levy M, Wexler MJ, Fechner C: Renal perfusion in dogs with experimental hepatic cirrhosis: Role of prostaglandins. Am J Physiol 1983;245:F521–F529.

106. Sola J, Camps J, Arroyo V, et al: Longitudinal study of renal prostaglandin excretion in cirrhotic rats: Relationship with the renin-aldosterone system. Clin Sci 1988;75:263–269.

107. Zipser RD, Kerlin P, Hoefs J, et al: Urinary kallikrein excretion in cirrhosis: Relationship to other vasoactive systems. Am J Gastroenterol 1981;75:183–187.

108. Brater DC. Pharmacokinetics and pharmacodynamics in cirrhosis. In Epstein M (ed): The Kidney in Liver Disease, 3rd ed. Baltimore: Williams & Wilkins, 1988; 551–571.

109. Laffi G, Daskalopoulos G, Kronborg I, et al: Effects of sulindac and ibuprofen in patients with cirrhosis and ascites: An explanation for the renal-sparing effect of sulindac. Gastroenterology 1986;90:182–187.

110. Kawasaki H, Nosaka Y, Yamada S, et al: Effect of renal prostaglandins on survival in patients with liver cirrhosis. Am J Gastroenterol 1989;84:285–289.

111. Planas R, Arroyo V, Rimola A, et al: Acetylsalicylic acid suppresses the renal hemodynamic effect and reduces the diuretic action of furosemide in cirrhosis with ascites. Gastroenterology 1983;84:247–252.

112. Daskalopoulos G, Kronborg I, Katkow W, et al: Sulindac and indomethacin suppress the diuretic action of furosemide in patients with cirrhosis and ascites: Evidence that sulindac affects renal prostaglandins. Am J Kidney Dis 1985;6:217–221.

113. Gentilini P, Romanelli RG, La Villa G, et al: Effects of low-dose captopril on renal hemodynamics and function in patients with cirrhosis of the liver. Gastroenterology 1993;104:588–594.

114. Mirouze D, Zipser RD, Reynolds TB: Effect of inhibitors of prostaglandin synthesis on induced diuresis in cirrhosis. Hepatology 1983;3:50–55.

115. Ciabattoni G, Cinotti GA, Pierucci A, et al: Effects of sulindac and ibuprofen in patients with chronic glomerular disease. Evidence for the dependence of renal function on prostacyclin. N Engl J Med 1984;310: 279–283.

116. Brater DC, Anderson S, Baird B, Campbell WB: Effects of ibuprofen, naproxen an sulindac on prostaglandins in men. Kidney Int 1985;27:66–73.

117. Whelton A, Stout RL, Spilman PS, Klassen DK: Renal effects of ibuprofen, piroxicam and sulindac in patients with asymptomatic renal failure. A prospective, randomized, crossover comparison. Ann Intern Med 1990; 112:568–576.

118. Zambraski EJ, Chremos AN, Dunn MJ: Comparison of the effects of sulindac with other cyclooxygenase inhibitors on prostaglandin excretion and renal function in normal and chronic bile duct-ligated dogs and swine. J Pharmacol Exp Ther 1984;228:560–566.

119. Quintero E, Gines P, Arroyo V, et al: Sulindac reduces the urinary excretion of prostaglandins and impairs renal function in cirrhosis with ascites. Nephron 1986; 42:298–303.

120. Juhl RP, Van Thiel BH, Dittert LW, et al: Ibuprofen and sulindac kinetics in alcoholic liver disease. Clin Pharmacol Ther 1983;34:104–109.

121. Antillon M, Cominelli F, Reynolds TB, Zipser RD: Comparative acute effects of diflunisal and indomethacin on renal function in patients with cirrhosis and ascites. Am J Gastroenterol 1989;84:153–155.

122. Zambraski EJ, Guidotti SM, Atkinson DC, Diamond J: Salicylic acid causes a diuresis and natriuresis in normal and common bile-duct-ligated cirrhotic miniature swine. J Pharmacol Exp Ther 1988;247:983–988.

123. Fantozzi R: Imidazole-2-hydroxybenzoate: A new anti-inflammatory drug. Interaction with the arachidonic acid cascade. Drugs Exp Clin Res 1984;10:853–856.

124. Lorenzano E, Badalamenti S, Scotti A, et al: Renal effects of imidazole-2-hydroxybenzoate in patients with compensated liver cirrhosis. Int J Clin Pharm Ther Toxicol 1992;30:225–229.

125. Salerno F, Lorenzano E, Maggi A, et al: Effects of imidazole-salicylate on renal function and the diuretic action of furosemide in cirrhotic patients with ascites. J Hepatol 1993;19:279–284.

126. Gentilini P: Cirrhosis, renal function and NSAIDs. J Hepatol 1993;19:200–203.

127. Ciabattoni G, Pugliese F, Cinotti GA, et al: Characterization of furosemide-induced activation of the renal prostaglandin system. Eur J Pharmacol 1979; 60:181–187.

128. Pinzani M, Daskalopoulos G, Laffi G, et al: Altered furosemide pharmacokinetics in chronic alcoholic liver disease with ascites contributes to diuretic resistance. Gastroenterology 1987;92:294–298.

129. Medina JF, Prieto J, Guarner F, et al: Effect of spironolactone on renal prostaglandin excretion in patients with liver cirrhosis and ascites. J Hepatol 1986;3:206–211.

130. Quiroga J, Zozaya JM, Labarga P, et al: Renal prostacyclin influences renal function in non-azotemic cirrhotic patients treated with furosemide. J Hepatol 1991;12:170–175.

131. Badr KF, Jacobson HR: Arachidonic acid metabolites and the kidney. In Brenner BM, Rector FC (eds): The Kidney, 4th ed. Philadelphia: W.B. Saunders, 1991; 584–619.

132. Burch RM, Halushka PV: Vasopressin stimulates prostaglandin and thromboxane synthesis in toad bladder epithelial cells. Am J Physiol 1982;243:F539–F597.

133. Burch RM, Knapp DR, Halushka PV: Vasopressin-stimulated water flow is decreased by thromboxane synthesis inhibition or antagonism. Am J Physiol 1980; 239:F160–F166.

134. Ahonen J, Isoniemi H, Eklund B, et al: Thromboxane-receptor antagonist in renal transplantation. Transplant Proc 1990;22:1370.

135. Benigni A, Rizzoni G, Antolini A, et al: Preliminary report: Renal thromboxane A_2 synthesis in children with frequent relapsing nephrotic syndrome. Lancet 1990;336:533–534.

136. Pierucci A, Simonetti BM, Pecci G, et al: Improvement of renal function with selective thromboxane antagonism in lupus nephritis. N Engl J Med 1989;320:421–425.

137. Gentilini P, Laffi G, Meacci E, et al: Effects of OKY 046, a thromboxane synthase inhibitor, on renal function in non-azotemic cirrhotic patients with ascites. Gastroenterology 1988;94:1470–1477.

138. Pinzani M, Laffi G, Meacci E, et al: Intrarenal thromboxane A_2 generation reduces the furosemide-induced sodium and water diuresis in cirrhosis with ascites. Gastroenterology 1988;95:1081–1087.

139. Laffi G, Marra F, Carloni V, et al: Thromboxane receptor blockade increases water diuresis cirrhotics with ascites. Gastroenterology 1992;103:1017–1021.

140. Epstein M: Hepatorenal syndrome. In Epstein M (ed): The Kidney in Liver Disease. Baltimore: Williams & Wilkins, 1988;89-118.

141. Zipser RD, Radvan GH, Kronborg IJ, et al: Urinary thromboxane B_2 and prostaglandin E_2 in the hepatorenal syndrome: Evidence for increased vasoconstrictor and decreased vasodilator factors. Gastroenterology 1983;84:697–703.

142. Zipser RD, Kronborg IJ, Rector W, et al: Therapeutic trial of thromboxane synthase inhibition in the hepatorenal syndrome. Gastroenterology 1984;87:1228–1232.

143. Guarner F, Guarner C, Prieto J, et al: Increased synthesis of systemic prostacyclin in cirrhotic patients. Gastroenterology 1986; 90:687–694.

144. Schrier RW, Caramelo C: Hemodynamics and hormonal alterations in hepatic cirrhosis. In Epstein M (ed): The Kidney in Liver Disease, 3rd ed. Baltimore: Williams & Wilkins, 1988;265–285.

145. Bruix J, Bosch J, Kravetz D, et al: Effects of prostaglandin inhibition on systemic and hepatic hemodynamics in patients with cirrhosis of the liver. Gastroenterology 1985;88:430–435.

146. Hamilton G, Phing RCF, Hutton RA, et al:. The relationship between prostacyclin activity and pressure in the portal vein. Hepatology 1982;2:236–242.

147. Guarner C, Soriano G, Such J, et al: Systemic prostacyclin in cirrhosis. Relationship with portal hypertension, and changes after intestinal decontamination. Gastroenterology 1992;102:303–309.

148. Goerig M, Wernze H, Kommerell B, Grun M: Increased bioavailability of enzymes of eicosanoid synthesis in hepatic and extrahepatic tissues after portacaval shunting. Hepatology 1989;10:154–162.

149. Laffi G, Marra F, Failli P, et al: Defective signal transduction in platelets from cirrhotics is associated with increased cyclic nucleotides. Gastroenterology 1993; 105:148–156.

150. Johnston DE: Is prostacyclin synthesis greater in cirrhotic patients? [letter]. Gastroenterology 1992;103:1369.

151. Gentilini P, Laffi G: Renal functional impairment and sodium retention in liver cirrhosis. Digestion 1989;43: 1–32.

152. Gentilini P: Hepatorenal syndrome: Differerential diagnosis and therapy. In Schmid R, Gerok W, Bianchi L, Maier KP (eds): Extrahepatic manifestations in liver diseases. Dordrecht: Kluwer, 1993;193–212.

153. Fichman MP, Littenburg G, Brooker G, et al: Effects of prostaglandin A_1 on renal and adrenal function in man. Circ Res 1972;31/31(Suppl 2):19–35.

154. Arieff AI, Chidsey CA: Renal function in cirrhosis and the effects of prostaglandin A_1. Am J Med 1974;56: 695–703.

155. Zusman RM, Axelrod L, Tolkoff-Rubin N: The treatment of the hepatorenal syndrome (HRS. with intrarenal administration of prostaglandin E_1. Prostaglandins 1977;13:819–830.

156. Gines A, Salmeron JM, Gines P, et al: Oral misoprostol or intravenous prostaglandin E_2 do not improve renal function in patients with cirrhosis and ascites with hyponatremia or renal failure. J Hepatol 1993;17:220–226.

157. Fevery J, Van Cutsem E, Nevens F, et al: Reversal of hepatorenal syndrome in four patients by peroral misoprostol (prostaglandin E_1 analogue) and albumin administration. J Hepatol 1990;11:153–158.

158. Antillon M, Cominelli F, Lo S, et al: Effects of oral prostaglandins on indomethacin-induced renal failure in patients with cirrhosis and ascites. J Rheumatol 1990;17:46–49.

159. Wong F, Massie D, Hsu P, Dudley F: Dose dependent effect of misoprostol on indomethacin induced renal dysfunction in alcoholic cirrhosis [abstract]. Hepatology 1991;14:134A.

160. Harry DS, McIntyre N: Plasma lipoproteins and the liver. In Millward-Sadler GH, Wright R, Arthur MJP (eds): Wright's Liver and Biliary Disease, 3rd ed. London: W.B. Saunders 1992;61–106.

161. Johnson SB, Gordon E, McClain C, et al: Abnormal polyunsaturated fatty acid pattern of serum lipids in alcoholism and cirrhosis: Arachidonic acid deficiency in cirrhosis. Proc Natl Acad Sci USA 1985;82:1815–1818.

162. Owen JS, Hutton RA, Day RC, et al: Platelet lipid composition and platelet aggregation in human liver disease. J Lipid Res 1981;22:423–430.

163. Palombo JD, Lopes SM, Zeisel SH, et al: Effectiveness of orthotopic liver transplantation on the restoration of cholesterol metabolism in patients with end-stage liver disease. Gastroenterology 1987;93:1170–1177.

164. Owen JS, Bruckdorfer KR, Day RC, McIntyre N: Decreased eritrocyte membrane fluidity and altered lipid composition in human liver disease. J Lipid Res 1982;23:124–132.

165. Kawata S, Chitranukroh A, Owen JS, McIntyre N: Membrane lipid changes in erytrocytes, liver and kidney in acute and chronic experimental liver disease in rats. Biochem Biophys Acta 1987;896:26–34.

166. Imai Y, Scoble JE, McIntyre N, Owen JS: Increased Na^+-dependent D-glucose transport and altered lipid composition in renal cortical brush border membrane vescicles from bile duct-ligated rats. J Lipid Res 1992; 33:473–483.

167. Epstein M, Lifschitz M, Rappaport K: Augmentation of prostaglandin production by linoleic acid in man. Clin Sci 1982;63:565–571.

168. Rimola A, Gines P, Cusï E, et al: Prostaglandin precursor fatty acid in cirrhosis with ascites: Effect of linoleic acid infusion in functional renal failure. Clin Sci 1988; 74:613–619.

169. Keppler D, Huber M, Baumert T: Leukotrienes as mediators in diseases of the liver. Semin Liver Dis 1988; 8:357–366.

170. Lewis RA, Austen KF, Soberman RJ: Leukotrienes and other products of the 5-lipoxygenase pathway. Biochemistry and relation to pathobiology in human diseases. N Engl J Med 1990;323:645–655.

171. Huber M, Kastner S, Scholmerich J, et al: Analysis of cysteinyl leukotrienes in human urine: Enhanced excretion in patients with liver cirrhosis and hepatorenal syndrome. Eur J Clin Invest 1989;19:53–60.

172. Moore KP, Taylor GW, Maltby NH, et al: Increased production of cysteinyl leukotrienes in hepatorenal syndrome. J Hepatol 1990;11:263–271.

173. Prescott SM, Zimmermann GA, McIntyre TM: Platelet activating factor. J Biol Chem 1990;265:17381–17384.

174. Laffi G, Carloni V, Baldi E, et al: Impaired superoxide anion, platelet activating factor and leukotriene B_4 synthesis by neutrophils in cirrhosis. Gastroenterology 1993;105:170–177.

175. Schondorff D, Neuwirth R: Platelet-activating factor and the kidney. Am J Physiol 1986;251:F1–F11.

176. Caramelo C, Fernandez-Gallardo S, Santos JC, et al: Increased levels of platelet-activating factor in blood from patients with cirrhosis of the liver. Eur J Clin Invest 1987;17:7–11.

177. Villamediana LM, Sans E, Fernandez-Gallardo S, et al: Effects of platelet-activating factor antagonist BN 52021 on the hemodynamics of rats with experimental cirrhosis of the liver. Life Sci 1986;39:201–205.

178. Kleber G, Braillon A, Gaudin C, et al: Hemodynamic effects of endotoxin and platelet activating factor in cirrhotic rats. Gastroenterology 1992;103:282–288.

179. Garrick RE: The renal eicosanoids. In Goldfarb S, Ziyadeh FN, Stein JH (eds): Hormones, Autacoids, and the Kidney. New York: Churchill Livingstone 1991; 231–261.

180. Sacerdoti D, Escalante BA, Schwartzman ML, et al: Renal cytochrome P-450-dependent metabolism of arachidonic acid in cirrhotic rats. J Hepatol 1991;12: 230–235.

181. Muredach PR, Lawson JA, FitzGerald GA: Human urinary levels of 5,6 epoxy-eicosatrienoic acid are raised in disorders of salt and water handling [abstract]. Circulation 1993; 88:I-514.

Chapter 15

ATRIAL NATRIURETIC FACTOR AND LIVER DISEASE

MURRAY EPSTEIN, M.D., F.A.C.P.

Overview of ANF Action
Alterations of ANF in Liver Disease
  ANF Levels During Spontaneous Natriuresis
  ANF Levels in Fulminant Hepatic Failure
Metabolism and Arteriovenous Extraction of ANF
Characterization of ANF
ANF Responsiveness to Volume Contraction
ANF Responsiveness to Volume Expansion
  Maneuvers
  Head-out Water Immersion (HWI)
  Saline-induced Volume Expansion
  Peritoneovenous Shunting

Response of ANF to Dietary Sodium Challenges
Renal Responsiveness to Infusion of Exogenous
  Peptide
Circadian Patterns
Relationship between Circulating ANF and Renal
  Excretory Function: Consideration of Resistance
  to Natriuretic Action of ANF
Endopeptidase and Other Urinary Peptide
  Cofactors
Additional Peptide Hormones Derived from ANF
  Prohormone
Summary

Atrial natriuretic factor (ANF) is the first well-defined natriuretic hormone. The best characterized pharmacologic and partly physiologic actions of ANF are natriuresis, diuresis, and smooth muscle relaxation. Recent evidence has been accrued that ANF might be involved in various biologic actions apart from its role in volume homeostasis, such as immune or reproductive functions. With the characterization of ANF and the demonstration that it participates in the regulation of volume homeostasis in both animals and humans,[1–6] theoretical considerations suggest a potential role for ANF in the pathogenesis of the impaired sodium homeostasis and possibly the decrements of GFR of decompensated cirrhosis.[7,8] On the one hand, patients with cirrhosis manifest clinical findings indicative of a reduction in effective circulating blood volume.[7–10] Furthermore, direct measurements indicate that the central blood volume is often reduced in cirrhotic patients.[11–14] Because atrial distention is considered to be a major stimulus for ANF release, a reduction in the effective circulating blood volume and a reduced filling pressure theoretically could lead to diminished ANF release. On the other hand, according to the overflow hypothesis,[7,15] the central hypervolemia that results from a primary disturbance in renal sodium

handling might tend to favor an increase in ANF release. Indeed, Rector et al.[16,17] reported that the heart, lung, and aortic root components of central blood volume may be expanded or normal in cirrhotic patients. The possible role of ANF in this disorder has been defined only recently.

The past decade has witnessed numerous studies investigating the role of ANF in regulating renal sodium and water handling in patients with liver disease. Initially, the majority of studies focused on determinations of circulating ANF levels. More recently, several investigators have utilized experimental maneuvers that acutely alter volume distribution, such as head-out water immersion (HWI) and peritoneovenous (PV) shunting, as a means of assessing the relationship between ANF and concomitant renal function.

The aims of this chapter are several-fold. The first is to review briefly the relationship of plasma ANF levels with the stage of liver disease. The second aim is to consider the effects of dietary sodium challenges and volume-expanding maneuvers such as HWI and PV shunting on ANF responsiveness. The third aim is to review the extensive experience with infusion of exogenous ANF on renal function and the implications of these studies in delineating a pathophysiologic role for abnormal responses to ANF in the salt and water retention of cirrhosis. The final aim is to consider the additional peptide hormones derived from ANF prohormone, including kaliuretic stimulator, that may play a role in mediating sodium and water homeostasis in patients with liver disease.

OVERVIEW OF ANF ACTION

In 1981 deBold et al.[18] reported that a crude protein extract derived from atrial myocytes could induce a rapid and reversible marked rise in renal sodium and water excretion. In a few short years, the factor responsible for this effect was identified as the circulating 28 amino acid polypeptide, atrial natriuretic factor. ANF is synthesized in the human heart as a 151 amino acid pre-prohormone and stored primarily as a 126 amino acid prohormone in atrial myocytes.[19] Upon appropriate stimulation, such as atrial stretch, the prohormone is cleaved into an N-terminal and C-terminal fragment. The latter has been identified as the circulating bioactive ANF-(99-126). ANF release is enhanced by atrial distention and possibly by vasoconstrictor hormones.[5,6] ANF receptors have been identified in vascular smooth muscle, kidney, adrenal gland, and brain.[20] More recently, three classes of ANF receptors have been characterized.[20] These include two biologically active receptors (A and B) and a C-type or clearance receptor that may serve as a reservoir for sequestration and release of ANF.[21] The second messenger signaling system in the cellular response to ANF has been identified as the particulate or membrane bound guanylate cyclase, which leads to the generation of cyclic guanosine monophosphate (GMP). A prompt rise in serum and urine cyclic GMP can be measured following stimulation with exogenous or endogenous ANF.[22] In fact, the type A biologically active ANF receptor has guanylate cyclase catalytic activity as part of its cytoplasmic domain and this is directly activated upon occupancy of the receptor.[20] There are numerous physiologic and cellular responses to ANF in different organ systems. Increased sodium excretion in the kidney is attributed to inhibition of sodium reabsorption in the inner medullary collecting duct.[23] Other renal effects include an increase in glomerular filtration rate;[24] inhibition of vasopressin action in the medullary collecting duct, which leads to increased solute-free water clearance;[25] and blockade of renin secretion.[26] In the adrenals, aldosterone secretion is inhibited.[26] In vascular tissues, ANF is both a direct vasorelaxant [27] and an antagonist of the vasoconstrictive

effects of angiotensin II.[28] ANF inhibits release of vasopressin in the brain.[29]

ALTERATIONS OF ANF IN LIVER DISEASE

In late stages of cirrhosis, patients manifest clinical findings indicative of a reduction in effective circulating volume.[7,8,10,11] Direct measurements indicate that central blood volume is often reduced.[10,11,14] Because atrial distention is a major stimulus for ANF release, a reduction in central filling pressure with a decreased effective circulating volume may lead to reduced ANF secretion. Despite these considerations, the available data indicate that ANF levels are not suppressed but rather are either normal or elevated.[10,30] In most studies, ANF concentrations in cirrhotic patients without ascites, as a group, do not differ significantly from those observed in normal control subjects.[31–36] In patients with ascites, plasma ANF values equal[10,32,36,37] or exceed[33–35,38–41] those of normal subjects. In functional renal failure of cirrhosis (hepatorenal syndrome), plasma ANF levels have been reported to be elevated compared with patients with liver disease and normal renal function or with normal subjects.[39] One study found that cirrhotic patients with ascites had reduced ANF levels; more than one-half of these patients were on diuretic therapy.[31] In general, the variability of plasma ANF levels may be attributable to several factors, including the technique of plasma extraction, radioimmunoassay, posture of the subjects, variations in dietary sodium intake, concomitant diuretic treatment, and possibly variations in hepatic and renal clearance of ANF.

In part, these discrepancies in plasma ANF levels may also be explained by the different stages of cirrhosis. ANF levels and their effects need not be the same in the early, preascitic phase of the disease as they are when ascites is far advanced. The demonstration that in most studies ANF levels are normal or elevated may be interpreted as supporting the overflow theory of ascites formation in cirrhosis. According to this formulation, slight degrees of hypervolemia and atrial enlargement might lead to an elevation of ANF levels or resetting of the threshold for ANF release. As the patients retain more sodium, ANF levels may continue to rise. In preascitic hepatic cirrhosis or fibrosis, Warner et al.[42] have shown that ANF levels rise in parallel with increases in intrasinusoidal pressure (Fig. 15.1) to the extent that ANF reflects a mild degree of volume expansion. This finding is also consistent with the overflow hypothesis in early stages of the disease. When ascites becomes massive and fluid that is translocated outside the intravascular compartment can no longer signal an ANF rise, ANF levels may have a tendency to fall toward the normal range.[40] However, atrial enlargement or elevated atrial pressures are not necessarily a feature of cirrhosis with ascites.

Recent careful studies by Henriksen et al.[10,11] add important information as well as complexity to this issue. They demonstrated that the estimated central blood volume (ECBV; i.e., blood volume in the heart cavities, lungs, and central arterial tree) is decreased in patients with cirrhosis.[10] More recently they assessed the relationship between ECBV, systemic and portal hemodynamics, and markers of overall and renal sympathetic nervous activity.[11] They measured the ECBV and the circulating and renal venous levels of norepinephrine, arterial epinephrine, and ANF in patients with cirrhosis and esophageal varices who were undergoing hemodynamic investigation. They observed that arterial norepinephrine levels, an index of overall sympathetic nervous activity, was negatively correlated with ECBV. Similarly, renal venous norepinephrine levels (an index of renal sympathetic tone) was inversely correlated with ECBV. In contrast to the significant relationship between decreased ECBV and enhanced sympathetic nervous tone, they failed to demonstrate a relationship between ECBV and circulating levels of ANF.[11] They proposed that the normal ANF levels and the absence of correlation with ECBV suggests that atrial volume is not affected substantially by ECBV reduction. This point of view is in keeping with recent reports by Rector et al.,[16,17] who actually found an insignificant decrease in right atrial volume (−5 ml) and a significant increase in left atrial volume (+16 ml) in patients with cirrhosis. Another possibility is that the presence of ascites alters spatial relationships in the heart,[12,13] thereby rendering the release of ANF more or less independent of the magnitude of ECBV.

Finally, additional factors besides mechanical atrial stretch may enhance ANF release, including alpha-adrenergic stimulation and stimulation by other vasoconstrictors.[43–47] It is also conceivable that the markedly enhanced lymph flow in patients with decompensated cirrhosis[15] may promote an increase in atrial stretch despite the

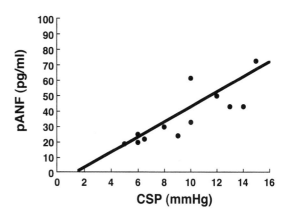

FIGURE 15.1   Correlation between plasma ANF and corrected sinusoidal pressure (CSP) (p < 0.01). (Adapted from Warner LC, et al: The role of resistance to atrial natriuretic peptide and the pathogenesis of sodium retention in hepatic cirrhosis. In Brenner BM, Laragh J (eds): Progress in Atrial Peptide Research. New York: Raven Press, 1989;3: 185–203, with permission.)

maldistribution of blood volume with relative central hypovolemia.[30]

An alternative explanation has been proposed.[30] A physiologic negative-feedback control loop has been postulated in which an ANF-induced volume correction (attributable to the natriuresis) leads to a diminished ANF secretion. Observations by Epstein et al.[34] and Campbell et al.[48] of an exaggerated augmentation of ANF in response to head-out water immersion (HWI) are consistent with this postulate. Thus, a decreased renal responsiveness to ANF due to interruption of the feedback mechanism might lead to an exaggerated augmentation of circulating ANF.

ANF Levels During Spontaneous Natriuresis

A study by Angeli et al.[49] suggests a possible role for ANF in mediating the spontaneous natriuresis observed in some patients with cirrhosis. They assessed ANF levels in a large heterogenous group of nonazotemic cirrhotic patients: (1) ascitic cirrhotic patients who underwent spontaneous diuresis, (2) ascitic cirrhotic patients who responded to spironolactone, and (3) ascitic cirrhotic patients who did not respond to 500 mg/day of spironolactone. The last group was then divided into two subgroups. Subgroup B-R (n = 25) included patients who responded to spironolactone alone, whereas subgroup B-NR (n = 19) included patients who did not respond to 500 mg/day of spironolactone. Patients and control subjects were maintained on a normocaloric diet containing 80 mEq/day of sodium throughout the study. Ascitic cirrhotic patients, as a whole, had higher ANF values than did controls. ANF values in group A (n = 7) and those in group B (n = 44) were greater than those in controls.

The data of Angeli et al.[49] are also consistent with the formulation that ANF may have a role in determining the negative sodium balance in cirrhotic patients who undergo spontaneous diuresis. They suggested that the mechanism may be an ANF-mediated escape from sodium retentive influences that is related to a supranormal recumbency-induced central redistribution of increased plasma volume.[50] This hypothesis is consistent with the report of Bernardi et al.,[51] who observed a supranormal recumbency-induced increase in cardiac output.

ANF Levels in Fulminant Hepatic Failure

Patients with fulminant hepatic failure frequently manifest sodium retention and a hyperdynamic state characterized by high cardiac output and a low systemic vascular resistance.[52,53] To assess the possibility that a deficiency of ANF may contribute to the sodium retention, Panos et al.[54] investigated alterations in ANF and its possible relation to the renin-aldosterone system in fulminant hepatic failure. They determined levels of h-ANF, PRA, and aldosterone concentration in 33 patients with fulminant hepatic failure due to paracetamol overdose and 12 healthy controls. Levels of h-ANF were raised only in patients with evidence of severe renal functional impairment (serum creatinine > 300 μmol/L and urine output < 100 ml/24 hours).

Additional studies were conducted to assess the responsiveness of ANF to alterations of volume and right atrial pressure, induced by either hemodialysis or by the infusion of 5% human albumin solution.[54] The changes in circulating ANF induced by hemodialysis correlated with changes in volume and right atrial pressure. In 6 patients with no or mild renal failure, infusion of 900 ml of 5% human albumin solution induced a significant increase in changes in circulating h-ANF, which correlated with volume and right atrial pressure changes (p < 0.001 and p < 0.05 respectively). The augmentation of ANF was not accompanied by a concomitant natriuresis or diuresis, a

finding compatible with the hypothesis that there may be resistance to h-ANF in this group. Collectively the above cited findings indicate that there is no deficiency of h-ANF in fulminant hepatic failure and that known mechanisms of h-ANF release are not impaired.

METABOLISM AND ARTERIOVENOUS EXTRACTION OF ANF

Plasma disappearance of ANF after intravenous infusion is rapid, indicating a substantial plasma turnover rate of this peptide.[55-57] Other peptides with a fast turnover rate, such as insulin, neurotensin, and vasoactive intestinal polypeptide, have a substantial hepatic degradation,[57-59] raising the possibility that splanchnic removal of ANF may be impaired in liver disease. Several investigators have assessed this possibility.

Ginés et al.[41] investigated ANF metabolism in patients with cirrhosis and ascites to assess the relative contribution of impaired degradation of ANF to the elevated plasma levels. Eleven patients with cirrhosis and ascites without renal failure and 11 control patients were studied. The plasma concentrations of immunoreactive ANF in coronary sinus, right atrium, pulmonary artery, hepatic vein and peripheral vein were significantly elevated in cirrhotic patients compared with controls. There were no significant differences in splanchnic and peripheral extraction between controls and cirrhotic patients. The cardiac release of ANF, calculated as the product of blood flow and immunoreactive ANF concentration in the coronary sinus, was 8 times greater in cirrhotic patients than in controls. These latter studies provide definitive evidence that elevated plasma ANF levels in cirrhotic patients are attributable to the increased cardiac release and not to an impaired splanchnic or peripheral extraction of the peptide.

Hollister and coworkers[60] suggested that reduced liver function as found in patients with cirrhosis is associated with reduced plasma ANF clearance. Their suggestion was based on the demonstration of a substantial hepatic-intestinal clearance of ANF in subjects without reduced liver function.

Henriksen et al.[61] investigated the hepatic-intestinal removal rate of endogenous circulating ANF in cirrhosis. Thirteen patients with cirrhosis (6 with Child-Turcotte class A, 5 with class B, and 2 with class C) and 8 controls. The Fick principle was applied during hepatic vein characterization.

They demonstrated that the arteriohepatic venous extraction ratio of ANF, hepatic-intestinal clearance, and the removal rate in cirrhotic patients were quite similar to those of controls.

Henriksen et al.[61] interpreted their data to indicate that hepatic-intestinal disposal of ANF in cirrhosis does not differ from that of controls; indeed, the values were similar. They concluded that patients with cirrhosis and decreased hepatic function do not have decreased disposal of circulating endogenous ANF.

The possibility that splanchnic disposal of ANF may be influenced by food intake has recently been addressed. Vierhapper et al.[62] found a basal splanchnic uptake of ANF of 8.5 pmol/min in healthy humans. Henriksen et al.[63] assessed the effect of food ingestion on splanchnic disposal of human alpha-atrial natriuretic peptide in 6 subjects referred for hepatic vein catheterization but without hepatic disease. Hepatic-intestinal removal of ANF was determined before and after a test meal. They observed enhanced splanchnic removal of ANF after food intake, which they attributed to increased hepatic-intestinal clearance of the peptide consequent to increased splanchnic blood flow rather than altered fractional extraction of ANF.

CHARACTERIZATION OF ANF

The paradoxical observation that patients with cirrhosis and ascites and sodium retention often manifest normal or increased levels of ANF has suggested the possibility of a dysregulation in the atrial natriuretic factor maturation process that may lead to abnormal forms of the peptide as occurs in other clinical disorders. Patients with congestive heart failure who have high circulating ANF levels also manifest a considerable amount of N-terminal pro-ANF, which increases with the severity of disease.[64] On the other hand, molecular weight heterogeneity of ANF has been noted in patients with hypertension[65] and chronic renal failure.[66] Trace amounts of high-molecular-weight material have been reported in a preliminary structural analysis of plasma ANF performed by gel permeation chromatography in 31 cirrhotic patients.[65] Previous studies aimed at characterizing immunoreactive ANF by high-pressure liquid chromatography (HPLC) techniques suggested the presence of an immunoreactive component of higher molecular weight in some of these patients.[67] Epstein et al.[34] carried out chromatographic analyses by reverse-phase HPLC in

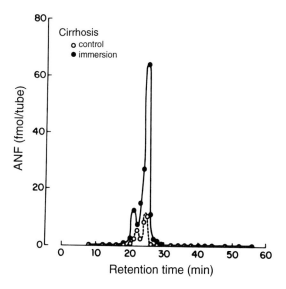

FIGURE 15.2. Reversed-phase HPLC of C_{18} Sep-Pak extracts of plasma obtained from a cirrhotic patient prior to (control, o) and during (immersion, ●) stimulation of ANF secretion by head-out water immersion. Samples were injected onto a 0.39 × 30-cm µBondapak C_{18} column and eluted at 1.0 ml/min with a linear gradient of 10–60% acetonitrile in 0.1% trifluoracetic acid over 50 minutes, as previously described[68]; the gradient was begun coincident with sample injection at 0 min. The major peak of irANF has a retention time (25 min) identical to that of synthetic ANF-(99-126). No immunoreactivity was detected in either sample at a retention time of 38 minutes, which corresponds to that of the ANF precursor, ANF-(1-126).[68] (From Epstein M, et al: Relationship between plasma ANF responsiveness and renal sodium handling in cirrhotic humans. Am J Nephrol 1989;9:133–143, with permission.)

extracts of plasma from several cirrhotic patients both under control conditions and following stimulation of ANF secretion by water immersion. They demonstrated that the pattern obtained was identical to that in normal humans (Fig. 15.2).[68]

Subsequently, Jiménez et al.[69] characterized the chromatographic patterns of ANF contained in plasma extracts from 10 patients with cirrhosis and ascites and 6 healthy subjects. They also tested the ANF from the cirrhotic patients in two different radioreceptor assays that detect the biologically active form(s) of this peptide. High performance liquid chromatography analysis of ANF disclosed an identical chromatographic pattern in cirrhotic patients and controls. Three peaks related to the atrial natriuretic factor prohormone were observed in cirrhotic patients and controls, accounting for 64%, 23%, and 11% of the total ANF factor in cirrhotic patients and 63%, 18%, and 8% of the total ANF in controls. The main peak eluted at the same position of synthetic human ANF (Ser 99-Tyr 126), which represents the major active form of the circulating hormone. ANF from cirrhotic patients displayed the same ability as synthetic human ANF to inhibit the binding of ^{125}I-atrial natriuretic factor to rat glomerular and bovine adrenal membrane receptors. The investigators concluded that ANF from patients with cirrhosis and ascites has an equipotent binding activity to its receptor as to that of synthetic human ANF and possesses the same molecular weight and biologically active forms as ANF of normal subjects .[69]

Collectively, the above studies indicate that elevated levels of ANF in cirrhosis cannot be attributed to release of an altered molecular species that is recognized by conventional radioimmunoassay.

ANF RESPONSIVENESS TO VOLUME CONTRACTION

Jespersen et al.[70] assessed the relationship between ANF and cyclic 3',5'-guanosine monophosphate (cGMP) in patients with cirrhosis, both with and without ascites, and in controls undergoing diuretic-induced volume contraction. Basal plasma levels of ANF and cGMP were higher in patients with cirrhosis than in controls, but the levels were similar in cirrhotic patients with and without ascites. Blood volume was reduced less after furosemide in cirrhotic patients (6.0%) than in healthy subjects (10.1%), but basal blood volume did not differ. In response to furosemide, ANF and cGMP decreased slightly in both groups.

ANF RESPONSIVENESS TO VOLUME EXPANSION MANEUVERS

Head-out Water Immersion

Although attempts have been undertaken to assess renal and hormonal responsiveness with saline infusion, several limitations of the study design confound interpretation of the results. As detailed previously,[71,72] rapid volume expansion of solutions such as saline have a number of drawbacks related to lack of specificity. For example, saline infusion increases the volume of all fluid compartments and induces concomitant alterations in plasma composition.

Studies from Epstein's laboratory over the past 27 years have circumvented many of these methodologic problems by applying a newly developed investigative tool—the model of head-out water immersion (HWI)—to the assessment of renal sodium and water homeostasis in both normal and diverse edematous states.[71,72] Earlier studies from our laboratory demonstrated that this maneuver produces prompt, sustained diuresis and natriuresis and markedly suppresses levels of PRA, plasma aldosterone (PA), and arginine vasopressin (AVP).[71,72]

Epstein et al.[73,74] and Warner et al.[75] demonstrated that HWI is a useful model for investigating the responsiveness of the ANF system to acute reversible central blood augmentation in normal subjects. This maneuver elicits a marked rise in ANF levels, natriuresis,[68,74] and a rise in plasma cGMP[75] and urinary excretion of cGMP.[68,74–76] Urinary excretion of cGMP is a marker of biochemical responsiveness to ANF signaling.[77,78]

Epstein et al[34] used HWI to determine whether the responsiveness of ANF to volume expansion is impaired in cirrhosis. Eight of the 9 patients in the study had marked ascites. Following equilibration on a 10-mEq sodium diet, during 3 hours of immersion, 5 of 9 cirrhotic patients manifested an exaggerated peak ANF response, whereas the remaining 4 manifested increases similar to those of normal subjects (Fig. 15.3). The concomitant natriuretic response varied widely, ranging from absent to markedly exaggerated. In contrast to normal subjects, the natriuretic responses of cirrhotic patients were dissociated from the concomitant increases in ANF. These observations indicate that there is no impairment in the release of ANF in cirrhosis.

A similar conclusion was reached by Skorecki et al.,[40] who studied 12 sodium-retaining cirrhotic patients during HWI. The patients were maintained for 7 days on 20-mEq sodium intake and then studied on both control and immersion days. In 6 patients, immersion resulted in a marked natriuresis sufficient to induce negative sodium balance by the third hour; these patients were termed responders. In the 6 responders, baseline preimmersion levels of plasma renin activity and serum aldosterone were below 3 ng/L/sec and 4 nmol/L, respectively. In the other 6 patients, the natriuretic response to immersion was markedly blunted and insufficient to induce negative sodium balance;

these patients were termed nonresponders. In contrast to responders, baseline preimmersion levels of plasma renin activity and aldosterone in nonresponders were above 3.5 ng/L/sec and 5 nmol/L, respectively. These levels were significantly elevated compared with responders and normal subjects consuming the same sodium intake. Furthermore, during HWI, none of the nonresponders suppressed to an aldosterone level below 1.4 nmol/L, a level that previously was proposed as permissive for a natriuretic response.[79] In both groups of cirrhotic patients, baseline levels of plasma ANF and urine cGMP excretion were significantly and comparably elevated compared with the normal range for controls ingesting the same sodium intake. Despite the marked difference in the natriuretic response to immersion between responders and nonresponders, there was significant and comparable further elevation of plasma ANF and urinary cGMP excretion during immersion compared with the control day in both groups. Such results indicate that even in nonresponders, there is no defect in ANF release or biochemical responsiveness, at least at the level of cGMP signaling.

The pattern of urine cGMP responses suggests that the relative renal resistance to the natriuretic action of ANF in nonresponders is mediated at a level parallel with or beyond coupling of ANF to its guanylate cyclase-linked receptor. However, it is possible that urinary cGMP excretion may predominantly reflect cGMP of glomerular origin and therefore may not reflect guanylate cyclase activation at tubule segments relevant to the natriuretic action of ANF. Resistance to the natriuretic action of ANF appears to be associated with activation of antinatriuretic factors, including the renin-angiotensin-aldosterone system, which is clearly activated in nonresponders. Epstein et al.[34] also observed significant elevation of basal plasma renin activity in nonresponders compared with responders.

Saline-induced Volume Expansion

As a more conventional volume-expanding maneuver, Tesar et al.[80] infused 2 L of saline solution per 70 kg of body weight during 2 hours into 6 normal subjects, 6 compensated cirrhotic patients and 6 decompensated cirrhotic patients. In the nonascitic cirrhotic patients and normal controls, infusion of saline was associated with a significant rise in ANF with a concomitant significant

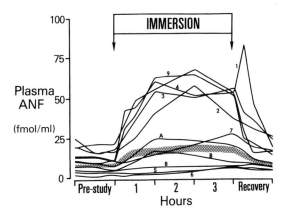

FIGURE 15.3. Effect of head-out water immersion on plasma ANF levels in 11 cirrhotic patients. The *shaded area* represents means ± SE for 13 normal subjects[74] undergoing an identical immersion study. Cirrhotic patients manifested a wide continuum of responses, with patients 1–4 and 9 manifesting a markedly exaggerated augmentation of ANF. (From Epstein M, et al: Relationship between ANF responsiveness and renal sodium handling in cirrhotic humans. Am J Nephrol 1989;9: 133–143, with permission.)

natriuresis and diuresis. The cirrhotic patients with ascites responded to infusion of saline with a rise in ANF comparable to nonascitic cirrhotic patients and controls. In contrast, the ascitic cirrhotic patients did not have a significant natriuresis or diuresis. In this group of ascitic cirrhotic patients, plasma renin activity and plasma aldosterone were incompletely suppressed by saline infusion. Tesar et al. also concluded that the renal resistance to the natriuretic action of ANF could be mediated, in part, by the incomplete suppression of the renin-angiotensin-aldosterone system.

Peritoneovenous Shunting

Another maneuver used to assess ANF responsiveness and its relationship with renal excretory function is peritoneovenous shunting (PVS). The physiologic consequences of PVS have been well documented[81] (see chapter 24). Acutely, there is a marked translocation of volume into the intravascular compartment, as demonstrated by an average 15% fall in hematocrit without a change in red cell mass. A rise in cardiac output, renal plasma flow, and creatinine clearance is accompanied by diuresis and natriuresis. Although the elevated levels of plasma renin activity (PRA), serum aldosterone, plasma catecholamines, and vasopressin eventually decline during the postoperative period, there are few if any changes in these parameters during the first 2–4 hours after PVS when changes in systemic hemodynamics and urinary sodium and water excretion are maximal. As an intravascular volume load is known to be a potent and rapid stimulus for ANF release, it was of interest to investigate the response of this hormone to PVS.

Campbell et al.[35] studied 6 cirrhotic patients with massive refractory ascites under strict metabolic conditions while they were receiving a 20-mEq sodium diet. Baseline ANF levels were significantly elevated compared with both normal subjects and cirrhotic patients without ascites on a 20-mEq sodium diet. Following shunt insertion, an immediate natriuresis and diuresis were observed in 5 of the 6 cirrhotic patients with refractory ascites. In these 5 patients, right atrial pressure and ANF rose immediately, followed by a rise in urinary cyclic GMP excretion. In the sixth patient, the rise in right atrial pressure was delayed by initial mechanical failure of shunt patency, and the rise in ANF, diuresis, and natriuresis were correspondingly delayed. The changes in ANF following PVS were positively correlated with changes in right atrial pressure, urinary cyclic GMP excretion, urine excretion of sodium, and urine volume. Such results suggested that a rise in ANF may contribute to the acute urinary response to PVS and confirm that even cirrhotic patients with severe sodium retention and refractory ascites do not have a defect in either ANF release or biochemical responsiveness at the level of cyclic GMP signaling. These studies suggest that a relative resistance to the natriuretic action of ANF can be overcome by the consequences of PVS.

Klepetko et al.[82] reported similar responses to PVS and measured the same parameters at subsequent intervals. Ten patients with cirrhosis and ascites underwent PVS, which resulted in an acute rise in plasma ANF levels. Mean preoperative plasma ANF levels of 82 ± 13.5 ng/L rose significantly to 308 ± 60 ng/L immediately after surgery. The ANF levels gradually fell but were still significantly elevated at 7 days after the operation (149 ± 28 ng/L). However, 3 months after shunt insertion, plasma ANF levels had fallen to the preoperative level (75 ± 9 ng/L).

Alternative explanations have been proposed for the augmented levels of ANF following PV shunting. Salerno et al.[83] have shown that immediately after a large volume paracentesis prior to colloid replacement, there is a significant rise in plasma ANF levels with a concomitant decrease in plasma renin activity and serum aldosterone. The authors concluded that the rapid relief of high intraabdominal pressure increases central venous blood return and cardiac output. It appears, therefore, that the acute rise in ANF following PV shunting is mediated initially by the relief of tense ascites as well as by intravascular fluid translocation. The potential role of ascites fluid in stimulating ANF release, over and above relief of elevated intraabdominal pressure and central volume expansion, has not been evaluated. Such evaluation requires an isovolemic infusion of ascites fluid.

RESPONSE OF ANF TO DIETARY SODIUM CHALLENGES

To delineate the role of ANF under more physiologic conditions, Warner et al.[42] studied the effect of ANF levels and urinary sodium excretion of varying dietary sodium intake in 11 patients with chronic liver disease (6 without and 5 with a history of clinical sodium retention [ascites or edema]).

The patients were placed on a 20-mmol constant sodium diet for 1 week, followed by a constant 100-mmol sodium diet under strict metabolic conditions. Following 5 days of equilibration on each diet, blood and urine samples were collected for plasma ANF levels and urinary sodium excretion. Normal controls (n = 6), as expected, remained in sodium balance on both the 20-mmol ($U_{Na}V$, 19±2) and the 100-mmol diet ($U_{Na}V$, 99 ± 7). ANF levels rose on the higher sodium diet (10 ± 4 pg/ml to 19 ± 4 pg/ml). Patients with no history of clinical sodium retention (n = 6) achieved near sodium balance in 5 days on both a 20-mmol sodium diet ($U_{Na}V$, 17 ± 3 mmol/day) and 100-mmol sodium diet ($U_{Na}V$, 80 ± 5 mmol/day). ANF levels rose on the 100-mmol diet (21 ± 7 to 30 ± 7 pg/ml) but were not significantly elevated compared with normal controls. In contrast, patients with a history of clinical sodium retention were in significant positive balance on both the 20-mmol sodium diet ($U_{Na}V$, 9.5 ± 3.3 mmol/day) and the 100-mmol sodium diet ($U_{Na}V$, 37 ± 13 mmol/day), despite significantly elevated plasma ANF levels on a 20-mmol diet (29 ± 4 pg/ml) and a significant increase in plasma ANF levels on a 100-mmol sodium diet (62 ± 9 pg/ml). These results are also consistent with renal resistance to the natriuretic actions of ANF in such patients.

As mentioned previously, the 6 patients without sodium retention were further studied on the 100-mmol sodium diet along with 7 other similar patients. The 13 patients underwent measurement of estimated portal pressures (corrected sinusoidal pressure), which was positively correlated with ANF levels (n = 13, p < 0.01, r = 0.75) (see Fig. 15.1). These results are consistent with the proposal that in patients with chronic liver disease intrasinusoidal hypertension may play a role in the initial development of sodium retention and that sodium retention is maintained on various sodium diets at the expense of a gradual elevation in ANF levels.

RENAL RESPONSIVENESS TO INFUSION OF EXOGENOUS PEPTIDE

The volume-expanding maneuvers described in the previous section induce complex shifts in multiple parameters involved in the regulation of sodium excretion. To assess the responsiveness to ANF per se, investigators have infused exogenous ANF into cirrhotic patients. The available reports indicate that many patients manifested a blunted natriuretic response to infusion of ANF.

Legault et al .(unpublished data) compared the natriuretic response to HWI with the response to infusion of α-human ANF in 12 cirrhotic patients. ANF was administered as an initial bolus of 35 ng/kg/min for 5 minutes, followed by a constant infusion of 15 ng/kg/min for 115 minutes. There was no significant change in mean arterial blood pressure with either maneuver in any patient. Five patients displayed a natriuretic response to HWI, sufficient to achieve negative sodium balance analogous to the responders in the previously cited study by Skorecki et al.[40] Each of these 5 patients also mounted a natriuretic response to ANF infusion. In contrast, the other 7 patients consistently failed to develop a natriuretic response to either maneuver. In these nonresponders, levels of plasma renin activity (PRA) and serum aldosterone were significantly elevated, and basal urinary sodium excretion and plasma sodium concentration were significantly depressed compared with responders. The congruency among patients in the response to ANF infusion on the one hand and HWI on the other hand indicates that resistance to the natriuretic effect of HWI indeed represents resistance to the natriuretic action of ANF. ANF levels achieved with infusion were comparable to peak levels achieved immediately following PVS. Failure of nonresponders to mount a natriuresis in response to this ANF infusion protocol clearly suggests that factors in addition to ANF release mediate the natriuretic response to PVS.

Salerno et al. also studied the effects of ANF infusion in cirrhotic patients.[84] Following a bolus injection of ANF (1 μg/kg), 7 patients with elevated baseline PRA and aldosterone levels demonstrated an attenuated or absent natriuretic response. Seven patients without sodium retention or with moderate sodium retention and normal baseline PRA and aldosterone levels had a marked natriuresis, as did normal controls. This supraphysiologic dose of ANF caused a transient drop in blood pressure in both cirrhotic patients and normal controls.

Fried et al.[85] evaluated the effects of anaritide, a 25-amino acid synthetic analog of ANF, in 28 cirrhotic patients with ascites and edema. Patients received infusions ranging from 0.015–0.300 μg/kg/min. There was a significant natriuresis at all doses of anaritide with the exception of the highest dose. With infusion rates of 0.60 μg/kg/min or greater there was a progressive significant decline in mean arterial pressure. The authors concluded that the therapeutic potential of anaritide could be limited by its hypotensive effect at high doses. Petrillo et al.[86] have shown that the hypotension caused by high-dose anaritide was associated with a rise in plasma catecholamines and plasma renin activity. Thus, it appears that the attenuated renal response to ANF infused at high doses may be mediated in turn by activation of the sympathetic nervous system and renin-angiotensin systems and possibly other factors, such as decrease in glomerular filtration rate, that abrogate the natriuretic activity of ANF.

Investigators have attempted to improve the therapeutic potential of intravenous ANF infusion in patients with cirrhosis by the simultaneous infusion of norepinephrine to prevent the hypotensive effects of ANF. However, two groups of investigators have observed that the blunted natriuretic response to ANF in patients with advanced cirrhosis could not be reversed by prevention or correction of hypotension with intravenous norepinephrine.[87,88] In both studies, norepinephrine infusion had no significant effect on plasma renin activity or aldosterone. Thus the systemic hypotensive state per se, which is characteristic of advanced cirrhosis, does not appear to be the critical determinant of sodium retention.

Beutler et al.[89] compared the response of patients with biopsy-proved cirrhosis but without ascites (proved by sonography) to normal controls to comparable infusions of ANF. The controls were studied on a 20-, 100-, or 200-mmol sodium/day diet, whereas the cirrhotic patients were ingesting either 40 or 120 mmol of sodium/day. Mean basal ANF levels in cirrhotic patients was 34.4 ± 4 pmol/L compared with 11.3 ± 3 pmol/L in controls. Blood pressure, GFR (inulin clearance), renal plasma flow (p-aminohippurate clearance), solute-free water clearance, and maximal urine flow were normal in cirrhotic patients. In response to a single injection of 100 μg of ANF, the normal subjects manifested a much greater proportional rise in sodium excretion at all levels of sodium intake compared with cirrhotic patients. In addition, no rise in the GFR occurred in cirrhotic patients, and the maximal urine flow was significantly less. Such observations suggest that the alterations in ANF levels and ANF response occur in the early, preascitic phase of cirrhosis as well as in established disease. An intriguing feature of this study—but one that potentially confounds interpretation of results—is that in patients with compensated cirrhosis, ANF administration caused a large drop in blood pressure (mean decrease of 22/13 mmHg) that was not seen in normal subjects. The concomitant drop in blood pressure could be explained by impending underfill or possibly by an abnormality in the regulation of systemic vascular tone, as recently proposed according to the peripheral arterial vasodilation hypothesis.[90] This hypothesis proposes that vasodilatation is the first hemodynamic abnormality to precede renal sodium retention in early cirrhosis.

Laffi et al.[91] found that in cirrhotic patients with refractory ascites and striking activation of the renin-angiotensin-aldosterone system, bolus infusion of α-human ANF (1 μg/kg IV every 3 hours for 4 doses) caused no appreciable natriuresis and diuresis. In contrast, when the α-human ANF was infused as a smaller initial bolus (50 ng/kg) followed by an infusion of 0.1 μg/kg/min for 45 minutes, there was a heterogeneous natriuretic response.[92] In responders, the extent of the natriuretic response paralleled the increase of effective renal plasma flow and glomerular filtration rate. In nonresponders the absent natriuretic response was associated with a reduction of these parameters. As noted by other investigators,[86] plasma renin activity was increased in nonresponders but not in responders to ANF infusion.

CIRCADIAN PATTERNS

In normal subjects, urine volume flow and sodium excretion are subject to diurnal variation with a reduction of both during the night.[93,94] This pattern is either reversed or lost in patients with liver cirrhosis.[95,96] In studies of circulating aldosterone concentration in cirrhosis during which patients remained supine over a 24-hour period, Bernardi et al.[97,98] demonstrated a loss of the circadian pattern of PRA and aldosterone and norepinephrine concentration in patients with cirrhosis and ascites. Colantonio et al.[99] reported the absence of variation of plasma atrial natriuretic peptide (ANP) in cirrhotic patients under similar conditions. Unfortunately, the investigators failed to report data about concomitant renal excretory function.

Recently, Panos et al.[100] investigated whether the circadian pattern of circulating ANF is altered in cirrhosis and whether ANF alterations contribute to the reversed nocturnal natriuretic and diuretic patterns observed in cirrhotic patients. They studied 21 patients with cirrhosis and moderate-to-marked ascites and compared them with 10 age-matched controls. In 8 of the cirrhotic patients, PRA, plasma aldosterone (PA), and urine sodium excretion (U_{Na}) were measured every 4 hours for 24 hours. Subjects were ambulatory between 0800–2300 hours and supine from 2300–0800 hours. In controls, U_{Na} was highest between 1600–2400 and lowest between 2400–0800 hours. In patients with cirrhosis, U_{Na} was 0.6 ± 0.1 mmol/min between 1600–2400 hours and 1.9 ± 0.7 mmol/min ($p < 0.08$) between 2400–0800 hours. Concomitantly, mean plasma ANF concentration did not change during the day, but there was a large, sustained rise in PRA and PA. There was a correlation between ANF and U_{Na} between 2400–0800 hours ($r = 0.65$; $p < 0.02$) and 1600–2400 hours ($r = 0.54$, $p < 0.05$) but not between 0800–1600 hours. PRA declined from 12.5 ± 2.5 at 2400 hours to 7.4 ± 0.9 pmol/h/ml at 0800 hours ($p < 0.05$) and PA from 1032 ± 101 to $798 + 56$ pmol/L ($p < 0.05$). Panos et al.[100] interpreted their findings as suggesting that ANF contributed to the nocturnal natriuresis of cirrhosis. They postulated that a suppression in the activity of the renin-aldosterone system during recumbency may allow the natriuretic effect of ANF to become manifest.

RELATIONSHIP BETWEEN CIRCULATING ANF AND RENAL EXCRETORY FUNCTION: CONSIDERATION OF RESISTANCE TO NATRIURETIC ACTION OF ANF

The above studies, on the whole, indicate that there is no deficiency in plasma ANF levels in cirrhosis and ascites. Neither is there an impairment in release of ANF following volume expansion maneuvers. There is no apparent impairment in generation of cGMP, as evidenced by the rise in urine cyclic GMP following HWI, even in nonresponders,[40] which indicates that relative resistance to the natriuretic action of ANF is likely mediated at a level beyond ANF release or coupling to its receptor.

Nevertheless, there is a clear dissociation between circulating levels of ANF and renal responsiveness to its natriuretic actions . What mediates the resistance to ANF? Possibilities include (1) impaired delivery of salt and water to distal nephron sites responsive to ANF mediated by antinatriuretic factors and a reduced glomerular filtration rate; (2) forces favoring sodium retention that override the natriuretic effects of ANF at its site of action in the medullary collecting duct; (3) downregulation of a population of ANF receptors at a distal nephron site, not reflected in urinary cGMP; (4) a biochemical defect beyond the level of cGMP production, such as cGMP-dependent kinase; and (5) decreased delivery of permissive cofactors that allow appropriate ANF action to be effected at the luminal distal tubule (see next section).

A review of the available evidence indicates that the presence of opposing antinatriuretic factors is likely an important factor in mediating the renal resistance to the natriuretic actions of ANF. Experiments using HWI have shown that nonresponders have significantly greater activation of the renin-angiotensin system than responders.[34,40] None of the nonresponders were able to reach a nadir of aldosterone less than 1.4 nmol/L following HWI[40]—values previously shown by others[79] to be permissive for a natriuretic response.

Gerbes et al.[101] have shown that neither ANF nor plasma renin activity nor aldosterone alone correlated with sodium excretion; rather, the ratio of atrial natriuretic factor to plasma aldosterone concentrations was closely correlated to basal and stimulated natriuresis in cirrhotic patients. Such results do not imply that activation of the renin-angiotensin-aldosterone system is the only

important antinatriuretic factor but rather that this system is a suitable marker for enhanced antinatriuretic activity caused by several efferent antinatriuretic factors. The finding that some sodium-retaining cirrhotic subjects show a hyperresponsiveness to HWI in terms of both enhanced ANF release and natriuresis compared with normal subjects[48] strongly suggests that there is no intrinsic biochemical resistance to ANF in cirrhosis. Once antinatriuretic factors have been adequately suppressed, the full effect of increased levels of ANF can be expressed by the kidney as an exaggerated natriuretic response.

The renal resistance to the natriuretic actions of ANF may be mediated in part by increased renal sympathetic nerve activity. Studies by Koepke et al.[102–104] implicate a role for heightened renal nerve activity in experimental animal models of ANF resistance, including cirrhosis. Nicholls et al.[105] have shown that HWI caused a significant suppression of norepinephrine in patients who developed natriuresis. Lumbar sympathetic block has been shown to increase sodium excretion in 6 of 8 sodium-retaining cirrhotic patients.[106]

A study by Morali et al.[107] is of interest in this regard. The authors studied the potential role of the sympathetic nervous system as a determinant of the responsiveness of ANF by using microneurography to measure muscle sympathetic nerve activity (SNA). Twenty-six patients with biopsy-proved cirrhosis and 7 age- and sex-matched normal volunteers were studied after 1 week of a 20-mmol sodium diet without diuretic administration. Muscle SNA was recorded from the peroneal nerve and correlated with responsiveness to a 2-hour ANF infusion. Lithium clearance was used as a marker for sodium reabsorption proximal to the intramedullary collecting duct, the main site of ANF action. Muscle SNA was greatly increased in the 12 ascitic patients who were nonresponders to ANF infusion compared with normal subjects (64 ± 4 vs. 27 ± 7 bursts/min, $p < 0.001$), moderately increased in 5 ascitic responders (47 ± 6 bursts/min, $p < 0.05$), but not significantly increased in 9 nonascitic patients with cirrhosis (34 ± 5 bursts/min). SNA correlated positively with plasma norepinephrine levels ($r = 0.69$, $p < 0.005$) and correlated inversely with peak sodium excretion during the ANF infusion ($r = 0.63$, $p < 0.0001$). Consistent with previous studies, plasma renin activity and aldosterone were markedly elevated in ascitic nonresponders and normal in ascitic responders and nonascitic patients. Lithium clearance was reduced in as-citic patients compared with nonascitic patients, did not change after ANF infusion, and correlated inversely with SNA (r = 0.61, p <0.01). Such results support the concept that the sympathetic nervous system is a factor in renal sodium handling in cirrhosis, and refractoriness to ANF might be explained, in part, by increased neurally mediated sodium reabsorption proximal to the intramedullary collecting duct, the main site of ANF action.

The mechanism whereby candidate antinatriuretic forces impair the response to ANF warrants consideration. One obvious potential mechanism is the action of angiotensin II and catecholamines to enhance fractional proximal reabsorption of filtered fluid and hence to diminish delivery to ANF-responsive sites in the distal nephron. In turn, this may result from direct effects on sodium handling by the proximal tubule as well as by perturbations in peritubule capillary Starling forces consequent to adjustments in glomerular hemodynamics.[108] Both micropuncture and clearance studies in humans and animals confirm that abnormal salt and water processing in cirrhosis occurs at multiple tubule sites even in the face of normal GFR[108] (also see chapter 1). The necessary and sufficient site for ANF-induced natriuresis is the medullary collecting tubule, although actions at more proximal segments may be contributory.[108–113] Indeed, there is indirect evidence from HWI studies that in some circumstances resistance to ANF action at the distal nephron contributes to the blunted natriuretic response.[40] In these studies, both nonresponders and responders demonstrated significant kaliuresis during HWI, but only the responders significantly increased solute-free water clearance. Thus, the delivery of sodium to distal nephron segments was at least adequate for a kaliuretic response, even in the nonresponders.

Another action of ANF in the collecting tubules is to antagonize the hydroosmotic action of vaso-pressin,[25] and it is tempting to speculate that there is resistance to both the diuretic and the natriuretic actions of ANF in the collecting tubule. It has been demonstrated that at peak natriuretic effect urinary potassium excretion is significantly greater in responders than nonresponders during both ANF infusion and HWI,[113a] despite lower aldosterone concentration in responders. This finding suggests that distal delivery may be limiting in nonresponders. The lack of a kaliuresis following

infusion of physiologic doses of ANF in responders suggests that the dominant effect of ANF is to reverse the antinatriuretic factors at the collecting tubule and that improved distal sodium delivery during HWI is mediated more by other factors associated with volume expansion besides the rise of ANF per se. Furthermore, the ability of an ANF infusion to cause a natriuresis only in responders without a concomitant change in lithium clearance confirms a distal site of ANF resistance in nonresponders.[107]

Morali et al.[114] studied 10 patients with massive, resistant ascites, off diuretics and on a 20-mmol/day sodium diet for 7 days. ANF responsiveness was confirmed by the failure of a 2-hour infusion of ANF to induce a natriuresis. The following day all patients received an infusion of 40 gm of mannitol and subsequently a combined infusion of mannitol and ANF. Six of the 10 patients responded to mannitol alone with an increased natriuresis (0.27 ± 0.05 mmol/hr to 1.65 ± 0.53 mmol/hr). The combination of ANF and mannitol induced a further significant increase in sodium excretion (3.28 ± 0.68 mmol/hr). Lithium clearance increased in the responders after mannitol infusion but did not increase further with ANF and mannitol. Inulin and PAH clearances were equally low in both mannitol responders and mannitol nonresponders and did not change with ANF and mannitol infusions. The mannitol responders had significantly lower plasma renin activity (PRA), aldosterone, and norepinephrine than the mannitol nonresponders. Thus ANF unresponsiveness in some cirrhotic patients was shown to be due in part to increased sodium reabsorption proximal to the distal site of ANF action as well as to resistance to the action of ANF in the collecting tubule. The increased proximal reabsorption could be mediated by perturbations in physical forces governing fluid reabsorption in the proximal tubule or by direct actions of angiotensin II or catecholamines.

A potential biochemical mechanism for resistance of the collecting tubule to ANF in cirrhosis remains to be clarified. The well-preserved cGMP responses might suggest that resistance to ANF is mediated in a pathway distal to or parallel with cGMP signaling. However, as noted previously, urinary cGMP appearance may be a predominant reflection of cGMP of glomerular origin; thus inhibition of guanylate cyclase at relevant downstream tubule sites might not be readily discerned with measurements of urinary cGMP excretion.

Relatively high concentrations of calcium are required to inhibit ANF-stimulated guanylate cyclase in cultured rat renal glomerular mesangial cells.[115] In these cells, activation of protein kinase C with phorbol esters also causes marked inhibition of guanylate cyclase activation. Such results are consistent with the studies of Jaiswal et al.,[116] who proposed that the guanylate cyclase coupled to the ANP receptor is partially under the regulation of protein kinase C-mediated phosphorylation. No vasoconstrictor hormones that inhibit cGMP production have been found in intact glomerular mesangial cells, in agreement with unaltered urinary cGMP responses in cirrhosis. In contrast, vasoconstrictor hormones have been shown to inhibit the cGMP response of vascular smooth muscle cells in culture.[117,118] There is a less likely possibility that resistance to ANF is mediated at the level of receptors not coupled to guanylate cyclase or at the level of cGMP kinase.

Another possible mechanism to account for renal resistance to elevated circulating ANF levels is of a change in "clearance" ANF receptors. Consistent with this formulation, Gerbes et al. recently reported a higher density of clearance ANF receptors and lower density of biologically active ANF receptors in bile duct-ligated rats compared with control animals.[119]

ENDOPEPTIDASE AND OTHER URINARY PEPTIDE COFACTORS

Two novel approaches have been proposed to enhance ANF activity without resorting to an infusion of ANF. As noted earlier, because ANF is a peptide, it can be administered only by the intravenous route. The rapid metabolic clearance[120,121] necessitates repeated bolus injections or continuous infusions. Alternatively, circulating ANF concentrations might be elevated by blocking its clearance through administration of truncated analogs that bind only to clearance receptors and thus augment the concentration of ANF reaching the B-receptors.[21,122,123] A second approach to enhancing ANF activity is to inhibit metabolism of the peptide. In vitro studies have demonstrated that ANF is a substrate for neutral endopeptidase (NEP; membrane metalloendopeptidase).[20] The major cleavage site is the Cys^{105}-Phe^{106} bond, which results in an inactive metabolite. The enzyme is widely distributed in the body but is most abundant in the renal cortex, in particular the proximal tubule.[124] Several inhibitors of NEP

are known; one such compound is thiorphan (DL-3mercapto-2benzylpropanoyl-glycine). Given alone to rats, it is natriuretic and diuretic.[125] Co-administered with ANF, it has been reported to enhance plasma ANF levels and to potentiate the renal response to the peptide.[125]

Wilkins et al.[126] investigated the effect of thiorphan in rats in which an aortavenocaval (AV) shunt was established distal to the renal arteries to create a model of high-output cardiac failure with chronically elevated plasma ANF and urinary cGMP levels. The authors demonstrated that thiorphan induced a natriuresis in AV fistula rats, which exceeded that in control animals receiving the same compounds and matched the peak natriuresis produced in sham-operated animals by high doses of ANF. The investigators speculated that the greater potency of thiorphan in heart failure compared with infusions of ANF may be attributable to the ability of thiorphan to protect filtered ANF from degradation in the kidney, thereby enabling ANF to reach normally inaccessible renal tubule sites. Consistent with this hypothesis was the appearance of ANF in the urine of animals treated with thiorphan. In contrast, very little ANF was detected in the urine of sham-operated or AV fistula rats under basal conditions or even when plasma ANF levels were greatly elevated by infusion.

Levy et al.[127] studied the effect of inhibition of neutral endopeptidase 24-11 on caval dogs that were unresponsive to a supraphysiologic dose of intravenous ANF. Inhibition of neutral endopeptidase 24-11 converted a nonresponder caval dog into a responder. The investigators found this exciting result after many previous strategies to convert nonresponder to responder caval dogs had been unsuccessful. Administration of ANF in the face of alpha-adrenergic blockade, saralasin (an angiotensin II antagonist), dypridamole (an inhibitor of adenosine uptake), and elevation of blood pressure could not alter the initial response to ANF.[128] Recently, Levy's group also observed that the provision of bradykinin allows nonresponding caval dogs to respond to ANF, urodilatin (see below), and 8-bromo cyclic GMP.[129] Conversely, pretreatment of caval dogs with either aprotinin or a specific bradykinin antagonist significantly attenuated the natriuretic action of ANF. Such results indicate that nonresponding caval dogs appeared to have a deficiency in kinins below some critical level. It is possible that the renal activity of ANF may be potentiated by inhibition of endopeptidase 24-11 by a mechanism that involves the accumulation of bradykinin.[130,131]

Urodilatin, a homologous natriuretic peptide of renal origin, was first discovered in 1988.[132] The prohormone produced by the kidney tubules may be identical to the 126-residue prohormone of atrial natriuretic peptide.[133] This prohormone is cleaved to urodilatin, a 32-residue peptide (identical to circulating ANF with the addition of four amino acids and an NH_2-terminal extension) that is found in urine but not in plasma. Urodilatin has a natriuretic potency at least equal to that of ANF. It is unclear whether under physiologic circumstances urodilatin has primacy over ANF in governing natriuretic responses.[133] It may be the physiologic ligand for more distal "ANF" receptors.

Drummer et al.[134] found that urodilatin excretion closely paralleled circadian renal sodium excretion in 9 healthy humans and also correlated well with the natriuresis following saline infusion. They found no similar correlation with plasma ANF and concluded that urodilatin was the important peptide in the physiologic regulation of natriuresis. It may well be that ANF is

predominantly active in terms of its vasoactive properties in the kidney and elsewhere in the body, whereas urodilatin may mediate the epithelial modulatory responses.

It has been postulated that brush border peptidases may prevent peptides such as ANF from reaching the distal nephron and causing an inappropriate natriuresis.[135] In contrast, urodilatin is resistant to degradation by these enzymes and is produced beyond their site of action.[134]

Recently, Norsk et al.[136] investigated the relationship between urodilatin and renal sodium and water handling during immersion in normal subjects. Immersion induced an increase in renal excretion of urodilatin and guanosine 3',5'-cyclic monophosphate (cGMP). Because they demonstrated a correlation between renal urodilatin excretion and both urine flow and sodium excretion, the investigators concluded that urodilatin may participate as one of the mechanisms mediating the natriuresis and diuresis of immersion in humans.

We are unaware of studies assessing urodilatin responsiveness in cirrhotic patients. Additional studies are needed to delineate the role of urodilatin in modulating sodium homeostasis in normal subjects and in mediating the sodium retention of cirrhosis.

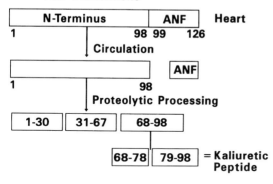

FIGURE 15.4. Origination of kaliuretic stimulator from atrial natriuretic factor prohormone. The 126-amino acid atrial natriuretic factor prohormone (pro ANF) is stored within granules in myocytes within the heart. Shortly before release pro ANF is processed into a 98-amino acid N-terminus and a 28-amino acid C-terminus (i.e., ANF), both of which circulate. The 98-amino acid N-terminus is further proteolytically processed in the circulation to three peptides consisting of amino acids 1-30, 31-67, and 68-98. The peptide consisting of amino acids 68-98 has its N-terminal amino acids proteolytically removed in the circulation to form a peptide consisting of amino acids 79-98 of this prohormone. This peptide is a kaliuretic stimulator.

ADDITIONAL PEPTIDE HORMONES DERIVED FROM ANF PROHORMONE

Kaliuretic stimulator is a new peptide hormone consisting of amino acids 79-98 of the 126-amino acid ANF prohormone[137] (Fig. 15.4). This peptide originates from the 98-amino acid N-terminus of ANF prohormone by proteolytic processing to a peptide consisting of amino acids 68-98; with further processing, pro-ANF 79-98 is formed (see Fig. 15.4). Kaliuretic stimulator has the strongest potassium-excreting properties of all the atrial natriuretic peptides in animals[140] and humans.[141] In addition to stimulating potassium excretion, it has blood pressure-lowering and diuretic properties,[140–142] Recently, kaliuretic stimulator was demonstrated to circulate in healthy humans.[137]

We recently conducted studies using water immersion, a well-defined model for reproducibly stimulating a marked and sustained release of the C-terminus[34,68,72–74] and the N-terminus of the ANF prohormone in healthy humans[138] to assess the responsiveness of kaliuretic peptide. We demonstrated that both kaliuretic stimulator and

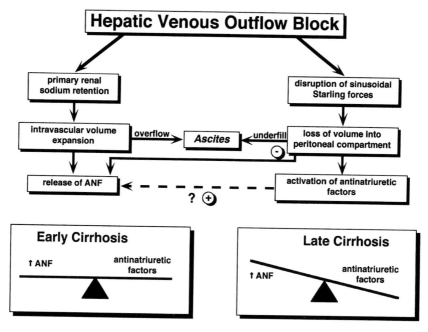

FIGURE 15.5. Working formulation for the role of ANF in the renal sodium retention of cirrhosis. The primary hepatic abnormality that is necessary and sufficient for renal sodium retention is hepatic venous overflow blockade. In early disease, this signals renal sodium retention with consequent intravascular volume expansion and a compensatory rise in plasma ANF level. At this stage of disease, the rise in ANF level is sufficient to counterbalance the primary antinatriuretic or renal sodium-retaining influences; however, it does so at the expense of an expanded intravascular volume with the potential for overflow ascites. Progressive disease is characterized by disruption of intrasinusoidal Starling forces and loss of volume from the vascular compartment into the peritoneal compartment. This underfilling of the circulation may attenuate further increases in ANF levels and promotes the activation of antinatriuretic factors. Whether the antinatriuretic factors activated by underfilling are the same as or different from those that promote primary renal sodium retention in early disease remains to be determined. At this later stage of disease, elevated levels of ANF may not be sufficient to counterbalance antinatriuretic influences. (From Warner LC, et al: The role of resistance to atrial natriuretic peptide and the pathogenesis of sodium retention in hepatic cirrhosis. In Brenner BM, Laragh J (eds): Progress in Atrial Peptide Research. New York: Raven Press, 1989;3:185–203, with permission.)

ANF increased promptly and markedly in response to immersion.[137]

Such studies have recently been extended to a group of decompensated cirrhotic patients.[143] We demonstrated that the response of circulating kaliuretic peptide and ANF to water immersion in 8 cirrhotic patients was significantly greater than in 7 healthy volunteers, suggesting that release of this peptide was not impaired in cirrhotic patients.

SUMMARY

A working formulation for the role of ANF in the sodium retention of cirrhosis is summarized in Figure 15.5. Sodium retention is initiated early in cirrhosis either as a result of hepatic venous outflow block[144–146] (see also chapter 8) or primary vasodilation.[90] The consequent intravascular volume expansion causes a rise in ANF levels. At this stage of disease, the rise in ANF level is sufficient to counterbalance the antinatriuretic influences. However, this balance occurs at the expense of an expanded intravascular volume with the potential for overflow ascites. Progressive disease is characterized by disruption of intrasinusoidal Starling forces and loss of volume from the vascular compartment into the peritoneal compartment[145] This underfilling of the circulation may attenuate further increases in plasma ANF and promotes the activation of antinatriuretic factors. At this later stage of disease, elevated levels of ANF are insufficient to counterbalance antinatriuretic influences. Thus, the role of ANF in cirrhosis is primarily beneficial in that it successfully attenuates the antinatriuretic forces in the compensated stage. There are, however, two potential deleterious effects of raised ANF levels:

1. ANF may exacerbate arterial vasodilation, leading to further sodium retention whose primacy in initiating renal sodium retention has been proposed as an alternate formulation to the overflow and underfill hypotheses.[90]

2. Epstein et al.[30] found higher basal ANF in cirrhotic patients with edema than in cirrhotic patients without edema. ANF is known to reduce plasma volume in anephric animals[147] and to increase the ultrafiltration coefficient of isolated capillaries.[148] Therefore, it is conceivable that in the clinical setting in which antinatriuretic factors limit renal responsiveness to elevated levels of ANF (i.e., cirrhosis, congestive heart failure, primary renal disease), ANF may contribute to edema formation at the level of the peripheral microcirculation. In general, ANF likely has no primary role in the sodium retention in cirrhosis. In early compensated cirrhosis, ANF may maintain sodium homeostasis despite the presence of mild antinatriuretic factors. In late ascitic cirrhosis renal resistance to ANF renders it ineffective.

Future studies should address the biochemical mechanisms that mediate ANF resistance. Hopefully more information is forthcoming about the interaction of bradykinin with ANF to cause a natriuresis. Deficiencies in renal kinins are possibly important in advanced cirrhosis and perhaps in other sodium-retaining states.

Another potential area of research involves the identification of antinatriuretic factors in early preascitic cirrhosis. The finding of an association between corrected sinusoidal pressures and steady-state plasma ANF levels[42] suggests that intrasinusoidal hypertension may stimulate sodium retention. In humans, preascitic cirrhosis has been associated with a trend toward elevated muscle sympathetic nerve activity compared with normal subjects.[107] It remains to be established in animal models whether intrasinusoidal hypertension leads to sodium retention initially through increased renal sympathetic nerve activity or other mechanisms. In portal vein-ligated rats, plasma ANF decreased by 50%.[149] A more appropriate model to investigate the relationship between ANF and cirrhosis might be hepatic vein ligation, which would lead to an increase in intrasinusoidal hypertension.

Insights gleaned from studies of ANF action in cirrhosis suggest a number of potential therapeutic prospects. Endopeptidase inhibitors that augment ANF and kinin delivery distally appear to show promise in some preliminary studies in nonresponders. ANF infusion alone has been disappointing; patients who could benefit the most are resistant. ANF may be much more effective when coupled with an endopeptidase inhibitor or other agents; such combined therapy may find a role as a temporary supportive measure in the management of patients with hepatorenal syndrome. Finally urodilatin, which is resistant to breakdown by brush border enzymes, may have added therapeutic potential when used with bradykinin.

Acknowledgments. The author thanks Elsa V. Reina for her expert secretarial help. Portions of this chapter have been adapted with permission from an earlier review by Warner L, Skorecki K, Blendis LM, Epstein M: Atrial natriuretic factor in liver disease. Hepatology 1993;17:500-513.

REFERENCES

1. Atlas SA, Laragh JH: Physiological actions of atrial natriuretic factor. In Mulrow PJ, Schrier R (eds): Atrial Hormones and Other Natriuretic Factors. Bethesda, MD: American Physiological Society, 1987;53–76.
2. Needleman P, Adams SP, Cole BR, et al: Atriopeptin as cardiac hormones. Hypertension (NY) 1985;7:469–482.
3. Cantin M, Genest J: The heart and the atrial natriuretic factor. Endocr Rev 1985;6:107–127.
4. Weidmann P, Saxenhofer H, Ferrier C, Shaw SG: Atrial natriuretic peptide in man. Am J Nephrol 1988; 8:1-14.
5. Goetz KL: Physiology and pathophysiology of atrial peptides. Am J Physiol 1988;254:E1–E15.
6. Vesely DL: Atrial natriuretic hormones. Englewood Cliffs, NJ: Prentice Hall, 1992; 1–256.
7. Epstein M: Hepatorenal syndrome: Emerging perspectives of pathophysiology and therapy. J Am Soc Nephrol, 1994;4:1735–1753.
8. Epstein M: The sodium retention of cirrhosis: A reappraisal. Hepatology 1986;6:312–315.
9. Better OS, Schrier RW: Disturbed volume homeostasis in patients with cirrhosis of the liver. Kidney Int 1983; 23:303–311.
10. Henriksen JH, Bendtsen F, Gerbes AL, et al: Estimated central blood volume in cirrhosis: Relationship to sympathetic nervous activity, β-adrenergic blockade and atrial natriuretic factor. Hepatology 1992;1163–1170.
11. Henriksen JH, Bendtsen F, Sørensen TIA, et al: Reduced central blood volume in cirrhosis. Gastroenterology 1989;97:1506–1513.
12. Panos MZ, Moore K, Vlavianos P, et al: Single, total paracentesis for tense ascites: Sequential hemodynamic changes and right atrial size. Hepatology 1990;11: 662–667.
13. Keller H, Bezjak V, Stegaru B, Buss J, et al: Ventricular function in cirrhosis and portasystemic shunt: A two-dimensional echocardiographic study. Hepatology 1988; 8:658–662.

14. Henriksen JH, Schutten HJ, Bendtsen F, Warberg J: Circulating atrial natriuretic peptide (ANP) and central blood volume (CBV) in cirrhosis. Liver 1986;6:361–368.

15. Levy M: Pathophysiology of ascites formation. In Epstein M(ed): The Kidney in Liver Disease, 3rd ed. Baltimore: Williams & Wilkins, 1988;209–243.

16. Rector WG, Hossack KF: Pathogenesis of sodium retention complicating cirrhosis: Is there room for diminished "effective" arterial blood volume? Gastroenterology 1988;95:1658–1663.

17. Rector WG Jr, Adair O, Hossack K, Painguet S: Atrial volume in cirrhosis: Relationship to blood volume and plasma concentration of atrial natriuretic factor. Gastroenterology 1990;99:766–770.

18. deBold AJ, Borenstein HB, Veress AT, Sonnenberg H: A rapid and potent natriuretic response to intravenous injection of atrial myocardial extract in rats. Life Sci 1981;28:89–94.

19. Seidman CE, Duby AD, Choi E, et al: The structure of rat preproatrial natriuretic factor as defined by a complementary DNA clone. Science 1986;225:324–326.

20. Ballerman BJ, Zeidel ML, Gunning ME, Brenner BM: Atrial natriuretic peptide. In Brenner and Rector (eds): The Kidney, 4th ed. Philadelphia: W.B. Saunders, 1991;1:537–558.

21. Maack T, Suzuki M, Almeida FA, et al: Physiological role of silent receptors of atrial natriuretic factor. Science 1987;238:675–679.

22. Hamet P, Tremblay J, Pan SC, et al: Cyclic GMP as a mediator and biological marker of atrial natriuretic factor. J Hypertension 1986;4(Suppl 2):S49–S56.

23. Sonnenberg H: Mechanisms of release and renal tubular actions of atrial natriuretic factor. Fed Proc 1986; 45:2106–2110.

24. Huang CL, Lewicki J, Johnson LK, Cogan MG: Renal mechanisms of action of rat atrial natriuretic factor. J Clin Invest 1985;75:769–773.

25. Dillingham MH, Anderson RJ: Inhibition of vasopressin action by atrial natriuretic factor. Science 1986; 231:1572–1573.

26. Maack T, Marion DN, Camargo MJ, et al: Effects of auriculin (atrial natriuretic factor) on blood pressure, renal function and the renin-aldosterone system in dogs. Am J Med 1984;77:1069–1075.

27. Bussien JP, Biollaz J, Waeber B, et al: Dose dependent effect of atrial natriuretic peptide on blood pressure, heart rate and skin blood flow of normal volunteers. J Cardiovasc Pharmacol 1986;8:216–220.

28. Kleinert HD, Maack T, Atlas SA, et al: Atrial natriuretic factor inhibits angiotensin-, norepinephrine-, and potassium-induced vascular contractility. Hypertension 1984;6(Suppl I):I143–I147.

29. Samson WK: Atrial natriuretic factor inhibits dehydration- and hemorrhage-induced vasopressin release. Neuroendocrinology 1985;40:277–279.

30. Epstein M: Atrial natriuretic factor in patients with liver disease. Am J Nephrol 1989;9:89–100.

31. Bonkovsky HL, Hartle DK, Mellen BG, et al: Plasma concentrations of immunoreactive atrial natriuretic peptide in hospitalized cirrhotic and non-cirrhotic patients: Evidence of a role of deficient atrial natriuretic peptide in pathogenesis of cirrhotic ascites. Am J Gastroenterology 1988;83:531–535.

32. Burghardt W, Wernze H, Diehl KL: Atrial natriuretic peptide in cirrhosis: Relation to stage of disease, sympathoadrenal system and renin-aldosterone axis. Klin Wochenschr 1986;64(Suppl 6):103–107.

33. Vinel JP, Denoyel PH, Chabrier PE, et al: Relationships between atrial natriuretic factor, plasma renin activity and plasma volume in cirrhotic patients with and without ascites. In Brenner BM, Laragh JH (eds): Advances in Atrial Peptide Research. New York: Raven Press, 1988;416–421.

34. Epstein M, Loutzenhiser R, Norsk P, Atlas S: Relationship between plasma ANF responsiveness and renal sodium handling in cirrhotic humans. Am J Nephrol 1989;9:133–143.

35. Campbell PJ, Skorecki KL, Logan AG, et al: Acute effects of peritoneovenous shunting on plasma atrial natriuretic peptide in cirrhotic patients with massive refractory ascites. Am J Med 1988;84:112–119.

36. Burghardt W, Muller R, Diehl KL, Wernze H: Interrelationship between atrial natriuretic peptide and plasma renin, aldosterone and catecholamines in hepatic cirrhosis: The effect of passive leg raising. S Kardiol 1988;77(Suppl 2):104–110.

37. Epstein M, Preston R, Aceto R, et al: Dissociation of plasma irANF and renal sodium handling in cirrhotic humans undergoing water immersion [abstract]. Kidney Int 1987;31:269.

38. Fernandez-Cruz A, Marco J, Cuadrado LM, et al: Plasma levels of atrial natriuretic peptide in cirrhotic patients [letter]. Lancet 1985;ii:1439–1440.

39. Morgan TR, Imada T, Hollister AS, Inagami T: Plasma human atrial natriuretic factor in cirrhosis and ascites with and without functional renal failure. Gastroenterology 1988;95:1641–1647.

40. Skorecki KL, Leung WM, Campbell P, et al: Role of atrial natriuretic peptide in the natriuretic response to central volume expansion induced by head-out water immersion in sodium retaining cirrhotic subjects. Am J Med 1988;85:375–382.

41. Ginés P, Jiménez W, Arroyo V, et al: Atrial natriuretic factor in cirrhosis with ascites: Plasma levels, cardiac release and splanchnic extraction. Hepatology 1988; 8:636–642.

42. Warner LC, Campbell PJ, Morali G, et al: The response of atrial natriuretic factor (ANF) and sodium excretion to dietary sodium challenges in patients with chronic liver disease. Hepatology 1990;12:460–466.

43. Sonnenberg H, Veress AT: Cellular mechanism of release of atrial natriuretic factor. Biochem Biophys Res Commun 1984;124:443–449.

44. Sonnenberg H, Krebs RF, Veress AT: Release of atrial natriuretic factor from incubated rat heart atria. IRCS Med Sci 1984;12:783–784.

45. Manning PT, Schwartz D, Katsube NC, et al: Vasopressin-stimulated release of atriopeptin: Endocrine antagonists in fluid homeostasis. Science 1985;229: 395–397.

46. Sanfield JA, Shenker Y, Grekin RJ, Rosen SG: Epinephrine increases plasma immunoreactive atrial natriuretic hormone levels in humans. Am J Physiol 1987; 252:E740–E745.

47. Rankin AJ: Mechanisms for the release of atrial natriuretic peptide. Can J Physiol Pharmacol. 1987;65:1673–1679.

48. Campbell PJ, Leung WM, Logan A, et al: Hyper-responsiveness to water immersion in sodium retaining cirrhotics: The role of atrial natriuretic peptide. Clin Invest Med 1988;11:392–395.

49. Angeli P, Caregaro L, Menon F, et al: Variability of atrial natriuretic peptide plasma levels in ascitic cirrhotics: Pathophysiological and clinical implications. Hepatology 1992;16:1389–1394.

50. Gonzalez-Campoy J, Romero JC, Knox FG: Escape from the sodium retaining effects of mineralcorticoids: Role of ANF and intrarenal hormone system. Kidney Int 1989;35:767–777.

51. Bernardi M, Di Marco C, Trevisani F, et al: Hemodynamic status and its neurohumoral control in pre-ascitic cirrhosis [abstract]. Ital J Gastroenterol 1991;23:507–508.

52. Wilkinson SP, Arroyo VA, Moodie H, et al: Abnormalities of sodium excretion and other disorders of renal function in fulminant hepatic failure. Gut 1976;17:501–505.

53. Guarner F, Hughes RD, Gimson AES, Williams R: Renal function in fulminant hepatic failure: Haemodynamics and renal prostaglandins. Gut 1987;28:1643–1647.

54. Panos MZ, Anderson JV, Forbes A, et al: Human atrial natriuretic factor and renin-aldosterone in paracetamol induced fulminant hepatic failure. Gut 1991;32:85–89.

55. Tikkanen I, Fyhrquist F, Metsärinne K, Leidenius R: Plasma atrial natriuretic peptide in cardiac disease and during infusion in healthy volunteers. Lancet 1985;2:66–69.

56. Yandle TG, Richards AM, Nicholls MG, et al: Metabolic clearance rate and plasma half life of alpha-human natriuretic peptide in man. Life Sci 1986;38:1827–1833.

57. Henriksen JH, Bülöw JB, Tronier B: Kinetics of circulating endogenous insulin, C-peptide, and proinsulin in fasting non-diabetic man. Metabolism 1987;26:463–468.

58. Holst-Pedersen J, Andersen H, Olsen SP, Henriksen JH: Pharmacokinetics and metabolism of neurotensin in man. J Clin Endocrinol Metab. 1989;68:294–300.

59. Henriksen JH, Staun-Olsen P, Mogensen NB, Fahrenkrug J: Circulating endogenous vasoactive intestinal polypeptide (VIP) in patients with uraemia and liver cirrhosis. Eur J Clin Invest 1986;16:211–216.

60. Hollister AS, Rodeheffer RJ, White FJ, et al: Clearance of atrial natriuretic factor by lung, liver and kidney in humans subjects and the dog. J Clin Invest 1989;83:623–628.

61. Henriksen JH, Bendtsen F, Schütten HJ, Warberg J: Hepatic-intestinal disposal of endogenous human alpha natriuretic factor[99-126] (ANF) in patients with cirrhosis. Am J Gastroenterol 1990;85:1155–1159.

62. Vierhapper H, Gasic S, Nowotny P, Waldhäusl W: Splanchnic disposal of human natriuretic peptide in humans. Metabolism 1988;37:973–975.

63. Henriksen JH, Bendtsen F, Gerbes AL: Splanchnic removal of atrial natriuretic factor (ANF) in man: Enhancement after food intake. Metabolism 1990;39:553–556.

64. Winters CJ, Sallman AL, Baker BJ, et al: The N-terminus and 4000-MW peptide from the midportion of the N-terminus of the atrial natriuretic factor prohormone each circulate in humans and increase in congestive heart failure. Circulation 1989;80:438–449.

65. Arendt RM, Gerbes AL, Ritter D, Stangl E: Molecular weight heterogeneity of plasma ANF in cardiovascular disease. Klin Wochenschr 1986;64(Suppl VI):97–102.

66. Ogawa K, Smith IA, Hodsman GP, et al: Plasma atrial natriuretic peptide: Concentration and circulating forms in normal man and patients with chronic renal failure. Clin Exp Pharmacol Physiol 1987;14:95–102.

67. Arendt RM, Gerbes AL, Ritter D, et al: Atrial natriuretic factor in plasma of patients with arterial hypertension, heart failure, or cirrhosis of the liver. J. Hypertension 1986;4(Suppl 2):S131-S135.

68. Epstein M, Loutzenhiser R, Friedland E, et al: Increases in circulating atrial natriuretic factor during immersion induced central hypervolemia in normal humans. J Hypertens 1986;4(Suppl 2):S93–S99.

69. Jiménez W, Gutkowska J, Ginés P, et al: Molecular forms and biological activity of atrial natriuretic factor in patients with cirrhosis and ascites. Hepatology 1991;14:601–607.

70. Jespersen B, Jensen L, Sorensen SS, Pedersen EB: Atrial natriuretic factor, cyclic 3',5'-guanosine monophosphate and prostaglandin E_2 in liver cirrhosis: Relation to blood volume and changes in blood volume after furosemide. Eur J Clin Invest 1990;20:632–641.

71. Epstein M: Renal effects of head-out water immersion in man: Implications for an understanding of volume homeostasis. Physiol Rev 1978;58:529–581.

72. Epstein M: Renal effects of head-out water immersion in humans: A 15-year update. Physiol Rev 1992;72:563–621.

73. Epstein M, Norsk P, Loutzenhiser R: Effects of water immersion on ANP release in humans. Am J Nephrol 1989;9:1–24.

74. Epstein M, Loutzenhiser R, Friedland E, et al: Relationship of increased plasma atrial natriuretic factor and renal sodium handling during immersion-induced central hypervolemia in normal humans. J Clin Invest 1987;76:1705–1709.

75. Warner LC, Morali GA, Miller JA, et al: Aldosterone, atrial natriuretic factor and sodium intake as determinants of the natriuretic response to head-out water immersion in healthy subjects. Clin Sci 1991;80:475–480.

76. Leung WH, Logan AG, Campbell PJ, et al: Role of atrial natriuretic peptide and urinary cGMP in the natriuretic and diuretic response to central hypervolemia in normal human subjects. Can J Physiol Pharmacol 1987;65:2076–2080.

77. Gerzer R, Witzgall H, Tremblay J, et al: Rapid increase in plasma and urine cGMP after bolus injection of atrial natriuretic factor in man. J Clin Endocrinol Metab 1985;61:1217–1219.

78. Tremblay J, Gerzer R, Vinay P, et al: The increase of cGMP by atrial natriuretic factor correlates with the distribution of particulate guanylate cyclase. FEBS Lett 1985;181(1):17–22.

79. Nicholls KM, Shapiro MD, Kluge R, et al: Sodium excretion in advanced cirrhosis: Effect of expansion of central blood volume and suppression of plasma aldosterone. Hepatology 1986;6:235–238.

80. Tesar V, Horky K, Petryl J, et al: Atrial natriuretic factor in liver cirrhosis—the influence of volume expansion. Horm Metab Res 1989;21:519–522.

81. Reznick RK, Langer B, Taylor BR, et al: Hyponatremia and arginine vasopressin secretion in patients with refractory hepatic ascites undergoing peritoneovenous shunting. Gastroenterology 1983;84:713–718.

82. Klepetko W, Muller CH, Hartter E, et al: Plasma atrial natriuretic factor in cirrhotic patients with ascites. Effect of peritoneovenous shunt implantation. Gastroenterology 1988;95:764–770.

83. Salerno F, Badalamenti S, Maser P, et al: Atrial natriuretic factor in cirrhotic patients with tense ascites. Effect of large-volume paracentesis. Gastroenterology 1990;98:1063–1070.

84. Salerno F, Badalamenti S, Incerti P, et al: Renal response to atrial natriuretic peptide in patients with advanced liver cirrhosis. Hepatology 1988;8:21–26.

85. Fried T, Aronoff GR, Benabe JE, et al: Renal and hemodynamic effects of atrial natriuretic peptide in patients with cirrhosis. Am J Med Sci 1990;299:2–9.

86. Petrillo A, Scherrer JJG, Nussberger J, et al: Atrial natriuretic peptide administered as intravenous infusion or bolus injection to patients with liver cirrhosis and ascites. J Cardiovasc Pharm.1988;12:279–285.

87. Badalamenti S, Borroni G, Lorenzano E, et al: Renal effects in cirrhotic patients with avid sodium retention of ANF injection during norepinephrine infusion. Hepatology 1992;15:824–829.

88. Ginés P, Tito L, Arroyo V, Llach J, et al: Renal insensitivity to atrial natriuretic peptide in patients with cirrhosis and ascites. Gastroenterology 1992;102:280–286.

89. Beutler JJ, Koomans HA, Rabelink TJ, et al: Blunted natriuretic response and low blood pressure after atrial natriuretic factor in early cirrhosis. Hepatology 1989;10:148–153.

90. Schrier RW, Arroyo V, Bernardi M, et al: Peripheral arterial vasodilation hypothesis: A proposal for the initiation of renal sodium and water retention in cirrhosis. Hepatology 1988;8:1151–1157.

91. Laffi G, Marra F, Pinzani M, et al: Effects of repeated atrial natriuretic peptide bolus injections in cirrhotic patients with refractory ascites. Liver 1989;9:315–321.

92. Laffi G, Pinzani M, Meacci E, et al: Renal hemodynamic and natriuretic effects of human atrial natriuretic factor infusion in cirrhosis with ascites. Gastroenterology 1989;96:167–177.

93. Wesson LG: Electrolyte excretion in relation to diurnal cycles of renal function. Medicine 1964;43:547–592.

94. Moore-Ede MC, Herd J: Renal electrolyte circadian rhythms: Independence from feeding and activity patterns. Am J Physiol 1977;232(Renal Fluid Electrolyte Physiol.):F128–F135.

95. Goldman R: Studies in diurnal variation of water and electrolyte excretion: Nocturnal diuresis of water and sodium in congestive cardiac failure and cirrhosis of the liver. J Clin Invest 1951;30:1191–1199.

96. Papper S, Rosenbaum JD: Abnormalities in the excretion of water and sodium in "compensated" cirrhosis of the liver. J Lab Clin Med. 1952;40:523–530.

97. Bernardi M, de Palma R, Trevisani F, et al: Chronobiological study of factors affecting plasma aldosterone concentration in cirrhosis. Gastroenterology 1986;91:683–691.

98. Bernardi M, Trevisani F, de Palma R, et al: Chronobiological evaluation of sympathoadrenergic function in cirrhosis. Gastroenterology 1987;93:1178–1186.

99. Colantonio D, Pasqualetti P, Casale R, et al: Atrial natriuretic peptide-renin-aldosterone system in cirrhosis of the liver: Circadian study. Life Sci 1989;45:631–635.

100. Panos MZ, Anderson JV, Payne N, et al: Plasma atrial natriuretic peptide and renin-aldosterone in patients with cirrhosis and ascites: Basal levels, changes during daily activity and nocturnal diuresis. Hepatology, 1992;16:82–87.

101. Gerbes AL, Wernze H, Arendt RM, et al: Atrial natriuretic factor and renin-aldosterone in volume regulation in patients with cirrhosis. Hepatology 1989;9:417–422.

102. Koepke JP, DiBona GF: Blunted natriuresis to atrial natriuretic peptide in chronic sodium retaining disorders. Am J Physiol 1987;252:F865–F871.

103. Koepke JP, Jones S, DiBona GF: Renal nerves mediate blunted natriuresis to atrial natriuretic peptide in cirrhotic rats. Am J Physiol 1987;252:R1019–R1023.

104. Morgan DA, Peuler JD, Koepke JP, et al: Renal sympathetic nerves attenuate the natriuretic effects of atrial peptide. J Lab Clin Med 1989;114:538–544.

105. Nicholls KM, Shapiro MD, Van Putten VJ, et al: Elevated plasma norepinephrine concentrations in decompensated cirrhosis. Association with increased secretion rates, normal clearance rates, and suppressibility by central blood expansion. Circ Res 1985;56:457–461.

106. Solis-Herruzo JA, Duran JA, Favela V, et al: Effects of lumbar sympathetic block on kidney function in cirrhotic patients with hepatorenal syndrome. J Hepatol 1987;5:167–173.

107. Morali G, Floras JS, Legault L, et al: Muscle sympathetic nerve activity and renal responsiveness to atrial natriuretic factor during the development of hepatic ascites. Am J Med 1991;91:383–392.

108. Moe GW, Legault L, Skorecki KL: Control of extracellular fluid volume and pathophysiology of edema formation. In Brenner BM, Rector JF (eds): The Kidney, 4th ed. Philadelphia: W.B. Saunders, 1991;623–676.

109. Sonnenberg H, Cupples WA, deBold AJ, Veress AT: Intrarenal localization of the effect of cardiac atrial extract. Can J Physiol Pharmacol 1982;60:1149–1152.

110. Baum M, Toto RD: Lack of a direct effect of atrial natriuretic factor in the rabbit proximal tubule. Am J Physiol 1986;250:F66–F69.

111. Sonnenberg H, Honrath U, Chung CK, Wilson DR: Atrial natriuretic factor inhibits sodium transport in medullary collecting duct. Am J Physiol 1986;250:F963–F966.

112. Liu FY, Cogan MG: Atrial natriuretic factor does not inhibit basal or angiotensin II stimulated proximal transport. Am J Physiol 1988;255:F434–F437.

113. Ziedel ML, Kikeri D, Silva P, et al: Atrial natriuretic peptides inhibit conductive sodium uptake by rabbit inner medullary collecting duct cells. J Clin Invest 1988;82:1067–1074.

113a. Legault L, unpublished data.

114. Morali GA, Tobe S, Skorecki KL, Blendis LM: Refractory ascites: Modulation of ANF unresponsiveness by mannitol. Hepatology 1992;16:42–48.

115. Kremer S, Troyer D, Kreisberg J, Skorecki KL: Interaction of atrial natriuretic peptide stimulated guanylate cyclase and vasopressin-stimulated calcium signalling pathways in glomerular mesangial cells. Arch Biochem Biophys 1988;269:763–770.

116. Jaiswal RK, Jaiswal N, Sharma RK: Negative regulation of atrial natriuretic factor receptor coupled membrane guanylate cyclase by phorbol ester. FEBS 1988;227: 47–50.

117. Nambi P, Whitman M, Gessner G, et al: Vasopressin-mediated inhibition of atrial natriuretic factor stimulated cGMP accumulation in an established smooth muscle cell line. Proc Natl Acad Sci USA 1986;83: 8492–8495.

118. Smith JB, Lincoln TM: Angiotensin decreases cGMP accumulation produced by atrial natriuretic factor. Am J Physiol 1987; 253:C147–C150.

119. Gerbes AL, Kollenda C, Vollmar AM, et al: Altered density of binding sites for atrial natriuretic factor in bile duct-ligated rats with ascites. Hepatology 1991;13:562–566.

120. Nakao K, Sugawara A, Morii N, et al: The pharmacokinetics of alpha-human atrial natriuretic polypeptide in healthy subjects. Eur J Clin Pharmacol 1986;31:101–103.

121. Luft FC, Lang RE, Aronoff GR, et al: Atriopeptin III kinetics and pharmacodynamics in normal and anephric rats. J Pharmacol Exp Ther 1986;236:416–418.

122. Almeida FA Suzuki M, Scarborough RM, et al: Clearance function of type C receptors of atrial natriuretic factor in rats. Am J Physiol 1989;256:R469–R475.

123. Koepke JP, Tyler LD, Trapani AJ, et al: Interaction of non-guanylate cyclase-linked atriopeptin receptor ligand and endopeptidase inhibitor in concious rats. J Pharmacol Exp Ther 1989;249:172–176.

124. Gee NS, Bowes MA, Buck P, Kenny AJ: An immunoradiometric assay for endopeptidase-24.11 shows it to be widely distributed enzyme in pig tissues. Biochem J 1985;228:119–126.

125. Trapani AJ, Smits GJ, McGraw DE, et al: Thiorphan, an inhibitor of endopeptidase 24.11, potentiates the natriuretic activity of atrial natriuretic peptide. J Cardiovasc Pharmacol 1989;14:419–424.

126. Wilkins MR, Settle SL, Stockmann PT, Needleman P: Maximizing the natriuretic effect of endogenous atriopeptin in a rat model of heart failure. Proc Natl Acad Sci 1990;87:6465–6469

127. Levy M, Cernacek P: Renal neutral endopeptidase (NEP 24:1) activity and natriuretic peptide (ANP) induced sodium excretion in chronic caval dogs with ascites (TIVC) [abstract]. Can J Invest Med 1994;17:B95.

128. Legault L, Cernacek P, Levy M: Attempts to alter the heterogenous response to ANP in sodium retaining caval dogs. Can J Physiol Pharmacol (in press).

129. Legault L, Cernacek P, Levy M, et al: Renal tubular responsiveness to atrial natriuretic peptide in sodium-retaining chronic caval dogs: A possible role for kinins and luminal actions of the peptide. J Clin Invest 1992; 90:1425–1435.

130. Smits GJ, McGraw DE, Trapani AJ: Interaction of ANP and bradykinin during endopeptidase 24.11 inhibition: Renal effects. Am J Physiol 1990;258:F1417–F1424.

131. Sybertz EJ Jr, Chiu PJS, Watkins RW, Vemulapalli S: Neutral metalloendopeptidase inhibitors as ANF potentiators: Sites and mechanisms of action. Can J Physiol Pharmacol 1991;69:1628–1635.

132. Schultz-Knappe P, Forssmann K, Herbst F, et al: Isolation and structural analysis of "urodilatin", a new peptide of the cardiodilatin-(ANP)-family, extracted from human urine. Klin Wochenschr 1988;66:752–759.

133. Goetz KL: Renal natriuretic peptide (urodilatin?) and atriopeptin: Evolving concepts. Am J Physiol 1991; 261:F921–F932.

134. Drummer C, Fiedler F, Konig A, Gerzer R: Urodilatin, a kidney-derived natriuretic factor, is excreted with a circadian rhythm and is stimulated by saline infusion in man. J Am Soc Nephrol 1991;1:1109–1113.

135. Kenny AJ, Stephenson SL: Role of endopeptidase -24.11 in the inactivation of atrial natriuretic peptide. FEBS Lett 1988;232:1–8.

136. Norsk P, Drummer C, Johansen LB, Gerzer R: Effect of water immersion on renal natriuretic peptide (urodilatin) excretion in humans. J Appl Physiol 1993;74:2881–2885.

137. Vesely DL, Norsk P, Gower WR Jr., Chiou S, Epstein M: Release of kaliuretic stimulator during immersion-induced central hypervolemia in healthy humans. Proc Soc Exp Biol Med 1995;209:20–26.

138. Vesely DL, Norsk P, Winters CJ, et al: Increased release of the N-terminal and C-terminal portions of the prohormone of atrial natriuretic factor during immersion-induced central hypervolemia in normal humans. Proc Soc Exp Biol Med 1989;192:230–235.

139. Vesely DL, Preston R, Winters CJ, et al: Increased release of the N-terminal and C-terminal portions of the atrial natriuretic factor prohormone during immersion-induced central hypervolemia in cirrhotic humans. Am J Nephrol 1991;11:207–216.

140. Martin DR, Pevahouse JB, Trigg DJ, et al: Three peptides from the ANF prohormone NH2-terminus are natriuretic and/or kaliuretic. Am J Physiol 1990;258: F1401–F1408.

141. Vesely DL, Douglass MA, Dietz JR, et al: Three peptides from the atrial natriuretic factor prohormone amino terminus lower blood pressure and produce a diuresis, natriuresis, and/or kaliuresis in humans. Circulation 1994;90:1129–1140.

142. Vesely DL, Douglass MA, Dietz JR, et al: Negative feedback of atrial natriuretic peptides. J Clin Endocrinol Metab 1994;78:1128–1134.

143. Vesely DL, Preston R, Gower WR, et al: Increased release of kaliuretic peptide during immersion-induced central hypervolemia in cirrhotic humans (in press).

144. Levy M: Sodium retention and ascites formation in dogs with experimental portal cirrhosis. Am J Physiol 1977;237:F572–F585.

145. Levy M, Allotey JB: Temporal relationships between urinary salt retention and altered systemic hemodynamics in dogs with experimental cirrhosis. J Lab Clin Med 1978;92:560–569.

146. Levy M: Pathogenesis of sodium retention in early cirrhosis of the liver: Evidence for vascular overfilling. Semin Liver Dis 1994;14:4–13.

147. Almeida FA, Muneya M, Maack T: Atrial natriuretic factor increases hematocrit and decreases plasma volume in nephrectomized rats. Life Sci 1986;38: 1193–1199.

148. Huxley VH, Tucker VL, Verburg KM, Freeman RH: Increased capillary hydraulic conductivity induced by atrial natriuretic peptide. Circ Res 1987;60:304–307.

149. Jonas GM, Morgan TR, Morgan K, et al: Atrial natriuretic peptide in portal vein-ligated rats: Alterations in cardiac production, plasma level and glomerular receptor density and affinity. Hepatology 1992;15:696–701.

Chapter 16

NATRIURETIC HORMONE

VARDAMAN M. BUCKALEW, JR., M.D.

On the Existence of Natriuretic Hormone
  Cross-circulation Studies
  Effect of Plasma, Plasma Extracts, and Urine
Biologic Activities of Natriuretic Hormone
  Sodium Pump Inhibition
  Digitalislike Activity
Characterization of digitalislike Factors
  Ouabain
  Ouabain Isomer
  19-Norbufalin
  Digoxin
  Other Steroids
Physiologic Significance of Digitalislike Factor

Other Humoral Natriuretic Factors
  Lysophosphatidyl Choline
Renal Paracrine Factors
Urinary Factors
  Urinary Peptides
  Urodiolenone
Unknown Tissue Factors
Role of Natriuretic Hormone in Extracellular Fluid
  Volume Regulation
  Normal Subjects
  Patients with Hepatic Disease
Summary

The volume of extracellular fluid (ECF) is regulated by a complex interaction of physiologic variables, including several "volume-sensitive" hormones that alter renal sodium and water excretion. The antinatriuretic and antidiuretic hormones activated by volume depletion— renin-angiotensin-aldosterone, antidiuretic hormone (ADH), and norepinephrine (NE)—have been well characterized with respect to both control of secretion and renal effects. Initial hypotheses suggested that ECF volume was regulated by changes in activity of antinatriuretic hormonal systems.[1] However, it is now recognized that volume regulation also involves natriuretic factors activated by volume expansion.

Atrial natriuretic factor (ANF), discovered in 1981, was the first natriuretic factor to be characterized completely and to meet the criteria for a natriuretic hormone. ANF is produced outside the kidney, its plasma concentration is increased by volume expansion, and it causes natriuresis in physiologic concentrations. This important humoral factor is discussed in detail in chapter 15. This chapter reviews the evidence for other humoral natriuretic systems that are also activated by volume expansion. This discussion is, of necessity, more speculative than that pertaining to ANF, because the exact nature of other systems has not yet been fully elucidated. As the title of this chapter indicates, we refer to non-ANF systems as natriuretic hormone (NH). This label is for expedience only and should not obscure the fact that NH is composed of multiple factors, which this chapter attempts to define.

ON THE EXISTENCE OF NATRIURETIC HORMONE

Cross-circulation Studies

The first solid evidence for the existence of a humoral natriuretic factor activated by ECF volume expansion was presented by De Wardener et al.[2] when they showed that blood circulated from a volume-expanded dog (donor) to a euvolemic (recipient) dog caused natriuresis in the recipient. Other investigators reported similar results in both dogs and rats.[3–7] The question now is whether the transferrable natriuresis observed in early cross circulation studies was due to ANF, NH, or both.

In early cross-circulation studies, the natriuresis observed in the recipient animal was far less impressive than that in the donor. This discrepancy was of concern at the time because of doubts concerning the existence of NH. In retrospect, studies of this phenomenon provide interesting clues to understanding the role of NH vs.

ANF in volume regulation. Blythe et al.[8] were able to increase the magnitude of the recipient response by delivering the donor blood into the aorta directly above the renal arteries. These studies suggested that the reduced response of the recipient was due to a short biologic half-life of the humoral natriuretic factor and are compatible with a role for ANF, a 28-amino acid peptide known to be removed rapidly from the circulation by clearance receptors and a neutral endopeptidase.[9] Sonnenberg recently tested this possibility.[10] He injected a maximally natriuretic dose of atrial extract into one of a pair of cross-circulated rats. The partner sharing the common circulation with the injected rat showed no increase in sodium excretion, despite a blood exchange of approximately one-tenth the cardiac output per minute. This suggests that the transferrable natriuresis observed in cross-circulation studies is not caused by ANF and argues for the existence of a second blood-borne natriuretic hormone.

The recipient response can be affected by conditions in the donor. Lichardus and Ponec[11] and Sonnenberg et al.[7] demonstrated marked enhancement of the recipient response by infusing the donor with its own urine[7,11] or with a volume of Ringer's solution similar to the volume of urine passed by the donor, or by nephrectomy in the donor rat.[7] These studies were designed to prevent the donor animal from excreting the volume load and suggest some as yet poorly defined effect of "sustained" volume expansion on the donor that allows the natriuretic effect of the hormone to be more fully expressed in the recipient.[12] The mechanism of this effect has not been elucidated but is not suggestive of a role for ANF.

Effect of Plasma, Plasma Extracts, and Urine

Another argument supporting the existence of a non-ANF humoral natriuretic factor is based on the pattern of the natriuretic effect of whole plasma, extracts of plasma, and urine in assay rats.[13] The typical response to bolus ANF injection was well illustrated by the initial studies of atrial extract by De Bold and coworkers.[14] Natriuresis begins immediately within 5 minutes, peaks in 10–15 minutes, and is completely dissipated after 20–30 minutes. No analog of ANF that deviates significantly from this pattern has yet been described. By contrast, the natriuresis of plasma, plasma extracts, and urine exhibits two

basic patterns that differ primarily with respect to peak time and duration of effect[13] (Fig. 16.1). The shorter-acting pattern shows an immediate onset, a peak effect in 40–60 minutes, and a duration of about 120 minutes. The longer-acting pattern exhibits a delay in onset of 10–60 minutes, a peak effect in 2–3 hours, and activity that persists longer than 2 hours. The short activity pattern is generally associated with extracts containing exclusively low-molecular-weight substances and sodium transport inhibitory activity,[15,16] whereas the long-acting pattern is generally associated with whole plasma[17] or extracts containing mostly high-molecular-weight substances.[18,19]

These contrasting patterns suggest the existence of two natriuretic factors other than ANF. Whether the longer-acting factor is a precursor of the shorter-acting one, as has been suggested,[20] is not known. However, together with the discovery of ANF, such studies suggest the existence of three natriuretic hormones with different durations of action: short (30 minutes), intermediate (60 minutes), and long (greater than 2 hours). The way in which the several factors interact to control renal sodium excretion in response to changes in ECF volume is of some importance for future studies.

The reason that natriuretic assays of plasma and plasma extracts do not demonstrate an effect resembling that of ANF is of some interest. The most likely explanation is that the assays are not sensitive enough to detect the amount of ANF that can be extracted from small amounts of blood. The intermediate and long-acting natriuretic factors can be demonstrated in as little as 1–2 ml of plasma from volume-expanded subjects.[13] It can be argued that the amount of ANF in 1–2 ml of plasma is insufficient to cause natriuresis in assay rats, even when the plasma is obtained from volume-expanded subjects.[21,22] The threshold dose for the natriuretic effect of bolus ANF in the rat is probably in the range of 20–200 ng in a 200- gram rat.[23–25] Using 400 pg/ml as an average plasma ANF concentration in acutely volume expanded rats,[22,26] more than 50 ml of rat plasma would have to be extracted to obtain sufficient ANF for detection. In humans, plasma ANF concentrations are in the range of 20–40 pg/ml and rise 2–8 fold following acute volume expansion.[22] Thus, more than 100 ml of human plasma would have to be extracted to obtain sufficient ANF to be detected in a rat bioassay for natriuresis.

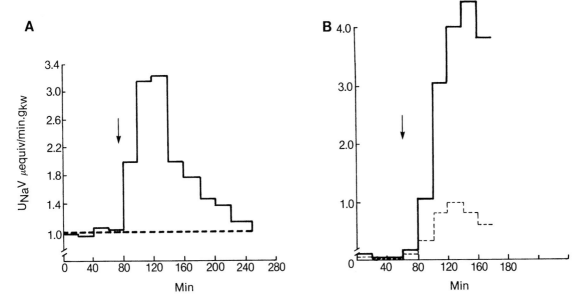

FIGURE 16.1. Time course of the natriuretic activities extracted from mammalian plasma. *A,* Low-molecular-weight fraction of plasma equivalent to 10 ml of original plasma from a volume-expanded dog was injected at the 80-minute time point. Peak sodium excretion occurred 40–60 minutes after injection, slowly returning to baseline over a 2–3 hour period. (From Buckalew VM Jr, Nelson DB: Natriuretic and sodium transport inhibitory activity in plasma of volume expanded dogs. Kidney Int 1974;5:12–22, with permission.) *B,* High-molecular-weight fraction of plasma equivalent to 6 ml of original plasma from a volume-expanded rat (*solid line*) and an euvolemic rat (*interrupted line*) was injected at the 60-minute time point. Peak sodium excretion 60 minutes after injection and did not return to baseline over a 2-hour period of observation. (From Pearce JW, Veress AT: Concentration and bioassay of a natriuretic factor in plasma of volume expanded rats. Can J Physiol Pharm 1975;53:742, with permission.)

BIOLOGIC ACTIVITIES OF NATRIURETIC HORMONE

Sodium Pump Inhibition

Because of the difficulties encountered with assays for natriuretic activity, various surrogates have been used in searching for the identity of NH. The most popular have been assays for inhibition of the sodium pump, including inhibition of microsomal Na-K-ATPase activity.[27–30] Such surrogate assays were introduced originally on the assumption that NH would inhibit sodium transport somewhere in the nephron.[27,31] The earliest studies were performed by testing extracts of plasma in tissues such as anuran membrane (short circuit current inhibition)[31] or isolated renal tubule preparations (intracellular sodium concentration).[30] These and other studies showed that both natriuretic and sodium pump inhibitory activities were found in the same partially purified extracts of various biologic fluids and tissue, thus supporting the transport inhibitor hypothesis.[27] Also supportive of this hypothesis was the demonstration that ECF volume expansion increased the bioassayable plasma and urine level of both natriuretic and sodium transport inhibitory activity.[13,15,19,27,28,31–33]

Digitalislike Activity

Because Na-K-ATPase is responsible for the majority of sodium reabsorption by the renal tubule, it seemed reasonable to postulate that the circulating sodium transport inhibitor might inhibit that enzyme. Kramer, Gonick, and coworkers were the first to show that plasma extracts inhibited an in vitro preparation of Na-K-ATPase and that the plasma level of this activity was increased by acute ECF volume expansion.[28,32] Subsequently, Hillyard et al. showed that extracts of kidneys removed from volume-expanded rats inhibited Na-K-ATPase and toad bladder sodium transport.[34] Consequently, the investigators suggested that NH might cause natriuresis by inhibiting renal tubular Na-K-ATPase.

TABLE 16.1. Na-K-ATPase Inhibitors Isolated from Mammalian Species

Species	Source/Subjects	Structure	Reference
Tissue			
Human	Cataracts	19-norbufalin	45
Bovine	Hypothalamus	Ouabain stereoisomer	46
Bovine	Hypothalamus	Unknown	47
Bovine	Adrenal	Digoxin	48
Porcine	Heart	Unknown	49
Rat	Hypothalamus	Choline analog	50
Mouse	Adrenal tumor cell line	Unknown steroid	51
Plasma			
Human	Normals	Ouabain	52,53
Human	Uremics	Unknown	54
Bovine	Normals	LPC; fatty acids	55,56
Bovine	Normals	11,13-dihydroxy-14-octadecaenoic acid	57
Urine			
Human	Normals	Digoxin	58
Pig	Normals	Unknown	59

LPC = lysophosphatidyl choline.

Flier et al., using a radioligand binding assay for ouabain and an antidigitalis antibody,[35,36] demonstrated an endogenous digitalislike substances in plasma and skin of the toad *Bufo marinus*. The investigators were unable to demonstrate such a substance in mammalian plasma using the same technique.[36] However, Gruber et al. showed that dog plasma extracts cross-reacted with antidigoxin antibodies and inhibited Na-K-ATPase and that plasma levels of this digitalislike activity increased with plasma volume expansion.[29]

Other investigators have used various assays for digitalislike activity in plasma of volume-expanded subjects, including a cytochemical assay for glucose-6-phosphate dehydrogenase stimulation; inhibition of particulate Na-K-ATPase; inhibition of ouabain-sensitive sodium or rubidium transport in tissues such as red cell and tail artery; and inhibition of ouabain binding to particulate Na-K-ATPase.[37–41] These studies showed digitalislike activity that increased following volume expansion or high sodium diet.

CHARACTERIZATION OF DIGITALISLIKE FACTORS

Numerous groups have reported attempts to isolate and characterize endogenous digitalislike factors from various tissues and body fluids. Most groups have not been successful in identifying a factor or have reported isolation of factors that are not truly digitalislike. Several complete catalogs of ongoing projects have recently been published.[22,42–44] Mammalian Na-K-ATPase inhibitors for which a structure has either been proposed or is under active investigation are shown in Table 16.1. The four factors that appear to be potentially important are discussed in more detail.

Ouabain

Hamlyn and colleagues reported the isolation from human plasma of a steroid that is indistinguishable from ouabain.[52,53] This finding is surprising, because it had been thought that ouabain was synthesized only by plants. Using an enzyme-linked assay (ELISA) with an anti-ouabain antibody, Hamlyn and collaborators originally reported ouabain concentrations in normal human plasma of about 0.1 nM.[60] Higher values (up to 1.0 nM) have been reported in more recent publications.[61,62] Ouabain levels appear to increase with increasing sodium intake and age[62] and are elevated in hypothyroidism[62] and congestive heart failure.[61] The source of ouabain appears to be the adrenal glands, because ouabain was secreted by bovine adrenal cells in tissue culture[53] and plasma levels declined following adrenalectomy in rats.[63]

Two biologic problems are associated with the hypothesis that ouabain is a naturally occurring endogenous steroid in mammalian species:

1. It has not been demonstrated that mammals can synthesize steroids in the same three-dimensional structure as cardiac glycosides that have the A:B and C:D ring junctions in the *cis* configuration[42] (Fig. 16.2). Mammalian steroids such as cortisol have the A:B and C:D ring junctions in the *trans* configuration.[42] The enzyme thought essential to generating the *cis* configuration, 14β hydroxylase, has not been demonstrated in mammalian adrenal glands.

2. Rhamnose, the sugar found in ouabain, had not been found until recently in mammalian species except in rabbit skin, where it might have been produced by bacteria.[64] The recently identified ouabain isomer isolated from bovine hypothalamus appears to contain rhamnose (see below), but the site of rhamnose synthesis has not yet been determined.

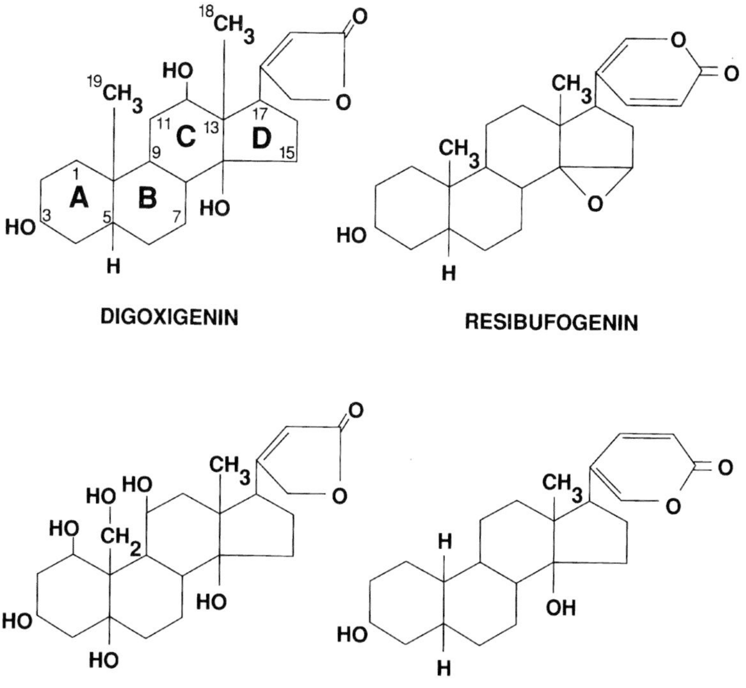

FIGURE 16.2. The aglycones (genins) of four steroids are shown. The classic cardiac glycosides ouabain and digoxin have rhamnose and three digitoxose, respectively, attached at positon 3. Both of these glycosides (or some closely related analog) have recently been isolated from body fluids and tissue sof nomrla mammalian species. Resibufogenin is one of a class of compounds isolated from skin and body fluids of toads. A similar compound, 19-norbufalin, has been isolated from human cataractous lens.

There are at least two experimental objections to the claim that endogenous ouabain originates in the adrenal gland and is a biologically important regulator of cell function:

1. Many of the studies published by Hamlyn and colleagues have not rigorously identified authentic ouabain as the endogenous substance cross-reacting with their antibody. Although the antibody used in their assay does not cross-react extensively with other known glycosides, its cross-reactivity with other putative endogenous digitalislike steroids is not known. In fact, Ludens et al.[63] showed that the antibody used by Hamlyn and colleagues identifies a number of compounds in adrenal extract other than authentic ouabain.

2. Doris et al.[65] recently failed to confirm the presence of significant amounts of authentic ouabain in human plasma or in culture medium conditioned by adrenocortical cells. Thus, although there is no reason to doubt that authentic ouabain can be isolated from mammalian tissues, much more work is necessary to establish its site of origin and biologic significance.

Ouabain Isomer

Haupert and colleagues reported a series of studies on a Na-K-ATPase inhibitor isolated from bovine hypothalamus.[66] Previous physiologic characterization of this factor using partially purified preparations indicated that it was distinct from ouabain, yet had inotropic[67] and vasoconstrictive properties.[68] In fact, further characterization has now identified the compound as a ouabain stereoisomer containing rhamnose.[46] Although the site of synthesis of this isomer has not been identified, the observation that hypothalami of Milan hypertensive rats contain 10 times more than normotensive controls on the same diet[69] suggests that it originates from endogenous synthesis rather than diet. Further studies of differences in physiologic effects between this isomer and authentic ouabain will be of considerable interest.

19-Norbufalin

A second class of steroids with digitalis-like activity which may be endogenous to humans has recently been reported by Lichtstein and colleagues.[45] Lichtstein's group chose to purify this factor from human cataracts, because an inhibitor of Na-K-ATPase had previously been demonstrated and implicated in the pathogenesis of cataracts.[70,71] A complete purification was achieved, and initial mass spectroscopic analysis suggests that the structure is 19-norbufalin, a compound closely related to resibufogenin, the digitalislike factor previously isolated by Lichtstein's group from toad skin[72] (see Fig. 16.2). Again, this finding is surprising, because it had previously been thought that bufodienolides were confined to amphibians such as the toad. It is not yet known whether this factor circulates in plasma or what its physiologic significance might be.

Digoxin

Many investigators have demonstrated that extracts of various mammalian tissues contain numerous substances that cross-react with digoxin antibodies, including a number of lipids and steroids that are clearly not endogenous digitalis-like substances.[22,73,74] However, two groups have recently isolated from human urine[58] and bovine adrenal gland[48] a compound that is indistinguishable from digoxin. The significance of such observations is uncertain, because the same caveats that apply to the demonstration of endogenous ouabain are relevant. In fact, a food source seems more likely for digoxin than for ouabain, because enteral absorption of the former is far greater than the latter. However, if mammalian species are shown to be capable of synthesizing ouabain, it would not be far-fetched to postulate their ability to synthesize digoxin (see Fig. 16.2).

Other Steroids

New evidence continues to suggest the presence of other substances with digoxin immunoreactivity. Doris recently reported partial isolation of a factor from culture media of an adrenocortical tumor cell line that cross-reacts with digoxin antibodies, inhibits ouabain binding, and is not digoxin or ouabain.[51] In addition, Naomi et al. recently used the different cross-reactivities exhibited by different digoxin antibodies to construct an immunochemical fingerprint of the endogenous substance in mammalian plasma.[75] This ingenious approach suggested that the endogenous immunoreactive substance resembled bufalin

more closely than digoxin or ouabain. This observation is interesting, because Flier et al. had shown originally that toad skin Na-K-ATPase inhibitors (bufodienolides) cross-reacted with digoxin antibodies.[36] Thus, the possibility still exists that digoxin antibodies recognize a novel endogenous substance, possibly a bufodienolide, with some physiologic or pathophysiologic significance.

PHYSIOLOGIC SIGNIFICANCE OF DIGITALISLIKE FACTOR

Digitalislike factors (DLFs) have been implicated in the control of renal sodium excretion and in the pathophysiology of hypertension.[13,76] The identification of four digitalislike steroids in mammals is important, but much work is required to determine their physiologic significance. For purposes of this discussion, the issue is whether any of the four could be NH. It has been known for many years that ouabain and digoxin are natriuretic, especially when given directly into the renal artery to avoid cardiac toxicity.[77–79] In addition, ouabain has been shown to stimulate ANF secretion.[80,81] The discovery of cardiac glycosides and bufodienolides in mammalian species has stimulated further investigation of their effects on renal function. Pamnani et al. demonstrated that bufalin, an aglycone that differs from resibufogenin by only one hydrogen (see Fig. 16.2), was a potent natriuretic and pressor agent when given systemically in low microgram doses in rats.[82] Ouabain in equimolar doses caused a much smaller natriuretic and pressor effect. Thus, the more potent natriuretic effect of bufalin might have been due to a pressure-induced natriuresis. This possibility is supported by the study of Yates and McDougall,[83] who infused equimolar doses of ouabain and bufalin directly into the renal artery of conscious ewes. Under these conditions, ouabain had a more potent natriuretic effect than bufalin; the main difference was that ouabain's effect persisted for more than 2 hours after infusion whereas bufalin's effect had returned to baseline by that time.

Both studies reaffirm the suggestion that circulating Na-K-ATPase inhibitors could be pressor and natriuretic factors. However, the doses used in the studies are in the pharmacologic range, producing blood levels higher than would be expected for an endogenous digitalislike factor. In fact, estimated blood levels in the experiments of Pamnani et al. and Yates and McDougall were about 1,000-fold higher than basal levels of the endogenous material that cross-reacts with ouabain antibodies.[82,83] Furthermore, Ludens et al. showed that acute volume expansion in dogs did not increase the plasma concentration of endogenous ouabain at a time when urine sodium excretion was markedly elevated.[84] Therefore, it seems unlikely that blood-borne, authentic ouabain is a physiologic regulator of blood pressure or renal sodium excretion. It remains to be seen whether any of the other endogenous steroids now under investigation might be more potent natriuretic factors.

It is also possible that endogenous digitalislike factors may be involved in regulation of blood pressure by the central nervous system (CNS), the evidence for which has recently been reviewed.[76] It has been known for many years that central administration of ouabain causes a rise in blood pressure.[85,86] In addition, central administration of CNS extracts containing endogenous digitalislike factors have been shown to raise blood pressure.[87–89] Therefore, the suggestion that increased CNS levels in critical brain areas might cause hypertension is reasonable. Because the regulation of blood pressure and renal sodium excretion are tightly linked through the mechanism of pressure natriuresis,[90] it is possible that the central effects of endogenous digitalislike factors also regulate renal sodium excretion.

OTHER HUMORAL NATRIURETIC FACTORS

Evidence suggesting the existence of endogenous natriuretic factors that are not digitalislike continues to accumulate.[43,91] Two such factors that may function as natriuretic hormones have been identified in blood.

Proopiomelanocortin Fragments

Proopiomelancortin (POMC) is a large peptide precursor of several anterior pituitary hormones with various biologic activities including adrenocorticotropic hormone (ACTH), melanocyte-stimulating hormone (MSH), endorphin, and lipotropin (LPH).[92] MSH has been classified into 3 types: α- and β-MSH, derived from the C-terminal portion of POMC, and γ-MSH derived from the N-terminal portion.[92] All three MSH peptides are natriuretic, but only γ-MSH has been

implicated in the physiologic regulation of renal sodium excretion.[93–97] A series of studies by Humphreys and colleagues suggested that γ-MSH may be the mediator of the natriuresis that follows acute unilateral nephrectomy and unilateral carotid artery traction.[95–97] Such results are intriguing, because the reflex natriuresis invoked by unilateral nephrectomy and carotid artery traction may be analogous to at least some part of the more complex reflex activated by acute volume expansion. The possibility that γ-MSH may be involved in the physiologic regulation of sodium balance is supported by the recent demonstration that the circulating concentration in rats is increased about two-fold by a high sodium diet.[98]

Lysophosphatidyl Choline

Several investigators have demonstrated that much of the plasma Na-K-ATPase inhibitory activity is due to lysophosphatidyl choline (LPC).[55,56,99,100] Although LPC is not truly digitalislike, it may be of some interest for two reasons: (1) its plasma concentration is increased by acute volume expansion, a phenomenon for which there is no obvious explanation,[55,100] and (2) LPC appears to be a mild natriuretic agent with a very longlasting effect when given in small doses intravenously in rats and dogs.[101–103] In addition, the O-alkyl class of phospholipids, such as platelet-activating factor (PAF), have been shown to be natriuretic in picomole quantities,[103,104] an effect that may be due in part to inhibition of proximal tubule Na-K-ATPase.[104] Together these observations suggest the possibility that circulating phospholipids function as NHs and may be, at least in part, responsible for the long-acting natriuretic principle observed in plasma isolates (see Fig. 16.1). This possibility requires further investigation.

RENAL PARACRINE FACTORS

A series of studies published more than 15 years ago called attention to the role of the kidney in the natriuretic response to volume expansion. Animals preconditioned with a high sodium and water intake responded more vigorously to acute volume expansion[105–107] or to injection of a natriuretic urine fraction.[108] Transplanted kidneys from preconditioned animals responded more vigorously to volume expansion than kidneys transplanted from nonpreconditioned animals,[107] and a natriuretic material could be recovered from renal venous effluent.[109] This suggested that the effect of preconditioning is due, at least in part, to some change in the kidney itself. These findings have taken on more significance in light of recent studies showing several paracrine natriuretic factors produced by the kidney.

Natriuretic factors identified in kidney tissue include dopamine,[110,111] epoxyeicosatetraenoic acids (EETs) and hydroxy-EETs,[112,113] prostaglandins,[114,115] nitric oxide,[116–118] ANF and urodilatin,[9,119] and more recently a newly discovered angiotensin peptide angiotensin [1-7]. Angiotensin [1-7], a 7-amino acid peptide produced in the kidney,[120–125] has recently been shown by Handa et al. and DelliPizzi et al. to be natriuretic in low nanomolar amounts.[123,124]

Some of the above renal natriuretic factors are thought to play a role in the abnormal control of renal sodium excretion in patients with hepatic disease and are discussed in detail elsewhere in this book. They are mentioned here only to point out that, as indicated by the early work of Nizet and colleagues,[106,107,109] the kidney makes its own natriuretic hormones. A full understanding of volume regulation in health and disease requires a better understanding not only of the intrarenal systems themselves but also of the way in which they interact with the circulating natriuretic factors. For example, the kidney in hepatic failure is refractory to the natriuretic effect of ANF (see chapter 15). Although the mechanism of this phenomenon is not known, it may be due, at least in part, to alteration in one or more of the renal paracrine natriuretic systems.

URINARY FACTORS

Several natriuretic factors identified in urine may play a role in regulating renal sodium excretion. It is not clear at this time whether these factors originate from a paracrine natriuretic system in the kidney or circulate in plasma and reach the urine by glomerular filtration.

Urinary Peptides

Kramer and colleagues recently reported the amino acid composition of a peptide derived from urine that causes a prolonged (2–3 hours) natriuresis in assay rats.[125] The compound contains aspartic acid, glutamine, glycine, and serine with a molecular weight of 640, is not a fragment of ANF, and does not inhibit Na-K-ATPase.[125]

Further work on this factor is needed to determine whether it has physiologic and/or pathophysiologic significance.

Urodiolenone

Neufeld et al. reported isolation of a urodiolenone from urine of 30% of hypertensive subjects that inhibits Na-K-ATPase in a concentration of 0.5 pg/ml and may be natriuretic.[126] Mass spectroscopy indicates that this compound is a bicyclic enone, possibly sesquiterpenoid in nature. It is similar to a compound in plants and soft coral known as phytoalexin. Further studies of the possible physiologic significance of this compound have not been reported.

UNKNOWN TISSUE FACTORS

Extracts of hypothalamus, kidney, and liver are natriuretic,[13,127] and hepatic venous blood contains increased amounts of a natriuretic factor compared with peripheral blood.[128] The natriuretic effect of kidney tissue is likely due to one or more of the factors discussed above. The identity of the natriuretic factor or factors found in the liver and hypothalamus is not yet known.

ROLE OF NATRIURETIC HORMONE IN EXTRACELLULAR FLUID VOLUME REGULATION

Normal Subjects

The discovery of ANF provided an impetus to studies of the mechanisms of ECF volume regulation in normal subjects and in patients with various edema states. Interest in this topic is also spurred by the view that essential hypertension is a condition of disordered volume regulation.[129]

We know that part of normal adaptation involves alterations in the humoral composition of plasma and that these humoral alterations result from—and may also influence—chemical mediators at the cellular level. A large body of information has accumulated about the alterations in plasma ANF associated with changes in ECF volume. Whereas a large body of evidence also documents changes in other humoral activities during changes in ECF volume,[13,16] most studies simply demonstrate that ECF volume expansion increases the plasma levels of other activities without attempting to define their exact physiologic role.

Buckalew and Lancaster attempted to correlate the daily excretion of sodium in dogs with plasma activity of a sodium transport inhibitor.[130,131] In both normal dogs and dogs given deoxycorticosterone acetate (DOCA) daily, counterbalancing natriuretic and antinatriuretic forces oscillated around the point of sodium balance. The transport inhibitor appeared to participate in returning sodium excretion to the point of balance when sodium excretion fell below intake either spontaneously or after administration of DOCA. The relationship of the factor detected by the toad bladder assay to factors discussed in this chapter is uncertain.

Numerous studies have demonstrated that acute volume expansion increases plasma concentration of Na-K-ATPase inhibitory activity.[13,27] Because most studies of the effect of ECF volume expansion on plasma digitalislike activity have not taken into account the effect of volume expansion on LPC and free fatty acids (FFA), many demonstrations of increased digitalislike activity in volume-expanded subjects[132] may be due to increased plasma FFA and LPC.

With this possibility in mind, Buckalew, Rauch, and colleagues demonstrated a nonlipid digitalislike factor in plasma,[41,133] levels of which are increased by both acute and chronic sodium loading. Although ANF and plasma digitalislike activity tend to be increased by many of the same physiologic maneuvers,[132] Rauch et al. found a difference between the effect of sodium chloride feeding on ANF and the water-soluble plasma ouabainlike factor. Atrial natriuretic factor was elevated only on day 7 of the high-salt diet, whereas the digitalislike factor slowly increased with time over 3 weeks of observation.[41] These studies suggest that ANF is involved in the more rapid adjustments of renal sodium excretion to increased sodium intake, whereas the digitalislike factor may be more important in the chronic phases. Rauch et al. have not identified the digitalislike factor under investigation, and its relation to previously discussed factors is uncertain.

The central nervous system involvement in the regulation of NH has yet to be explored extensively. Rats with lesions of the anteroventral third-ventricle (AV3V) area showed a blunted renal response to acute salt loading.[134] Assays of plasma from lesioned animals do not show the inhibitor of sodium transport found during acute volume expansion in normal animals.[134] Rauch et al. also demonstrated that AV3V lesions in rats blocked the release of ANF associated with acute volume expansion with saline[135] Thus, it seems possible that the AV3V area of the brain has some control over release of both ANF and a digitalislike factor. More recently, Lichardus and colleagues failed to confirm that the blunted natriuresis of AV3V lesions in sheep might be due to decreased release of NH.[136] Lack of natriuresis apparently was due to increased plasma renin activity and increased catecholamines, probably secondary to volume depletion. Normal volume regulation was restored by administration of the angiotensin-converting enzyme inhibitor captopril.

Patients with Hepatic Disease

Various abnormalities in the putative natriuretic hormones discussed in this chapter have been reported in patients and experimental models of hepatic disease. Plasma digoxinlike immunoreactivity is increased in patients with various hepatic diseases,[137–143] and some attempt has been made to relate these levels to volume status. Nanji and Greenway demonstrated significantly higher levels in cirrhotic patients with ascites and edema compared with patients who had no evidence of volume overload,[144] and Yang et al. showed that plasma digoxinlike activity correlated with central venous pressure in patients with acute liver disease secondary to viral hepatitis or acetaminophen overdose.[142] More recently, La Villa et al. found increased levels of urinary Na-K-ATPase inhibitory activity and digoxinlike immunoreactivity in cirrhosis with ascites and functional renal failure but not in compensated cirrhosis.[145] The investigators found that Na-K-ATPase inhibitory activity and digoxin immunoreactivity correlated with the degree of hepatic and renal impairment, plasma renin activity, and plasma levels of aldosterone and norepinephrine. Interpretation of these studies is complicated by the fact that bile acids have been shown to have digoxinlike immunoreactivity.[137,146] However, no correlation was found between bile acid concentrations and digitalislike activity in the study of La Villa et al.[145] Such studies are compatible with increased digoxinlike factor in volume-expanded patients with hepatic disease, although its role in the pathophysiology of hepatic failure is not clear.

On the other hand, Buckalew and Lancaster, using the toad bladder assay, found that plasma of dogs with inferior vena cava ligation and ascites had no detectable sodium transport inhibitory activity either in the basal state or after acute ECF volume expansion with normal saline.[130] Similarly, Tejedor et al. found that dialysates of renal microsomes of normal rats inhibited Na-K-ATPase activity, whereas dialysates of rats with carbon tetrachloride-induced cirrhosis did not.[147] These studies suggest that absence of a Na-K-ATPase inhibitor might contribute to sodium retention in hepatic disease.

Studies of urinary natriuretic activity in liver disease have also yielded conflicting results. Naccarato et al. found decreased urinary natriuretic activity in 8 cirrhotic patients with no history of edema or ascites.[148] Favre found decreased urinary natriuretic factor in 8 cirrhotic patients with edema.[149] However, when Favre's patients were expanded with albumin, 4 had an increase in sodium excretion and 4 did not; the 4 patients with natriuresis had increased excretion of urinary natriuretic activity. In the study of La Villa et al., increased urinary natriuretic activity was found in patients with decompensated cirrhosis and in patients with cirrhosis and functional renal failure.[145] Urine natriuretic activity was not increased in patients with compensated cirrhosis.

Such studies, although intriguing, are obviously confounded by the probability that several factors are assayed, the identity and function of which are unknown. The studies suggest, however, that a better understanding of the putative natriuretic factors discussed in this chapter is required before the complex disorder of volume regulation in patients with hepatic disease is fully understood.

SUMMARY

Evidence for the existence of endogenous natriuretic factors other than ANF continues to mount. Mammalian plasma contains various digitalislike factors, including a compound that is indistinguishable from ouabain. Several lines of reasoning suggest that ouabain is unlikely to play a role in regulating renal sodium excretion. There are indications for the existence of several other endogenous digitalislike factors, one or more of which may be the putative NH. In addition, good evidence suggests that renal sodium excretion is regulated by several factors produced locally in the kidney, several of which inhibit Na-K-ATPase. It has not been clearly shown, however, that their natriuretic effect is due to digitalislike activity.

Some evidence suggests that various factors with digitalislike activity play a role in ECF volume regulation in normal subjects and in the dysregulation of ECF volume in hypertension and generalized edema states such as hepatic cirrhosis. Their exact role in complex regulatory systems must await full characterization of their biochemical structure and biologic activities.

REFERENCES

1. Smith HW: Salt and water volume receptors: An exercise in physiologic apologetics. Am J Med 1957;23:623–652.
2. De Wardener HE, Mills IH, Clapham WF, Hayter CJ: Studies on the efferent mechanism of the sodium diuresis which follows the administration of intravenous saline in the dog. Clin Sci 1961;21:249–258.
3. Johnston CI, Davis JO: Evidence from cross circulation studies for a humoral mechanism in the natriuresis of saline loading. Proc Soc Exp Biol Med 1966;121:1058–1063.
4. Tobian L, Coffee K, McCrea P: Evidence for a humoral factor of non-renal and non-adrenal origin which influences renal sodium excretion. Trans Assoc Am Phys 1967;80:200–206.
5. Kaloyanides GJ, Azer M: Evidence for a humoral mechanism in volume expansion natriuresis. J Clin Invest 1971;50:1603–1612.
6. Pearce JW, Sonnenberg H, Veress AT, Ackermann U: Evidence for a humoral factor modifying the renal response to blood volume expansion in the rat. Can J Physiol Pharmacol 1969;47:377–386.
7. Sonnenberg H, Veress AT, Pearce JW: A humoral component of the natriuretic mechanism in sustained blood volume expansion. J Clin Invest 1972;51:2631–2644.
8. Blythe WB, D'Avila D, Gitelman HJ, Welt LG: Further evidence for a humoral natriuretic factor. Circ Res 1971;28:II-21–II-31.
9. Ballermann BJ, Zeidel ML, Gunning ME, Brenner BM: Vasoactive peptides and the kidney. In Brenner BM, Rector FC (eds): The Kidney, 4th ed. Philadelphia: WB Saunders, 1991;510–583.
10. Sonnenberg, H: Hormonal control of sodium excretion. In Lote CJ (ed): Advances in Renal Physiology. London: Croom Helm, 1986;180–217.
11. Lichardus B, Ponec J: Conditions for biological evidence of a natriuretic hormone: Experiments with rat cross circulation. Physiol Bohemoslov 1970;19:33.
12. Pearce JW, Veress AT, Sonnenberg H: Time course of onset and decay of humoral natriuretic activity in the rat. Can J Physiol Pharmacol 1975;53:734–741.
13. De Wardener HE, Clarkson EM: Concept of natriuretic hormone. Physiol Rev 1985;65:658–759.
14. De Bold AJ, Borenstein HB, Veress AT, Sonnenberg H: A rapid and potent natriuretic response to intravenous injection of atrial myocardial extract in rats. Life Sci 1981;28:89–94.
15. Buckalew VM Jr, Nelson DB: Natriuretic and sodium transport inhibitory activity in plasma of volume expanded dogs. Kidney Int 1974;5:12–22.

16. Buckalew VM Jr, Gruber KA: Natriuretic hormone. In Epstein M (ed): The Kidney in Liver Disease, 2nd ed. New York: Elsevier, 1983;479–499.

17. Knock CA: Further evidence in vivo for a circulating natriuretic substance after expanding the blood volume in rats. Clin Sci 1980;59:423–433.

18. Sealey JE, Kirshman JD, Laragh JH: Natriuretic activity in plasma and urine of salt loaded man and sheep. J Clin Invest 1969;48:2210–2224.

19. Pearce JW, Veress AT: Concentration and bioassay of a natriuretic factor in plasma of volume expanded rats. Can J Physiol Pharmacol 1975;53:742–747.

20. Gruber KA, Buckalew VM Jr: Further characterization and evidence for a precursor in the formation of plasma antinatriferic factor. Proc Soc Exp Biol Med 1978;159: 463–467.

21. Buckalew VM Jr: The natriuretic hormones. AKF Nephrol Lett 1987;4:1–12.

22. Buckalew VM Jr, Paschal-McCormick C: Natriuretic hormone: Current status. Am J Nephrol 1989;9:329–342.

23. Blaine EH, Heinel LA, Schorn TW, et al: The character of the atrial natriuretic response: Pressure and volume effects. J Hypertens 1986;4(Suppl 2):S17–S24.

24. Sonnenberg C, Muir AC, Criscione L, et al: Is the natriuretic effect of atrial natriuretic factor in conscious rats mediated by renal vasodilatation? J Hypertens 1985;3: S303–S305.

25. Seidah NG, Lazure C, Chretien M, et al: Amino acid sequence of homologous rat atrial peptides: Natriuretic activity of native and synthetic forms. Proc Natl Acad Sci USA 1984;81:2640–2644.

26. Eskay R, Zukowska-Grojec Z, Haass M, et al: Circulating atrial natriuretic peptides in conscious rats: Regulation of release by multiple factors. Science 1986;232:636–639.

27. Buckalew VM Jr, Gruber KA: Natriuretic hormone. Annu Rev Physiol 1984;46:343–358.

28. Gonick HC, Kramer HJ, Paul W, Lu E: Circulating inhibitor of sodium-potassium activated adenosine triphosphatase after expansion of extracellular fluid volume in rats. Clin Sci Mol Med 1977;53:329–334.

29. Gruber KA, Whitaker JM, Buckalew VM Jr: Endogenous digitalis-like substance in plasma of volume-expanded dogs. Nature 1980;287:743–745.

30. Clarkson EM, Talner LB, deWardener HE: The effect of plasma from blood volume expanded dogs on sodium, potassium and PAH transport of renal tubule fragments. Clin Sci 1970;38:617–627.

31. Buckalew VM Jr, Martinez J, Green WS: The effect of dialysates and ultrafiltrates of plasma of saline-loaded dogs on toad bladder sodium transport. J Clin Invest 1970;49:926–935.

32. Kramer HJ, Gonick HC, Krück F: Natriuretic hormone. Klin Wochenschr 1972;50:893–897.

33. Kramer HJ, Backer A, Krück F: Antinatriferic activity following acute and chronic salt-loading. Kidney Int 1977;12:214–222.

34. Hillyard SD, Lu E, Gonick HC: Further characterization of the natriuretic factor derived from kidney tissue of volume-expanded rats: Effects on short-circuit current and sodium-potassium-adenosine triphosphatase activity. Circ Res 1976;38:250–255.

35. Flier JS: Ouabain-like activity in toad skin and its implications for endogenous regulation of ion transport. Nature 1978;274:285–286.

36. Flier JS, Maratos-Flier E, Pallotta JA, McIssac D: Endogenous digitalis-like activity in the plasma of the toad Bufo marinus. Nature 1979;279:341–343.

37. De Wardener HE, Clarkson EM, Bitensky L, et al: Effect of sodium intake on ability of human plasma to inhibit renal Na+-K+-adenosine triphosphatase in vitro. Lancet 1981;1:411–412.

38. Poston L, Wilkinson S, Sewell RB, Williams R: Sodium transport during the natriuresis of volume expansion: A study using peripheral blood leucocytes. Clin Sci 1982;63:243–249.

39. Price MB, Pamnani MB, Burris JF, et al: Acute volume expansion in humans releases a factor which inhibits the vascular Na+-K+ pump. J Hypertens 1984;2:S471–S472.

40. Swann AC: (Na+,K+)-ATPase regulation and NaCl intake: Effects on circulating inhibitor and sensitivity to noradrenaline. Clin Sci 1985;69:441–447.

41. Buckalew VM Jr, Morris M, Rauch AL: Plasma inhibitors of Na,K-ATPase: Relation to salt balance and hypertension. Klin Wochenschr 1987;65:133–138.

42. Goto A, Yamada K, Yagi N, et al: Physiology and pharmacology of endogenous digitalis-like factors. Pharmacol Rev 1992;44:377–399.

43. Wechter WJ, Benaksas EJ: Natriuretic hormones. Prog Drug Res 1990;34:231–260.

44. Lichtstein D, Samuelov S, Gati I, Wechter WJ: Digitalis-like compounds in animal tissue. J Basic Clin Physiol Pharmacol 1992;3(4):269–292.

45. Lichtstein D, Gati I, Samuelov S, et al: Identification of digitalis-like compounds in human cataractous lenses. Eur J Biochem 1993;216:261–268.

46. Tymiak AA, Norman JA, Bolgar M, et al: Physicochemical characterization of a ouabain isomer isolated from bovine hypothalamus. Proc Natl Acad Sci 1993; 90:8189–8193.

47. Illescas M, Ricote M, Mendez E, et al: Complete purification of two identical (Na(+)-pump inhibitors isolated from bovine hypothalamus and hypophysis. FEBS Lett 1990;261:436–440.

48. Shaikh IM, Lau BWC, Siegfried BA, Valdes R: Isolation of digoxin-like immunoreactive factors from mammalian adrenal cortex. J Biol Chem 1991;266: 13672–13678.

49. Agbanyo M, Khatter JC: Purification and characterization of endogenous digitalis-like substance (DLS) from pig heart. Res Commun Chem Pathol Pharmacol 1990;68:41–54.

50. De Wardener HE, Holland S, Alaghband-Zadeh J, et al: A possible connection between an increased concentration of cytochemically detectable substance in the hypothalamus of the spontaneously hypertensive rat and certain cerebral cholinergic disturbances. J Cardiovasc Pharmacol 1993;22(Suppl 2):S109–111.

51. Doris PA: Characterization and Scatchard binding analysis of adrenal digitalis-like material. Life Sci 1992;50:1935–1941.

52. Mathews WR, DuCharme DW, Hamlyn JM, et al: Mass spectral characterization of an endogenous digitalislike factor from human plasma. Hypertension 1991;17: 930–935.

53. Hamlyn JM, Blaustein MP, Bova S, Det al: Identification and characterization of a ouabain-like compound from human plasma. Proc Natl Acad Sci 1991; 88:6259–6263.

54. Schoner W, Heidrich-Lorsbach E, Kirch U, et al: Purification and properties of endogenous ouabain-like substances from hemofiltrate and adrenal glands. J Cardiovasc Pharmacol 1993;22(Suppl 2):S29–S31.

55. Tamura M, Harris TM, Higashimori K, et al: Lysophosphatidylcholines containing polyunsatured fatty acids were found as Na+,K+-ATPase inhibitors in acutely volume-expanded hog. Biochemistry 1987;26:2797–2806.

56. Kelly RA, O'Hara DS, Mitch WE, Smith TW: Identification of Na K-ATPase inhibitors in human plasma as nonesterified fatty acids and lysophospholipids. J Biol Chem 1986;261:11704–11711.

57. Lichtstein D, Samuelov S, Gati I, et al: Identification of 11,13-dihidroxy-14-octadecaenoic acid as a circulating Na+,K+-ATPase inhibitor. J Endocrinol 1991;128:71–78.

58. Goto A, Ishiguro T, Yamada K, et al: Isolation of a urinary digitalis-like factor indistinguishable from digoxin. Biochem Biophys Res Commun 1990;173:1093–1101.

59. Tamura M, Konishi F, Inagami T: A novel endogenous sodium-pump inhibitor in pig urine: Purification and comparison with the inhibitor purified from bovine adrenal glands. J Cardiovasc Pharmacol 1993;22(Suppl 2):S47–S50.

60. Harris DW, Clark MA, Fisher JF, et al: Development of an immunoassay for endogenous digitalislike factor. Hypertension 1991;17:936–943.

61. Gottlieb SS, Rogowski AC, Weinberg M, et al: Elevated concentrations of endogenous ouabain in patients with congestive heart failure. Circulation 1992;86:420–425.

62. Hamlyn JM, Manuta P: Ouabain, digitalis-like factors and hypertension. J Hypertens 1992;10(Suppl 7):S99–S111.

63. Ludens JH, Clark MA, Robinson FG, DuCharme DW: Rat adrenal cortex is a source of a circulating ouabain-like compound. Hypertension 1992;19:721 724.

64. Malawista I, Davidson EA: Isolation and identification of rhamnose from rabbit skin. Nature (Lond) 1961;192:871–872.

65. Doris PA, Jenkins LA, Stocco DM: Is ouabain an authentic endogenous mammalian substance derived from the adrenal? Hypertension 1994;23:632–638.

66. Haupert GT: Physiological inhibitors of Na,K-ATPase: Concept and status. In The Na+,K+-Pump, Part B: Cellular Aspects. New York: Alan R. Liss, 1988;297–320.

67. Hallaq HA, Haupert GT Jr: Positive inotropic effects of the endogenous Na+/K+-transporting ATPase inhibitor from the hypothalamus. Proc Natl Acad Sci 1989;86:10080–10084.

68. Janssens SP, Kachoris C, Parker WL, et al: Hypothalamic Na+-K+-ATPase inhibitor constricts pulmonary arteries of spontaneously hypertensive rats. J Cardiovasc Pharmacol 1993;22:S42–S46.

69. Ferrandi M, Minotti E, Salardi S, et al: Ouabainlike factor in Milan hypertensive rats. Am J Physiol 1992;32:F739–F748.

70. Fukui HN, Merola LO , Kinoshita JH: A possible cataractogenic factor in the Nakano mouse lens. Exp Eye Res 1978;26:1–9.

71. Russell P, Fukui HN, Kinoshita JH: Properties of a Na+,K+-ATPase inhibitor in cultured lens epithelial cells. Vision Res 1981;21:37–39.

72. Lichtstein D, Kachalsky S, Deutsch J: Identification of a ouabain-like compound in toad skin and plasma as a bufodienolide derivative. Life Sci 1986;38:1261–1270.

73. Buckalew VM Jr, Kramer HJ: Natriuretic hormones and sodium homeostasis: Roles of digitalis-like factors and atrial natriuretic peptide. In Gonick HC (ed): Current Nephrology, vol. 15. Baltimore: Mosby Year Book, 1992:207–244.

74. Goto A, Yamada K, Yagi N, et al: Digoxin-like immunoreactivity: Is it still worth measuring? Life Sci 1991;49:1667–1678.

75. Naomi S, Graves S, Lazarus M, et al: Variation in apparent serum digitalis-like factor levels with different digoxin antibodies: The 'immunochemical fingerprint.' Am J Hypertens 1991;4:795–801.

76. Haddy FJ, Buckalew VM Jr: Endogenous digitalis-like factors in hypertension. In Laragh JH, Brenner BM (eds): Hypertension: Pathophysiology, Diagnosis, and Management. New York: Raven Press, 1995;1055–1068.

77. Martinez-Maldonado M, Allen JC, Inagaki C, et al: Renal sodium-potassium-activated adenosine triphosphatase and sodium reabsorption. J Clin Invest 1972; 51:2544–2551.

78. Torretti J, Hendler E, Weinstein E, et al: Functional significance of Na-K-ATPase in the kidney: Effects of ouabain inhibition. Am J Physiol 1972;222(6):1398–1405.

79. Ross B, Leaf A, Silva P, Epstein FH: Na-K-ATPase in sodium transport by the perfused rat kidney. Am J Physiol 1974;226(3):624–629.

80. Yamamoto A, Shouji T, Kimura S, et al: Effects of hypercalcemia and ouabain on plasma atrial natriuretic polypeptide in anesthetized dogs. Am J Physiol 1988; 255:E437–E441.

81. Schiebinger RJ, Cragoe EJ: Ouabain. A stimulator of atrial natriuretic peptide secretion and its mechanism of action. Circ Res 1993;72:1035–1043.

82. Pamnani MB, Chen S, Bryant HJ, et al: Effects of three sodium-potassium adenosine triphosphatase inhibitors. Hypertension 1991;18:316–324.

83. Yates NA, McDougall JG: Effects of direct renal arterial infusion of bufalin and ouabain in conscious sheep. Br J Pharmacol 1993;108:627–630.

84. Ludens JH, Clark MA, Kolbasa KP, Hamlyn JM: Digitalis-like factor and ouabain-like compound in plasma of volume-expanded dogs. J Cardiovasc Pharmacol 1993;22(Suppl 2):S38–S41.

85. Takahashi H, Iyoda I, Takeda K, et al: Centrally-induced vasopressor responses to oubain are augmented in spontaneously hypertensive rats. Clin Exp Hypertens 1984;A6:1499–1515.

86. Jandhyala BS, Hom G, Kivlighn SD: Studies on the role of intracellular sodium and calcium in the centrally mediated pressor effects of CSF[Na+], ouabain and angiotensin II in anesthetized dogs. Clin Exp Hypertens 1985;A7:793–807.

87. Devynck MA, Pernollet MG, Cloix JF, et al: Circulating digitalis-like compounds in essential hypertension. Clin Exp Hypertens 1984;A6:441–453.

88. Takahashi H, Matsuzawa M, Okabayashi H, et al: Evidence for a digitalis-like substance in the hypothalamopituitary axis in rats: Implications in the central cardiovascular regulation associated with an excess intake of sodium. Jpn Circ J 1987;51:1199–1207.

89. Huang BS, Harmsen E, Yu H, Leenen FHH: Brain ouabain-like activity and the sympathoexcitatory and pressor effects of central sodium in rats. Circ Res 1992;71:1059–1066.

90. Guyton AC: Arterial Pressure and Hypertension. Philadelphia: WB Saunders, 1980;117.

91. Benaksas EJ, Murray ED, Rodgers CL, et al: Endogenous natriuretic factors 1: Sodium pump inhibition does not correlate with natriuretic or pressor activities from uremic urine. Life Sci 1993;52:1045–1054.

92. Humphreys MH, Lin SY: Peptide hormones and the regulation of sodium excretion. Hypertension 1988;11: 397–410.

93. Lymangrover JR, Buckalew VM, Harris J, et al: Gamma-2 MSH is natriuretic in the rat. Endocrinology 1985;116:1227–1229.

94. Gruber KA, Callahan MF: ACTH-(4-10) through γ-MSH: Evidence for a new class of central autonomic system-regulating peptides. Am J Physiol 1989;257: R681–694.

95. Mazbar SA, Wiedemann E, Humphreys MH: Mechanism of the natriuretic effect of unilateral carotid artery traction in the rat. J Am Soc Nephrol 1990;1:266–271.

96. Humphreys MH, Lin SY, Wiedemann E: Renal nerves and the natriuresis following unilateral renal exclusion in the rat. Kidney Int 1991;39:63–70.

97. Qiu C, Valentin JP, Chen XW, et al: Acute unilateral nephrectomy elicits a specific increase in plasma of peptides derived from the N-terminal region of proopiomelanocortin. J Am Soc Nephrol 1992;3:1105–1112.

98. Mayan H, Ling KT, Kalinyak JE, et al: Modulation by dietary salt intake of pituitary proopiomelanocortin (POMC) messenger RNA (mRNA) abundance in normotensive and hypertensive rats. Proceedings of the XII International Congress of Nephrology, Jerusalem, Israel, 1993.

99. Hamlyn JM, Schenden JA, Zyren J, Baczynskyj L: Purification and characterization of digitalislike factors from human plasma. Hypertension 1987;10(Suppl I): I71–I77.

100. Rauch AL, Buckalew VM Jr: Plasma volume expansion increases lysophosphatidyl-choline and digitalis-like activity in rat plasma. Life Sci 1988;42:1189–1197.

101. Rauch AL, Buckalew VM Jr. Lysophospholipids are natriuretic and diuretic in rats. Am J Physiol 1988;254: F824–F827.

102. Handa RK, Buckalew VM: Effect of lysophosphatidyl-choline on renal hemo-dynamics and excretory function in anesthetized rats. Life Sci 1992;51:1571–1575.

103. Buckalew VM Jr, Strandhoy JW, Handa RK: Effects of phospholipids on renal function. J Cardiovasc Pharmacol 1993;22(Suppl 2):S79–S81.

104. Handa RK, Giammattei CE, Whitehead TD, Strandhoy JW: Platelet-activating factor (L-PAF) inhibits renal sodium transport in vivo and in vitro. J Am Soc Nephrol 1993;4:454.

105. Sonnenberg H, Pearce JW: Renal response to measured blood volume expansion in differently hydrated dogs. Am J Physiol 1962;203:344–352.

106. Nizet A: Excretion of sodium and water by kidneys in situ and by transplanted kidneys following isotonic, hypotonic, iso-oncotic and hyperoncotic intravenous infusions in sodium-loaded and sodium-deprived dogs. Arch Int Physiol Biochim 1976;84:997–1015.

107. Nizet A: Comparative evaluation of fractional excretion of sodium following saline infusion in transplanted kidneys and in isolated perfused kidneys in conditions of previous high or low dietary sodium intake. Pflugers Arch 1976;361:121–126.

108. Favre H, Louis F, Gourjon M: Role of the basal sodium intake in the rats on their response to a natriuretic factor. Pflugers Arch 1979;382:73–79.

109. Godon JP, Nizet A: Release by isolated dog kidney of a natriuretic material following saline loading. Arch Int Physiol Biochim 82:309-311, 1974.

110. Bertorello A, Aperia A: Short-term regulation of Na+,K+-ATPase activity by dopamine. Am J Hypertens 1990;3:52

111. Bertorello A, Hökfelt T, Goldstein M, Aperia A: Proximal tubule Na+,K+-ATPase activity is inhibited during high-salt diet: Evidence for DA-mediated effect. Am J Physiol 1988;254:F795-F801.

112. Carroll MA, Schwartzman M, Sacerdoti D, McGiff JC: Novel renal arachidonate metabolites. Am J Med Sci 1988;295:268–274.

113. Quilley J, Quilley CP, McGiff JC: Eicosanoids and hypertension. In Laragh JH, Brenner BM (eds): Hypertension: Pathophysiology, Diagnosis, and Management. New York: Raven Press, 1990;829–840.

114. Cordova HR, Kokko JP, Marver D: Chronic indomethacin increases rabbit cortical collecting tubule Na+,K+-ATPase activity. Am J Physiol 1989;256: F570–F576.

115. Jabs K, Zeidel ML, Silva P: Prostaglandin E2 inhibits Na+,K+-ATPase activity in the inner medullary collecting duct. Am J Physiol 1989;257:F424–F430.

116. Lahera V, Salazar J, Salom MG, Romero JC: Deficient production of nitric oxide induces volume-dependent hypertension. J Hypertens 1992;10(Suppl 7):S173–S177.

117. Alberola A, Pinilla JM, Quesada T, et al: Role of nitric oxide in mediating renal response to volume expansion. Hypertension 1992;19:780-784.

118. Salazar FJ, Alberola A, Pinilla JM, et al: Salt-induced increase in arterial pressure during nitric oxide synthesis inhibition. Hypertension 1993; 22:49–55.

119. Awazu M, Ichikawa I: Biological significance of atrial natriuretic peptide in the kidney. Nephron 1993;63:1–14.

120. Kohara K, Brosnihan KB, Chappell MC, et al: Angiotensin-(1-7): A member of circulating angiotensin peptides. Hypertension 1991;17:131–138.

121. Ferrario CM, Brosnihan KB, Diz DI, et al: Angiotensin-(1-7): A new hormone of the angiotensin system. Hypertension 1991;18(Suppl III):III126–III133.

122. Ferrario CM: Biological roles of angiotensin (1-7). Hypertens Res 1992;15:61–66.

123. Handa RK, Handa SE, Ferrario CM, Strandhoy JW: In vivo actions of angiotensin (1-7) in the rat kidney. FASEB J 1993;7:A221.

124. DelliPizzi AM, Hilchey SD, McGiff JC, Quilley CP: Renal actions of angiotensin-[1-7]: Comparison with angiotensin II. Pharmacologist 1992;34:93.

125. Kramer HJ, Bäcker A, Michel H, Meyer-Lehnert H: Human urinary natriuretic factor: A peptide distinct from ouabain-like activity. Proceedings of the XII International Congress of Nephrology, Jerusalem, Israel, 1993.

126. Neufeld E, Sklarz B, Goldberg S, et al: Observations on the chemical and physiological properties of urodiolenone, an urinary compound found in hypertension. Nephron 1985;39:146-148.

127. Clarkson EM, Koutsaimanis KG, Davidman M, et al: The effect of brain extracts on urinary sodium excretion of the rat and the intracellular sodium concentration of renal tubule fragments. Clin Sci Mol Med 1974;47:201–213.

128. Zubiaur M, Peces R, Mombiela MT, et al: Study on the natriuretic activity in the suprahepatic plasma after portal hypertonic NaCl infusion in dogs. Acta Physiol Lat Am 1981;31:129–137.

129. Coleman TG, Guyton AC: Hypertension caused by salt loading in the dog. III. Onset transients of cardiac output and other circulatory variables. Circ Res 1969;25:153–160.

130. Buckalew VM Jr, Lancaster CD Jr: Studies of a humoral sodium transport inhibitory activity in normal dogs and dogs with ligation of the inferior vena cava. Circ Res 1971;29:II-44–II-52.

131. Buckalew VM Jr, Lancaster CD Jr: The association of a humoral sodium transport inhibitory activity with renal escape from chronic mineralocorticoid administration in the dog. Clin Sci 1972;42:69–78.

132. Haddy FJ, Pamnani MB: Natriuretic hormones in low renin hypertension. Klin Wochenschr 1987;65:154–160.

133. Rauch AL, Buckalew VM Jr: Characterization of a competitive and reversible ligand to E2 conformation of Na,K ATPase molecule. Biochem Biophys Res Commun 1988;150:648–654.

134. Bealer SL, Haywood JR, Gruber KA, et al: Preoptic-hypothalamic periventricular lesions reduce natriuresis to volume expansion. Am J Physiol 1983;244:R51–R57.

135. Rauch AL, Callahan MF, Buckalew VM Jr, Morris M: Regulation of plasma atrial natriuretic peptide by the central nervous system. Am J Physiol 1990;27:R531–R535.

136. Lichardus B: Natriuretic hormone: A contribution to the development of a hypothesis. NIPS 1991;6:114–118.

137. Gault MH, Vasdev SC, Longerich LL: Endogenous digoxin like substance(s) and combined hepatic and renal failure. Ann Intern Med 1984;101:567–568.

138. Nanji AA, Greenway DC: Falsely raised plasma digoxin concentrations in liver disease. Br J Med 1985;290:432–433.

139. Greenway DC, Nanji AA: Falsely increased results for digoxin in sera from patients with liver disease: Ten immunoassay kits compared. Clin Chem 1985;31:1078–1079.

140. Pudek MR, Seccombe DW, Humphries K: Digoxin-like immunoreactive substances and bile acids in the serum of patients with liver disease. Clin Chem 1986;32:2005–2006.

141. Wickramasinghe LSP, Bansal SK, Dillon RDS: 'Digoxin-like' substance in serum of elderly patients. Age Ageing 1986;15:271–277.

142. Yang SS, Hughes RD, Williams R: Digoxin-like immunoreactive substances in severe acute liver disease due to viral hepatitis and paracetamol overdose. Hepatology 1988;8:93–97.

143. Day CP, James OFW: Digoxin-like factors in liver disease. J Hepatol 1989;9:281–284.

144. Nanji AA, Greenway DC: Correlation between serum albumin and digoxin-like immunoreactive substance in liver disease. J Clin Pharmacol 1986;26:152–153.

145. La Villa G, Asbert M, Jimenez W, et al: Natriuretic hormone activity in the urine of cirrhotic patients. Hepatology 1990;12:467–475.

146. Vasdev SC, Longerich LL, Ittel TH, et al: Bile salts as endogenous digitalis-like factors. Clin Invest Med 1986;9:201–208.

147. Tejedor A, Conesa D, Hernando N, et al: Absence of a regulatory endogenous factor of Na+,K+ ATPase activity during experimental cirrhosis in the rat. Biochem Cell Biol 1988;66:218–230.

148. Naccarato R, Messa P, D'Angelo A, et al: Renal handling of sodium and water in early chronic liver disease: Evidence for a reduced natriuretic activity of the cirrhotic urinary extracts in rats. Gastroenterology 1981;81:205–210.

149. Favre H: Role of the natriuretic factor in the disorders of sodium balance. Adv Nephrol 1983;11:3–23.

Chapter 17

NITRIC OXIDE AND RENAL FUNCTION: THE CONTROL OF BLOOD PRESSURE UNDER NORMAL CONDITIONS AND DURING CIRRHOSIS

J. C. ROMERO, M.D.
JOAQUÍN GARCÍA-ESTAÑ, M.D.
NOEMÍ M. ATUCHA, M.D.

General Principles of the Synthesis of Nitric Oxide
Specific Effects of Nitric Oxide in the Kidney
  Pressure-induced Natriuresis and Regulation of
    Blood Pressure
  Regulation of Glomerular-tubular Dynamics
    by Nitric Oxide

Nitric Oxide in Cirrhotic Hemodynamic and
** Renal Alterations**
  Increased Production
  Hyperdynamic Circulation
  Renal Alterations
Summary

In 1980, Furchgott and Zawadzki[1] reported that the vasodilator effects of acetylcholine were mediated by the release of a smooth muscle-relaxing factor from the endothelial cells, which was called endothelium-derived relaxing factor (EDRF). In the years that followed this discovery, significant advances were made on the chemical characterization of EDRF, which was identified as nitric oxide (NO)[2–4]; its synthesis precursors[2,4]; the pharmacologic and physiologic alterations that stimulate the release of NO[2,5]; and the mechanism of NO vasodilation.[3,5] Furthermore, attempts have been made to characterize the pathophysiologic consequences of deficient production of NO in endothelial cells. Such a condition, which has been experimentally achieved by the systemic administration of potent inhibitors of NO synthesis, has invariably resulted in a significant increase in mean arterial pressure.[6] In contrast, no effective method producing sustained enhancement of NO synthesis has been yet developed, although transient stimulation with intravenous injections of acetylcholine or bradykinin has resulted in a marked fall in blood pressure. These changes were associated with renal vasodilatation and natriuresis.[7]

The identification of pathologic conditions characterized by a continuous enhancement of NO synthesis awaits further experimentation. However, recent studies appear to support the notion that increased synthesis of NO may be mainly responsible for the marked vasodilatation during the development of cirrhosis with and without ascites.[8,9] This chapter reviews the supporting evidence. Furthermore, an important aspect of the consequences of either deficient or excessive production of NO is that the earliest and most immediate repercussions appear in the kidney.[6] For these reasons, we examine first the role of NO in renal function, its interaction with prostaglandins and the renin-angiotensin system, and the manner in which disruption of the interaction among these three mediators may affect sodium retention in patients with portal hypertension.

GENERAL PRINCIPLES OF THE SYNTHESIS OF NITRIC OXIDE

EDRF appears to be represented mainly by NO (Fig. 17.1), which is synthesized in endothelial cells from a nitrogen atom contained in the guanidine group of the amino acid L-arginine.[2,4] Such a reaction does not appear to consist of a simple process of deamination with the formation of NH_3, because exogenous NH_3 cannot be used

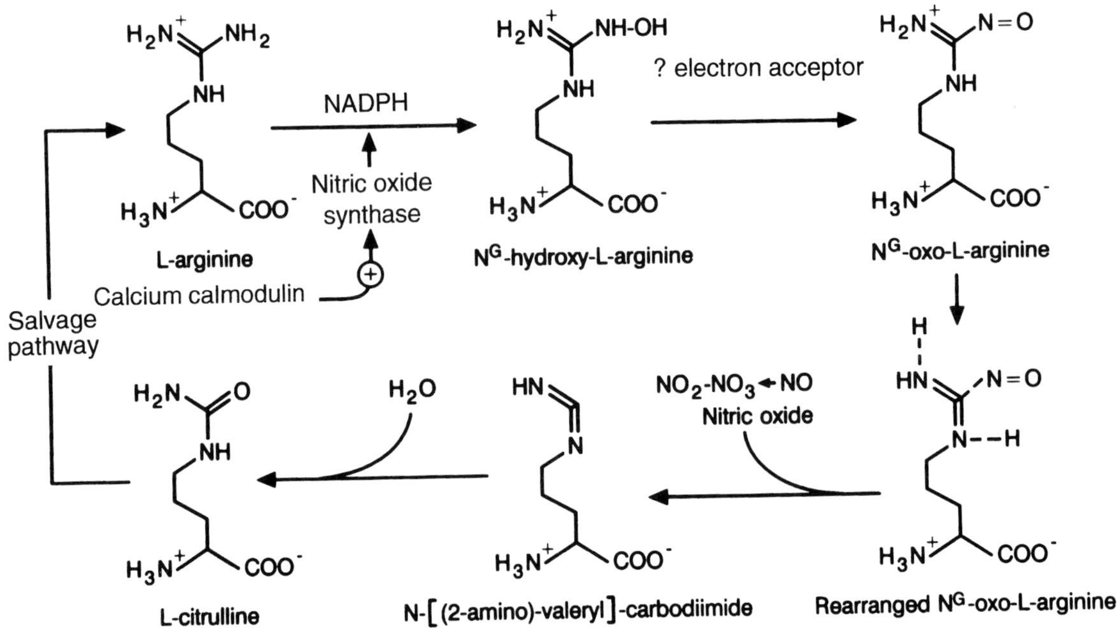

FIGURE 17.1. Possible synthesis pathway of nitric oxide from a single amino acid precursor, L-arginine. (Adapted from Pearson PJ: Mechanism of coronary vasospasm following reperfusion injury: Role of vaso-active factors produced by the endothelium [thesis]. Rochester, MN: Mayo Graduate School of Medicine, 1991, with permission.)

as a precursor of NO in macrophages.[10] The most plausible pathway, as indicated by Marletta,[11] involves first a monooxygenase type of hydroxylation-generating N[G]-hydroxy-L-arginine, which is subsequently converted to N[G]-oxo-L-arginine by oxidation of the hydroxylamine group. The amino acid radical generated in this last step is so unstable that it fragments to yield NO and a stable compound, N-[(2-amino)-valeryl]-carbodiimide.[11] This amino acid reacts with H_2O, yielding citrulline. In support of this pathway of NO formation are the findings that N[G]-hydroxy-L-arginine serves as a precursor for NO_2 and NO_3[12] and that endothelial cells convert L-arginine to citrulline by a process that depends on reduced nicotinamide adenine dinucleoide (NADH).[13] Endothelial cells can also metabolize citrulline to L-arginine.[13] These findings have raised the notion of the so-called L-arginine salvage pathway, by which citrulline is recycled to generate L-arginine.[14]

Two distinctive NO monooxygenases (NO synthases), a constitutive form[15] and an inducible form,[10,16] have been isolated. The constitutive form is activated by the increase in Ca^{2+} in the cytosol and the resultant binding of Ca^{2+} to calmodulin (Fig. 17.2). The reaction depends on reduced

NADH phosphate.[13,17–20] The constitutive form of the enzyme is found mostly in endothelial cells,[1,2] although it also has been found in other tissues such as the central nervous system[12,21,22] and the tubular epithelium.[23]

The inducible form of the enzyme was first discovered in macrophages,[10,16] in which its activity was found to be induced by factors such as endotoxin, tumor necrosis factor, and cytokines.[24] This enzyme, which is not calcium-dependent, also may be induced in vascular smooth muscle and endothelial cells,[25] particularly by the administration of cytokine.[26–28] Such observations suggest that the inducible form may be responsible for hypotension during endotoxic shock.[29] The inducible enzyme is also activated in cultured mesangial cells by lipopolysaccharides,[30] but the significance of this finding remains unknown. It has also been shown that induction of nitric oxide synthase can be markedly reduced by administration of steroids.[31] This observation has raised the question of the extent to which corticosteroids also inhibit the activity of the constitutive form. This issue is important, because it may largely account for the increase in total peripheral resistance and hypertension during continuous administration of mineralocorticoids.[32]

NO also can be synthesized from L-homoarginine, methyl and ethyl ester analogs of L-arginine, and certain dipeptide analogs of L-arginine such as L-arginine-L-alanine.[5] All of these analogs have been shown to be highly active in inducing the relaxation of L-arginine–depleted arterial rings. In contrast, substitution of one or both of the two basic amino nitrogen atoms in the guanidine group (N^G) of L-arginine (see Fig. 17.1) results in analogs that competitively antagonize endothelium-dependent relaxation.[18] This substitution of guanidine nitrogen atoms with allyl, ethyl, succinyl, or nitro groups confers pronounced inhibitory activity.[5] Of all these compounds, the most commonly used have been N^G-monomethyl-L-arginine (L-NMMA) and N^G-nitro-L-arginine methylester (L-NAME). The most likely mechanism of action of the N^G-substituted analogs of L-arginine is competitive inhibition of the conversion of L-arginine or an arginine-containing substance to NO.[18] In support of this concept is the demonstration that the inhibitory effect is reversed by increasing the concentration of the precursor L-arginine but not that of the enantiomer D-arginine.[18]

A recent finding of considerable interest was that an inhibitor of NO synthesis appears to be synthesized in vivo. This inhibitor, known as N^G-D-methylarginine or asymmetric dimethylarginine,[33] consists of two methyl groups bound to the nitrogen atom of the guanidine group of L-arginine and has been isolated from human plasma. More than 10 mg is excreted in urine over 24 hours. However, in patients with end-stage chronic renal failure and little or no urine output, elimination of the inhibitor is impaired, and circulating concentrations presumably rise sufficiently to inhibit NO synthesis. Accumulation of endogenous asymmetric dimethylarginine may thus contribute to the hypertension and immune system dysfunction associated with chronic renal failure. More studies are needed to determine the mechanism of action of the inhibitor (e.g., whether it regulates the activity of NO synthase).

Another mechanism of regulation of the biologic activity of NO is production of substances that protect NO from rapid degradation. For example, NO is rapidly transformed to NO_2 and NO_3.[11] However, the half-life of NO may be prolonged by the presence of protector molecules or adductors. Among the chemical species thought to be of potential importance as NO adductors are S-nitrosothiol adducts of the sulfhydryl groups of

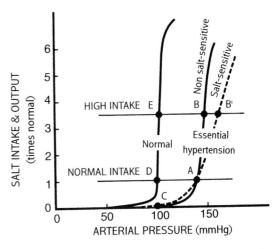

FIGURE 17.2. Characteristic steady-state relationships between mean arterial pressure and sodium intake and output for normal kidneys and kidneys in non–salt-sensitive and salt-sensitive hypertension. (From Guyton AC: Arterial Pressure and Hypertension. Philadelphia: W.B. Saunders, 1980, with permission.)

amino acids, peptides, and proteins. Recently it was shown that NO reacts with free thiol groups of proteins in vitro to form S-nitroso-protein-NO adducts with bioactivities comparable to those of endothelium-derived vasodilating factor but with half-lives on the order of hours.[34] Analytic methods that determine plasma levels of free NO and S-nitrosothiols have shown that the concentration of S-nitrosothiols is 3–4 orders of magnitude greater than that of free NO in mammalian plasma and is mostly composed of the S-nitrosothiol adduct of serum albumin.[35] Of interest, it was also observed that inhibition of NO synthesis by L-N^G-monomethyl-arginine (L-NMMA) in rabbits causes a significant decrease in the circulating level of S-nitrosothiol-serum albumin to 60% of the initial values by 1 hour after administration of L-NMMA. Within that time, blood pressure increased significantly by approximately 25 mmHg.[35] The study suggests that changes in the rate of NO synthesis may be reflected in the plasma levels of S-nitrosothiols. The biologic activity of endogenous NO also may be enhanced by the administration of pharmacologic agents that are thiol donors. Lahera et al.[36] demonstrated that N-acetyl cysteine or N-thiol salicylic acid produced a 20–40% potentiation of the hypotensive response to acetylcholine.

Under the physiologic condition of neutral pH, NO is not highly reactive, but its paramagnetic properties (odd number of electrons) account for its remarkable binding affinity for heme iron[4] and thereby for the inactivation produced by hemoglobin or many other hemoproteins.[5] This affinity is closely related to the mechanism of guanylate cyclase activation, because NO binds the heme group of this enzyme. The requirement of reduced iron (Fe^{2+}) in the form of heme for the activation of cytosolic guanylate cyclase[37] has been regarded by Ignarro "as a novel and widespread signal transduction mechanism" that links endothelial signals to the effects of cyclic guanosine monophosphate (GMP) generated in neighboring cells.[5] Such a relationship may play a major role in coupling renal hemodynamic events to changes in tubular reabsorption of sodium.

SPECIFIC EFFECTS OF NITRIC OXIDE IN THE KIDNEY

In the kidney the administration of endothelium-dependent vasodilators such as bradykinin[38] or acetylcholine[39] produces vasodilatation and natriuresis which are mediated by both prostaglandins and NO. The inhibition of NO synthesis alone by L-NMMA does not alter the vasodilatation induced by acetylcholine.[40] Similarly, inhibiting only prostaglandin synthesis leaves all of the renal responses to acetylcholine unaltered[40]; that is, the intrarenal actions of acetylcholine are blocked effectively only when both NO and prostaglandin synthesis are blocked simultaneously.[40] Furthermore, increases in total renal blood flow are not systematically followed by natriuresis. For example, substances such as secretion[41] and synthetic prostaglandin E_2 (PGE$_2$) analogs[42] that produce vasodilatation of a magnitude comparable to that produced by bradykinin[38] have minimal effects on urinary sodium excretion. It has been suggested[43] that the ability of a renal vasodilator to increase urinary sodium excretion is intimately linked to its ability to redistribute the total renal blood flow and, specifically, to increase renal medullary blood flow[44] and renal interstitial hydrostatic pressure.[44–45] These effects are produced by bradykinin.[44,45] In contrast, secretin may not increase medullary blood flow[45] or alter renal interstitial pressure.[41]

Evidence from several studies suggests that the mechanism coupling changes in medullary blood flow and interstitial pressure to natriuresis may involve NO. Biondi et al.[46] showed that 85–90% of NO-dependent formation of cGMP

takes place in the inner renal medulla. Stoos et al.[47] demonstrated that NO released from cultured endothelial cells decreased sodium transport (as measured by short circuit currents) through isolated collecting ducts. Increases in medullary blood flow conceivably may increase shear stress on medullary vascular endothelial cells (a signal for NO synthesis and release). The NO may then couple the changes in medullary hemodynamics to alterations in sodium excretion. This coupling mechanism not only may be activated by pharmacologic interventions but also may underlie the manifestation of pressure- and volume-induced natriuresis .[43,61,64]

Pressure-induced Natriuresis and Regulation of Blood Pressure

Increasing renal perfusion pressure results in proportional increases in medullary blood flow and interstitial pressure, which precede natriuresis[48–50] and may be mediated by decreased interstitial levels of renin and angiotensin.[43] Under such conditions, blood flow to the renal cortex remains unchanged because of an efficient autoregulatory response.[43,48] The increases in interstitial pressure, however, are often quite modest (only 2–3 mmHg[48–50]) and may be too small to signal a decrease in renal tubular reabsorption. For these reasons, it has been suggested[43,51] that the effect of changes in interstitial pressure may be amplified significantly by release of intrarenal natriuretic factors such as PGE$_2$ or NO. This concept is based on evidence that blockade of prostaglandin synthesis with nonsteroidal antiinflammatory drugs decreases pressure-induced natriuresis.[52,53] The natriuresis is restored by infusions of small amounts of synthetic PGE$_2$ analogs that produce no hemodynamic effects.[53] Intrarenal infusions of comparable amounts of PGI$_2$ do not restore the response.[53] Similarly, the blockade of NO also decreases pressure-induced natriuresis, and the response is restored by the administration of L-arginine, the precursor of NO synthesis.[54]

The significance of NO as a mediator of pressure-induced natriuresis was explored by Lahera et al.,[55] who systemically induced progressively greater inhibition of NO synthesis in rats. The earliest (60 minutes after infusion was started) and most sensitive alterations produced by small doses of L-NAME (0.1–1.0 µg/kg/min) were decreases in water and sodium excretion. By 120 minutes after beginning the infusion, intrarenal vascular resistance was found to be increased. All such changes took place with no alteration in systemic blood pressure. Inhibition of NO synthesis with a higher dose of L-NAME (10 µg/kg/min) was needed to produce increases in systemic blood pressure and urinary sodium excretion rates that overcame the initial antinatriuretic effect of NO synthesis inhibition.

Ito et al.[56] and DeNicola et al.[57] presented data suggesting that at least part of the systemic and renal effects produced by inhibition of NO synthesis are not due to the cessation of the actions of NO but to the biologic activity of angiotensin II, which becomes manifested after NO tissue concentrations are lowered. In fact, Sigmon et al.[58] showed that the antinatriuresis during NO synthesis inhibition with L-NAME was significantly decreased by prior administration of an angiotensin II receptor antagonist, whereas the increase in systemic blood pressure remained unaltered.

Regardless of the mechanism responsible for mediating the antinatriuretic effect of L-NAME, a decrease in NO synthesis should shift the pressure natriuresis curve toward a higher level of renal perfusion pressure,[55] thereby inducing a positive balance of sodium and fostering the development of hypertension.[51] This concept is supported by results showing that the administration of a very low dose of L-NAME during 5 consecutive days to normal dogs decreased urinary sodium excretion without increasing blood pressure. Blood pressure was markedly increased, however, when sodium intake in L-NAME–treated animals was increased from 80 to 300 mEq/day.[59] Such observations have important clinical implications, because they show that the blockade of the synthesis of a single endogenous vasodilator may render blood pressure volume-dependent. The importance of NO in regulating sodium excretion was further supported by studies [60,61] showing that blockade of NO synthesis impaired natriuresis induced by volume expansion.

The manner in which alterations in renal function shift the pressure natriuresis curve and whether such changes induce a condition known as salt sensitivity have been examined by Hall.[62] According to Hall, maneuvers that increase tubular sodium reabsorption, such as administration of aldosterone or blockade of NO, displace the pressure natriuresis curve in a salt-sensitive manner[62]; that is, not only is the curve shifted toward higher pressures, but the slope is also altered so that urinary sodium excretion becomes strictly proportional to the level of renal perfusion pressure (see Fig. 17.2).[114] In contrast, an increase in afferent glomerular arteriolar resistance displaces the pressure natriuresis curve toward higher pressures—but in a manner parallel to normal conditions,[62] because once the increase in systemic arterial pressure restores the glomerular pressure to original levels, the magnitude of increase in sodium excretion in response to increased sodium intake does not differ from the magnitude of increase under normal conditions.

Of interest, parallel displacement of the pressure natriuresis curve may also result from decreased NO synthesis by endothelial cells of the preglomerular renal vasculature. The "rubbing" action of blood against the vascular endothelium, known as shear stress, is a major stimulus for the release of NO.[63] At high levels of renal perfusion pressure such a mechanism of NO release may be important, because NO conceivably modulates the autoregulatory (i.e., vasoconstrictor) response of renal vasculature.[51] This concept is supported by experimental evidence that the blockade of NO synthesis induces exaggerated renal vasoconstriction and results in the loss of autoregulation at high levels of renal perfusion pressure.[54,65] Other investigators, however,[66,67] have shown that decreased NO synthesis produces only a decrease in blood flow without altering the efficiency of renal blood flow autoregulation. In either case, there is an increase in preglomerular resistance, which, if sustained, may displace the pressure natriuresis curve with respect to the normal curve. Together the induction of salt sensitivity and a shift of the pressure natriuresis curve in response to even partial inhibition of NO synthesis may create conditions conducive to development of severe forms of hypertension.

Regulation of Glomerular-tubular Dynamics by Nitric Oxide

The regulation of glomerular filtration rate is a complex process that involves the participation of at least three redundant systems[68]: (1) autoregulation of renal blood flow, which is controlled by myogenic responses[43] limited to preglomerular vessels[69]; (2) changes in the glomerular surface area available for filtration, as determined by the myogenic contraction of mesangial microfilaments[70]; and (3) the tubuloglomerular feedback response, which regulates afferent glomerular tone[71] to keep glomerular capillary pressure and the volume of glomerular filtrate proportional to the volume of fluid flowing in the distal tubules. The influence of NO on these homeostatic mechanisms is summarized below.

Renal Blood Flow Autoregulation and Renin Release

An important phenomenon, characteristics of which were demonstrated about 30 years ago, is the fact that increments in renal perfusion pressure significantly decrease the release of renin, whereas the opposite occurs when renal perfusion pressure is decreased.[72] On the basis of this relationship, it has been suggested that the release of nitric oxide at high levels of renal perfusion pressure may modulate not only the smooth muscle contractility triggered by autoregulation but also the arterial pressure-induced decreases of renin release.[51] Studies conducted in vitro support this notion, because incubation of cultured endothelial cells with renal cortical slices for 30 minutes in the presence of indomethacin decreased renin release when the production of NO was stimulated with bradykinin (acetylcholine is a poor stimulator of NO by cultured endothelial cells).[73] Such effects were not seen when bradykinin was added to cortical slices in the absence of endothelial cells or when bradykinin was added to endothelial cells in the presence of oxyhemoglobin, an inactivator of NO.

The inhibitory effects of EDRF on renin were confirmed in additional studies in which the rate of secretion of renin from renal cortical slices was significantly decreased in the perfusate from an acetylcholine-stimulated carotid artery (a rich source of NO).[74] This inhibitory effect continued when carotid arteries were treated with indomethacin, but it was abolished by hemoglobin or when carotid arteries without endothelial cells were exposed to acetylcholine.[74] More recently, Henrich et al.[75] provided strong experimental evidence that the inhibitory effect of NO on renin release is mediated by formation of cGMP. For example, other agents that increase cGMP accumulation, such as atriopeptins, sodium nitroprusside, and 8-bromo-cGMP, also inhibit the release of renin. Furthermore, inhibition of guanylate cyclase with methylene blue blocks the inhibition of renin release and the increase in cGMP by atriopeptins and sodium nitroprusside.

Consistent with the described effects of NO on renin release is the finding by Beierwaltes and Carretero[76] that incubation of rat kidney slices with L-NMMA (10^{-4} M) enhanced renin release by more than 50% of control, most probably by removing the inhibitory action of NO. Inhibition of prostaglandin synthesis with meclofenamate (1.6×10^{-5} M) did not alter the stimulatory effect of L-NMMA on renin release. Furthermore, the stimulation of renin release produced by isoproterenol (a β-adrenergic agonist) was not potentiated by L-NMMA but was blocked by incubation with the NO precursor L-arginine. In agreement with this demonstration are the studies of Kurtz et al., who showed that the release of renin under basal conditions or stimulation by forskolin or isoproterenol is markedly attenuated in the presence of endothelial cells.[77]

In vitro demonstrations that NO inhibits renin release correlate to a certain extent with in vivo studies. Sigmon et al. proved that in rats inhibition of NO synthesis produces a significant elevation of plasma renin activity.[78] More recently, Lahera et al. showed that in anesthetized rats the blockade of NO synthesis produces an increase in blood pressure but no decrease in renin release.[113] However, these findings have not been confirmed by other investigators. Johnson and Freeman[79,80] observed that inhibition of NO synthesis with L-NAME in rats is followed by a decrease of renin release, even when renal perfusion pressure is maintained constant.[80] Studies conducted in rat isolated perfused kidney[81,82] are also congruent with a notion that NO produces a strong stimulation of renin release. At present such contradictory results have no logical explanation.

Glomerular Mesangium

The exact circumstances under which the regulation of glomerular filtration rate is altered by changes in the total glomerular surface area remain undefined. It appears that such a mechanism does not act independently, but rather in concert with factors that affect afferent and efferent glomerular arteriolar tone. Schultz et al.[83] and Marsden et al.[84] provided evidence from in vitro studies that NO released from the endothelial cells of glomerular capillaries can modulate the production of cGMP in mesangial cells and thereby affect the contractility of mesangial cells. More recently, Schultz et al.[85] demonstrated that mesangial cells are also capable of synthesizing significant amounts of NO in the absence of endothelial cells.

Tubuloglomerular Feedback Response

The specialized cells of the nephron located at the junction of the ascending limb of the loop of Henle and the distal convoluted tubule, termed the macula densa, release substances that cause vasoconstriction of the adjacent afferent arterioles. Activation of this tubuloglomerular feedback response reduces the glomerular capillary pressure of the nephron and hence the glomerular filtration rate. Consequently, the tubuloglomerular feedback response should be regarded as a negative feedback mechanism that relates glomerular capillary pressure to distal tubule fluid delivery and reabsorption. In a recent study, Wilcox et al.[86] showed that inhibition of NO synthesis with N[w]-methyl-L-arginine enhanced afferent arteriole tone when tubuloglomerular responses were stimulated by infusing artificial fluid into the loop of Henle. It was concluded that NO synthase in the cells of the macula densa is activated by tubular fluid reabsorption and mediates a novel vasodilating component of the tubuloglomerular feedback response. The modulatory role of NO in glomerular dynamics resembles the role previously described for NO in mediation of the vasoconstrictor responses triggered by renal blood flow autoregulation.[51]

Many more studies are needed to establish the roles of NO in the regulatory mechanisms mentioned above. However, two outstanding contributions from earlier experimental observations deserve to be emphasized: (1) NO appears to exert a continuous or tonic vasodilatory influence on the systemic vasculature, and (2) NO plays a major role in coupling changes in renal hemodynamics to tubular sodium reabsorption. From these two effects, it is easy to realize that a deficiency in NO synthesis may foster the optimal conditions that produce hypertension experimentally.

Nitric Oxide in Cirrhotic Hemodynamic and Renal Alterations

Reduced arterial pressure and vascular resistances, combined with an increase in cardiac output, are important characteristics of cirrhosis that define a hyperdynamic circulatory state. This hyperdynamic state is believed to play a primary role in the activation of antinatriuretic systems (e.g., vasopressin and sympathetic nervous and renin-angiotensin-aldosterone systems) that leads to sodium and water retention. Although the origin of the hemodynamic alteration is unclear, systemic vasodilation in cirrhosis is probably related to an imbalance between endogenous vasodilator and vasoconstrictor substances. In fact, the tendency toward arterial hypotension in cirrhosis is surprising when one considers the high plasma levels of catecholamines, vasopressin, and angiotensin II of cirrhotic animals and patients.[87] However, vascular responses to these vasoconstrictors are reduced in cirrhosis, perhaps by elevated levels of a vasodilator substance. Hemodynamic alterations in cirrhosis are similar to those produced by infusion of exogenous vasodilators; therefore, they may be secondary to increased synthesis of endogenous vasodilator substances. However, numerous investigations of the roles of prostaglandins, kinins, and atrial natriuretic peptide have not indicated a clearly predominant role for any one of the three as the mediator of increased vasodilator mediator in cirrhosis. NO, a recently discovered vasodilator of endothelial origin, has been proposed as an important mediator of the systemic and local alterations of liver cirrhosis.[88,89] The following sections review here the evidence supporting a role for NO in cirrhosis.

Increased Production

Production of NO in cirrhosis may be elevated by at least two different mechanisms:

1. NO may be released from endothelial cells by an increase in blood flow. Elevated blood flow is thought to release NO through a mechanism related to shear stress.[90,91] In liver cirrhosis and portal hypertensive states, elevated blood flows have been described in the splanchnic, renal, and systemic circulations.[87,88] However, whether elevated blood flows are the cause or consequence of increased NO production is not known.

2. Elevated endotoxin levels in cirrhosis[92] may increase endothelial synthesis of NO. Endotoxin has been shown to stimulate an inducible NO synthase in endothelium and smooth muscle. An endotoxin-induced increase in NO production leads to vasodilation and to decreased responsiveness to vasoconstrictors; both effects can be reversed by treatment with NO synthesis inhibitors .[88,93,94]

Most published studies dealing with the role of NO in cirrhosis provide only indirect evidence of increased NO production. Thus, conscious or anesthetized animals with cirrhosis induced by carbon tetrachloride (CCl_4),[9,95] anesthetized portal vein-ligated rats,[8] and anesthetized bile duct-ligated rats[96] show increased pressor sensitivity to inhibition of endogenous NO synthesis. However, in one study in conscious bile duct-ligated rats, the pressor response to a single dose of NO synthesis inhibitor was similar to that of controls.[97] In an interesting case report, methylene blue, a blocker of NO action, elevated blood pressure in a patient with advanced decompensated cirrhosis and severe hypotension.[98] Reduced vascular reactivity to vasoconstrictors in several models of animal cirrhosis can be corrected by treatment with NO synthesis inhibitors.[99–102] Cirrhotic animals also show an increased renal vasodilatory response to the endothelium-dependent vasodilator, acetylcholine.[103] Finally, direct measures of increased NO synthase activity in portal hypertensive and cirrhotic rats have been described recently.[104,105] Other authors, however, found no elevation of NO activity in splanchnic organs from two models of portal hypertensive rats.[106] Therefore, although most studies support the idea of excessive production of NO in liver cirrhosis, much more work still needs to be done to clarify the origin of the elevated production of NO in cirrhosis.

Hyperdynamic Circulation

Acute intravenous administration of NO synthesis inhibitors in experimental animals with CCl_4-induced cirrhosis,[9,95] portal hypertension induced by partial portal vein ligation,[8] or cirrhosis induced by bile duct ligation[96] increases blood pressure in a dose-dependent manner. This hypertensive effect is more pronounced in cirrhotic than in control animals,[8,9,95] although total peripheral, splanchnic, and renal vascular resistance is elevated to the same level in both cirrhotic and control animals.[8,95]

Several studies have also investigated the role of NO as a mediator of the vascular hyporesponsiveness to vasoconstrictors and found that pretreatment with NO synthesis inhibitors abolishes the reduced pressor response to methoxamine ,[99] norepinephrine, vasopressin and potassium chloride,[100,101] and angiotensin II.[102]

Chronic treatment of portal hypertensive rats with the NO synthesis inhibitor, N^w-nitro-L-arginine, also increased blood pressure and vascular resistance, decreased cardiac output and plasma

volume, and corrected the decreased systemic capillary pressure (another index of peripheral vasodilation) in the portal vein-ligated rats.[107] Therefore, the studies indicate that increased activity of NO plays an important role as a mediator of the hyperdynamic circulation and the reduced sensitivity of vasoconstrictors in cirrhosis.

Renal Alterations

According to the peripheral arterial vasodilation hypothesis,[87] sodium and water retention in cirrhosis is secondary to decreased filling of the arterial vascular tree, which activates antinatriuretic hormonal and nervous systems as a compensatory response to maintain arterial pressure. As reviewed above, NO is a vasodilator contributing to normal renal hemodynamic and tubular function. In control animals, stimulation of NO production with acetylcholine produces renal vasodilation and increases in urine output.[39] Moreover, inhibition of NO synthesis at nonpressor doses reduces renal blood flow (RBF), urine flow rate, and sodium excretion.[55] The fact that GFR did not change indicates that NO inhibits sodium and water reabsorption at some point in the nephron. According to such findings, the blockade of NO in cirrhotic animals should produce vasoconstriction and sodium and water retention. Thus it is possible that reduced intrarenal levels of NO may contribute to sodium retention in cirrhosis. However, the few studies performed in cirrhotic animals so far suggest that inhibition of NO synthesis may have a beneficial effect on volume homeostasis.

Inhibition of NO synthesis at pressor doses in conscious cirrhotic animals with ascites increased sodium excretion. The direct mechanism was an increase in the filtered load of sodium, since GFR also increased.[9] To avoid the confounding influence of the increase of blood pressure elicited by high doses of the NO blockers, experiments were done in cirrhotic animals infused with nonpressor doses of a NO synthesis inhibitor (Fig. 17.3).[108] Infusing 10 μg/kg/min of L-NAME in cirrhotic nonascitic animals and 1 μg/kg/min in cirrhotic ascitic animals increased urine flow and sodium excretion up to levels similar to those of control animals infused with saline. This increase in urine output was not due to an increase in GFR, which remained unchanged even when the cirrhotic animals experienced a decrease in RBF. More evidence for a role of NO as a mediator of sodium and water hyperreabsorption in cirrhosis comes from studies in portal

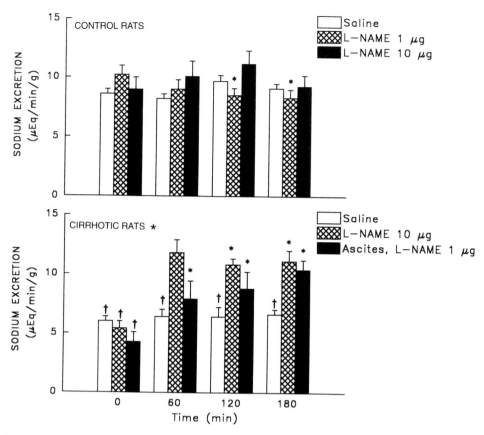

FIGURE 17.3. Effect of administration of two doses of L-NAME to control rats and cirrhotic rats with and without ascites. (For explanation, see text.)

vein-ligated animals.[105] In such experiments, chronic inhibition of NO synthesis reduced—but did not completely abolish—the increased sodium space, an index of sodium retention.

Experimental evidence allows no clear conclusion about the contribution of NO to the renal hyperemia usually found in cirrhotic and portal hypertensive animals. Thus, infusion of pressor doses of NO inhibitors significantly reduced RBF in cirrhotic animals[8,95–97,108] and in portal hypertensive rats,[8] but the responses were similar to those in control animals. However, in experiments using nonpressor doses of NO inhibitor, the decreases in RBF were higher in cirrhotic rats than in controls.[108] In only one case was it concluded that NO does not contribute to the control of renal hemodynamics after administration of a NO blocker in conscious cirrhotic rats; this exception may be due to the important pressor effect elicited by the NO synthesis inhibitor.[9]

The mechanisms involved in the beneficial effect of NO synthesis inhibition on sodium and water excretion are not clear. Inhibition of the renin-angiotensin system may contribute to this response; a decrease in plasma renin activity was found when a pressor bolus of an NO blocker was injected in conscious cirrhotic rats.[9] However, the important pressor effect (20 mmHg) may decrease PRA by itself. Prostaglandins are of major importance in maintaining renal function in cirrhosis and in settings in which the antinatriuretic systems are activated.[109,112] L-NAME infusion may have stimulated release and/or action of prostaglandins. This idea is supported by experiments showing that NO inhibits prostacyclin release in endothelial cells cultured in vitro.[110] Thus, NO inhibition in cirrhotic rats with ascites increases the urinary excretion of 6-keto-PGF_{1a},[9] and the simultaneous inhibition of NO and prostaglandin synthesis markedly reduced renal hemodynamics in conscious cirrhotic rats.[111] In another study, the vasodilatory effects of acetylcholine were enhanced in the kidneys of anesthetized animals, and treatment with an NO blocker reduced but did not abolish the higher vasodilatory effect of acetylcholine. However, when prostaglandin and NO synthesis were simultaneously inhibited in isolated perfused kidneys, no differences in the acetylcholine response of control and cirrhotic kidneys were observed.[103] Such results support the idea[51] that under normal conditions the major compound synthesized by endothelium is NO, which keeps the synthesis of prostaglandins significantly reduced. In contrast, the inhibition of NO leads to a full synthesis of prostaglandin, which in fact may not only compensate for the natriuretic actions of NO but also enhance further sodium excretion. This action may could explain the natriuretic effects that followed the withdrawal of NO in cirrhotic animals. Such results also indicate that complete inhibition of NO synthesis is not necessary to improve sodium and water homeostasis and may produce detrimental effects.[115] Clearly, more studies are needed to elucidate the manner in which the NO-prostaglandins synthesis interaction may influence renal function during the development of cirrhosis with and without ascites.

SUMMARY

Despite an apparent elevation of renal and systemic NO activity in cirrhotic animals and patients, the cirrhotic kidney seems to be refractory to its natriuretic effect. Intrarenal elevation of NO may be produced as a compensatory mechanism against the stimulation of antinatriuretic systems, which seem to predominate and are responsible for sodium retention in cirrhosis. The increase of NO would not be enough, however, to compensate for the antinatriuretic influences. Other possibilities also should be studied to elucidate the role of NO in the sodium and water retention of cirrhosis.

REFERENCES

1. Furchgott RF, Zawadzki JV: The obligatory role of endothelial cells in the relaxation of arterial smooth muscle by acetylcholine. Nature 1980;299:373–376.
2. Moncada S, Palmer RMJ, Higgs EA: The discovery of nitric oxide as the endogenous nitrovasodilator. Hypertension 1988;12:365–372.
3. Furchgott RF, Vanhoutte PM: Endothelium-derived relaxing and contracting factors. FASEB J 1989;3:2007–2018.
4. Ignarro LJ: Biosynthesis and metabolism of endothelium-derived nitric oxide. Annu Rev Pharmacol Toxicol 1990;30:535–560.
5. Ignarro LJ: Nitric oxide: A novel signal transduction mechanism for transcellular communication. Hypertension 1990;16:477–483.
6. Romero JC, Lahera V, Salom MG, Biondi ML: Role of the endothelium-dependent relaxing factor nitric oxide on renal function. J Am Soc Nephrol 1992;2:1371–1387.
7. Tolins JP, Palmer RM, Moncada S, Raij L: Role of endothelium-derived relaxing factor in regulation of renal hemodynamic responses. Am J Physiol 1990;258:H655–662.
8. Pizcueta MP, Piqué JM, Bosch J, et al: Effects of inhibiting nitric oxide biosynthesis on the systemic and splanchnic circulation of rats with portal hypertension. Br J Pharmacol 1992;105:184–190.
9. Clària J, Jiménez W, Ros J, et al: Pathogenesis of arterial hypotension in cirrhotic rats with ascites: Role of endogenous nitric oxide. Hepatology 1992;15:343–349.
10. Hibbs JC, Taintor RR, Vavrin Z: Macrophage cytotoxicity: Role for L-arginine deiminase and imino nitrogen oxidation to nitrite. Science 1987;235:473–476.
11. Marletta MA: Nitric oxide: Biosynthesis and biological significance. Trends Pharmacol Sci 1989;14:488–492.
12. Garthwaite J, Charles SL, Chess-Williams R: Endothelium-derived relaxing factor release on activation of NMDA receptors suggests role as intercellular messenger in the brain. Nature 1988;336:385–388.
13. Palmer RMJ, Moncada S: A novel citrulline-forming enzyme implicated in the formation of nitric oxide by vascular endothelial cells. Biochem Biophys Res Comm 1989;158:348–352.
14. Hecker M, Mitchell JA, Harris HJ, et al: Endothelial cells metabolize N^G-monomethyl-L-arginine to L-citrulline and subsequently to L-arginine. Biochem Biophys Res Comm 1990;167:1037-1043.
15. Leone AM, Palmer RM, Knowles RG, et al: Constitutive and inducible nitric oxide synthases incorporate molecular oxygen into both nitric oxide and citrulline. J Biol Chem 1991;266:23790–23795.
16. Iyengar R, Stuehr DJ, Marletta MA: Macrophage synthesis of nitrite, nitrate, and N-nitrosamines: Precursors and role of the respiratory burst. Proc Natl Acad Sci 1987;84:6369-6373.
17. Lopez-Jaramillo P, Gonzalez MC, Palmer RM, Moncada S: The crucial role of physiological Ca^{2+} concentrations in the production of endothelial nitric oxide and the control of vascular tone. Br J Pharmacol 1990;101:489–493.
18. Palmer RM, Rees DD, Ashton DS, Moncada S: L-arginine is the physiological precursor for the formation of nitric oxide in endothelium-dependent relaxation. Biochem Biophys Res Comm 1988;153:1251–1256.
19. Moore PK, al-Swayeh OA, Chong NS, et al: L-N^G-nitro arginine (L-NOARG), a novel, L-arginine-reversible inhibitor of endothelium-dependent vasodilatation in vitro. Br J Pharmacol 1990;99:408–412.
20. Ishii K, Chang B, Kerwin JF, et al: N^w-nitro-L-arginine: A potent inhibitor of endothelium-derived relaxing factor formation. Eur J Pharmacol 1990;176:219–223.
21. Knowles GK, Palacios M, Palmer RM, Moncada S: Formation of nitric oxide from L-arginine in the central nervous system: A transduction mechanism for stimulation of the soluble guanylate cyclase. Proc Nat Acad Sci 1989;86:5159–5162.
22. Bredt DS, Snyder SH: Nitric oxide mediates glutamate-linked enhancement of cGMP levels in the cerebellum. Proc Nat Acad Sci 1989;86:9030–9033.

23. Ishii K, Chang B, Kerwin JF Jr, et al: Formation of endothelium-derived relaxing factor in porcine kidney epithelial LLC-PK1 cells: An intra- and intercellular messenger for activation of soluble guanylate cyclase. J Pharmacol Exp Ther 1991;256(1):38–43.

24. Nathan CF, Hibbs JB Jr: Role of nitric oxide synthesis in macrophage antimicrobial activity. Curr Opin Immunol 1991;3:65–70.

25. Moncada S, Palmer RMJ, Higgs EA: Nitric oxide physiology, pathophysiology, and pharmacology. Pharmacol Rev 1991;43:109–142.

26. Busse R, Mulsch A: Induction of nitric oxide synthase by cytokines in vascular smooth muscle cells. FEBS Lett 1990;275:87–90.

27. Lamas S, Michel T, Brenner BM, Marsden PA: Nitric oxide synthesis in endothelial cells: Evidence for a pathway inducible by TNF-α. Am J Physiol 1991; C634–641.

28. Beasley D, Schwartz JH, Brenner BM: Interleukin 1 induces prolonged L-arginine–dependent cyclic guanosine monophosphate and nitrite production in rat vascular smooth muscle cells. J Clin Invest 1991;87: 602–608.

29. Baker CH, Sutton ET: Arteriolar endothelium-dependent vasodilation occurs during endotoxin shock. Am J Physiol 1993;264:1118–1123.

30. Shultz PJ, Tayeh MA, Marletta MA, Raij L: Synthesis and action of nitric oxide in rat glomerular mesangial cells. Am J Physiol 1991;261:F600–F606.

31. Radomski MW, Palmer RM, Moncada S: Glucocorticoids inhibit the expression of an inducible, but not the constitutive, nitric oxide synthase in vascular endothlial cells. Proc Natl Acad Sci 1990;87:10043–10047.

32. Dananberg J, Sider RS, Grekin RJ: Deoxycorticosterone suppresses the pressor response to nitroarginine [abstract]. Clin Res 1992;40:172A.

33. Vallance P, Leone A, Calver A, et al: Accumulation of an endogenous inhibitor of nitric oxide synthesis in chronic renal failure. Lancet 1992;339:572–575.

34. Stamler JS, Simon DI, Osborne JA, et al: S-nitrosylation of proteins with nitric oxide: Synthesis and characterization of biologically active compounds. Proc Natl Acad Sci USA 1992;89:444–448.

35. Stamler JS, Jaraki O, Osborne J, et al: Nitric oxide circulates in mammalian plasma primarily as an S-nitroso adduct of serum albumin. Proc Natl Acad Sci USA 1992;89:7674–7677.

36. Lahera V, Khraibi AA, Romero JC: Sulfhydryl group donors potentiate the hypotensive effect of acetylcholine in rats. Hypertension 1993;22:156–160.

37. Craven PA, DeRubertis FR: Restoration of the responsiveness of purified guanylate cyclase to nitrosoguanidine, nitric oxide, and related activators by heme and heme proteins: Evidence of the involvement of the paramagnetic nitrosylheme complex in enzyme activation. J Biol Chem 1978;253:8433–8443.

38. Lahera V, Salom MG, Fiksen-Olsen MJ, Romero JC: Mediatory role of endothelium-derived nitric oxide in renal vasodilatory and excretory effects of bradykinin. Am J Hypertens 1991; 4:260–262.

39. Lahera V, Salom MG, Fiksen-Olsen MJ, et al: Effects of NG-monomethyl-L-arginine and L-arginine on acetylcholine renal response. Hypertension 1990;15:659–663.

40. Salom MG, Lahera V, Romero JC: Role of prostaglandins and endothelium-derived relaxing factor on the renal response to acetylcholine. Am J Physiol 1991; 260:F145–F149.

41. Marchand GR, Ott CE, Lang FC, et al: Effect of secretin on renal blood flow, interstitial pressure, and sodium excretion. Am J Physiol 1977;232:F147–F151.

42. Haas JA, Hammond TG, Granger JP, et al: Mechanism of natriuresis during intrarenal infusion of prostaglandins. Am J Physiol 1984;247:F475–F479.

43. Romero JC, Knox FG: Mechanisms underlying pressure-related natriuresis: The role of the renin-angiotensin and prostaglandin systems: State of the art lecture. Hypertension 1988;11:724–738.

44. Lameire N, Vanholder R, Ringoir S, Leusen I: Role of medullary hemodynamics in the natriuresis of drug-induced renal vasodilation in the rat. Circ Res 1980; 47:839–844.

45. Fadem SZ, Hernandez-Llamas G, Patak RV, et al: Studies on the mechanism of sodium excretion during drug-induced vasodilatation in the dog. J Clin Invest 1982;69:604–610.

46. Biondi ML, Bolterman RJ, Romero JC: Zonal changes of guanidine 3',5'-cyclic monophosphate related to endothelium-derived relaxing factor in dog renal medulla. Renal Physiol Biochem 1992;15:1–7.

47. Stoos BA, Carretero OA, Farhy RD, et al: Endothelium-derived relaxing factor inhibits transport and increases cGMP content in cultured mouse cortical collecting duct cells. J Clin Invest 1992;89(3):761–765.

48. Roman RJ, Cowley AW, Garcia-Estañ J, Lombard JH: Pressure-diuresis in volume-expanded rats: Cortical and medullary hemodynamics. Hypertension 1988;12:168–176.

49. Garcia-Estañ J, Roman RJ: Role of renal interstitial hydrostatic pressure in the pressure diuresis response. Am J Physiol 1989;256:F63–F70.

50. Khraibi AA, Haas JA, Knox FG: Effect of renal perfusion pressure on renal interstitial hydrostatic pressure in rats. Am J Physiol 1989;256:F165–F170.

51. Romero JC, Lahera V, Salom MG, Biondi ML: Role of the endothelium-dependent relaxing factor nitric oxide on renal function. J Am Soc Nephrol 1992;2:1371–1387.

52. Carmines PK, Bell PD, Roman RJ, et al: Prostaglandins in the sodium excretory response to altered renal arterial pressure in dogs. Am J Physiol 1985;248:F8–F14.

53. Gonzalez-Campoy JM, Long C, Roberts D, et al: Renal interstitial hydrostatic pressure and PGE$_2$ in pressure natriuresis. Am J Physiol 1991;260:F643–F649.

54. Salom MG, Lahera V, Guardiola F, Romero JC: Blockade of pressure natriuresis induced by the inhibition of the renal synthesis of nitric oxide in dogs. Am J Physiol 1992;262:F718–F722.

55. Lahera V, Salom MG, Miranda-Guardiola F, et al: Effects of NG-nitro-L-arginine methylester on renal function and blood pressure. Am J Physiol 1991;261: F1033–F1037.

56. Ito S, Johnson CS, Carretero OA: Modulation of angiotensin II-induced vasoconstriction by endothelium-derived relaxing factor in the isolated microperfused rabbit afferent arteriole. J Clin Invest 1991;87(5): 1656–1663.

57. DeNicola L, Blantz RC, Gabbai FB: Nitric oxide and angiotensin II. Glomerular and tubular interaction in the rat. J Clin Invest 1992;89(4):1248–1256.

58. Sigmon DH, Carretero OA, Beierwaltes WH: Angiotensin dependence of endothelium-mediated renal hemodynamics. Hypertension 1992;20:643–650.

59. Lahera V, Salazar J, Salom MG, Romero JC: Deficient production of nitric oxide induces volume-dependent hypertension. J Hypertens 1992;10(Suppl 7):S173–S177.

60. Alberola A, Pinilla JM, Quesada T, et al: Role of nitric oxide in mediating renal response to volume expansion. Hypertension 1992;19:780–784.

61. Atucha NM, Ramírez A, Quesada T, García-Estañ J: Effects of nitric oxide inhibition on rat renal papillary blood flow response to volume expansion. Clin Sci 1994;86:405–409.

62. Hall JE: Renal function in one-kidney, one-clip hypertension and low renin essential hypertension. Am J Hypertens 1991;4:523S–533S.

63. Olesen S-P, Clapham DE, Davies PF: Haemodynamic shear stress activates a K+ current in vascular endothelial cells. Nature (Lond) 1988;331:168–170.

64. Lockhart JC, Larson TS, Knox FG: Perfusion pressure and volume status determine the microvascular response of the rat kidney to NG-monomethyl-L-arginine. Circ Res 1994;75:829–835.

65. Imig JD, Roman RJ: Nitric oxide modulates vascular tone in preglomerular arterioles. Hypertension 1992;19:770–774.

66. Majid DS, Navar LG: Suppression of blood flow autoregulation plateau during nitric oxide blockade in canine kidney. Am J Physiol 1992;262:F40–46.

67. Beierwaltes WH, Sigmon DH, Carretero OA: Endothelium modulates renal blood flow but not autoregulation. Am J Physiol 1992;262:F943–F949.

68. Romero JC, Bentley MD, Vanhoutte PM, Knox FG: Intrarenal mechanisms that regulate sodium excretion in relation to changes in blood pressure. Mayo Clin Proc 1989;64:1406–1424.

69. Gilmore JP, Cornish KG, Rogers SD, Joyner WL: Direct evidence for myogenic autoregulation of the renal microcirculation in the hamster. Circ Res 1980;47:226–250.

70. Michielsen P, Creemers F: The structure and function of the glomerular mesangium. In Dalton AJ, Hauguenau F (eds): Ultrastructure of the Kidney. New York: Academic Press, 1967;57–72.

71. Thurau K, Schnermann J: Die Natriumkonzentration an den Macula denas-zellen als regulierender Factor fur das Glomerulumfiltrat (mikropunktionszersuche). Klin Wochesnschr 1965;43:410–413.

72. Romero JC: El riñón en la regulación de la presión arterial. In Martinez-Maldonado M, Rodicio JL (eds): Tratado de Nefrologia. Barcelona, Spain: Salvat, 1982;172–213.

73. Boulanger C, Vidal-Ragout M, Fiksen-Olsen M, et al: Cultured endothelial cells release a non-prostanoid inhibitor of renin release [abstract]. Clin Res 1988,36:539A.

74. Vidal MJ, Romero JC, Vanhoutte PM: Endothelium-derived relaxing factor inhibits renin release. Eur J Pharmacol 1988;149:401–402.

75. Henrich WL, McAllister EA, Smith PB, Campbell WB: Guanosine 3'-5'-cyclic monophosphate as a mediator of inhibition of renin release. Am J Physiol 1988;255: F474–F478.

76. Beierwaltes WH, Carretero OA: Nonprostanoid endothelium-derived factors inhibit renin release. Hypertension 1992;19(Suppl 2):II68-II73.

77. Kurtz A, Kaissling B, Busse R, Baier W: Endothelial cells modulate renin secretion from isolated mouse juxtaglomerular cells. J Clin Invest 1991;88:1147–1154.

78. Sigmon DH, Carretero OA, Beierwaltes WH: Endothelium-derived relaxing factor regulates renin release in vivo. Am J Physiol 1992;263:F256-F261.

79. Johnson RA, Freeman RH: Pressure natriuresis in rats during blockade of the L-arginine/nitric oxide pathway. Hypertension 1992;19:333–338.

80. Johnson RA, Freeman RH: Sustained hypertension in the rat induced by chronic blockade of nitric oxide production. Am J Hypertension 1992;5:919–922.

81. Gardes J, Poux J-M, Gonzalez M-F, et al: Decreased renin release and constant kallikrein secretion after injection of L-NAME in isolated perfused rat kidney. Life Sci 1992;50:987–993.

82. Münter K, Hackenthal E: The participation of the endothelium in the control of renin release. J Hypertension 1991;9(Suppl 6):S236–S237.

83. Schultz PJ, Schorer AE, Raij L: Effects of endothelium-derived relaxing factor and nitric oxide on rat mesangial cells. Am J Physiol 1990;258:F162–F167.

84. Marsden PA, Brock TA, Ballermann FJ: Glomerular endothelial cells respond to calcium-mobilizing agonists with release of EDRF. Am J Physiol 1990;258: F1295–F1303.

85. Shultz PJ, Tayeh MA, Marletta MA, Raij L: Synthesis and action of nitric oxide in rat glomerular mesangial cells. Am J Physiol 1991;261:F600–F606.

86. Wilcox CS, Welch WJ, Murad F, et al: Nitric oxide synthase in macula densa regulates glomerular capillary pressure. Proc Natl Acad Sci USA 1992;89(24):11993–11997.

87. Schrier RW, Arroyo V, Bernardi M, et al: Peripheral arterial vasodilation hypothesis: A proposal for the initiation of renal sodium and water retention in cirrhosis. Hepatology 1988;8:1151–1157.

88. Vallance P, Moncada S: Hyperdynamic circulation in cirrhosis: A role for nitric oxide? Lancet 1991;337: 776–777.

89. Stark ME, Szurskewki JH: Role of nitric oxide in gastrointestinal and hepatic function and disease. Gastroenterology 1992;103:1928–1949.

90. Rubanyi GM, Romero JC, Vanhoutte PM: Flow-induced release of endothelium-derived relaxing factor. Am J Physiol 1986;250:H1145–H1149.

91. Miller VM, Vanhoutte PM: Enhanced release of endothelium-derived factor(s) by chronic increases in blood flow. Am J Physiol 1988;255:H446–H451.

92. Lumsden AB, Henderson JM, Kutner MH: Endotoxin levels measured by a chromogenic assay in portal, hepatic and peripheral venous blood in patients with cirrhosis. Hepatology 1988;8:232–236.

93. Rees DD, Cellek S, Palmer RMJ, Moncada S: Dexamethasone prevents the induction by endotoxin of a nitric oxide synthase and the associated effects on vascular tone: An insight into endotoxin shock. Biochem Biophys Res Commun 1990;173:541–547.

94. Gray GA, Schott C, Julou-Schaeffer G, et al: The effect of inhibitors of the L-arginine/nitric oxide pathway on endotoxin-induced loss of vascular responsiveness in anesthetized rats. Br J Pharmacol 1991;103:1218–1224.

95. Pizcueta MP, Piqué JM, Fernández M, et al: Modulation of the hyperdynamic circulation of cirrhotic rats by nitric oxide inhibition. Gastroenterology 1992;103:1909–1915.

96. Ramírez A, Atucha NM, Quesada T, et al: Efectos de la inhibición de la síntesis de óxido nítrico en la hemodinámica y excreción renal de ratas con cirrosis biliar crónica. Nefrología 1994;14:656–662.

97. Sogni P, Moreau R, Ohsuga M, et al: Evidence for normal nitric oxide-mediated vasodilator tone in conscious rats with cirrhosis. Hepatology 1992;16:980–983.

98. Midgley S, Grant IS, Haynes WG, Webb DJ: Nitric oxide in liver failure (letter). Lancet 1991;338:1590.

99. Lee F-Y, Albillos A, Colombato LA, Groszmann RJ: The role of nitric oxide in the vascular hyporesponsiveness to methoxamine in portal hypertensive rats. Hepatology 1992;16:1043-1048.

100. Sieber CC, Groszmann RJ: Nitric oxide mediates hyporeactivity to vasopressors in mesenteric vessels of portal hypertensive rats. Gastroenterology 1992;103:235–239.

101. Sieber CC, López-Talavera JC, Groszmann RJ: Role of nitric oxide in the in vitro splanchnic vascular hyporeactivity in ascitic cirrhotic rats. Gastroenterology 1993;104:1750–1754.

102. Castro A, Jiménez W, Clària J, et al: Impaired responsiveness to angiotensin II in experimental cirrhosis: Role of nitric oxide. Hepatology 1993;18:367–372.

103. García-Estañ J, Atucha NM, Sabio JM, et al: Increased endothelium-dependent renal vasodilation in cirrhotic rats. Am J Physiol 1994;267:R549–R553.

104. Ros J, Jiménez W, Lamas S, et al: Increased vascular nitric oxide synthase activity in aortic segments of rats with cirrhosis and ascites [abstract]. J Hepatol 1993;18:S14.

105. Cahill PA, Wu YP, Sitzmann JV: Nitric oxide synthase activity in portal hypertension [abstract]. Hepatology 1993;18:141A.

106. Fernández M, Rovira H, Piqué JM, et al: Activity of Ca^{2+}-dependent and independent nitric oxide synthase in tissues from portal hypertensive and cirrhotic rats [abstract]. Gastroenterology 1994;106:A892.

107. Lee F-Y, Colombato LA, Albillos A, Groszmann RJ: N^w-nitro-L-arginine administration corrects peripheral vasodilation and systemic capillary hypotension and ameliorates plasma volume expansion and sodium retention in portal hypertensive rats. Hepatology 1993;17:84–90.

108. Atucha NM, Ramírez A, Quesada T, et al: Renal effects of nitric oxide synthesis inhibition in cirrhotic rats. Am J Physiol 1994;267:R1454–R1460.

109. Zipser RD, Lifschitz MD: Prostaglandins and related compounds. In Epstein M, (ed): The Kidney in Liver Disease, 3rd ed. Baltimore: Williams & Wilkins, 1988;393–415.

110. Doni MG, Whittle BJR, Palmer RMJ, Moncada S: Actions of nitric oxide on the release of prostacyclin from bovine endothelial cells in culture. Eur J Pharmacol 1988;151:19–25.

111. Ros J, Clària J, Jiménez W, et al: Role of nitric oxide and prostaglandins in the regulation of renal perfusion in conscious rats with cirrhosis and ascites. J Hepatol 1992;16(Suppl 1):S5.

112. Wong F, Massie D, Hsu P, Dudley F: Indomethacin-induced renal dysfunction in patients with well-compensated cirrhosis. Gastroenterology 1993;104:869–876.

113. Navarro J, Sánchez A, Sáiz J, et al: Hormonal, renal and metabolic alterations during the hypertension induced by chronic inhibition of nitric oxide in rats. Am J Physiol 1994;267:R1516–R1521.

114. Guyton AC: Arterial Pressure and Hypertension. Philadelphia, W.B. Saunders, 1980.

115. Nava E, Palmer RMJ, Moncada S: Inhibition of nitric oxide synthesis in septic shock: How much is beneficial? Lancet 1991;338:1555-1557.

116. Pearson PJ: Mechanism of coronary vasospasm following reperfusion injury: Role of vasoactive factors produced by the endothelium [thesis]. Rochester, MN, Mayo Graduate School of Medicine, 1991.

Chapter 18

ENDOTHELIN AND RENAL DYSFUNCTION IN LIVER DISEASE

MICHAEL S. GOLIGORSKY, M.D., Ph.D.
EDWARD P. NORD, M.D.

Endothelin Synthesis
  Structure
  Endothelin-converting Enzyme
Sites of Endothelin Production
  ET Production by the Kidney
  ET Production by the Liver
  Regulation of Endothelin Synthesis and Degradation
Endothelin Receptors
  Distribution of ET Receptors along the Nephron
  Endothelin Receptors in the Liver
Physiologic Role of Endothelin in Renal and Liver Function

Physiologic Role of ET in Renal Function
Physiologic Role of ET in Liver Function
Cellular Mechanisms of Endothelin Action
  Effects of ET-1 on Cells of the Vasculature
  Pharmacologic Tools for Modulation of ET
    Synthesis, Conversion, Action, and Degradation
Putative Role of Endothelin in Acute Renal Failure
  Evidence for a Role of ET-1 in ARF
  Emerging Evidence for a Possible Role of
    Endothelin in HRS
Summary and Future Directions

The development of renal failure in advanced liver cirrhosis is well established, and its peculiar features have been extensively reviewed in previous chapters. This chapter provides a foray into the newly described family of vasoactive peptides, endothelins, focusing on their structure, sites of production, modes of action, structure-function relationships, and emerging role as potentially important mediators of renal failure, both in general and in the specific setting of advanced irreversible hepatic dysfunction.

The current view of the local regulation of blood flow in various vascular beds has been shaped to a considerable degree by two major discoveries of the past decade: specific endothelium-derived relaxing and constricting factors.[1,2] The relaxing factor has been identified as nitric oxide,[3] the constricting factor as a member of the endothelin family.[4] As described below, the synthesis, release, and action of these two factors are frequently mutually interactive.

ENDOTHELIN SYNTHESIS

Structure

Endothelin (ET) is a novel 21-amino acid peptide, originally purified from the supernatant of cultured porcine aortic endothelial cells, that exhibits potent vasoconstrictor activity.[4] To date, three isoforms of human ET have been identified: ET-1, ET-2, and ET-3, each encoded by a distinct gene.[5] The 21 residue peptides display highly homologous amino acid sequences (Fig.18.1), which include four cysteine residues connected by two internal disulfide bridges.[5] The major variation in amino acid sequences occurs between residues 4–7, suggesting that this variable region may determine the functional characteristics of the different isopeptides. Of interest, endothelins share significant structural homologies with the sarafotoxins found in the venom of the Israeli burrowing asp.[6]

Sequence analysis of cloned cDNA for human ET-1 precursor[7] demonstrated that, much like other peptide hormones and neuropeptides, ET is translated as a 212-amino acid precursor, preproET. PreproET-1 mRNA is constitutively expressed in cultured endothelial cells and levels of transcripts can be modulated.[8] PreproET-1 mRNA is extremely unstable with a half-life of about 15 minutes.[9] It has been suggested that the instability of preproET-1 mRNA results from the presence of two conserved AUUUA sequences in the 3'-untranslated region that mediate selective

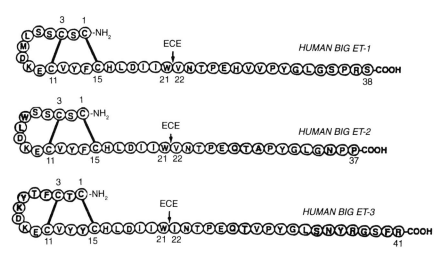

FIGURE 18.1. Amino acid sequences of the three isoforms of "big" endothelin and the respective sites of their cleavage by endothelin-converting enzyme (ECE) yielding active isoforms of endothelin. (From Opgenorth T, Wu-Wong J, Shiosaki K: Endothelin-converting enzyme. FASEB J 1992;6:1653–2659, with permission.)

mRNA degradation. Shortly after translation, cleavage of this peptide yields a 38-amino acid intermediate termed "big" ET,[8,10] which has been shown to possess minimal vasoconstrictor properties. The 38-amino acid residue, in turn, is further cleaved by a putative endothelin-converting enzyme (ECE) to yield the mature, physiologically active 21-amino acid peptide (see Fig. 18.1 and below).

Endothelin-converting Enzyme

Several putative enzymes have been identified that may function as endothelin-converting enzyme (ECE) in the cleavage of the Trp^{21}-Val^{22} bond of big ET-1 to yield ET-1.[11] The initial hypothesis that ECE was a serine protease with chymotrypsinlike activity was later superseded by other putative candidates with either aspartic or metalloprotease characteristics. The universal aspartic protease inhibitor pepstatin-A has been shown to inhibit the production of ET-1 from porcine big ET incubated with an extract from cultured endothelial cells.[12] An antibody raised against cathepsin D (bovine spleen) was able to adsorb this ECE activity.[13] A more likely candidate, however, was later identified as cathepsin E, which was able to cleave big ET to yield only ET-1 and the carboxyl-terminal fragment.[14] The major conceptual drawback for the cathepsins as ECE candidates has been the low-pH optimum required for the activity of these lysosomal enzymes. Thus it has been suggested that the enzymes instead may participate in the metabolism of ETs. However, in human polymorphonuclear leukocytes, ECE activity was significantly blunted by the serine protease inhibitor, 3,4-dichloroisocumarin (50 µM) or the elastase inhibitor ONO-5046 (100 µM), suggesting that in these cells a chymotrypsin-like ECE may be present.[15]

ECE activity with pH optimum in the neutral range has been identified in the cytosolic fraction of endothelial cells.[16] Enzyme activity was inhibited by the neutral (metallo) endopeptidase inhibitor phosphoramidone and by the metal-chelator ethylenediamine tetraacetic acid (EDTA) but was resistant to other neutral endopeptidase (NEP) inhibitors, such as captopril. Experiments in cultured endothelial cells and whole animal studies with regional and systemic administration of phosphoramidon support the role of NEP in converting big ET to ET-1.[17-22] An ECE more recently purified to homogeneity from rat lung microsomes[23] has remarkably similar properties to the enzyme identified in endothelial cells The purified enzyme showed a single band at a molecular mass of 130 kDa by SDS-PAGE analysis, similar to that described in endothelial cells (100–120 kDa). Of interest, the lung ECE converted big ET-1 to ET-1, big ET-2 to ET-2 and big ET-3 to ET-3; big ET-1 was the preferred substrate. Thus there are several candidate ECEs that may indicate tissue-specific enzymes. Alternatively, a uniform mechanism of conversion remains masked by the inadequate selectivity of the inhibitor probes of involved peptidases.

SITES OF ENDOTHELIN PRODUCTION

In initial studies, endothelial cells of large vessels were identified as a site of ET production,[4,24] but firm evidence now indicates that certain non-endothelial cells synthesize the peptide. For example, cultured rat and bovine parathyroid cells (but not endothelial cells) and cultured human breast epithelial cells (but not stromal cells) produce the peptide.[25,26] Of great interest is the observation that ET-like immunoreactivity has been identified by immunohistochemistry in the paraventricular and supraoptic nuclear neurons and their terminals in the posterior pituitary of pigs and rats.[27] Furthermore, in situ hybridization localized ET mRNA to paraventricular nuclear neurons.[27] These are the identical sites at which arginine vasopressin (AVP) is synthesized and stored. Indeed, ET-like immunoreactive products in the posterior pituitary of the rat were depleted by water deprivation, raising the intriguing possibility that ET and AVP are released under conditions of a common stimulus and that ET, in some manner, may be involved in water homeostasis. The combined evidence firmly establishes that ET production is not confined to endothelial cells. The precise physiologic role of ET and factors that elicit its production in extra-vasculature sites remains to be elucidated.

ET Production by the Kidney

Overwhelming evidence indicates that ET is produced in the kidney both by endothelial and non-endothelial cells. Using a polyclonal antibody raised in rabbit, ET-like immunoreactivity was found to be widely distributed in normal rat kidney.[28] Immunostaining density was greatest in the renal papilla, where it was localized to the vasae rectae and epithelial cells of the inner medullary collecting duct (IMCD). Cortical immunostaining was localized to the endothelial surface of arcuate arteries, veins, arterioles and peritubular capillaries. Glomerular immunostaining followed a capillary loop distribution and appeared to be localized primarily to endothelial cells; smaller amounts of staining were observed in mesangial cells. The brush border membrane of the most proximal portion of the proximal tubule demonstrated focal immunostaining. On the basis of these observations a more precise cellular localization of ET production has been forthcoming.

With regard to the glomerulus, ET has been shown to be synthesized by all resident cells of the glomerular tuft, namely, mesangial, endothelial, and epithelial cells.[29–31] Human mesangial cells in culture produce ET-1 as measured by radioimmunoassay, and the production was augmented by vasopressin.[29] Bovine glomerular capillary endothelial cells in culture released ET-1 in a time-dependent fashion, which was further enhanced by exposure of cultures to bradykinin.[30] PreproET-1 mRNA levels rose in a biphasic manner in response to challenge with bradykinin; the early phase increment was not dependent on new protein synthesis, whereas the late rise appeared to be dependent on the de novo protein synthesis. More recently, cultured bovine glomerular epithelial cells also have been shown to synthesize ET-1 and ET-3 as measured by RIA and Northern analysis.[31] The physiologic relevance of these findings awaits clarification.

Of the different nephron segments studied, the inner medullary collecting duct (IMCD) appears to be the predominant if not sole site of ET production. Using microdissected nephron segments, Ujiie and coworkers[32] measured ET-1 production by radioimmunoassay and ET-1 mRNA by the polymerase chain reaction technique coupled with reverse transcription (RT-PCR). IMCD—but neither medullary thick ascending limb (MTAL) nor proximal convoluted tubule (PCT)—produced ET-1. In parallel studies ET-1 mRNA was detected only in IMCD but not in MTAL, PCT, cortical collecting duct (CCD) or outer medullary collecting duct (OMCD). The authors did not investigate ET-3 synthesis. Both freshly isolated and cultured human IMCD cells synthesize significant amounts of ET-1.[33] ET-3 and ET-3 mRNA were also reported in the same study but at barely detectable levels. In cultured rat IMCD cells ET-1 and ET-3 were detected by immunostaining.[34] Of interest, brief exposure of cells to hyperosmolar solutions (NaCl, mannitol and urea) strikingly enhanced ET-1 immunostaining, whereas concomitant exposure of cells to a hypoosmolar solution essentially eliminated the baseline signal. Similar observations have been made using the isolated perfused IMCD.[35] The most recent survey of the microdissected rat nephron using RT-PCR[36] demonstrated that, although ET-1 mRNA expression was highest in the IMCD, the product was also found in the proximal nephron, thick ascending limbs, and outer medullary collecting ducts. In homozygous Brattleboro rats, the increase in

TABLE 18.1. Stimulators and Inhibitors of ET-1 Synthesis

Agent	Stimulation	Inhibition
Heparin		+
Nitric oxide*		+
Arginine vasopressin*	+	
Angiotensin II*	+	
Norepinephrine	+?	
Transforming growth factor-β*	+	
Tumor necrosing factor-α*	+	
Interleukin-1	+	
Alcohol*	+	
Thrombin*	+	
Atrial natriuretic peptide		+
Ca-ionophores	+	
Phorbol esters	+?	
Glucose*	+	
Shear stress	+	
Cyclic guanosine monophosphate		+
Ischemia	+	

* Indicates that the particular agonist may have a functional role in hepatic failure.

ET-1 mRNA along the corticomedullary axis and its preponderance in IMCD were not found, further raising an intriguing possibility that ET-1 plays a crucial role in urinary concentration.

ET Production by the Liver

Sinusoidal endothelial cells represent an established site of ET-1 production. Rieder et al.[37] have isolated guinea pig sinusoidal endothelial cells (separated from Kupffer cells by centrifugal elutriation) and examined the release of ET-1 into the culture medium by radioimmunoassay. Under resting conditions, approximately 900 pg/µg DNA/24 hr of ET-1 were released, a value comparable to the synthetic rate reported for the more extensively studied human umbilical vein endothelial cells (HUVEC). When sinusoidal endothelial cells were exposed to Kupffer cell-conditioned culture medium, accumulation of immunoreactive ET increased by 50%. Under identical culture conditions, transforming growth factor (TGF)-β evoked a comparable increment in ET-1 production. Perhaps the most intriguing observation was that ET-1 production by sinusoidal endothelial cells was further augmented by conditioned medium derived from Kupffer cells exposed to endotoxin, whereas endotoxin itself had no effect on ET-1 production by the sinusoidal cells. Such studies bring out several important points: (1) humoral messenger(s) produced by activated Kupffer cells may be viewed as a paracrine modulator of sinusoidal endothelial cell function; (2) TGF-β appears to exert a direct effect on sinusoidal endothelial cell production of ET-1; and (3) endotoxin induces the release of a paracrine substance from Kupffer cells that stimulates ET-1 production. The paracrine substance has been tentatively identified as TGF-β. No other data are available regarding the regulation of ET-1 release from sinusoidal cells.

Regulation of Endothelin Synthesis and Degradation

A large body of information has accrued over the past few years regarding factors that regulate endothelin synthesis in vascular endothelial cells. Such data are comprehensively summarized in several excellent reviews.[38–41] The paucity of data pertaining to potential mechanisms operative in liver or kidney necessitates analogies with the better studied vascular endothelium. Several well established regulators are summarized in Table 18.1

The degradation pathway for ET involves a phosphoramidone-sensitive neutral endopeptidase 24.[11] which was purified from rat kidneys and aortic smooth muscle cells.[11,42] In polymorphonuclear leukocytes, elastase may play an important role in degradation of ET-1.[15]

ENDOTHELIN RECEPTORS

To date, three types of ET receptors (ET-R) have been cloned, sequenced, and designated A, B, and C (i.e., ET_A-R, ET_B-R and ET_C-R). ET_A-R displays preferential recognition for ET-1,[43,44] ET_C-R recognizes ET-3 with highest affinity,[45] and ET_B-R is a non–isopeptide-selective receptor that recognizes all three peptides with equal affinity.[46] Both ET_A-R and ET_B-R have been identified in a wide range of mammalian tissues. The newly discovered ET_C-R, identified on *Xenopus laevis* dermal melanophores, has now been cloned and characterized.[45] Its activation induced the dispersion of pigment granules within the melanophores. The abundance and location of ET_C-R in mammalian tissues is currently not known.

Recent studies from Masaki's laboratory have established potential models for molecular recognition by ET_A-R and ET_B-R for their ligands.[47] It has been postulated that both the C- and N-termini of ET-1 are engaged in high-affinity binding to

ET_A-R, whereas ET_B-R binds only the C-terminal portion of the peptide, especially the Glu10-Trp21 amino acid residues (Fig. 18.2). Because the major structural differences between ET isopeptides are located primarily toward the N-terminus, this schema provides an elegant explanation for the selective and nonselective types of ET receptors for their ligands. The mode of molecular recognition by the ET_C-R remains to be identified, along with its existence in mammals.

Distribution of ET Receptors along the Nephron

The seminal observation regarding the distribution of ET receptors in the kidney comes from the work of Kohzuki and coworkers[48] in a simple but convincing autoradiogram of rat kidney slice exposed to ^{125}I-endothelin. Details of the molecular nature of the different ET receptor subtypes delineated above were not available at that time. ^{125}I-endothelin binding to glomeruli, PCT, vasa recta bundles, and inner medulla was noted. The most important if not surprising observation was that the vast majority of ET receptors were located in the inner medulla. Subsequent more detailed studies followed up on this observation to provide important information about the precise cellular location of ET receptors along different nephron segments and other intrarenal structures.

Using microdissected tubular and vascular fragments and RT-PCR, Terada and coworkers[49] recently localized mRNA coding for ET_A-R and ET_B-R. ET_A-R mRNA was found primarily in the microvasculature, notably the arcuate arteries, vasae rectae, and glomeruli, whereas ET_B-R mRNA was identified in the epithelial cells of the collecting duct, with the greatest preponderance in the IMCD. ET_B-R mRNA was also detected in the glomeruli. With regard to the glomerulus, these findings are in broad agreement with earlier radioligand binding data from several laboratories that detected two classes of ET receptors on mesangial cell preparations.[50–53] We have observed only ET_B-R both in cultured IMCD cells using a radioligand binding assay[54] and in slices of rat medulla using in situ RT-PCR.[55] On the other hand, other workers have detected both ET_A-R and ET_B-R mRNA in the IMCD.[56] The nature of the discrepancy is currently unresolved. Another area of dispute is the presence of ET receptors on the proximal tubule, where physiologic responses have been detected[57] yet no ET receptor has been

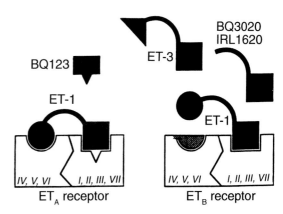

FIGURE 18.2. Proposed mode of interaction of endothelins or endothelin receptor agonists or antagonists with their receptors. The carboxyl-terminal sequence of all natural and synthetic agonists (*filled squares*) are recognized by both types of receptors. Selectivity of the ET_AR resides in the region spanning transmembrane loops IV–VI and interacting with the amino-terminal address domain of ET-1. The amino-terminal domain of ET-3 can interact only weakly with the address-recognition site of the ET_AR. The corresponding address-recognition domain of the ET_BR can interact with a much wider spectrum of ligands' address portions. Alternatively, the ET_BR has an internal, self-content address domain (depicted with a striped hemisphere) so that it requires no external address sequence. BQ123 = cyclic pentapeptide antagonist; BQ3020 and IRL1620 = selective ET_BR agonists. (From Sakamoto A, Yanagisawa M, Sawamura T, et al: Distinct subdomains of endothelin receptors determine their selectivity to endothelin$_A$-selective antagonist and endothelin$_B$-selective agonists. J Biol Chem 1993; 268:8547–8553, with permission.)

clearly discerned to date. In medullary interstitial cells we have detected a single population of the ET_A-R.[58] Of interest, cells with a common mesenchymal origin (mesangial cells, vascular smooth muscle cells, and renal medullary interstitial cells) possess ET_A receptors, whereas cells of epithelial origin possess ET_B receptors.

Endothelin Receptors in the Liver

Radioligand-binding studies using rat liver plasma membranes indicate the presence of a single class of high affinity and high capacity binding sites (K_d 32.4 pM, B_{max} 1084 fmol/mg protein).[59] Because both ET-1 and ET-3 displaced ^{125}I-ET-1, albeit with different IC_{50} values, it can be concluded that the major if not sole hepatic ET receptor is of the ET_B-R variety. Of note, the Hill coefficient of displacement by ET-3 suggested the presence of a second, low-affinity binding site for ET in this preparation. Further studies are required to resolve this issue. The precise location of ET receptors within the hepatic parenchyma awaits resolution.

PHYSIOLOGIC ROLE OF ENDOTHELIN IN RENAL AND LIVER FUNCTION

Physiologic Role of ET in Renal Function

Early studies on the potential role of ET in renal physiology were performed on the intact organ. Infusion of ET into the renal artery of rats within a range of 5–40 pmol/hr decreased renal plasma flow (RPF), glomerular filtration rate (GFR), and urine volume,[60] with no appreciable change in the fractional excretion of sodium (FENa). Mean arterial pressure (MAP) did not substantially change, implicating a direct action of the peptide on the kidney. Such observations are best explained by the potent vasoconstrictor effect of ET. In addition, the calcium channel blocker, nicardipine, diminished ET-induced reduction in urine volume, GFR, and RBF in keeping with the concept that the peptide mediates its profound vasoconstrictor effects via voltage-operated calcium channels. These observations also predict that ET has a direct tubular effect, because FENa was unaffected despite a decrement in GFR. Essentially identical results have been reported in canine models.[61]

Micropuncture studies have further elucidated the mechanism(s) by which ET decreases GFR. Both afferent and efferent arteriolar resistances were increased (afferent somewhat more than efferent), thereby reducing nephron plasma flow rate.[62] In addition, ET reduced glomerular ultrafiltration coefficient (KF) and hence diminished single nephron GFR (SNGFR).[62] Other studies are in general accord with these observations. In one such study, afferent and efferent arteriolar resistances were increased and KF was decreased, but SNGFR was not significantly diminished, because the decrement in KF was offset by a concomitant increase in glomerular capillary hydrostatic pressure.[63] In another study, afferent arteriolar resistance was increased to a greater extent than efferent arteriolar resistance and KF was unchanged, but SNGFR was diminished because of the profound reduction in RPF.[64] The somewhat discrepant findings in such studies are probably related to differences in specific experimental protocols. Edwards and coworkers examined the sensitivity to ET of microdissected afferent and efferent glomerular arterioles from rabbits.[65] Afferent as well as efferent vessels responded to ET-1 and ET-2; similar EC50 values were found for both peptides in both structures. ET-3, on the other hand, was considerably less potent. Of interest, inhibition of the ET-mediated vasoconstrictor effect by dihydropyridines was observed exclusively in afferent arterioles. Whether efferent vessels possess dihydropyridine-insensitive or phenylalkylamine-insensitive calcium channels was not determined; however, the results are in keeping with the previous videomicroscopic studies of the afferent and efferent arterioles that suggested the absence of voltage-dependent calcium channels in the efferent vessels.[66] The combined evidence strongly indicates that vasoconstriction of the afferent and, to a lesser extent, efferent glomerular arterioles plays a predominant role in ET modulation of glomerular function.

Perhaps the most firmly established tubular action of ET is its ability to inhibit the hydroosmotic effect of arginine vasopressin (AVP), particularly in the IMCD. Using the isolated perfused IMCD preparation, Oishi and coworkers demonstrated that ET (10^{-10}M–10^{-8}M) reversibly inhibited AVP-stimulated water permeability.[67] AVP-stimulated urea permeability was not augmented. Nadler and coworkers confirmed and expanded this observation by demonstrating that ET blunted the hydroosmotic effect in IMCD via a pertussis toxin-sensitive pathway that was only partially dependent on protein kinase C.[68] The observation that changes in osmolarity modulate ET production in the IMCD[34] supports the notion that ET may be an autocrine regulator of water flux in distal nephron segments. An autocrine and paracrine role for ET within the inner medulla is schematically depicted in Figure 18.3. According to this schema, ET synthesis induced by changes in osmolarity or other yet-to-be-identified trigger mechanisms results in the paracrine (RMIC) or autocrine (IMCD) action of the peptide. In this manner ET may serve as an important local modulator of water absorption at the major site of AVP action. The precise mechanism by which ET blunts the hydroosmotic effect of AVP remains to be determined. One potential but untested mechanism may be the phosphorylation of a phosphoprotein recently identified in cultured human umbilical cord vein endothelial cells.[69]

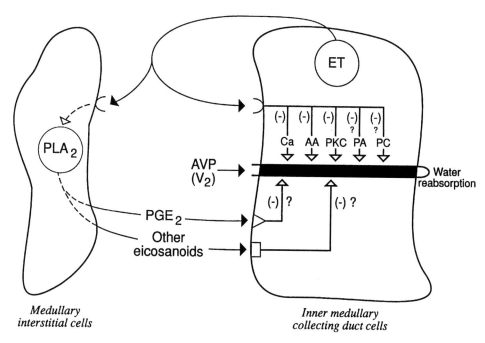

FIGURE 18.3.   Depiction of an autocrine and/or paracrine role of endothelin (ET) in blunting the hydro-osmotic effect of arginine vasopressin (AVP) acting via its V_2 receptor. Ca = increments in intracellular calcium, AA = arachidonic acid or its metabolites, PKC = protein kinase C, PA = phosphatidic acid, PC = other product of phosphatidylcholine hydrolysis. (From Nord EP: Renal actions of endothelin. Kidney Int 1993; 44:451–463, with permission.)

Hyperosmotic conditions (cell shrinkage) were associated with increased phosphorylation, and hypoosmotic conditions (cell swelling) were associated with decreased phosphorylation of a 16.5 kDa band. Further analysis will be required to reveal whether a similar mechanism modulates IMCD production of ET.

In a preliminary study using rabbit cortical collecting duct, ET has been reported to inhibit luminal amiloride-sensitive sodium channels.[70] It was suggested that the process was calcium-dependent. Further studies are required to confirm this observation, which in part may explain the natriuretic effect of ET observed by some workers.

The proximal tubule has been identified most recently as a site of ET action. ET (10^{-9} M) diminished fluid absorption, blunted bicarbonate absorption, and inhibited activity of sodium-potassium adenosine triphosphatase (Na^+-K^+ ATPase) in rat proximal straight tubule, leading the authors to conclude that the peptide mediated its effect on fluid and bicarbonate absorption via inhibition of Na^+-K^+-ATPase.[57] Although sodium pump activity was statistically significantly inhibited by ET, the reduction was a modest 20% of oubain-sensitive enzyme activity. However,

experiments performed on basolateral membrane vesicles prepared from rabbit renal cortex[71] demonstrated that ET accelerated sodium bicarbonate cotransport (increase in V_{max} but no change in K_m), suggesting that ET modulates bicarbonate reabsorption independently of actions on the sodium pump. The latter study also reported that ET directly stimulates the Na^+/H^+ antiporter (increase in V_{max} but no change in K_m) in brush border membrane vesicles, a finding that is in keeping with ET stimulation of bicarbonate reabsorption. Indeed, in the intact rabbit proximal tubule ET was found to be without effect on Na^+-K^+-ATPase activity.[72] In summary, data about the precise role of ET in proximal tubule function are conflicting. Interpretation of these findings is further complicated by the fact that no ET receptors have been identified on the proximal nephron to date.[49] Whether the proximal tubule possess a unique ET receptor is currently not known.

Physiologic Role of ET in Liver Function

Whole organ studies have shown that ET plays an important role in modulating a number of important hepatic functions. In the isolated perfused

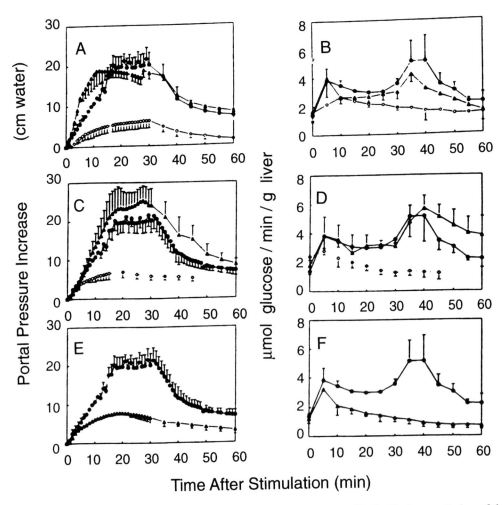

FIGURE 18.4. Changes in portal pressure (*A, C, E*) and glucose output (*B, D, F*) after perfusion of the liver with ET-1. *A* and *B*, Livers were perfused with various concentrations of ET-1 for 30 minutes, followed by an additional 30-minute perfusion with no effector. The *closed circles* refer to stimulation with 1 mM ET-1, *closed triangles* show 10 nM ET-1, and *open diamonds* depict the effects of 0.1 nM ET-1. *C* and *D*, Stimulation was performed for 30 minutes in the presence of 1 nM ET-1 and 50 μM indomethacin (*closed triangles*) or for 15 minutes in the presence of 1 nM ET-1 and 1 μM Iloprost (*open diamonds*). *E* and *F*, Livers were perfused with 1 nM ET-1 and 100 μM SIN-1 (*closed triangles*). (From Tran-Thi T, Kawada N, Decker K: Regulation of endothelin-1 action on the perfused rat liver. FEBS Lett 1993;318:353–357, with permission.)

rat liver, infusion of physiologic concentrations of both ET-1 and ET-3 produced severe vasoconstriction with ensuing portal hypertension (EC50 1 nM), suggesting that the target for the infused peptides was localized on contractile cells.[73] Such effects were accompanied by an increase in oxygen consumption and augmented glycogenolysis, suggesting that hepatocytes were the target cells. Of interest, the effects of ET on portal pressure were characterized by slow onset and delayed recovery phase compared with the response evoked by phenylephrine. In keeping with such findings, Tran-Thi and coworkers[74] reported that 1 nM ET-1

elevated portal pressure by 22.1 cm water and enhanced glucose output by up to threefold in the perfused rat liver preparation (Fig. 18.4). The elevation in portal pressure was accompanied by a concomitant decrease in bile flow. Furthermore, the effects of ET-1 were attenuated by Iloprost, a prostaglandin I_2 analog (but not by other eicosinoids), as well as by a nitric oxide donor, SIN-1.

Application of ET-1 to cultured sinusoidal stellate cells (also known as Ito cells, hepatic perisinusoidal lipocytes, or fat-storing cells) has been shown to enhance cell contraction and elevate cytosolic calcium in a concentration-dependent manner.[75] Curiously, Iloprost, PGE$_2$, and sodium nitroprusside promoted relaxation of the same cells, which was associated with the disappearance of stress fibers. Pinzani et al.[76] have also observed increased fura-2 fluorescence in Ito cells stimulated with ET-1. Nifedipine, at concentrations of up to 10 µM, did not blunt the ET-1-induced increase in cytosolic calcium, unlike its effect on thrombin- and angiotensin II-mediated calcium increments.

Several investigators have examined the effects of ET on hepatocytes. Gandhi et al. reported increased turnover of phosphatidyl inositol in hepatocytes (a similar effect was detected also in Kupffer cells) stimulated with ET-3.[73] Tran-Thi et al.[74] observed stimulation of glycogenolysis by rat hepatocytes exposed to ET-1. These effects of ET-1 were dependent on the presence of extracellular calcium and protein kinase C (similar dependency was observed for ET-1 effects on portal pressure).

In summary, at least three cell types resident in the liver have been shown to be responsive to ET: Ito cells, hepatocytes, and Kupffer cells. Although the detailed nature of their interactive responses has not yet emerged, the hemodynamic effects of ET appear to predominate. Taking into consideration the actions of endotoxin, TGF-β, and Kupffer cell-conditioned medium on sinusoidal endothelial cells described earlier, it is possible to envisage a cascade of paracrine interactions between Kupffer cells, sinusoidal endothelial cells, and liver-specific pericytes, Ito cells (Fig. 18.5.)

CELLULAR MECHANISMS OF ENDOTHELIN ACTION

Effects of ET-1 on Cells of the Vasculature

A plethora of information exists regarding the mode of ET-1 action on vascular smooth muscle cells. Based on the structural resemblance of ET-1 to scorpion toxin, the initial supposition was that ET-1 acted on sodium channels.[4] This view was subsequently supplanted by the realization that ET-1 augments turnover of phosphoinositol and releases calcium from intracellular stores.[62,77] To explain the unusually sustained contractile effect of ET-1, several investigators invoked persistent elevation of cytosolic calcium as the putative mechanism.[78,79] However, this explanation accounts only for about 50–70% of smooth muscle contraction, depending on the origin of the smooth muscle cell.[78,79] The sustained elevation of cytosolic calcium concentration is a result of activation

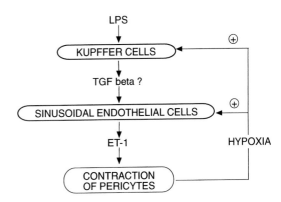

FIGURE 18.5. Hypothetical schema of intercellular communications between the Kupffer cells, sinusoidal endothelial cells, and pericytes. Paracrine signals from the Kupffer cells induce ET-1 production by the endothelial cells of sinusoids, which, in turn, acts on pericytes (Ito cells), resulting in their contraction. The resulting decrease in the blood flow may provide a positive feedback mechanism for further stimulation of Kupffer and endothelial cells. LPS = lipopolysaccharide; circled + denotes the positive feedback loop. (Adapted from Rieder H, Ramadori G: Sinusoidal endothelial liver cells in vitro release endothelin—augmentation by transforming growth factor beta and Kupffer cell-conditioned media. Klin Wochenschr 1991;69:387–391.)

of voltage-sensitive calcium channels, chloride channels, and/or nonselective cationic channels.

Our previous findings in cultured rat aortic smooth muscle cells[78] recently were buttressed by observations in vascular smooth muscle cells freshly isolated from rat renal resistance vessels (arcuate and interlobar arteries).[80] Whole-cell patch-clamp recordings in the current-clamp mode demonstrated that ET-1 challenge results in membrane depolarization (Fig. 18.6). This phenomenon was explained by the finding of a calcium-sensitive inward current that was identified as a chloride current. Furthermore, we observed late activation (after a delay of about 1 minute) of L-type calcium channels in the smooth muscle cells. Collectively, such data are consistent with the model whereby ET-1 induces intracellular calcium release, followed by activation of chloride channels with subsequent membrane depolarization and activation of L-type (but not T-type) calcium channels (see Fig. 18.6). Such findings are further supported by the observations that a chloride channel inhibitor, IAA 94, blunted both the ET-1–induced elevation of cytosolic calcium concentration and contraction of the afferent arterioles

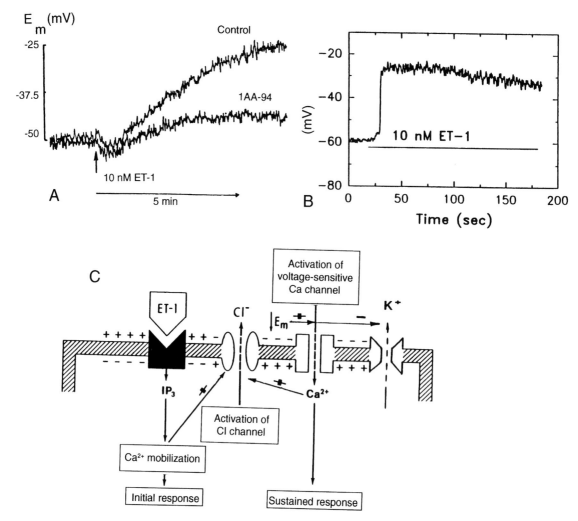

FIGURE 18.6. ET-1–induced membrane depolarization in smooth muscle cells. The similar results were obtained by two independent techniques: membrane potential-sensitive fluorescent probe, DiBAC$_4$(3), in cultured rat aortic smooth muscle cells *(A)*, and the patch-clamp technique (current clamp mode) in freshly isolated smooth muscle cells obtained from microdissected and collagenase-digested rat renal intralobular and arcuate arteries *(B)*. Both techniques brought about comparable results for amplitude and duration of membrane depolarization in response to the application of ET-1. *C*, Hypothetical schema of ET-1 action on smooth muscle cell. (Adapted from Iijima K, Lin L, Nasjletti A, Goligorsky MS: Intracellular ramification of endothelin signal. Am J Physiol 1991;260:C982–C992; Takenaka T, Epstein M, Forster H, et al: Attenuation of endothelin effects by a chloride channel inhibitor, indanyloxyacetic acid. Am J Physiol 1992; 262:F799–F806; and Gordienko D, Clausen C, Goligorsky MS: Ion currents and endothelin signaling in smooth muscle cells from rat renal resistance arteries. Am J Physiol 1994;266:F325–F341, with permission.)

in the hydronephrotic rat kidney model.[79] Such data, nevertheless, do not preclude the possibility of the involvement of receptor-operated and/or nonselective cationic channels in smooth muscle responses to ET-1.

The effect of nitric oxide on ET-1 binding to the ET$_A$ receptors was studied in CHO cells stably expressing the receptor.[81] We have demonstrated that donors of nitric oxide—SIN-1 or sodium nitroprusside—rapidly displace the biotinylated ligand from its binding sites, suggesting that nitric oxide changes the affinity of ligand-receptor binding. In addition to this site of nitric oxide action, we have suggested another postreceptoral site, distal from the G protein, where nitric oxide can disrupt ET-1 signal transduction. These two actions of nitric oxide do not seem to require activation of guanylate cyclase and production of cGMP. The second mechanism of nitric oxide action, together with the above receptoral and postreceptoral targets, underlies the well-known vasodilatory properties of nitric oxide.

The mode of ET-1 action on vascular endothelial cells seems to be even more complex. Growing evidence suggests that endothelial cells express non–isopeptide-selective ET_B receptors.[82] It has been postulated that ET binding to these receptors results in increased production of nitric oxide. Using an NO-selective electrode in double transfected CHO cells (cDNA for the ETB receptor and for endothelial nitric oxide synthase), we demonstrated a direct coupling of the receptor to the enzyme.[83] ET-1 or a selective ETB receptor agonist (IRL 1620) induced an immediate elevation of nitric oxide in the culture medium. Similar effects were observed in cultured endothelial cells.

The studies exploring the properties of the ET_A and ET_B receptors lead to a hypothetical schema of interactions between the vascular endothelial cells and smooth muscle cells via an interplay of two messengers produced by the endothelium, ET-1 and nitric oxide. Production of ET-1 leads to the activation of both types of receptors in an autocrine and paracrine fashion (Fig. 18.7): activation of the ET_A receptor induces the contraction of smooth muscle cells, whereas ligand binding to the ET_B receptor on the endothelial cells results in the activation of nitric oxide synthase, production of nitric oxide, and its action on three targets in smooth muscle cells: the ET_A receptor, postreceptoral signaling cascade, and soluble guanylate cyclase. Combined action of nitric oxide leads to the restoration of smooth muscle tone.

Pharmacologic Tools for Modulation of ET Synthesis, Conversion, Action, and Degradation

Diverse physiologically active substances modulate synthesis of ETs (see Table 18.1). Stimuli that may be relevant to the state of hepatic insufficiency are emphasized, and the reader is referred to companion chapters for details.

ECE represents another potentially exciting target for pharmacological modulation of ET synthesis. Despite considerable efforts to identify ECE(s), it remains elusive (vide supra). Furthermore, some ECE inhibitors, like phosphoramidone, also block the degradative pathway via the endopeptidase 24.11, thus limiting the applicability of ECEs. Future development of more

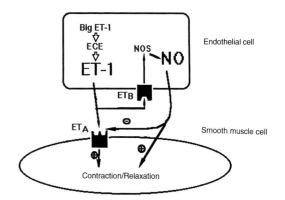

FIGURE 18.7. Interplay between endothelium-derived constricting (ET-1) and relaxing (NO) activities that may underscore self-regulation of the vascular tone and its spontaneous oscillations. + or – denotes the positive or negative regulatory signals, respectively. (Adapted from Goligorsky MS, Tsukahara H, Magazine H, et al: Termination of endothelin signaling: Role of nitric oxide. J Cell Physiol 1994;158:485–496; Hirata Y, Emori T, Eguchi S, et al: Endothelin receptor subtype B synthesis of nitric oxide by cultured bovine endothelial cells. J Clin Invest 1993;91:1367–1373; and Goligorsky MS, Tsukahara H, Ende H, et al: Functional characterization of the non–isopeptide-selective ET_B receptor in endothelial cells. J Biol Chem 1994;269:21778–21785, with permission.)

selective inhibitors undoubtedly will become an important experimental and clinical tool in the modulation of ET production.

Synthesis of the peptides with ET-agonistic and ET-antagonistic properties has advanced more rapidly. The compound BE18257B, a cyclic pentapeptide resembling the C-terminal portion of ET, has ET_A-R–antagonistic properties [84] It competitively inhibits binding of ET-1 to the ET_A receptor (IC50=1.4 µM) but has little effect on binding to the ET_B receptor. Further derivation of BE18257B produced a highly potent ET_A-R–selective inhibitor, BQ123 (IC50 = 22 nM),[85] which was used extensively in evaluation of ET-1 effects on renal hemodynamics (vide infra).

Recent studies on the design of an orally active ET-R antagonist culminated in the discovery of a pyrimidinyl sulphonamide derivative, 4-tert-butyl-N-[6-(2-hydroxyethoxy)-5-(3-methoxy-phenoxy)-4-pyrimidinyl]-benzene-sulphonamide (Ro 46-2005).[86] This nonpeptide, low-molecular-weight compound competitively inhibited ^{125}I-ET-1 binding to human vascular smooth muscle cells and rat aortic endothelial cells

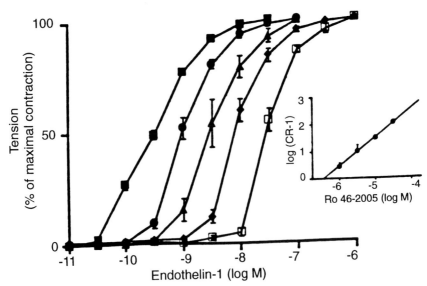

FIGURE 18.8. In vitro antagonism of ET_A-R and ET_B-R by the orally active nonpeptidic ET receptor antagonist, Ro 46-2005. Effects of Ro 46-2005 on the constrictor effect of ET-1 in isolated deendothelialized rat aortic rings. After 10 minutes of incubation with various concentrations of Ro 46-2005, cumulative doses of ET-1 were added. Inset: Schild plot of log [concentration ratio (CR)-1] as a function of antagonist concentration. Closed square = control, closed circle = 10^{-6} M, closed diamond = 10^{-5} M, open square = 3×10^{-5} M. (From Clozel M, Breu V, Burri K, et al: Pathophysiological role of endothelin revealed by the first orally active endothelin receptor antagonist. Nature 1993;365:759–761, with permission.)

with IC50 = 2.2×10^{-7}M and 1×10^{-6}M, respectively. In deendothelialized rat aortic rings, Ro 46-2005 dose-dependently inhibited ET-1–induced contraction (Fig. 18.8). In addition, the antagonist also inhibited endothelium-dependent vasorelaxation produced by sarafotoxin S6c in rat mesenteric arteries. Ro 46-2005 significantly improved renal and cerebral perfusion in the ischemic model of acute renal failure and post-subarachnoid hemorrhage, respectively (see below), further establishing its therapeutic potential.

PUTATIVE ROLE OF ENDOTHELIN IN ACUTE RENAL FAILURE

Evidence for a Role of ET-1

The first indication for a potential role for ET-1 in acute renal failure (ARF) was provided by Kon et al.[48] These investigators infused antibodies to ET-1 into a branch of the renal artery of a kidney subjected to ischemia and established the reversibility of vasoconstriction in the vascular bed of the infused branch but not in the branches that served as controls.[87] More recently, Bock et al.[88] showed that *Pseudomonas* endotoxin increased the resistance of in vitro perfused rabbit glomeruli

by about 50%. This effect was attenuated by the TXA_2/PGH_2 receptor antagonist SQ-29548; the PAF receptor antagonist, BN-52021; and the ET_A receptor antagonist, BQ123. Gellai et al.[89] reached similar conclusions in whole animal experiments. The investigators demonstrated that a single infusion of BQ123 (100 µg/kg/min for 3 hr) reversed severe ischemic renal failure. Although these initial observations require more extensive confirmation, it seems reasonable to speculate that acute renal failure is associated with an elevated production of ET-1 which in turn may precipitate the hemodynamic consequences of ischemia.

The demonstration by Chintala et al.[90] that ET-1 message in a kidney subjected to 40 minutes of ischemia and 30 minutes of reperfusion was upregulated compared with the contralateral, non-clamped kidney complements the above findings. In addition, the ET_A receptor message was down-regulated without detectable changes in the abundance of ET_B receptor message. The investigators speculated that increased production of ET-1 combined with the decreased expression of ET_A receptors leads to preferential ET-1 binding to the ET_B receptor subtype and results in enhanced production of nitric oxide, which may be responsible to some extent for the nephrotoxic sequelae of ARF.

On the other hand, Schramm et al.[91] observed a beneficial effect from L-arginine in toxic ARF, which contradicts the previous speculation. Perhaps the most compelling observation about the role of ETs in ARF was provided by Clozel et al.,[86] who demonstrated an improvement in renal perfusion after a 45-minute clamp of one renal artery in rats pretreated with a potent ET-antagonist, Ro 46-2005 (Fig. 18.9). Although the detailed picture of pathophysiologically relevant steps leading to ARF is far from clear, emerging evidence supports a role for ET-1. The possible mechanisms for the induction of ET-1 in acute renal failure are schematically presented in Figure 18.10. This deliberately oversimplified schema does not include vasorelaxant mediators which are released simultaneously.[87] However, both local systems of control of vascular tone—i.e., vasoconstriction and vasodilatation—are tightly interconnected, and any acutely imposed imbalance between them tends to be restored, unless crucial communication elements are impaired.

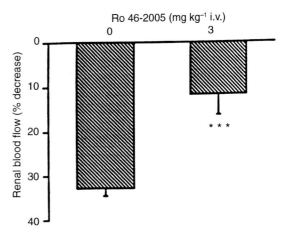

FIGURE 18.9.   In vivo effect of th ET receptor antagonist, Ro 46-2005, on renal blood flow in ischemic acute renal failure. Values depicted are percent decreases in renal blood flow expressed as mean ± SEM. Asterisks denote p < 0.001 by unpaired Student's t-test. (From Clozel M, Breu V, Burri K, et al: Pathophysiological role of endothelin revealed by the first orally active endothelin receptor antagonist. Nature 1993;365:759–761, with permission.)

Emerging Evidence for a Possible Role of Endothelin in Hepatorenal Syndrome

Although it is tempting to speculate that ET may be important in the pathogenesis of hepatorenal syndrome (HRS), as yet no firm evidence indicates that this is indeed the case. There are no published data about the local production of ET-1 by the liver or kidney in HRS, nor are data available about the status of hepatic and/or renal ET receptors. Studies performed by several groups of investigators examining humans with HRS have documented elevated circulating plasma levels of ET-1 (Fig. 18.11).[92–94] However, plasma ET-1 levels documented in such studies were not of a magnitude that merits consideration for pathophysiologic consequence. Furthermore, cause and effect have not been established. Although the exact source(s) of elevated plasma ET-1 values in HRS has not been determined, it is safe to speculate (1) that ET is produced throughout the vasculature and (2) that the plasma level represents an integrated sum of the rates of generation, degradation, and excretion of the peptide.

Although the test has rather limited diagnostic value, it may nevertheless provide some clue to the pathophysiology of renal failure. In addition, an elevation in plasma ET-1 level is associated with various stress situations, including endotoxic shock, myocardial infarction, adult respiratory

distress, and disseminated intravascular coagulation.[95] Such associations cast further doubt on the specificity of the test. Furthermore, plasma level of ET-1 may be elevated in acute and chronic renal failure of diverse etiologies, although different laboratories have reported controversial results.[95] An important example of dissociation between plasma and urinary concentrations of ET has been reported recently by Benigni et al.[96] The authors observed that plasma levels of the immunoreactive peptide were decreased in rats with reduced renal mass compared with sham-operated rats, yet urinary excretion of ET-1 was significantly elevated in the experimental group compared with control, sham-operated animals. Such data tend to suggest a renal source for the increased ET-1 production. To the best of our knowledge, no equivalent studies have been performed in the ARF model. Hence, a carefully conducted investigation into the exact role of endothelins in the pathophysiology of acute renal failure—and in HRS in particular—is still forthcoming.

The significance of elevated plasma ET levels is further complicated by the observation that plasma ET levels have been found to be significantly higher in cirrhotic patients with ascites than in cirrhotic patients without ascites or patients with chronic liver disease without cirrhosis.[97] As noted earlier, the absolute increment in plasma ET level,

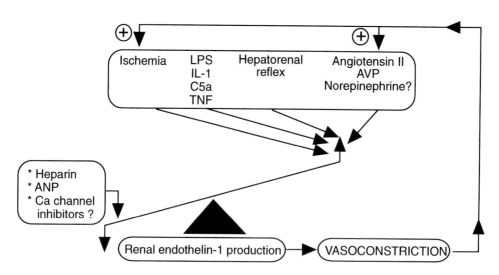

FIGURE 18.10. The possible mechanisms of induction of ET-1 synthesis in acute renal failure. Renal ET production is stimulated by ischemia, cytokines and complement components, vasoactive peptides (angiotensin II, AVP, and norepinephrine), and, possibly, activation of the hepatorenal reflex (*upper panel*). Resulting renal vasoconstriction may serve as a positive feedback loop for the aggravation of ischemia and increased activity of sympathetic and renin-angiotensin systems. Several potential inhibitors of ET-1 production are depicted in the left panel (heparin, ANP, calcium channel inhibitors). This schema does not incorporate the negative feedback mechanism provided by vasorelaxing substances.

although statistically significant compared with the control group, was extremely modest. Of interest was the fact that the plasma ET level showed a significant negative correlation with creatinine clearance but no significant correlation with fractional excretion of sodium. Furthermore, in only 2 of the 20 patients with cirrhosis was creatinine clearance below 20 ml/min. Such data argue that in the setting of intact or moderately impaired renal function, elevated ET levels in patients with cirrhosis and ascites are unlikely to play a causative role in the pathogenesis of renal dysfunction in HRS.

Plasma endothelin levels also have been monitored in patients before and after orthotopic liver transplantation.[98] In a cohort of 32 patients with advanced liver disease secondary to various disorders (primary biliary cirrhosis, primary sclerosing cholangitis, chronic active hepatitis or cryptogenic cirrhosis, and alcoholic cirrhosis) plasma ET levels before transplantation were found to be no different from those in a pool of 75 normal subjects. GFR in all patients was remarkably normal, and the presence or absence of ascites was not specified. Of interest, plasma ET levels doubled during the first week after transplantation and by 4 weeks after transplantation returned to pretransplant levels. Whereas the complexities of hepatic and renal function under such arduous

conditions are readily appreciated, these findings further emphasize the lack of correlation between cause and effect of elevated ET levels in the setting of profound liver dysfunction.

Theoretically, endotoxemia may serve as a common denominator for the induction of endothelium-derived vasoactive substances. The role of the complement-derived anaphylotoxin, a major circulating mediator of acute renal failure in endotoxemia, has recently been investigated in normal and split hydronephrotic kidneys.[99] A profound decrease in RBF and GFR in response to the intravenous infusion of a recombinant C5a was noted. The hemodynamic changes were prevented by the competitive leukotriene D4/E4 antagonist, ICI-198615, and attenuated by the competitive thromboxane A_2 antagonist, daltroban. The authors concluded that cysteinyl leukotrienes, as well as TxA_2, produced largely by polymorphonuclear leukocytes, play an important role in mediating vasoconstriction of endotoxemia. Of note, urinary excretion of cysteinyl leukotrienes increased approximately 5.5-fold in patients with liver cirrhosis compared with healthy individuals and exhibited a 60-fold elevation in patients with HRS.[100] Such findings have subsequently been confirmed by others.[101] A separate study examined the effect of leukotriene D4 on

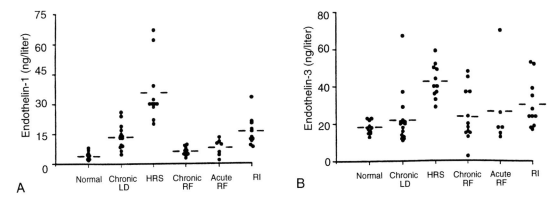

FIGURE 18.11.   Plasma immunoreactive ET-1 *(A)* and ET-3 *(B)* concentration in hepatorenal syndrome. LD = liver disease, RF = renal failure, RI = renal impairment and liver dysfunction not due to hepatorenal syndrome. (From Moore K, Wendon J, Frazer M, et al: Plasma endothelin immunoreactivity in liver disease and the hepatorenal syndrome. N Engl J Med 1992;327:1774–1778, with permission.)

canine renal artery.[102] The cytokine was found to stimulate the release of a labile vasorelaxing substance, similar to EDRF, from vessels with intact endothelium. It is interesting, therefore, that endotoxemia and its major mediators of hemodynamic disturbances are accompanied by elevated production of ET-1.[103] It is quite possible that the increased production of these vasoactive substances has either a common denominator or reflects an intrinsic cooperativity in their generation.

SUMMARY AND FUTURE DIRECTIONS

Two main conclusions may be drawn from the current state of knowledge about the role of ET in the pathophysiology of HRS: (1) emerging evidence indicates that endothelins may be involved in some manner in the pathophysiology of acute renal failure in general and HRS in particular, and (2) a precise role for ET in the pathophysiology of HRS awaits elucidation

The first conclusion is based on a substantial body of data incriminating endothelins in the pathophysiology of the renal vasculature in ARF. Studies using anti-ET antibodies or the first orally active nonpeptidic ET receptor antagonist[86,87] have provided convincing information that ET-induced vasoconstriction of the renal vasculature is an important factor in the course of ischemic acute renal failure. Based on such data, it is reasonable to speculate that pharmacologic manipulations of ET synthesis, processing, and/or binding to their receptors may alleviate ARF. Three general directions in this field of investigation are rapidly evolving: (1) strategies to inhibit ET production (e.g., nitric

oxide or heparin), (2) design and evaluation of ECE inhibitors, and (3) in vivo studies using ET receptor antagonists, e.g., Ro 46-2005. The tailoring of these strategies to different pathophysiologic situations requires a more profound understanding of the role of ET in the development of ARF.

In regard to the second conclusion, information about the precise role of ET in ARF and HRS in particular is currently scarce. As the renowned detective Sherlock Holmes once declared, "It is a capital mistake to theorize before one has data" (A.C. Doyle, *A Scandal in Bohemia*). Clearly, with the advent of knowledge about the specific role of ET in the course of renal insufficiency associated with HRS, new strategies to alter the course of this perplexing entity will evolve.

NOTE ADDED IN PROOF

After the submission of the manuscript, several important and pertinent studies were published. Yanagisawa's laboratory reported on the targeted disruption of the mouse endothelin-3 and endothelin-B receptor genes.[a,b] Y. Kurihara et al. performed targeted disruption of Edn1 locus encoding endothelin-1.[c] Furthermore, Yanagisawa and colleagues have cloned and characterized endothelin-converting-enzyme-1 and 2.[d,e] A novel nonpeptide antagonist of endothelin receptors has been synthesized and characterized.[f] The effects of this antagonist on GFR and RBF in control dogs and in animals with ischemic acute renal failure have been examined.[g] Growth-inhibitory effect of endothelin-1 in human hepatic Ito cells have been shown.[h]

a Hosoda K, Hammer J Richardson J, et al: Targeted and natural (piebald-lethal) mutations of endothelin-B receptor gene produce megacolon associated with spotted coat color in mice. Cell 1994;79:1267–1276.

b Greenstein Baynash A, Hosoda K, Giaid A, et al: Interaction of endothelin-3 with endothelin-B receptor is essential for development of epidermal melanocytes and enteric neurons. Cell 1994;79:1277–1285.

c Kurihara Y, Kurihara H, Oda H, et al: Aortic arch malformations and ventricular septal defect in mice deficient in endothelin-1. J Clin Invest 1995;96:293–300.

d Xu D, Emoto N, Giaid A, et al: ECE-1: A membrane-bound metalloprotease that catalyzes the proteolytic activation of big endothelin-1. Cell 1994;78:473–485.

e Emoto N, Yanagisawa M: Endothelin-converting-enzyme-2 is a membrane-bound, phosphoramidone-sensitive metalloprotease with acidic pH optimum. J Biol Chem 1995;270:15262–15268.

f Nambi P, Elshourbagy N, Wu H-L, et al: Nonpeptide endothelin receptor antagonists. J Pharmacol Exp Ther 1994;271:755–761.

g Brooks D, DePalma D, Gellai M, et al: Nonpeptide endothelin receptor antagonists. III. Effect of SB209670 and BQ123 on acute renal failure in anesthetized dogs. J Pharmacol Exp Ther 1994;271:769–775.

h Mallat A, Fouassier L, Preaux A-M, et al: Growth-inhibitory properties of endothelin-1 in human hepatic myofibroblastic Ito cells. J Clin Invest 1995;96:42–49.

Acknowledgments. The studies from the authors' laboratories were supported in part by NIH grants DK45695, DK45462, DK41573, and DK36351.

REFERENCES

1. Furchgott R, Zawadzki J: The obligatory role of endothelial cells in the relaxation of arterial smooth muscle by acetylcholine. Nature 1984;288:373–376.
2. O'Brien R, Robins R, McMurtry I: J Cell Physiol 132:263–270, 1987.
3. Palmer RM, Ferridge AG, Moncada S: Nitric oxide release accounts for the biological activity of endothelium-derived relaxing factor. Nature 1987;327:524–526.
4. Yanagisawa M, Kurihara H, Kimura H, et al: A novel potent vasoconstrictor peptide produced by vascular endothelial cells. Nature 1988;332:411–415.
5. Inoue A, Yanagisawa M, Kimura S, et al: The human endothelin family: Three structurally and pharmacologically distinct isopeptides predicted by three separate genes. Proc Natl Acad Sci USA 1989;86:2863–2867.
6. Kloog Y, Ambar I, Sokolovsky M, et al: Sarafotoxin, a novel vasoconstrictor peptide: Phosphoinositide hydrolysis in rat heart and brain. Science 1988;242:268–270.
7. Itho Y, Yanagasawa M, Ohkuba S, et al: Cloning and sequence analysis of cDNA encoding the precursor of a human endothelium-derived vasoconstrictor peptide, endothelin: Identity of human and porcine endothelin. FEBS Lett 1988;231:440–444.
8. Emori T, Hirata Y, Ohta K, et al: Secretory mechanism of immunoreactive endothelin in cultured bovine endothelial cells. Biochem Biophys Res Commun 1989;169:93–100.
9. Inoue A, Yanagisawa M, Takuwa Y, et al: The human preproendothelin-1 gene. J Biol Chem 1993;264:14954–14959.
10. Sawamura T, Kimura S, Shinmi O, et al: Analysis of endothelin related peptides in culture supernatant of porcine aortic endothelial cells: Evidence for biosynthetic pathway of endothelin-1. Biochem Biophys Res Commun 1989;162:1287–1294.
11. Opgenorth T, Wu-Wong J, Shiosaki K: Endothelin-converting enzymes. FASEB J 1992;6:2653–2659.
12. Matsumura Y, Ikegawa R, Takaoka M, Morimoto S: Conversion of porcine big endothelin to endothelin by an extract from the porcine aortic endothelial cells. Biochem Biophys Res Commun 1990,167:203–210.
13. Sawamura T, Kimura T, Shinmi O, et al: Purification and characterization of putative endothelin converting enzyme in bovine adrenal medulla: Evidence for a cathepsin D-like enzyme. Biochem Biophys Res Commun 1990;168:1230–1236.
14. Lees W, Kalinka S, Meech J, et al: Generation of human endothelin by cathepsin E. FEBS Lett 1990;273:99–102.
15. Kaw S, Hecker M, Vane JR: Two-step conversion of big endothelin 1 to endothelin 1 and degradation of endothelin 1 by subcellular fractions from human polymorphonuclear leukocytes. Proc Natl Acad Sci USA 1992;89:6886–6890.
16. Ohnaka K, Takayanagi R, Yamauchi T, et al: Identification and characterization of endothelin converting activity in cultured bovine endothelial cells. Biochem Biophys Res Commun 1990;168:1128–1136.
17. Shields P, Gonzales T, Charles C, et al: Accumulation of pepstatin in cultured endothelial cells and its effect on endothelin processing. Biochem Biophys Res Commun 1991;177:1006–1012.
18. Ikegawa R., Matsumura Y, Tsukahara, et al: Phosphoramidon, a metalloproteinase inhibitor, suppresses the secretion of endothelin-1 from cultured endothelial cells by inhibiting a big endothelin-1 converting enzyme. Biochem Biophys Res Commun 1990;171:669–675.
19. Matsumura Y., Hisaki K, Takaoka M, Morimoto S: Phosphoramidone, a metalloproteinase inhibitor, suppresses the hypertensive effect of big endothelin-1. Eur J Pharmacol 1990;185:103–106.
20. McMahon E, Palomo M, Moore W, et al: Phosphoramidon blocks the pressor activity of porcine big endothelin-1 (1-39) in vivo and conversion of big endothelin-1-(1-39) to endothelin-1-(1-21) in vitro. Proc Natl Acad Sci 1991;88:703–707.
21. Pollock D, Opgenorth T: Evidence for metalloprotease involvement in the in vivo effects of big endothelin. Am J Physiol 1991;261:R257–R263.
22. Gardiner S, Compton A, Kemp P, Bennett T: The effects of phosphoramidon on the regional haemodynamic responses to human proendothelin [1-38] in conscious rats. Br J Pharmacol 1991;103:2009–2015.
23. Takahashi M, Matsushita Y, Iijima Y, Tanazawa K: Purification and characterization of endothelin-converting enzyme from rat lung. J Biol Chem 1993;268:21394–21398.
24. Yanagisawa M, Inoue T, Isikawa T, et al: Primary structure, synthesis, and biological activity of rat endothelin, an endothelium-derived vaso-constrictor peptide. Proc Natl Acad Sci 1988;85:6964–6967.
25. Fujii Y, Moriera JE, Orlando C, et al: Endothelin as an autocrine factor in the regulation of parathyroid cells. Proc Nat Acad Sci 1991;88:4235–4239.

26. Baley PA, Resnik TJ, Eppenberger U, Hahn WA: Endothelin messenger RNA and receptors are differentially expressed in cultured human breast epithelial and stromal cells. J Clin Invest 1990;85:1320–1323.

27. Yoshizawa T, Shinmi O, Giaid A, et al: Endothelin: A novel peptide in the posterior pituitary system. Science 1990;247:462–464

28. Wilkes BM, Susan M, Mento PF, et al: Localization of endothelin like immunoreactivity in rat kidneys. Am J Physiol 1991;260:F913–F920.

29. Bakris GL, Fairbankes R, Troish AM: Arginine vasopressin stimulates human mesangial cell production of endothelin. J Clin Invest 1991;87:1158–1164.

30. Marsden PA, Dorfman DM, Collins T, et al: Regulated expression of endothelin-1 in glomerular capillary endothelial cells. Am J Physiol 1991;261:F117-F125.

31. Kasinath BS, Fried TA, Davalath S, Marsden PA: Glomerular epithelial cells synthesis endothelin peptides. Am J Pathol 1992;141:279–283

32. Ujiie K, Terada Y, Nonoguchi H, et al: Messenger RNA expression and synthesis of endothelin-1 along rat nephron segments. J Clin Invest 1992;90:1043–1048.

33. Kohan DE: Endothelin production by human inner medullary collecting duct cells. J Am Soc Nephrol 1993; 3:1719–1721.

34. Hart D, Goligorsky MS, Nord EP: Osmolar regulation of endothelin-1 synthesis by rat inner medullary collecting duct cells in primary culture. J Am Soc Nephrol 1991;2:402A.

35. Schnermann J, Urbanes A, Briggs J: Effect of endothelin on renal water transport. J Am Soc Nephrol 1991;2:416A.

36. Chen M., Todd-Turla K, Wang W-H, et al: Endothelin-1 mRNA in glomerular and epithelial cells of kidney. Am J Physiol 1993;265:F542–F550.

37. Rieder H., Ramadori G: Sinusoidal endothelial liver cells in vitro release endothelin—augmentation by transforming growth factor beta and Kupffer cell-conditioned media. Klin Wochenschr 1991;69:387–391.

38. Marsden P, Goligorsky MS, Brenner BM: Endothelial cell biology in relation to current concepts of vessel wall structure and function. J Am Soc Nephrol 1991;1:931–948.

39. Simonson M: Endothelins: Multifunctional renal peptides. Physiol Rev 1993;73:375–398.

40. Kon V, Badr K: Biological actions and pathophysiologic significance of endothelin in the kidney. Kidney Int 1991;40:1-12.

41. Nord EP: Renal actions of endothelin. Kidney Int 1993; 44:451–463.

42. Kimura SY, Kaysuya T, Sawamura O, et al: Conversion of big endothelin-1 to 21-residue endothelin-1 is essential for expression of full vasoconstrictor activity: Structure-activity relationships of big endothelin-1. J Cardiovasc Pharmacol 1989;13:S5–S7.

43. Sakurai T, Yanagisawa M, Masaki T: Molecular characterization of endothelin receptors. Trends Pharmacol Sci 1992;13:103–108.

44. Arai H, Hori S, Aramoni I, et al: Cloning and expression of a cDNA encoding an endothelin receptor. Nature 1990;348:730–732.

45. Karne S, Jayawickreme, Lerner M: Cloning and characterization of an endothelin-3 specific receptor (ETc receptor) from Xenopus laevis dermal melanophores. J Biol Chem 1993;268:19126–19133.

46. Sakurai T, Yanagisawa M, Takuwa Y, et al: Cloning of a DNA encoding a non-isopeptide selective subtype of the endothelin receptor. Nature 1990;348:732–735.

47. Sakamoto A, Yanagisawa M, Sawamura T, et al: Distinct subdomains of endothelin receptors determine their selectivity to endothelin$_A$—selective antagonist and endothelin$_B$-selective agonists. J Biol Chem 1993;268:8547–8553.

48. Kon V, Yoshioka T, Fogo A, Ichikawa I: Glomerular actions of endothelin in vivo. J Clin Invest 1989;83:1762–1767.

49. Terada Y, Tomita K, Nonoguchi H, Marumo F: Different localization of two types of endothelin receptor mRNA in microdissected rat nephron segments using reverse transcription and polymerase chain reaction assay. J Clin Invest 1992;90:107–112, 1992.

50. Martin ER, Marsden PA, Brenner BM, Ballermann BJ: Identification and characterization of endothelin binding sites in rat renal papillary and glomerular membranes. Biochem Biophys Res Comm 1989;162:130–137.

51. Gauquelin G, Thibault G, Garcia R: Characterization of renal glomerular endothelin receptors in the rat. Biochem Biophys Res Comm 1989;164:54–57.

52. Badr KF, Manger KA, Saguira M, et al: High and low affinity binding sites for endothelin on cultured rat glomerular mesangial cells. Biochem Biophys Res Commun 1989;161:776–781.

53. Martin ER, Brenner BM, Ballermann BJ: Heterogeneity of cell surface endothelin receptors. J Biol Chem 1990; 265:14044–14049.

54. Cassals M, Wilkes BM, Hart D, et al: Mechanism of endothelin action in inner medullary collecting duct cells. J Am Soc Nephrol 1990;l:467A.

55. Chow L, Subrumanian S, Nuovo J, et al: Endothelin receptor mRNA expression in the renal medulla identified by in situ RT-PCR. Am J Physiol (in press).

56. Kohan DE, Hughs AK, Perkins SL: Characterization of endothelin receptors in the inner medullary collecting duct of the rat. J Biol Chem 1992;267:12336–12340.

57. Garvin J, Sanders K: Endothelin inhibits fluid and bicarbonate transport in part by reducing Na/K-ATPase activity in the rat proximal straight tubule. J Am Soc Nephrol 1991;2:976–982.

58. Wlkes BM, Ruston AS, Mento P, et al: Characterization of the endothelin-1 receptor and signal transduction mechanisms in rat renal medullary interstitial cells. Am J Physiol 1991;260:F579–F589.

59. Serradiel-Le Gal C, Jouneaux C, Sanchez-Bueno A, et al: Endothelin action in rat liver. Receptors, free Ca^{2+} oscillations, and activation of glycogenolysis. J Clin Invest 1991;87:133–138.

60. Katoh T, Chang H, Uchida S, et al: Direct effects of endothelin in the rat kidney. Am J Physiol 1990;258:397–403.

61. Stacy DL, Scott JW, Granger JP: Control of renal function during intra renal infusion of endothelin. Am J Physiol 1990;258:F1232–F1236.

62. Badr KF, Murray JJ, Breyer MD, et al: Mesangial cell, glomerular and renal vascular responses to endothelin in the rat kidney. J Clin Invest 1989;83:336–342.

63. King AJ, Brenner BM, Anderson S: Endothelin: A potent renal and systemic vasoconstrictor peptide. Am J Physiol 1989;256:F1051–F1058

64. Kon V, Yoshioka T, Fogo A, Ichikawa I: Glomerular actions of endothelin in vivo. J Clin Invest 1989;83:1762–1767.

65. Edwards RM, Trinza W, Ohlstrin EH: Renal microvascular effects of endothelin. Am J Physiol 1990;259: F217–F221.

66. Loutzenhiser R, Hayashi K, Epstein M: Divergent effects of KCl induced depolarization on afferent and efferent arterioles. Am J Physiol 1989;257:F561–F564.

67. Oishi R, Nonoguchi H, Tomita K, Marumo F: Endothelin-1 inhibits AVP stimulated osmotic water permeability in rat inner medullary collecting duct. Am J Physiol 1991;261:F951–F956.

68. Nadler SP, Zimpelmann J, Hebert RC: Pertussis toxin sensitive signalling pathway for endothelin in rat inner medullary collecting duct. J Am Soc Nephrol 1991; 2:410A.

69. Santell L, Rubin RL, Levin EG: Enhanced phosphorylation and dephosphorylation of a histone-like protein in response to hyperosmotic and hypoosmotic conditions. J Biol Chem 1993;268:21443–21447.

70. Yoshitomi K, Naruse M, Uchida S, Kurokawa K: Endothelin inhibits luminal Na+ channel in rabbit cortical collecting duct. J Am Soc Nephrol 1991;2:423A.

71. Eiam-Ong S, Hilden SA, King AJ, et al: Endothelin-1 stimulation of the apical Na+/H+ exchanger and the basolateral Na/HCO$_3$ cotransporter in rabbit renal cortex. J Am Soc Nephrol 1991;2:699A.

72. Zeidel ML, Brady HR, Kone BC, et al: Endothelin, a peptide inhibitor of Na+K+-ATPase in intact renal tubular epithelial cells. Am J Physiol 1989;257:C1101–C1107.

73. Gandhi C, Stephenson K, Olson M: Endothelin, a potent peptide agonist in the liver. J Biol Chem 1990;265: 17432-17435.

74. Tran-Thi T, Kawada N, Decker K: Regulation of endothelin-1 action on the perfused rat liver. FEBS Lett 1993; 318:353–357.

75. Kawada N, Tran-Thi T, Klein H, Decker K: The contraction of hepatic stellate (Ito) cells stimulated with vasoactive substances. Possible involvement of endothelin-1 and nitric oxide in the regulation of the sinusoidal tonus. Eur J Biochem 1993; 213:815–823.

76. Pinzani M, Failli P, Ruocco C, et al: Fat-storing cells as liver-specific pericytes. Spatial dynamics of agonist-stimulated intracellular calcium transients. J Clin Invest 1992;90:642-646.

77. Simonson M, Wann S, Mene P, et al: Endothelin stimulates phospholipase C, Na/H exchange, c-fos expression and mitogenesis in rat mesangial cells. J Clin Invest 1989;83:702–712.

78. Iijima K, Lin L, Nasjletti A, Goligorsky MS: Intracellular ramification of endothelin signal. Am J Physiol 1991; 260:C982–C992.

79. Takenaka T, Epstein M, Forster H, et al: Attenuation of endothelin effects by a chloride channel inhibitor, indanyloxyacetic acid. Am J Physiol 1992;262:F799–F806.

80. Gordienko D, Clausen D, Goligorsky MS: Ion currents and endothelin signaling in smooth muscle cells from rat renal resistance arteries. Am J Physiol 1994;266:F325–F341.

81. Goligorsky MS, Tsukahara H, Magazine H, et al: Termination of endothelin signaling: Role of nitric oxide. J Cell Physiol 1994;158:485–496.

82. Hirata Y., Emori T, Eguchi S, et al: Endothelin receptor subtype B mediates synthesis of nitric oxide by cultured bovine endothelial cells. J Clin Invest 1993;91:1367–1373.

83. Goligorsky MS, Tsukahara H, Ende H, et al: Molecular and functional characterization of the non-isopeptide-selective ET$_B$ receptor in endothelial cells. J Biol Chem 1994;269:21778–21785.

84. Ihara M, Fukuroda M, Saeki T, et al: Biochem Biophys Res Commun 1991;178:132–137.

85. Ihara M, Noguchi K, Saeki T, et al: Biological profiles of highly potent novel endothelin antagonists selective for the ETA receptor. Life Sci 1992;50:247–255.

86. Clozel M, Breu V, Burri K, et al: Pathophysiological role of endothelin revealed by the first orally active endothelin receptor antagonist. Nature 1993;365:759– 761.

87. Vallance P, Moncada S: Hyperdynamic circulation in cirrhosis: A role for nitric oxide? Lancet 1991;337: 776–778.

88. Bock H, Muller V, Hermle M et al: Endotoxin increases glomerular heamodynamic resistance via PAF and endothelin-1 [abstract] J Am Soc Nephrol 1993;4:732.

89. Gellai M, Jugus M, Fletcher T: Reversal of acute renal failure by BQ123, an ETA receptor antagonist [abstract]. J Am Soc Nephrol 1993;4:735.

90. Chintala M, Rudinski M: Modulation of ET-1, ET receptor subtypes and c-fos protooncogene mRNA's in early ischemic acute renal failure in rats [abstract]. J Am Soc Nephrol 1993;4:733.

91. Schramm L, Lopau K, Schaar J, et al: Beneficial effect of L-arginine and methy-L-arginine on renal function in toxic acute renal failure [abstract] J Am Soc Nephrol 1993;4:744.

92. Schrader J, Tebbe U, Borries M, et al: Plasma endothelin in normal probands and patients with nephrologic-rheumatologic and cardiovascular diseaeses. Klin Wochenschr 1990;68:774–779.

93. Moore K, Wendon J, Frazer M, et al: Plasma endothelin immunoreactivity in liver disease and the hepatorenal syndrome. N Engl J Med 1992;327:1774–1778.

94. Moller S, Emmeluth C, Henriksen J: Elevated circulating plasma endothelin-1 concentrations in cirrhosis. J Hepatol 1993;19:285–290.

95. Battistini B, D'Orleans-Juste P, Sirois P: Endothelins: circulating plasma levels and presence in other biological fluids. Lab Invest 1993;68:600–628.

96. Benigni A, Perico N, Gaspari F, et al: Increased renal endothelin production in rats with reduced renal mass. Am J Physiol 1991;260:F331–F339.

97. Uchihara M, Izumi N, Sato C, Marumo F: Clinical significance of elevated plasma endothelin concentration in patients with cirrhosis. Hepatology 1992;16:95–99.

98. Textor SC, Wilson D, Lerman A, et al: Renal hemodynamics, urinary eicosanoids and endothelin after liver transplantation. Transplantation 1992;54:73–80.

99. Gulbins E, Schlottmann K, Rauterberg E, Steinhausen M: Effects of rC5a on the circulation of normal and split hydronephrotic rat kidneys. Am J Physiol 1993;265: F96–F103.

100. Huber M, Kastner S, Scholmerich J, et al: Analysis of cysteinyl leukotrienes in human urine: Enhanced excretion in patients with liver cirrhosis and hepatorenal syndrome. Eur J Clin Invest 1989;19:53–60.

101. Moore K., Taylor G, Maltby N, et al: Increased production of cysteinyl leukotrienes in hepatorenal syndrome. J Hepatol 1990;11:263–271.

102. Pawloski J, Chapnick B: Release of EDRF from canine renal artery by leukotriene D4. Am.J.Physiol. 1990; 258:H1449–H1456.

103. Sugiura M, Inagami T, Kon V: Endotoxin stimulates endothelin release in vivo and in vitro as determined by radioimmunoassay. Biochem Biophys Res Commun 1989; 161:1220–1227.

RENAL SYMPATHETIC NERVOUS SYSTEM IN HEPATIC CIRRHOSIS

EDWARD J. ZAMBRASKI, Ph.D.
GERALD DiBONA, M.D.

Characterization of the Disease State
Measurement of Activity of the Sympathetic Nervous System
Activation of the Sympathetic System in Cirrhosis
  Arterial Baroreceptors
  Cardiac Baroreceptors
  Renal Sensory Receptors
  Intrahepatic Baroreceptors and Chemoreceptors
Evidence for Increased Sympathetic Activity in Cirrhosis
  Plasma Norepinephrine Concentration
  Renal Sympathetic Nerve Activity
  Muscle Sympathetic Nerve Activity
Mechanisms Responsible for Increased Sympathetic Nerve Activity

Influence of Sympathetic Nervous System on Renal Function
  Renal Hemodynamics
  Renal Sodium Handling
  Sympathetic Nervous System Activity and Basal Urinary Sodium Excretion
  Acute Decreases in Sympathetic Nervous System Activity—Relationship to Changes in Urinary Sodium Excretion
  Interruption of Renal Sympathetic Nerve Activity—Acute Effect on Renal Sodium Handling
  Role of Renal Sympathetic Nerve Activity in Long-Term Sodium and Volume Control
Summary and Unanswered Questions

The importance of the sympathetic nervous system (SNS) in cirrhosis is derived from the fact that activation of the SNS has the capacity to alter many aspects of renal function (hemodynamic, tubular transport, hormonal release) in a manner consistent with what is observed in cirrhosis. Thus, the SNS has the potential to play a primary or causative role in the renal functional abnormalities of cirrhosis. Certain conditions in the early stages of cirrhosis have the potential to activate the SNS. In addition, many of the systemic changes observed in the advanced stages of cirrhosis also would be predicted to activate the SNS. Consequently, a secondary or reactive increase in SNS activity may interact with other renal regulatory mechanisms to intensify the abnormalities of renal function in cirrhotic patients.

This chapter discusses the potential role of the SNS, particularly renal sympathetic nerve activity (SNA),[1] as both a primary and a secondary mechanism in determining the alterations in renal function in cirrhosis.

CHARACTERIZATION OF THE DISEASE STATE

Knowledge of regulation of the SNS in cirrhosis has been greatly enhanced by advances in analytic methodologies, experimental techniques, and animal models of cirrhosis. A clear understanding of the role of the SNS is complicated by the fact that cirrhosis is a progressive disease in which various stages demonstrate different changes in renal and cardiovascular function that, depending on the time point, may be mediated by different mechanisms. Studies that have not defined precisely the exact stage of the disease have produced results that are difficult to incorporate into a cohesive pathogenic scheme. It is clear that the subjects (patients, experimental animals) must be characterized as to whether they are compensated (i.e., without edema or ascites) or decompensated (i.e., with ascites or edema). Even the compensated stage shows evidence of neutral sodium balance as opposed to a sodium-retaining (preascitic) state.[2] In addition, in the decompensated phase it is essential to distinguish between patients without renal vasoconstriction and decreases in renal blood flow (RBF) and glomerular filtration rate (GFR) and patients with marked decreases in both GFR and RBF. The decompensated stage also shows evidence of differences in SNS activity in patients who normally excrete a water load (excretors) and patients who do not (nonexcretors). It is clear that the SNS is differentially activated and influences kidney function to a varied degree during the heterogenous stages of cirrhosis. Despite such complexities, many studies of SNS activity in cirrhosis have characterized accurately the subjects under investigation and thus have provided new, interpretable, and important information.

MEASUREMENT OF ACTIVITY OF THE SYMPATHETIC NERVOUS SYSTEM

The measurement of peripheral and, more specifically, renal SNA has been greatly improved by new methodologies and approaches. New analytic methods for measurement of plasma norepinephrine (NE) concentrations (radioenzymatic and high-performance liquid chromatographic assays) have replaced the fluorometric assays. The newer methods are extremely sensitive and can detect approximately 0.02 ng/ml of NE in plasma[3]; they also are reliable, with interassay coefficients of variation in the range of 10% or less.

The majority of NE circulating in plasma is released as a transmitter at postsynaptic sympathetic nerve terminals.[4] With the availability of sensitive methods for the measurement of NE, it may be reasonable to assume that plasma NE concentration reflects the status of the SNS (i.e., increased plasma NE concentration signifies elevated SNA). Unfortunately, this may not be the case; the issue is much more complex. The plasma represents a large compartment for NE released from various sources. At any point, the steady-state plasma NE concentration is a function of the rate of transmitter release from sympathetic nerve terminals (i.e., peripheral SNA) into plasma and the rate of clearance of NE from plasma. A major site of metabolic clearance of NE is the liver. There is also an intraneuronal uptake and metabolism pathway for the storage and degradation of NE released from nerve terminals. Consequently, an increase in plasma NE concentration may be due to an increase in SNA, with more NE released into the circulation and/or a decrease in plasma clearance. The interpretation

of measurements of plasma NE concentrations is further complicated by the fact that different organs may be heterogenous in terms of their release and clearance of NE.[5]

In dealing with the question of whether peripheral and renal SNA is elevated in cirrhosis, such considerations have led to various experimental approaches that go beyond the measurement of plasma NE concentration. Examples include the measurement of renal venous NE concentration, which appears to be proportional to renal SNA[6]; differences in arteriovenous catecholamine concentration across the kidney and other organs[5–7]; and NE extraction ratios of kidney, liver, and other organs.[7–10] In addition, simultaneous measurements of cardiac output and organ blood (plasma) flow rates permit calculation of total body and individual organ NE spillover rates,[4,7,9,11–13] which reflect total SNS activity and organ-specific SNA, respectively.

In addition to NE measurements, there are ways to estimate the magnitude of renal SNA. Recording electrodes allow direct measurements of renal SNA, both acutely in anesthetized animals and chronically in instrumented conscious animals. In measuring activity in a multifiber nerve preparation, it is not possible to compare quantitatively total nerve activity between animals. Therefore, repeated measurements must be made in the same animal. A limitation of applying this technique to cirrhosis is that the experimentally induced cirrhotic conditions may require several weeks or months to develop. Currently it is not possible to make chronic recordings of renal nerve activity for longer than a few days in rats and approximately 2 weeks in dogs, cats, and rabbits. Consequently, at the present time, changes in renal nerve activity cannot be followed throughout the development of cirrhosis, including the various stages (ie., compensated, decompensated). Nerve recording techniques, however, have been extremely important in defining specific reflex pathways that may be responsible for influencing renal SNA in cirrhosis.[14]

Renal denervation may be used to assess the dependence of various renal functional responses on intact innervation, with the implication that the response depends on alteration (increase or decrease) in renal SNA. Both surgical and pharmacologic renal denervation have been used in cirrhotic animals.[15–21] Anesthetic techniques have been used to denervate the kidney in cirrhotic patients.[22] Sympathetic ganglion-blocking agents and adrenoceptor

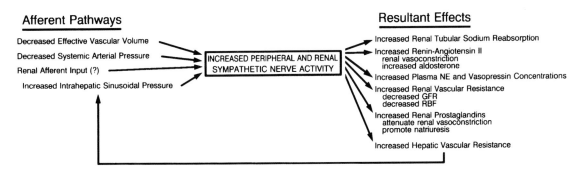

FIGURE 19.1. Afferent mechanisms that increase peripheral and renal sympathetic nerve activity and the resultant renal effects.

antagonists[15] may be used to assess the magnitude of the contribution of renal SNA and its influence on various renal functional responses.

In addition to the importance of increases in peripheral or renal SNA in cirrhosis, the influence of the SNS on renal function relates to alterations in the sensitivity of the renal response elements (vessels, tubules, juxtaglomerualr granular cells) to renal nerve activity and NE. To address this issue, studies have examined the responsiveness of the SNS and renal function to specific stimuli in cirrhotic subjects.[23] Studies to identify and characterize specific renal adrenoceptor number and type, although available for other disease states, have not been performed in cirrhosis.

ACTIVATION OF THE SYMPATHETIC SYSTEM IN CIRRHOSIS

Several pathways may be responsible for an increase in peripheral and renal SNA in cirrhosis (Fig. 19.1). Sympathetic outflow may be increased because of volume, pressure, and/or chemoreceptor input to the central nervous system as part of reflex responses that maintain homeostatic conditions. The pathways and specific stimuli responsible for an increase in peripheral and renal SNA have been described in detail elsewhere,[24] but a brief review in the context of the systemic conditions associated with cirrhosis is appropriate.

Arterial Baroreceptors

High-pressure arterial baroreceptors respond to a pressure-derived increase in transmural wall tension by increasing afferent neural activity.

Afferent impulses, arising from the carotid sinus, travel via the glossopharyngeal nerve to the medulla, where they converge with similar afferent impulses transmitted from the aortic arch through the vagus nerves. At an integrative site within the medulla, increased afferent input from arterial baroreceptors has inhibitory effects on sympathetic efferent outflow. A decrease in peripheral SNA lowers peripheral vascular resistance and cardiac performance, thereby decreasing arterial pressure and stimulation of the sinoaortic baroreceptors. As part of this reflex arc to normalize blood pressure, a decrease in systemic arterial pressure results in less baroreceptor afferent input, which in turn increases peripheral sympathetic outflow.

Mean arterial pressure is significantly lower in most cirrhotic patients than in normal subjects.[3,25–29] The decrease in pressure, which may range from approximately 8–20 mmHg, is still within the renal autoregulatory range. The lower pressure is due to a decrease in peripheral vascular resistance while cardiac output is increased.[26] This decreased arterial pressure increases peripheral and renal SNA acutely. There is considerable discussion over the extent to which arterial baroreceptors adapt or reset to a higher or lower than "normal" pressure over a long period.[30] In cirrhotic patients it is not known whether complete adaptation of the arterial baroreceptors occurs. Anything less than complete resetting would be predicted to increase peripheral/renal SNA.

Cardiac Baroreceptors

The left atrial wall contains mechanoreceptors (unencapsulated neural elements) that, based on discharge characteristics, have been classified as type A or B.[31] Type A receptors discharge during atrial systole, whereas type B receptors discharge during atrial filling. Increased left atrial pressure increases atrial receptor discharge, whereas decreased left atrial pressure decreases atrial receptor discharge. Afferent impulses are conducted via the vagus nerve to the medulla and the supraoptic and paraventricular nuclei of the hypothalamus. The consequence of an increase in afferent vagal nerve activity from these receptors is a decrease in the release of antidiuretic hormone[32] and in peripheral and renal SNA.[33,34]

Several studies in conscious animals have directly measured renal SNA during experimentally manipulated changes in atrial pressure induced by balloon inflation,[3–36] whole animal volume depletion and expansion,[37] head-out water immersion,[38] or head-up tilt.[39] The relationship between atrial pressure and renal SNA is both linear and bidirectional[1,37]; that is, increases in atrial pressure decrease renal SNA, and decrease in atrial pressure increase renal SNA. The gain of the relationship is approximately –20%/mmHg; that is, for each 1-mmHg change in atrial pressure, there is an inverse change in renal SNA of 20%. Such studies provide strong evidence for a cardiorenal neural reflex that transduces changes in blood volume sensed as changes in atrial pressure into appropriate adjustment in urinary sodium excretion that are mediated by changes in renal SNA. For example, both head-out water immersion[38] and left atrial balloon inflation[34–36] produced increases in left atrial pressure and decreases in renal SNA that were associated with a natriuresis in the presence of unchanged GFR. Renal[36,38] or cardiac denervation[36] completely prevented the natriuresis, demonstrating that it was mediated by a vagal afferent-dependent decrease in SNA, which caused a decrease in renal tubular sodium reabsorption. Because renal denervation completely prevented the natriuresis without affecting the hormonal alterations accompanying head-out water immersion and left atrial balloon inflation (decreases in plasma concentrations of renin-angiotensin-aldosterone, vasopressin, NE), it is apparent that withdrawal of renal SNA plays the major role in mediating the observed natriuresis.

In cirrhotic patients a decrease in effective arterial volume has been well characterized.[40] With this decrease in volume and a relatively fixed intrathoracic vascular compliance, atrial pressures are decreased in cirrhotic patients.[3,25,26] This decrease in atrial pressures provides an important stimulus for both nonosmotic release of antidiuretic hormone and an increase in renal SNA in cirrhotic patients. The importance of this pathway has been identified in studies using acute volume expansion, head-out water immersion, or peritoneovenous shunting to increase central blood volume and atrial pressure.[25,27–29] Such maneuvers, which decrease peripheral and renal SNA, result in decreased circulating antidiuretic hormone and plasma NE concentrations and improved renal function (increased sodium and water excretion) in some cirrhotic patients.[13,25,27–29]

Renal Sensory Receptors

The kidney contains renal sensory receptors that respond both to alterations in intrarenal pressure (mechanoreceptors) produced by increasing ureteral or renal venous pressure and to alterations in intrarenal chemical milieu (chemoreceptors) produced by renal ischemia and anoxia or retrograde ureteropelvic perfusion of hypertonic saline or capsaicin.[24,41,42]

In cirrhotic patients, it is possible that the development of portal hypertension and ascites may increase renal venous pressure via transmission of generally increased intraperitoneal pressure. Kostreva et al.[43] showed that increased renal venous pressure in dogs elicited a decrease in contralateral renal vascular resistance and a decrease in cardiac SNA that was associated with a decrease in right but not left ventricular contractile force. However, Kopp et al.[44] found no effect on any aspect of contralateral renal hemodynamic or excretory function during ipsilateral renal venous pressure elevation in dogs. Moreover, in the rat, Kopp et al.[45] observed that in rats elevation of renal venous pressure elicits a contralateral inhibitory renorenal reflex wherein a decrease in contralateral efferent renal SNA produces a diuresis and natriuresis without changes in renal hemodynamics.

Thus, in cirrhotic patients, afferent renal input, possibly derived from renal mechanoreceptor activation, may contribute to an increase in peripheral SNA, but the observations yield no consensus as to an important effect on renal SNA.

Intrahepatic Baroreceptors and Chemoreceptors

The existence of a hepatorenal reflex arc was first suggested by experiments of Anderson et al.[46] When hepatic portal pressure was increased experimentally, renal vasoconstriction and sodium excretion decreased, whereas renin release increased. The renal vasoconstriction and renin responses were abolished by renal denervation. The strongest evidence for a hepatorenal reflex, involving directly measured afferent hepatic and efferent renal SNA, derived initially from the work of Kostreva et al.[14] The authors found that increasing intrahepatic sinusoidal pressure increased measured renal SNA; the increase in renal SNA was prevented by hepatic denervation. In cirrhotic patients with hepatic fibrous bridging and regenerative nodules, resistance to hepatic venous outflow is increased. The resultant increase in intrahepatic intrasinusoidal pressure is usually greater than inferior vena cava pressure by 5 mmHg or more. This degree of intrahepatic hypertension appears to be of sufficient magnitude to stimulate an intrahepatic baroreceptor with activation of a hepatorenal reflex that causes an increase in efferent renal SNA.

Lang et al.[47,48] reported that portal vein (but not jugular or femoral vein) infusions of serotonin, glutamine, or serine markedly decreased GFR, renal plasma flow, and urinary flow rate in rats. The renal functional responses were abolished by prior renal denervation or sectioning of the hepatic vagal nerves and by the serotonin antagonist, methysergide. It was proposed that, since the amino acid infusions can produce hepatocyte swelling, intrahepatic intrasinusoidal pressure is increased and that this hepatorenal reflex regulates renal function via alterations in renal SNA. It was further speculated that this reflex may explain the renal vasoconstriction observed in the presence of primary liver disease and the evolution of hepatorenal syndrome.[49] Because intrahepatic sinusoidal pressure was not determined in these studies, it is possible that the amino acids resulted in activation of intrahepatic chemoreceptors. However, in anesthetized dogs, Levy found that portal vein infusion of glutamine had no effect on portal vein pressure, renal hemodynamics, or excretory function.[50]

Other studies have proposed a role for hepatic NaCl receptors in the hepatic and renal neural responses to a hypertonic saline load in both rabbits and dogs. Intrahepatic infusion of 9.0% NaCl but not 6.5% LiCl decreased renal SNA in conscious rabbits; this response was not seen after sectioning of the anterior and posterior hepatic nerves.[51] In response to an intravenous hypertonic saline load, renal SNA was markedly reduced; the natriuretic response was greater from the innervated than the denervated kidney. The decrease in renal SNA was partially blocked by prior sinoaortic denervation plus either vagotomy or sectioning of the anterior and posterior hepatic nerves but was completely blocked only by a combination of all three denervation procedures.[52] The physiologic significance of this hepatorenal control system was extended in studies demonstrating that oral intake of a high NaCl meal, sufficient to increase plasma sodium and chloride concentrations by approximately 3–4 mEq/L each, decreased renal SNA and produced natriuresis (36 ± 5% of the load) and chloruresis (36 ± 4% of the load). Prior hepatic denervation prevented the decrease in renal SNA and attenuated the postprandial natriuresis (9 ± 5%) and chloruresis (7 ± 3%). Prior renal denervation also attenuated the postprandial natriuresis (15 ± 5%) and chloruresis (9 ± 3%). These observations indicate that the high NaCl meal elicits a decrease in renal SNA that is mediated predominantly by the hepatic nerves and that the decrease in renal SNA contributes importantly to augmentation of urinary sodium and chloride excretion. Thus, hepatorenal reflexes are capable of regulating renal SNA, thereby influencing renal excretory function, and may play an important role in controlling extracellular fluid homeostasis during food intake.[53]

Summary

Renal SNA is regulated by afferent input derived from renal afferent nerves at the level of the spinal cord. Reflex mechanisms involving arterial baroreceptors (carotid sinus, aortic arch), cardiac baroreceptors (atria), and intrahepatic baroreceptors are capable of increasing renal SNA. In cirrhotic patients, overfill is predicted to increase renal SNA via a hepatorenal reflex, whereas underfill is predicted to increase renal SNA via stimuli provided by intrahepatic hypertension and excitatory stimuli from both arterial and cardiac baroreceptors.

EVIDENCE FOR INCREASED SYMPATHETIC ACTIVITY IN CIRRHOSIS

Plasma Norepinephrine Concentration

Henriksen, Ring-Larsen, and Christensen[54] reviewed the studies of norepinephrine measurements in cirrhosis. Plasma NE concentrations are nearly normal in compensated cirrhotic patients,[9,55,56] whereas they are increased in most decompensated cirrhotic patients.[10,55,56] Moreover, plasma NE concentrations may be normal in a cirrhotic patient who through dietary sodium restriction and/or diuretic treatment has become recompensated.[9] This finding emphasizes that the decompensated stage or the presence of ascites or edema is associated with increased plasma NE concentration. However, there appears to be no correlation between the degree of ascites and plasma NE concentrations in decompensated cirrhotic patients.[57] In addition, Bichet et al.[58] found that cirrhotic patients with an impaired ability to excrete an acute water load have higher plasma NE concentrations than those who excrete a water load appropriately.

The increase in plasma NE is due to increased release of NE from postganglionic sympathetic nerve fibers into the circulation and not to diminished clearance of NE from the circulation by the diseased liver or other organs.[7–9] In fact, evidence suggests that clearance of NE from the circulation may be increased rather than decreased. Willet et et al. [59] reported that total body plasma NE clearance was significantly increased in cirrhotic patients. This observation was confirmed by MacGilchrist et al.,[60] who found that, whereas total body spillover of NE to plasma increased by 272% in ascitic cirrhotic patients, total body plasma NE clearance also increased by 67%. Plasma NE concentrations were also increased.[60] Therefore, plasma NE concentrations, which represent the difference between total body spillover into plasma and total body clearance from plasma, may underestimate the degree of SNS activation. Of interest, the authors[60] detected increases in SNS activity in cirrhotic patients before the onset of ascites.

Renal Sympathetic Nerve Activity

The important question of whether renal SNA is elevated in cirrhosis has been addressed by measurements of renal venous NE concentration, renal venoarterial NE concentration differences, and assessment of renal NE secretion and extraction. Such studies indicate that renal SNA is substantially increased and that the kidneys contribute significantly to the increase in circulating NE concentrations. Compared with controls, decompensated cirrhotic patients have (1) increased renal venous NE concentrations; (2) increased and

significantly positive renal venoarterial NE differences (normally slightly negative or zero); and (3) increased renal NE spillover to plasma.[7,9–11,59] Whether renal SNA is preferentially elevated in cirrhotic patients, however, is still debated. The release of large amounts of NE into the circulation by the kidney suggests that renal SNA may be preferentially elevated,[10,61] whereas measurements of the ratio of renal to total body NE release show no differences between controls ($23 \pm 5\%$) and cirrhotics ($26 \pm 7\%$).[59] Although this issue requires definitive resolution, available data clearly indicate that renal SNA is increased in cirrhotic patients.

Muscle Sympathetic Nerve Activity

Microneurographic measurements of activity in sympathetic nerves to skeletal muscles, most commonly the peroneal nerve, permits direct measurement of SNA in humans. Floras et al.[62] found that muscle SNA was increased in decompensated cirrhotic patients compared with compensated cirrhotic patients, whose muscle SNA was similar to controls (Figs. 19.2 and 19.3). Muscle SNA showed a significant positive correlation with plasma NE concentration, plasma renin activity, and heart rate and an inverse correlation with fractional sodium excretion, suggesting that the increase in central sympathetic outflow is generalized and not limited to muscle nerves. Decompensated cirrhotic patients also demonstrated an abnormal response of muscle SNA to the Valsalva maneuver: fixed high levels of muscle SNA neither increased during the strain phase nor suppressed during the release phase (Fig. 19.4). In a single decompensated patient, both muscle SNA and plasma NE concentration fell by over 90% 1 month after successful liver transplantation. Such studies provide direct evidence that increased plasma NE concentrations in decompensated cirrhotic patients are due to a generalized increase in central sympathetic outflow.

MECHANISMS RESPONSIBLE FOR INCREASED SYMPATHETIC NERVE ACTIVITY

Several studies implicate specific mechanisms as responsible for the increase in peripheral and renal SNA in cirrhotic patients. If arterial hypotension initiated an increase in SNA, plasma NE concentration might be inversely correlated

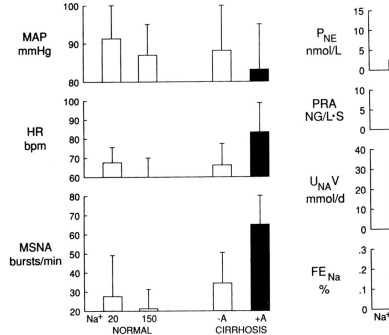

FIGURE 19.2. Mean arterial pressure (MAP), heart rate (HR), and muscle SNA (MSNA) in normal subjects on daily dietary sodium intake of either 20 or 150 mEq/day and cirrhotic patients without (−A) or with (+A) ascites. (Data from Floras JS, Legault L, Morali GA, et al: Increased sympathetic outflow in cirrhosis and ascites: direct evidence from intraneural recordings. Ann Intern Med 1991;114:373–380, with permission.)

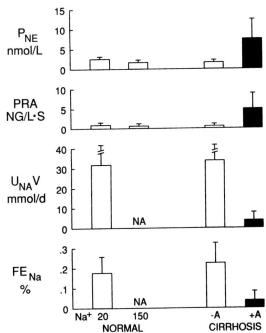

FIGURE 19.3. Plasma norepinephrine concentrations (P_{NE}), plasma renin activity (PRA), and absolute ($U_{NA}V$) and fractional (FE_{NA}) urinary sodium excretion in the same groups as shown in Figure 19.2. (Data from Floras JS, Legault L, Morali GA, et al: Increased sympathetic outflow in cirrhosis and ascites: direct evidence from intraneural recordings. Ann Intern Med 1991;114:373–380, with permission.)

with arterial pressure. Henriksen et al. found no significant correlation between blood pressure and plasma NE concentration.[3,9,10] Thus, cirrhotic patients have decreased blood pressure and increased plasma NE concentrations, but the two are not tightly linked.

Strong evidence suggests that decreases in central blood volume or effective blood volume are coupled to the increase in plasma NE concentration. Henriksen et al.[10] reported that in cirrhotic patients plasma NE concentration correlated negatively with plasma volume. The effective blood volume as determined by central and arterial blood volume is decreased in cirrhotic patients,[40] and the arterial and renal venous NE concentrations correlated inversely with the size of the central and arterial blood volume.[54] Such findings suggest that unloaded arterial and cardiac baroreceptors may be the stimuli for the increase in peripheral and renal SNA. In agreement with these findings, it has been proposed that arteriolar vasodilation and arterial hypovolemia are initiators of the increased peripheral and renal SNA and renal sodium retention in cirrhosis.[63,64]

To evaluate this hypothesis, the effects of maneuvers designed to increase central blood volume have been studied. Head-out water immersion[28] and peritoneovenous shunting,[29] both of which increase central blood volume, result in a decrease in plasma NE concentrations. In studies using head-out water immersion, plasma NE concentration correlated significantly with plasma antidiuretic hormone concentration, suggesting interaction via a common stimulus-receptor interaction via cardiac baroreceptors.[58] Furthermore, the researchers found a negative correlation between plasma NE correlation and urinary sodium excretion.[58] However, the suppression of of plasma NE concentration during head-out water immersion has not been found in all cirrhotic patients. Epstein et al.[57] observed suppression in only 7 of 16 decompensated cirrhotic patients. In addition,

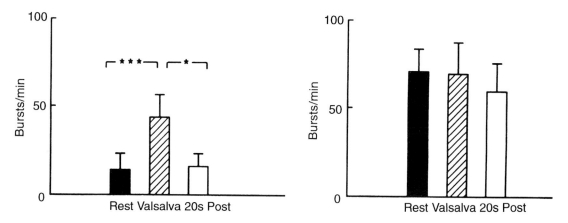

FIGURE 19.4. Response to Valsalva maneuver in normal subjects (*left*) and cirrhotic patients (*right*). Compared with normal subjects, cirrhotic patients have increased muscle SNA (bursts/min) that fails to increase further in response to Valsalva or to suppress upon release of Valsalva (20s Post). (Data from Floras JS, Legault L, Morali GA, et al: Increased sympathetic outflow in cirrhosis and ascites: direct evidence from intraneural recordings. Ann Intern Med 1991;114:373–380, with permission.)

in a series wherein head-out water immersion decreased plasma NE concentration in each 7 decompensated cirrhotic patients, the change was from 704 ± 72 to 475 ± 70 pg/ml; the second value was still substantially higher than the value in control subjects.13 These studies suggest that stimuli in addition to decreased central blood volume contribute to the increased peripheral and renal SNA represented by the increased plasma NE concentration.

In the aggregate, such studies support the concept that in decompensated cirrhotics a decrease in effective vascular volume, presumably sensed by both cardiac and arterial baroreceptors, is an important but not sole stimulus for increased peripheral and renal SNA.

As indicated earlier, a hepatorenal reflex may be responsible for increasing renal SNA. Because of the difficulty of measuring intrahepatic pressure, or manipulating it experimentally, relatively few studies have evaluated this pathway for increased renal SNA in cirrhotic subjects. Henriksen et al.[10] reported that elevated plasma NE concentration correlated significantly with wedged hepatic vein pressure in cirrhotic patients. The same group subsequently reported[9] that wedge minus free hepatic venous pressure correlated significantly with differences in renal arteriovenous NE concentration. Data about the effect of a primary decrease in intrahepatic sinusoidal pressure on peripheral and renal SNA in cirrhosis are required. However, changes observed in renal function with the lowering of intrahepatic pressure in cirrhotic

animals[65] are consistent with the existence of a hepatorenal reflex that contributes to an increase in renal SNA.[65–67]

INFLUENCE OF SYMPATHETIC NERVOUS SYSTEM ON RENAL FUNCTION

An increase in peripheral and renal SNA may potentially influence many aspects of kidney function in a manner consistent with the renal functional abnormalities observed in cirrhotic patients (see Fig. 19.1). Indirectly, kidney function can be altered by sympathetically mediated changes in circulatory parameters. Cirrhosis is characterized by a hyperkinetic state of the systemic circulation with increased cardiac output; however, systemic vascular resistance is decreased so that arterial and renal perfusion pressures are lower than in normal subjects.[3] Even though the arterial resistance vasculature is dilated, the SNS and renin-angiotensin systems are important in maintaining systemic arterial pressure. Pharmacologic interventions to interrupt or decrease peripheral SNA, such as the administration of propranolol,[68] clonidine,[69–72] or low doses of phentolamine,[73] may decrease arterial pressure in cirrhotic patients even when given into the kidney.

It is clear that the SNS has the capacity to stimulate directly the release of renin,[24] which indirectly influences kidney function because of the resultant production of angiotensin II and aldosterone. Plasma NE concentration is correlated with plasma renin activity as well as concentrations of plasma aldosterone and plasma vasopressin in cirrhotic patients.[23,54–56] Whether the SNS is primarily or solely responsible for the elevation in plasma renin activity in decompensated cirrhotic patients remains unresolved.

Renal Hemodynamics

Alteration in renal hemodynamics may be another effect of the SNS on kidney function. To evaluate this possibility, Gatta et al.[74] injected the α-adrenoreceptor antagonist dihydroergocristine into the renal artery of 13 cirrhotic patients (10 compensated, 3 decompensated). Baseline mean renal and cortical RBFs, as measured by xenon washout, were significantly lower in cirrhotic patients than in controls. Alpha-adrenoceptor blockade significantly increased both RBFs but also decreased GFR. Baldus[75] found that systemic phenoxybenzamine administration increased RBF if systemic arterial pressure was maintained by albumin infusion. In 4 cirrhotic patients who showed active renal vasoconstriction and renal hemodynamic instability, intrarenal α-adrenoreceptor blockade with phentolamine did not consistently increase RBF.[73] RBF is decreased in cirrhotic patients, more so in decompensated than compensated patients, and is inversely correlated with both arterial and renal venous NE concentrations.[54,76]

When decompensated cirrhotic patients are divided into those with or without functional renal failure (hepatorenal syndrome), an important interaction between systemic and renal hemodynamics becomes evident.[77] Patients without functional renal failure exhibit increased cardiac index, decreased total peripheral vascular resistance, normal arterial pressure, normal RBF, and increased femoral blood flow, whereas patients with functional renal failure show a further increase in cardiac index, a further decrease in total peripheral vascular resistance, a decrease in arterial pressure, a decrease in RBF, and a decrease in femoral blood flow to normal levels. When expressed as a fraction of cardiac output, patients without functional renal failure have a decrease in renal and an increase in femoral fraction of cardiac output, whereas patients with functional renal failure have a further marked decrease in renal and a decrease in femoral fraction of cardiac output. Femoral and renal fractions of cardiac output were directly correlated, and each independently was directly correlated with total vascular

resistance. Thus, the transition of the decompensated cirrhotic patient into functional and renal failure involves a progressive increase in the hyperdynamic circulatory status with a reduction in the renal vascular resistance as well as a reversal of extrasplanchnic vasodilation. In cirrhotic patients, functional renal failure due to renal vasoconstriction is associated with striking increases in plasma NE concentrations.[55,78] GFR was inversely correlated with plasma NE concentration and plasma renin activity and directly correlated with urinary excretion of prostaglandin E_2.[55] Thus alterations in the activities of multiple vasoactive systems, alone or in concert, may decrease GFR.

Melman and Massry[79] observed that in cirrhotic dogs the renal vasodilator response to acute volume loading is blunted. Chaimovitz et al.[15] reported that in cirrhotic dogs surgical or pharmacologic renal denervation failed to alter baseline GFR or RBF and did not restore the blunted renal vasodilator response. In the miniature swine model of cirrhosis due to common bile-duct ligation,[19] surgical renal denervation had no effect on RBF or GFR in either compensated or decompensated animals.

Such data indicate that marked renal vasoconstriction in cirrhosis is associated with increases in arterial and renal venous NE concentration. However, removal of SNA by renal denervation does not reverse the renal vasoconstriction, indicating that other mechanisms contribute importantly to the renal vasoconstriction.

Renal Sodium Handling

In the past decade studies from various laboratories have demonstrated that the renal sympathetic nerves have the capacity to alter directly the renal handling of sodium.[24] Increased renal SNA directly increases renal tubular sodium reabsorption. This neurogenic effect has been shown to occur throughout the nephron and is mediated by renal tubular α_1-adrenoceptors. Consequently, renal SNA has the potential to be a major factor in causing renal sodium retention in cirrhosis.

Three approaches can be used to evaluate whether an increase in renal SNA alters renal sodium handling in cirrhosis. The first approach is to attempt to correlate basal urinary sodium excretion with some index of renal SNA. Second, if renal SNA is responsible for a significant amount of renal tubular sodium reabsorption, maneuvers known to decrease renal SNA acutely should alter urinary sodium excretion. The third approach is to demonstrate that elimination of renal SNA increases urinary sodium excretion. A major limitation with the first two approaches has been the measurement selected as an index of renal SNA. In humans, this index has generally been plasma NE concentration, which provides limited information about renal SNA; the more precise (but more difficult) measurements of renal vein NE concentration or renal NE spillover have been used less often. Only through the third approach can a direct cause-and-effect relationship be established.

Sympathetic Nervous System Activity and Basal Urinary Sodium Excretion

In contrast to excretor cirrhotic patients, nonexcretor cirrhotic patients have significantly elevated plasma NE concentrations and, during excretion of a water load, exhibited a significant negative correlation between plasma NE concentration and urinary sodium excretion.[58] Cirrhotics without functional renal impairment demonstrate increases in plasma NE concentration as daily basal urinary sodium excretion decreases, whereas cirrhotic patients with functional renal failure and decreased GFR had the highest plasma NE concentrations and markedly reduced urinary sodium excretion.[55,78] Both the tubular rejection fraction and the urinary excretion of sodium showed a significant inverse correlation with plasma NE and aldosterone concentrations in decompensated cirrhotic patients.[23]

Simon et al.[80] studied the relationship between plasma concentration and fractional proximal tubular sodium reabsorption (FPR, by lithium clearance) during the adaptive change from an unrestricted sodium diet to a 40-mEq/day sodium diet in three groups of subjects: controls, compensated cirrhotics (without ascites), and decompensated cirrhotics (with ascites). The three groups exhibited different patterns of response to modest dietary sodium restriction. Controls displayed no change in plasma NE concentration of FPR. Compensated cirrhotics had normal plasma NE concentration and FPR during the unrestricted sodium diet and showed significantly correlated, parallel increases during restriction of dietary sodium. Decompensated cirrhotics had increased plasma NE concentration and FPR and decreased urinary sodium excretion during the unrestricted sodium diet that did not increase further during restriction of dietary sodium. Because

dietary sodium restriction increases renal SNA,[37,81] which directly increases tubular sodium and water reabsorption, such studies suggest that the evolution from the control to the compensated state is characterized by an enhanced activation or renal SNA with increased tubular sodium and water reabsorption in response to the stimulus of dietary sodium restriction with blood volume contraction. The evolution from the compensated to the decompensated state is characterized by the appearance of high fixed levels of renal SNA, tubular sodium, and water reabsorption before dietary sodium is restricted. Such studies suggest that ineffective circulatory volume is detected in compensated cirrhotics only under conditions of dietary sodium restriction but is always present in decompensated cirrhotics. The results are compatible with the existence of fixed arterial vasodilation in cirrhosis with activation of renal SNA in response to progressive reductions in effective circulatory volume.

Acute Decreases in Sympathetic Nervous System Activity—Relationship to Changes in Urinary Sodium Excretion

Many studies have used acute volume expansion or head-out water immersion to suppress reflexly both peripheral and renal SNA. Several such studies have evaluated the changes in renal handling of sodium in response to these interventions.

Epstein et al.[57] reported that in 16 cirrhotic subjects head-out water immersion caused a diuresis in 15 and a natriuresis in 12 but a decrease in plasma NE concentration in only 7. Such data were interpreted as indicating that the increased urinary sodium and water excretion with immersion was not due primarily to withdrawal of peripheral or renal SNA. Bichet et al.[19] subjected 8 decompensated cirrhotic patients to head-out water immersion and observed a significant increase in urinary sodium excretion. The increased fractional excretion of sodium was directly correlated with the increase in right atrial pressure. Although plasma NE concentrations were not consistently decreased, the change in plasma NE concentration inversely correlated with the increase in right atrial pressure. Shapiro et al.[27] used NE infusion during head-out water immersion to prevent the usual decrease in systemic vascular resistance and arterial pressure; this combination resulted in a greater natriuresis than either intervention alone. The combination of increased central blood volume and sustained arterial pressure may have resulted in a greater degree of inhibition of renal SNA than the combination of increased central blood volume and decreased arterial pressure.

Studies designed to stimulate the SNS and renin-angiotensin system in relation to renal sodium handling disclose differences between controls and cirrhotic patients.[23] Assumption of the upright posture increased plasma renin activity, aldosterone, and NE concentrations to a much greater extent in cirrhotics than in controls. Urinary sodium excretion decreased, but the decrements did not correlate with the increases in plasma NE concentration and were related more to the increases in plasma aldosterone concentration. A relatively more important role for aldosterone than SNA in the regulation of urinary sodium excretion has been suggested by head-out water immersion as well.[28]

Direct measurements of renal SNA have been made in the common bile-duct ligation model of cirrhosis in rats.[17,18] In conscious decompensated cirrhotic rats, bilateral renal denervation normalized the markedly attenuated diuretic and natriuretic responses to administration of atrial natriuretic peptide.[17] In addition, in response to administration of atrial natriuretic peptide, renal SNA decreased in control rats, whereas it increased in cirrhotic rats. Such results suggest that baseline renal SNA was increased in cirrhotic rats and opposed the diuretic and natriuretic actions of atrial natriuretic peptide by increasing renal tubular sodium and water reabsorption upstream from the tubular site of action of atrial natriuretic peptide in the medullary collecting duct. Furthermore, the abnormal renal SNA response to atrial natriuretic peptide administration suggested that cirrhotic rats display abnormal regulation of renal SNA in response to acute volume loading stimuli, which are known to increase circulating atrial natriuretic peptide concentrations. Conscious decompensated cirrhotic rats displayed attenuated diuretic and natriuretic responses to both oral and intravenous acute loading of isotonic saline, which was associated with early paradoxical increases in renal SNA and an overall failure of renal SNA to suppress normally as seen in control rats.[18] Bilateral renal denervation markedly improved the diuretic and natriuretic responses (Fig. 19.5). Thus decompensated cirrhotic rats have increased basal levels of renal SNA that fail to suppress normally in response to

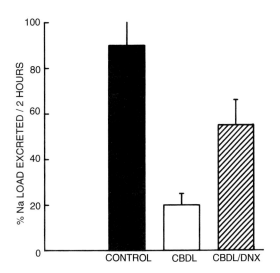

FIGURE 19.5. Compared with control rats, rats with decompensated cirrhosis due to common bile duct ligation (CBDL) exhibit a decreased natriuretic response to an intravenous isotonic saline load (% of infused sodium excreted over subsequent 2 hours).Bilateral renal denervation (DNX) significantly improves the natriuretic response of the CBDL rats. (Data from DiBona GF, Herman PJ, Sawin LL: Neural control of renal function in edema forming states. Am J Physiol 1988;254:R1017–R1024, with permission.)

acute volume loading. Such abnormalities in renal SNA account for the concomitantly impaired diuretic and natriuretic responses, which are reversed by bilateral renal denervation.

Studies using the technique of recording SNA in human muscle have extended these observations to cirrhotic patients. Morali et al.[82] studied the response to atrial natriuretic peptide administration in normal subjects and both compensated and decompensated cirrhotic patients. The decompensated cirrhotic patients were further classified into responders (> 0.833 mmol/hr) and nonresponders (≤ 0.833 mol/hr) according to peak hourly natriuresis after atrial natriuretic peptide administration. Muscle SNA was markedly increased in decompensated cirrhotic nonresponders (64 ± 4 bursts/min), moderately increased in decompensated cirrhotic responders (47 ± 6 bursts/min) and not increased in compensated cirrhotics (34 ± 5 bursts/min) compared with normal subjects (24 ± 7 bursts/min) (Fig. 19.6). Muscle SNA was positively correlated with plasma NE concentrations and inversely correlated with peak natriuresis during atrial natriuretic peptide administration (Fig. 19.7). Plasma

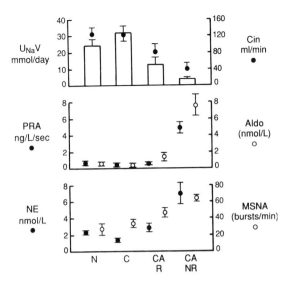

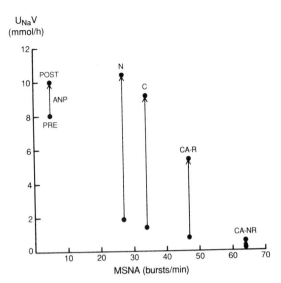

FIGURE 19.6. Urinary sodium excretion ($U_{Na}V$), inulin clearance (C_{in}), plasma renin activity (PRA), plasma aldosterone concentration (Aldo), plasma norepinephrine concentration (NE), and muscle sympathetic nerve activity (MSNA) in normal subjects (N), cirrhotic patients (C), and cirrhotic patients with ascites (CA) who were responders (R) or nonresponders (NR) to atrial natriuretic peptide administration. (Data from Morali GA, Floras JS, Legault L, et al: Muscle sympathetic nerve activity and renal responsiveness to atrial natriuretic factor during the development of hepatic ascites. Am J Med 1991;91:383–392, with permission.)

FIGURE 19.7. The natriuretic response to atrial natriuretic peptide (ANP) administration as a function of the level of of muscle sympathetic nerve activity (MSNA) in the same groups as shown in Figure 19.6. The basal $U_{Na}V$ before AMP administration is shown is as the solid circle at the tail of the arrow, and the $U_{Na}V$ after ANP administration as the solid circle at the head of the arrow. The magnitude of the natriuretic response to ANP administration, represented by the length of the arrow, is inversely related to the level of MSNA. (Data from Morali GA, Floras JS, Legault L, et al: Muscle sympathetic nerve activity and renal responsiveness to atrial natriuretic factor during the development of hepatic ascites. Am J Med 1991;91:383–392, with permission.)

renin activity and aldosterone concentrations were markedly increased in decompensated nonresponders and normal in decompensated responders and compensated cirrhotics.

Interruption of Renal Sympathetic Nerve Activity—Acute Effect on Renal Sodium Handing

A limited number of studies have attempted to inhibit renal SNA directly and to evaluate changes in urinary sodium excretion in cirrhotic subjects. The administration of β-adrenoreceptor antagonists (propranolol, practolol) in patients with decompensated cirrhosis produced no consistent changes in urinary sodium excretion,[68,84] but it improved ability to excrete an intravenous sodium load, an effect that could not be ascribed to changes in the renin-angiotensin system. Accumulated evidence indicates that the direct effect of renal SNA on renal tubular sodium and water reabsorption is mediated by α_1-adrenoreceptors.[27]

Solis Herruzo et al.[22] showed that this maneuver increased GFR, renal plasma flow, and absolute and fractional urinary sodium excretion in decompensated cirrhotic patients with hepatorenal syndrome and an initial GFR less than 24 ml/min. This study demonstrates that increased renal SNA contributes to the impaired renal hemodynamics and excretory function characteristic of cirrhotic patients with hepatorenal syndrome.

Three studies have evaluated the effects of renal denervation in a bile-duct-ligated cirrhotic animal model. Chaimovitz et al.[14] assessed the effects of surgical denervation and intrarenal α-adrenoreceptor blockade in cirrhotic dogs. Renal denervation increased urinary sodium excretion to a similar extent in cirrhotic and control dogs. An explanation of this finding may lie in the fact that it is not clear whether the cirrhotic dogs were compensated or decompensated, as reflected by presence of ascites or renal sodium retention.

This point is crucial in light of the demonstration that a natriuretic effect of renal denervation in miniature swine with cirrhosis due to common bile duct ligation was observed only in decompensated animals and not in compensated animals.[16,19,20]. Consequently, the failure of the cirrhotic dogs to demonstrate a significant natriuresis with renal denervation in the study of Chaimovitz et al.[15] may have been due to the fact that the animals were not retaining sodium. As noted above, in conscious rats with decompensated cirrhosis due to common bile duct ligation, bilateral renal denervation significantly improved the ability to excrete both an intravenous and an oral acute isotonic saline load.[18]

Renal Sympathetic Nerve Activity in Long-term Sodium and Volume Control

To explore the contribution of renal SNA to the chronic renal sodium and water retention that results in the ascites and edema of fully developed decompensated cirrhosis, the effect of chronic bilateral denervation on sodium balance has been examined in both miniature swine[20] and rats[21] with cirrhosis due to common bile duct ligation. In cirrhotic miniature swine[20] (Fig. 19.8),

bilateral renal denervation was performed 4–5 weeks following common bile duct ligation. Renal denervation reversed the increased renal sodium retention observed with both normal and 2.5-fold increased dietary intake of sodium and prevented the development of ascites. In cirrhotic rats[21] (Fig. 19.9), bilateral renal denervation was performed 2 weeks following common bile duct ligation, and cumulative sodium balance was examined over the subsequent 26 days. Cumulative sodium balance was 36% less in cirrhotic rats with bilateral renal denervation than in cirrhotic rats with intact renal innervation. Bilateral renal denervation did not affect cumulative sodium balance in sham control (noncirrhotic) rats. Therefore, studies in two different cirrhotic animal models indicate that renal SNA is increased above normal and that increased renal SNA constitutes an important mechanism contributing to the chronic progressive renal sodium retention that leads to ascites and edema in cirrhosis.

Additional studies focused on the contribution of a hepatorenal reflex to the increased renal SNA and the ensuing renal sodium retention and ascites in cirrhosis. Unikowsky et al.[65] demonstrated that dogs with cirrhosis due to common

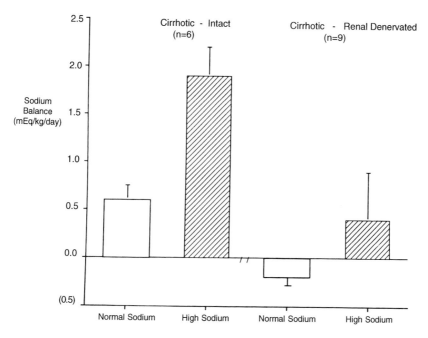

FIGURE 19.8. Sodium balance in intact and renal denervated cirrhotic miniature swine on normal and high dietary sodium intake. Bilateral renal denervation reversed the sodium retention in cirrhotic animals and prevented the development of ascites. (Data from Zambraski EJ, O'Hagan K, Thomas G, Hora D: Chronic renal denervation prevents sodium retention in cirrhotic miniature swine [abstract]. J Am Soc Nephrol 1990;1:322.)

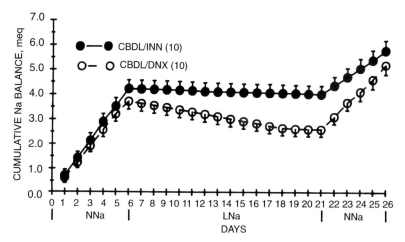

FIGURE 19.9. Cumulative sodium balance in rats with cirrhosis due to common bile duct ligation (CBDL) with intact renal innervation (INN) or bilateral renal denervation (DNX) studied over 26 days during periods of normal (NNA) or low (LNa) dietary sodium intake. (Data from DiBona GF, Sawin LL: Role of renal nerves in sodium retention of cirrhosis and congestive heart failure. Am J Physiol 1991;260:R298–R305, with permission.)

bile duct ligation do not develop ascites if a functional side-to-side portacaval anastomosis keeps intrahepatic sinusoidal pressure at normal levels. The dogs maintain a normal sodium balance even on increased dietary sodium intake and exhibit normal mineralocorticoid escape. Intrahepatic sinusoidal pressure rather than portal venous pressure appears to be the initiating stimulus, because the creation of an end-to-side portacaval anastomosis that reduced portal venous but not intrahepatic sinusoidal pressure did not prevent renal sodium retention and ascites. Such experiments strongly implicate involvement of a possible hepatorenal reflex in the long-term control of renal sodium handling in the development of decompensated cirrhosis. Subsequent studies demonstrated that hepatic denervation prevents renal sodium retention in dogs with cirrhosis due to common bile duct ligation[66] and in dogs with thoracic inferior vena cava ligation,[67] both of which increase intrahepatic sinusoidal pressure. Such studies add additional support to the view that, in cirrhosis, increased intrahepatic sinusoidal pressure stimulates intraheaptic baroreceptors and results in the activation of a hepatorenal reflex via afferent hepatic nerves and efferent renal sympathetic nerves that plays a significant role in renal sodium retention and formation of edema.

Another factor related to long-term involvement of the SNS in the abnormalities of renal sodium handling is the possibility that the SNS is responsible or capable of self-activation in a progressive, ever-increasing manner. To explore this issue, the effects of both acute and chronic administration of clonidine (an α_2-adrenoceptor agonist that decreases peripheral and renal SNA) to cirrhotic patients have been studied. Willet et al.[69]

and Albillos et al.[70] reported that acute administration of clonidine decreased intrahepatic sinusoidal pressure (corrected wedged hepatic venous pressure) and hepatic vascular resistance, whereas hepatic blood flow was unchanged. Chronic administration of clonidine (mean of 7[69] or 64[70] days) yielded similar hepatic hemodynamic results with no adverse effects on hepatic function and no patient withdrawal due to side effects. In addition, plasma NE concentration in the right renal vein was decreased, whereas neither RBF nor GFR was affected. Although urinary flow rate increased 35% and urinary sodium excretion increased 49%, such changes did not achieve statistical significance. In studies combining measurements of regional NE overflow to plasma and muscle SNA, acute administration of clonidine decreased the elevated NE overflow rates for the whole body, kidney, and hepatomesenteric circulation.[72] The changes in peripheral and renal SNA were associated with decreased intrahepatic sinusoidal pressure (corrected wedged hepatic venous pressure) and hepatic vascular resistance, whereas hepatic blood flow was unchanged. In addition, renal vascular resistance was decreased, glomerular filtration increased, and, despite the substantial reduction in mean arterial pressure, urinary flow rate was significantly increased, whereas urinary sodium excretion was unchanged.

Such findings imply that, regardless of what early event may initiate an increase in peripheral and renal SNA, increases in efferent hepatic SNA may increase intrahepatic sinusoidal pressure, and subsequent activation of a hepatorenal reflex may further increase renal SNA. This reflex would establish a positive feedback loop between the liver and peripheral and renal SNA (see Fig. 19.1) and, unless intrahepatic sinusoidal pressure was reduced or afferent/efferent hepatic nerves were interrupted, would continue to support a progressive increase in renal SNA. It is important to define the role of this feedback loop in cirrhosis.

SUMMARY AND UNANSWERED QUESTIONS

The SNS must be considered to be of prime importance in determining renal function in cirrhosis. During various stages of cirrhosis at least three afferent pathways known to increase peripheral and renal SNA are activated: high-pressure arterial baroreceptors, low-pressure cardiac (atrial) volume receptors, and intrahepatic baroreceptors. Muscle and renal SNA is increased in decompensated cirrhotic patients and animals. The increase in renal SNA may contribute to abnormalities in renal sodium handling and renal hemodynamics as well as activation of the renin-angiotensin-aldosterone system. Studies in cirrhotic patients demonstrate strong association between increased muscle and renal SNA and renal function abnormalities. Studies in cirrhotic animals demonstrate that renal SNA is increased, that it mediates the attenuated natriuretic response to acute volume expansion, and that it contributes importantly to the chronic progressive renal sodium retention that leads to ascites.

The exact stimulus or stimuli for the increase in peripheral and renal SNA at the various stages of cirrhosis remain to be identified. At any point the relative importance of a given afferent pathway must be ascertained. It also is essential to determine possible redundancy among the various afferent pathways capable of increasing peripheral and renal SNA and to characterize the effect of elimination of one pathway on the function of the other pathways.

The data indicate that peripheral and renal SNA are increased mainly in the decompensated stage of cirrhosis. Studies must examine more closely the role of peripheral and renal SNA during the development of and the transition from the compensated to the decompensated stage of cirrhosis. A sequence whereby increased intraheaptic sinusoidal pressure elicits increases in renal SNA via a hepatorenal reflex before the development of ascites and decrease in effective vascular volume supports a primary or causative role for increased renal SNA in renal sodium retention and ascites formation. Conversely, if increased renal SNA occurs only after the development of decreased effective vascular volume, the response is secondary or reactive.

The hypothesis that increased renal SNA contributes to the intense renal vasoconstriction of hepatorenal syndrome requires testing. The inability to predict which cirrhotic patient will develop hepatorenal syndrome and the lack of a simple and reliable approach to either precise quantitation of renal SNA or renal denervation in humans have limited progress in this area. Whereas the animal models of cirrhosis faithfully reproduce much of the pathophysiology of the human condition, they do not exhibit readily detectable hepatorenal syndrome. A further complicating factor is the potential involvement of multiple other factors in the renal vasoconstriction of hepatorenal syndrome.

Acknowledgment. The research from the authors' laboratories was supported by National Institutes of Health grant HL 25255 and American Heart Association Grant-in-Aid no. 880972 (EJZ) and by National Institutes of Health grants DK 15843, HL 44546, and HL 14388 and Veterans Administration Merit Review (GFD).

REFERENCES

1. DiBona G: Renal neural activity in hepatorenal syndrome. Kidney Int 1984;25:841–853.
2. Levy M: Sodium retention and ascites formation in dogs with portal cirrhosis. Am J Physiol 1977;233:F572–F585.
3. Henriksen J, Ring-Larsen H, Christensen N: Circulating noradrenaline and central hemodynamics in patients with cirrhosis. Scand J Gastroenterol 1985;20:1185–1190.
4. Esler M, Jennings G, Lambert G, et al: Overflow of catecholamine neurotransmitters to the circulation: Source, fate and functions. Physiol Rev 1990; 70:963–985.
5. Folkow B, DiBona G, Hjemdahl P, et al: Measurement of plasma norepinephrine concentrations in hypertension—a word of caution concerning their applicability for assessing neurogenic contribution. Hypertension 1983;5:399–403.
6. Oliver J, Pinto J, Sciacca R, et al: Basal norepinephrine overflow into the renal vein: Effect of renal nerve stimulation. Am J Physiol 1980;239:F371–377.
7. Ring-Larsen H, Hesse B, Henriksen J, et al: Sympathetic nervous activity and renal and systemic hemodynamics in cirrhosis: Plasma norepinephrine concentration, hepatic extraction, and renal release. Hepatology 1982;2:304–310.
8. Henriksen J, Ring-Larsen H, Christensen N, et al: Catecholamines in plasma from artery, cubital vein, and femoral vein in patients with cirrhosis. Significance of sampling site. Scand J Clin Lab Invest 1986;46:39–44.
9. Henriksen J, Ring-Larsen H, Kanstrup I, et al: Splanchnic and renal elimination and release of catecholamines in cirrhosis. Evidence of enhanced sympathetic nervous activity in patients with decompensated cirrhosis. Gut 1984;25:1034–1043.

10. Henriksen J, Christensen N, Ring-Larsen H: Noradrenaline and adrenaline concentrations in various vascular beds in patients with cirrhosis. Relation to haemodynamics. Clin Physiol 1981;1:293–304.

11. Henriksen J, Christensen NJ, Ring-Larsen H: Continuous infusion of tracer norepinephrine may miscalculate unidirectional nerve uptake of norepinephrine in humans. Circ Res 1989;65:388–395.

12. Bendtsen F, Christensen NJ, Sørensen TIA, Henriksen JH: Effects of oral propranolol administration on azygos, renal and hepatic uptake and output of catecholamines in cirrhosis. Hepatology 1991;14:237–243.

13. Nicholls K, Shapiro M, VanPutten V, et al: Elevated plasma norepinephrine concentrations in decompensated cirrhosis. Association with increased secretion rates, normal clearance rates, and suppressibility by central blood volume expansion. Circ Res 1985;56: 457–461.

14. Kostreva D, Castaner A, Kampine J:Reflex effects of hepatic baroreceptors on renal and cardiac sympathetic nerve activity Am J Physiol 1980;238:R390–R394.

15. Chaimovitz C, Massry S, Friedler R, et al: Effect of renal denervation and α-adrenergic blockade on sodium excretion in dogs with chronic ligation of the common bile duct. Proc Soc Exp Biol Med 1974;146:764–770.

16. Zambraski E: Effects of acute renal denervation on sodium excretion in miniature swine with cirrhosis and ascites. Physiologist 1985;28:268.

17. Koepke J, Jones S, DiBona G: Renal nerves mediate blunted natriuresis to atrial natriuretic peptide in cirrhotic rats. Am J Physiol 1987;252:R1010–R1023.

18. DiBona GF, Herman PJ, Sawin LL: Neural control of renal function in edema forming states. Am J Physiol 1988;254:R1017–R1024.

19. Zambraski EJ: Renal nerves in renal sodium retaining states: Cirrhotic ascites, congestive heart failure, nephrotic syndrome. Miner Electrolyte Metab 1989;15:88–96.

20. Zambraski EJ, O'Hagan K, Thomas G, Hora D: Chronic renal denervation prevents sodium retention in cirrhotic miniature swine [abstract]. J Am Soc Nephrol 1990; 1:322.

21. DiBona GF, Sawin LL: Role of renal nerves in sodium retention of cirrhosis and congestive heart failure. Am J Physiol 1991;260:R298–R305.

22. Solis-Herruzo JA, Duran A, Favela V, et al: Effects of lumbar sympathetic block on kidney function in cirrhotic patients with hepatorenal syndrome. J Hepatol 1987;5:167–173.

23. Bernardi M, Santini C, Trevisani F: Renal function impairment induced by change in posture in patients with cirrhosis and ascites. Gut 1985;26:629–635.

24. Kopp UC, DiBona GF: The neural control of renal function. In Seldin DW, Giebisch G (eds): The Kidney—Physiology and Pathophysiology, 2nd ed. New York: Raven, 1992;1157–1204.

25. Bichet D, Groves B, Schrier R: Mechanisms of improvement of water and sodium excretion by immersion in decompensated cirrhotic patients. Kidney Int 1983;24: 788–794.

26. Gentilini P, Giacomo L, Fantini F, et al: Systemic hemodynamics and renal function in cirrhotic patients during plasma volume expansion. Digestion 1983;27: 138–145.

27. Shapiro M, Nicholls K, Groves B, et al: Interrelationship between cardiac output and vascular resistance as determinants of effective arterial blood volume in cirrhotic patients. Kidney Int 1985;28:206–211.

28. Nicholls K, Shapiro M, Kluge R, et al: Sodium excretion in advanced cirrhosis: Effect of expansion of central blood volume and suppression of plasma aldosterone. Hepatology 1986;6:235–238.

29. Blendis LM, Sole DP, Campbell P: The effect of peritoneovenous shunting on catecholamine metabolism in patients with hepatic ascites. Hepatology 1987;7:143–148.

30. Dorward P, Riedel W, Burke S, et al: The renal sympathetic baroreflex in the rabbit. Arterial and cardiac baroreceptor influences, resetting, and effect of anesthesia. Circ Res 1985;57:618–633.

31. Paintal A: Vagal sensory receptors and their reflex effects. Physiol Rev 1973;53:159–227.

32. DeTorrente A, Robertson D, McDonald G, et al: Mechanism of diuretic response to increased left atrial pressure in the anesthetized dog. Kidney Int 1975;8:355–361.

33. Karim F, Kidd C, Malpus C, et al: Effect of stimulation of the left atrial receptors on sympathetic efferent nerve activity. J Physiol (Lond) 1972;227:243–260.

34. Prosnitz E, DiBona G: Effect of decreased renal sympathetic nerve activity on renal tubular sodium reabsorption. Am J Physiol 1978;235:F557–F563.

35. Miki K, Hayashida Y, Shiraki K: Quantitative and sustained suppression of renal sympathetic nerve activity by left atrial distension in conscious dogs. Pflugers Arch 1991;419:610–615.

36. Miki H, Hayashida Y, Shiraki K: Cardiac-renal-neural reflex plays a major role in natriuresis induced by left atrial distension. Am J Physiol 1992;264:R369–R375.

37. DiBona G, Sawin L: Renal nerve activity in conscious rats during volume expansion and depletion. Am J Physiol 1985;248:F15–F23.

38. Miki K, Harashida Y, Sagawa S, Shiraki K: Renal sympathetic nerve activity and natriuresis during water immersion in conscious dogs. Am J Physiol 1989;256:R299–R305.

39. Miki K, Hayashida Y, Tajima F, et al: Renal sympathetic nerve activity and renal responses during head-up tilt in conscious dogs. Am J Physiol 1989;257:R337–R343.

40. Henriksen JH, Bendtsen F, Sørensen TIA, et al: Reduced central blood volume in cirrhosis. Gastorenterology 1989;97:1506–1513.

41. Kopp UC: Renorenal reflexes: Interaction between efferent and afferent renal neural activity. Can J Physiol Pharmacol 1992;70:750–758.

42. Kopp UC: Renorenal reflex. J Hypertens 1993;11:765–773.

43. Kostreva D, Seagard J, Castaner A, et al: Reflex effects of renal afferents on the heart and kidney. Am J Physiol 1981;241:R286–R292.

44. Kopp U, Olson L, DiBona G: Renorenal reflex responses to mechano- and chemoreceptor stimulation in the dog and rat. Am J Physiol 1984;246:F67–F77.

45. Kopp U, Smith L, DiBona G: Renorenal reflexes: Neural components of ipsilateral and contralateral renal responses. Am J Physiol 1985;249:F507–F517.

46. Anderson R, Cronin R, McDonald K, et al: Mechanisms of portal hypertension-induced alterations in renal hemodynamics, renal water excretion, and renin secretion. J Clin Invest 1976;58:964–970.

47. Lang F, Öttl I, Freundenschuss K, et al: Serotoninergic hepatorenal reflex regulating glomerular filtration rate. Pflugers Arch 1991;419:111–113.

48. Lang F, Tshernko E, Schulze E, et al: Hepatorenal reflex regulating kidney function. Hepatology 1991;14:590–594.

49. Levitt MF, Safirstein R: Hepatorenal reflex regulating kidney function. Hepatology 1991;14:734–735.

50. Levy M: Portal venous infusions of L-glutamine in anesthetized dogs, do not influence renal function. Can J Physiol Pharmacol 1992;70:1432–1435.

51. Morita H, Ishiki K, Hosomi H: Effects of hepatic NaCl receptor stimulation on renal nerve activity in conscious rabbits. Neurosci Lett 1991;123:1–3.

52. Morita H, Nishida Y, Hosomi H: Neural control of urinary sodium excretion during hypertonic NaCl load in conscious rabbits: Role of renal and hepatic nerves and baroreceptors. J Auton Nerv Sys 1991;34:157–170.

53. Morita H, Matsuda T, Furuya F, et al: Hepatorenal reflex plays an important role in natriuresis after high NaCl food intake in conscious dogs. Circ Res 1993;72:552–559.

54. Henriksen J, Ring-Larsen H, Christensen N: Sympathetic nervous activity in cirrhosis. A survey of plasma catecholamine studies. J Hepatol 1984;1:55–65.

55. Arroyo V, Planas R, Gaya J, et al: Sympathetic nervous activity, renin-angiotensin system and renal excretion of prostaglandin E_2 in cirrhosis. Relationship to functional renal failure and sodium and water excretion. Eur J Clin Invest 1983;13:271–278.

56. Burghardt W, Wernze H, Deihl K: Atrial natriuretic peptide in hepatic cirrhosis: Relation to stage of disease, sympathoadrenal system and renin-aldosterone axis. Klin Wochenschr 1986;64 (Suppl 6):103–107.

57. Epstein M, Larios O, Johnson G: Effects of water immersion on plasma catecholamines in decompensated cirrhosis. Miner Electrolyte Metab 1985;11:25–34.

58. Bichet D, Van Putten V, Schrier R: Potential role of increased sympathetic activity in impaired sodium and water excretion in cirrhosis. N Engl J Med 1982;307:1552–1557.

59. Willett I, Esler M, Burke F, et al: Total and renal sympathetic nervous system activity in alcoholic cirrhosis. J Hepatol 1985;1:639–648.

60. MacGilchrist AJ, Howes G, Hawksby C, Reid JL: Plasma noradrenaline in cirrhosis: A study of kinetics and temporal relationship to ascites formation. Eur J Clin Invest 1991;21:238–243.

61. Henriksen J, Ring-Larsen, Christensen N: Sympathetic nervous activity in cirrhosis: A survey of plasma catecholamine studies. J Hepatol 1984;1:55–65.

62. Floras JS, Legault L, Morali GA, et al: Increased sympathetic outflow in cirrhosis and ascites: Direct evidence from intraneural recordings. Ann Intern Med 1991;114:373–380.

63. Schrier RW, Arroyo V, Bernardi M, et al: Peripheral arterial vasodilation hypothesis: A proposal for the initiation of renal sodium and water retention in cirrhosis. Hepatology 1988;8:1151–1157.

64. Schrier RW: An odyssey into the milieu interieur: Pondering the enigmas. J Am Soc Nephrol 1992;2:1549–1559.

65. Unikowsky B, Wexler M, Levy M: Dogs with experimental cirrhosis of the liver but without intrahepatic hypertension do not retain sodium or form ascites. J Clin Invest 1983;72:1594–1604.

66. Wexler MJ, Levy M: Hepatic denervation alters first-phase urinary sodium excretion in dogs with cirrhosis. Am J Physiol 1987;253:F664–F671.

67. Levy M, Wexler MJ: Sodium excretion in dogs with low-grade caval constriction: Role of hepatic nerves. Am J Physiol 1987;253:F672–F678.

68. Wilkinson S, Bernardi M, Smith I, et al: Effect of β-adrenergic blocking drugs on the renin-aldosterone system, sodium excretion, and renal hemodynamics in cirrhosis with ascites. Gastroenterology 1977;73:659–663.

69. Willet I, Esler M, Jennings G, et al: Sympathetic tone modulates portal venous pressure in alcoholic cirrhosis. Lancet 1986;2:939–943.

70. Albillos A, Banares R, Barrios C, et al: Oral administration of clonidine in patients with alcoholic cirrhosis. Gastroenterology 1992;102:248–254.

71. Roulot D, Moreau R, Gaudin C, et al: Increased sympathetic and hemodynamic responses to clonidine in patients with cirrhosis and ascites. Gastroenterology 1992;102:1309–1318.

72. Esler M, Dudley F, Jennings G, et al: Increased sympathetic nervous activity and the effects of its inhibition with clonidine in alcoholic cirrhosis. Ann Intern Med 1992;116:446–455.

73. Epstein M, Berk D, Hollenberg N, et al: Renal failure in the patient with cirrhosis. The role of active vasoconstriction. Am J Med 1970;49:175–185.

74. Gatta A, Merkel C, Grassertto M, et al: Enhanced renal sympathetic tone in liver cirrhosis: Evaluation by intrarenal administration of dihydroergocristine. Nephron 1982;30:364-367.

75. Baldus W: Etiology and management of renal failure in cirrhosis. Ann NY Acad Sci 1970;170:267-279.

76. Ring-Larsen H, Henriksen JH, Christensen NJ: Prerenal failure. N Engl J Med 1989;320:393–398.

77. Fernandez-Seara J, Prieto J, Quiroga J, et al: Systemic and regional hemodynamics in patients with liver cirrhosis and ascites with and without functional renal failure. Gastroenterology 1989;97:1304–1312.

78. Rimola A, Gines P, Arroyo V, et al: Urinary excretion of 6-keto-prostaglandin $F_{1\alpha}$, thromboxane B_2 and prostaglandin E_2 in cirrhosis with ascites: Relationship to functional renal failure (hepatorenal syndrome). J Hepatol 1986;3:111–117.

79. Melman A, Massry S: Role of renal vasodilation in the blunted natriuresis of saline infusion in dogs with chronic bile duct obstruction. J Lab Clin Med 1977;89:1053-1065.

80. Simon M-A, Diez J, Prieto J: Abnormal sympathetic and renal response to sodium restriction in compensated cirrhosis. Gastroenterology 1991;101:1354–1360.

81. Friberg P, Meredith I, Jennings G, et al: Evidence for increased renal norepinephrine overflow during sodium restriction in humans. Hypertension 1990;16:121–130.

82. Morali GA, Floras JS, Legault L, et al: Muscle sympathetic nerve activity and renal responsiveness to atrial natriuretic factor during the development of hepatic ascites. Am J Med 1991;91:383–392.

83. Morali GA, Tobe SW, Skorecki KL, Blendis LM: Refractory ascites: Modulation of atrial natriuretic factor unresponsiveness by mannitol. Hepatology 1992;16:42–48.

84. Shohat J, Iaina A, Serban E, et al: The effect of propranolol on renal sodium handling in patients with cirrhosis. Biomedicine 1979;31:128–131.

Chapter 20

JAUNDICE AND THE KIDNEY

ARIEH BOMZON, Ph.D.
GIRIS JACOB, M.D.
ORI S. BETTER, M.D.

Jaundice and Renal Failure
  Renal Perfusion
  Tubular Function
  Conclusions
**Extrarenal and Predisposing Factors in the
  Pathogenesis of Renal Failure**
  Cardiovascular System
  Anemia
  Malnutrition
  Concomitant Bacteremia and Endotoxemia

Impaired Stress Response
  Hemorrhage
  Anesthesia and Preanesthetic Medications
Bile Constituents and Renal Failure
  Bile Acids
  Bilirubin
General Conclusion
  Prophylactic Treatment of Renal Failure in Jaundice
  Postoperative Management of Jaundiced Patients

Three of every four surgical patients who develop acute renal failure die, and the jaundiced patient is considered to be at a higher risk than the nonjaundiced patient.[1–4] Despite advances in perioperative care, the incidence rates for clinical association between jaundice and acute renal failure have changed little over the past 25 years.[5] Wait and Kahng found that the mean operative mortality rate in patients with obstructive jaundice was 16%, and the incidence of postoperative renal failure was approximately 9%. The mortality rate in the subgroup developing acute renal failure was 76%. The mortality rate from acute renal failure following biliary tract surgery in nonjaundiced patients is approximately 0.1%. Although such figures do not indicate a causal relationship, they emphasize the increased propensity of jaundiced patients undergoing surgical procedures to develop and die from acute renal failure.

The biliary tract is an important excretory route for many compounds that are potentially toxic. When this route is obstructed, such compounds accumulate in the plasma, and the kidney becomes the main excretory organ. Thus, in cholestatic liver disease, the patient becomes dependent on the kidney for survival, because it is the only route available for disposal of bile constituents.

Walker was one of the first to recognize an association between jaundice and renal function.[6]

He described his observations in 11 jaundiced patients who developed renal failure. Each patient had acute tubular necrosis with blood urea levels over 200 mg/dl. The causes of jaundice were obstructive jaundice (7 patients), acute liver necrosis from inhalation of the hepatotoxin, carbon tetrachloride (2 patients), and traumatic shock (2 patients). Walker observed a 40% reduction in renal blood flow, and the transit time for red blood cells through the oliguric kidneys was increased. The urine contained high concentrations of sodium, and the endogenous creatinine clearance was less than 1 ml/min. Renal biopsy showed normal glomeruli with either mild degenerative changes and dilatation of the distal tubules with bile casts or an acute tubular necrosis with bile casts. Dehydration, hemorrhage, hypotension, and sepsis were present in each case. Walker was unable to correlate the severity of renal disease with the degree of hepatic damage; thus he was unable to present direct evidence for the existence of a hepatorenal syndrome. However, he hypothesized that the presence of bile or some toxic metabolite from the damaged liver cells rendered the kidney more susceptible to damage.

At postmortem examination, the kidneys of jaundiced patients are swollen and discolored because of the accumulation of bile constituents such as bile acids and bilirubin; renal enlargement is an inflammatory reaction characterized by disruption of the tubular epithelium, cellular infiltration, and edema induced by accumulation of bile constituents.[7] In addition, cardiovascular dysfunction also is present in jaundiced patients. Cardiovascular features include a tendency to hypotension, hypovolemia, bradycardia, and increased risk of peri- and postoperative hemorrhagic shock. Because the kidney lesion is not unlike that seen in acute tubular necrosis following hemorrhagic shock, such cardiovascular factors may well predispose the kidney to shut down.

This chapter describes jaundice-induced renal failure and delineates some of the pathophysiologic mechanisms that contribute to onset of this life-threatening complication by answering three questions:

1. What is the effect of jaundice on renal function?

2. Is renal failure a consequence of the effects of jaundice on extrarenal factors such as the cardiovascular system (prerenal failure)?

3. Are bile constituents, such as bile acids and bilirubin, nephrotoxic?

Although the same three questions were addressed in a previous edition of this book, additional information derived from studies in jaundiced patients and animal experiments has become available since its publication in 1988.[8] This information has expanded our knowledge base and led to a greater understanding of why the jaundiced patient is more likely to develop postoperative renal failure, and to become more susceptible to hemorrhagic shock.

JAUNDICE AND RENAL FAILURE

Studies on the effect of jaundice on renal function are few and have failed to provide unequivocal answers. For example, Thompson and colleagues,[9] using ^{99m}Tc-DTPA renal scintigraphy, measured the changes in renal blood flow and glomerular filtration in 6 patients with obstructive jaundice before and 8 weeks after elective hepatobiliary surgery. They compared the results with those observed in 6 nonjaundiced patients undergoing the same procedure. There was no significant difference in preoperative renal mean transit time between the jaundiced and control patients. In the jaundiced patients they found no significant difference in mean renal transit times before and after surgery, whereas in the control patients postoperative renal transit times were increased from preoperative values. Postoperative glomerular filtration rates in the jaundiced patients were lower than in the controls preoperatively. After surgery glomerular filtration rates rose in the jaundiced patients and fell in the control patients, but postoperative values were not significantly different from each other. Thompson and colleagues proposed that the changes in glomerular filtration rate may simply reflect altered renal perfusion and that the changes in renal blood flow may be the underlying mechanism of increased renal susceptibility to injury (Fig. 20.1).

Unfortunately, clinical studies are difficult to undertake and do not always address the question in its entirety. The study by Thompson et al. is no exception; its shortcoming is failure to monitor changes in tubular function, such as sodium excretion, when blood flow and glomerular filtration were measured.

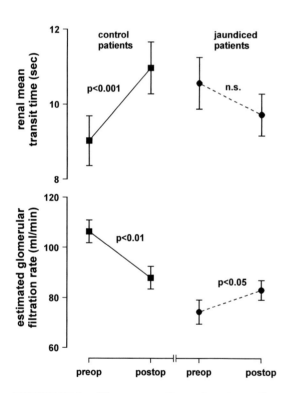

FIGURE 20.1. The preoperative and postoperative mean renal transit times (*top*) and estimated glomerular filtration rates (*bottom*) for 6 nonjaundiced control patients and 6 patients with obstructive jaundice. Mean values with standard error are shown. (Modified from Thompson JN, Carolan G, Myers MJ, Blumgart LH: The perioperative changes in glomerular function and renal blood flow in patients with obstructive jaundice. Acta Chir Scand 1989; 155:465–470, with permission.)

Many of the limitations of clinical investigation can be overcome by using experimental animals. The recently published study of Monasterolo et al.[10] in bile duct-ligated rats neatly summarizes the renal events following the onset of cholestasis. The authors found that the fractional excretion of water, sodium, and potassium increased as the total serum bilirubin levels rose over the 6 days of bile duct ligation. Over the same period, renal plasma flow decreased, whereas glomerular filtration rate remained essentially unchanged, slightly above normal values despite reduction in renal plasma flow from the second postoperative day (Fig. 20.2). The authors also demonstrated that the reduction in renal blood flow was due to active renal vasoconstriction, because the effects could be reversed by dopamine. Moreover, they demonstrated that diuresis and natriuresis in the face of reduced renal blood flow could be reversed by the renal vasodilator, dopamine.

Clinical vs. Animal Studies. A brief review of study design highlights important differences between clinical studies in jaundiced patients and experimental studies in bile duct-ligated animals:

1. Clinical studies are always conducted with jaundiced patients before and after decompression of the biliary obstruction. In animal experiments, the order of measurements is reversed; that is, biliary obstruction is produced in healthy animals, and it is assumed that the development of jaundice and its complications reflects the changes as they occur in the clinical environment but in reverse order.

2. Experimental results do not always agree with clinical observations. For example, renal blood or plasma flow and glomerular filtration rate are reduced in jaundiced patients. In the animal study renal blood flow was reduced, but glomerular filtration rate remained normal and then tended to increase.

3. Usually only one measurement is made after decompressive surgery when the patient is no longer jaundiced, and it is often performed after a considerable time lapse. In the study of Thompson et al.,[9] measurements were made 8 weeks later; and the investigators assumed that the clinical end-points were representative of the changes that took place over the observation period when measurements were not made. In animal studies, repeated measurements are easy to make, regardless of whether the design is longitudinal or cross-sectional. Hence, day-to-day measurements can be made, and it is possible to

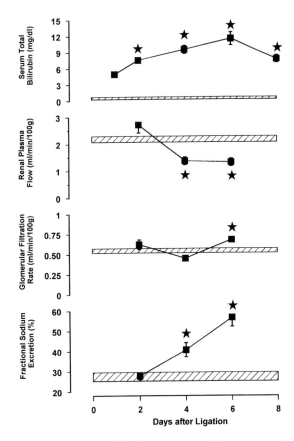

FIGURE 20.2. The time course of serum total bilirubin, renal plasma flow, glomerular filtration rate, and fractional sodium excretion in bile duct-ligated rats. The hatched areas represent the estimated normal ranges for each variable. Mean values with standard error are show. * = significance of differences from control. (Modified from Monasterolo L, Peiretti A, Elias MM: Rat renal functions during the first days post-bile duct ligation. Ren Fail 1993; 15:461–467, with permission.)

conduct research into the underlying mechanism and to evaluate the efficacy of potential therapy.

4. Clinical studies are usually performed with noninvasive techniques when the patient is conscious, whereas highly invasive techniques, usually under anesthesia, are used in animal experiments.

5. Interpretation of data from such studies, whether clinical or experimental, is often difficult, because the times at which the measurements were made differ preoperatively and postoperatively and do not always correspond to the peaks of jaundice and hepatocellular damage which themselves may vary between man and animals and from species to species.

6. There are both quantitative and qualitative differences within and between species in jaundice secondary to bile duct ligation. In animals the duration and severity of jaundice and hepatocellular damage are markedly influenced by whether the bile duct was ligated only or ligated and divided or resected between the ligatures. Such factors (reviewed by Better and Bomzon[8] and Bomzon and Blendis[11] influence the rate of onset of complications in liver disease. The significance of the different rates or onset of change to the clinical population is not known.

Renal Perfusion

What is the effect of jaundice on the kidney? The short answer is that jaundice appears to promote diuresis and natriuresis in the face of renal vasoconstriction and an essentially unchanged glomerular filtration rate. The mechanism of such changes is not clearly understood, and the following section discusses possible mediators (Table 20.1). The role of many of these mediators in cholestasis is not known.

Norepinephrine is the best studied mediator in bile duct-ligated animals. Angiotensin and prostaglandins have been studied to a far lesser extent. Studies of the effects of atrial natriuretic factor in jaundice have begun only recently. Of the remainder, bile constituents, bile acids, and bilirubin are discussed elsewhere in this chapter. The role of endotoxin was discussed previously in an earlier edition of this book.[8,12] No information about the roles in obstructive jaundice of endothelium-derived vasoactive compounds, nitric

oxide, endothelin and endothelium-derived hyperpolarizing factor, kallikrein-kinin system, and glomerulopressin has been published.

Renal Sympathetic Nerves and Norepinephrine

The physiologic role in renal blood flow of the sympathetic nerves and their neurotransmitter, norepinephrine, has been extensively studied and reviewed.[13–15] Of all the mediators, norepinephrine has been the most widely studied in jaundice but the results are conflicting.

Some studies indicate that sympathetic nervous system hyperactivity or excessive norepinephrine mediates renal vasoconstriction. One of the first groups to examine the effects of norepinephrine on renal blood flow was Bomzon and colleagues in a study of bile duct-ligated baboons.[16,17] Using xenon wash-out, Bomzon and colleagues observed a time-dependent reduction in renal blood flow and its intrarenal distribution with no change in systemic blood pressure.[16,17] Their data suggested that reduced renal perfusion was associated with an enhanced renovascular reactivity to norepinephrine due to increased activity of renal vascular α-adrenoceptors. Their results were confirmed by Wait and Kahng, who studied the effects of renal nerve stimulation and norepinephrine on renal blood flow in experimentally induced extrahepatic cholestasis. Using an in vivo technique to measure renal blood flow in bile duct-ligated rats, Wait and Kahng also demonstrated enhanced renovascular reactivity to norepinephrine and renal nerve stimulation.[18,19] Moreover, they showed that renovascular changes were associated with decreased creatinine clearance, decreased sodium excretion, and increased renal prostaglandin production.

On the basis of such data, one may hypothesize that jaundice reduces renal blood flow and that the reduction is mediated by hyperactivity of the renal sympathetic nerves and hyperresponsiveness of the renal vascular α-adrenoceptors. The consequences of reduced renal perfusion are a reduction in glomerular filtration, reduced sodium excretion, and compensatory increase in the synthesis of renal prostaglandins. Some support for this hypothesis was provided by Schroeder and colleagues, who showed that incubating vascular tissue with jaundiced serum increased the vascular sensitivity to catecholamines by suppressing the synthesis of vascular prostacyclin.[20] Moreover, the authors claimed that the enhanced

TABLE 20.1. Known Mechanisms that May Contribute to the Renal Vasoconstriction and Diuresis and Natriuresis of Cholestasis

Humoral mechanisms
  Renin-angiotensin system
  Renal prostaglandins
  Endotoxin
  Endothelium-derived vasoactive factors
  Kallikrein-kinin system
  Bile constitutents
    Bile acids
    Bilirubin
    Cholesterol
  Glomerulopressin
  Atrial natriuretic peptide
Neural mechanisms
  Sympathetic nervous system
  Norepinephrine

renovascular response to catecholamines and the reduced synthesis of prostacyclin were associated with high levels of serum lipid peroxidases, which are elevated in jaundiced patients.[21]

In contrast, other data demonstrate vascular and renovascular hyporesponsiveness to norepinephrine in vessels isolated from jaundiced animals. Bomzon and coworkers observed that isolated vessels from bile duct-ligated rats exhibited hyporeactivity to norepinephrine.[22–25] Cioffi et al.[26] also found that the dose-response curves of renal and interlobar arteries from bile duct-ligated rabbits to norepinephrine were attenuated. They also showed that the norepinephrine response of segments of the renal and interlobar arteries from normal rabbits was blunted when incubated with jaundiced serum; this attenuation could be reversed by indomethacin.[26] Cioffi and colleagues concluded that obstructive jaundice induces a decreased renovascular response to norepinephrine and that this effect is modified by prostaglandins.

Finally, some data suggest that the renal nerves and norepinephrine have little or no effect on renal blood flow in cholestasis. Hishida and colleagues[27] showed normal renovascular reactivity to norepinephrine in bile duct-ligated rabbits. A later study by Bomzon et al.[28] showed that isolated blood vessels from bile duct-ligated dogs have normal responsiveness to norepinephrine. Because the same group also demonstrated that the number and binding affinity of α_1-adrenoceptors in rat kidneys were unaffected by jaundice,[29] it is not altogether surprising that renovascular reactivity to norepinephrine was normal.

Using another approach, Bomzon and colleagues showed that the urinary excretion of norepinephrine and its metabolites was unchanged in jaundiced rats compared with normals.[30] In an unpublished study, Bomzon and Lebrec were unable to demonstrate significant elevations in plasma norepinephrine and epinephrine levels in bile duct-ligated rats (Table 20.2). O'Neill et al.[31] also found that the perturbations in renal function in bile duct-ligated rats were not mediated by the renal sympathetic nerves.

Renin-Angiotensin System

Equally intriguing but less extensively investigated is the effect of jaundice on the renin-angiotensin system, which is also an important determinant of renal blood flow. Numerous studies have shown that 1 week after bile duct ligation, jaundiced animals have attenuated pressor responsiveness to angiotensin II[32] and that the attenuation is due to blunted responsiveness of the peripheral vasculature.[28] In the same animals, plasma renin substrate was decreased despite increases in plasma renin activity and plasma angiotensin II levels.[27] O'Neill and others found normal plasma renin activity in bile duct-ligated rats and concluded that the renin-angiotensin system was not involved in changes in renal function after bile duct ligation.[19] Their observations support the earlier findings of Hishida et al.,[27] who found normal renovascular responsiveness to angiotensin in bile duct-ligated rabbits. Finally, it is worth noting that angiotensinase activity in the plasma of jaundiced patients is higher than in normal controls[33]; this may explain angiotensin hyporesponsiveness and why no definitive role for the renin-angiotensin system in renal perfusion has been identified.

Because the above studies indicate that angiotensin is not responsible for the renal vasoconstriction of cholestasis, they also provide additional but indirect evidence that renal nerve hyperactivity and norepinephrine cannot be the causative mechanisms.

Renal Prostaglandins

Renal prostaglandins are synthesized and released in response to renal vasoconstriction,[34] and obstructive jaundice does not modify this response.[18,19] However, in studies of kidneys of jaundiced animals, it was not clear whether increased synthesis was of vascular or tubular origin (see chapter 14).

Tubular Function

Based on the initial observations by Walker[6] of tubular damage in jaundiced patients, it became widely accepted that jaundice was nephrotoxic. The nephrotoxicity manifested itself clinically as

TABLE 20.2. Plasma Norepinephrine and Epinephrine Concentrations in Sham-Operated and Bile Duct-ligated Rats*

	Norepinephrine (pg.ml)	Epinephrine (pg/ml)
Sham-operated	544 ± 126	768 ± 185
Bile duct-ligated	405 ± 54	462 ± 61

* Values are given as mean ± standard error of the mean. n = 7–9 (Bomzon and Lebrec, unpublished data.)

a reduction in glomerular filtration rate and reduced sodium excretion and was not secondary to renal vasoconstriction. In 1980 Masumoto and Masuoka[35] confirmed Walker's observations in various experimental models of jaundice by demonstrating reductions in glomerular filtration rate and tubular damage. However, this dogma was questioned after the observations of Hishida et al. and Alon and colleagues in 1982. Using bile duct-ligated rabbits, Hishida and colleagues failed to observe reductions in urine volume and urinary sodium excretion despite reduced renal perfusion and glomerular filtration rates.[27,36] Alon et al.[37] showed that cholemic dogs have normal glomerular filtration rates with an impaired ability to concentrate and dilute urine. In a subsequent study the same investigators showed that an intrarenal infusion of bile increased the mean fractional excretion of sodium and potassium in the face of unchanged clearances of inulin and para-aminohippuric acid.[38] Such results suggested that jaundice per se is not nephrotoxic but may cause diuresis, natriuresis, and kaliuresis. Additional support that jaundice was a salt losing syndrome was provided by Levy and Finestone,[39] Sitprija et al.,[40] and Monasterolo et al.[10]

The mechanism of diuresis is unknown, but several mediators have been suggested (see Table 20.1), including renal prostaglandins, atrial natriuretic factor, bile acids, and bilirubin. The physiologic role of prostaglandins and related compounds in kidney function is discussed in chapter 14. The effect of bilirubin and bile acids on tubular function is discussed below. Endotoxin was discussed in a previous edition of this book.[12]

Atrial Natriuretic Factor

Recent studies report that plasma levels of atrial natriuretic factor (ANF) are increased after bile duct ligation in rabbits.[41,42] This increase is associated with an increased amount of cardiac ANF content and a higher percentage of atrial cells that stain for ANF activity.[42] The investigators concluded that ANF may be involved in the pathogenesis of the renal tubular disturbances of water and sodium handling in obstructive jaundice.

Conclusion

What is the effect of jaundice on renal function? In the face of reduced renal perfusion, it seems that the kidney still attempts to fulfill it function as the main excretory organ for bile constituents by attempting to maintain the glomerular filtration rate and normal tubular function. The mechanism of renal vasoconstriction is unclear, but current evidence does not support a prominent role for either the renal nerves, its neurotransmitter, or angiotensin. The role of other vasoconstrictor mediators has not been investigated; therefore, it would be worthwhile to explore the role of factors such as endothelin on renal blood flow in obstructive jaundice. Regardless of the mechanism, prostaglandin synthesis is increased to counterbalance or minimize the yet undescribed mechanisms that promote renal vasoconstriction and may participate in the processes that lead to diuresis and natriuresis.

Despite the need to evaluate the role of other mediators, it is not clear how the combination of renal vasoconstriction and diuresis and natriuresis leads to renal failure. Neither clinical nor animal studies describe renal failure. Yet, as noted initially, the incidence of postoperative renal failure in jaundiced patients is high despite improvements in perioperative care. This suggests that other factors may be involved, some of which are discussed below.

EXTRARENAL AND PREDISPOSING FACTORS IN THE PATHOGENESIS OF RENAL FAILURE

The effect of jaundice on extrarenal factors need to be considered in any discussion of the development of renal failure in cholestatic patients. Factors other than the effects of jaundice on the cardiovascular system that predispose the cholestatic patient to renal failure may be classified into two categories: (1) factors related to the preoperative status of the jaundiced patient and (2) factors attributable to abdominal surgery (see Table 20.5).[43]

Cardiovascular System

In 1932 Meakins[44] described his observations of a patient with essential hypertension who developed "catarrhal jaundice" with complete biliary obstruction. He noted that with the onset of jaundice, blood pressure fell rapidly to normal and returned to the elevated value only long after the jaundice had dissipated. This observation stimulated considerable personal interest, and Meakins extracted from records of the local public hospital the blood pressure readings from

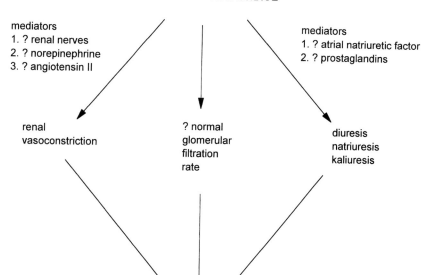

FIGURE 20.3. Summary of the known effects of obstructive jaundice on renal function and the possible mediators of the dysfunction.

100 cases of "catarrhal jaundice." He found that systolic, diastolic, and pulse pressures tended to be lower than in the normal population. Bradycardia was also a common clinical finding. In 1956 Zollinger and Williams[1] observed that jaundiced patients were more susceptible to hypotensive crises after intraoperative hemorrhage than nonjaundiced patients. In a subsequent study the same investigators recommended amelioration of the increased susceptibility by volume expansion prior to surgery.[45] In 1966 and 1967 Morandini and colleagues[46,47] observed that jaundiced patients were hypotensive and had attenuated pressor and flow responses to exogenous angiotensin II and norepinephrine. Collectively, such observations established that jaundice adversely affects cardiovascular function, but only recently has the pathophysiologic basis of jaundiced-induced cardiodepression been investigated.

In attempting to explain the tendency toward hypotension in jaundiced patients, pressor responsiveness to endogenous vasoactive compounds has been measured in bile duct-ligated animals. Such studies have demonstrated attenuated pressor responses to norepinephrine, α_1-adrenoceptor agonists,[25,28,48,49] and angiotensin II[28] but not to 5-hydroxytryptamine (serotonin)[50] or vasopressin.[50a] From such studies it was hypothesized that the hypotension of cholestasis was mediated by attenuated responsiveness to

sympathomimetic stimulation and angiotensin. Furthermore, the studies showed that the mechanisms of hypotension and pressor hyporesponsiveness are species-dependent; the effect of jaundice on the heart and blood vessels is different in the two widely used animal models of obstructive jaundice, bile duct-ligated dogs and rats.

Heart

The effect of jaundice on the heart has not been extensively studied. Several studies have shown that jaundice leads to cardiomyopathy, which in all likelihood is functional because the myocardium of bile duct-ligated dogs is histologically normal.[51]

One of the first experimental indications of such a myopathy was made by Better and Bomzon,[8] who reanalyzed the cardiac output data published by Sasha et al.[52] in chronic bile duct-ligated dogs. Reanalysis established that the increase in cardiac output after intravascular volume loading correlated with the serum bilirubin concentration. Since then, several studies in conscious and anesthetized bile duct ligated animals have described a jaundiced-induced cardiomyopathy characterized by impaired indices of contractility, such as the rate force of contraction and relaxation (dP/dt) and altered cardiac responsiveness to β-adrenoceptor stimulation.[28,53–55] Table 20.3 and Figure 20.4 describe the characteristics of

TABLE 20.3. Characteristics of a Single Cardiac Twitch from Sham-operated and 3-Day Bile Duct-ligated Rats*

Twitch Characteristics	Sham-operated Rats (n = 5)	Bile Duct-ligated Rats (n = 5)
Peak tension (mm Hg)	54 ± 4	44 ± 3†
+dP/dt (mm Hg/s)	1206 ± 97	807 ±25†
–dP/dt (mm Hg/s)	1186 ± 76	753 ± 53†
Time to peak tension (ms)	78 ± 4	78 ± 3
Twitch duration (ms)	146 ± 12	160 ± 10

* Values are mean ± standard error.
† Significance of difference between two groups, p < 0.05.
Modified from Jacob G, Nassar N, Hayam G, et al: Cardiac function and responsiveness to β-adrenoreceptor in rats with obstructive jaundice. Am J Physiol 1993;265:G314–G320, with permission.

single cardiac twitch measured from an intracardiac pressure recording in sham-operated and bile duct-ligated rats.[55]

To date, only one clinical study confirms the existence of jaundice-induced cardiomyopathy in patients. Lumlertgol et al.[56] described reduced left ventricular rate force of contraction as well as reduced cardiac responsiveness to dobutamine, the selective β₁-adrenoceptor agonist.

Peripheral Vasculature

The effect of jaundice on vascular reactivity to vasoactive amines and in particular to norepinephrine and α-adrenoceptor agonists has been extensively investigated by Bomzon and colleagues in bile duct-ligated rats.[22–25] The investigators showed that reduced contractile responsiveness to norepinephrine in jaundiced rats is reversible as the jaundice dissipates[23,24] (Fig. 20.5). Moreover,

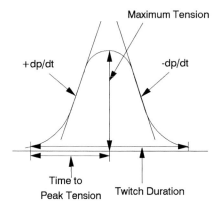

FIGURE 20.4. A schematic explanation of expressions used to characterize the single cardiac twitch, as outlined in Table 20.3.

they showed that bile duct ligation in the rat induces a functional defect in the expression of cardiovascular α₁-adrenoceptors with no effect on the activity of α₂-adrenoceptors or neuronal and extraneuronal uptake of norepinephrine.[25] In contrast, they also demonstrated that pressor and contractile responsiveness to 5-hydroxytryptamine[50] or pressor responsiveness to vasopressin[50a] was unaffected by bile duct ligation in rats.

Such findings indicate that bile duct ligation in rats exerts a deleterious effect on cardiovascular α₁-adrenoceptors. This effect is selective; it does not adversely affect other receptor systems that also use inositol phospholipid metabolism as the second messenger in the signal transduction process. Furthermore, the effect may have important therapeutic implications (see below) discussed later in this chapter. In jaundiced dogs, on the other hand, in vitro contractile vascular reactivity to norepinephrine was unaffected by jaundice,[28] although in both bile duct-ligated dogs and rats, the reactivity to angiotensin II was blunted.[28,49]

Finally, diminished responsiveness in rats is transient; loss of response is maximal at the peak of jaundice and disappears as the jaundice dissipates.[23,24] The effect of time on responsiveness has not been studied in other species. Table 20.4 summarizes the effects of jaundice on the different receptor systems; it is not obvious why they behave differently in different animal models of obstructive jaundice.

Blood Volume

The status of blood volume in jaundiced patients and animals is controversial. Williams, Elliott, and Zollinger[45] claimed that intravascular blood volume was reduced in bile duct-ligated dogs if the calculations were based on preoperative or preligation weight, rather than postoperative weight. Later studies by Yarger,[57] Aarseth et al.,[58] and Gillett[59] also described reduced blood volume in bile duct-ligated rats. Cattell and Birstingl calculated that absolute blood and plasma volumes were altered by bile duct ligation, even if they were corrected for the pre- and postoperative weights.[60]

Using hematocrit as an index of plasma volume, some investigators have reported reductions in packed cell volume,[57,61,62] whereas others have reported no change.[58] The interpretation of hematocrit as a measure of blood cell volume is hazardous, because survival time and membrane

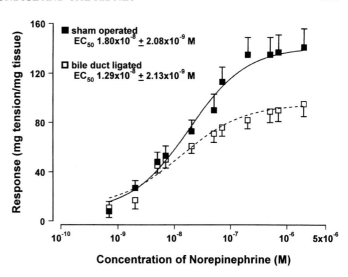

FIGURE 20.5. The effect of increasing concentrations of norepinephrine on isolated rat arterial rings prepared from sham-operated and 3-day bile duct-ligated rats. (Modified from Gali D, Blendis LM, Bomzon A: Vascular reactivity in reversible experimental obstructive jaundice. J Surg Res 1987;42:242–246.)

integrity of red blood cells may be compromised in jaundice by plasma accumulation of bile acids.[63]

We recently measured blood volume using ^{125}I-labeled albumin in 3-day bile duct-ligated rats and compared the results with unoperated control and bile duct-manipulated (sham-operated) rats.[50a] No significant differences in absolute blood volumes and hematocrit were found among the three groups. However, when blood volume was adjusted to postoperative body weight, the ml/g blood volume was significantly lower in bile duct-ligated rats than in the other two groups.

Clearly there is a tendency toward hypotension and depression of cardiovascular function in jaundice. The hypotension is due to (1) functional cardiomyopathy that may be associated with down-regulation of β-adrenoceptors, (2) impaired function of α[1]-adrenoceptors in the vasculature and attenuated responsiveness to angiotensin II, and (3) relative hypovolemia.

In addition, one cannot overlook the role of additional factors that are considered to predispose the jaundiced patient to develop postoperative acute renal failure (Table 20.5).

Anemia

The evidence that jaundiced patients are anemic dates back to the studies of Jordan and coworkers in 1930.[64,65] Since then little has been done to establish the origin of anemia or to explain how it relates to development of renal failure. Much of the recent evidence for anemia is based on the finding of reduced hematocrit in jaundiced patients and bile duct-ligated animals. However, it has been shown that survival time of red blood cells in jaundiced rats is reduced and that the fragility of the red blood cell membrane is increased.[63] The plasma accumulation of bile salts has been proposed to account for such disturbances in red blood cell function.[63]

Malnutrition

Jaundiced patients lose weight because of (1) reduced appetite and food intake, (2) fat malabsorption due to absence or decreased amounts of bile acids in the intestine, or (3) both. We have recorded up to 15% weight loss after 3 days of

TABLE 20.4. Summary of Certain Experiments that Measured Vascular Reactivity of Isolated Vessels to Different Agonists Prepared from Bile Duct-ligated Animals

Model	Agonist	Preparation	Response	Reference
3-Day BDL rat	NE	Portal vein	Diminished	22
3-Day BDL rat	NE	Aortic ring	Diminished	23
6-Day BDL rat	NE	Aortic ring and portal vein	Normal	24
3-Week BDL dog	NE	Arterial strips	Normal	28
3-Week BDL dog	AII	Arterial strips	Diminished	28
3-Day BDL rat	5-HT	Aortic ring and portal vein	Normal	50

BDL = bile duct-ligated, NE = norepinephrine, AII = angiotensin II, 5-HT = serotonin

TABLE 20.5. Factors Predisposing to Postoperative Renal Failure in Jaundiced Patients

Patient factors
  Anemia
  Degree of jaundice
  Concomitant bacteremia
  Coexisting cholangitis
  Coexisting pancreatitis
  Malnutrition
  Malignancy
  Impaired stress response

Perioperative factors
  Hemorrhage
  Laparotomy
  Preanesthetic medicants
  Anesthetic agents

bile duct ligation in laboratory rats.[23] Reduced fluid intake probably contributes to weight loss and relative hypovolemia. There are also alterations in the body water compartments.[66] Other studies have shown that cellular energy metabolism is reduced by jaundice.[67] Finally, in obstructive jaundice hepatic extraction of insulin is increased, whereas pancreatic secretion is decreased.[68] This too contributes to malnutrition by reducing the availability of intracellular glucose for cellular energy metabolism.

Concomitant Bacteremia and Endotoxemia

Jaundiced patients have a concomitant portal and systemic endotoxemia and bacteremia.[69–74] The many causative factors include gastric mucosal

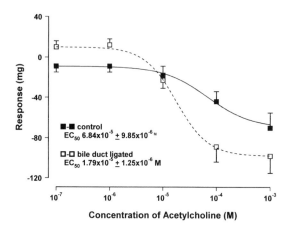

FIGURE 20.6. Response of isolated arterial rings to increasing concentrations of acetylcholine. Values are mean ± standard error of the mean; n = 6–9. (Mor and Bomzon A, unpublished data.)

barrier breakdown,[71] increased bacterial translocation,[75,76] reduced amounts of intestinal bile salt and increased endotoxin absorption,[77] impaired gastrointestinal bile flow and Kupffer cell function,[78] and impaired bactericidal capacity.[79] In addition, immune suppression is associated with serum and cellular factors,[80,81] lymphocyte function is reduced,[82] and response to alloantigens is blunted.[83] Collectively, such data indicate that a functional deficit in the endogenous protective systems renders the jaundiced patient more susceptible to infection and endotoxins.

Many authors believe that endotoxin is the most important causative factor in the development of renal and cardiovascular complications of jaundice. Endotoxin induces the enzyme, nitric oxide synthase, to enhance the secretion of the endothelial-derived vasorelaxant, nitric oxide.[84] This labile vasodilator may contribute to the hypotension of jaundice but in all likelihood has little effect in the renal vasculature, where vasoconstriction is present. The vasodilator response of isolated endothelium-intact rat arterial rings to acetylcholine (which stimulates the release of nitric oxide from the vascular endothelium) was unaffected by bile duct ligation (Fig. 20.6).

Impaired Stress Response

Experimental evidence suggests that jaundice blunts the response to stress. We have shown that laparotomy and bile duct manipulation cause upregulation of renal α_1-adrenoceptors[29] and central and peripheral binding sites of benzodiazepines.[85] Because of functional downregulation of cardiovascular adrenoceptors in surgically induced extrahepatic cholestasis,[25,30,86] such data indicate that jaundice may impair the compensatory cardiovascular response by suppression of the upregulatory response of receptors induced by surgery. If this is so, the stress response to abdominal surgery in jaundiced patients would be expected to be suppressed. Recently, Swain et al.[87] observed that suppression of the stress response is mediated by the hypothalamic–pituitary–adrenal axis in bile duct-ligated rats. We believe that the "natural" surgically-induced stress is suppressed after biliary surgery in jaundiced patients. Obviously, this idea needs validation by clinical and experimental investigations that compare the responses of the renal and cardiovascular systems to various identical stimuli in normal and jaundiced patients.

Hemorrhage

Although the causes of blood coagulation disorders in patients with hepatobiliary disease are particularly complex,[7] it is easy to understand why jaundiced patients have a tendency to bleeding episodes. The consequences of moderate hemorrhage during surgery may reduce renal perfusion; in nonjaundiced patients, this event is well tolerated. In jaundiced patients, however, even minor hemorrhage during surgery often has fatal consequences, in part perhaps because anesthesia exacerbates the preoperative relative hypovolemia in jaundiced patients. The different studies that emphasize the importance of anesthesia in enhancing the susceptibility of jaundiced patients to hemorrhagic shock were reviewed by Better and Bomzon.[8]

Levy [87a] reduced the blood pressure by 30–40 mmHg by removing up to 500 ml of blood from conscious and anesthetized sham-operated and bile duct-ligated dogs for 5 consecutive days. This procedure predisposed the anesthetized bile duct-ligated dogs but not the conscious dogs to acute renal insufficiency. A recent study by Bomzon and coworkers showed that the rate of onset of hypotension and mortality following a controlled hemorrhage in conscious bile duct-ligated rats was not significantly different from that in unoperated control or sham-operated rats.[49] Using the same rat model, we found that the volume of removed blood necessary to drop mean arterial blood pressure in pentobarbitone-anesthetized rats to 60 mmHg was 25% less than the volume necessary to cause the identical effect in control and sham-operated rats.[50a] This finding agrees with the earlier observations of Aarseth et al.,[58,88] who demonstrated that anesthetized bile duct-ligated rats were sensitive to hemorrhage because the different partitioning of plasma volume impaired compensatory response to bleeding.

Anesthesia and Preanesthetic Medications

Anesthesia in jaundiced patients necessitates evaluation of three factors: (1) the extent to which the particular anesthetic agent depends on the liver for inactivation or elimination, (2) the effect of the agent on liver function, and (3) the effect of the agent on renal and cardiovascular function. The third factor is probably more important than the other two in selecting an anesthetic agent. These same considerations need to be assessed in the selection of anesthetic premedications, which also affect the renal and cardiovascular systems. In practical terms, the roles of individual anesthetic agents and anesthetic premedications in determining the postoperative incidence of renal and cardiovascular side effects are by and large unknown despite extensive knowledge of the pharmacologic effects of individual agents on renal and vascular function.

We recently compared the effects of three different anesthetic agents—halothane, sodium pentobarbitone, and fentanyl—on pressor responsiveness in bile duct ligated-dogs.[89] We found no synergistic or antagonistic effects of anesthesia and jaundice on cardiovascular responsiveness. Data showed that halothane- and barbiturate-induced anesthesia did not alter blood pressure in unoperated dogs. The negative results, however, do not exclude other potential adverse effects of other anesthetic agents on different aspects of cardiovascular and renal function.

Clearly prerenal factors are important in the development of postoperative renal failure. Based on existing knowledge, we propose that the mechanism of postoperative renal failure and hemorrhagic shock is multifactorial in origin. The contributory factors are jaundice-induced derangements of renal and cardiovascular function, diminished intracellular energy metabolism, and a functional deficit or suppression of the protective and defense systems of the body. The confounding influences of surgery, anesthesia, and minor surgical bleeding may exacerbate the precarious state of the jaundiced patient; 9% succumb to postoperative renal failure, which has fatal consequences in 3 of 4 cases (Fig. 20.7).

BILE CONSTITUENTS AND RENAL FAILURE

The plasma accumulation of bile constituents that are normally secreted via the biliary and gastrointestinal tracts has long been thought to be involved in the pathogenesis of renal failure in cholestatic liver disease. Of the many substances, two compounds, bile acids and bilirubin, have been considered pathogenic because they accumulate in the plasma of jaundiced patients and both are known to be toxic (Fig. 20.8).

Bile Acids

The role of bile acids in the pathogenesis of renal failure in jaundiced patients has fascinating

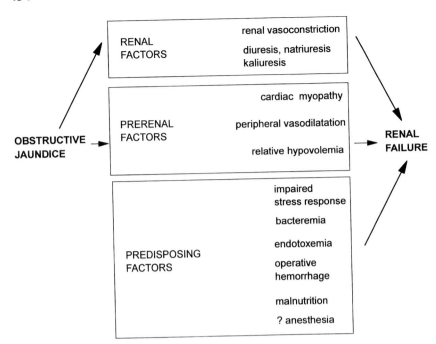

FIGURE 20.7. A summary of the renal, prerenal, and predisposing factors that contribute to the development of postoperative renal failure in jaundiced patients.

aspects: (1) they have been implicated as nephrotoxins, because they reduce glomerular filtration rate and sodium excretion after transient ischemia[90]; (2) they are cardiodepressants[91] and hence are thought to be one of the prerenal mediators that contribute to the development of renal failure[92-96]; and (3) they are renoprotectants, because they are vasodilators,[22,97] promote diuresis,[38,98-100] and reduce intestinal absorption of endotoxin.[77] Understanding of these features is facilitated by basic information about the biosynthesis and physicochemical properties of bile acids. Additional and more specific information can be found in the comprehensive review by Radominska et al.[101]

Biosynthesis

Bile acids are steroids synthesized from free cholesterol in hepatocytes; the conversion of cholesterol into bile acids represents the major pathway for elimination of cholesterol from the body. Bile acids are essential for the solubilization of lipids in bile, the induction and possible maintenance of bile flow, and the absorption of fat from the gastrointestinal tract. Initially, they are synthesized into two primary types—cholic acid and chenodeoxycholic acid. The primary bile acids may be conjugated by amidation with amino acids (glycine and taurine), sulfated, or glucuronidated within the liver to give rise to conjugated bile acids; they also may undergo bacterial

transformation or dehydroxylation in the intestine to give rise to secondary bile acids such as deoxycholic acid. Hence, the bile acid pool contains a mixture of primary bile acids, conjugated bile acids, and secondary bile acids.

Conjugation and presence of hydroxyl groups on the steroid nucleus increase hydrophilicity; thus it is common to refer to the hydrophobic-hydrophilic balance of an individual bile acid.[102] The relative balance between the hydrophobic and hydrophilic properties of naturally occurring bile acids is determined by state of ionization, orientation, position and number of hydroxyl groups, and presence or absence of side-chain esters, be they taurine, glycine, sulfate, or glucuronate (Fig. 20.9).

The highest plasma concentrations of bile acids are found in the portal vasculature because of their enterohepatic circulation. The total systemic concentration of bile acids is less than 1 μM, and they are usually bound to albumin and lipoproteins. The total free plasma concentration of bile acids is low, probably in the order of nM. In liver disease, the total systemic concentration of bile acids rises as high as 100 μM, and the ratio between free and bound bile acids increases as the concentrations rise. Because the bile acid pool contains a mixture of bile acids, the plasma bile acid profiles vary with the different types of liver disease, depending on the nature of hepatocellular damage, degree of biliary obstruction,

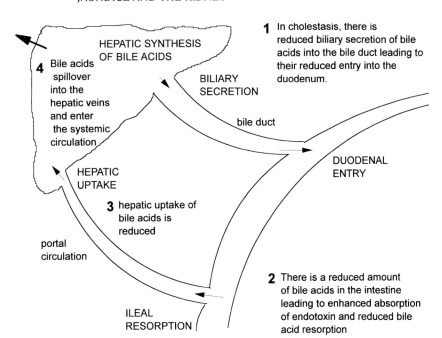

FIGURE 20.8. The derangement in the bile acid pool that occurs in cholestasis.

and presence of portosystemic shunts. In cholestatic liver disease such as obstructive jaundice, urinary excretion of bile acids increases, the ratio of trihydroxy- to dihydroxy-bile acids decreases, and sulfation and glucuronidation become the significant modes of conjugation.

As a group, the bile acids are amphipathic compounds with physicochemical properties that enable them to interact with biologic membranes, including insertion into the lipid bilayer and solubilization. Such effects depend to a great extent on the hydrophobic-hydrophilic balance and con-

centration of the bile acid. Moreover, the effects are observed predominantly with the hydrophobic bile acids at low concentrations and are less likely to occur with more hydrophilic bile acids, even at high concentrations. Hydrophobic bile acid-induced membrane damage appears to involve the production of oxygen free radicals. In epithelial cells, hydrophobic bile acids such as deoxycholic acid and chenodeoxycholic acid increase membrane turnover of phospholipids and production of oxygen free radicals. Free radicals injure tissue by attacking membrane lipids, thiol

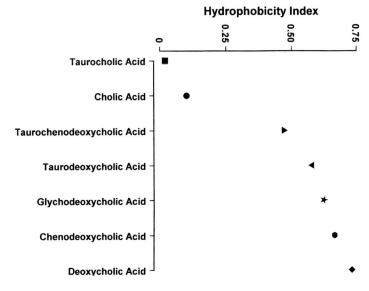

FIGURE 20.9. The hydrophobicity index of several different bile acids. (Modified from Heuman DM: Quantitative estimates of mixed bile salt solutions. J Lipid Res 1989;30:719–730, with permission.)

proteins, or nucleic acid and causing lipid peroxidation, which in turn leads to accumulation of highly toxic lipoxides, such as malondialdehyde and 4-hydroxynonal.[103] Evidence for the mediation role of oxygen free radicals in bile acid-induced membrane damage was recently provided by Sokol et al.,[104] who showed that bile acids, especially the hydrophobic species, enhance lipid peroxidation. In cholestatic liver disease, the bile acid pool shifts in favor of hydrophobic bile acids; this shift tends to promote tissue damage mediated by oxygen free radicals. Several studies have reported increases in the activity of plasma and tissue peroxidases[20,21]; the plasma accumulation of bile acids may account for this increase.

Nephrotoxicity

In 1962 Walker[6] suggested that a bile constituent from damaged liver cells rendered the kidney more sensitive to damage. Bile acids seem likely culprits, because they can inhibit cellular

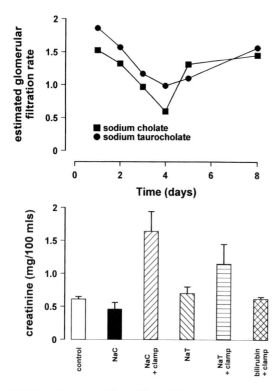

metabolism,[105–109] disrupt cell membranes, and cause hemolysis.[110–112]

In 1968 Aoyago and Lowenstein[90] attempted to validate the hypothesis of bile acid nephrotoxicity by intravenously infusing 5 µmol/min sodium cholate (NaC) and sodium taurocholate (NaT) into the femoral artery of anesthetized rats. At the end of the 30-minute infusion period, the renal pedicle was clamped for 30 minutes, and the animals were allowed to recover in metabolic cages. Over the next 8 days the investigators measured serum and urinary creatinine as well as urinary water and sodium excretion. Results were compared among different groups of rats who had (1) the two bile acids infused without clamping, (2) a saline infusion with clamping, (3) a 2.5% albumin infusion with clamping, and (4) an infusion of bilirubin with clamping. The rats that received the infusions of the two bile acids followed by clamping showed a decrease in glomerular filtration rate and water and sodium excretion over the first 4 days (Fig. 20.10). Thereafter, all three variables began to return to normal, and by the eighth day glomerular filtration and water and sodium excretion had reached normal values. Such changes were associated with increases in serum creatinine levels (Fig. 20.10). Because no changes in glomerular filtration rate, water and sodium excretion, or serum creatinine levels were observed in control groups, the authors concluded that bile acids in combination with renal ischemia rendered the kidney susceptible to renal insufficiency.

For many years this conclusion was accepted dogma until it was realized that the results were not consistent with observations in bile duct-ligated animals or after intrarenal infusions of bile or bile salts. Using the experiment of Monasterolo et al.[10] (see Fig. 20.2) as the representative example and assuming that renal ischemia represents maximal renal vasoconstriction, one can see obvious differences between the two experiments. By the end of the fourth day after bile duct ligation, water and sodium excretion increased without significant change in the glomerular filtration rate. Over the same period, bile acid infusion and renal ischemia reduced glomerular filtration rate and excretion of water and sodium.

Another approach used to test the Walker hypothesis was evaluation of the effect of bile acids by intrarenal infusion of different bile acids at pathophysiologic plasma concentrations. Using anesthetized baboons, Bomzon et al.[113] were unable

FIGURE 20.10. The effect of 5-µmol/min intravenous infusion of sodium cholate (NaC) and sodium taurocholate (NaT) on glomerular filtration rate and serum creatinine levels in anesthetized rats. (Modified from Aoyagi T, Lowenstein LM: The effect of bile acids and renal ischemia on renal perfusion. J Lab Clin Med 1968;71:686–692, with permission.)

to show that sodium taurocholate modified renal blood flow, its intrarenal distribution, or renovascular reactivity to norepinephrine; these in vivo findings were confirmed in isolated perfused rabbit kidneys (Fig. 20.11).

The study by Aoyagi and Lowenstein established that bile acids are nephrotoxic. In fact, their experiment is one of renal ischemia and reperfusion. This procedure is a potent stimulus for releasing reactive oxygen species, and such oxygen free radicals play a major role in causing microvascular and cellular injury.[114] The end result of oxidative attack is cell swelling, and interstitial edema with ultimate cell death and tissue necrosis. This description is similar to that of jaundiced kidney.[6,7] In the experiment of Aoyagi and Lowenstein,[90] endogenous oxygen radical scavengers in kidneys from the control groups overcame the oxidative attack resulting from 30 minutes of ischemia and reperfusion. We propose that with the addition of a second mediator that generates oxygen free radicals—i.e., infusion of bile acid—the kidney was unable to overcome the two-pronged oxidative attack; hence the transient loss of tubular function. In the same vein, it is not altogether surprising that the results of the experiment of Bomzon and colleagues[113] was negative. The oxidative attack was minimal, because the investigators used taurocholic acid, a hydrophilic bile acid; any free radical generation stimulated by this acid was easily overcome by endogenous renal scavenger systems.

Cardiac Function

As noted earlier, prerenal factors may be important in the development of postoperative renal failure in jaundiced patients. Bile acids exert a negative inotropic and chronotropic action on the heart at plasma concentrations within the pathophysiologic range.[91–96,115,116] The mechanism whereby bile acids exert their cardiac effects is unclear, but several mechanisms have been proposed. Joubert[116] suggested that bile acids interfere with cardiac β-adrenoceptors, whereas several studies have shown that bile acids reduce the slow inward current of calcium in ventricular muscle,[96] the sinoatrial node,[117] and the time-dependent outward potassium current.[117]

The effects of bile acids on cardiac function are equivocal. Moreover, cardiodepression appears to be independent of bile acid type; the effects were observed with both hydrophobic and hydrophilic forms.

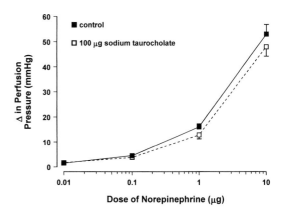

FIGURE 20.11. The effect of constant infusion of sodium taurocholate on renovascular responsiveness to norepinephrine in isolated perfused kidneys. (Modified from Bomzon L, Wilton PB, Mendelsohn D, Kew MC: Bile salts, obstructive jaundice and renal blood flow. Isr J Med Sci 1979;15:169–171, with permission.)

Peripheral Vasculature

A tendency to hypotension is observed in jaundiced patients. Bile acids have been implicated since an intravenous infusion of the hydrophobic deoxycholic acid can significantly reduce blood pressure in spontaneously hypertensive rats.[118] In the early 1980s, several groups showed that bile acids are vasodilators,[22,97] and this finding has been confirmed by others.[118–120] The mechanism whereby bile acids cause vasodilatation is not clear, but several groups have shown that bile acids (1) attenuate the contractile response to norepinephrine[22,118] as well as other agonists,[121,122] (2) relax precontracted blood vessels,[121,122] and (3) block calcium channels.[121,122] Furthermore, the vasorelaxant action is not endothelium-dependent,[121,122] as suggested by experiments demonstrating the vasorelaxant action of deoxycholic acid in endothelium-intact and endothelium-denuded arterial rings (Fig. 20.12). The EC_{50} values of the two response curves were not different, suggesting that the vasorelaxant effects of bile acids is not dependent on the presence of endothelium. Such effects on blood vessels are more apparent with hydrophobic bile acids and are not observed with hydrophilic bile acids.[122]

Oxygen free radicals may be one of the mediators of such effects on receptors and ion channels in vascular smooth muscle membrane. Recently, Kaneko et al.[123] and Ghosh et al.[124] found that the affinity of cardiac α- and β-adrenoceptors and neuronal muscarinic receptors, respectively, were

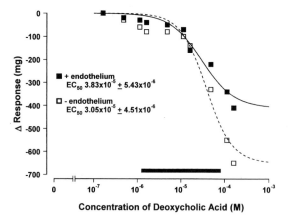

FIGURE 20.12. A representative experiment showing the vasorelaxant action of the hydrophobic bile acid, deoxycholic acid, on the precontracted endothelium-intact and endothelium-denuded arterial ring. The black line represents the pathophysiologic plasma concentration range for total serum bile acids. (Ehrlich and Bomzon, unpublished data.)

depressed by oxygen free radicals. They speculated that the mechanism by which oxygen free radicals may modify receptors or membrane proteins was initiated by membrane lipid peroxidation and production of acyl derivatives and malondialdehyde. As noted previously, hydrophobic bile acids have the potential to initiate this process.

Hence, the mechanism of systemic hypotension in jaundiced patients may be due to cardiodepressant and vasorelaxant actions of bile acids. This conclusion needs clinical corroboration; all the experiments involving bile acids on cardiac and vascular function were undertaken in experimental animals.

Tubular Function

Obstructive jaundice is associated with diuresis and natriuresis. Several studies have shown that bile acids may account for both effects. Topuzlu and Stahl[98] observed that small amounts of bile infused into anesthetized dogs produced natriuresis and diuresis, apparently due to a decrease in proximal tubular resorption of sodium and water. Others have observed that bile acids per se promote diuresis, natriuresis, and kaliuresis.[38,99,100] The effects are not bile acid type-dependent, although sulfated conjugates appear to be potent inhibitors of such processes.[40]

How do bile acids mediate diuretic and natriuretic action? Recently, Jourd'Heuil et al.[125]

demonstrated that oxidative attack decreased sodium-dependent glucose uptake in brush border membrane vesicles by damaging the glucose carrier. Similar findings were reported by Cogan and coworkers.[126] Thus it is not unreasonable to assume that the mechanism by which bile acids cause diuresis and natriuresis is oxidative attack on the ion cotransporter in the proximal convoluted tubule.

Bile acids and bile duct ligation have the same effect on water and sodium excretion. Accordingly, bile acids may be viewed as salt-losing substances because of their diuretic-like action. In view of this action, bile acids are now considered to be renoprotective rather than nephrotoxic.

Renoprotection

The rationale behind the use of bile acids for renoprotection assumes that endotoxemia causes acute renal failure in jaundiced patients because intestinal absorption of endotoxin is enhanced by reduced amounts of bile acids in the gastrointestinal tract.[77] Hence, prophylactic treatment with bile acids, administered orally, should reduce endotoxin absorption in the intestine and thus prevent postoperative renal failure.

Several clinical trials have been conducted to determine whether prophylactic use of hydrophobic and hydrophilic bile acids prevents deterioration of renal function in patients with obstructive jaundice. The results have been mixed.[72,127–129] The obvious question is why this line of treatment has not been as successful as one would expect. This question has become more pertinent since the recent demonstration that hydrophobic bile acids significantly inhibit the growth of the intestinal pathogen, *Escherichia coli*, a source of intestinal endotoxin.[130]

All of the evidence suggests that renal vasoconstriction is the principal pathophysiologic effect of jaundice in the kidney. We speculate that bile acids failed to prevent renal failure, or to reverse renal vasoconstriction for several reasons:

1. Endotoxin is not the factor causing renal vasoconstriction in jaundice. As already noted, endotoxin causes vasodilatation mediated by induction of nitric oxide synthase, which increases generation of the endothelium-derived vasorelaxant, nitric oxide.[84]

2. Vasodilator or vasorelaxant action is observed primarily with the hydrophobic bile acids, such as deoxycholic acid. Even if hydrophobic

bile acids could reverse renal vasoconstriction, their beneficial effect on the kidney would be offset by their negative inotropic and chronotropic action on the heart and generalized vasodilatation, which may redistribute reduced cardiac output away from the kidney.

3. Organizers of the clinical trails often used ursodeoxycholic acid. Although this acid is hydrophilic, it still may depress cardiac output and cause vasodilatation. As noted earlier, the bile acid pool in cholestatic patients favors the deleterious hydrophobic bile acids. Thus, the use of ursodeoxycholic acid shifts the balance of the pool in favor of the hydrophilic acids, thereby minimizing the oxidative attack on cell membranes by hydrophobic bile acids and possibly improving cardiac function. However, it is the hydrophobic bile acids that relax smooth muscle and even their vasodilator action is not sufficient to overcome renal vasoconstriction, possibly mediated by norepinephrine and/or angiotensin II. Thus, treatment with ursodeoxycholic acid is even less likely to be of benefit in reversing vasoconstriction.

4. Regardless of which bile acid is used, natriuresis and diuresis occur because all bile acids, endogenous and exogenous, are filtered at the glomerulus and the high tubular concentration of bile acids inhibits sodium and water reabsorption in the proximal tubule.

Conclusion

Much of our current knowledge about the role of bile acids in the pathogenesis of renal failure is based on experiments in laboratory animals rather than in patients. As amphiphilic compounds, bile acids are expected to have cytotoxic effects, and with their plasma accumulation and ubiquitous presence in jaundiced patients, it is not surprising that they are considered to be one of the pathogenetic factors in the development of postoperative renal failure. Their role in the pathogenesis of renal failure is complex, because they influence both renal and prerenal elements involving different mediators. They may account for the prerenal tendency to hypotension by depressing cardiac output and promoting vasodilatation, both of which are probably mediated by oxygen free radicals. This effect leads to renal vasoconstriction caused by redistribution of cardiac output away from the kidney and by reflex stimulation of the renal sympathetic nerves. In the kidney bile acids tend to promote

renal vasodilatation, but this action is not an effective counterbalance to prerenal actions such as peripheral vasodilatation.

Because they cross the glomerular filter to the proximal convoluted tubule, bile acids promote diuresis and natriuresis by attacking the proximal tubule ion cotransporter through generation of oxygen free radicals. Although this response is viewed as renoprotective, in fact it is nephrotoxic or cytotoxic, leading to less efficient resorption of sodium and water. In all likelihood, the glomerular membrane is also damaged by bile acids, but it appears that such damage does not adversely affect the rate of glomerular filtration. As mentioned earlier, cholestasis leads to enhanced intestinal absorption of endotoxin,[12] which also mediates its effects in part through the generation of oxygen free radicals.[84] Thus, the cardiovascular system and kidney are subjected to oxidative attack from plasma accumulation of bile acids and endotoxin. Increased synthesis of eicosanoids also may influence the renal vasculature and tubular function. This hypothetical pathway is outlined in Figure 20.13.

If oxidative attack is the underlying mediator for the development of renal failure, alternate prophylactic treatments with free radical scavengers may prove to be more effective than previously used regimens. This option, along with existing treatment modalities, is discussed in the general conclusion to this chapter.

Bilirubin

Biosynthesis

Bilirubin also accumulates in the plasma of jaundiced patients and also has been implicated in the etiology of renal failure. In jaundiced patients bilirubin is present in two forms—conjugated or soluble bilirubin and unconjugated or insoluble bilirubin. Unconjugated bilirubin is derived from the breakdown of hemoglobin and conjugated in the liver by the enzyme glucuronyl transferase. Both types of bilirubin are excreted principally in bile, although the conjugated form also is excreted in urine. The total concentration of bilirubin is normally low (< 1 mg/dl), and both forms are bound to plasma albumin. In cholestatic liver disease with hepatocellular damage and biliary obstruction, conjugated and unconjugated bilirubin spill over into the plasma and the plasma level of free bilirubin rises. In humans the total bilirubin concentration may rise to 30 mg/dl,

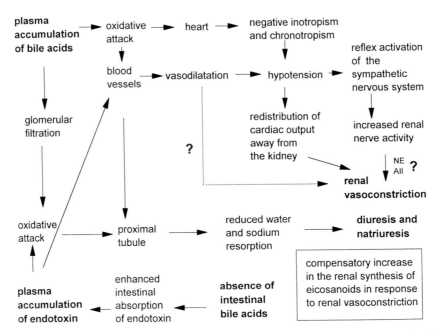

FIGURE 20.13. The possible mechanisms whereby plasma accumulation of bile acids and endotoxin promotes oxygen free radical production and oxidative attack in the kidney and cardiovascular system and thus
leads to renal vasoconstriction, diuresis, and natriuresis in obstructive jaundice.

whereas in bile duct-ligated rats levels as high as
15 mg/dl have been reported.

Nephrotoxicity

In their previously described experiment in
which bile acids were infused and the kidney
subjected to transient ischemia, Aoyagi and
Lowenstein[90] also infused unconjugated bilirubin
(see Fig. 20.10). They concluded that bilirubin
did not cause renal damage. In 1969 Baum and
colleagues[4] assessed the nephrotoxicity of bilirubin in bile duct-ligated rats with elevated plasma
concentrations of unconjugated bilirubin due to
congenital glucuronyl transferase deficiency
(Gunn rats) by subjecting the kidney to 60 minutes of ischemia. The mortality rate was higher
than in sham-operated Gunn rats, but the investigators found no significant differences in blood
urea concentrations or degree of renal damage, as
assessed histologically. They concluded that high
levels of conjugated bilirubin were responsible
for sensitizing the renal tubules to ischemia.

The two experiments raise several questions
that have not yet been adequately addressed: (1)
Is bilirubin nephrotoxic? (2) If so, which form is
nephrotoxic—the unconjugated or conjugated
form? (3) Is bilirubin-induced nephrotoxicity a
renovascular or tubular lesion? (4) Does bilirubin

exert its nephrotoxicity directly or through a mediator such as generation of oxygen free radicals?

Is bilirubin nephrotoxic? If so, which form is
responsible? Alon and colleagues[38] infused unconjugated bilirubin intrarenally into anesthetized
dogs and measured glomerular filtration rate, renal
plasma flow, urine flow, and excretion of sodium
and potassium. The found no evidence to suggest
that bilirubin was nephrotoxic. In 1984, using a
similar protocol, Finestone et al.[131] also found
that unconjugated bilirubin had no effect on renal
function except at high doses (400 mg/ml/min),
which resulted in arterial hypotension.

Does bilirubin cause vasoconstriction? The
studies of Alon et al.[38] and Finestone et al.[131]
showed that unconjugated bilirubin did not
affect renal blood flow. In recent years, the effects of bilirubin on the cerebral vasculature
following subarachnoid hemorrhage have been
investigated, and it appears that bilirubin causes
vasoconstriction by a yet-undescribed mechanism.[132–135] Although this observation may explain renal vasoconstriction, the concentrations
of unconjugated bilirubin in these experiments
were much higher concentrations than one normally sees in the plasma of jaundiced patients.

Does bilirubin cause tubular damage? With
the exception of the study by Baum, Stirling, and

Dawson,[4] none of the above described studies indicates that bilirubin causes tubular damage. In fact, it must be noted that both types of bilirubin are antioxidants since they can prevent oxidative damage to lipids and proteins and protect tissues such as the myocardium where the antioxidant defenses are less than in the liver.[136–139]

Conclusion

The potential deleterious effects of bilirubin on cellular integrity and function have been summarized by Better and Berl.[140] Hence, it is reasonable to speculate that bilirubin may account, in part, for the high incidence of renal failure in jaundiced patients. Regrettably, the evidence supporting a pathogenetic role for bilirubin is not convincing; additional experiments are needed to clarify the effects of bilirubin on all aspects of renal function.

GENERAL CONCLUSION

The overall well-being of patients with cholestasis is compromised. Symptoms include reduced appetite, depressed cellular metabolism due to reduced availability of glucose, increased susceptibility to infection, and apparent loss of immune responsiveness. In addition, both renal and cardiovascular systems are affected. In the kidney vasoconstriction is the prominent event. Glomerular filtration rates are maintained and, in the initial stages, diuresis and natriuresis, which may exacerbate the relative hypovolemia into an absolute hypovolemia. In the cardiovascular system a tendency to hypotension is mediated by cardiac myopathy and functional α1-adrenoceptor antagonism. Considerable evidence indicates that plasma accumulation of endotoxin and hydrophobic bile acids may be responsible for many of these effects in the renal and cardiovascular systems. Depending on the duration and severity of disease, such factors contribute to the increased susceptibility of hemorrhagic shock and postoperative renal failure during and after surgery in jaundiced patients.

Prophylactic Treatment of Renal Failure in Jaundice

Renal complications can be prevented theoretically by improving the physical and physiologic status of the jaundiced patient before surgery. Several methods have been used, including biliary drainage; prophylactic treatment with bile acids and other compounds, such as polymyxin B and lactulose, to reduce intestinal absorption of endotoxin; parenteral nutrition; and plasma volume expansion.

Biliary Drainage. Theoretically, the insertion of a biliary drain should reduce the incidence of renal failure in jaundiced patients. However, this procedure has not proved as effective as it should for two reasons:

1. Regardless of the cause of renal failure, all evidence indicates involvement of the renal and cardiovascular systems, whether damage is mediated by an endogenous circulating factor or by abnormal renal and cardiovascular function. Although the drain ensures effective removal of newly synthesized or accumulated bile, the renal and cardiovascular systems and the blood-borne elements are not influenced by this procedure.

2. Insertion of the drain is often complicated by infection, which may be exacerbated in the jaundiced patients.[75,76]

Antiendotoxin Therapy. The prophylactic use of polymyxin B, bile acids, and lactulose is based on the concept that endotoxin plays a major role in the development of postoperative renal failure in obstructive jaundice. The prophylactic use of bile acids has been already discussed. Pain and colleagues found that prophylactic treatment with lactulose, a nonabsorbable disaccharide, minimized intestinal absorption of endotoxin and reduced the incidence of renal dysfunction in jaundiced patients.[141] However, a recent study using a combined prophylactic therapy of lactulose or bile acids with preoperative hydration[129] concluded that preoperative hydration was more valuable than either lactulose or bile acids in preventing renal dysfunction, despite some benefit from the latter.

Parenteral Nutrition. Parenteral nutrition to improve the nutritional status of jaundiced patients has been tried but is not without risks. Although it was shown recently that parenteral nutrition decreases bacterial translocation in bile duct-ligated animals,[142] it unfortunately promotes cholestasis,[143,144] which obviously is not desirable in cholestatic patients.

Plasma Volume Expansion. The use of preoperative plasma volume expansion to prevent postoperative renal failure was suggested first in 1960 by Williams et al.[45] and again in 1964 by Dawson.[145] Using a protocol of transient ischemia and reperfusion of the kidney by clamping the renal pedicle for 60 minutes in unilateral nephrectomized bile duct-ligated rats, Dawson showed that 10% mannitol reduced the mortality rate and the subsequent rise in blood urea. On the basis of these data, he suggested that the preoperative use of mannitol would be useful in preventing renal failure in jaundiced patients. Later he added that other solutions given in larger volumes, such as Ringer's lactate or glucose saline, probably would have the same effect as mannitol.[146] He cautioned, however, that it would be difficult to maintain high urine flows and that fluid retention may occur with use of other solutions. Regardless of which fluid is used, plasma volume expansion is cost-effective and cheaper than other modalities that change the internal milieu, such as dialysis.

Such comments, made in 1970, highlight the immediate obvious advantages of preoperative plasma volume expansion, especially if mannitol is used: (1) it corrects preexisting volume deficits; (2) it lowers plasma concentrations of endotoxin, hydrophobic bile acids, and other toxic compounds that contribute to depression of cardiovascular and renal function; (3) it improves cardiovascular function by increasing cardiac output and distribution of cardiac output to the kidney; and (4) it increases renal clearance of accumulated bile constituents through improved renal perfusion. More recently, Pain et al.[129] also found that the use of preoperative hydration with mannitol reduced the incidence of impaired renal function in jaundiced patients.

There are also less obvious advantages in using mannitol as opposed to other solutions: (1) one needs smaller volumes, and (2) mannitol is protective. We emphasize the second point. As noted previously, we propose that the renal complications of obstructive jaundice may be due to increased generation of oxygen free radicals through plasma accumulation of bile acids. Mannitol is a potent scavenger of oxygen free radicals,[114] and this action probably explains why Dawson's experiments found mannitol to be renoprotective in obstructive jaundice.

Vasoactive Sympathomimetic Drugs. The perioperative use of positive inotropic drugs, such as dopamine, in managing hypotensive crises in jaundiced patients deserves comment. In addition to its positive inotropic action, dopamine is a renal vasodilator and has been used to reverse the renal vasoconstriction of obstructive jaundice.[10,147–149] As noted previously, patients have cardiac myopathy and attenuated pressor, cardiac, and vascular reactivity to both α- and β-adrenoceptor

agonists[86,91] as well as deranged cellular energy metabolism.[67,68] Because it excites both receptor subtypes, one should be cautious in using dopamine and other drugs with a similar mechanism of action. Large doses, which probably are required to overcome the functional defect of the adrenoceptors, may exacerbate renal vasoconstriction by stimulating the renal α-adrenoceptors and leading to more rapid depletion of cardiac myocyte energy stores. Hence, we suggest that the preferential use of nonadrenergic drugs to control perioperative hypotensive crises. Again, preoperative hydration may serve this purpose. Preoperative hydration also may be used to deliver metabolites such as glucose to the cell. In addition, hydration also has a positive inotropic action through intrinsic cardiac mechanisms, such as an increase in end-diastolic volume; this action increases the distribution of cardiac output to the kidney and hence assists in overcoming renal vasoconstriction.

Postoperative Management of Jaundiced Patients

In the postoperative phase hydration should be maintained because of its beneficial effect on renal perfusion and cardiovascular function. In this phase it helps to reduce the effective concentrations of endotoxin and bile acids to negligible levels and encourages the return of normal cardiovascular function after surgery. Furthermore, it contributes to more rapid elimination of unwanted bile constituents and facilitates their efflux into the plasma for ultimate elimination by the kidney.

Acknowledgments. The authors thank Samuel Lee, M.D., and Murray Epstein, M.D., for their constructive comments in the preparation of the manuscript. This work was supported by grants from the Chief Scientist, Ministry of Health, Jerusalem, Israel; the Technion Vice-President Fund for the Promotion of Research, Technion-Israel Institute of Technology, Haifa, Israel; and the David Ben-Gurion Research Fund, Israel Labor Federation, Tel Aviv, Israel.

REFERENCES

1. Zollinger RM, Williams RD: Surgical aspects of jaundice. Surgery 1956;39:1016–1030.
2. Dawson JL: The incidence of postoperative renal failure in obstructive jaundice. Br J Surg 1965;52:663–665.
3. Dawson JL: Acute post-operative renal failure in obstructive jaundice. Ann R Coll Surg Engl 1968;42:163–181.

4. Baum M, Stirling GA, Dawson JL: Further study into obstructive jaundice and ischemic renal damage. BMJ 1969;2:229–231.

5. Wait RB, Kahng KU: Renal failure complicating obstructive jaundice. Am J Surg 1989;157:256–263.

6. Walker JG: Renal failure in jaundice. Proc R Soc Med 1962;55:30–30.

7. Sherlock S: Diseases of the Liver and Biliary System, 5th ed. Oxford: Blackwell Scientific Publications, 1978.

8. Better OS, Bomzon A: Effects of jaundice on the renal and cardiovascular systems. In Epstein M (ed): The Kidney and Liver Disease, 3rd ed. Baltimore: Williams & Wilkins, 1988;508–536.

9. Thompson JN, Carolan G, Myers MJ, Blumgart LH: The perioperative changes in glomerular filtration and renal blood flow in patients with obstructive jaundice. Acta Chir Scand 1989;155:465–470.

10. Monasterolo L, Peiretti A, Elias MM: Rat renal functions during the first days post-bile duct ligation. Ren Fail 1993;15:461–467.

11. Bomzon A, Blendis LM: Animal models of liver disease. In Bomzon A, Blendis LM (eds): Cardiovascular Complications of Liver Disease. Boca Raton, FL: CRC Press, 1990;9–28.

12. Bourgoignie JJ, Valle GA: Endotoxin and renal dysfunction in liver disease. In Epstein M (ed): The Kidney and Liver Disease, 3rd ed. Baltimore: Williams & Wilkins, 1988;486–507.

13. DiBona GF: The functions of the renal nerves. Rev Physiol Biochem Pharmacol 1982;94:75–181.

14. Bomzon A: Sympathetic control of the renal circulation. J Auton Pharmac 1983;3:37–46.

15. Zambraski EJ, DiBona GF: Sympathetic nervous system in hepatic cirrhosis. In Epstein M (ed): The Kidney in Liver Disease, 3rd ed. Baltimore: Williams & Wilkins, 1988;469–485.

16. Bloom DS, Bomzon L, Rosendorff C, Kew MC: Renal blood flow in obstructive jaundice: An experimental study in baboons. Clin Exp Pharmacol Physiol 1976;3: 461–472.

17. Bomzon L, Kew MC: Renal blood flow in experimental obstructive jaundice. In Epstein M (ed): The Kidney in Liver Disease, 2nd ed. Amsterdam: Elsevier Science, 1983;313–326.

18. Kahng KU, Monaco DO, Schnabel FR, Wait RB: Renal vascular reactivity in the bile duct-ligated rat. Surgery 1988;104:250–256.

19. O'Neill P, Wait RB, Kahng KU: Obstructive jaundice and renal failure in the rat: The role of renal prostaglandins and the renin-angiotensin system. Surgery 1990;108:356–362.

20. Schroeder ET, Finn AF Jr, Hueber P: Suppression of vascular prostacyclin generation by jaundiced serum: Relation to lipid peroxides. J Lab Clin Med 1988;112: 784–791.

21. Tsai LY, Lee KT, Tsai SM, et al: Changes of lipid peroxide levels in blood and liver tissue of patients with obstructive jaundice. Clin Chim Acta 1993;215: 41–50.

22. Bomzon A, Finberg JP, Tovbin D, et al: Bile salts, hypotension and obstructive jaundice. Clin Sci 1984;67: 177–183.

23. Bomzon A, Gali D, Better OS, Blendis LM: Reversible suppression of the vascular contractile response in rats with obstructive jaundice. J Lab Clin Med 1985;105: 568–572.

24. Gali D, Blendis LM, Bomzon A: Vascular reactivity in reversible experimental obstructive jaundice. J Surg Res 1987;42:242–246.

25. Jacob G, Said O, Finberg J, Bomzon A: Peripheral vascular neuroeffector mechanisms in experimental cholestasis. Am J Physiol 1993;265:G579–G586.

26. Cioffi WG, DeMeules JE, Kahng KU, Wait RB: Renal vascular reactivity in jaundice. Surgery 1986;100: 356–362.

27. Hishida A, Honda N, Sudo M, Nagase M: Mechanism of altered renal perfusion in the early stage of obstructive jaundice. Kidney Int 1980;17:223–230.

28. Bomzon A, Rosenberg M, Gali D, et al: Systemic hypotension and decreased pressor response in dogs with chronic bile duct ligation. Hepatology 1986;6:595–600.

29. Bomzon A, Better OS, Blendis LM: Renal alpha-1-adrenoreceptors in rats with obstructive jaundice. Nephron 1986;42:258–261.

30. Bomzon A, Better OS, Blendis LM: Cardiovascular function and amine metabolism in liver disease. Rev Clin Basic Pharmacol 1985;5:71–98.

31. O'Neill PA, Wait RB, Kahng KU: Role of renal sympathetic nerve activity in renal failure associated with obstructive jaundice in the rat. Am J Surg 1991;161: 662–667.

32. Naveh Y, Finberg JP, Kahana L, Better OS: Renin-angiotensin system in dogs following chronic bile-duct ligation. Relation to vascular reactivity. J Hepatol 1988;6:57–62.

33. Kokube T, Ueda E, Fujimoto S, et al: Plasma angiotensinase activity in liver disease. Clin Chim Acta 1965;12:484–488.

34. Zipser RD, Lifschitz MD: Prostaglandins and related compounds. In Epstein M (ed): The Kidney in Liver Disease, 3rd ed. Baltimore: Williams & Wilkins, 1988; 393–416.

35. Masumoto T, Masuoka S: Kidney function in the severely jaundiced dog. Am J Surg 1980;140:426–430.

36. Hishida A, Honda N, Sudo M, et al: Renal handling of salt and water in the early stage of obstructive jaundice in rabbits. Nephron 1982;30:368–373.

37. Alon U, Berant M, Mordechovitz D, et al: Effect of isolated cholaemia on systemic haemodynamics and kidney function in conscious dogs. Clin Sci 1982;63: 59–64.

38. Alon U, Berant M, Mordechovitz D, Better OS: The effect of intrarenal infusion of bile on kidney function in the dog. Clin Sci 1982;62:431–433.

39. Levy M, Finestone H: Renal response to four hours of biliary obstruction in the dog. Am J Physiol 1983;244: F516–F425.

40. Sitprija V, Kashemsant U, Sriratanaban A, et al: Renal function in obstructive jaundice in man: Cholangiocarcinoma model. Kidney Int 1990;38:948–955.

41. Valverde J, Martínez-Ródenas F, Pereira JA, et al: Rapid increase in plasma levels of atrial natriuretic peptide after common bile duct ligation in the rabbit. Ann Surg 1992;216:554–559.

42. Pereira JA, Torregrosa MA, Martínez-Ródenas F, et al: Increased cardiac endocrine activity after common bile duct ligation in the rabbit: Atrial endocrine cells in obstructive jaundice. Ann Surg 1994;219:73–78.

43. Dixon JM, Armstrong CP, Duffy SW, Davies GC: Factors affecting morbidity and mortality after obstructive jaundice: A review of 373 patients. Gut 1983;24:845–852.

44. Meakins JC: Jaundice and blood pressure. Med Clin North Am 1932;16:715–726.

45. Williams RD, Elliott DW, Zollinger RM: The effect of hypotension in obstructive jaundice. Arch Surg 1960;87:334–340.

46. Morandini G, Spanedda M, Spanedda L: La resposta pressoria all'angiotensina e alla noradrenalina in soggetti con affezioni epatiche. Minerva Med 1967;58:1794–1798.

47. Morandini G, Spanedda M: Contributo allo studio della reattività vascolare periferica all'angiotensina ed alla noradrenalina in corso di affezioni epatiche. Minerva Med 1966;57:2175–2180.

48. Finberg JP, Syrop HA, Better OS: Blunted pressor response to angiotensin and sympathomimetic amines in bile-duct ligated dogs. Clin Sci 1981;61:535–539.

49. Bomzon A, Weinbroum A, Kamenetz L: Systemic hypotension and pressor responsiveness in cholestasis. A study in conscious 3-day bile duct ligated rats. J Hepatol 1990;11:70–76.

50. Jacob G, Bishara B, Lee SS, et al: Cardiovascular responses to serotonin in experimental liver disease. Hepatology 1991;14:1235–1242.

50a. Bomzon A, Jacob G: Unpublished observations.

51. Ludatscher RM, Binah O, Bomzon A, et al: Ultrastructure of the myocardium in dogs with induced jaundice. Acta Anatom 1987;130:242–246.

52. Shasha SM, Better OS, Chaimovitz C, et al: Haemodynamic studies in dogs with chronic bile-duct ligation. Clin Sci Mol Med 1976;50:533–537.

53. Green J, Beyar R, Sideman S, et al: The "jaundiced heart." a possible explanation for postoperative shock in obstructive jaundice. Surgery 1986;100:14–20.

54. Binah O, Bomzon A, Blendis LM, et al: Obstructive jaundice blunts myocardial contractile response to isoprenaline in the dog: A clue to the susceptibility of jaundiced patients to shock? Clin Sci 1985;69:647–653.

55. Jacob G, Nassar N, Hayam G, et al: Cardiac function and responsiveness to β-adrenoceptor agonists in rats with obstructive jaundice. Am J Physiol 1993;265:G314–G320.

56. Lumlertgol D, Boonyaprapa S, Bunnachek D, et al: The jaundiced heart: Evidence of blunted response to positive inotropic stimulation. Ren Fail 1991;13:15–22.

57. Yarger WE: Intrarenal mechanisms of salt retention after bile duct ligation in rats. J Clin Invest 1976;57:408–418.

58. Aarseth P, Aarseth S, Bergan A: Blood volume partition after acute cholestasis in the rat. Eur Surg Res 1976;8:61–70.

59. Gillett DJ: The effect of obstructive jaundice on the blood volume in rats. J Surg Res 1971;11:447–449.

60. Cattell WR, Birnstingl MA: Blood-volume and hypotension in obstructive jaundice. Brit J Surg 1967;54:272–277.

61. Allison MEM, Moss NG, Fraser MM, et al: Renal function in chronic obstructive jaundice: A micropuncture study in rats. Clin Sci Mol Med 1978;54:649–659.

62. Bank N, Aynedjian HS: A micropuncture study of renal salt and water retention in chronic bile duct ligation. J Clin Invest 1975;55:994–1002.

63. Stevenson DK, Salomon WL, Moore LY, et al: Pulmonary excretion rate of carbon monoxide as an index of total bilirubin formation in adult male Wistar rats with common bile duct ligation. J Pediatr Gastroenterol Nutr 1984;3:790–794.

64. Jordan FM, McVicar CS: Anemia in jaundice. I. A clinical study of cases in which jaundice was of the obstructive or intrahepatic types. Am J Med Sci 1930;179:654–659.

65. Jordan FM, Greene CH: Anemia in jaundice. II. The formation of hemoglobin in experimental obstructive jaundice. Am J Physiol 1930;91:409–422.

66. Martínez-Ródenas F, Oms LM, Carulla X, et al: Measurement of body water compartments after ligation of the common bile duct in the rabbit. Br J Surg 1989;76:461–464.

67. Heidenreich S, Brinkema E, Martin A, et al: The kidney and cardiovascular system in obstructive jaundice: Functional and metabolic studies in conscious rats. Clin Sci 1987;73:593–599.

68. Yoshiya K, Kishimotor T, Ishikawa Y, Utsunomiya J: Insulin response following intravenous glucose administration in dogs with obstructive jaundice. J Surg Res 1987;43:271–277.

69. Wardle EN, Wright NA: Endotoxin and acute renal failure associated with obstructive jaundice. BMJ 1970;4:472–474.

70. Wardle NE: Endotoxin and acute renal failure. Nephron 1975;14:321–332.

71. Kostakoglu N, Mentes A, Topuzlu C, et al: The effect of bile on the gastric mucosal barrier in the presence after blockade of normal gastric acidity. J Pak Med Assoc 1989;39:231–234.

72. Cahill CJ, Pain JA, Bailey ME: Bile salts, endotoxin and renal function in obstructive jaundice. Surg Gynecol Obstet 1987;165:519–522.

73. Pain JA, Bailey ME: Measurement of operative plasma endotoxin levels in jaundiced and non-jaundiced patients. Eur J Surg 1987;19:207–216.

74. Ennis M, Clements B, Campbell GR, et al: The effect of obstructive jaundice on systemic concentrations of bile acids, histamine and antibodies to the core region of endotoxin glycolipid. Agents Actions 1993;38 (Suppl C):C283–C285.

75. Ding JW, Andersson R, Soltesz V, et al: The role of bile and bile acids in bacterial translocation in obstructive jaundice in rats. Eur Surg Res 1993;25:11–19.

76. Ding JW, Andersson R, Soltesz V, et al: The role of bile and bile acids in bacterial translocaton in obstructive jaundice in rats. Eur Surg Res 1993;25:11–19.

77. Bailey ME: Endotoxin, bile salts and renal function in obstructive jaundice. Br J Surg 1976;63:774–778.

78. Diamond T, Dolan S, Thompson RL, Rowlands BJ: Development and reversal of endotoxemia and endotoxin-related death in obstructive jaundice. Surgery 1990;108:370–374.

79. Scott-Conner CEH, Grogan JB, Scher KS, et al: Impaired bacterial killing in early obstructive jaundice. Am J Surg 1993;166:308–310.

80. Greve JWM, Gouma DJ, Buurman WA: Complications in obstructive jaundice: Role of endotoxins. Scand J Gastroenterol 1992;27(Suppl 194):8–12.

81. Scott-Conner CEH, Grogan JB: Serum and cellular factors in murine obstructive jaundice. Surgery 1994; 115:77–84.

82. Li H, Xiong ST, Zhang SZ, et al: Effect of arginine on immune function in rats with obstructive jaundice. J Tongji Med Univ 1991;11:150–154.

83. Nie CH, Grogan JB, Crick MP, Scott-Conner CEH: Impaired response to alloantigens in murine biliary obstruction. J Surg Res 1993;54:145–149.

84. Moncada S, Palmer RMJ, Higgs EA: Nitric oxide: Physiology, pathophysiology, and pharmacology. Pharmacol Rev 1991;43:109–142.

85. Okun F, Weizman R, Katz Y, et al: Increase in central and peripheral benzodiazepine receptors following surgery. Brain Res 1988;458:31–36.

86. Bomzon A: Vascular reactivity in liver disease. In Bomzon A, Blendis LM (eds): Cardiovascular Complications of Liver Disease. Boca Raton, FL: CRC Press, 1990;207–224.

87. Swain MG, Patchev V, Vergalla J, et al: Suppression of hypothalamic-pituitary-adrenal axis responsiveness to stress in a rat model of acute cholestasis. J Clin Invest 1993;91:1903–1908.

87a. Levy M, personal communication.

88. Aarseth S, Bergan A, Aarseth P: Circulatory homeostasis in rats after bile duct ligation. Scand J Clin Lab Invest 12979;39:93–97.

89. Bomzon A, Monies-Chass I, Kamenetz L, Blendis LM: Anesthesia and pressor responsiveness in chronic bile-duct-ligated dogs. Hepatology 1990;11:551–556.

90. Aoyagi T, Lowenstein LM: The effect of bile acids and renal ischemia on renal function. J Lab Clin Med 1968; 71:686–692.

91. Lee S, Bomzon A: The heart in liver disease. In Bomzon A, Blendis LM (eds): Cardiovascular Complications of Liver Disease. Boca Raton, FL: CRC Press, 1990;81–102.

92. Wakim KG, Essex HE, Mann FC: The effects of whole bile and bile salts on the perfused heart. Am Heart J 1939;18:171–175.

93. Joubert P: Cholic acid and the heart: In vitro studies of the effect on heart rate and myocardial contractility in the heart. Clin Exp Pharmacol Physiol 1978;5:9–16.

94. Bogin E, Better O, Harari I: The effect of jaundiced sera and bile salts on cultured beating rat heart cells. Experientia 1983;39:1307–1308.

95. Enriquez de Salamanca E, Toni P, Montes MJ, et al: Negative chronotropic effect of cholic acid in isolated rat heart. Med Chir Dig 1985;14:585–589.

96. Binah O, Rubinstein I, Bomzon A, Better OS: Effects of bile acids on ventricular muscle contraction and electrophysiological properties: Studies in rat papillary muscle and isolated ventricular myocytes. Naunyn-Schmiedeberg's Arch Pharmacol 1987;335:160–165.

97. Kvietys PR, McLendon JM, Granger DN: Postprandial intestinal hyperemia: Role of bile salts in the ileum. Am J Physiol 1981;241:G469–G477.

98. Topuzlu C, Stahl WM: Effect of bile infusion on the dog kidney. N Engl J Med 1966;274:760–763.

99. Better OS, Guckian V, Giebisch G, Green R: The effect of sodium taurocholate on proximal tubular reabsorption in the rat kidney. Clin Sci 1987;72: 139–141.

100. Dillingham MA, Better OS, Anderson RJ: Sodium taurocholate increases hydraulic conductivity in rabbit collecting tubule. Kidney Int 1988;33:782–786.

101. Radominska A, Treat S, Little J: Bile acid metabolism and the pathophysiology of cholestasis. Semin Liv Dis 1993;13:219–234.

102. Heuman DM: Quantitative estimation of the hydrophilic-hydrophobic balance of mixed bile salt solutions. J Lipid Res 1989;30:719–730.

103. Halliwell B: Reactive oxygen species in living systems: Source, biochemistry, and role in human disease. Am J Med 1991;91:145–225.

104. Sokol RJ, Devereaux M, Khandwala R, O'Brien K: Evidence for involvement of oxygen free radicals in bile acid toxicity to isolated rat hepatocytes. Hepatology 1993;17:869–881.

105. Parkinson TM, Olson JA: Inhibitory effects of bile acids on adenosine tryphosphatase. oxygen consumption, and the transport and diffusion of water soluble substances in the small intestine of the rat. Life Sci 1964;3:107–112.

106. Krähenbühl S, Krähenbühl-Glauser S, Stucki J, et al: Stereological and functional analysis of liver mitochondria from rats with secondary biliary cirrhosis: Impaired mitochondrial metabolism and increased mitochondrial content per hepatocyte. Hepatology 1992;15:1167–1172.

107. Dietschy JM: Effects of bile salts on intermediate metabolism of the intestinal mucosa. Fed Proc 1967;26: 1589–1598.

108. Chadwick VS, Gaginella TS, Carlson GL, et al: Effect of molecular structure on bile acid-induced alterations in absorptive function, permeability, and morphology in the perfused rat colon. J Lab Clin Med 1979;94: 661–674.

109. Krähenbühl S, Talos C, Fischer S, Reichen J: Toxicity of bile acids on the electron transport chain of isolated rat liver mitochondria. Hepatology 1994;19:471–479.

110. Weissmann G, Keiser H: Hemolysis and the augmentation of hemolysis by neutral steroids and bile acids. Biochem Pharmacol 1965;14:525–535.

111. Schubert R, Schmidt K-H: Structural changes in vesicle membranes and mixed micelles of various lipid compositions after binding of different bile salts. Biochemistry 1988;27:8787–8794.

112. Ilani A, Granoth R: The pH dependence of the hemolytic potency of bile salts. Biochim Biophys Acta 1990;1027:199–204.

113. Bomzon L, Wilton PB, Mendelsohn D, Kew MC: Bile salts, obstructive jaundice and renal blood flow. Isr J Med Sci 1979;15:169–171.

114. Odeh M: The role of reperfusion-induced injury in the pathogenesis of the crush syndrome. N Engl J Med 1991;324:1417–1422.

115. Wakim KG, Essex HE, Mann FC: The effects of whole bile and bile salts on the innervated and the denervated heart. Am Heart J 1940;19:487–491.

116. Joubert P: An in vivo investigation of the negative chronotropic effect of cholic acid in the rat. Clin Exp Pharmacol Physiol 1978;5:1–8.

117. Kotake H, Itoh T, Watanabe M, et al: Effect of bile acid on electrophysiological properties of rabbit sino-atrial node in vivo. Br J Pharmacol 1989;98:357–360.

118. Tominaga T, Suzuki H, Ogata Y, et al: Bile acids are able to reduce blood pressure by attenuating vascular reactivity in spontaneously hypertensive rats. Life Sci 1988;42:1861–1868.

119. Thomas SH, Joh T, Benoit JN: Role of bile acids in splanchnic hemodynamic response to chronic portal hypertension. Dig Dis Sci 1991;36:1243–1248.

120. Pak J-M, Lee SS: Vasoactive effects of bile salts in cirrhotic rats. In vivo and in vitro studies. Hepatology 1993;18:1175–1181.

121. Pak J-M, Adeagbo ASO, Triggle CR, et al: Mechanism of bile salt vasoactivity: Dependence on calcium channels in vascular smooth muscle. Br J Pharmacol 1994; 112:1209–1215.

122. Bomzon A, Ljubuncic P: Bile acids as endogenous vasodilators? Biochem Pharmacol 1995;49:581–589.

123. Kaneko M, Chapman DC, Ganguly PK, et al: Modification of cardiac adrenergic receptors by oxygen free radicals. Am J Physiol 1991;260:H821–H826.

124. Ghosh C, Dick RM, Ali SF: Iron/ascorbate-induced lipid peroxidation changes membrane fluidity and muscarinic cholinergic receptor binding in rat frontal cortex. Neurochem Int 1993;23:479–484.

125. Jourd'Heuil D, Vaananen P, Meddings JB: Lipid peroxidation of the brush-border membrane: Membrane physical properties and glucose transport. Am J Physiol 1993;264:G1009–G1015.

126. Hayam I, Cogan U, Mokady S: Dietary oxidized oil enhances the activity of (Na^+K^+) ATPase and acetylcholinesterase and lowers the fluidity of rat erythrocyte membrane. J Nutr Biochem 1993;4:563–568.

127. Thompson JN, Cohen J, Blenkharn JI, et al: A randomized clinical trial of oral ursodeoxycholic acid in obstructive jaundice. Br J Surg 1986;73:634–636.

128. Pain JA, Bailey ME: Prevention of endotoxaemia in obstructive jaundice—a comparative study of bile salts. HPB Surg 1988;1:21–27.

129. Pain JA, Cahill CJ, Gilbert JM, et al: Prevention of postoperative renal dysfunction in patients with obstructive jaundice: A multicentre study of bile salts and lactulose. Br J Surg 1991;78:467–469.

130. Sung JY, Shaffer EA, Costerton JW: Antibacterial activity of bile salts against common biliary pathogens: Effects of hydrophobicity of the molecule and in the presence of phospholipids. Dig Dis Sci 1993;38:2104–2112.

131. Finestone H, Fechner C, Levy M: Effects of bile and bile salt infusion on renal function in dogs. Can J Physiol Pharmacol 1984;62:762–768.

132. Miao FJ, Lee TJ: Effects of bilirubin on cerebral arterial tone in vitro. J Cereb Blood Flow Metab 1989;9:666–674.

133. Macdonald RL, Weir BK, Chen MH, Grace MG: Scanning electron microscopy of normal and vasospastic monkey cerebrovascular smooth muscle cells. Neurosurgery 1991;29:544–550.

134. Tanaka Y, Kassell NF, Machi T, et al: Effect of bilirubin on rabbit cerebral arteries in vivo and in vitro. Neurosurgery 1992;30:195–201.

135. Trost GR, Nagatani K, Goknur AB, et al: Bilirubin levels in subarachnoid clot and effects on canine arterial smooth muscle cells. Stroke 1993;24:1241–1245.

136. Wu TW, Wu J, Li RK, Mickle D, Carey D: Albumin-bound albumin bilirubins protect human ventricular myocytes against oxyradical damage. Biochem Cell Biol 1991;69:683–688.

137. Neuzil J, Stocker R: Bilirubin attenuates radical-mediated damage to serum albumin. FEBS Lett 1993;331: 281–284.

138. Neuzil J, Stocker R: Free and albumin-bound bilirubin are efficient co-antioxidants for alpha-tocopherol, inhibiting plasma and low density lipoprotein lipid peroxidation. J Biol Chem 1994;269:1612–1619.

139. Farrera JA, Jauma A, Ribo JM, et al: The antioxidant role of bile pigments evaluated by chemical tests. Biorganic Med Chem 1994;2:181–185.

140. Better OS, Berl T: Jaundice and the kidney. In Suki WN, Eknoyan G (eds): The Kidney in Systemic Disease, 2nd ed. New York: John Wiley & Sons, 1981;521–537.

141. Pain JA, Bailey ME: Experimental and clinical study of lactulose in obstructive jaundice. Br J Surg 1986;73: 775–778.

142. Chuang J-H, Shieh C-S, Chang N-K, et al: Role of parenteral nutrition in preventing malnutrition and decreasing bacterial translocation to liver in obstructive jaundice. World J Surg 1993;17:580–585.

143. Merritt RJ: Cholestasis associated with total parenteral nutrition. J Parenter Enteral Nutr 1986;5:9–13.

144. Sax HC, Bower RH: Hepatic complications of total parenteral nutrition. J Parenter Enteral Nutr 1988;12:615–620.

145. Dawson JL: Jaundice and anoxic renal damage. BMJ 1964;1:810–811.

146. Dawson JL: Surgical aspects: Recent advances in jaundice. BMJ 1970;1:228–230.

147. Benko H, Mostbeck A, Peschl L, et al: The effect of dopamine on the renal function in dogs with chronic ligation of the common bile duct. Wien Klin Wochenschr 1977;89:562–566.

148. Bomzon L, Wilton PB, Kew MC: The effect of dopamine on renal cortical blood flow in baboons with experimentally induced obstructive jaundice. Isr J Med Sci 1978;14:1069–1072.

149. Levy M, Finestone H, Fechner C: Action of renal vasodilators in dogs following acute biliary obstruction. J Surg Res 1984;36:163–171.

Chapter 21

DIURETIC THERAPY IN LIVER DISEASE

MURRAY EPSTEIN, M.D., F.A.C.P.

Management of Ascites and Edema in Liver Disease
  The Morbidity of Ascites
  Recommendations for Medical Therapy of Ascites
  Role of Diuretics
Physiology and Control of Renal Sodium Handling
Diuretic Agents
  Acetazolamide
  Thiazide-type Drugs
  Organomercurials

Furosemide, Ethacrynic Acid, and Bumetanide
Potassium-sparing Diuretics
Choice of Diuretic Agent
Combined Therapy with Thiazide-type and Loop
  Diuretic Agents for Resistant Sodium Retention
Role of Albumin
Rapid Diuresis with Intravenous Diuretic Therapy
Ancillary Measures
Future Prospects
Summary

There's always an easy solution to every human problem—neat, plausible, wrong.

H. L. Mencken

MANAGEMENT OF ASCITES AND EDEMA IN LIVER DISEASE

The question of when and how to mobilize the ascites and edema of liver disease and the rapidity with which to accomplish this goal remains a subject of continuing controversy.

Aside from questions of when to intervene and the vigor with which such intervention should be accomplished, clinicians presently have at their disposal a considerable armamentarium consisting of several techniques for rapidly mobilizing ascites and edema. These include diuretic therapy, paracentesis, peritoneovenous shunting, and extracorporeal techniques such as continuous arteriovenous ultrafiltration (CAVU). This chapter reviews current concepts of the role of diuretic therapy. The other techniques for mobilization of excess fluid are reviewed in chapters 23, 24, and 26.

The Morbidity of Ascites

Ascites is associated with unwanted side effects in patients with liver disease.[1,2] Clearly the marked accumulation of ascites is associated with significant discomfort. Some observers have proposed a causal relationship between ascites and the subsequent development of both high portal pressure and gastroesophageal reflux.[1]

According to this formulation, ascites enhances the possibility of variceal bleeding by favoring both rupture of varices and reflux with a resultant erosion of the varices. Although this theory has not been clearly established, it underscores the general clinical notion that ascites per se is detrimental and requires relief. Furthermore, it has been suggested that ascites is the sine qua non of spontaneous bacterial peritonitis.[2]

Ascites indeed may be the "root of much evil,"[1] but the decision to relieve ascites with diuretic agents should not be automatic. Several older studies showed that diuretic therapy in the cirrhotic patient may be associated with a substantial risk of adverse effects[3] (Table 21.1). Reports of prospective drug surveillance programs suggest that diuretic-induced complications in the cirrhotic patient still constitute a formidable problem even today.[4] Given these drawbacks, what should our approach be? The following sections outline a rational approach to the management of ascites.

Recommendations for Medical Therapy of Ascites

The general principles for the medical therapy of hospitalized patients with ascites are outlined

447

TABLE 21.1. Potential Major Complications of
Diuretics in Cirrhotic Patients

Complication	Diuretic
Azotemia	All
Hyponatremia	All
Hypokalemia	All except spironolactone, amiloride, and triamterene (Dyrenium)
Hyperkalemia	Spironolactone, amiloride, and triamterene
Metabolic acidosis	Spironolactone, amiloride, and triamterene
Metabolic alkalosis	Loop of Henle and distal diuretics (except spironolactone, amiloride, and triamterene)

in Table 21.2. The initial goal should be weight loss resulting from a spontaneous diuresis in association with consistent and scrupulous adherence to a well-balanced diet with rigid dietary sodium restriction (250 mg/day or about 10 mEq). It should be emphasized that the sodium intake prescribed for cardiac patients (1200–1500 mg/day) is often not sufficiently restrictive for cirrhotic patients, who often continue to gain weight on such a regimen. Since cirrhotic patients frequently excrete as little as 5–10 mEq of sodium per day or less, it is evident that a 1500-mg sodium diet (i.e., 65 mEq of sodium) may result in a net positive sodium balance exceeding 420 mEq/week with an attendant weight gain of approximately 3 kg. Although the frequency with which dietary management successfully relieves ascites is unsettled, a sodium-restricted diet should be prescribed to all hospitalized patients since it is impossible to predict which patients will respond.

In occasional symptomatic patients, however, less rigid sodium restriction may be advisable for two major reasons: (1) as a consequence of the anorexia, such patients will eat only part of the meals offered to them and thus only a fraction of the daily sodium allowance and (2) in malnourished patients, nutrition must have a priority over rigid sodium restriction.

The level of fluid intake must also be carefully adjusted, because most edematous patients with liver disease also are prone to develop dilutional hyponatremia. To avoid this abnormality, the daily fluid intake should be adjusted to equal insensible losses (approximately 500–700 ml/day) plus daily urinary losses.

Role of Diuretics

Historical Note

Currently diuretics constitute the mainstay of the therapeutic armamentarium in managing ascites in patients with liver disease. In light of the long history of this florid complication of liver disease, it is surprising to note that diuretics are a relatively new class of drugs in the management of such patients. Some consider the observations of Alfred Boge as the seminal event in the subsequent development and widespread adoption of diuretics in managing ascites.[5] While a third-year medical student in the Wenckebach Clinic in Vienna, Boge noticed the diuretic activity of the organic mercurial compound Novasurol on the bedside chart of a nonedematous patient with congenital syphilis. Fortunately, a nurse had taken the initiative to report the vital signs, including the urine volume. In 1924, mersalyl (Salyrgan) and subsequently other mercurial diuretics with fewer side effects were introduced, eventuating in the widespread use of these drugs in the management of patients with cirrhosis and ascites.

Use of Diuretics

When the response to dietary management is inadequate, or when the imposition of rigid dietary sodium restriction is not feasible because of cost or unpalatability of the diet, the use of diuretic

TABLE 21.2. General Principles in the Treatment of Ascites

1. Daily measurement of the patient's weight and careful clinical monitoring are mandatory.
2. Biochemical parameters (blood urea nitrogen, serum creatinine, serum electrolytes) should be monitored at appropriate intervals.
3. Make sure that liver and renal functions are stable before instituting diuretic therapy.
4. Attempt to mobilize ascites and edema initially via rest and restriction of dietary sodium before instituting diuretic therapy.
5. Aim for a daily weight loss of 0.5–1.0 kg in patients who have ascites with edema and of 0.3 kg in patients who have ascites without edema.
6. Maintain as the end point of therapy the greatest degree of patient comfort possible with the minimum of drug-induced complications.

TABLE 21.3. Indications for Use of Diuretics in the Ascites of Liver Disease

1. Impaired cardiovascular function due to fluid overload
2. Impaired respiratory function
   (a) Incipient or overt pulmonary edema
   (b) Elevated diaphragms with resultant ascites (incipient or overt)
3. Tense ascites resulting in eventration of umbilicus
4. Tense edema resulting in skin breakdown
5. Excessive fluid that limits physical activity
6. Excessive fluid that causes significant discomfort
7. Inability to restrict sodium intake
8. Anorexia related to massive ascites

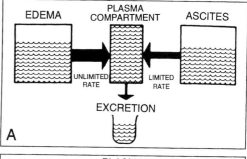

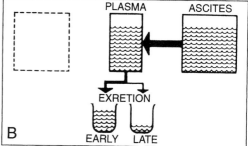

FIGURE 21.1. The mobilization and formation of fluid in ECF compartments in patients with fluid retention. Understanding of this diagram is enhanced by the realization that the rate of ascites mobilization is limited, whereas that of edema is relatively unlimited. *A,* In the presence of ascites and edema, edema is recruited in an unlimited manner to equal the rate of diuresis. *B,* In the ascitic patient without edema, the rate of mobilization of ascitic fluid is limited (700–900 ml/day). Thus, any diuresis that exceeds 900 ml/day must be mobilized at the expense of the plasma compartment. (Adapted from a drawing by A. Miller in Gabuzda GJ: Cirrhotic ascites: An etiologic approach to management. Hosp Pract 1973;8(8):67–74, with permission.)

agents may be considered if there are definite indications (Table 21.3). The presence of fluid retention per se is not a definite indication for administration of diuretics. Rather, as indicated in Table 21.3, diuretics should be used primarily in situations in which fluid accumulation produces impairment of cardiac and/or respiratory function or physical discomfort. In the absence of such discrete indications, *diuretics merely subvert the compensatory process and do not alter the underlying abnormality.*

The rational basis of diuretic therapy lies in an understanding of mechanism(s) and sites of action of the diuretic agent, coupled with an understanding of the kinetics of ascites absorption in cirrhosis. The attributes and efficacy of the varying diuretic agents are reviewed in detail in chapter 22; this chapter focuses solely on therapeutic considerations that are unique to cirrhotic patients.

An understanding of the efficacy and limitations of various therapies in the mobilization of ascites is provided by a classic study of Shear et al.[6] of the kinetics of ascites absorption and formation in patients with hepatic cirrhosis. The hallmark of their study was the observation that various extracellular fluid compartments—vascular, interstitial, and peritoneal—can change in disproportion to each other. They further demonstrated that ascites absorption averages about 300 to 500 ml/day during spontaneous diuresis and has as its upper limits 700 to 900 ml/day. Implicit in these findings is the realization that when diuretics are used, the therapeutic aim is to induce a slow and gradual diuresis not exceeding the capacity for mobilization of ascitic fluid. The major findings of their study are summarized in schematic fashion in Figure 21.1. When diuretics are administered to the patient with ascites and edema, optimal

therapy results when the rates of mobilization of edema and ascites equal (and are not less than) the rate of diuresis (Fig. 21.1A). In essence, the edema reservoir acts as a buffer preventing a contraction of plasma volume. In contrast, in ascitic patients without edema (Fig. 21.1B), any diuresis that exceeds 900 ml/day must perforce be mobilized at the expense of the plasma compartment, with resultant volume contraction and eventually oliguria, azotemia, and electrolyte abnormalities.

In planning a diuretic regimen, a number of principles should be kept in mind. Diuretic drugs should be viewed as adjuncts to other measures, including bed rest and nutritional supplementation, in the therapy of patients with advanced liver disease. Diuretic treatment may have two distinct

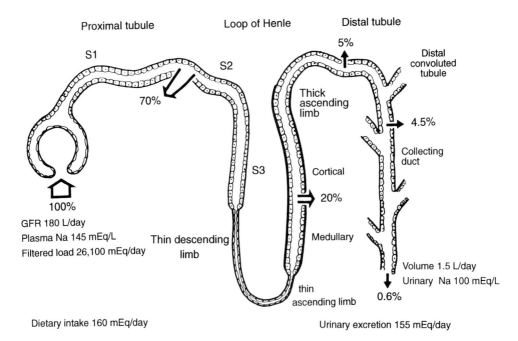

FIGURE 21.2. Summary of sodium reabsorption in a normal sodium-replete subject. In this idealized example, urinary sodium excretion approximates 155 mEq/day, which equals the dietary salt intake. The arrows indicate the percent of the filtered load of sodium that is reabsorbed in each segment of the nephron. GFR is glomerular filtration rate. (From Quamme GA: Loop diuretics. In Dirks JH, Sutton RAL (eds): Diuretics: Physiology, Pharmacology and Clinical Use. Philadelphia: W.B. Saunders, 1986, pp 86–116, with permission.)

goals: (1) to mobilize large surpluses of salt and water from the interstitial fluid space and the peritoneal cavity and (2) to maintain a "normal" sodium balance in edema-free patients in whom additional reduction of sodium intake is not feasible because of cost or unpalatability of the diet. It should be remembered that the drugs initially chosen to mobilize edema fluid may be different from diuretic agents required subsequently to maintain a normal sodium balance. Given the diversity of the underlying liver disease and the degree of fluid retention, it is apparent that any diuretic regimen must be individualized for the needs of each patient. Finally, as noted earlier, the goal of diuretic administration in the cirrhotic patient with ascites is not to render the patient edema- and ascites-free but rather to remove only enough retained fluid to ensure patient comfort. The overriding consideration in diuretic therapy, however, is that its use solely for cosmetic improvement is clearly contraindicated.

In addition to the hazards of an overly rapid diuresis, the dangers of hypokalemia should be emphasized. Since cirrhotic patients are at great risk for diuretic-induced potassium depletion,[7] the use of any diuretic that acts proximal to the distal

potassium-secretory site may result in profound hypokalemia. Because of (1) the frequently observed temporal relationship between diuretic therapy and induction of hepatic encephalopathy and (2) the probability that the enhanced renal ammonia production of hypokalemia may be related to the encephalopathy,[7,8] great care should be exercised in monitoring potassium derangements in cirrhotic patients receiving diuretics.

PHYSIOLOGY AND CONTROL OF RENAL SODIUM HANDLING

A clear understanding of the normal function of the kidney is essential in the rational use of diuretics and is important in the anticipation of possible complications. Figure 21.2 schematically illustrates the normal segmental absorptive pattern of the nephron. About 70% of the glomerular filtrate—including sodium, calcium, and chloride—is reabsorbed in the proximal tubule. The loop reabsorbs 20–30% of the filtered sodium, potassium, calcium, and chloride. The reabsorption of the major electrolytes by the loop thus amounts to 80% of the delivered load. Of the remaining 10% of salt delivered to the distal

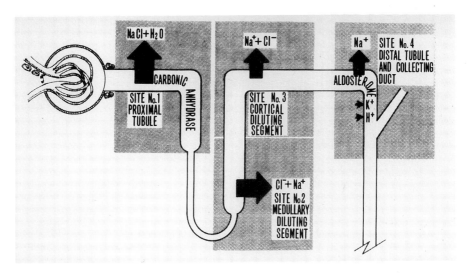

FIGURE 21.3. Sites of action of the major diuretics. Although the bulk of sodium reabsorption occurs in the proximal tubule (site 1), site 1 diuretics induce only a modest natriuresis.

nephron, including the distal convoluted tubule and the collecting duct, about 5–9% is reabsorbed. Net secretion is normally present in the case of potassium. Under normal conditions the serial arrangements of these segments accounts for the reabsorption of about 99% of the filtered sodium, calcium, and chloride and 90% of the filtered potassium; the remainder appears in the final urine.

The different tubule segments are characterized by markedly different transport systems. The linking of these systems in series provides an ideal arrangement by which the glomerular filtrate may be modified as it traverses the nephron from the glomerulus to the final urine. Specific agents may act in each segment to alter specific transport processes. Tubule segments distal to the site of action of a specific diuretic agent, however, are able to compensate to a limited extent for the inhibition at the more proximal sites. For instance, the increase in distal salt and water flow resulting from the loop diuretics may be altered before the final urine. Because the loop diuretics are potent agents, the distal nephron can modify only partially the additional effluent spilling over from the loop of Henle, and the urine generally reflects events within the loop.

DIURETIC AGENTS

The effectiveness of diuretics depends on their site of action within the nephron and on the potency of their inhibitory effect on electrolyte reabsorption. The proper use of diuretics, therefore, requires an understanding of the normal renal handling of salt and water, the site in the nephron at which reabsorption is inhibited by each of the diuretics, and the relative potency and pharmacokinetics of each agent. The anatomic and functional subdivisions of the nephron and the tubular site of action of diuretics are shown schematically in Figures 21.2 and 21.3.

Diuretics are best classified by the site in the nephron at which they inhibit reabsorption of sodium salts (Fig. 21.3). Their effect on renal electrolyte excretion, mechanism, duration, and site of action are summarized in Table 21.4; usual dosages are presented in Table 21.5. The salient features of the commonly prescribed diuretics are summarized briefly below.

Acetazolamide

Acetazolamide was the first orally effective diuretic agent, developed as an outgrowth of sulfanilamide therapy. It is of limited usefulness in the treatment of edema, because it ceases to be effective within 48–72 hours when metabolic acidosis develops as a result of excretion of bicarbonate caused by inhibition of tubular carbonic anhydrase activity.

Thiazide-type Drugs

Since their introduction in 1958, thiazide-type drugs have become the cornerstone for the therapy

TABLE 21.4. Site, Mechanism, and Duration of Action of Diuretics*

	Site of Action	Mechanism of Action	Action (hr) Onset	Peak	Duration
Acetazolamide	1	Inhibition of carbonic anhydrase	1–2	2	4–6
Thiazide and related drugs					
Moderate	3, 1	Inhibition of Na reabsorption	1–2	4–6	12–24
Long-acting	3, 1	Inhibition of Na reabsorption	2	6	24–36
Loop diuretics					
Ethacrynic acid	2	Inhibition of NaCl reabsorption	0.5–1	2–4	6–8
Furosemide	2, 1	Inhibition of NaCl reabsorption	0.5–1	2–4	6–8
Bumetanide	2, 1	Inhibition of NaCl reabsorption	0.5–1	2–3	4–6
Potassium-sparing agents					
Spironolactone	4	Competitive inhibition of aldosterone	8–24	24–48	48–72
Triamterene	4	Direct effect by reducing electrical potential between tubular cell and lumen	2–4	6–8	6–12
Amiloride	4	Direct effect by reducing electrical potential between tubular cell and lumen	2–4	4–6	6–12

* For illustration of site of action, see Figure 21.3.

of edema and hypertension. These halogenated organic compounds do not depend on carbonic anhydrase inhibition to induce diuresis, but rather directly inhibit sodium reabsorption in the cortical diluting segment—site 3 in Figure 21.3. Not all agents in this group are thiazides; for example, chlorthalidone, quinethazone, and metolazone are longer-acting phthalmidine derivatives. Independently of their structural formula and duration of action (Tables 21.4 and 21.5), this group of compounds exerts the same effect in the cortical diluting segment.

Whereas the major side effects of thiazide-type drugs are similar to those of most other diuretics, the hypokalemia and hyperuricemia that they produce may be more prominent; their relatively long duration of action does not allow a "recovery" period during which the kidney may reclaim some of the lost potassium or excrete the urate that has been retained. Other side effects include hyperglycemia in prediabetic patients with limited insulin stores, light-sensitive dermatologic lesions in susceptible patients, and hyperlipidemia, which recently has become a major focus of interest in hypertensive patients chronically treated with thiazide-related diuretics.

Organomercurials

Organomercurials are the oldest diuretics. They produce a predictable diuresis without excessive potassium losses by inhibiting chloride reabsorption in the medullary diluting segment (site 2 in Fig. 21.3). Unfortunately, their administration

TABLE 21.5. Usual Dosage of Diuretic Drugs

Generic Name	Brand Name	Usual Dosage
Acetazolamide	Diamox	250 mg 3–4 × daily
Thiazide and related drugs		
Hydrochlorothiazide	Hydrodiuril, Esidrix, Oretic	25–50 mg 1–2 × daily
Chlorthalidone	Hygroton, Thalitone	25–100 mg once daily
Indapamide	Lozol	2.5–5.0 mg once daily
Metolazone	Zaroyxlyn, Diulo	2.5–20 mg once daily
Loop diuretics		
Ethacrynic acid	Edecrin	50–200 mg 1–2 × daily
Furosemide	Lasix	40–240 mg 1–2 × daily
Bumetanide	Bumex	0.5–2 mg 1–2 × daily
Potassium-sparing agents		
Spironolactone	Aldactone	25–100 mg 1–4 × daily
Triamterene	Dyrenium	50–100 mg 1–2 × daily
Amiloride	Midamor	5–10 mg 1–2 × daily

TABLE 21.6. Classification of Site 2 (Loop) Diuretics

Chemical Structure	Major Examples
Sulfanyl benzoic acids	Furosemide, bumetanide, piretanide
Phenoxyacetic acids	Ethacrynic acid
Organomercurials	Mersalyl
Thiazolidones	Etozoline, 1-ozolinone
Aminopyrazolinones	Muzolimine
Aminomethylphenols	MK 447

requires intramuscular injection, and they are potentially nephrotoxic. With the availability of orally effective, similarly acting safer agents, the organomercurials are no longer used in the United States.

Furosemide, Ethacrynic Acid, and Bumetanide

The diuretics that inhibit sodium chloride absorption in the thick ascending portion of the loop of Henle (site 2, Fig. 21.2) are the most powerful natriuretic drugs in clinical use and are referred to as "loop" or "high-ceiling" diuretics. This group of diuretics consists of a variety of different medications that may be divided into six chemical classes (Table 21.6). The sulfamyl benzoates, such as furosemide, bumetanide, azosemide, and piretanide, have the greatest natriuretic efficacy and are capable of increasing fractional sodium excretion to as high as 20–25%. Compared with furosemide, bumetanide has a rapid onset and short duration of action. Both agents (and ethacrynic acid) accumulate in the cochlea, and toxicity is encountered when large doses are used in patients with reduced renal function. Ethacrynic acid is chemically unrelated to other diuretics. Patients with a history of sulfonamide sensitivity or photosensitive skin reactions should be treated with ethacrynic acid rather than furosemide or bumetanide. Muzolimine is a new nonsulfonamide diuretic drug of the pyrazolinone group.

Furosemide, bumetanide, and ethacrynic acid may be administered intravenously or orally. The magnitude of the diuresis produced by these agents greatly exceeds that of other diuretic agents (see Table 21.1), as does the amount of potassium loss that may occur if the medications are given repeatedly several times a day. On the other hand, their relatively short duration of action permits restoration of potassium losses when they are given once or twice a day. Thus,

the magnitude of hypokalemia may not be as severe as with the longer-acting thiazides. Finally, the steep dose-response curve of these agents and their duration of action (Table 21.5) permits a stepwise increase in dosage and frequency of administration until the desired effect is obtained.

Bernardi et al.[9] compared furosemide and muzolimine in a group of cirrhotic patients and reported that although muzolimine induced a natriuresis equivalent to that of furosemide, Unfortunately, development of this diuretic was discontinued because of adverse neurologic effects.

Potassium-sparing Diuretics

Because of their distal site of action (site 4, Fig. 21.3), beyond the sites of reabsorption of most of the filtered sodium, potassium-sparing diuretics are not potent diuretics when used alone (see Table 21.4). These agents, however, amplify the degree of diuresis obtained by other drugs. They are therefore particularly effective when combined with other diuretics that impair sodium reabsorption more proximally, thereby delivering more sodium to site 4. Obviously, their administration not only increases sodium excretion but also reduces potassium and magnesium losses.

Before prescribing potassium-sparing diuretics, one must review the patient's dietary habits and medications and counsel against the excessive intake of foods high in potassium content. All low-sodium foods, especially salt substitutes, contain large amounts of potassium. Inhibition of potassium excretion in the face of increased dietary intake may result in fatal hyperkalemia, particularly in patients in whom potassium homeostasis is concomitantly perturbed by other agents. Patients with reduced renal function are particularly susceptible to this complication and should not receive potassium-sparing diuretics when the glomerular filtration rate is less than

30 ml/min or the serum creatinine is greater than 3.0 mg/dl.

Finally, attention should be directed to the potential interaction between potassium-sparing diuretics and other agents that perturb potassium homeostasis, either external or internal.[10] Particularly important, because of the frequency with which they are prescribed, are the nonsteroidal antiinflammatory drugs and the angiotensin-converting enzyme inhibitors. Both classes of medications may limit the ability of the kidney to excrete potassium, and when they are used together with potassium-sparing diuretics, the risk of hyperkalemia appears to be markedly enhanced.

Choice of a Diuretic Agent

As previously discussed, there is considerable sodium retention at both proximal and distal tubular sits in patients with liver disease (see chapter 1). Although at first glance one may consider the therapeutic use of agents that act primarily by inhibiting proximal tubular reabsorption (site 1, Fig. 21.3) (e.g., carbonic anhydrase inhibitors or osmotic diuretics), their use is not advocated. In general, despite their ability to promote proximal tubular rejection of filtrate, these agents, when administered alone, are only weakly natriuretic. This relates primarily to an enhancement of sodium reabsorption at distal tubular sites that tends to counteract the proximal tubular effect of the drug. Finally, carbonic anhydrase inhibitors have potential side effects that are unique to the patient with liver disease. As an example, by causing a marked increase in urinary pH, acetazolamide favors decreased ammonium excretion so that ammonia is diverted into the systemic circulation. In patients with severe hepatic dysfunction, this may precipitate hepatic encephalopathy.

If there is no compelling reason for rapidly mobilizing excessive fluid, therapy may be initiated with one of the distal potassium-sparing diuretics. Although such diuretics usually induce merely a modest natriuresis, this feature does not necessarily apply to patients with severe hepatic disease. As an example, Perez-Ayuso et al.[11] reported that of 40 patients with stable cirrhosis and ascites, only 11 of 21 had an adequate diuresis with furosemide (80–160 mg/day). In comparison, 18 of 19 patients and 9 of the 10 furosemide-resistant patients responded well to relatively high doses of spironolactone (150–300 mg/day). The authors attributed this apparently paradoxical response to the marked hyperaldosteronism that may occur in cirrhotic patients. As a result, the aldosterone-sensitive site in the cortical collecting tubule can reclaim most of the furosemide-induced increase in fluid delivered out of the loop of Henle, thereby diminishing the diuretic effect. The observation by Perez-Ayuso et al. that the furosemide-resistant patients had a very high plasma renin activity and tended to become hypokalemic (suggesting an enhanced distal exchange of sodium for potassium) are consistent with this hypothesis.

In addition to being more effective, the potassium-sparing diuretics may be safer in patients with cirrhosis. They prevent the development of hypokalemia and metabolic alkalosis, which occasionally precipitate hepatic coma.[7,8]

It is reasonable to start with spironolactone, 200 mg/day in two doses. This drug is an inhibitor of aldosterone-mediated distal tubular sodium reabsorption and in effective dosage can be roughly titrated to urinary sodium excretion and overall diuretic response. If this dosage of spironolactone does not induce a natriuresis, it may be increased in stepwise fashion every 3–5 days until the peak effect becomes manifest; thus a natriuresis does not occur during the initial 2–3 days of therapy. Such a regimen results in a natriuresis in approximately 50% of patients.

Disposition studies of spironolactone have provided a basis for rational dosing of this diuretic. Canrenone and/or canrenoate, the major active metabolites of spironolactone, have a long plasma half-life of 17–22 hours. Furthermore, evidence suggests that the mean half-life of canrenone is further prolonged in patients with hepatic cirrhosis; estimates as high as 60 hours have been reported.[12] These observations permit daily or twice-daily dosing.

Unfortunately, spironolactone is not free of side effects. It causes gynecomastia in a large fraction of cirrhotic patients who receive large doses. To circumvent this problem, it has been suggested that the other potassium-sparing diuretics, triamterene or amiloride, may constitute alternative medications for such patients. Both are nonsteroidal, natriuretic, potassium-sparing agents that both promote sodium excretion and limit potassium excretion even in the absence of mineralocorticoids. Both triamterene and amiloride are less potent natriuretic agents than spironolactone

TABLE 21.7. Treatment of Refractory Edema According to Underlying Mechanism

Problem	Treatment
Excessive sodium intake	Measure urinary sodium excretion; if greater than 75–100 mEq/day, attempt more rigorous dietary restriction.
Decreased intestinal drug absorption	Switch to intravenous loop diuretic.
Increased distal resabsorption	Add thiazide-type diuretic and/or potassium-sparing diuretic.
Decreased loop delivery	Try to increase delivery out of proximal tubule with albumin.
Reduced delivery of furosemide to kidney because of severe hypoalbuminemia	Injection of furosemide-albumin complex.
Decreased drug entry into tubule lumen	Massive doses of loop diuretic. If unresponsive, initiate extracorporeal techniques or the peritoneovenous shunt.

or thiazide-type agents.13 All three potassium-sparing diuretics have the potential to induce hyperkalemia and hyperchloremic acidosis, sometimes of serious proportions.

If no natriuresis occurs with the maximum dosage of spironolactone, one can add a loop diuretic. If no natriuresis is observed on this regimen, the physician should reassess dietary intake to ensure that the patient is not cheating. If dietary sodium intake is being restricted, and if hepatic and renal function show no deterioration, one may consider increasing the dosage of furosemide in a stepwise fashion to a maximum of 200 mg/day.

As noted in chapter 22, the usual custom of increasing the dosage of loop diuretics in a stepwise fashion to a maximum of 400 mg/day for furosemide and 10 mg/day for bumetanide appears to be without merit. Brater has shown that if the natriuretic response after administration of a loop diuretic is inadequate, increasing the dose to $2\frac{1}{2}$ times the usual clinical dose should more than compensate for any changes in the disposition of loop diuretics in patients with liver disease. Some patients are truly refractory to diuretics and do not respond to any dose. Aggressive escalation to doses greater than $2\frac{1}{2}$ times normal in such patients offers no hope of inducing a further natriuresis but entails the risk of toxicity.

Finally, in an attempt to minimize the complications of diuretic therapy, it has been proposed that intermittent administration is safer than continuous treatment.[14,15] From the limited data available, such rest periods appear advisable. At the very least, they provide the clinician adequate time to observe and detect any adverse effects and to discontinue the therapy if so indicated.

Infrequently, a patient does not respond to conventional diuretic therapy even when a loop diuretic is used. Several possible mechanisms

may mediate such refractoriness, and each can be treated in a specific way (Table 21.7).

The initial step in the management of refractory edema is to quantitate the natriuresis. If sodium excretion is greater than 75–100 mEq/day, more rigorous dietary sodium restriction should allow a net fluid loss to occur (see chapter 1). If, however, the natriuresis is inadequate, the orally administered loop diuretic should be given in increasing doses. It is important to note that the size of the dose rather than the frequency of administration should be changed. For example, 40 mg of furosemide may be ineffective in a given patient, in part because the rate of drug delivery to the tubules is too low.[16] In this setting, a diuresis may be induced by raising the single dose to 80 mg, but probably not by repeating the 40-mg dose 8 hours later.

If the patient is resistant to high doses of an oral loop diuretic (such as 240 mg of furosemide), one possibility is that interstitial edema in the bowel wall is impairing drug absorption.[17,18] This will decrease the peak urinary drug concentration and thus the net diuresis. Some patients who are refractory to 200–240 mg of oral furosemide may respond to as little as 40 mg of the drug intravenously.[17] This altered responsiveness is reversible, since removal of the bowel edema with intravenous therapy can improve intestinal absorption, thereby restoring the effectiveness of oral diuretics.[17] An additional approach merits consideration. Recent evidence indicates that binding to albumin is essential for the delivery of sufficient furosemide to the kidney[19] and that injection of a furosemide-albumin complex may overcome the resistance to large doses of furosemide in severely hypoalbuminemic patients. Even though success with this approach has been reported in patients with nephrotic syndrome,[19] it is reasonable to assume that the same principle pertains to hypoalbuminemic cirrhotic patients. Finally, patients who manifest resistance to the natriuretic effect of one of the loop diuretics may respond to another. Thus, some furosemide-resistant patients may be managed successfully with bumetanide and vice versa.

Combined Therapy with Thiazide-type and Loop Diuretic Agents for Resistant Sodium Retention

As noted previously, true resistance to conventional diuretic regimens is unusual.[20] When true resistance is encountered, one approach to management is the combined use of a thiazide-type diuretic with a loop diuretic. The addition of a relatively small dose of a diuretic agent that acts mainly in the cortical diluting segment of the distal nephron (e.g., metolazone or thiazides) to a very large but apparently ineffective dose of a potent loop diuretic (i.e., furosemide or ethacrynic acid) may not be expected to produce a massive natriuretic response. Nevertheless, a synergistic effect of such a combination has been documented in several reports, and successful fluid removal has occurred in patients with previously resistant severe sodium retention associated with diverse disorders, including hepatic cirrhosis.[20]

The mechanism for the diuretic-diuretic potentiation is unknown. It has been proposed that the thiazide-type diuretic agent acts to counter the enhanced distal tubular sodium reabsorption that limits the natriuresis induced by the loop-active agents.[21,22] Thus, the addition of a relatively small dose of another, less potent diuretic agent to furosemide can induce a profound natriuretic and kaliuretic response.

There is no question that diuretic combinations can constitute a highly efficacious means to relieve refractory edema. Nevertheless, despite the positive aspects of these regimens, increasing experience has resulted in disturbing observations about morbidity. Specifically, there is a growing awareness that the use of such combinations may be attended by a wide array of complications, including massive fluid and electrolyte losses and circulatory collapse.[21] Of particular concern in the cirrhotic patient, there is a major risk of profound hypokalemia that may occur with alarming rapidity. Furthermore, such patients with a diminished effective volume are at risk of developing the hepatorenal syndrome, acute renal failure (ATN), and hepatic encephalopathy if an overly rapid diuresis occurs. As we explained in a recent editorial,[21] the potential risk may be only rarely justifiable in patients with liver disease. Rather, if there are compelling reasons for mobilizing excessive fluid (as discussed above), one should resort to the use of the peritoneovenous shunt (for a detailed discussion, see chapter 24).

Role of Albumin

Because hypoalbuminemia is considered a major factor in the pathogenesis of ascites, many physicians administer albumin solutions to mobilize ascites. In my opinion, the indiscriminate administration of albumin solutions has a highly limited role in the mobilization of ascites and edema in patients with liver disease. The intravenous administration of albumin causes, at best, a transient increase in plasma volume and urine output, but rapid equilibration with ascitic albumin quickly blunts these effects. In addition, the degradation of albumin accelerates as its concentration increases. To be effective, albumin must be given in large amounts; its expense and the potential hazards of hemorrhage as plasma volume increases make its use impractical.

Albumin infusion should be reserved for (1) patients with liver disease and extreme hypoalbuminemia (< 2.0 gm/dl) in whom intravascular volume depletion is markedly evident (e.g., a fall in orthostatic blood pressure) and (2) selected patients with very tense ascites in whom a rapid diuresis is desirable, particularly if they have an umbilical hernia or if the ascites is producing respiratory embarrassment. In the second instance, intravenous albumin should be used in conjunction with intravenous diuretic therapy Table 21.3).

Rapid Diuresis with Intravenous Diuretic Therapy

Selected patients may be candidates for rapid diuresis with the so-called "Galambos' cocktail."[23] In essence, this regimen is a variant of the combined diuretic-albumin infusion, and the indications for its use are similar. The regimen, as outlined by Galambos,[23] consists of the following:
1. Two hundred fifty or 500 ml of either 5% albumin in saline or fresh frozen plasma is infused at 4 ml/min.
2. This is followed by intravenous injection of 20–60 mg of furosemide.

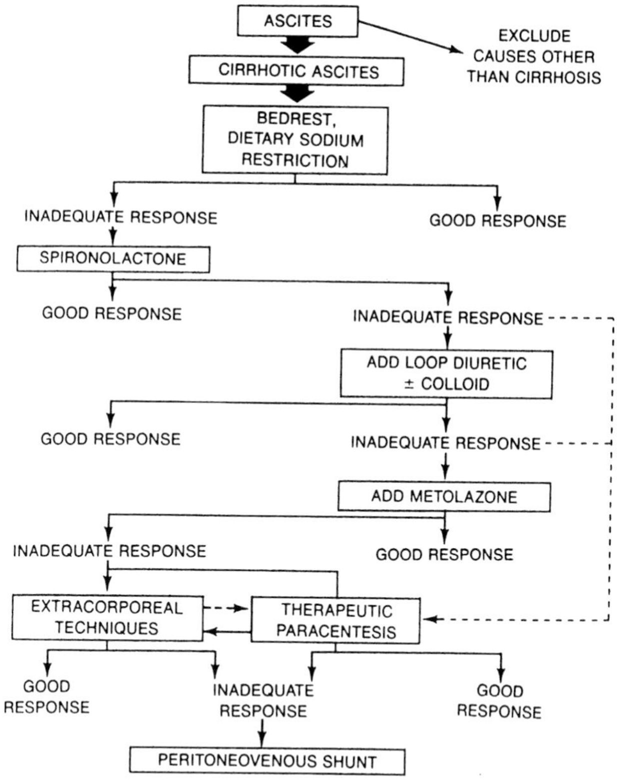

FIGURE 21.4. Algorithm for the comprehensive management of cirrhotic ascites and edema. The solid lines represent therapeutic options and sequences believed to be well established. The interrupted lines indicate uncertainty about the appropriate position of paracentesis in the therapeutic sequence.

3. This is followed promptly by infusion of 20% mannitol at 5.6 ml/min. With the advent of large volume paracentesis, this regimen has been supplanted and now is rarely used.

Ancillary Measures

Another measure that may be helpful in severely edematous patients is tight wrapping of the legs. Bank reported that this maneuver, which enhances venous return to the heart and thus produces effective volume expansion, enhances sodium excretion.[24]

FUTURE PROSPECTS

Spironolactone is the most commonly used antimineralocorticoid drug in the management of cirrhotic patients with ascites, but the value of its prolonged administration may be diminished by the appearance of side effects related to its anti-androgenic action.[25] It is well established that the sexual endocrine effects of spironolactone are due largely to this compound's strong affinity for the androgen and progesterone receptors.[26–28] Recently, an epoxy-derivative of spironolactone has been developed that has less affinity for the androgen

and progesterone receptors. Studies to assess the anti-mineralocorticoid potency of this new agent are currently undergoing clinical investigation.

SUMMARY

After a review of the specific attributes and usage of various diuretics used to mobilize ascites and edema in patients with liver disease, it is helpful to consider the appropriate role of diuretics in the overall management of sodium retention associated with liver disease. The algorithm in Figure 21.4 is recommended as a guide to management of cirrhotic ascites. Approximately 10% of cirrhotic patients with ascites can be managed with bed rest and sodium restriction. The importance of good nutrition and abstention from alcohol should be emphasized. The next step is the use of spironolactone in doses up to 400–600 mg/day. Cautiously used, a combination of diuretic therapy with spironolactone and loop diuretics (with or without addition of metolazone) may induce a response in many patients. Simultaneous administration of colloid may help to reduce the risk of hyponatremia and volume contraction. In some patients, especially those with peripheral edema, therapeutic paracentesis may be a reasonable alternative. For the patient truly refractory to the above maneuvers, the therapeutic choices include extracorporeal techniques (see chapter 26) and the peritoneovenous shunt (see chapter 24). Extracorporeal techniques include ascites reinfusion, dialytic ultrafiltration of ascites, or continuous arteriovenous hemofiltration (CAVH). In my opinion, CAVH is currently the best extracorporeal technique. Additional experience with CAVH may suggest that it should be tried before the peritoneous shunt, which carries a higher rate of complications.

REFERENCES

1. Conn HO: Diuresis of ascites: Fraught with or free from hazard. Gastroenterology 1977;73:619–621.
2. Conn HO, Fessell JM: Spontaneous bacterial peritonitis in cirrhosis. Variations on a theme. Medicine 1971; 50:161–167.
3. Sherlock S: Ascites formation in cirrhosis and its management. Scand J Gastroenterol 1970;7(Suppl):9–15.
4. Naranjo CA, Pontigo E, Valdenegro C, et al: Furosemide-induced adverse reactions in cirrhosis of the liver. Clin Pharmacol Ther 1979;25:154–160.
5. Muschaweck R: Discovery and development of furosemide: Historical remarks. In Puschett JB, Greenberg A (eds): Diuretics: Chemistry, Pharmacology, and Clinical Applications. New York: Elsevier, 1984;4–11.
6. Shear L, Ching S, Gabuzda GJ: Compartmentalization of ascites and edema in patients with hepatic cirrhosis. N Engl J Med 1970;282:1391–1396.
7. Perez GO, Oster JR: Altered potassium metabolism in liver disease. In Epstein M (ed): The Kidney in Liver Disease, 2nd ed. New York: Elsevier, 1983;147–182.
8. Baertl JM, Sancetta SM, Gabuzda GJ: Relation of acute potassium depletion to renal ammonium metabolism in patients with cirrhosis. J Clin Invest 1963;42:696.
9. Bernardi M, De Palma R, Trevisani F, et al: Effects of a new loop diuretic (muzolimine) in cirrhosis with ascites: Comparison with furosemide. Hepatology 1986;6:400–405.
10. Ponce SP, Jennings AE, Madis NE, Harrington JT: Drug-induced hyperkalemia. Medicine 1985;64:357–370.
11. Perez-Ayuso RM, Arroyo V, Planas R, et al: Randomized comparative study of efficacy of furosemide versus spironolactone in nonazotemic cirrhosis with ascites. Relationship between the diuretic response and the activity of the renin-aldosterone system. Gastroenterology 1983;84:961–968.
12. Jackson L, Branch R, Levine D, Ramsay L: Elimination of canrenone in congestive heart failure and chronic liver disease. Eur J Clin Pharmacol 1977;11:177–179.
13. DeCarvalho JG, Emery AC Jr, Frohlich ED: Spironolactone and triamterene in volume-dependent essential hypertension. Clin Pharmacol Ther 1980;27:53–56.
14. Lieberman FL, Reynolds TB: The use of ethacrynic acid in patients with cirrhosis and ascites. Gastroenterology 1965;49:531–538.
15. Fuller RK, Khambatta PB, Gobezie GC: An optimal diuretic regimen for cirrhotic ascites. A controlled trial evaluating safety and efficacy of spironolactone and furosemide. JAMA 1977;237:972–975.
16. Kaojarern S, Day B, Brater DC: The time course of delivery of furosemide into the urine: An independent determinant of overall response. Kidney Int 1982;22: 69–74.
17. Odlind BOG, Beermann B: Diuretic resistance: Reduced bioavailability and effect of oral furosemide. BMJ 1980; 280:1577.
18. Vasko MR, Brown-Cartwright D, Knochel JP, et al: Furosemide absorption altered in decompensated congestive heart failure. Ann Intern Med 1985;102:314–318.
19. Inoue M, Okajima K, Itch K, et al: Mechanisms of furosemide resistance in analbuminemic rats and hypoalbuminemic patients. Kidney Int 1987;32:198–203.
20. Epstein M, Lepp BA, Hoffman DS, Levinson R: Potentiation of furosemide by metolazone in refractory edema. Curr Ther Res 1977;21:656–667.
21. Oster JR, Epstein M, Smoller S: Combined therapy with thiazide-type and loop diuretic agents for resistant sodium retention. Ann Intern Med 1983;99:405–406.
22. Sigurd B, Olesen KH, Wennevold A: The supra-additive natriuretic effect of addition of bendroflumethiazide and bumetanide in congestive heart failure. Am Heart J 1975; 89:163–170.
23. Galambos JT: Cirrhosis. Philadelphia: W.B. Saunders, 1979;349–350.
24. Bank N: External compression for treatment of resistant edema [letter]. N Engl J Med 1980;302:969.
25. Loriaux DL, Menard R, Taylor A, et al: Spironolactone and endocrine dysfunction. Ann Intern Med 1976;85:630–636.
26. Corvol P, Michaud A, Menard J, et al: Antiandrogenic effect of spirolactones: Mechanism of action. Endocrinology 1975;97:52–58.
27. Cutler GB, Pita JC, Rifka SM, et al: A potent mineralcorticoid antagonist with affinity for the 5α-dihydrotestosterone receptor of human and rat prostate. J Clin Endocrinol Metab 1978;47:171–175.
28. Huffman DH, Kampmann JP, Hignite CE, et al: Gynecomastia induced in normal males by spironolactone. Clin Pharmacol Ther 1978;24:465–473.

Chapter 22

PHARMACOKINETICS AND PHARMACODYNAMICS IN CIRRHOSIS

D. CRAIG BRATER, M.D.

Pharmacokinetic Principles in Liver Disease
  Absorption and First-pass Effect
  Distribution
  Elimination

Specific Drugs Used in Patients with Liver Disease and Affecting the Kidney
  Nonsteroidal Antiinflammatory Drugs
  Diuretics

PHARMACOKINETIC PRINCIPLES IN LIVER DISEASE

The liver metabolizes a vast number of drugs that are then eliminated either by the liver via excretion in bile or by the kidney. Thus, hepatic impairment with its attendant effects on metabolic capacity and blood flow distribution within the liver may have profound effects on elimination of numerous drugs.[1,2] In addition, an important determinant of the disposition of some drugs is binding to serum proteins, the concentrations of which may be influenced by liver disease. The multiplicity of potential effects of hepatic impairment on disposition of drugs requires an understanding of the changes that occur and the drugs for which hepatic elimination is important.

This chapter emphasizes the influence of liver disease on the pharmacokinetics of drugs and the implications of changes in drug disposition for dosing strategies. Liver disease also may influence the response to drugs over and above any changes in disposition. Two classes of drugs that have important effects on the kidney in liver disease are reviewed: (1) nonsteroidal antiinflammatory drugs (NSAIDs), which are metabolized by the liver and may adversely affect the kidney, and (2) diuretics, which are frequently used in patients with severe liver disease and to which response is often subnormal.

Absorption and First-pass Effect

Severe cirrhosis is associated with ascites and peripheral edema, and it has been presumed that edema of the intestinal wall is also present. Because of decreased oncotic pressure due to hypoalbuminemia and increased portal venous pressures, this assumption seems tenable. In turn, it has been postulated that edematous states in general are associated with altered absorption of drugs due to local edema, changed intestinal perfusion, and/or altered gastrointestinal motility. Unfortunately, there is a paucity of direct evaluation of this general question, particularly in patients with liver disease.

Detailed studies of digoxin and furosemide absorption have been performed in other edematous disorders. Furosemide absorption has been evaluated in patients with heart failure.[3–5] In such studies, quantitative absorption (bioavailability) did not differ from that in normal subjects. Moreover, no difference in bioavailability was found in patients with heart failure when data from the same patient were compared in the decompensated state and after attainment of dry weight.[5] Similar studies of digoxin absorption in patients with heart failure have shown normal bioavailability.[6] In contrast, one case report described a patient with idiopathic edema in whom bioavailability of furosemide was decreased.[7] One study specifically assessed bioavailability of furosemide in patients with cirrhosis.[8] In both compensated and decompensated patients bioavailability was normal.[8] From these data it seems reasonable to conclude that the edematous state per se does not adversely affect quantitative drug absorption. In rare circumstances diminished absorption may occur, but this mechanism of abnormal response to an orally administered drug should be entertained only after other causes are excluded.

Despite the absence of quantitative effects on drug absorption, there are changes in rate of absorption in patients with liver disease and other edematous states.[1–6] The mechanism(s) of these effects is unknown but may relate to factors such as altered gastric emptying and changed intestinal motility. Such effects on rate of absorption, which do not affect bioavailability, have no effect on average serum concentrations of a drug and simply decrease the magnitude of swing between peak and trough concentrations. Conceptually, this type of change is similar to the difference between standard and slow-release formulations of a drug. Clinically, the effects do not alter dosing strategies, although with initial doses the onset of effect may be slower than in patients whose absorption rate is more rapid.

Although historically drug absorption in patients with liver disease has focused on decreased bioavailability, paradoxically, the reverse occurs more often. Once a drug crosses the gastrointestinal epithelium and enters the portal circulation, it reaches the liver, where it can be metabolized before entering the systemic circulation. This process is called presystemic elimination or the first-pass effect. In patients with liver disease, hepatic metabolic capacity may be diminished and/or portosystemic shunts may bypass hepatocytes. Both effects result in diminished presystemic elimination and increased access of drug to the systemic circulation; in other words, increased bioavailability. This phenomenon has been described for the drugs listed in Table 22.1.[9–33] In patients with cirrhosis, the increase in bioavailability requires a decrease in dose over and above the decrease needed to compensate for diminished ability to eliminate the drugs (see below).

The degree of hepatic dysfunction needed to change bioavailability is unknown, but probably severe cirrhosis is required. On the other hand, a patient with moderate disease who is administered other drugs that inhibit hepatic metabolism may be expected to need the same dose modifications as a patient with severe disease. Drugs other than those listed in Table 22.1 may also be subject to the same phenomenon, but studies have not been performed. Clinicians should be aware that drugs with a large first-pass effect may demonstrate increased bioavailability in patients with cirrhosis; such drugs should be used cautiously, beginning with low doses and titrating slowly upward with close monitoring of the patient.

Overall, then, liver disease affects the time course of drug absorption, most commonly by slowing rates of absorption with consequent decreases in the magnitude of difference between peak and trough serum concentrations. Bioavailability does not seem to be decreased; in contrast, a greater concern is increased bioavailability of drugs with a large first-pass effect. With such drugs, downward dose adjustment is necessary.

Distribution

Determinants of Drug Distribution and Influence of Liver Disease

The precise determinants of distribution of drugs to tissues are not well known. Molecular size, lipid solubility, pKa, and protein binding are important. Of these, liver disease may considerably influence protein binding by affecting circulating concentrations of binding proteins. The effects of hepatic dysfunction on other determinants of distribution remain speculative. Early studies with cimetidine in patients with liver disease noted disproportionate adverse central nervous system effects relative to circulating concentrations.[34] Subsequent studies showed that liver disease was associated with increased distribution of cimetidine into the brain, the mechanism of which is unclear but may relate to breakdown in the blood-brain barrier.[35] Whether this occurs with other drugs and accounts for the increased susceptibility of patients with cirrhosis to central nervous system depressant effects is unknown. Similarly, whether liver disease invokes differences in distribution of drugs to other tissue sites is unknown.

Binding of drugs to serum proteins restricts them to the vascular compartment. Hence, drugs that are highly protein-bound have small volumes of distribution. Drug binding in turn is a function of affinity of the drug for protein-binding sites and concentration of the binding protein.[36,37]

It is important to examine in detail the effects of changes in protein binding on the volume in which a drug distributes, for this subject has been a source of considerable confusion. As discussed below, the volume of distribution (Vd) of a drug is clinically important for determining the

TABLE 22.1. Drugs with Diminished Presystemic Elimination (Increased Bioavailability) in Liver Disease

Drug	Bioavailability (%)		
	Normal Hepatic Function	Cirrhosis	Reference
Beta-adrenergic antagonists			
Labetalol	30	60	9
Metoprolol	50	85	10
Propranolol	36	75	11
Calcium channel antagonists			
Isradipine	15–20	40	12, 13
Nifedipine	40–50	90	14, 15
Nisoldipine	4	15	16, 17
Verapamil	35	70	18, 19
Analgesics			
Meperidine	56	87	20
Morphine	24–50	100	21
Pentazocine	20	70	20
Histamine H_2 antagnoists			
Cimetidine	60	75	22
Ranitidine	50	70	23
Antianxiety agents			
Buspirone	1–13	Increased	24
Chlormethiazole	10	100	25
Flumazenil	16–28	65	26, 27
Midazolam	40–50	75	28
Miscellaneous			
Metoclopramide	60–75	80	29
Encainide	14–38	83–88	29–31
Perindopril	17–20	30	32
Pentoxifyline	30	60	33

loading dose. A proportionality factor relates the dose of a drug to its serum concentration:

$$\text{Concentration attained} = \frac{\text{Loading dose}}{\text{Volume of distribution}}$$

Consequently, a drug with a large Vd requires a larger loading dose to attain the same serum concentration as a drug with a lower Vd. Similarly, if a disease affects Vd, then a concomitant change in loading dose must be made to reach the same serum concentration.

Confusion occurs in conditions in which protein binding is changed. For example, the Vd of a drug with a total serum concentration (protein-bound plus free) of 10 mg/L after a 100-mg loading dose may be calculated on the basis of total drug concentration:

$$\text{Concentration attained} = \frac{\text{Loading dose}}{\text{Vd}}$$

$$10 \text{ mg/L} = \frac{100 \text{ mg}}{\text{Vd}}$$

$$\text{Vd} = 10 \text{ L}$$

If the drug is 90% bound to serum proteins, the unbound or free concentration that is pharmacologically active is 1 mg/L. One can also calculate the Vd of the free drug:

$$1 \text{ mg/L} = \frac{100 \text{ mg}}{\text{Vd}_{\text{free}}}$$

$$\text{Vd}_{\text{free}} = 100 \text{ L}$$

If changes in protein binding occur, one must assess effects on the volume of distribution relative to both total and unbound drug. If, for example, a patient has liver disease sufficient to decrease the concentration of binding protein, the percent of bound drug may decrease from 90% to 60%. This does not appear to be a large quantitative change; however, it represents a quadrupling of the free, pharmacologically active drug from 10% to 40%. The influence of such a change on the Vd of total compared with free drug is different. For total drug, the serum concentration is still 10 mg/L; thus the Vd is still 10 L. In contrast, for free drug the concentration is 4 mg/L and the

Vd_{free} is thus one-fourth the value before the change in binding:

$$4 \text{ mg/L} = \frac{100 \text{ mg}}{Vd_{free}}$$

Vd_{free} = 25 L (compared with 100 L before the change in binding)

Which of these values is more important clinically? Because the free drug is pharmacologically active, Vd_{free} should be used to guide dosing. If the goal of therapy were to maintain the same level of pharmacologic activity, one would need to decrease the loading dose to one-fourth of the previous dose to attain a free concentration of 1 mg/L in the setting of decreased protein binding. A corollary is that dosing based on the Vd for total drug would result in a free concentration 4 times as high as that desired. Hence, basing dosing strategy on the Vd of the total drug leads to dosing errors.

To elaborate the effect of protein binding on volume of distribution, it is useful to consider another common scenario. Frequently a decrease in binding has no effect on free drug concentration. This scenario is explained by the fact a decrease in binding provides increased amounts of drug not only to interact with sites of pharmacologic activity but also to be metabolized, excreted, and/or distributed into tissues. In fact, in most settings distribution and elimination pathways are sufficient to keep free drug concentration the same as in the state of normal binding.[38]

Consider the influence of this common scenario on the Vds of total and unbound drug. If, as in the normal state, the total concentration of a drug after a 100-mg dose is 10 mg/L, of which 90% is bound, the Vd for total drug is 10 L and Vd_{free} is 100 L. If protein binding decreases, but the concentration of free drug does not change, the following concentrations and volumes of distribution would be found:

Bound drug	+	Free drug	=	Total drug concentration
6 mg/L		1 mg/L		7 mg/L

$$1 \text{ mg/L} = \frac{100 \text{ mg}}{Vd_{free}} \qquad 7 \text{ mg/L} = \frac{100 \text{ mg}}{Vd}$$

$$Vd_{free} = 100 \text{ L} \qquad Vd = 14.3 \text{ L}$$

Although Vd_{free} has not changed, Vd for total drug increased from 10 L to 14.3 L. If dosing were based on Vd for total drug, a larger loading dose would be administered, resulting in increased free concentrations and potential toxicity. Again, focusing strictly on total drug concentration is misleading.

In normal people the usual scenario is that decreased protein binding does not change free drug concentration. The scenario may be quite different in patients with liver disease, because impaired metabolic capacity may not allow a compensatory increase in elimination. Hence, it is particularly important in patients with hepatic disease to be wary of increased free drug concentrations when protein binding is diminished.

The preceding considerations are important in patients with liver disease because of frequent changes in concentrations of binding proteins. The major drug-binding proteins are albumin and alpha$_1$-acid glycoprotein. In patients with severe liver disease, hepatic synthesis of albumin is decreased, and hypoalbuminemia is frequent. The result is diminished binding of a number of acidic drugs. Many basic drugs are highly bound to alpha$_1$-acid glycoprotein, the concentration of which is also affected by hepatic disease. Alpha$_1$-acid glycoprotein is an acute phase reactant and thereby increases in a number of settings, including inflammatory liver diseases. On the other hand, patients with severe cirrhosis have diminished alpha$_1$-acid glycoprotein production and decreased serum concentrations. However, the severity of liver disease that is necessary to suppress synthesis of this protein is unknown. Because alpha$_1$-acid glycoprotein is not routinely measured in clinical settings, it is difficult to predict its concentration in individual patients. When using basic drugs with high protein binding, clinicians should be aware that altered concentrations of this protein may involve concomitant changes in binding.

In summary, liver disease is the prototypic clinical condition in which changed protein binding of drugs occurs. This effect can profoundly influence free, pharmacologically active drug. Many data and clinical recommendations for dosing are based on total drug concentration, which can be misleading. For drugs with binding less than about 80%, the magnitude of change in unbound drug concentration is not sufficient to cause clinical concern. With such drugs, basing dosage on Vd for total drug is sufficient. For drugs that are highly protein-bound, one should focus on unbound drug concentrations.

Loading Dose

As implied above, the volume of distribution is important clinically as a determinant of loading dose. Not all patients or all drugs require a loading-dose strategy, depending on how quickly attainment of a therapeutic concentration is needed. If a loading dose is not administered, a period 4–5 times the drug's half-life is needed to attain steady-state serum concentrations. If this period is too long, a loading dose should be administered. The size of the loading dose is determined from the relationships presented above:

$$\text{Concentration attained} = \frac{\text{Loading dose}}{\text{Volume of distribution}}$$

For example, if one desires a concentration of 10 mg/L and the Vd is 10 L, the loading dose required is easily calculated:

$$10 \text{ mg/dl} = \frac{\text{Loading dose}}{10 \text{ L}}$$

$$\text{Loading dose} = 100 \text{ mg}$$

In some settings one can use the Vd for total drug, whereas in others Vd_{free} must be used.

Table 22.2 presents drugs for which the volume of distribution is changed in patients with liver disease.[39] For a number of highly bound drugs there are changes in protein binding, but whether Vd_{free} is changed is unclear. Even when crucial data are lacking, the drug is included in the table to emphasize that caution is needed. Other drugs in Table 22.2 demonstrate changes in Vd unrelated to altered protein binding. The mechanism of such effects is unknown.

Elimination

Influence on Bioavailability

The relationship between hepatic metabolic capacities for drugs and bioavailability relates to effects on presystemic elimination (see Table 22.1). The impact of this process on circulating concentrations can be addressed in a quantitative sense. At steady state, by definition, the rate of drug entering the body equals the rate of elimination:

$$\text{Rate of drug in} = \text{Rate of drug elimination}$$

In turn, the "rate in" is a function of the maintenance dose, the fraction of that dose absorbed (bioavailability), and the frequency of dosing:

$$\text{Rate of drug in} = \frac{\text{Bioavailability} \times \text{Maintenance dose}}{\text{Dosing interval}}$$

TABLE 22.2. Drugs with Changed Volume of Distribution in Patients with Cirrhosis

Drug	Total Drug	Free Drug
Carvedilol	2½ Normal	?
Cefodizime	2½ Normal	?
Cefpiramide		¼ Normal
Ceftriaxone		½ Normal
Cimetidine	½ Normal	Decreased
Clofibrate	Increased	No change
Clotiazepam	⅔ Normal	?
Erythromycin	Increased	No change
Guanabenz	⅓ Normal	?
Hydroxyzine	1⅓ Normal	?
Indoramin	1⅓ Normal	Probably no change
Ketansirin	¾ Normal	?
Lidocaine	1½ Normal	Increased
Miconazole	Decreased	?
Nisoldipine	2¼ Normal	?
Oxaprozin	Increased	No change
Phenytoin	Increased	No change
Pinacidil	⅔ Normal	?
Propranolol	Increased	No change
Tolbutamide	Increased	No change
Valproate	Increased	No change
Verapamil	½ Normal	?

TABLE 22.3.   Clearance and Half-life Values of Drugs for Which Liver Disease Requires Dose Adjustment

Drug	Clearance (ml/min/kg)		Half-life (hr)	
	Normal	Cirrhosis	Normal	Cirrhosis
Alfentanil	4.4–6.5	1.6	1.4–2.2	3.5
Amlodipine			34–50	60
Azapropazone	0.14	0.03	10–15	60
Azithromycin			41	68
Aztreonam	1.0	0.8	1.7	3.2
Bevantolol			1.5–2.0	7
Bisoprolol	1.8–3.4	2.6	9–12	13–17
Brotizolam	1.5–2.5	0.75	3.6–7.9	13
Carvedilol	8.7	5.5		
Cefoperazone			1.5–2.5	11
Cefotaxime	3.6–4.5	2.7	1–1.5	4.8
Cefpiramide	0.27	0.38	4.5	6.2
Cefprozil		0.38	1.2–1.7	1.5–2.2
Ceftriaxone		½ normal for free drug		
Chloramphenicol	2.5–3.2	0.7–2.1	3–5	7–11
Chlordiazepoxide	0.25–0.5	0.12	6–28	
Chlormethiazole	16	11	5	9
Cimetidine	8–10	4	1–5	
Clindamycin	2.1–3.5	1.7	2.5–3.5	4.5
Clofibrate		½ normal for free drug		
Clotiazepam	3–4	2	9–10	32
Cyclosporine	6–10	2–5	3–16	35
Dapsone	0.6	0.4	10–30	
Diphenhydramine	8	4	3.5–9	
Disopyramide		¾ normal for free drug		
Encainide	25	17	2.5	3.7
ODE			2.8	8.7
Felodipine	12–24	7	10–25	16
Flecainide	16	4	7	50
Fleroxacin	1.2–1.4	0.6		
Flumazenil	10–17	9–10	0.7–1.3	1.4
Fluoxetine	9.6	4.2	2.2–4	6.6
Guanabenz	9	2	6–10	
Iloprost	16–20	10		
Indoramin	20	12	4–5.5	9–12
Isradipine			1.9–4.8	6.5–12
Josamycin			0.9–2	5.4
Ketansirin	6–10	4.6	6–14	10
Lidocaine	10	6	1.8	4.9
Lorcainide	14–21	12	7–8	12
Meperidine	7.5–12	8	3–7	11
Metoclopramide	8–11	2.7–6	2.5–5	10–15
Metoprolol	10–20	9	2.5–5	7
Metronidazole	0.7–1.3	0.25	8	20

(Continued)

TABLE 22.3. Clearance and Half-life Values for Drugs in Which Liver Disease Requires Dose Adjustment (*Continued*)

Drug	Clearance (ml/min/kg)		Half-life (hr)	
	Normal	Cirrhosis	Normal	Cirrhosis
Mexiletine	6.3–8.3	2.3	8–12	29
Mezlocillin	4.0	1.8	1	2.6
Midazolam	4–9	3.3	1.5–5.1	7.4
Mitoxantrone		Decreased		Increased
Moclobemide	7–14	3.5	1–2	4
Morphine	8–27	11	1.7–4.5	4
Nicardipine			3.5–4.8	14
Nicorandil			0.8–1.5	1.7
Nifedipine	6–15	3	3.5–4	7
Nimodipine			1–6	8–22
Nisoldipine	8–16	7	10–15	17–19
Omeprazole	2.9	1.0	0.5–1.5	2.8
Pefloxacin	1.7–2.1	0.6	7.5–11	29–35
Pentazocine	17–20	9.5	3–5	7
Pentobarbital			20–25	40
Pentoxifylline			0.8	2.1
Pinacidil	9.5	4.9	1.5–3	6
Prednisone		⅔ normal for free drug		
Propranolol	12	8	2.5–5	12
Roxithromycin			10–13	19–36
Theophylline	1.0	0.7	4–12	26
Tolbutamide			4–6	8–12
Urapadil			1.8–3.9	8–20
Vecuronium	3.0–6.4	2.7	0.5–1.3	1.4
Verapamil	14–20	5	3–5	14
Zidovudine	17–30	6.6	1–1.5	2.4
Zolpidem			1.5–2.4	10

The rate of drug elimination is a function of the average drug concentration at steady state (Cp_{ss}) and clearance of the drug:

Rate of drug elimination = Cp_{ss} × Clearance

Hence,

$$Cp_{ss} \times Clearance = \frac{Bioavailability \times Maintenance\ dose}{Dosing\ interval}$$

or

$$Cp_{ss} \times Clearance = \frac{Bioavailability \times Maintenance\ dose}{Dosing\ interval \times Clearance}$$

As should be readily apparent from this relationship, a decrease in presystemic elimination associated with increased bioavailability directly and proportionally increases the steady-state drug concentration. To avoid drug accumulation, the dose must be reduced.

Influence on Clearance

Since the liver is responsible for the elimination of so many drugs, it is to be expected that hepatic disease impairs their clearance. Drugs cleared by hepatic metabolism are frequently characterized in terms of the hepatic extraction ratio, which allows classification into two categories: (1) flow-limited drugs, clearance of which relates to hepatic blood flow, and (2) capacity-limited drugs, clearance of which is a function of hepatic metabolic capacity.[1,2,40] In simplistic terms one may think of flow-limited drugs as having a very high metabolic capacity so that the liver is able to metabolize all of the drug that reaches it, which is a function of hepatic blood flow. With such drugs, changes in protein binding do not influence clearance. In contrast, capacity-limited drugs depend on the liver's metabolic capabilities and have lower extraction ratios; hepatic perfusion does not influence clearance. Instead, the determinants of clearance are metabolic capacity and access of drug to hepatocytes, which is a function of unbound drug concentration. Thus, changes in protein binding influence clearance of capacity-limited drugs.[1,2,40]

Whether the distinction between capacity- and flow-limited drugs is maintained in patients with liver disease is debated. Clinically, the specifics of this argument may be superfluous, for in terms of dosing strategy one simply needs to know whether or not clearance is changed in patients with liver disease. As with volume of distribution, one must distinguish between clearance of total versus unbound drug. Table 22.3 lists drugs for which clearance is reduced in patients with hepatic impairment.[39] These data can be used to modify dosing in such patients.

Maintenance Doses

The quantitative relationships presented above can be used to illustrate the relationship between clearance and maintenance dose of a drug:

$$Cp_{ss} = \frac{Bioavailability \times Maintenance\ dose}{Dosing\ interval \times Clearance}$$

Hence, clearance is a determinant of the average drug concentration at steady state. In turn, changes in clearance must be compensated by proportional changes in the dosing regimen, either the amount or the frequency of drug administration.

Particular caution must be exercised with drugs in which both presystemic elimination (see Table 22.1) and clearance (see Table 22.3) are affected by liver disease. With such drugs both parameters are usually affected simultaneously, resulting in a multiplier effect. For example, if bioavailability doubles while clearance simultaneously decreases to one-half normal, the combined effect is a quadrupling of steady-state drug serum concentrations. Clearly, cautious dosing is mandatory.

Overall, hepatic elimination of drugs is important in determining the maintenance dose. In patients with liver disease, the clearance of many drugs declines, mandating changes in dosing strategy (see Table 22.3). Clinicians should remember the caveats concerning effects on unbound drug concentrations and should exercise great caution with drugs in which bioavailability is also affected (see Table 22.1).

SPECIFIC DRUGS USED IN PATIENTS WITH LIVER DISEASE AND AFFECTING THE KIDNEY

Patients with liver disease show increased sensitivity to various drugs, including central nervous system depressants, although the mechanism(s) is not understood. Two classes of drugs with altered kinetics and response are NSAIDs and diuretics. Because of their importance in such patients, they are discussed in detail.

Nonsteroidal Antiinflammatory Drugs

NSAIDs inhibit cyclooxygenase and thereby decrease prostaglandin (PG) synthesis throughout the body, including the kidney. The currently known physiologic roles of PGs in the kidney include hemodynamic effects in certain clinical conditions (see below); inhibition of tubular reabsorption of sodium, which appears to occur at the medullary segment of the thick ascending limb of the loop of Henle; inhibition of the hydroosmotic effect of antidiuretic hormone (ADH); and stimulation of renin release.[41–44]

Prostaglandins help to maintain renal blood flow in states of diminished actual or effective circulating volume, such as sodium depletion,[45–47] hemorrhage,[48] decreased cardiac output,[49,50] and cirrhosis.[51–53] The altered circulatory state results in release of various vasoconstricting autacoids, including catecholamines, angiotensin II, and vasopressin. To maintain renal perfusion, the kidney synthesizes vasodilating PGs (PGE_2 and PGI_2) that blunt the effects of the endogenous vasoconstrictors, thereby preventing declines in renal blood flow (Fig 22.1).

Because of the known renal physiology of PGs, NSAIDs have predictable effects on renal function.[41–44] In patients with cirrhosis, they may cause abrupt and substantial declines in renal perfusion (Fig 22.1), sodium retention, retention of free water, and hyporeninemic hypoaldosteronism with hyperkalemia. The effect on renal hemodynamics is particularly hazardous; although usually reversible, it can be associated with considerable morbidity, especially in severely ill patients. The sodium and water retention attendant to severe cirrhosis may be sufficient that an incremental effect of NSAIDs is negligible. On the other hand, in patients with less severe disease, NSAIDs may cause enough sodium retention to result in development of new peripheral edema (and presumably ascites) and sufficient free water accumulation to contribute to hyponatremia. The potential for hyponatremia is enhanced by the nonosmotic ADH release that often occurs in patients with cirrhosis.[54,55] Hence, many patients have pathologically increased plasma concentrations of ADH relative to serum osmolality, the renal effects of which may be accentuated by inhibition of PGs with NSAIDs.

Disposition

NSAIDs have various effects on renal function in patients with liver disease. In addition, liver disease may affect the disposition of NSAIDs. Consequently, patients not only manifest increased susceptibility to this class of drugs from a pharmacodynamic perspective but also experience changes in pharmacokinetics.

All NSAIDs are highly bound to serum albumin and have small volumes of distribution. Because patients with liver disease often have diminished albumin concentrations, the potential for changes in free, pharmacologically active concentrations is considerable. Hence, considerations discussed above need particular emphasis. Studies of NSAID disposition in patients with liver disease should assess concentrations of unbound rather than total drug, particularly since the vast majority of NSAIDs are eliminated by hepatic metabolism; thus patients with liver disease are at particular risk for changes in drug disposition. Although a number of NSAIDs have been studied in patients with cirrhosis, in many studies only total drug concentrations were measured; therefore, the data are uninformative if not misleading. Drugs that have been assessed in cirrhosis include azapropazone, carprofen, ibuprofen, nabumetone, naproxen, oxaproxen, sulindac, tenoxicam, tolfenamic acid, and ximoprofen.

Azapropazone. Azapropazone is one of the few NSAIDs with a component of renal elimination. Because a substantial portion is excreted by the liver, however, studies have appropriately addressed the influence of cirrhosis on disposition. Protein binding is considerably decreased in patients with cirrhosis, with a 5-fold increase in percent of free drug from 0.44 ± 0.09% to 2.1 ± 2.4%.[56] Clearance of total drug was not affected by cirrhosis, but clearance of unbound drug was half that in healthy subjects (15.8 ± 10.5 vs. 32.4 ± 8.8 ml/min/kg, respectively).[57] Such patients should receive half the normally administered dose of azapropazone. The data emphasize the

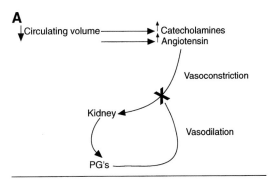

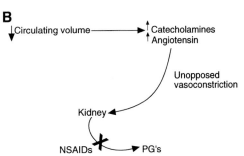

FIGURE 22.1. *A*, The role of prostaglandins (PG) in maintaining renal perfusion in patients with diminished actual or effective circulating blood volume, including those with cirrhosis. *B*, If nonsteroidal antiinflammatory drugs are administered to such patients, unopposed vasoconstriction ensues.

importance of measuring unbound drug concentrations. Total azapropazone concentrations suggest that disposition is unchanged in patients with cirrhosis. Clearly, this conclusion is erroneous and may result in inappropriate dosing. A normal dose in patients with cirrhosis results in an unbound concentration twice that expected, along with risk of toxicity.

Of considerable clinical importance were observations in 7 patients with severe impairment of liver function, defined as 50% of normal prothrombin complex activity and total serum bilirubin of more than 7 mg/dl. The clearance of free drug was markedly decreased to 0.5 ± 0.3 ml/min/kg.[57] Purely on the basis of pharmacokinetic considerations, therefore, azapropazone should be avoided in patients with severe liver disease.

Carprofen. The disposition of carprofen has been assessed in 12 patients with cirrhosis compared with 6 healthy volunteers.[58] Pharmacokinetics of total drug did not differ. However, potential changes in the pharmacokinetics of free drug were not determined. Therefore, whether the effects of cirrhosis on disposition of carprofen are clinically important is uncertain.

Ibuprofen. Studies of ibuprofen in cirrhosis are similarly flawed by the fact that only total drug concentrations have been quantified. In 15 patients with cirrhosis, the pharmacokinetics of total ibuprofen did not differ from normal controls.[59,60] Whether protein binding and/or handling of unbound drug differs in such patients is unknown. Therefore, the effect of cirrhosis on the disposition of ibuprofen cannot be confidently predicted.

Nabumetone. Nabumetone is a prodrug for the active compound, 6-methoxy-2-naphthylacetic acid (6-MNA). It has a bioavailability of 35–40%. The metabolite is highly bound to albumin (>99%) and eliminated by metabolism and has a long half-life of 24 hours. Studies in patients with cirrhosis have presumably shown no change from healthy subjects, except a slight prolongation in the time at which peak concentrations occur. However, the studies assessed only total and not unbound 6-MNA.[61,62]

Naproxen. Naproxen pharmacokinetics have been evaluated in 10 patients with cirrhosis compared with 10 normal volunteers.[63] The results were similar to those with azapropazone in that volume of distribution and clearance of total drug after oral administration were the same in both groups. In contrast, when free drug concentrations were assessed, clearance in patients with cirrhosis was about 40% of that in the control group (149 ± 68 vs. 396 ± 155 L/hr). Hence, such patients should receive half as much naproxen as patients with normal hepatic function. The potential for incorrect conclusions based on measurement of total drug concentration is again illustrated.

Oxaprozin. Oxaprozin is a long-acting arylpropionic NSAID with a half-life of 50–60 hours. In patients with cirrhosis, decreased binding to albumin caused an increase in both volume of distribution and clearance.[64] There were no changes in pharmacokinetic parameters of unbound drug.[64] Thus, dose adjustment is not necessary.

Sulindac. Sulindac is a prodrug converted by the liver to the active metabolite sulindac sulfide. In addition, the sulfide can be reconverted to the parent drug, and the liver also forms an inactive sulfone. All three compounds appear to be subject to enterohepatic recirculation.[65] Hence, liver disease may affect sulindac disposition at many steps. Juhl et al.[59] assessed the disposition of sulindac in 15 patients with cirrhosis and found delayed formation of both sulfide and sulfone. However, elimination of sulfide was considerably delayed, resulting in an area under the curve for the active drug that was approximately 4 times greater than in normal controls. The data were verified by Quintero et al.[66] Patients with liver disease who receive sulindac should be administered one-fourth the usual dose.

Tenoxicam. Tenoxicam disposition has been studied in 6 patients with cirrhosis compared with 14 healthy volunteers.[67] The half-life was not different in cirrhotic patients (53 ± 19 hr) and healthy controls (69 ± 19 hr). The area under the serum concentration vs. time curve was less in cirrhotic patients (159 ± 65 vs. 254 ± 92 μg·hr/ml). Such findings suggest decreased protein binding in cirrhotic patients with an increase in both clearance and volume of distribution of total drug. However, no difference in binding was found. If, in fact, the binding data are accurate, one can best explain such results by decreased bioavailability of tenoxicam in patients with cirrhosis. This scenario seems unlikely. More data are clearly needed.

Tolfenamic Acid. The disposition of tolfenamic acid has been studied in 6 patients with cirrhosis.[68] Because the pharmacokinetics of total drug were not different from those in patients with liver disease and historical controls, it was concluded that no change in dosing was warranted. The disconcerting nature of this conclusion is increased by data from other investigators showing that patients with liver disease had a 4-fold increase in the fraction of tolfenamic acid that was free in serum.[69] The disposition of free drug may well be altered in patients with cirrhosis. Consequently, data are insufficient to allow conclusions about tolfenamic acid in patients with liver disease.

Ximoprofen. Ximoprofen disposition has been studied in 10 patients with cirrhosis and compared with 12 healthy volunteers.[70] Half-life was little changed in cirrhotic patients (2.2 ± 0.7 vs. 1.6 ± 0.4 hr), whereas protein binding decreased from 93 ± 20% to 82 ± 33%. Despite this decrease, which ordinarily would be expected to decrease total serum concentrations of ximoprofen, the area under the curve of total drug was markedly increased (6.1 ± 2.9 vs. 3.5 ± 1.5 μg·hr/ml). Thus the clearance of unbound ximoprofen in cirrhotic patients is about one-half that in healthy subjects, indicating that cirrhotic patients should receive doses one-half of normal.

The pharmacokinetics of only a few NSAIDs have been evaluated in patients with liver disease

(Table 22.4), and even fewer studies have properly examined the concentration of unbound drug. The data about total drug concentrations lead to the incorrect conclusion that disposition is not affected in patients with cirrhosis. In other words, the only studies that have assessed free drug concentration have found substantial changes in elimination that require dosage adjustments. Better, definitive studies are needed with other NSAIDs. In lieu of such information, clinicians should exercise great caution when using NSAIDs in cirrhotic patients, who may have not only increased susceptibility to the effects of NSAIDs but also a diminished capacity to eliminate them.

Response

The mechanisms by which NSAIDs can affect renal function are discussed above.[41–44] Of particular interest is the recent controversy concerning differences among NSAIDs in their potential to inhibit renal PGs. Specifically, some investigators have suggested that sulindac spares renal PGs and thereby has less potential to cause adverse effects on renal function than other NSAIDs.[71–76] The proposed mechanism for this disparity in renal effects is that the active sulfide congener of sulindac can be metabolized to the inactive sulfone by the kidney.[76] Thereby, the kidney has been postulated to be capable of protecting itself from the PG-inhibiting effects of sulindac. The putative unique action of sulindac is based on initial studies by Ciabattoni et al.,[71] who performed several different protocols. In each, however, the number of patients was small. In one study, the authors assessed the effects of 300 mg/day of sulindac on basal 24-hour urinary PGE_2 excretion and on serum thromboxane (TxB_2) production in 3 healthy women. One woman was reevaluated on 150 mg/day of indomethacin. At such doses, sulindac did not affect urinary PGs or plasma renin activity (PRA), whereas both decreased in patients who received indomethacin. Both drugs decreased serum TxB_2. A similar pattern was observed in 1 patient with Bartter's syndrome. The final protocol involved measurement of PRA and serum TxB_2 production in 4 men administered furosemide with and without pretreatment with 800 mg of sulindac. Sulindac had no effect on either basal or furosemide-stimulated PRA but markedly suppressed TxB_2. No comparison was made with other NSAIDs, and effects on renal function were not reported.

In another report, Ciabattoni et al. demonstrated a renal-sparing effect of sulindac compared with ibuprofen in 20 women with chronic glomerular disease, 2 of whom were nephrotic and 5 of whom had systemic lupus erythematosus.[72] One week of treatment with 1.2 gm/day of ibuprofen was compared with 1 week of treatment with 400 mg/day of sulindac. Sulindac did not affect urinary excretion of PGE_2 or 6 keto-PGF_1 or cause renal function to deteriorate, and serum TxB_2 decreased by 85%. In contrast, ibuprofen caused 80% decreases in both urinary PGs, a 30% decrease in creatinine clearance, and a 35% decrease in paraaminohippurate clearance. Such results were interpreted to mean that prostacyclin maintains renal function in patients with chronic glomerular disease and that sulindac spares renal synthesis of this PG.

Similar results were found by Vriesendorp et al., who compared the effects of indomethacin (150 mg/day), diclofenac (200 mg/day), and flurbiprofen (200 mg/day) with the effects of sulindac (400 mg/day) in salt-depleted patients with nephrotic syndrome.[98] Sulindac had no effect on any renal parameter that was assessed, whereas the other NSAIDs decreased urinary protein excretion, glomerular filtration rate, plasma renin activity, and urinary PGE_2 excretion.

In a randomized controlled trial, Puddey et al. compared the effects of indomethacin (75 mg/day) and sulindac (400 mg/day) on the blood pressure of patients treated for essential hypertension.[99] Indomethacin inhibited urinary PGE_2 excretion, plasma renin activity, and serum TxB_2 production and caused an increase in blood pressure. In contrast, sulindac decreased serum TxB_2 but had no effect on renal function or blood pressure.

Finally, Bunning and Barth reported 3 patients who suffered acute renal insufficiency with ibuprofen or naproxen but were able to receive sulindac with no adverse effects.[97]

TABLE 22.4. Dosing Changes Required for Nonsteroidal Antiinflammatory Drugs in Patients with Cirrhosis

Azapropazone	Mild—half of normal dose Severe—avoid
Carprofen	Insufficient data
Etodolac	No change
Ibuprofen	Insufficient data
Naproxen	One-half of normal dose
Oxaprozin	No change
Sulindac	One-fourth of normal dose
Tolfenamic acid	Insufficient data
Ximoprofen	One-half of normal dose

The above studies indicate that sulindac has no effect on renal PGs. Thus, in patients susceptible to adverse renal effects of NSAIDs related to PG inhibition, sulindac is expected to involve less risk than other NSAIDs. Unfortunately, other studies have cast doubts about the renal-sparing effects of sulindac.[77–86]

Three studies compared the effects of sulindac and other NSAIDs on renal function in healthy people.[77–79] All showed that sulindac affected renal functional parameters. The authors postulated that conventional doses of sulindac were less potent than conventional doses of other NSAIDs.[77] A clinical corollary of this hypothesis was that the same cautions exercised with other NSAIDs in susceptible patients should also be used with sulindac. Studies in additional patient groups seem to support this hypothesis.

Three groups of investigators examined the effects of sulindac on renal function in patients with renal insufficiency.[80–82] All showed an effect of sulindac and suggested that it differed from other NSAIDs in being less potent at conventional doses. In addition, a study by Koopmans et al. in patients with hypertension found that indomethacin and sulindac have similar effects.[83]

The renal effects of sulindac also have been examined in patients with cirrhosis who, as discussed above, have increased sensitivity to the adverse renal effects of NSAIDs.[66,84–86] All of these studies showed decrements in renal function due to sulindac. Two of the studies were confounded by chronic dosing with sulindac.[66,85] In the setting of chronic administration, the changed disposition of sulindac in patients with liver disease allows accumulation of sulindac sulfide to concentrations higher than normal.[59] Hence, an adverse effect may represent attainment of toxic concentrations of sulindac. Of importance, however, two of the studies examined the effects of 1[86] or 2 doses[84] of sulindac, in which circumstance serum concentrations of sulindac sulfide are comparable to those in normal subjects. In both studies sulindac caused a decline in renal function and PGs.

The reasons for the discrepancies among studies assessing the renal effects of sulindac remain unexplained, as do similar differences in results from studies in animal models. Different study designs, experimental conditions, and severity of diseases may play a role. At the least, the renal-sparing effect of sulindac is uncertain; therefore, one must apply the same cautions to its use in susceptible patients as with any other NSAID.

Diuretics

The principles of use of diuretics in patients with liver disease are discussed in chapter 21. Here the focus is on their pharmacokinetics and pharmacodynamics and implications thereof for dosing strategies.

Potassium-sparing Agents

Aldosterone Antagonists. Because cirrhosis is commonly associated with secondary hyperaldosteronism and because the usual goal of diuretic use in such patients is to induce a gradual diuresis, aldosterone antagonists are used first. Their mechanism of action is desirable because they reverse an element of the pathophysiology and their low potency means that overly rapid diuresis is unlikely.

Spironolactone is the only potassium-sparing diuretic that directly inhibits the effects of aldosterone. Although considerable research has focused on the disposition and determinants of response to spironolactone, little definitive information is available. Earlier studies used nonspecific assay techniques and concluded that the majority of spironolactone was converted to canrenone, which constituted the active moiety.[87] In fact, these conclusions have prompted use of canrenone as a diuretic.

Such concepts have been revised substantially since the development of a more specific assay for spironolactone and its metabolites. Spironolactone is rapidly converted to a 7-alpha-thiol that is then metabolized to canrenone.[88,89] Prior evidence suggested that the 7-alpha metabolite and spironolactone itself constituted the active compounds.[90] However, this intermediate can be degraded to 6α–hydroxy-7α-thiol and yet unidentified compounds that also appear to be active and may account for a substantial portion of the biologic effects of spironolactone.[91] Studies in normal subjects indicate that canrenone accounts for only about one-tenth of the antimineralocorticoid effect after acute dosing and at most one-third after chronic dosing.[88–90] The pharmacokinetics of the 7-alpha-thiol and other potentially active moieties await elucidation. Clearly, only limited pharmacokinetic information is available about spironolactone, much less how its disposition may be affected in patients with liver disease.

Because of the lack of pharmacokinetic data, one must rely on clinical observation to design dosing strategies for spironolactone. Clinically this diuretic must be titrated to a dose sufficient to block the effects of circulating aldosterone. The dose necessary to do so may vary widely among patients, may be quite large in patients with cirrhosis, and can be determined only by titration in individual patients. What appear to be long half-lives of the active species fit well with clinical observations of slow onset of peak effect with chronic dosing, i.e., 3–4 days. Clinically this means that a change in spironolactone dose will not extrapolate to peak effect until 3–4 days. Dosage alterations on a more frequent basis should be avoided.

Amiloride and Triamterene. In contrast to spironolactone, amiloride and triamterene inhibit distal nephron sodium reabsorption by non–aldosterone-dependent mechanisms. Amiloride, and most likely triamterene, act from the urine side of the nephron. Both drugs are basic compounds and therefore are secreted into the urine by the organic base pathway. Consequently, other basic drugs such as cimetidine, procainamide, and trimethoprim may compete for secretion of these diuretics into the tubular lumen and thereby diminish their effect. Whether they do so has not been assessed clinically.

Very few pharmacokinetic data are available concerning amiloride. In normal subjects, peak concentrations occurred at 4 hours with elimination half-lives ranging from 7–11 hours.[92] This study employed radio-labeled compounds and therefore lacks specificity. Because most amiloride is eliminated unchanged in the urine, one would predict a prolonged half-life and decreased clearance in azotemic patients. Conversely, one would predict little or no effect of hepatic disease on the disposition of amiloride, although no data have been reported.

No pharmacodynamic studies have been performed with amiloride. From its pharmacokinetic parameters one would predict a relatively quick onset of effect, and its half-life suggests attainment of steady-state effects within 1–2 days. This seems to correspond well with clinical experience.

Triamterene has low activity, and approximately 80% is converted first to parahydroxytriamterene and then to the sulfuric acid ester of the parahydroxy metabolite.[93] This latter compound accounts for the major, if not total, diuretic effect. In normal subjects after oral dosing, peak concentrations of the parent compound occurred within 0.8–2.3 hours and of the active metabolite within 1.1–1.6 hours.[94] Consequently, onset of diuretic effect is rapid. The elimination half-lives of the parent drug and metabolite range from 3.3–5.1 hours and from 2.1–5.3 hours, respectively.[94] Clearance of parent drug is 0.06 ± 0.02 ml/min/kg with a volume of distribution of 13.4 ± 4.9 L/kg.[94] Because the drug is both absorbed[95] and eliminated quickly, 2–3 daily doses are needed.

Because of its complex handling, one would predict important influences of hepatic and renal disease on the disposition of triamterene. Because of impaired biotransformation to the active metabolite in liver disease, the half-life of the parent drug is prolonged to approximately 13 hours, with no change in elimination of the metabolite.[93] This may require larger doses of triamterene in such patients to achieve needed amounts of the active metabolite. This strategy, however, would result in elevated and potentially toxic concentrations of the parent drug. A better alternative is to use a different agent. In contrast, renal insufficiency does not affect excretion of the parent drug but dramatically prolongs elimination of the active metabolite.[93,96] For this and other reasons, triamterene should be avoided in patients with renal impairment. Pharmacodynamic data are not available for triamterene.

Spironolactone is usually tried first in patients with liver disease, because it directly counteracts secondary hyperaldosteronism. If it cannot be used successfully, amiloride and triamterene may be considered. In patients with hepatic disease, amiloride seems preferable to triamterene to avoid problems associated with conversion of triamterene to its active metabolite.

Thiazide Diuretics

A host of thiazide and thiazide-like diuretics (e.g., chlorthalidone, metolazone, indapamide) are available for clinical use. Although distinctions among them have been promulgated, all have the same site and mechanism of action and the same maximal effect. They differ in certain pharmacokinetic parameters, which from a practical perspective mean different durations of action; differences in potency mean simply that the doses of the various preparations differ. The choice of thiazide, then, should be determined by desired duration of action (Table 22.5) and cost. Alternatively, if the duration of effect does not matter, choice of drug should be dictated by which is least expensive for the patient.

Little is known about the disposition and determinants of response to the thiazide diuretics.[97]

TABLE 22.5. Durations of Effect of Thiazide and Thiazide-like Diuretics

Short duration of effect (6–12 hr)
    Chlorothiazide
    Hydrochlorothiazide

Medium duration of effect (12–24 hr)
    Bendroflumethiazide
    Benzthiazide
    Cyclothiazide
    Hydroflumethiazide
    Metolazone
    Quinethazone
    Trichloromethiazide

Long duration of effect (24–48 hr)
    Chlorthalidone
    Indapamide
    Methyclothiazide
    Polythiazide

Their site of action at the cortical segment of the thick ascending limb of the loop of Henle is reached from the lumen. In turn, the drugs reach the tubular lumen by being actively secreted via the organic acid transport pump of the proximal tubule. Other organic acids such as probenecid can interfere with this secretion and thereby affect the amounts of thiazide reaching the tubular site of action.

In healthy subjects, the onset of effect of thiazide diuretics is fairly rapid—within about 1.5–4 hours with no differences among agents. After an oral dose, the amount of drug appearing unchanged in urine varies greatly among the various agents, with indapamide the least at approximately 5%; amounts range upward to 40-70% for chlorthalidone, hydrochlorothiazide, hydroflumethiazide, and trichlormethiazide. Whether the variability among drugs represents differences in absorption from the gastrointestinal tract, differences in metabolic as opposed to renal clearance, or a combination of both is unclear for most of the thiazides. As a result, it is impossible to make predictions about the influence of liver disease (or other clinical conditions) on their disposition.

Patients with decreased renal function have been shown to have decreased clearance of trichlormethiazide.[74] Presumably, this effect results in a diminished peak diuresis and a prolonged response compared with normal subjects. No studies have assessed this hypothesis, probably because thiazides are relatively ineffective in patients with decreased renal function. Rather than attempt to discern what may be needed to effect a response, it is clinically simpler to use a more potent agent, namely, a loop diuretic.

One study has quantified the time at which the peak concentration of chlorothiazide occurred in patients with cirrhosis.[75] It was not different from normal. In fact, this parameter has not been shown to be affected by renal or cardiac disease or hypertension for a variety of the thiazides.[73]

In summary, from a mechanistic perspective additional data about the pharmacokinetics and pharmacodynamics of thiazide diuretics would be useful. However, from a clinical perspective, how additional data might influence our use of these drugs in liver disease is unclear. Because they are relatively weak diuretics, if resistance to a thiazide occurs in a patient with cirrhosis, more potent agents can be used instead. It is unlikely that additional data would alter this strategy. Similarly, one selects a thiazide according to whether it is a long- or short-acting agent. Such decisions are made on clinical grounds, and it is unlikely that additional pharmacokinetic data would influence the selection process.

Loop Diuretics

Occasional patients with cirrhosis do not respond to spironolactone, amiloride, or thiazide diuretics; thus loop diuretics become necessary. Considerable data have been generated to assess the determinants of response to loop diuretics in patients with liver disease.

Like thiazides, loop diuretics require delivery into the lumen of the renal tubule to produce a pharmacologic effect.[97,100] Loop diuretics are highly bound to serum albumin and are thereby minimally filtered at the glomerulus. As a result, they reach the urine by active secretion from the peritubular capillary via the organic acid transport pathway of the proximal tubule. As with thiazide diuretics, this system transports a number of endogenous and exogenous weak acids, some of which compete with loop diuretics for secretion.

Thus a major determinant of response to a loop diuretic is access of the agent to the urine, where it can then interact at the thick ascending limb of the loop of Henle (TALH). As a result, urinary diuretic excretion rate can be used to construct and assess dose-response relationships to loop diuretics. Doing so reveals a sigmoid-shaped curve with a distinct upper plateau of response. The sigmoid nature of this relationship indicates that response does not occur until sufficient drug is delivered to its site of action; in other words, until there is enough drug to reach the steep portion of the dose-response curve. Excretion rates beyond this value result in a disproportionate rise in response until an upper plateau is reached. Dosing strategies therefore need to entail administration of large enough doses to reach an effective part of the dose-response curve. In turn, a possible mechanism for abnormal response to a loop diuretic is disease that limits the amount of drug delivered into the urine. On the other hand, doses of diuretic that produce rates of drug excretion greater than those needed to reach the upper plateau do little to improve response but may subject the patient to drug toxicity. Consequently, if one defines the dose sufficient to reach the upper plateau of the dose-response curve, one has also defined the maximal dose to be administered, i.e., a ceiling dose. Such characteristics of the dose-response curve are of fundamental importance in treating a patient with subnormal response (i.e., resistance) to a loop diuretic.

Because delivery of sufficient drug into the urine is of major importance, one must first assess whether the patient's clinical condition alters this determinant of response. For example, it is clear that azotemic patients have impaired delivery of loop diuretics into the urine.[100] As a consequence, large doses must be administered to attain "normal" amounts of diuretic at the site of action. Whether similar changes occur in patients with cirrhosis has also been examined.[101–107]

Of the seven published reports evaluating the disposition of furosemide in patients with cirrhosis, four found no alteration in delivery of diuretic into the urine,[010–104] whereas the remaining three found differences in some patients.[105–107] Wide variability in response correlated well with delivery of diuretic into the urine. Hence, some patients clearly have diminished ability to attain sufficient drug in the urine to cause a response. In one of these studies, the decreased furosemide in the urine was caused by decreased renal function,[106] but in another report no such relationship was found.[107] At present the possible mechanism of decreased delivery of furosemide into the urine of cirrhotic patients, the degree to which it occurs, and the proportion of such patients to which this concern may apply remain unresolved. How, then, does one collate the data to arrive at reasonable clinical guidelines for use of loop diuretics in such patients?

My interpretation is that some patients may require 2–2½ times greater doses of loop diuretics

to attain "normal" amounts at the site of action. Hence, a reasonable therapeutic strategy is first to administer conventional doses of a loop diuretic (e.g., 40 mg of intravenous furosemide = 80 mg of oral furosemide = 1 mg of intravenous or oral bumetanide = 15–20 mg of intravenous or oral torsemide).[108] If no response or an inadequate response ensues, the dose may be increased by at most 2½-fold. There appears to be no justification for higher doses. Such a strategy should compensate for any changes in the disposition of loop diuretics in patients with liver disease and still be safe.

Even though one may deliver normal amounts of diuretic to the site of action, the response that ensues may be blunted. This phenomenon constitutes pharmacodynamic rather than pharmacokinetic.

Response to a loop diuretic is defined in terms of the drug's effect on the overall rate of sodium excretion measured in the final urine. As such, tubular reabsorption of sodium at sites other than the thick ascending limb can affect overall sodium excretion and influence dose-response relationships. Both delivery of sodium to the thick ascending limb and reabsorption by more distal segments contribute to the final natriuresis. Therefore, conditions associated with excessive sodium reabsorption at sites either proximal or distal (e.g., secondary hyperaldosteronism) to the thick ascending limb predictably have a reduced response. The different mechanisms of subnormal response cannot be readily distinguished clinically; however, strategies for coping with pharmacodynamic mechanisms for diuretic resistance can still be formulated.

Figure 22.2 illustrates two types of abnormal pharmacodynamics of response that may result from enhanced sodium reabsorption by non-TALH segments or that also may be due to tubular insensitivity to the diuretic. Curve A represents a subnormal response to adequate amounts of diuretic in the urine and is similar to the response in patients with cirrhosis.[101–108] A dose can be defined that will elicit a response in such patients by ascending the steep portion of the curve and reaching the plateau. However, the therapeutic expectations from such a dose are less in the patient with a suppressed dose-response curve than in one with normal pharmacodynamics of response.

Consequently, patients with cirrhosis who respond to the dose titration scheme outlined above do not manifest the same intensity of natriuresis

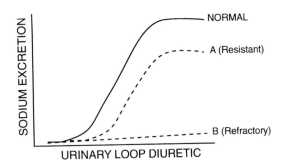

FIGURE 22.2. Relationship between urinary loop diuretic excretion rate ("dose") and response measured as sodium excretion. Curve A depicts a patient "resistant" to diuretics in whom a response occurs but is always subnormal.Curve B depicts a patient "refractory" to diuretics, in whom no response occurs.

as someone with a normal response. For example, a normal subject may excrete 200 mEq or more of sodium after receiving a 40-mg dose of furosemide. A patient with severe cirrhosis, on the other hand, may need 100 mg of furosemide to achieve maximal response, but the total amount of sodium excreted may be only 50 mEq. In such a patient, increasing the single effective dose causes no greater natriuresis; instead, to increase overall response, one must administer the effective dose of the diuretic more frequently (i.e., on 4 separate occasions in the above example).

In summary, when using loop diuretics in patients with liver disease, one should first identify a single dose that is effective, but there is no rationale for administering doses more than 2½ times normal. Once an effective dose is identified, the abnormal pharmacodynamic response in many patients dictates that the effective dose be administered on multiple occasions to achieve the desired level of sodium loss.

Some patients are truly refractory to diuretics and do not respond to any dose (Fig 22.2, curve B). Aggressive dose escalation in such patients has no hope of inducing a natriuresis but entails the risk of toxicity. For this reason, doses greater than 2½ times normal should not be exceeded. In such a patient addition of thiazides or thiazide-like agents should be attempted. Caution is mandatory, for a substantial response to combined diuretics may cause volume depletion and electrolyte abnormalities with attendant hazards.

If combinations of diuretics prove ineffective, alternative treatment modalities must be invoked, such as peritoneovenous shunts. Of interest, after a successful shunt is created in patients with severe cirrhosis, the response to furosemide (and presumably other loop diuretics) has been shown to increase.[109] This increase probably is due to reversal of hemodynamic abnormalities and secondarily to changes in responsivity of the nephron to loop diuretics. In effect, a refractory patient is converted to a patient who is only resistant.

REFERENCES

1. Williams RL, Mamelok RD: Hepatic disease and drug pharmacokinetics. Clin Pharmacokinet 1980;5:528–547.
2. Williams RL: Drug administration in hepatic disease. N Engl J Med 31983;09:1616–1622.
3. Greither A, Goldman S, Edelen JS, et al: Pharmacokinetics of furosemide in patients with congestive heart failure. Pharmacology 1979;19:121–131.
4. Brater DC, Seiwell R, Anderson S, et al: Absorption and disposition of furosemide in congestive heart failure. Kidney Int 1982;22:171–176.
5. Vasko MR, Brown-Cartwright D, Knochel JP, et al: Furosemide absorption altered in decompensated congestive heart failure. Ann Intern Med 1985;102:314–318.
6. Korhonen UR, Jounela AJ, Pakarinen AJ, P et al: Pharmacokinetics of digoxin in patients with acute myocardial infarction. Am J Cardiol 1979;44:1190–1194.
7. Odlind BG, Beermann B: Diuretic resistance: Reduced bioavailability and effect of oral furosemide. BMJ 1980;208:1577.
8. Fredrick MJ, Pound DC, Hall SD, Brater DC: Furosemide absorption in patients with cirrhosis. Clin Pharmacol Ther 1991;49:241–247.
9. Homeida M, Jackson L, Roberts CJC: Decreased first-pass metabolism of labetalol in chronic liver disease. BMJ 1978;2:1048–1050.
10. Regardh C-G, Jordo L, Ervik M, et al: Pharmacokinetics of metoprolol in patients with hepatic cirrhosis. Clin Pharmacokinet 1981;6:375–388.
11. Wood AJJ, Kornhauser DM, Wilkinson GR, et al: The influence of cirrhosis on steady-state blood concentrations of unbound propranolol after oral administration. Clin Pharmacokinet 1978;3:478–487.
12. Cotting J, Reichen J, Kutz K, et al: Pharmacokinetics of isradipine in patients with chronic liver disease. Eur J Clin Pharmacol 1990;38:599–603.
13. Fitton A, Benfield P: Isradipine: A review of its pharmacodynamic and pharmacokinetic properties, and therapeutic use in cardiovascular disease. Drugs 1990;40:31–74.
14. Kleinbloesem CH, van Harten J, Wilson JPH, et al: Nifedipine: Kinetics and hemodynamic effects in patients with liver cirrhosis after intravenous and oral administration. Clin Pharmacol Ther 1986;40:21–28.
15. Kleinbloesem CH, van Brummelen P, Breimer DD: Nifedipine: Relationship between pharmacokinetics and pharmacodynamics. Clin Pharmacokinet 1987;12:12–29.
16. van Harten J, van Brummelen P, Wilson JHP, et al: Nisoldipine: Kinetics and effects on blood pressure and heart rate in patients with liver cirrhosis after intravenous and oral administration. Eur J Clin Pharmacol 1988;34:387–394.

17. Friedel HA, Sorkin EM: Nisoldipine: A preliminary review of its pharmacodynamic and pharmacokinetic properties, and therapeutic efficacy in the treatment of angina pectoris, hypertension and related cardiovascular disorders. Drugs 1988;36:682–731.

18. McTavish D, Sorkin EM: Verapamil: An updated review of its pharmacodynamic and pharmacokinetic properties, and therapeutic use in hypertension. Drugs 1989; 38:19–76.

19. Hamann SR, Blouin RA, McAllister RG: Clinical pharmacokinetics of verapamil. Clin Pharmacokinet 1984; 9:26–41

20. Neal EA, Meffin PJ, Gregory PB, Blaschke TF: Enhanced bioavailability and decreased clearance of analgesics in patients with cirrhosis. Gastroenterology 1979;77:96–102.

21. Hasselström J, Eriksson S, Persson A, Ret al: The metabolism and bioavailability of morphine in patients with severe liver cirrhosis. Br J Clin Pharmacol 1990; 29:289–297.

22. Grahnen A, Jameson S, Loof L, et al: Pharmacokinetics of cimetidine in advanced cirrhosis. Eur J Clin Pharmacol 1984;26:347–355.

23. Smith IL, Ziemniak JA, Bernhard H, et al: Ranitidine disposition and systemic availability in hepatic cirrhosis. Clin Pharmacol Ther 1984;35:487–494.

24. Goa KL, Ward A: Buspirone: A preliminary review of its pharmacological properties and therapeutic efficacy as an anxiolytic. Drugs 1986;32:114–129.

25. Pentikäinen PJ, Neuvonen PJ, Jostell K-G: Pharmacokinetics of chlormethiazole in healthy volunteers and patients with cirrhosis of the liver. Eur J Clin Pharmacol 1980;17:275–284.

26. Janssen U, Walker S, Maier K, von Gaisberg U, Klotz U: Flumazenil disposition and elimination in cirrhosis. Clin Pharmacol Ther 1989;46:317–323.

27. Brogden RN, Goa KL: Flumazenil: A reappraisal of its pharmacological properties and therapeutic efficacy as a benzodiazepine antagonist. Drugs 1991;42:1061–1089.

28. Pentikäinen PJ, Välisalmi L, Himberg J-J, Crevoisier C: Pharmacokinetics of midazolam following intravenous and oral administration in patients with chronic liver disease and in healthy subjects. J Clin Pharmacol 1989;29:272–277.

29. Magueur E, Hagege H, Attali P, et al: Pharmacokinetics of metoclopramide in patients with liver cirrhosis. Br J Clin Pharmacol 31:185–187, 1991.

30. Brogden RN, Todd PA: Encainide: A review of its pharmacological properties and therapeutic efficacy. Drugs 1987;34:519–538.

31. Bergstrand RH, Wang T, Roden DM, et al: Encainide disposition in patients with chronic cirrhosis. Clin Pharmacol Ther 1986;40:148–154.

32. Thiollet M, Funck-Brentano C, Grange J-D, et al: The pharmacokinetics of perindopril in patients with liver cirrhosis. Br J Clin Pharmacol 1992;33:326–328.

33. Rames A, Poirier J-M, LeCoz F, et al: Pharmacokinetics of intravenous and oral pentoxifylline in healthy volunteers and in cirrhotic patients. Clin Pharmacol Ther 1990;47:354–359.

34. Schentag JJ, Calleri G, Rose JQ, et al: Pharmacokinetic and clinical studies in patients with cimetidine-associated mental confusion. Lancet 1979;1:177–181.

35. Schentag JJ, Cerra FB, Calleri GM, et al: Age, disease, and cimetidine disposition in healthy subjects and chronically ill patients. Clin Pharmacol Ther 1981;29:737–743.

36. Jusko WJ, Gretch M: Plasma and tissue protein binding of drugs in pharmacokinetics. Drug Metab Rev 1976;5: 43–140.

37. Oie S: Drug distribution and binding. J Clin Pharmacol 1986;26:583–586.

38. Sellers EM: Plasma protein displacement interactions are rarely of clinical significance. Pharmacology 1979; 18:225–227.

39. Brater DC: Pocket Manual of Drug Use in Clinical Medicine. Indianapolis: Improved Therapeutics, 1993.

40. Blaschke TF: Protein binding and kinetics of drugs in liver diseases. Clin Pharmacokinet 1977;2:32–44.

41. Clive DM, Stoff JS: Renal syndromes associated with nonsteroidal anti-inflammatory drugs. N Engl J Med 1984;310:563–572.

42. Dunn MJ, Zambraski ED: Renal effects of drugs that inhibit prostaglandin synthesis. Kidney Int 1980;19: 609–622.

43. Dunn MJ: Nonsteroidal anti-inflammatory drugs and renal function. Annu Rev Med 1984;35:411–428.

44. Garella S, Matarese RA: Renal effects of prostaglandins and clinical adverse effects of nonsteroidal anti-inflammatory agents. Medicine (Baltimore) 1984; 63:165–181.

45. Muther RS, Bennett WM: Effects of aspirin on glomerular filtration rate in normal humans. Ann Intern Med 1980;92:386–387.

46. Muther RS, Potter DM, Bennett WM: Aspirin-induced depression of glomerular filtration rate in normal humans: Role of sodium balance. Ann Intern Med 1981; 94:317–321.

47. Oliver JA, Pinto J, Sciacca RR, Cannon PJ: Increased renal secretion of norepinephrine and prostaglandin E_2 during sodium depletion in the dog. J Clin Invest 1980;61:748–756.

48. Henrich WL, Anderson RJ, Berns AS, et al: The role of renal nerves and prostaglandins in control of renal hemodynamics and plasma renin activity during hypotensive hemorrhage in the dog. J Clin Invest 1978;61:744–750.

49. Oliver JA, Sciacca RR, Pinto J, Cannon PJ: Participation of the prostaglandins in the control of renal blood flow during acute reduction of cardiac output in the dog. J Clin Invest 1981;67:229–237.

50. Dzau VJ, Packer M, Lilly LS, et al: Prostaglandins in severe congestive heart failure. Relation to activation of the renin-angiotensin system and hyponatremia. N Engl J Med 1984;310:347–352.

51. Boyer TD, Zia P, Reynolds TB: Effect of indomethacin and prostaglandin A_1 on renal function and plasma renin activity in alcoholic liver disease. Gastroenterology 1979;77:215–222.

52. Zambraski EJ, Dunn MJ: Importance of renal prostaglandins in control of renal function after chronic ligation of the common bile duct in dogs. J Lab Clin Med 1984;103:549–559.

53. Zipser RD, Hoefs JC, Speckart PF, et al: Prostaglandins: Modulators of renal function and pressor resistance in chronic liver disease. J Clin Endocrinol Metab 1979;48:895–900.

54. Schrier RW, Berl T: Nonosmolar factors affecting renal water excretion. N Engl J Med 1975;292:81–87,141–145.

55. Better OS, Schrier RW: Disturbed volume homeostasis in patients with cirrhosis of the liver. Kidney Int 1983; 23:303–311.

56. Jahnchen E, Blanck KJ, Breuing KH, et al: Plasma protein binding of azapropazone in patients with kidney and liver disease. Br J Clin Pharmacol 1981;11: 361–367.

57. Breuing KH, Gilfrich HJ, Meinertz T, et al: Disposition of azapropazone in chronic renal and hepatic failure. Eur J Clin Pharmacol 1981;20:147–155.

58. Holazo AA, Chen SS, McMahon FG, et al: The influence of liver dysfunction on the pharmacokinetics of carprofen. J Clin Pharmacol 1985;25:109–114.

59. Juhl RP, Van Thiel DH, Dittert LW, et al: Ibuprofen and sulindac kinetics in alcoholic liver disease. Clin Pharmacol Ther 1983;34:104–109.

60. Albert KS, Gernaat CM: Pharmacokinetics of ibuprofen. Am J Med 1984;77:40–46.

61. Friedel HA, Todd PA: Nabumetone: A preliminary review of its pharmacodynamic and pharmacokinetic properties, and therapeutic efficacy in rheumatic diseases. Drugs 1988;35:504–524.

62. Friedel HA, Langtry HD, Buckley MM: Nabumetone: A reappraisal of its pharmacology and therapeutic use in rheumatic diseases. Drugs 1993;45:131–156.

63. Williams RL, Upton RA, Cello JP, et al: Naproxen disposition in patients with alcoholic cirrhosis. Eur J Clin Pharmacol 1984;27:291–296.

64. Todd PA, Brogden RN: Oxaprozin: A preliminary review of its pharmacodynamic and pharmacokinetic properties, and therapeutic efficacy. Drugs 1986;32: 291–312.

65. Duggan DE: Therapeutic implications of the prodrug-pharmacophore equilibrium. Drug Metab Rev 1981;12: 325–337.

66. Quintero E, Gines P, Arroyo V, et al: Sulindac reduces the urinary excretion of prostaglandins and impairs renal function in cirrhosis with ascites. Nephron 1986; 42:298–303.

67. Crevoisier CH, Zaugg PY, Heizmann P, Meyer J: Influence of liver cirrhosis upon the pharmacokinetics of tenoxicam. Int J Clin Pharm Res 1989;9:327–334.

68. Stenderup J, Eriksen J, Pedersen SB, Christiansen LV: Pharmacokinetics of tolfenamic acid in patients with cirrhosis of the liver. Eur J Clin Pharmacol 1985;28: 573–579.

69. Laznicek M, Senius KEO: Protein binding of tolfenamic acid in the plasma from patients with renal and hepatic disease. Eur J Clin Pharmacol 1986;30:591–596.

70. Taylor IW, Taylor T, James I, et al: Pharmacokinetics of the anti-inflammatory drug ximoprofen in healthy subjects and in disease states. Eur J Clin Pharmacol 1991;40:101–106.

71. Ciabattoni G, Pugliese F, Cinotti GA, Patrono C: Renal effects of anti-inflammatory drugs. Eur J Rheumatol 1980;3:210–221.

72. Ciabattoni G, Cinotti GA, Pierucci A, et al: Effects of sulindac and ibuprofen in patients with chronic glomerular disease: Evidence for the dependence of renal function on prostacyclin. N Engl J Med 1984;310:279–283.

73. Bunning RD, Barth WF: Sulindac. A potentially renal-sparing nonsteroidal anti-inflammatory drug. JAMA 1982;248:2864–2867.

74. Vriesendorp R, deZeeuw D, deJong PE, et al: Reduction of urinary protein and prostaglandin E_2 excretion in the nephrotic syndrome by non-steroidal anti-inflammatory drugs. Clin Nephrol 1986;25:105–110.

75. Puddey IB, Beilin LJ, Vandongen R, et al: Differential effects of sulindac and indomethacin on blood pressure in treated essential hypertensive subjects. Clin Sci 1985;69:327–336.

76. Miller MJS, Bednar MM, McGiff JC: Renal metabolism of sulindac: Functional implications. J Pharmacol Exp Ther 1984;231:449–456.

77. Brater DC, Anderson S, Baird B, Campbell WB: Effects of ibuprofen, naproxen, and sulindac on prostaglandins in men. Kidney Int 1985;27:66–73.

78. Roberts DG, Gerber JG, Barnes JS, et al: Sulindac is not renal sparing in man. Clin Pharmacol Ther 1985; 38:258–265.

79. Riley LJ, Vlasses PH, Rotmensch HH, et al: Sulindac and ibuprofen inhibit furosemide-stimulated renin release but not natriuresis in men on a normal sodium diet. Nephron 1985;41:283–288.

80. Berg KJ, Talseth T: Acute renal effects of sulindac and indomethacin in chronic renal failure. Clin Pharmacol Ther 1985;37:447–452.

81. Swainson CP, Griffiths P, Watson ML: Chronic effects of oral sulindac on renal hemodynamics and hormones in subjects with chronic renal disease. Clin Sci 1986; 70:243–247.

82. Mistry CD, Lote CJ, Gokal R, et al: Effects of sulindac on renal function and prostaglandin synthesis in patients with moderate chronic renal insufficiency. Clin Sci 1986;70:501–505.

83. Koopmans PP, Thien TH, Thomas CMG, et al: The effects of sulindac and indomethacin on the antihypertensive and diuretic action of hydrochlorothiazide in patients with mild to moderate essential hypertension. Br J Clin Pharmacol 1986;21:417–423.

84. Daskalopoulos G, Kronborg I, Katkov W, et al: Sulindac and indomethacin suppress the diuretic action of furosemide in patients with cirrhosis and ascites: Evidence that sulindac affects renal prostaglandins. Am J Kidney Dis 1985;6:217–221.

85. Laffi G, Daskalopoulos G, Kronborg I, et al: Effects of sulindac and ibuprofen in patients with cirrhosis and ascites. Gastroenterology 1986;90:182–187.

86. Brater DC, Anderson SA, Brown-Cartwright D: Reversible acute decrease in renal function by NSAIDs in cirrhosis. Am J Med Sci 1987;294:168–174.

87. Karim A: Spironolactone: Disposition, metabolism, pharmacodynamics, and bioavailability. Drug Metab Rev 1978;8:151–188.

88. Dahlof CG, Lundborg P, Persson BA, Regardh CG: Re-evaluation of the antimineralocorticoid effect of the spironolactone metabolite, canrenone, from plasma concentrations determined by a new high-pressure liquid-chromatographic method. Drug Metab Dispos 1979;7:103–107.

89. Merkus FWHM, Overdiek JWPM, Cilissen J, Zuidema J: Pharmacokinetics of spironolactone after a single dose: Evaluation of the true canrenone serum concentrations during 24 hours. Clin Exp Hypertens [A] 1983;5:239–248.

90. Overdiek HWPM, Hermens WAJJ, Merkus FWHM: New insights into the pharmacokinetics of spironolactone. Clin Pharmacol Ther 1985;38:469–474.

91. Gardiner P, Schrode K, Quinlan D, et al: Spironolactone metabolism: Steady-state serum levels of the sulfur-containing metabolites. J Clin Pharmacol 1989; 29:342–347.

92. Smith AJ, Smith RN: Kinetics and bioavailability of two formulations of amiloride in man. Br J Pharmacol 48:646–649, 1973.

93. Mutschler E, Gilfrich HJ, Knauf H, et al: Pharmacokinetics of triamterene. Clin Exp Hypertens [A] 1983; 5:249–269.

94. Hasegawa J, Lin ET, Williams RL, et al: Pharmacokinetics of triamterene and its metabolite in man. J Pharmacokinet Biopharm 1982;10:507–523.

95. Gilfrich HJ, Kremer G, Mohrke W, et al: Pharmacokinetics of triamterene after i.v. administration to man: Determination of bioavailability. Eur J Clin Pharmacol 1983;25:237–241.

96. Knauf H, Mohrke W, Mutschler E: Delayed elimination of triamterene and its active metabolite in chronic renal failure. Eur J Clin Pharmacol 1983;24: 453–456.

97. Beermann B, Groschinsky-Grind M: Clinical pharmacokinetics of diuretics. Clin Pharmacokinet 1980;5: 221–245.

98. Sketris IS, Skoutakis VA, Acchiardo SR, Meyer MC: The pharmacokinetics of trichlormethiazide in hypertensive patients with normal and compromised renal failure. Eur J Clin Pharmacol 1981;20:453–457.

99. Brettell HR, Aikawa JK, Gordon GS: Studies with chlorothiazide tagged with radioactive carbon (C14) in human beings. Arch Intern Med 1960;106:109–115.

100. Brater DC: Resistance to loop diuretics. Why it happens and what to do about it. Drugs 1985;30:427–443.

101. Keller E, Hoppe-Seyler G, Mumm R, Schollmeyer P: Influence of hepatic cirrhosis and end-stage renal disease on pharmacokinetics and pharmacodynamics of furosemide. Eur J Clin Pharmacol 1981;20:27–33.

102. Sawhney VK, Gregory PB, Swezey SE, Blaschke TF: Furosemide disposition in cirrhotic patients. Gastroenterology 1981;81:1012–1016.

103. Verbeeck RK, Patwardhan RV, Villeneuve J-P, et al: Furosemide disposition in cirrhosis. Clin Pharmacol Ther 1982;31:719–725.

104. Traeger A, Hantze R, Penzlin M, et al: Pharmacokinetics and pharmacodynamic effects of furosemide in patients with liver cirrhosis. Int J Clin Pharmacol Ther Toxicol 1985;23:129–133.

105. Fuller R, Hoppel C, Ingalls ST: Furosemide kinetics in patients with hepatic cirrhosis with ascites. Clin Pharmacol Ther 1981;30:461–467.

106. Villeneuve J-P, Verbeeck RK, Wilkinson GR, Branch RA: Furosemide kinetics and dynamics in patients with cirrhosis. Clin Pharmacol Ther 1986;40:14–20.

107. Pinzani M, Daskalopoulos G, Laffi G, et al: Altered furosemide pharmacokinetics in chronic alcoholic liver disease with ascites contributes to diuretic resistance. Gastroenterology 1987;92:294–298.

108. Schwartz S, Brater DC, Pound D, et al: Bioavailability, pharmacokinetics, and pharmacodynamics of torsemide in patients with cirrhosis. Clin Pharmacol Ther 1993; 54:90–97.

109. Blendis LM, Greig PD, Langer B, et al: The renal and hemodynamic effects of the peritoneovenous shunt for intractable hepatic ascites. Gastroenterology 1979;77: 250–257.

Chapter 23

PARACENTESIS IN THE MANAGEMENT OF CIRRHOTICS WITH ASCITES

RAMON PLANAS, M.D.
PERE GINÈS, M.D.
ANGELS GINÈS, M.D.
VICENTE ARROYO, M.D.

Comparison of Paracentesis plus Intravenous
  Albumin with Diuretics in the Treatment of
  Tense Ascites
Importance of Intravenous Albumin Infusion in the
  Treatment of Cirrhotics with Large-Volume
  Paracentesis
Use of Other Types of Plasma Expanders in
  Cirrhotic Patients Treated with Paracentesis

Comparison of Peritoneovenous Shunting with
  Paracentesis plus Intravenous Albumin Infusion
  in the Management of Patients with Refractory
  Ascites
Technical Considerations
Conclusions

Ascites is the first sign of decompensation in most cirrhotic patients, and is associated with a poor prognosis.[1] The probability rate for 1-year survival among patients admitted to hospital for treatment of an episode of ascites has been reported to be only 56%.[2]

Since the introduction of modern diuretics in the 1960s, the treatment of ascites in patients with cirrhosis has been based on the combination of low-sodium diet and administration of these drugs.[3] This therapeutic schedule, however, is not entirely satisfactory, because it is frequently associated with complications, particularly hepatic encephalopathy, renal failure, and dilutional hyponatremia.[4] To minimize the incidence of such side effects, diuretic dosage must be adjusted to cause a loss of ascitic fluid of less than 500 ml/day. Treatment of tense ascites with diuretics is, therefore, a slow process, requiring prolonged hospitalization. Finally, 5–10% of cirrhotics admitted to hospital for the treatment of an episode of tense ascites do not respond to diuretics, a condition known as refractory or diuretic resistant ascites.[5]

Most cirrhotics with refractory ascites have functional renal failure (FRF), as manifested by increased levels of blood urea nitrogen and serum creatinine concentration. The mechanism whereby ascites is refractory to diuretic therapy in such patients is probably related to alterations in both pharmacokinetics and pharmacodynamics of diuretics. The access of loop diuretics to the organic acid secretory site and of spironolactone to the aldosterone receptors may be impaired in cirrhotics with FRF because of low renal perfusion.[6] Moreover, the delivery of sodium chloride to Henle's loop and distal nephron, the sites at which furosemide and spironolactone inhibit sodium reabsorption, may be markedly reduced in cirrhotic patients with FRF secondary to low glomerular filtration rate and enhanced sodium reabsorption in the proximal tubule.[7]

Until recently, the prosthesis designed by LeVeen et al. in 1974[8] to shunt ascitic fluid to the general circulation was the only alternative treatment to diuretics for cirrhotic patients with ascites. However, the procedure may induce serious complications, is associated with a high rate of obstruction of the prosthesis, and does not improve survival.[9–11] In 1983, Ginès et al. reevaluated therapeutic paracentesis in the management of patients with cirrhosis and ascites. The most important reason cited by the authors for reevaluation was the lack of consistent evidence indicating that paracentesis could be dangerous. The traditional assumption that paracentesis adversely influences systemic hemodynamics and renal function in patients with cirrhosis had been substantiated not by carefully controlled prospective investigations but rather by individual observations or studies with few patients. In addition, it was difficult to ascertain whether complications attributed to paracentesis were caused by the procedure or by conditional events. Finally, several studies performed during the 1970s failed to observe major complications after large-volume paracentesis.[12-18]

Following the initial study by Ginès et al.[19] in 1987, numerous investigations have demonstrated that paracentesis is a rapid, effective, and safe therapy for tense ascites in patients with cirrhosis. It is, therefore, not surprising that at present therapeutic paracentesis is widely used. In fact, the results of a survey recently carried out in 121 hospitals throughout the world[20] disclosed that therapeutic paracentesis has become an accepted treatment for ascites, contrary to previous clinical practice, which was dictated by fear of complications.

COMPARISON OF PARACENTESIS PLUS INTRAVENOUS ALBUMIN WITH DIURETICS IN THE TREATMENT OF TENSE ASCITES (Table 23.1)

The first study reevaluating paracentesis was a randomized controlled trial comparing repeated large-volume paracentesis (4–6 L/day until the disappearance of ascites) plus intravenous albumin infusion (40 gm after each tap) with standard diuretic therapy (furosemide plus spironolactone at increasing doses) in 117 cirrhotic patients with tense ascites and avid sodium retention who were admitted to several hospitals in the Barcelona area.[19,21] Patients who did not respond to the highest scheduled doses of diuretics (furosemide, 240 mg/day, and spironolactone, 400 mg/day) were treated with a LeVeen shunt. Randomization was independent in each participating hospital and patients with and without renal failure (serum creatinine > 1.5 mg/dl) were randomized separately to ensure a similar number of cases with renal failure in both treatment groups. Patients with severe liver impairment (hepatic encephalopathy, serum bilirubin > 10 mg/dl, and prothrombin activity < 40%) or renal failure (serum creatinine > 3 mg/dl) were not included in the study. Once ascites disappeared, patients were discharged from hospital with diuretics to prevent reaccumulation. Cases developing tense

ascites during follow-up were treated according to their initial schedule.

The main results of this study were as follows:

1. Paracentesis was more effective than diuretics in eliminating ascites (96.5% vs. 72.8%).

2. Paracentesis plus intravenous albumin had no deleterious effect on systemic hemodynamics and renal function in the entire group of 58 patients treated with the procedure or in subgroups of patients with functional renal failure or without peripheral edema (Table 23.2). Large-volume paracentesis until disappearance of ascites was not associated with significant changes in blood urea nitrogen, serum creatinine concentration, glomerular filtration rate, free water clearance, or serum sodium concentration. On the other hand, although mean arterial pressure decreased slightly but significantly after paracentesis treatment in most patients, no significant changes were observed in plasma volume, cardiac output, or peripheral vascular resistances. The observation that paracentesis did not significantly modify the plasma levels of renin, norepinephrine, and antidiuretic hormone, which are highly sensitive to changes in effective intravascular volume, further supports this contention. As expected, ascites removal was associated with a marked reduction in free and wedged hepatic venous pressure (Fig. 23.1).

3. The incidence of hyponatremia, renal impairment, and hepatic encephalopathy was much lower in patients treated with paracentesis (5.1%, 3.4%, and 10.2%, respectively) than in patients receiving diuretics (30%, 27%, and 29%). Other complications occurred with similar frequency in both groups of patients (Table 23.3). The high incidence of hyponatremia, renal impairment, and encephalopathy in the diuretic group was comparable with that reported by Sherlock at et al.[22] (41%, 34%, and 29%) and by Strauss et al.[23] (22%, 24%, and 27%) in two large series of 112 and 100 patients, respectively, with nonazotemic normonatremic cirrhosis and ascites treated with various combinations of diuretics.

4. The duration of hospital stay and therefore the cost of treatment were lower in patients treated with paracentesis.

5. During follow-up there were no significant differences between the two groups in probability of readmission to the hospital, causes of readmission, probability of survival, or causes of death. Most of the results of this study were later confirmed in three further controlled trials,

TABLE 23.1. Incidence of Complications in Cirrhotic Patients with Tense Ascites Treated with Diuretics, Paracentesis without Plasma Volume Expansion, and Paracentesis with Different Plasma Expanders

Treatment	Study	n	Renal Impairment Number (%)	Hypo-natremia Number (%)	Hepatic Encephalopathy Number (%)	Plasma Renin Activity (ng/ml/hr) Before/After	p
Diuretics	Sherlock et al.[22]	112	38 (34)	46 (41)	32 (29)		
	Strauss et al.[23]	100	24 (24)	22 (22)	27 (27)		
	Ginès et al.[19]	59	16 (27)	18 (30)	17 (29)		
	Solá et al.[26]	40	5 (12)	8 (20)	12 (30)		
	Salerno et al.[24]	21	1 (5)	?	1 (5)		
RLVP; no VE	Ginès et al.[28]	53	6 (11)	9 (17)	3 (6)	$5.4 \pm 1.3/10.8 \pm 1.6$ (SE)*	< 0.001
TP + dextran-40	Solá et al.[26]	40	1 (2)	5 (12)	1 (2)	$5.3 \pm 1.4/10.9 \pm 3$ (SD)§	< 0.01
TP + dextran-70	Planas et al.[36]	45	1 (2)	4 (9)	3 (7)	$11 \pm 2/14.4 \pm 3$ (SE)§	<0.02
TP + hemaccel	Salerno et al.[37]	27	1 (4)	5 (18)	2 (7)	$11.9 \pm 1.5/12.4 \pm 1.4$ (SE)§	NS
RLVP + albumin	Ginès et al.[19]	58	2 (3)	3 (5)	6 (10)	$7.7 \pm 3.3/8.7 \pm 2.5$ (SE)*	NS
	Ginès et al.[28]	52	0	1 (2)	6 (11)	$6.2 \pm 1.3/6.5 \pm 1.4$ (SE)*	NS
	Ginès et al.[40]	41	2 (5)	3 (7)	6 (15)	$22.7 \pm 13.8/26.7 \pm 15.5$ (SD)*	NS
	Salerno et al.[24]	20	1 (5)	?	2 (10)	$12.6 \pm 1.5/13.1 \pm 1.6$ (SE)‡	NS
	Fassio et al.[38]	21	1 (5)	4 (19)	1 (5)	$7.7 \pm 5/7.9 \pm 7$ (SD)†	NS
TP + albumin	Planas et al.[36]	43	1 (2)	3 (7)	3 (7)	$9.3 \pm 1.8/10.8 \pm 1.8$ (SE)§	N S
	Tító et al.[27]	38	0	1 (3)	2 (5)	$8.2 \pm 1.6/7.8 \pm 1.5$ (SE)§	N S
	Salerno et al.[37]	27	1 (4)	4 (15)	2 (7)	$13.2 \pm 1.9/14.3 \pm 2.1$ (SE)§	NS

RLVP = repeated large-volume paracentesis, TP = total paracentesis, VE = volume expansion, NS = not significant. Plasma renin activity was measured: * 48 hr; † 4 days; ‡ 5 days; § 6 days after paracentesis, respectively.

reported by Salerno et al.,[24] Hagève et al.,[25] and Solà et al.[26]

Salerno et al.[24] in Milan randomized 41 cirrhotic patients with tense ascites, using the same inclusion criteria as Ginès et al.[19] Twenty cases were treated with repeated large-volume paracentesis (2–6 L/day until disappearance of ascites) and intravenous albumin infusion (20–60 gm after each tap, depending on the amount lost during ascites evacuation), and 21 with increasing doses of diuretics (spironolactone, 200 mg/day initially and 400 mg/day if no response; furosemide, 40 mg/day, was added for patients not responding to spironolactone). Both treatments were equally effective in mobilizing the intraabdominal fluid (95% and 90.4%, respectively; mean loss of body weight: 9.7 ± 0.6 and 8.9 ± 2.1 kg) with few side effects (two episodes of hepatic encephalopathy and one of renal failure in the paracentesis group; three episodes of hepatic encephalopathy and one of renal failure in the diuretic group). No significant changes in hepatic and renal function, serum sodium concentration, or plasma levels of renin and aldosterone were observed in any group. Of

interest, only 5 of the 20 cases treated with paracentesis reaccumulated more than 300ml/day of ascitic fluid, as estimated by the change in body weight, over a 15-day period during which patients were kept in hospital without diuretics; 4 patients did not reaccumulate ascites, as confirmed by ultrasonography.

Hagève et al.[25] in Bicêtre studied 53 nonazotemic, normonatremic cirrhotics with tense ascites. Twenty-six cases (group 1) were treated with repeated large-volume paracentesis (4 L/day until disappearance of ascites) and intravenous albumin infusion (10 gm/L of ascites removed), whereas 27 (group 2) were treated with spironolactone (225–300 mg/day), either alone or combined with furosemide (40–80 mg/day). Ascites and peripheral edema disappeared more rapidly in group 1 than in group 2 (8.6 ± 9.6 vs. $13/5 \pm 6.7$ days and 4.1 ± 2.6 vs. 10.5 ± 6.5, respectively). During hospitalization, the incidence of complications was significantly higher in group 1 than in group 2 (56% vs. 26%). Hyponatremia occurred in 30% of patients treated with diuretics and in only 4% of patients treated with paracentesis. The duration of

TABLE 23.2. Effects of Paracentesis Plus Intravenous Albumin on Plasma Volume, Renal Function, Endogenous Vasoactive Systems, and Systemic and Hepatic Hemodynamics*

Parameter	Before Treatment (mean + SEM)	After Treatment (mean ± SEM)
Plasma volume (ml)	3767 ± 160	3442 ± 170
Glomerular filtration rate (ml/min)	65 ± 7	73 ± 8
Free water clearance (ml/min)	2.5 ± 0.6	2.9 ± 0.7
Plasma renin activity (ng/ml/hr)	7.7 ± 3.3	8.7 ± 2.5
Norepinephrine (pg/ml)	630 ± 87	539 ± 70
Antidiuretic hormone (pg/ml)	4.6 ± 0.4	4.4 ± 0.5
Urinary PGE_2 (ng/day)	84 ± 19	105 ± 24
Urinary 6-keto-PGF_1 (ng/day)	257 ± 38	278 ± 46
Cardiac output (L/min)[†]	6.3 ± 0.6	6.1 ± 0.6
Peripheral resistance (dynes/sec/cm^{-5})[†]	1110 ± 104	1061 ± 1084
Hepatic venous pressure gradient (mmHG)[†]	19.2 ± 1.9	20.3 ± 1.9

* All values are nonsignificant.

[†] Measured in 7 patients; remaining parameters were measured in 24 patients.

hospital stay was shorter in group 1 (15.0 ± 10.4 days) than in group 2 (21.0 ± 11.7 days; p = 0.0007). Survival was similar in both groups.

Solà et al.26 in Barcelona compared total paracentesis (see below) associated with dextran-40 (8 gm/L of ascitic fluid removed) vs. diuretics (increasing doses of spironolactone, 100–400 mg/day, alone or combined with furosemide, 40–240 mg/day) in 80 cirrhotic patients with tense ascites (8 with renal failure and 11 with hyponatremia). Paracentesis was more effective than diuretics in mobilizing the ascitic fluid (100% vs .80%) and significantly reduced the duration of hospitalization (13 ± 1 vs. 19 ± 1 days). The incidence of complications during hospital stay was significantly higher in the diuretic group (38%) than in the paracentesis group (15%). This difference was due mainly to the higher incidence of hepatic encephalopathy in the former group (30% vs. 2.5%). There were no significant differences between treatment groups in the probability of survival after inclusion.

Finally, in 38 cirrhotic patients with tense ascites (6 with renal failure and 16 without peripheral edema), Tito et al.[27] investigated whether ascites can be safely mobilized in only one paracentesis session ("total paracentesis") plus intravenous albumin infusion (6–8 gm/L ascites removed). The aim of this study was to assess whether cirrhotic patients with tense ascites could be treated in a single-day hospitalization regimen. With the aid of a suction pump, the volume of ascitic fluid removed and the duration of the procedure were 10.7 ± 0.5L (mean ± SEM) and 60 ± 3 minutes, respectively. No significant changes in renal and hepatic function or in plasma levels of norepinephrine, renin, and aldosterone were observed over a 6-day period during which patients were kept in hospital without diuretics. The incidence of hyponatremia, renal impairment, and hepatic encephalopathy in this series of patients (3%, 0%, and 10%, respectively) and the clinical course of the disease, as estimated by the probability of readmission to hospital, causes of readmission, probability of survival, and causes of death, were comparable with results reported by the same group of investigators in patients treated with repeated large-volume paracentesis.[19]

Table 23.1 illustrates the main findings of all studies assessing the therapeutic paracentesis in cirrhosis. These studies demonstrate that mobilization of ascitic fluid by repeated large-volume paracentesis or total paracentesis associated with intravenous albumin infusion does not impair systemic hemodynamics and renal function in patients with cirrhosis and tense ascites. Because therapeutic paracentesis is more effective than conventional diuretic therapy in mobilizing the ascitic fluid, is associated with a lower incidence of complications, and considerably reduces the duration of hospitalization, it should be considered as the treatment of choice for cirrhotic patients admitted to hospital with tense ascites. Therapeutic paracentesis, however, does not improve systemic and renal hemodynamics or sodium retention. Therefore, to prevent reaccumulation of ascites, patients treated with paracentesis require dietary sodium restriction and administration of diuretics after the procedure.

IMPORTANCE OF INTRAVENOUS ALBUMIN INFUSION IN THE TREATMENT OF CIRRHOTICS WITH LARGE-VOLUME PARACENTESIS

A second randomized controlled trial from the Barcelona group was aimed at investigating whether intravenous albumin administration is necessary after therapeutic paracentesis.[28] Fifty-two cirrhotic patients with tense ascites (group 1) were treated by repeated large-volume paracentesis with intravenous albumin (40 gm after each tap) and 53 (group 2) by paracentesis without albumin. There were no differences between the two groups in the number of patients with "complete" removal of ascites (50 of 52 vs. 48 of 53 patients), loss of body weight (9.7 ± 0.6 vs. 9.4 ± 0.5 kg), and number of paracentesis procedures per patient (2.8 ± 0.1 vs. 2.9 ± 0.1). Confirming previous studies, paracentesis plus intravenous albumin did not induce significant changes in standard renal function tests, plasma renin activity, and plasma aldosterone concentration. In contrast, paracentesis without albumin was associated with significant increase in blood urea nitrogen, constant and marked elevation in plasma renin activity (Fig. 23.2) and plasma aldosterone concentration, and significant reduction in serum sodium concentration (see Table 23.3). Side effects occurred in 9 patients of group 1 and 16 of group 2. This difference was due to a significantly higher incidence of hyponatremia and/or renal impairment in group 2 (20% vs. 2%). The incidence of other complications was similar in the two groups. Serum sodium concentration returned to pretreatment values during follow-up in 6 of the 10 patients developing hyponatremia. However, renal function did no improve in any of the 5 patients developing renal impairment after paracentesis. Although the probability of survival was similar in the two groups, a multivariate analysis identified the development of hyponatremia, renal impairment, or both after paracentesis and the occurrence of other complications during the first hospitalization (encephalopathy, gastrointestinal bleeding, and severe infections) as the only independent predictors of mortality.

Four different groups of investigators have performed more detailed studies assessing the effects of complete mobilization of ascites by large-volume paracentesis without albumin infusion on systemic hemodynamics, vasoactive hormones, and renal function.

Simon et al.[29] in Atlanta studied 13 patients with cirrhosis and tense ascites before and 1 and 24 hours after total paracentesis (mean volume of ascitic fluid removed: 8.07 L; range: 4–15 L) without colloid replacement. The only change observed 1 hour after paracentesis was an increase

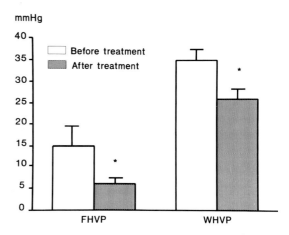

FIGURE 23.1. Effects of paracentesis on free hepatic venous pressure (FHVP) and wedged hepatic venous pressure (WHVP) in 7 cirrhotic patients with tense ascites. * $p < 0.001$ with respect to values before treatment.

in cardiac function, as indicated by elevation of cardiac output and decrease in pulmonary wedged capillary pressure and central venous pressure. However, 24 hours after mobilization of ascites there were significant decreases in cardiac output, central venous pressure, pulmonary wedged capillary pressure, creatinine clearance, serum sodium concentration, and plasma concentration of atrial natriuretic factor and significant increases in plasma renin activity and aldosterone concentration with respect to baseline values.

Panos et al.[30] in London, performed similar measurements before and 0.5, 1, 2, 3, 6, 24, 36, and 48 hours after total paracentesis without albumin infusion (the volume of ascitic fluid removed

TABLE 23.3. Complications During the First Hospital Stay in Patients Treated with Paracentesis plus Intravenous Albumin (Group 1) and Patients Treated with Diuretics (Group 2)

	Group 1 (n = 58)	Group 2 (n = 59)	p
Patients with complications	10	36	<0.001
Hyponatremia	3	18	<0.001
Encephalopathy	6	17	<0.002
Renal impairment	2	16	<0.001
Hyperkalemia	1	7	NS
Gastrointestinal bleeding	2	6	NS
Peritonitis	0	4	NS
Bacteremia	2	0	NS
Others	0	4	NS

NS = not significant.

PRA (ng/ml.h)

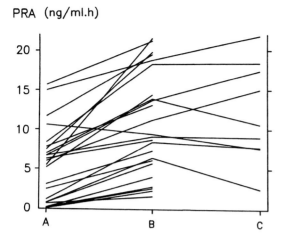

FIGURE 23.2. Changes in plasma renin activity (PRA) in patients treated with paracentesis without intravenous albumin. *A*, Before treatment (n = 24). *B*, 48 hr after treatment (n = 24). *C*, Five days after treatment (n = 9). (From Ginès P, Titó Ll, Arroyo V, et al: Randomized comparative study of therapeutic paracentesis with and without intravenous albumin in cirrhosis. Gastroenterology 1988;94:1493–1502, with permission.)

ranged from 4–16 L) in 21 cirrhotic patients with tense ascites. A significant increase in cardiac output was observed 1 hour after treatment. However, between 3 and 12 hours later there was a significant drop in cardiac output, pulmonary wedged capillary pressure, and central venous pressure with respect to baseline values. Plasma renin activity increased by 60% and plasma atrial natriuretic peptide concentration decreased by 33% 48 hours after paracentesis (Table 23.4).

Terg et al.[31] in Buenos Aires studied 10 cirrhotic patients with tense ascites treated with repeated large-volume (5 L) paracentesis associated with dextran-70 infusion. Hemodynamic evaluation was performed in basal conditions, 12 hours after paracentesis without plasma volume expansion, and following dextran infusion. Twelve hours after each paracentesis without expansion, significant drops in pulmonary wedged capillary pressure (from 9.5 ± 1.0 to 7.1 ± 1.7) and reductions in cardiac output (from 6.6 ± 1.0 to 5.0 ± 1.9) were observed. These parameters returned to baseline values after the administration of 84 ± 14 ml of dextran-70 for each liter of ascites removed. The mean volume of ascites removed was 12.3 ± 4.6 L.

Finally, Luca et al.[32] in Barcelona investigated in a randomized trial the hemodynamic and humoral changes before and 1 and 24 hours after total paracentesis in 18 cirrhotic patients with tense ascites. In 9 patients (group 1) total paracentesis was associated with albumin infusion (8 gm/L of ascitic fluid removed; half of the albumin was administered immediately after paracentesis and the other half 1 hour after). In the other 9 patients treated by total paracentesis (group 2) albumin infusion was administered after the hemodynamic investigation was completed (24 hours after paracentesis). In both groups, a significant increase in cardiac output (+17% in group 1 and +8% in group 2) and significant reductions in plasma renin activity (–59% and –58%), plasma aldosterone concentration (–25% and –49%), BUN (–3.7 and –3.7 mg/dl), and serum creatinine (–0.3 and –0.2 mg/dl) with respect to baseline values were observed 1 hour after paracentesis. Furthermore, a significant increase in plasma volume (+0.82 L) and in atrial natriuretic peptide (+189%) was observed in group 1. Twenty-four hours after paracentesis the beneficial effects persisted only in group 1 patients. In group 2 patients, cardiac output, plasma renin activity, and plasma aldosterone concentration returned to baseline values, with significant decreases in sodium serum concentration (–4 mEq/L), mean arterial pressure (–11%), pulmonary capillary wedged pressure (–33%), and atrial natriuretic peptide (–24%).

Kao et al.[33] and Pinto et al.[34] in Los Angeles and Gentile et al.[35] in Rome have shown that the extraction of 5 L of ascitic fluid by paracentesis without intravenous albumin infusion in cirrhotic patients with tense ascites is not associated with significant changes in plasma volume, plasma renin activity, or renal function. Therefore, it appears that impairment in systemic hemodynamics and renal function after paracentesis without albumin expansion occurs only inpatients in whom ascites is completely mobilized.

In conclusion, the above studies demonstrate that complete mobilization of ascites by paracentesis without plasma volume expansion is followed by reduction in effective intravascular volume, which leads to activation of the renin-aldosterone system and suppression of cardiac release of atrial natriuretic peptide. This impairment of effective circulating blood volume starts within the first hours after complete mobilization of ascites and is constantly detected 48 hours after treatment, as indicated by an increase in plasma renin activity and aldosterone concentration.

TABLE 23.4. Hemodynamic and Hormonal Changes after Total Paracentesis without Albumin Infusion in 21 Cirrhotic Patients with Tense Ascites

Time	0 Min	30 Min	60 Min	120 Min	180 Min	6 Hr	24 Hr	36 Hr	48 Hr
RAP	9 ± 0.8	7.6 ± 0.8	7.4 ± 0.8	7.4 ± 0.8	7.0 ± 0.8	$6.4 \pm 0.7*$	$6.3 \pm 0.7*$	5.9 ± 0.6	$5.8 \pm 0.8*$
PCWP	10.9 ± 0.9	10.7 ± 0.8	10.4 ± 0.9	10.2 ± 0.9	10.2 ± 0.9	$8.7 \pm 0.8*$	$8.3 \pm 0.9*$	$6.7 \pm 0.7*$	$7.2 \pm 0.8*$
CO	7.7 ± 0.5	8.2 ± 0.5	$8.5 \pm 0.6*$	$8.7 \pm 0.6*$	$9.03 \pm 0.7*$	$8.7 \pm 0.6*$	7.9 ± 0.7	7.7 ± 0.8	7.8 ± 0.7
ANP[†]	8.09 ± 1.18	—	—	10.25 ± 1.2	—	—	$5.9 \pm 0.84*$	—	$5.41 \pm 0.69*$
PRA[†]	10.85 ± 2.06	—	—	9.21 ± 2.48	—	—	13.18 ± 2.35	—	16.6 ± 2.76

RAP = right atrial pressure (mmHg), PCWP = pulmonary capillary wedge pressure (mmHG), CO = cardiac output (L/min), ANP = atrial natriuretic peptide (pmol/L), PRA = plasma renin activity (pmol/hr/ml).
* $p < 0.05$
[†] Measured in 12 patients.

Despite this deterioration of systemic hemodynamics in almost all patients treated with paracentesis without albumin infusion, only 20% develop renal or electrolyte complications, probably because of intrarenal compensatory mechanisms (i.e., renal prostaglandins) that antagonize the effects of circulating hypovolemia on kidney function. Because renal impairment and dilutional hyponatremia following paracentesis are not reversible in many cases and are associated with a poor prognosis, the prevention of impairment of effective blood volume by intravenous infusion of albumin is an important measure in cirrhotic patients with tense ascites treated with repeated large-volume or total paracentesis.

USE OF OTHER TYPES OF PLASMA EXPANDERS IN CIRRHOTIC PATIENTS TREATED WITH PARACENTESIS

The use of human serum albumin in cirrhotic patients treated with large-volume paracentesis is limited by its high price. In Spain, it represents more than 50% of the total cost of therapy for patients treated with total paracentesis, which requires only 1 day of hospitalization. On the other hand, in underdeveloped countries human serum albumin cannot be routinely prescribed in public hospitals. It is, therefore, not surprising that several groups investigated whether less expensive plasma expanders can be substituted for albumin. To date, four randomized controlled trials and one prospective study have investigated whether albumin can be replaced by dextran-70, dextran-40, hemaccel, or isotonic saline.

In a randomized trial Planas et al.[36] in Barcelona compared albumin vs. dextran-70 (6 gm/ml 100 ml of dextrose solution) as plasma expanders in 88 cirrhotic patients (16 with renal failure)

with tense ascites treated by total paracentesis. Both substances were given at a dose of 8 gm/L of ascitic fluid removed. After mobilization of ascites, patients were discharged from hospital with diuretics, and patients developing tense ascites during follow-up were treated according to their initial schedule. Neither paracentesis plus intravenous albumin nor paracentesis plus dextran-70 infusion was associated with significant changes in renal and hepatic function or serum electrolytes. The incidence of renal impairment (1 case in each therapeutic group), hyponatremia (3 and 4 cases, respectively), and other complications after paracentesis and the clinical course of the disease, as estimated by probability of readmission to hospital, causes of readmission, probability of survival, and causes of death, were similar in the two groups. The effect of paracentesis on effective intravascular volume was indirectly assessed by measuring plasma renin activity and aldosterone concentration before and 2 and 6 days after treatment during hospitalization without diuretics. In patients treated with albumin, no significant changes in these parameters were observed during the entire period. In contrast, both parameters increased significantly at the sixth day of treatment in patients receiving dextran-70 (Fig. 23.3). A significant increase in renin and aldosterone (30% over baseline values) was observed in 51% of the 45 patients treated with dextran-70 and in only 15% of the 43 patients receiving albumin, suggesting the lower efficacy of dextran-70 in preventing impairment in systemic hemodynamics induced by paracentesis.

Salerno et al.[37] in Milan performed a randomized controlled trial in 54 cirrhotic patients with refractory ascites treated by total paracentesis. Twenty-seven patients were given intravenous

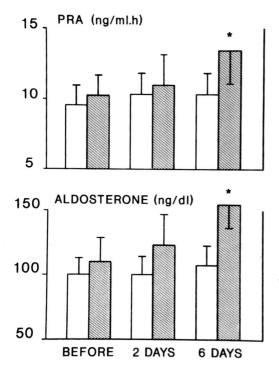

FIGURE 23.3. Plasmin renin activity (PRA) and plasma aldosterone concentration in patients treated with total paracentesis and intravenous albumin *(open bars)* and in patients treated with total paracentesis and intravenous dextran-70 *(shaded bars)* before and 2 and 6 days after treatment. (* p < 0.02 with respect to values obtained before treatment). Normal values in our laboratory: PRA, 1.3 ± 0.2 ng.ml^{-1}; aldosterone, 10.5 ± 1.1 ng/dl. (From Planas R, Ginès P, Arroyo V, et al: Dextran-70 versus albumin as plasma expanders in cirrhotic patients with tense ascites treated with total paracentesis: results of a randomized study. Gastroenterology 1990;99: 1736–1744, with permission.)

albumin (6 gm/L of ascitic fluid removed) and 27 received an intravenous infusion of hemaccel (Emagel, 3.5%, 150 ml/L of ascites evacuated). The mobilization of ascites in both groups was associated with no significant changes in renal and hepatic function, serum sodium concentration, plasma renin activity, or plasma concentrations of aldosterone and atrial natriuretic peptide, which were determined 1, 3 and 6 days after treatment. Nine patients (4 in the albumin group and 5 in the hemaccel group) developed hyponatremia and 2 (one from each group) developed renal impairment. The probability of recurrence of massive ascites and the probability of survival during follow-up were similar in both groups.

Fassio et al.[38] in Buenos Aires performed a randomized, controlled trial comparing dextran-70 (6 gm/100 ml isotonic saline solution) with human albumin in 41 cirrhotic patients treated daily with 5-L paracentesis until resolution of ascites. The criteria for inclusion were similar to those in previous trials assessing the safety of paracentesis associated with albumin infusion. Dextran-70 was infused in the same amount as human albumin (6 gm/L of ascites drained). Although the number of patients was relatively small, results indicate that dextran-70 was indeed a good substitute for albumin. This conclusion was based on the absence of significant changes in renal and hepatic function, serum electrolytes, and plasma renin activity 1 and 4 days after the last paracentesis in both groups. Four patients developed complications in each group, mainly hyponatremia, whereas one patient in each group developed renal impairment. Because dextran-70 can adversely affect platelet activity or clotting factors, both parameters were checked in short-term follow-up and found to be stable. The probability of survival and readmission to the hospital because of tense ascites were similar in both groups during follow-up.

Solà et al.[26] in Barcelona treated 49 cirrhotic patients with tense ascites (7 with renal failure) with total paracentesis plus intravenous dextran-40 infusion (10 gm/100 ml of dextrose solution; 8 gm/L of ascitic fluid removed) and measured hepatic and renal function and plasma levels of renin and aldosterone before and 2 and 6 days after treatment. Patients were subsequently discharged from hospital with diuretics, and patients developing tense ascites during follow-up were again treated with total paracentesis plus intravenous dextran-40 infusion. Plasma renin activity and plasma aldosterone concentration markedly increased after treatment in 70%. Of the 77 episodes of tense ascites treated with total paracentesis plus dextran-40 infusion during first hospitalization and follow-up, hyponatremia and/or renal impairment developed after treatment in 16 (21%) (hyponatremia in 14 and renal impairment in 6).

In a study of 14 patients, Cabrera et al.[39] in Las Palmas suggested that intravenous isotonic saline infusion can also be a safe and cost-effective alternative plasma expander in cirrhotic patients with tense ascites treated with paracentesis. Further studies are obviously needed to confirm their findings.

Such studies suggest that dextran-70 and hemaccel but not dextran-40 are as effective as albumin in preventing renal and electrolyte complications after therapeutic paracentesis in cirrhotic patients with tense ascites. They also suggest that plasma expanders may be more effective in saline solution than in dextrose solution for preventing impairment of systemic hemodynamics induced by paracentesis. Nevertheless, further studies including large number of patients are necessary to confirm such contentions.

COMPARISON OF PERITONEOVENOUS SHUNTING WITH PARACENTESIS PLUS INTRAVENOUS ALBUMIN INFUSION IN THE MANAGEMENT OF PATIENTS WITH REFRACTORY ASCITES

Recently, a Spanish multicenter, randomized trial[40] compared therapeutic paracentesis with peritoneovenous shunting in cirrhotic patients with refractory ascites. Forty-one patients were treated with repeated large-volume paracentesis plus intravenous albumin and 48 with a LeVeen shunt. Diuretics were subsequently given to avoid reaccumulation of ascites. Patients who were treated with paracentesis and developed tense ascites during follow-up were treated again by paracentesis, whereas patients originally treated with peritoneovenous shunting were retreated either with a new prosthesis (in case of shunt obstruction) or with diuretics. During first hospitalization, both treatments were equally effective in mobilizing the ascites, although the duration of stay was significantly longer in the shunt group (19 ± 1 vs. 11 ± 1 days). There were no significant differences between groups in the number of patients who developed complications (9 and 15) or died (3 and 6). During follow-up, 37 patients from each group were readmitted to hospital. The number of readmissions for any reason (174 vs. 97) or for ascites (125 vs. 38) was significantly higher in the shunt group, and the time to first readmission for any reason (1 ± 0.2 vs. 2.3 ± 0.3 months) and for ascites (2.4 ± 0.3 vs 8 ± 2.6 months) was significantly shorter in the paracentesis group than in the shunt group. However, the total time in hospital during follow-up was similar in the two groups (48 ± 8 and 44 ± 6 days; 19% ± 3% and 22% ± 4% of the follow-up period). Because the number of readmissions was higher among patients treated with paracentesis, the mean duration of hospital stays during follow-up was significantly shorter in that group than in the peritoneovenous shunt group (11 ± 8 vs. 18 ± 14 days). The peritoneovenous shunt was obstructed in 20 readmissions for ascites among 15 patients. The site of obstruction was the valve in 12 readmissions, the venous tube in 4, and thrombosis of the superior vena cava in 4; a superior vena cava syndrome developed in 2 patients. The probability of survival was similar in both groups (Fig. 23.4). The probabilities of obstruction of the shunt after 1 and 2 years were 40 and 52%, respectively (Fig. 23.5).

A recent study in a large series of cirrhotic patients with ascites treated with a LeVeen shunt demonstrated that the insertion of a 3-cm titanium tip into the venous end of the LeVeen shunt prevents thrombotic obstruction of the venous limb of the prosthesis and development of superior vena cava thrombosis.[41] This finding, however, was not confirmed in an European multicenter, randomized study comparing total paracentesis combined with intravenous albumin vs. LeVeen shunt with titanium tip.[42] Seventy-three cirrhotic patients with refractory or recidivant ascites (more than three episodes of ascites within 9 months despite adequate diuretic treatment) were included in the trial. Thirty six patients were treated with total paracentesis plus intravenous albumin infusion (8 gm/L of ascites removed) and 37 with a LeVeen shunt with titanium tip. Patients were discharged with diuretics to avoid reaccumulation of ascites. If tense ascites recurred, patients in the paracentesis group were again treated with total paracentesis, whereas patients in the LeVeen were treated with diuretics or a new prosthesis (if the shun was obstructed). Both types of treatment were equally effective in mobilizing ascites. During first hospitalization 8 patients in the paracentesis group and 19 in the LeVeen group had complications (p < 0.05), and 1 and 3 patients died, respectively. During follow-up (7.1 ± 1 vs. 7.4 ± 1 months), the number of readmissions was significantly greater in the paracentesis group (155 vs. 58) because of a higher recurrence of ascites (111 vs. 20). Total time spent in hospital, however, was similar in both groups (28 ± 5 vs. 30 ± 5 days/patient) because of a significantly lower mean duration of hospitalizations in the paracentesis group. There were 18 cases of shunt obstruction in 13 patients (43%), of which 50% occurred at the venous end. The probability of survival was similar in both groups.

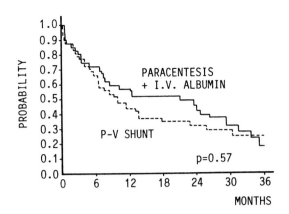

FIGURE 23.4. Probability of survival after entry into the study in the two study groups. (From Ginès P, Arroyo V, Vargas V, et al: Paracentesis with intravenous infusion of albumin as compared with peritoneovenous shunting in cirrhosis with refractory ascites. N Engl J Med 1991;325:829–835, with permission.)

The above trials show that although the LeVeen shunt is more effective than paracentesis in the long-term control of ascites, it does not reduce the total time in hospital or prolong survival. Patients treated with peritoneovenous shunt require frequent reoperations due to obstruction of the prosthesis. This complication is not prevented by insertion of a titanium tip at the venous end of the shunt. Therapeutic paracentesis is an alternative treatment to LeVeen shunt in cirrhotic patients with refractory ascites.

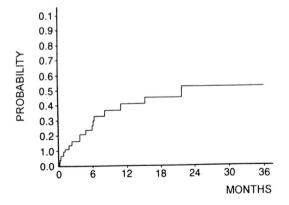

FIGURE 23.5. Probability of a peritoneovenous shunt obstruction after entry into the study in patients with cirrhosis and ascites. (From Ginès P, Arroyo V, Vargas V, et al: Paracentesis with intravenous infusion of albumin as compared with peritoneovenous shunting in cirrhosis with refractory ascites. N Engl J Med 1991;325:829–835, with permission.)

TECHNICAL CONSIDERATIONS

Although paracentesis is a simple procedure, several precautions should be taken to avoid local complications. It is advisable to perform the paracentesis under strict sterile conditions. The abdomen should be cleaned, disinfected, and draped in a sterile fashion, and the physician should wear sterile gown and gloves during the entire procedure. We use a modified Kuss needle, which is a sharp-pointed, blind, metal needle, within a 7-cm 17-G metal, blunt-edged cannula with side holes (Fig.23.6). Under local anesthesia, the Kuss needle is inserted in the left lower abdominal quadrant. Once the needle enters the peritoneal cavity, the inner part is removed and the cannula is connected to a large-volume suction pump. The physician remains at bedside throughout the treatment. Duration of treatment ranges from 20–90 minutes, depending on the amount of ascitic fluid removed.

In patients submitted to total paracentesis, the procedure is finished when the flow from the cannula becomes intermittent, despite gentle mobilization within the abdominal cavity and turning the patient to his or her left. After paracentesis, patients should recline for at least 2 hours on the site opposite the paracentesis to prevent leakage of ascitic fluid. Samples of ascitic fluid should be routinely taken for cell count, biochemical examination, and culture. The intravenous administration of albumin or other plasma expanders is initiated at the end of the procedure. In cases of massive ascites treated by total paracentesis (> 8 L), half of the dose of plasma expanders should be administered at the end of the procedure and half 6 hours later to prevent excessively rapid plasma volume expansion, which may lead to variceal bleeding. In most patients peripheral edema rapidly reabsorbs following mobilization of ascites and usually disappears within the first 2 days after treatment. Most of the fluid goes to the intraperitoneal cavity in the form of ascites. It is, therefore, not uncommon for patients with massive peripheral edema to require a second paracentesis to remove the fluid shifted from the interstitial space to the intraperitoneal compartment.

CONCLUSIONS

Therapeutic paracentesis, either repeated large-volume paracentesis or total paracentesis, combined with intravenous infusion of plasma expanders (albumin, dextran-70, hemaccel) is a rapid, effective, and safe treatment for ascites in patients with cirrhosis. Because therapeutic paracentesis is associated with a lower incidence of complications than standard diuretic therapy and considerably shortens the duration of hospital stay, it is the first-choice treatment for patients with marked sodium retention and tense ascites.

The mobilization of ascites by paracentesis without intravenous colloid administration is constantly associated with impairment of the effective circulating blood volume, as estimated by plasma levels of renin and aldosterone, and induces renal impairment and/or dilutional hyponatremia in approximately 20% of patients. Although albumin is probably the best plasma expander for cirrhotic patients with tense ascites treated with paracentesis, dextran-70 or hemaccel in saline solution seems to be as effective as albumin in preventing renal and electrolyte complications.

Therapeutic paracentesis does not improve systemic and renal hemodynamics or sodium retention. Therefore, cirrhotic patients treated with paracentesis require the administration of diuretics to avoid reaccumulation of ascites.

Although peritoneovenous shunting is more effective than therapeutic paracentesis in the long-term control of ascites in cirrhotic patients with refractory or recidivant ascites, a high proportion of patients treated with LeVeen shunt need reoperation due to obstruction of the prosthesis. The time spent in hospital and the probability of survival are identical with both procedures. Therefore, paracentesis is an alternative treatment to peritoneovenous shunting in cirrhotic patients with refractory or recidivant ascites.

Further research should (1) investigate in larger series of patients whether other, less expensive plasma expanders can be safely substituted for albumin, (2) assess the mechanism and clinical relevance of postparacentesis circulatory dysfunction, and (3) evaluate the safety of therapeutic paracentesis in patients with severe hepatic and/or renal dysfunction.

Acknowledgments. The authors are indebted to Drs. E. Quintero, J. Panes, J. Viver, J. Cabrera, J. Salo, A. Rimola, F. Rivera, J. Gaya, L. Tito, M. Torres, S. Badalamenti, W. Jimenez, P. Humbert, E. Domenech, and M.A. Gassull for their participation in the studies reported in this chapter. The work was funded by a grant from the Direccion General de Investigacion Cientifica y Tecnica (DGICYT PM 91-0216).

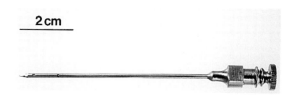

FIGURE 23.6. Modified Kuss needle used for paracentesis.

REFERENCES

1. Ginès P, Qunitero E, Arroyo V, et al: Compensated cirrhosis: Natural history and prognostic factors. Hepatology 1987;7:122–128.
2. Llach J Ginès P, Arroyo V, et al: Prognostic value of arterial pressure, endogenous vasoactive systems, and renal function in cirrhotic patients admitted to the hospital for the treatment of ascites. Gastroenterology 1988; 94:482–487.
3. Pérez-Ayuso RM, Arroyo V, Planas R, et al: Randomized comparative study of efficacy of furosemide versus spironolactone in nonazotemic cirrhosis with ascites. Gastroenterology 1983;84:961–968.
4. Arroyo V, Ginès P, Planas R, et al: Management of patients with cirrhosis and ascites. Semin Liver Dis 1986; 6:353–369.
5. Arroyo V, Ginès P, Planas R: Treatment of ascites in cirrhosis. Gastroenterol Clin North Am 1992;21:237–256.
6. Brater DC: Resistance to loop diuretics. Why it happens and what to do about it. Drugs 1985;30:327–433.
7. Chiandusi L, Bartoli E, Arras S: Reabsorption of sodium in the proximal renal tubule in cirrhosis of the liver. Gut 1978;19:497–503.
8. LeVeen HH, Christoudias G, Moon JP, et al: Peritoneovenous shunting for ascites. Ann Surg 1974;180:580–591.
9. Smajda C, Franco D: The LeVeen shunt in the elective treatment of intractable ascites in cirrhosis: A prospective study on 140 patients. Ann Surg 1985;201:488.
10. Stanley MM, Ochi S, Lee KK, et al: Peritoneovenous shunting as compared with medical treatment in patients with alcoholic cirrhosis and massive ascites. N Engl J Med 1989;321:1632–1638.
11. Linas SL, Schaefer JW, Moore EE, et al: Peritoneovenous shunt in the management of hepatorenal syndrome. Kidney Int 1986;30:736–740.
12. Gordon ME: The acute effects of abdominal paracentesis in Laennec's cirrhosis upon exchanges of electrolytes and water, renal function, and hemodynamics. Am J Gastroenterol 1960;33:15–37.
13. Kowalski HJ, Abelmann WH, McNeely WF: The cardiac output in patients with cirrhosis of the liver and tense ascites with observations on the effect of paracentesis. J Clin Invest 1954;33:768–773.
14. Shear L, Ching S, Gabuzda GJ: Compartmentalization of ascites and edema in patients with hepatic cirrhosis. N Engl J Med 1970;282:1391–1396.
15. Knauer CM, Lowe HM: Hemodynamics in the cirrhotic patient during paracentesis. N Engl J Med 1967;276: 491–496.

16. Gauzzi M, Polese A, Magrini F: Negative influences of ascites on the cardiac function of cirrhotic patients. Am J Med 1975;59:165–170.

17. Iwatsuki S, Reynolds TB: Effect of increased intraabdominal pressure on hepatic hemodynamics in patients with chronic liver disease and portal hypertension. Gastroenterology 1973;65:294–299.

18. Carey WD, Kohne JC, Leatherman J, Paradis K: Ascitic fluid removal: Does it cause renal or hemodynamic decompensation? Cleve Clin Q 1983;50:397–400.

19. Ginés P, Arroyo V, Qunitero E, et al: Comparison of paracentesis and diuretics in the treatment of cirrhotics with tense ascites. Results of a randomized study. Gastroenterology 1987;93:234–241.

20. Ascione A, Burroughs AK: Paracentesis for ascites in cirrhotic patients. Gastroenterol Int 1990;3:120–123.

21. Quintero E, Ginés P, Arroyo V, et al: Paracentesis versus diuretics in the treatment of cirrhotics with tense ascites. Lancet 1985;i:611–612.

22. Sherlock S, Senewiratne B, Scott A Walker JG: Complications of diuretic therapy in hepatic cirrhosis. Lancet 1966;i:1049–1053.

23. Strauss E, De Sa MF, Laut CM, et al: Standardization of a therapeutic approach for ascites due to chronic liver disease. A prospective study of 100 cases. Gastroenterol Endosc Dig 1985;4:79–86.

24. Salerno F, Badalamenti S, Incerti P, et al: Repeated paracentesis and IV albumin infusion to treat "tense" ascites in cirrhotic patients: A safe alternative therapy. J Hepatol 1987;5:102–108.

25. Hagève H, Ink O, Ducreux G, et al: Traitement de l'ascite chez les malades atteints de cirrhose sans hyponatrémie ni insuffisance rénale. Gastroenterol Clin Biol 1992;16:751–755.

26. Solà R, Villa C, Andreu M, et al: Total paracentesis with dextran-40 vs diuretics in the treatment of ascites in cirrhosis. A randomized controlled trial. J Hepatol 1994;20:282–288.

27. Tító Ll, Ginés P, Arroyo V, et al: Total paracentesis associated with intravenous albumin in the management of patients with cirrhosis and ascites. Gastroenterology 1990;98:146–151.

28. Ginés P, Tító Ll, Arroyo V, et al: Randomized comparative study of therapeutic paracentesis with and without intravenous albumin in cirrhosis. Gastroenterology 1988;94:1493–1502.

29. Simon DM, McCain JR, Bonkovsky HL, et al: Effects of therapeutic paracentesis on systemic and hepatic hemodynamics and on the renal and hormonal function. Hepatology 1988;7:423–429.

30. Panos MZ, Moore K, Vlavianos P, et al: Single, total paracentesis for tense ascites: Sequential hemodynamic changes and right atrial size. Hepatology 1990;11:662–667.

31. Terg R, Berreta J, Abecasis R, et al: Dextran administration avoids hemodynamic changes following paracentesis in cirrhotic patients. A safe and inexpensive option. Dig Dis Sci 1992;37:79–83.

32. Luca A, Feu F, García-Pagán JC, et al: Hemodynamic and humoral changes after total paracentesis with and without albumin infusion. J Hepatol 1993;18(Suppl 1):S60.

33. Kao HW, Rakov NE, Savage E, Reynolds TB: The effect of large volume paracentesis on plasma volume: A cause of hypovolemia? Hepatology 1985;5:403–407.

34. Pinto PC, Amerian J, Reynolds TB: Large-volume paracentesis in nonedematous patients with tense ascites: Its effects on intravascular volume. Hepatology 1988;8:207–210.

35. Gentile S, Angelico M, Bologna E, Capocaccia L: Clinical, biochemical, and hormonal changes after a single, large-volume paracentesis in cirrhosis with ascites. Am J Gatroenterol 1989;84:279–284.

36. Planas R, Ginés P, Arroyo V, et al: Dextran-70 versus albumin as plasma expanders in cirrhotic patients with tense ascites treated with total paracentesis: Results of a randomized study. Gastroenterology 1990;99:1736–1744.

37. Salerno F, Badalamenti S, Lorenza E, et al: Randomized comparative study of hemaccel vs albumin infusion after total paracentesis in cirrhotic patients with refractory ascites. Hepatology 1991;13:707–713.

38. Fassio E, Terg R, Landeire G, et al: Paracentesis with dextran-70 vs paracentesis with albumin in cirrhosis with tense ascites. Results of a randomized study. J Hepatol 1992;14:310–316.

39. Cabrera J, Inglada L, Quintero E, et al: Large-volume paracentesis and intravenous saline: Effects on the renin-angiotensin system. Hepatology 1991;14:1025–1028.

40. Ginés P, Arroyo V, Vargas V, et al: Paracentesis with intravenous infusion of albumin as compared with peritoneovenous shunting in cirrhosis with refractory ascites. N Engl J Med 1991;325:829–835.

41. Hillaire S, Labianca M, Smajda C, et al: Dérivation péritonéo-veineuse dans l'ascite irréductible de la cirrhose. Résultats d'une étude prospective sur les facteurs d'amélioration du pronostic. Gastroenterol Clin Biol 1988;12:681–686.

42. Ginés A, Planas R, Angeli P, et al: Treatment of patients with cirrhosis and refractory ascites using LeVeen shunt with titanium tip: Comparison with therapeutic paracentesis. Hepatology 1995;22:124–131.

Chapter 24

PERITONEOVENOUS SHUNT IN THE MANAGEMENT OF ASCITES AND THE HEPATORENAL SYNDROME

MURRAY EPSTEIN, M.D., F.A.C.P.

Characteristics of Peritoneovenous Shunt
  LeVeen Shunt
  Denver Shunt
  Shunt Patency
Physiological Consequences of Shunting
  Hemodynamic and Renal Effects
  Characterization of Renal Function by Metabolic
    Balance Studies
  Mechanisms Underlying the Natriuresis and
    Diuresis
  Effects on Body Composition
  Morbidity Associated with Peritoneovenous
    Shunting

Coagulation Abnormalities
Sepsis
Small Bowel Obstruction
Additional Adverse Effects
Differences in Frequency of Complications with
  Different Shunts
Differences in Morbidity of Peritoneovenous
  Shunting for Cirrhotic versus Malignant Ascites
Peritoneovenous Shunt in Clinical Practice
  Management of Ascites
  Management of the Hepatorenal Syndrome
Summary

As noted in chapter 1, the avid sodium retention and accumulation of ascites that often complicate the course of advanced liver disease are among the most difficult problems to manage in clinical medicine. Although diuretics are used commonly to decrease ascites, it is time-consuming and arduous to manage the sodium retention of liver disease with diuretics and dietary sodium restriction. Furthermore, such an approach may be fraught with hazards. If the forces acting to promote ascites are sufficiently strong, ascites may form at a rat exceeding its reabsorption rate, even when the vascular volume has been reduced to the point that azotemia supervenes. Such patients are considered to have intractable ascites, and they pose formidable problems in management. The administration of more potent diuretics in increasing doses is of no avail because, in essence, the problem is not renal refractoriness but rather maldistribution of fluid.

Because the underlying abnormality in such patients is not solely an excess of fluid, but rather a maldistribution of extracellular fluid, much attention has been focused on a mechanical solution to the problem. Various approaches have

been tried (Table 24.1). Perhaps the oldest known form of therapy for ascites is paracentesis, which was used as early as the Graeco-Roman period.[1]

During the first half of the 20th century, surgeons resorted to omentopexy to alleviate ascites. An additional approach has been the use of "buttons" that direct ascitic fluid into the subcutaneous tissue of the abdominal wall to be absorbed.[2] Although occasionally successful, the technique is only a transient approach and absorption ceases readily. Neumann et al.[3] described the operation known as "ileoentectropy," in which an ileal loop is implanted into the parietal peritoneum for purposes of absorbing the ascitic fluid. This approach is usually self-defeating, because the mucosal surface secretes mucus and local infection ensues.

Additional methods have included direct attempts at removal of ascitic fluid, such as peritoneo-ureterostomy and vesicocoelomic drainage,[4]

Portions of this chapter have been adapted from Epstein M: The peritoneovenous shunt in the management of ascites and the hepatorenal syndrome. Gastroenterology 1982; 82: 790–799, with permission.

TABLE 24.1. Surgical Approaches for the Relief of Ascites

Year	Procedure
Graeco-Roman era	Multiple paracentesis
1898–1943	Omentopexy
1943	Peritoneo-ureterostomy
1946	Subcutaneous drainage using "buttons"
1955	Vesicocoelomic drainage
1955	Ileal entectropy
1959	Side-to-side portacaval shunt
1962–1968	Peritoneocaval shunt with Holter valve
1961–1974	Ascites reinfusion
1974	Peritoneovenous (LeVeen) shunt

whereby the peritoneal cavity and bladder are connected by a length of tubing and thereby divert the flow of ascites out of the peritoneal cavity. While differing somewhat in detail, the experience of all investigators with the above techniques has been negative.

As noted earlier, there has been an increasing awareness that the underlying abnormality is not solely an excess of fluid, but rather a maldistribution of extracellular fluid. Consequently, much attention has been focused on developing procedures that might redistribute body fluids between compartments, so that the central compartment is replenished at a time when ascites is decreasing. Thus, many clinicians undertook the reinfusion of ascitic fluid into the circulation.[5–9] Although acute (and occasionally quite dramatic) benefits have followed ascites reinfusion, no long-term benefits have accrued from this form of therapy, and the survival of patients so treated was not prolonged. The general opinion of virtually all investigators was that the short-term gains did not warrant the risks and effort involved in this relatively cumbersome form of therapy.

In contrast to the above interventions, it may be surprising to the reader that the surgical approach recognized today as the peritoneovenous (PV) shunt was actually conceived near the turn of the century. In 1907, Ruotte addressed the Surgical Society of Lyon relating his experience with two patients in whom he had anastomosed the cephalad end of the saphenous vein into the peritoneal cavity to mobilize cirrhotic ascites. A few years later, Leuret described his experience with a peritoneal saphenous vein shunt to mobilize ascites.[9a] It is intriguing to note that over 70 years ago Leuret was aware that "one must eliminate without doubt ascites that contains infected germs." In view of the achievements of Ruotte and Leuret, the current technology that has been considered to be the cutting edge in management of intractable ascites is not as new as we had thought.

Previous attempts to establish permanent PV shunts with flow-activated valves such as the Holter valve have been unsuccessful, primarily because of the technical problems associated with maintaining shunt patency. In 1974, this hurdle was overcome with a technical breakthrough reported by LeVeen and associates.[10] The investigators developed a new device designed to function as a one-way valve activated by a pressure gradient. The success of the new valve in facilitating continuous PV shunting of ascitic fluid and the technical simplicity of its insertion resulted in a flurry of enthusiasm. Here at last seemed to be a rational and effective means of managing ascites. The medical community was quick to embrace the apparently promising technique. Precise figures are not available, but it may be estimated that over 80,000 LeVeen shunts have been inserted worldwide since this technique was introduced in 1974.[11] The majority of PV shunts available today are LeVeen shunts. However, other types include the Denver shunt[12] and the Cordis-Hakim shunt have been introduced.[13] Since 1977, over 65,000 Denver shunts have been implanted. At the time of this writing, only the former two shunts are commercially available.

CHARACTERISTICS OF PERITONEOVENOUS SHUNT

LeVeen Shunt

The characteristics and design of the LeVeen valve have been reviewed by the inventor.[14,15] LeVeen appreciated that the high failure rate of previous valves was attributable chiefly to backflow of blood into the connecting tubes, with subsequent clotting. In order for the valve to function indefinitely as a PV shunt, its design must satisfy several criteria. The valve must remain competent at all pressures to ensure patency. The valve must remain normally in the closed position. Finally, when the gradient pressure between the abdomen and central venous pressure rises above 3 cm H_2O, the valve must open. The new mechanism introduced by LeVeen in 1974 and released commercially in 1977 (Becton Dickinson Co., Franklin Lakes, NJ) fulfills these criteria. Figure 24.1 is a

FIGURE 24.1. Cross-section of the LeVeen valve. The diaphragm and struts are made of silicone rubber. The struts are attached to a ring that in turn attaches to the valve casing. The valve is normally in the closed position unless a pressure gradient of greater than 3–4 cm of water opens it. (From LeVeen H: Ann Surg 1976;184:574, with permission.)

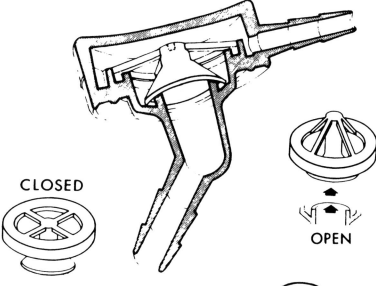

CLOSED

OPEN

schematic diagram of the valve. The valve is a sensitive silicone bell that sets like a "seat valve," closing a large orifice with modest pressure. The silicone rubber itself acts as the spring. The valve is kept closed by the tensile force exerted by the silicone struts. A pressure of 3 cm H_2O is required to overcome this force and to elevate the diaphragm and allow flow through the valve. One limb of the shunt lies free in the peritoneal space and is connected to the valve, which is placed extraperitoneally but beneath the abdominal wall muscles (Fig. 24.2).

The venous limb is burrowed subcutaneously up the chest wall and inserted into one of the jugular veins (usually the internal jugular vein) and positioned to lie in the superior vena cava near the opening into the right atrium. Whenever a pressure gradient of 3 cm H_2O exists between the peritoneal cavity and the superior vena cava, the valve will remain open and ascitic fluid will flow into the vein. If this pressure gradient diminishes, the valve will close. Blood is thus prevented from refluxing into the venous limb of the shunt and clotting.

Some investigators maintain that the operation is technically simple and can be performed under local anesthesia. Nevertheless, various observers have emphasized that several modifications are necessary to prevent technical failures and to maintain the patency of the shunt. The Toronto group[16] suggests that the internal jugular vein be used routinely, because the use of the cephalic vein or external jugular vein has led to kinking and the occlusion of the venous limb. Second, to

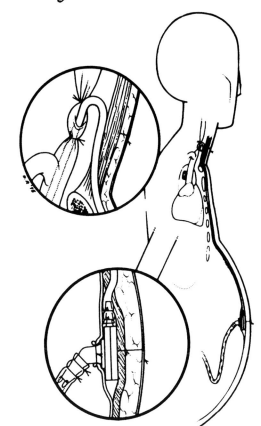

FIGURE 24.2. LeVeen shunt after implantation. The valve lies outside the peritoneum, deep to the abdominal muscles. The venous collecting tube traverses the subcutaneous tissue of the chest wall into the neck, where it enters the internal jugular vein. The two detailed views show the valve lying subcutaneously and the tip of the shunt tube entering the internal jugular vein. (From LeVeen H: Ann Surg 1976;184:574, with permission.)

minimize ascites leak, they propose that the valve be placed deep to the rectus muscle. Finally, they recommend that a shuntogram be routinely performed while the patient is on the operating table to confirm the correct positioning of the end of the venous limb in the superior vena cava above the right atrium.

Greenlee et al.[17] have emphasized that proper placement of the venous end of the shunt is critical to ensure proper function and to minimize subsequent outflow obstruction from clotting about the venus tip. They advocate the use of the right internal jugular vein (RIJV) for access and to verify placement of the outflow tip in the distal superior vena cava or preferably the right atrium.

Postoperatively, it is important that the pressure gradient be maintained to keep the valve open. Most patients with chronic ascites have stretched and thinned abdominal walls. When only a small volume of fluid is removed from the peritoneal cavity, the intraabdominal pressure falls to low levels because of the lax abdominal musculature. The normal abdominothoracic pressure gradient induced by inspiration may not develop adequately in such patients. Two maneuvers are used to assist in keeping the valve open:

1. An abdominal binder may be used to raise the intraabdominal pressure by compression. The degree of pressure generated is varied by altering the tightness with which the binder is applied. This technique has particular application for patients with large abdominal hernias, which rule out other means of increasing intraabdominal pressure.

2. The second technique involves exercises that require inspiration against resistance. Lying supine, the patient sucks on the tubing to draw air through a 15- to 20-cm column of water. This exercise increases the negative intrathoracic pressure and increases intraabdominal pressure. Patients are instructed to repeat these 10- to 20-minute exercises 3–6 times/day.

Denver Shunt

The observation that the LeVeen shunt frequently occludes has prompted a search for a new shunting system that would circumvent or reduce the incidence of this problem. This search has led to the introduction of a shunt with a pumping mechanism—the Denver shunt (Denver Biomaterials Inc., Evergreen, CO). In contrast to the laminar flow associated with the LeVeen shunt, this valve creates turbulence about the valve when pumped, thereby cleaning the valve mechanisms and minimizing the chance of occlusion.

The Denver shunt[12] is based on the hydrocephalus shunt. It consists of a peritoneovenous catheter to drain ascitic fluid from the abdominal cavity, a flexible pump body, and a distal catheter to infuse ascitic fluid into the cardiovascular system. The pumping chamber of the Denver valve presently consists of one or two duck-bill or miter (so termed because of its resemblance to the liturgical headdress) valves located at the entry (peritoneal end) of the pump body. The Denver shunt has recently been modified so that it contains a double valve rather than a single valve. With the earlier single-valve model, blood would sometimes reflux into the distal catheter during the release phase of the pumping cycle. The double-valve modification was designed to avoid this problem.

Opening Pressure. The Denver valve opens when a positive pressure of approximately 1 cm H_2O exists across the pumping chamber.

Pumping Mechanism. Ascitic fluid will flow uniformly through each system under the influence of a constant positive hydraulic pressure unless the tubing between the valve housings is deliberately pumped. When the pump body of the Denver shunt is sharply pressed, liquid is rapidly forced through the distal catheter. This manipulation allows the surgeon, attendant, or patient to clear the valve system of accumulating solid matter.

Detection on Radiograph. The LeVeen and Denver shunts have a radiopaque stripe running throughout the length of the venous tube for accurate location after insertion. The Denver system incorporates a barium sulfate line throughout the entire system, except for the pump body, to assist during placement at surgery and to confirm its location postoperatively. The entry tip of the peritoneal catheter and opposite ends of the valve pump body are thus radiographically detectable.

Shunt Patency

Successful management of the patient with persistent intractable ascites depends on continued PV shunt performance. Implicit with maintained PV shunt function is continued patency; however, data about patency duration after PV shunt implantation are few.

In a randomized, prospective study, Fulenwider et al.[18] compared the duration of patency of

TABLE 24.2.   Effects of Peritoneovenous Shunting*

	Perioperative (3 days after insertion)	Postoperative (2 weeks after insertion)	Late Postoperative
Hemodynamic parameters			
Cardiac output	↑	↑	↑
Pulmonary artery wedge pressure	—		
Mean arterial pressure	↓		
Calculated peripheral vascular resistance	↓		
Renal parameters			
p-Aminohippuric acid clearance	↑	↑ or —	
Creatinine clearance	↑	↑	↑
Urinary volume	↑	↑	
Sodium excretion	↑	↑	
Hormonal parameters			
Plasma renin activity	↓	↓	
Plasma aldosterone	↓	↓	↓

* As compared with preoperative levels.
Hemodynamic data based on observations of Blendis et al: The renal and hemodynamic effects of the peritoneovenous shunt for intractable hepatic ascites. Gastroenterology 1976;77:250–257, and Greig et al: Renal and hemodynamic effects of the peritoneovenous shunt. II. Long-term effects. Gastroenterology 1981;80:119–125.

the two most popular PV shunts for intractable ascites of cirrhotic patients: the LeVeen and the Denver (the single-valve model). Determinations of patency included contrast shuntogram, technitium Tc 99m albumin scintigraphy, sequential manual compression of the Denver shunt, and operative or autopsy observation.

The investigators observed that the patency of the LeVeen PV shunt exceeded that of the Denver shunt. Nevertheless, survival did not differ significantly with the two. Because the complications other than closure were similar, the authors concluded on the basis of their small prospective series that in cirrhotic patients with intractable ascites, the LeVeen shunt may be preferred. A caveat, however, is in order. Because the present model of the Denver PV shunt contains two valves, it may occlude less often. Additional studies are required to ascertain this possibility.

For a detailed review of the diagnosis and management of PV shunt occlusion, the reader is referred to a review by LeVeen et al.[18a]

PHYSIOLOGIC CONSEQUENCES OF SHUNTING

Hemodynamic and Renal Effects

Although over 80,000 LeVeen shunts have been implanted since 1977 in patients with ascites, relatively few of these patients have been studied in an effective manner that permits critical assessment of the results. Furthermore, with rare exceptions, the clinical results have not been described in a manner that permits adequate quantitative assessment of the benefits and risks in various subpopulations.

Many observers have documented a marked diuresis and augmentation in glomerular filtration rate (GFR) and a suppression of plasma renin activity (PRA), plasma aldosterone, and arginine vasopressin levels after PV shunting.[19–24] Few investigators, however, have carried out sequential determinations of renal, hormonal, and hemodynamic parameters over a prolonged period. Among the few well-conceived and accomplished studies is that of Blendis et al.[20] The investigators reported careful physiologic measurements of 15 patients with chronic liver disease and intractable ascites who were studied the 6 days immediately before shunt insertion and the first 3 days after insertion, and then 2 weeks after insertion (Table 24.2). Immediate and dramatic increases in cardiac output (38%) and decreases in calculated peripheral vascular resistance (33%) were reported.

In association with the increase in cardiac output, renal perfusion was augmented as indicated by an increase in clearance of both p-aminohippuric acid (89%) and creatinine (50%). Concomitantly, all patients, manifested an immediate marked natriuresis and diuresis. Indeed, some investigators have reported dramatic initial diureses with urine volume as high as 8–12 L/day. To a great extent, this extraordinarily rapid (and potentially dangerous) rate of diuresis can be modified by relatively simple measures such as a more judicious use of furosemide (or its omission altogether) during the immediate postoperative period and the avoidance of abdominal binders in the early postoperative period. The hemodynamic and renal effects are accompanied by dramatic reductions in both PRA and plasma aldosterone levels[19–24] and marked increases in plasma atrial natriuretic peptide.[24a]

The Toronto group has assessed the late postoperative status of their patients.[21] They determined changes in cardiac output, renal function, and plasma renin and aldosterone levels in 11 of the 24 patients who had received a PV shunt for intractable ascites. These late postoperative studies were carried out at intervals ranging from 3 to 29 months after shunt insertion. In comparison with the preoperative studies, it was observed that the cardiac output was still increased in 4 of 5 patients in whom hemodynamic studies were determined. The creatinine clearance remained increased over the preoperative values. Concomitantly, the normalization of PRA and plasma aldosterone levels persisted in most patients.

These results agree with the observations of Greenlee et al.,[17] who carried out serial studies in 19 of their initial 25 shunted patients and observed that creatinine clearance increased from a preshunt mean of 74 ± 8 ml/min to a mean of 112 ± 10 ml/min at 30 days after shunt insertion. Six months after shunting, the augmentation in creatinine clearance persisted (119 ± 8 ml/min).

Recently the Toronto group extended their observations of renal sodium handling and also characterized ANF responsiveness PV shunt insertion.[24b] They compared the response to ANF infusion before and 1 month after PV shunt insertion in 6 patients with massive ascites. The infusion of ANF after PV shunting induced a significant increase in both GFR and filtration fraction and also in distal delivery of sodium. Changes in renal sodium handling were accompanied by a significant decrease in antinatriuretic forces after PV shunting (i.e., baseline aldosterone of 2079 ± 507 vs. 647 ± 17 nmol/L after PV shunting; p < 0.04).

Of note, the improvement in natriuretic ability was accompanied by a return to diuretic responsiveness after shunt insertion. The investigators attributed the improvement in sodium homeostasis and response to ANF infusion after PV shunting to the decrease in antinatriuretic forces with the loss of massive refractory ascites. Thus, PV

shunting appears to restore the balance toward ANF responsiveness.

Characterization of Renal Function by Metabolic Balance Studies

Despite extensive experience with the placement of LeVeen shunts in cirrhotic patients with ascites, the alterations in renal sodium and water handling have not been characterized extensively in a systematic, prospective manner. Virtually all observations have been approximations made in the context of uncontrolled sodium and fluid access and with concomitant diuretic administration. There has been a dearth of metabolic balance studies before and after shunt insertion. In the only such study of which I am aware, Blendis et al.[20] studied 15 patients during the preoperative, perioperative, and postoperative periods. The preoperative period was defined as the 6 days before shunt insertion. The perioperative period consisted of the initial 72 hours after insertion of the shunt, and the postoperative period consisted of the subsequent 2 weeks, during which dietary sodium was maintained constant. At the time of study, patients were ingesting 20 mEq of sodium/day with fluid restricted to 1 L/day.

Perioperatively, daily sodium excretion increased from a mean of 7 mEq/day to a peak mean of 174 ± 44 mEq/day; daily urine volume increased from 0.8 ± 0.1 to 2.2 ± 0.2 L/day. At 2 weeks postoperatively, the daily urinary output was 1.0 ± 0.1 L/day, exceeding the average preoperative value of 0.76 L/day on an identical fluid intake. The daily sodium excretion was 16 ± 7 mEq/day—less than the levels during the perioperative period but exceeding the levels during the preoperative period. Although intake of sodium and fluid was unchanged during all three study periods, the patients received diuretics (furosemide and spironolactone), thereby confounding the interpretation of the data.

Subsequently, the Toronto group assessed renal sodium handling during the late postoperative period (at intervals ranging from 3 to 29 months after shunt insertion). Greig et al.[21] carried out sodium balance studies in 7 of the patients after discontinuation of diuretics. Each patient was investigated while equilibrating on 20 mEq sodium/day and subsequently on 100 mEq sodium/day. On the 20-mEq sodium diet, mean daily sodium excretion was 17 ± 5 mEq/day, exceeding the preoperative mean value of 2 ± 4 mEq/day with identical sodium intake. Nevertheless, when placed on the 100-mEq sodium diet, most patients were unable to adapt and manifested sodium retention. Sodium excretion ranged from 4 to 130 mEq/day, with a mean of 56 ± 27 mEq/day; 6 of the 7 patients displayed sodium retention. Of interest, despite the marked augmentation in creatinine clearance, renal sodium handling varied independently of GFR.

Mechanisms Underlying the Natriuresis and Diuresis

Although the PV shunt has been demonstrated repeatedly to induce a marked natriuresis and diuresis,[14–22] the mechanism(s) responsible for such effects remains undefined. Most (but not all) investigators have observed that insertion of the shunt per se was insufficient to sustain a natriuresis and diuresis and that concomitant diuretic therapy was a prerequisite to maintain the therapeutic response. If, as has been proposed, the shunt succeeds in repleting a diminished effective volume, it is difficult to understand why some (but not all) observers report that successful shunt insertion alone is incapable of inducing a natriuresis and diuresis. Such observations suggest that alternative mechanisms may account for the natriuresis and diuresis of the PV shunt.

Effects on Body Composition

The available literature concentrates primarily on the beneficial effects of PV shunting, both short-term and long-term, on sodium and water balance and renal function. It has been noted anecdotally that after successful PV shunting cirrhotic patients often regain their muscle mass in addition to losing excessive fluid. To examine this apparent improvement in protein status, Blendis et al.[25] measured total body nitrogen (TBN) and total body potassium (TBK) in 7 male cirrhotic patients before and after successful elective PV shunting for massive ascites. The results were compared with data from 3 patients with an unsuccessful shunt. Patients with functioning shunts manifested a decrease in TBK but not TBN. This resulted in a significant decrease in the TBK/TBN ratio. By a mean of 14 months, the 7 patients showed a significant increase in mean TBN associated with an improvement in the mean nitrogen index. The changes were associated with a significant increase in nonalcoholic calories, a nonsignificant increase in protein consumption, and a positive nitrogen balance. The authors interpreted such data as confirming the clinical observation that successful shunting is associated with a repletion of body protein.

Morbidity Associated with Peritoneovenous Shunting

Despite many encouraging reports of immediate and dramatic increases in renal blood flow, GFR, and renal salt and water excretion after shunt insertion, observations about morbidity are disturbing to an equal degree. Increasing experience with the LeVeen shunt has led to a growing awareness that its widespread use may be attended by a wide array of complications (Table 24.3).[16,26–63] Several recent reports involving over 300 patients have put the technique into perspective.[45–48] In patients with cirrhotic (nonmalignant) ascites, the operative mortality rate approaches 25%. Potential complications include fever, disseminated intravascular coagulation (DIC), shunt occlusion, hypokalemia, infection, and ascites leak. Among the less common but more challenging complications are variceal hemorrhage, bowel obstruction, pulmonary edema, air embolism, and pneumothorax. The incidence of shunt-related complications is formidable. Thus, Greig et al.[16] reported that 6 of 23 patients died within the fist month after surgery, for an operative mortality rate of 26%, with morbid events occurring in over two-thirds of patients with shunts. Fry et al.[26] surveyed the experience with peritoneal shunting of a number of surgical centers in Canada. Among the 60 patients for whom data were provided, the operative mortality rate was 20% (within 30 days of shunting).

Bernhoft et al.[49] reviewed their experience in 35 patients with refractory ascites who underwent 51 shunt placements over a 4-year period and reported a high rate of both operative (57%) and late (34%) complications.

Smadja and Franco reported their experience with PV shunting in 140 patients with intractable ascites.[48] The operative mortality rate was lower than in other large series. They attributed the lower rate to the external drainage of ascites at operation. Of note, despite such modifications, the authors encountered a high rate of recurrences by thrombosis at the tip of the venous catheter (24 patients). In another 10 patients the valve was obstructed by fiber and deposits.

TABLE 24.3.   Complications Associated with Peritoneovenous Shunting for Ascites

Technical problems	Coagulopathy
Occlusion of the venous limb	Asymptomatic
Neck hematoma	Disseminated intravascular coagulation
Migration of venous limb out of vein	Cardiorespiratory complications
Ascites leak	Elevation of central venous pressure
Bowel obstruction	Pulmonary edema
Air embolism	Renal complications
Pneumothorax	Hypokalemia
Trauma to recurrent laryngeal nerve	Hepatic complications
	Variceal hemorrhage
Infection	Hepatic failure
Peritonitis	General problems
Septicemia	"Allergic fever" associated with ascites auto infusion
Urinary tract infection	

Recently Hillaire et al.[50] investigated the possibility that a modified LeVeen shunt could obviate many of these problems. Based on an earlier suggestion by Franco,[51] they proposed that the addition of a nonthrombogenic titanium tip to the end of the venous catheter would obviate shunt patency problems due to catheter occlusion. The authors investigated the effects of elective insertion of the modified LeVeen shunt in 56 patients with cirrhosis and intractable ascites. Occlusion in the venous catheter was observed in only 2 patients during follow-up. This figure was much lower than that noted by the same group previously[48] and in most published series.[52,64] The cumulative rate of shunt blockage was 5.6% at 1 year and 12% at 2 years.

Coagulation Abnormalities

Consumption coagulopathy is probably the most worrisome complication encountered after shunt insertion.[27–33] Although precise figures are not available, it appears that this complication may occur in as many as one-third of patients with shunts. Tawes et al.[53] reviewed their experience in 24 patients and reported clinical coagulopathy in 37%. Affected patients bled profusely from wounds, intravenous lines, and venous puncture sites. Five other patients manifested laboratory evidence of early disseminated intravascular clotting. Ragni et al.[54] observed DIC in 10 of 11 patients after LeVeen shunt insertion.

An obstacle in ascertaining the frequency of DIC is the difficulty of establishing this diagnosis in patients with liver disease who have received the PV shunt.[28] Many, if not all, of the laboratory features of DIC are also encountered in other conditions that complicate the course of liver disease (Table 24.4).

The association of DIC with shunt insertion is not wholly unanticipated. A number of features unique to cirrhotic patients predispose them to the development of coagulopathy in general. As an example, Lerner et al.[31] reported that the cells in ascitic fluid (peritoneal macrophages and mesothelial cells) are thromboplastic. Furthermore, cirrhotic patients have low levels of a naturally occurring coagulation inhibitor, antithrombin III. Finally, ascitic fluid has been reported to exhibit procoagulant properties (an activator of factor X is present).[34]

Earlier attempts to manage refractory ascites with ultrafiltration and reinfusion of concentrated ascites (using the Rhodiascit apparatus) support these suggestions about coagulopathies. The infusion of ascites was attended by frequent and significant changes in the coagulation status of the patients.[7,8]

The precise pathophysiology of the coagulopathy is unknown, although triggering of the coagulation mechanism has been ascribed variously to activated tissue thromboplastin, activated clotting factors,[32,34] bacterial endotoxin,[30,35] and/or activator.[55] Other contributing factors include the severity of liver disease, a low plasma antithrombin III level, and decreased capacity of the reticuloendothelial system to clear activated clotting factors.[35] The coagulopathies that attend shunting vary widely from life-threatening DIC to asymptomatic changes in laboratory tests of clotting.

Although procoagulants, particularly thromboplastin, are considered major mediators of this complication,[31] the failure of other studies to detect such substances in ascitic fluid[32,56] suggests that alternative factors may be involved. Ascitic fluid contains a platelet aggregating factor identified as collagen.[56] By activating both platelets and

TABLE 24.4. Differential Diagnosis of Coagulopathy Following LeVeen Shunt

Condition	Platelet Count	Prothrombin Time	Fibrinogen Concentration	Fibrin Degradation Products
Massive transfusion	Decreased	Normal or increased	Normal	None*
Primary fibrinolysis	Normal	Increased	Normal or decreased	Increased
Disseminated intravascular coagulation	Decreased	Increased	Decreased	Increased
Liver disease				
Without hypersplenism	Normal	Normal or increased	Normal or decreased	None or increased
With hypersplenism	Decreased	Normal or increased	Normal or decreased	None or increased
Coagulopathy following LeVeen shunt	Decreased	Increased	Decreased	Increased

* Usually < 10μg/ml.
From Lewis RT: Severe coagulopathy following insertion of the LeVeen shunt: A potentially fatal complication. Can J Surg 1979;22:361–363, with permission.

clotting factors, collagen may be etiologically significant in the pathogenesis of disseminated intravascular coagulation complicating peritoneovenous shunt. To examine this possibility, Salem et al.[56] infused collagen, partially purified from ascitic fluid, into rabbits. All animals developed changes in hemostatic profile consistent with intravascular coagulation. Aspirin therapy for 5 days before the collagen infusion prevented these changes.

In addition to animal studies, clinical studies were undertaken. Seven patients undergoing a total of 8 peritoneovenous shunts for intractable ascites received antiplatelet therapy (aspirin and dipyridamole) in the immediate pre- and postoperative periods. After 6 shunts no thrombocytopenia or prolongation of clotting times developed to suggest decompensated consumptive coagulopathy. The authors interpreted their results as supporting the hypothesis that ascitic fluid collagen is important in the pathogenesis of shunt-associated disseminated intravascular coagulation. They suggest that antiplatelet drugs may be of value in preventing this complication.

The proper management of postoperative coagulopathy has not been established. The clinical threat may be minimized by complete ascites evacuation at operation with postoperative infusions of fresh-frozen plasma and platelet concentrates to keep the prolongation of prothrombin time less than 6 seconds and the platelet count higher than 50,000 per cubic millimeter. Fulenwider et al.[57] reported that adherence to this protocol appears to decrease drastically the incidence of postoperative hemorrhagic complications secondary to consumptive coagulopathy.

Biagini et al.[58] undertook a study to evaluate the efficacy of replacement of the ascitic fluid by normal saline as a means of ameliorating the prevalence and severity of postoperative DIC. Patients were divided into two groups: group I consisted of patients without replacement of ascites, and group II consisted of 10 patients in whom insertion of a LeVeen shunt was preceded by replacement of all ascitic fluid with normal saline. All patients in group I had laboratory evidence of coagulopathy; 4 had clinical signs of coagulopathy; and 2 died. In group II laboratory signs of consumptive coagulopathy were less marked, and no patient developed clinical bleeding.

Despite the widespread acceptance of evacuating ascites preoperatively to prevent DIC, occasional reports raise disturbing questions about the efficacy of this approach. Thus, Ragni et al.[54] reported that when they compared fibrin split product (FSP) titers of intraoperative ascitic fluid samples with those of plasma, they found no correlation between the ascitic and plasma FSP levels. They interpreted this lack of correlation as suggesting that systemic FSPs are not acquired passively from the ascitic fluid. Perhaps the widespread practice of replacing discarded ascitic fluid with saline during operation, before opening the shunt, does not prevent the postoperative coagulopathy. Furthermore, the investigators reported the development of postoperative DIC in a patient who underwent saline replacement at surgery. Additional therapeutic suggestions for managing the coagulopathy include administration of aminocaproic acid[59] and antithrombin III. The reader is referred to the review by LeVeen et al.[59] for a comprehensive discussion of this subject.

Sepsis

Infection constitutes a major problem in the experience of most surgeons. The immunocompromised state of cirrhosis and protein-calorie malnutrition predispose the patient to septic complications after implantation of foreign material. The critical status of these patients is reflected by reports of operative mortality rates generally in the range of 10–20%, with early morbidity in many series approaching 50%. Greig et al.[16] and Wexler[36] report an infectious complication rate of over 25%. When it occurs, septicemia is often devastating, as illustrated by the experience of Wexler, who observed two cases of staphylococcal peritonitis resistant to all antibiotics, numerous cases of septicemia, bacterial endocarditis, and a case of candidal septicemia in which *Candida* sp. was cultured only in the ascitic fluid and was not present before shunting.

Wormser and Hubbard[37] reported the important observation that *Staphylococcus aureus*, a rare cause of spontaneous peritonitis, was the etiologic organism in one-half of their cirrhotic patients who developed peritonitis after insertion of a PV shunt. All 6 patients had concomitant bacteremia that appeared to be attributable to the direct peritoneovenous connection. Appropriate systemic antimicrobial therapy without shunt removal failed to eradicate the infection, regardless of the state of the patency of the shunt or absence of inflammation at the sites of insertion. The authors recommend that the treatment for suspected peritonitis in patients with shunts should include, in addition to an aminoglycoside, an agent active against staphylococci. Initiation of parenteral antibiotic therapy should be followed by removal of the shunt if the diagnosis is confirmed.

Small Bowel Obstruction

Another complication is a unique type of small bowel obstruction. In a series of 60 patients with PV shunts for cirrhotic ascites at Hines Veterans Administration Hospital, Greenlee et al.[38] encountered small bowel obstruction in 7 patients. In each case, the small bowel was compressed and kinked inside multiple "cocoons" and cysts consequent to marked peritoneal fibrosis. In no patient was the shunt cannula ensnared in the fibrosed area; it remained free. The etiology is unknown.

Although predisposing factors are not fully elucidated, the emerging consensus is that patients with associated acute liver disease with jaundice and encephalopathic patients are at highest risk for complications such as symptomatic DIC and sepsis.

Additional Adverse Effects

In addition to the more common complications, bizarre and problematic complications such as pulmonary embolizations of ascitic fluid containing cholesterol crystals have been reported.[39–44,60–62]

Differences in Frequency of Complications with Different Shunts

In light of the formidable incidence of complications with the LeVeen shunt, investigators have questioned whether adverse effects are less common with the Denver shunt. Lund and Moritz[63] reviewed their experience with Denver PV shunting in 49 consecutive patients and suggested that the Denver shunt may be associated with a lower failure rate and a lower incidence of complications than the LeVeen shunt. Unfortunately, no rigorous studies examine this important question, which remains unresolved.

Differences in Morbidity of Peritoneovenous Shunting for Cirrhotic vs. Malignant Ascites

It appears that the complication rate of PV shunting is less with malignant ascites than with cirrhotic ascites. As an example, Kostroff et al.[46] carried out a retrospective study of 55 patients who underwent PV shunting for the management of ascites, 24 with cirrhosis and 31 with disseminated malignancies. The investigators noted that the cirrhotic patients had a complication rate of 84% compared with only 32% in the patients with cancer.

PERITONEOVENOUS SHUNT IN CLINICAL PRACTICE

Management of Ascites

PV shunting has been demonstrated to be a highly efficacious means of rapid relief of massive ascites. Nevertheless, the role of PV shunt in altering the natural history of refractory ascites is unclear. The difficulty of assessing the efficacy of PV shunting in managing the patient with refractory ascites is underscored by a report from Grischkan et al.[66] The investigators attempted to correlate the long-term (mean of 26 months) clinical response with shunt patency. Of the 6 responders (marked clinical loss of fluid after shunting), 3 had patent shunts and 3 had occluded shunts. Despite nonfunctioning shunts, the 3 patients with occlusion were able to maintain an average weight loss of 15.8 kg. Because the reliability of the radionuclide method used by the authors for assessing shunt patency has not been clearly defined, some observers have questioned their conclusions. Additional studies are clearly indicated.

The dilemma of rationally managing ascites has not yet been resolved.[67–69] Despite widespread usage of the PV shunt, few *specific* data about either its efficacy or its appropriate use in the treatment of ascites are currently available. As I noted in an earlier editorial,[69] once again we seem to have erred. We are quick enough to develop and apply new techniques but in no hurry to evaluate them rigorously.

Although it is clear that PV shunting has a role in the management of patients with tense ascites refractory to an optimal medical regimen, its use in the management of ascites otherwise amenable to medical therapy is open to question. Unfortunately, many patients with nonrefractory ascites undergo PV shunting because of an increasing tendency to liberalize the indications for its use.

Another factor that should be weighed in any decision about the suitability of shunting is the question of patient compliance. The patient's cooperation and compliance are requisite for successful functioning of the PV shunt. Patients with intractable ascites due to noncompliance are unlikely to benefit from PV shunting; rather, they are very likely to have recurrent "intractable" ascites aggravated by the superimposed complications of an intraperitoneal and intravenous foreign body. Furthermore, a functioning PV shunt does not constitute a "cure." For most patients, diuretics and dietary sodium restriction remain requisite parts of the therapeutic regimen. Respiratory exercises initiated in the postoperative period may have to be continued for an indefinite period, even after the patient's abdominal muscles regain their tone. An abdominal binder may be necessary for a prolonged period. Failure to comply with any of these facets of the regimen

may obviate completely the benefits of PV shunting with a recurrence of ascites.

In light of the significant morbidity and mortality associated with PV shunting,[68,69] it may be possible to do as well or even better with less expensive, conservative medical management. Such questions must be answered by carefully designed, randomized, prospective studies.

Wapnick et al.[70] assessed prospectively the benefits of the PV shunt. Although they suggest that PV shunting is superior to conventional therapy in the management of ascites,[70] their study leaves enough unanswered questions to preclude acceptance of their conclusions.[71] The intent was laudable, but the study fails to show whether PV shunting constitutes a safer and more efficacious treatment of ascites than more conventional therapy.

A randomized, multicenter trial of the LeVeen shunt vs. conventional medical therapy was carried out in France.[72] Of 57 patients with alcoholic cirrhosis and refractory ascites, 29 received a LeVeen shunt and 28 were treated by conventional medical therapy. Although the LeVeen shunt effectively mobilized ascites by the end of the first month, comparison of the two groups at the end of 1 year failed to show an advantage to the LeVeen shunt. Of the 29 patients in the surgical group, 25 (86%) developed one or more complications compared with 8 of 28 patients in the medical group (29%). The mortality rate at the end of the first month was higher in the surgical than in the medical group (41% vs. 18%, respectively). By the end of 1 year, the mortality rate of the two groups was almost identical: 23 (79%) and 21 (75%), respectively.[72] In light of the numerous complications in the group receiving the LeVeen shunt and the lack of increased survival after 1 year, the authors concluded that it was inadvisable to treat refractory ascites with LeVeen shunt implantation.

A randomized prospective study comparing PV shunt with medical treatment in 299 patients with cirrhosis and refractory or recurrent ascites suggested that the shunt may be more effective in the management of ascites.[52]

In the meanwhile, what should the approach be? In my opinion, given the constraints mentioned above, the PV shunt should be used less frequently and with greater forethought than is the case today.

Table 24.5 lists tentative indications for PV shunting in patients with ascites. Table 24.6 presents a tentative list of conditions that tend to militate against its use. The PV shunt should be

TABLE 24.5. Indications for Peritoneovenous Shunting in Portal Hypertension

Indication	Definition
Definite	
Completely refractory ascites	Refractory to maximal doses of diuretics
Relatively refractory ascites	Responds to maximal doses but only with development of complications
Possible	
Resistance to compliance	Massive ascites, responds in hospital but repeatedly relapses at home
Hepatorenal syndrome	Not resulting from intravascular depletion triggered by aggressive diuretic therapy

Modified from L. Blendis, with permission.

reserved for ascitic patients whose conditions remain truly refractory after an adequate trial of moderate doses of diuretics and dietary sodium restriction.

Such patients with refractory ascites may be less common than we have been led to believe. Greenlee et al.[18] reported their extensive experience in the management of ascites over a 40-month period and observed that only 4.5% of cirrhotic patients with ascites failed to respond to intensive medical therapy (diuretics and dietary sodium restriction) with a decrease in ascites.

PV shunting is indicated more commonly in patients who respond to optimal diuretic regimens in the hospital but rapidly reaccumulate ascites after discharge. After this cycle has been repeated several times, both physician and patient may think that an alternative therapy should be tried. Because of the associated risks, however, PV shunting should be carefully weighed before it is undertaken.

Management of Hepatorenal Syndrome

Although LeVeen and associates initially advocated the use of the LeVeen shunt in the management of refractory ascites,[10] the broadening indications for its use have encompassed "reversal" of the hepatorenal syndrome. Indeed, PV shunting has been advocated as established therapy for the hepatorenal syndrome.[14,15,68] The demonstration that shunt insertion may be associated with a dramatic increase in glomerular filtration rate has provided a rationale for considering such an approach.

Despite the exorbitant claims made for use of the PV shunt in this setting, a review of the available literature discloses few reports of reversal of *well-documented* hepatorenal syndrome. Grosberg and Wapnick[74] reported the results of a retrospective analysis of cirrhotic patients with azotemia treated with the shunt compared with similar patients treated medically. A review of the report raises questions about the true diagnoses of their patients. Although the mean creatinine of the PV shunt group was 4.3 ± 2.8 mg/dl and the average urinary sodium concentration was 10 mEq/L, the authors failed to exclude volume contraction as a cause of the azotemia and oliguria. Although the authors state that they excluded patients who developed azotemia as a result of diuretic treatment, bleeding, diarrhea, and vomiting, experience clearly dictates that relying solely on such florid evidence is insufficient to

TABLE 24.6. Contraindications for Peritoneovenous Shunting in Portal Hypertension

Contraindication	Definition
Definite	
Decompensated liver disease	Serum bilirubin 4 mg/dl (68 μmol/L); prothrombin time prolonged > 4 sec and hepatic encephalopathy
Underlying coagulopathy	Prothrombin time increased, platelets and fibrinogen decreased, fibrinogen degradation products increased
Infected ascites	Positive cultures
Loculated ascites	Previous abdominal surgery and demonstration of loculation using radionuclide peritoneogram
Relative	
Variceal bleeding	Documented bleeding in the absence of another cause
Large pleural effusion	No underlying pleuropulmonary pathology; fluid characteristics identical to ascites
Myocardial dysfunction	History, physical examination, electrocardiogram, 2-dimensional echocardiography, etc.

Modified from L. Blendis, with permission.

exclude volume contraction as a cause of the azotemia. As noted in chapter 3, the diagnosis of hepatorenal syndrome can be entertained only when attempts at volume repletion fail to reverse the azotemia. In summary, although the authors demonstrated a reversal of azotemia in their patients, the improvement may represent merely an anticipated effect in volume-contracted cirrhotic patients without hepatorenal syndrome.

Fullen observed reversal of the "hepatorenal syndrome" after insertion of the PV shunt in two patients.[75] As in the report by Grosberg and Wapnick, the difficulties reside in the diagnosis of the hepatorenal syndrome. Although both patients were azotemic and oliguric, both signs may be attributable to conditions other than the hepatorenal syndrome. Patient 1 developed relatively modest azotemia (blood urea nitrogen of 41 mg/dl and serum creatinine of 2.5 mg/dl) after long-term and vigorous diuretic therapy. Patient 2 had a stormy course that required numerous interventions, including an end-to-side portacaval shunt. He was noted to be oliguric, but clinically important azotemia was not documented. Success of the shunt was gauged solely by a marked diuresis and mobilization of ascitic fluid after shunting.

Schwartz and Vogel[76] reported the results of inserting a LeVeen shunt in 5 patients with the presumptive diagnosis of hepatorenal syndrome. Four of the 5 patients responded with a diuresis, natriuresis, and a decrease in serum creatinine from a preoperative mean of 4.0 ± 0.8 to a mean of 1.8 ± 0.4 mg/dl 1 week after surgery. Although the probable diagnosis was hepatorenal syndrome (all patients had oliguria, azotemia, and low urinary sodium concentrations), no attempts were made to assess the response to volume repletion. Thus, uncertainty persists as to whether the azotemia was attributable to marked volume contraction rather than to hepatorenal syndrome.

Pladson and Parrish[77] also reported successful reversal of renal failure in a patient whose clinical constellation supported the diagnosis of hepatorenal syndrome. The patient developed progressive oliguric renal failure that was unresponsive to volume repletion with massive infusions of fresh frozen plasma. At the time of shunt insertion, the patient's blood urea nitrogen was 144 mg/dl and his creatinine was 6.4 mg/dl. After insertion of the shunt, the decline in both values was dramatic (blood urea nitrogen, 16 mg/dl; creatinine, 1.0 mg/dl).

The study of Schroeder et al.[78] is an example of careful investigation of this important topic. The authors assessed the effects of PV shunting on renal function in 5 patients with the hepatorenal syndrome. In contrast to most other researchers, they were careful to ensure that the diagnosis was based on appropriate criteria (see chapter 3). All patients showed appropriate changes in urinary sodium concentration and osmolality. Furthermore, the renal failure was unresponsive to plasma volume expansion with intravenous saline (2–6 L) and albumin (50–200 gm) administered over 24–36 hours. Although renal function improved in all patients, the authors were careful to conclude that "the efficacy of these procedures in prolonging the survival of patients with the hepatorenal syndrome remains to be proven by controlled prospective study."[78]

Linas et al.[79] recently carried out a prospective study comparing the PV shunt (n = 10) with medical therapy in 20 patients with well-documented hepatorenal syndrome associated with alcoholic liver disease. The insertion of a PV shunt resulted in an increase in pulmonary capillary wedge pressure and in cardiac index with a concomitant decrease in serum creatinine (from 3.6 ± 0.4 to 3.0 ± 0.5; $p < 0.05$). Despite improvement in renal function, survival was prolonged significantly (210 days) in only 1 patient. In the remainder, survival was 13.8 ± 2.2 days compared with 4.1 ± 0.6 days with medical therapy. The investigators concluded that whereas the PV shunt often stabilizes renal function, it does not prolong life in patients with hepatorenal syndrome.

In addressing the discrepancy between the marginal improvement in life expectancy and the beneficial effect on systemic hemodynamics and renal function, the authors marshalled evidence that the results were related to the progressive nature of the severe liver disease rather than to problems of study design. They concluded, "Insertion of a PV shunt should not be utilized as a standard therapy for the treatment of patients with the HRS [hepatorenal syndrome]."[79]

In a preliminary report, Daskalopoulos et al.[80] summarized the results of a randomized trial of PV shunting in patients with hepatorenal syndrome. Twenty-eight patients with alcoholic liver disease and serum creatinine greater than 5 mg/dl were randomized to either PV shunting (13 patients) or medical management (15 patients). The patients were followed until death or discharge from the hospital. Three of 11 shunted patients survived compared with 2 of 15 in the control group. Serum creatinine tended to decrease (from 5.6 ± 0.2 to 4.9 ± 1.4 mg/dl; $p > 0.3$) in the shunted group, but increased further (from 6.1 ± 2.7 to 8.9 ± 1.1 mg/dl; $p < 0.02$) in the control group. The authors concluded that although PV shunting appears to prevent further progression of renal functional impairment, it does not alter survival in patients with hepatorenal syndrome.

Aside from the question of success in reversing hepatorenal syndrome, one must consider whether morbidity and mortality are increased. Smith et al.[65] reported that mean duration of shunt function was significantly less in patients with hepatorenal syndrome (15 ± 5 days) compared with the patients with refractory ascites alone (45 ± 13 days) or patients with nonrefractory ascites (64 ± 34 days). Survival of patients with nonrefractory ascites (767 ± 214 days) was significantly longer ($p < 0.05$) than in patients with hepatorenal syndrome (28 ± 5 days) or in patients with refractory ascites alone (256 ± 148 days). In-hospital mortality was significantly greater ($p < 0.05$) in patients with hepatorenal syndrome (70%) than in patients with refractory ascites alone (14%) or in patients with nonrefractory ascites (0%).

We must conclude that a number of putative "successes" occurred in patients who were not clearly documented to have hepatorenal syndrome; rather, many patients probably had reversible azotemia secondary to a diminished effective blood volume. Furthermore, even when the diagnosis of hepatorenal syndrome was established by appropriate criteria, the results are not encouraging. Collectively, the results of the available randomized trials suggest that although PV shunting may prevent progression of renal functional impairment, it does not prolong patient survival. A few well-documented cases in which the PV shunt was successful in reversing the hepatorenal syndrome and prolonging survival do not justify the growing and uncritical trend to resort to this procedure in the treatment of virtually any cirrhotic patient with azotemia. The PV shunt cannot be viewed as established therapy until its value is determined by appropriate peer-reviewed clinical trials such as those carried out by Linas et al.[79]

SUMMARY

The initial enthusiasm for the PV shunt has been tempered by our long-term experience. Reports involving almost 500 patients have put the technique into perspective. In malignant ascites, the PV shunt provides effective palliative relief with few complications. In cirrhotic ascites, however, an operative mortality rate as high as 25% has been reported, due largely to septicemia, disseminated intravascular coagulation, cardiac failure, hepatic failure, and variceal hemorrhage. The PV shunt as a means of relieving ascites offers benefit to appropriately selected patients. It has serious complications, however, and should not be used indiscriminately. The frequency and severity of the risks are formidable, mandating that the procedure be reserved for patients whose major medical problems will be addressed by relief of ascites and in whom more conservative forms of therapy have been ineffective after an *adequate* trial. In contrast to its role in the management of ascites, the PV shunt cannot be viewed presently as established therapy for patients with the hepatorenal syndrome. Its use should be considered in selected patients with this syndrome. Because the PV shunt conveys only a marginal improvement in life expectancy in the setting of severe liver disease,[79] PV shunt insertion may be considered for patients who develop hepatorenal syndrome in the setting of mild jaundice or at a time when liver function is improving.

REFERENCES

1. Dawson AD: Historical notes on ascites. Gastroenterology 1960;39:790–791.
2. Crosby RC, Cooney EA: Surgical treatment of ascites. N Engl J Med 1946;235:581–585.
3. Neumann CG, Braunwald NS, Hinton JW: The absorption of ascitic fluid following the eversion of a segment of intestinal mucosa within the peritoneal cavity. Surg Forum 1955;6:374–376.
4. Mulvaney D: Vesico-coelomic drainage for relief of ascites. Lancet 1955;2:748–749.
5. Yamahiro HS, Reynolds TB: Effects of ascitic fluid infusion on sodium excretion, blood volume, and creatinine clearance in cirrhosis. Gastroenterology 1961;40:497–503.
6. Villeneuve JP, Thuot C, Marleau D, et al: Treatment of resistant ascites by continuous ultrafiltration-reinfusion of ascitic fluid. Can Med Assoc J 1977;117:1296–1298.
7. Levy VG, Opolon P, Pauleau N, Caroli J: Treatment of ascites by reinfusion of concentrated peritoneal fluid—review of 318 procedures in 210 patients. Postgrad Med J 1975;51:564–566.
8. Wilkinson SP, Davidson AR, Henderson J, Williams R: Ascites reinfusion using the Rhodiascit apparatus—clinical experience and coagulation abnormalities. Postgrad Med J 1975;51:583–587.

9. Moult PJA, Parbhoo SP, Sherlock S: Clinical experience with the Rhone-Poulenc ascites reinfusion apparatus. Postgrad Med J 1975;51:574–576.

9a. Leuret M: Le traitement chirurgical de l'ascite des cirrhotiques. Un cas de drainage du peritoine par la saphene. Societe des Chirurgiens de Paris 1911;3:380.

10. LeVeen H, Christoudias G, Moon JP, et al: Peritoneovenous shunting for ascites. Ann Surg 1974;180:580–591.

11. Minutes of the Gastroenterology and Urology Section of the General Medical Devices Panel, Food and Drug Administration. Washington, DC, October 26, 1979;68–69.

12. Lund RH, Newkirk JB: Peritoneo-venous shunting system for surgical management of ascites. Contemp Surg 1979;14:31–45.

13. Patino JF, Hakim S, Sanclemente E, et al: El uso del "shunt" peritoneo-venoso de Hakim en el tratamiento de la ascitis. Rev Argentina Cir 1979;37:304–313.

14. LeVeen HH, Brown T, D'Ovidio NG: Surgical treatment of ascites. Adv Surg 1980;14:107–149.

15. LeVeen HH, Wapnick S, Diaz C, et al: Ascites: Its correction by peritoneovenous shunting. Curr Probl Surg 1979;16:1–61(Feb).

16. Greig PD, Langer B, Blendis LM, et al: Complications after peritoneovenous shunting for ascites. Am J Surg 1980;139:125–131.

17. Greenlee HB, Stanley MM, Reinhardt GF: Intractable ascites treated with peritoneovenous shunts (LeVeen): A 24- to 64-month follow up of results in 52 alcoholic cirrhotics. Arch Surg 1981;116:518–526.

18. Fulenwider JT, Galambos JD, Smith RB III, et al: LeVeen vs Denver peritoneovenous shunts for intractable ascites of cirrhosis. Arch Surg 1986;121:351–355.

18a. LeVeen HH, Vujic I, d'Ovidio NG, Hutto RB: Peritoneovenous shunt occlusion: Etiology, diagnosis, therapy. Ann Surg 1984;200:212–223.

19. Stanley MM: Treatment of intractable ascites in patients with alcoholic cirrhosis by peritoneovenous shunting (LeVeen). Med Clin North Am 1979;63:523–535.

20. Blendis LM, Greig PD, Langer B, et al: The renal and hemodynamic effects of the peritoneovenous shunt for intractable hepatic ascites. Gastroenterology 1979;77:250–257.

21. Greig PD, Blendis LM, Langer B, et al: Renal and hemodynamic effects of the peritoneovenous shunt. II. Long-term effects. Gastroenterology 1981;80:119–125.

22. Reinhardt GF, Stanley MM: Peritoneovenous shunting for ascites. Surg Gynecol Obstet 1977;145:419–424.

23. Berkowitz HD, Mullen JL, Miller LD, Rosato EF: Improved renal function and inhibition of renin and aldosterone secretion following peritoneovenous (LeVeen) shunt. Surgery 1978;84:120–126.

24. Witte MH, Witte CL, Jacobs S, Kut R: Peritoneovenous (LeVeen) shunt. Control of renin aldosterone system in cirrhotic ascites. JAMA 1978;239:31–33.

24a. Campbell PJ, Skorecki KL, Logan AG, et al: Acute effects of peritoneovenous shunting on plasma atrial natriuretic peptide in cirrhotic patients with massive refractory ascites. Am J Med 1988;84:112–119.

24b. Tobe SW, Morali GA, Greig PD, et al: Peritoneovenous shunting restores atrial natriuretic factor responsiveness in refractory hepatic ascites. Gastroenterology 1993;105:202–207.

25. Blendis LM, Harrison JE, Russell DM, et al: Effects of peritoneovenous shunting on body composition. Gastroenterology 1986;90:127–134.

26. Fry PD, Hallgren R, Robertson ME: Current status of the peritoneovenous shunt for the management of intractable ascites. Can J Surg 1979;22:557–559.

27. Ansley JD, Bethel RA, Bowen PA II, Warren WD: Effect of peritoneovenous shunting with the LeVeen valve on ascites, renal function and coagulation in six patients with intractable ascites. Surgery 1978;83:181–187.

28. Lewis RT: Severe coagulopathy following insertion of the LeVeen shunt: A potentially fatal complication. Can J Surg 1979;22:361–363.

29. Mateske JW, Beart RW Jr, Bartholomew LC, Baldus WP: Fatal disseminated intravascular coagulation after peritoneovenous shunt for intractable ascites. Mayo Clin Proc 1978;53:526–528.

30. Harmon DC, Demirjian Z, Ellman L, Fischer JE: Disseminated intravascular coagulation with the peritoneovenous shunt. Ann Intern Med 1979;90:774–776.

31. Lerner RG, Nelson JC, Corines P, del Guercio LRM: Disseminated intravascular coagulation. Complication of LeVeen peritoneovenous shunts. JAMA 1978;240:2064–2066.

32. Giles AR, Saunders D, Seaton TL, et al: Changes in the coagulation status of patients undergoing autotransfusion of concentrated ascitic fluid as treatment in refractory ascites. Blood 1977;50(Suppl 1):267.

33. Schwartz ML, Swaim WR, Vogel SB: Coagulopathy following peritoneovenous shunting. Surgery 1979;85:671–676.

34. Phillips LL, Rodgers JB: Procoagulant properties of ascitic fluid in hepatic cirrhosis. Presented at the 7th International Congress on Thrombosis and Haemostasis, London, July 15–20, 1979. Abstract P6-110.

35. Puig JG, Anton FM, Gonzalez JM, Vazquez JO: Peritoneovenous shunt and bacterial endotoxin [letter]. Mayo Clin Proc 1979;54:133.

36. Wexler MJ: Discussion of Greig paper. Am J Surg 1980;139:128–129.

37. Wormser GP, Hubbard RC: Peritonitis in cirrhotic patients with LeVeen shunts. Am J Med 1981;71:358–362.

38. Greenlee HB, Stanley MM, Reinhardt GF, Chejfec G: Small bowel obstruction (SBO) from compression and kinking of intestine by thickened peritoneum in cirrhotics with ascites treated with LeVeen shunt [abstract]. Gastroenterology 1979;76:1282.

39. Dupas JL, Remond A, Vermynck JP, et al: Superior vena cava thrombosis as a complication of peritoneovenous shunt. Gastroenterology 1978;75:899–900.

40. Van Deventer GM, Snyder N III, Patterson M: The superior vena cava syndrome. A complication of the LeVeen shunt. JAMA 1979;242:1655–1656.

41. Eckhauser FE, Strodel WE, Knol JA, Turcotte JG: Superior vena caval obstruction associated with long-term peritoneovenous shunting. Ann Surg 1979;190:758–760.

42. O'Laughlin JC, Hoftiezer JW, Gerhardt DC: Saccular dilatations in the LeVeen shunt [letter]. Ann Intern Med 1979;91:928–929.

43. Maat B, Oosterlee J, Spaas JA, et al: Dissemination of tumor cells via LeVeen shunt [letter]. Lancet 1979;1:988.

44. Markey W, Payne JA, Straus A: Hemorrhage from esophageal varices after placement of the LeVeen shunt. Gastroenterology 1979;77:341–343.

45. Rubinstein D, McInnes I, Dudley FJ: Morbidity and mortality after peritoneo-venous shunt surgery for refractory ascites. Gut 1985;26:1070–1073.

46. Kostroff KM, Ross DW, Davis JM: Peritoneovenous shunting for cirrhotic versus malignant ascites. Surg Gynecol Obstet 1985;161:204–208.

47. Lossing A, Greig PD, Blendis L, et al: The LeVeen shunt: A nine-year experience [abstract]. Hepatology 1984;4:1092.

48. Smadja C, Franco D: The LeVeen shunt in the elective treatment of intractable ascites in cirrhosis. A prospective study on 140 patients. Ann Surg 1985;201:488–493.

49. Bernhoft RA, Pellegrini CA, Way LW: Peritoneovenous shunt for refractory ascites: Operative complications and long-term results. Arch Surg 1982;117:631–634.

50. Hillaire S, Labianca M, Borgonovo G, et al: Peritoneovenous shunting of intractable ascites in patients with cirrhosis: Improving results and predictive factors of failure. Surgery 1993;113:373–379.

51. Franco D, Labianca M, Smadja C, Fragosos J: A titanium catheter tip for peritoneovenous shunts. Artif Organ 1988;12:81–82.

52. Stanley MM, Ochi S, Lee KK, et al: Peritoneovenous shunting as compared with medical treatment in patients with alcoholic cirrhosis and massive ascites. N Engl J Med 1989;321:1632–1638.

53. Tawes RL Jr, Sydorak GR, Kennedy PA, et al: Coagulopathy associated with peritoneovenous shunting. Am J Surg 1981;142:51–54.

54. Ragni MV, Lewis JH, Spero JA: Ascites-induced LeVeen shunt coagulopathy. Ann Surg 1985;198:91–95.

55. Henderson JM, Stein SF, Kutner M: Analysis of twenty-three plasma proteins in ascites. Ann Surg 1980;192:738–742.

56. Salem HH, Dudley FJ, Merrett A, et al: Coagulopathy of peritoneovenous shunts: Studies on the pathogenic role of ascitic fluid MB, collagen and value of antiplatelet therapy. Gut 1983;24:412–417.

57. Fulenwider JT, Smith RB III, Reed SC, et al: Peritoneovenous shunts. Lessons learned from an eight-year experience with 70 patients. Arch Surg 1984;119:1133–1173.

58. Biagini JR, Belghiti J, Fekete F: Prevention of coagulopathy after placement of peritoneovenous shunt with replacement of ascitic fluid by normal saline solution. Surg Gynecol Obstet 1986;163:315–318.

59. LeVeen HH, Ip M, Ahmed N, et al: Coagulopathy post peritoneovenous shunt. Ann Surg 1987;205:305–311.

60. Gilas T, Langer B, Taylor BR, et al: Hematogenous infection of peritoneovenous shunts after dental procedures. Can J Surg 1982;25:215–216.

61. Fenster LF, Wheelis RF, Ryan JA Jr: Acute respiratory distress syndrome after peritoneovenous shunt. Am Rev Respir Dis 1982;125:244–245.

62. Pozen RG, Covert M, Rozanski JJ, et al: Peritoneovenous shunt-induced ventricular tachycardia. Crit Care Med 1982;10:65–66.

63. Lund RH, Mortiz MW: Complications of Denver peritoneovenous shunting. Arch Surg 1982; 117:924–928.

64. Gleysteen JJ, Klamer TW: Peritoneovenous shunts: Predictive factors of early treatment failure. Am J Gastroenterol 1984;79:654–658.

65. Smith RE, Nostrant TT, Eckhauser FE, et al: Patient selection and survival after peritoneovenous shunting for nonmalignant ascites. Am J Gastroenterol 1984;79:659–662.

66. Grischkan DM, Cooperman AM, Hermann RE, et al: Failure of LeVeen shunting in refractory ascites—a view from the other side. Surgery 1981;89:304–308.

67. Treatment of refractory ascites [editorial]. Lancet 1985; 2:1164–1165.

68. Epstein M: The peritoneovenous shunt in the management of ascites and the hepatorenal syndrome. Gastroenterology 1982;82:790–799.

69. Epstein M: The LeVeen shunt for ascites and hepatorenal syndrome. N Engl J Med 1980;302:628–630.

70. Wapnick S, Grosberg SJ, Evans MI: Randomized prospective matched pair study comparing peritoneovenous shunt and conventional therapy in massive ascites Br J Surg 1979;66:667–670.

71. Epstein M: Peritoneovenous shunting for ascites [letter to the editor]. N Engl J Med 1980;303:461–462.

72. Bories P, Garcia Compean D, Michel H, et al: The treatment of refractory ascites by the LeVeen shunt. A multicentre controlled trial (57 patients). J Hepatol 1986; 3:212–218.

73. A randomized comparison of the peritoneovenous shunt (LeVeen) and conventional medical treatment alone for ascites in patients with alcoholic cirrhosis. Veterans Administration Cooperative Study. Washington, DC, Veterans Administration, 1979.

74. Grosberg SJ, Wapnick S: A retrospective comparison of functional renal failure in cirrhosis treated by conventional therapy or the peritoneo-venous shunt (LeVeen). Am J Med Sci 1978;276:287–291.

75. Fullen WD: Hepatorenal syndrome: Reversal by peritoneovenous shunt. Surgery 1977;82:337–341.

76. Schwartz ML, Vogel SB: Treatment of hepatorenal syndrome. Am J Surg 1980;139:370–373.

77. Pladson TR, Parrish RM: Hepatorenal syndrome: Recovery after peritoneovenous shunt. Arch Intern Med 1977;137:1248–1249.

78. Schroeder ET, Anderson GH Jr, Smulyan H: Effects of a portacaval or peritoneovenous shunt on renin in the hepatorenal syndrome. Kidney Int 1979;15:54–61.

79. Linas SL, Schaffer JW, Moore EE, et al: Peritoneovenous shunt in the management of the hepatorenal syndrome. Kidney Int 1986;30:736–740.

80. Daskalopoulos G, Jordan DR, Reynolds TB: Randomized trial of peritoneovenous shunt (PVS) in the treatment of hepatorenal syndrome (HRS) [abstract]. Gastroenterology 1985;88:1655.

TRANSJUGULAR INTRAHEPATIC PORTOSYSTEMIC SHUNT IN THE TREATMENT OF REFRACTORY ASCITES AND HEPATORENAL SYNDROME

KENNETH A. SOMBERG, M.D.

Theoretical Basis
  Pathogenesis
  Historical Data
Historical Development and Technique
Early Experience with Variceal Hemorrhage
Physiologic Assessment in Refractory Ascites
Clinical Efficacy in Refractory Ascites
Hepatorenal Syndrome

Current Issues and Future Directions
  Mechanism of Response
  Systemic Hemodynamics
  Complications
  Technical Issues
  Appropriate Use
Summary

Refractory ascites and hepatorenal syndrome represent important and potentially devastating complications of cirrhosis. This chapter focuses primarily on the use of the transjugular intrahepatic portosystemic shunt (TIPS) in the treatment of refractory ascites. The role of TIPS in hepatorenal syndrome (HRS) is also discussed, although there is substantially less information regarding the use of TIPS in this setting.

For the purpose of this discussion, ascites is considered to be refractory to diuretic therapy when it remains tense despite maximal diuretic therapy (typically furosemide, ≥ 160mg/day, and spironolactone, ≥ 200 mg/day, or equivalent doses of an alternative potassium-sparing diuretic). In addition, ascites is considered to be refractory if the serum creatinine rises and limits diuretic therapy at lower dosages or if the patient develops complications, such as symptomatic hyponatremia, that preclude effective use of diuretic therapy.

Various options exist for the treatment of refractory ascites. However, all of the currently available techniques have significant limitations. For example, although therapeutic paracentesis has been shown to be safe and effective,[1,2] it is time-consuming for both patient and physician and leaves the patient with the discomfort of reaccumulated ascites between treatments. In addition, large-volume paracentesis may predispose patients to bacterial infections due to the loss of ascitic fluid opsonic activity.[3] Peritoneovenous shunting has also been demonstrated to be effective in relieving ascites but is associated with an approximately 40% rate of shunt occlusion at 1 year.[4] Extracorporeal ascites ultrafiltration and reinfusion require specialized equipment that is not widely available.[5,6] Furthermore, although liver transplantation cures refractory ascites, therapy is still needed for patients awaiting transplantation and patients who are not considered to be acceptable candidates for transplantation. Side-to-side portacaval anastomosis provides another alternative in the treatment of refractory ascites. Although effective in more than 90% of cases, perioperative mortality and postoperative encephalopathy have limited its clinical utility.[7,8]

The drawbacks of the above therapies have prompted investigation of TIPS as a possible alternative. This chapter reviews the theoretical basis for using a portosystemic shunt. Further discussion highlights the historical development of TIPS and the technique for creating this intrahepatic shunt. In addition, a body of experimental and empirical data supports the use of TIPS for the treatment of ascites. The number of studies directly addressing the use of TIPS for refractory ascites is relatively small. However, some exciting physiologic and clinical data are emerging. Finally, the potential utility of TIPS in the treatment of hepatorenal syndrome is discussed.

THEORETICAL BASIS

Pathogenesis

Chapter 1 reviewed comprehensively the varying theories of ascites formation. Traditionally, it has been proposed that a contraction of the effective blood volume constitutes a pivotal event in cirrhotic patients who accumulate ascites.[9] This traditional underfill formulation suggests that the renal retention of sodium is a secondary rather than primary event. A variant of the underfill theory is the peripheral vasodilatation theory. The principal distinguishing feature of this theory is that the decrease in effective blood volume is attributable primarily to an early increase in vascular capacitance.[10] Thus, peripheral vasodilatation is the initial determinant of intravascular underfilling, and an imbalance between the expanded capacitance and available volume constitutes a diminished effective volume.

An alternative hypothesis to the two underfill theories is the overflow theory of ascites formation,[11] which postulates that the initial primary event is the inappropriate retention of excessive amounts of sodium by the kidneys, unrelated to defense of the plasma volume (and thought to be due to intrahepatic hypertension).

Although the pathophysiology of ascites formation is not fully defined, certain concepts (see chapter 1) provide a basis for designing therapy. The relief of sinusoidal hypertension may lead to decreased spillage of lymph, both hepatic and intestinal in origin, and interrupt a hepatorenal reflex arc responsible for renal sodium retention[12] In addition, a procedure that improves the effective arterial volume by redistributing splanchnic blood into the central circulation has the potential to normalize the neurohumoral response that promotes salt and fluid retention. A side-to-side portosystemic shunt potentially meets both of these hemodynamic objectives.

Historical Data

Surgical side-to-side portacaval shunts have been used in the past to treat refractory ascites. In 1968 Burchell and colleagues noted resolution of intractable ascites in 89% of 63 patients treated with a side-to-side portacaval shunt.[7] Of the 7 patients who did not have successful relief of ascites, two had technical complications with occlusion of the shunts. Five others were described as having cardiac, hepatic, and renal failure. The authors believed that the complication rate was too high to justify this procedure. The perioperative mortality was 12%, one-third of the patients developed encephalopathy, and approximately one-third had congestive heart failure at some time during the postoperative course.

The procedure was reevaluated by Franco et al. in a more recent study that noted resolution of ascites in 98% of 54 patients.[8] One patient failed to improve because of congestive heart failure. Perioperative mortality was reasonably low at 5%. However, the incidence of encephalopathy was noted to be 50%. Based on these and other studies, it is reasonable to conclude that a side-to-side portacaval shunt can be highly effective in relieving ascites. However, when performed surgically, portosystemic shunting leads to unacceptable morbidity and mortality rates, which preclude its use as a routine treatment of refractory ascites.

The transjugular intrahepatic portosystemic shunt was developed as a means of providing portal decompression while obviating the need for surgery. TIPS has several attractive features, including the fact that it can be placed under local anesthesia. TIPS also avoids postoperative morbidity associated with a surgical procedure, such as wound infection and ascites leaks. In addition, TIPS does not alter the extrahepatic vascular anatomy, which is important in potential candidates for liver transplantation.

HISTORICAL DEVELOPMENT AND TECHNIQUE

The development of TIPS represents an important advance in the treatment of complications of portal hypertension. The idea of creating a portosystemic shunt within the liver is not new; however, the technology to make such a technique clinically applicable has been available only in recent years. A percutaneous method of creating a portosystemic shunt was first developed by Rosch and Hanafee in 1969.[13] They introduced a long needle into the jugular vein, advanced it into the hepatic vein, and then passed it through the hepatic parenchyma into an intrahepatic branch of the portal vein. The resulting transparenchymal tract was then dilated to create a functional portosystemic shunt. The procedure was successful in dogs; however, all of the shunts thrombosed within a few days.

In 1986 Palmaz et al. described the first experimental use of a balloon-expandable metallic stent to perform TIPS.[14] They found that in dogs with induced portal hypertension, shunts remained patent up to 48 weeks. Richter first applied this technique to humans in 1990 using an implantable metallic stent.[15] Palmaz stents (Johnson & Johnson Interventional Systems, Warren, NJ) were used to line the intrahepatic channel, and excellent portal decompression was achieved in all cases. Subsequent larger series by Richter et al.,[16] who reported their experience in 9 patients, and by Zemel et al.,[17] who reported their experience in 8 patients, established the feasibility of this technique as a reliable means of portal decompression. However, the procedure times were quite long, in some cases requiring 8–12 hours. Procedural modifications introduced by Ring, et al., such as use of the more flexible Wallstent (Schneider USA, Minneapolis), led to significant reductions in procedure time, thereby making TIPS a practical therapeutic option.[18]

Subsequently clinical trials of TIPS were begun at numerous institutions. Different types of stents and different techniques are used around the world; what follows is a brief description of how TIPS is performed at the University of California, San Francisco (UCSF). The TIPS technique is illustrated in Figure 25.1, and a representative case is shown in Figure 25.2. Under conscious sedation, the right internal jugular vein is percutaneously punctured, and a 9-French sheath is advanced into the inferior vena cava, where a pressure measurement is obtained. The sheath is then selectively advanced into an hepatic vein and a transjugular needle is positioned through the sheath and advanced caudally and anteriorly 4–5 cm into the liver parenchyma. A syringe is attached and aspirated as the needle is slowly withdrawn. When blood fills the syringe, contrast medium is injected to determine the vascular structure entered. When a branch of the portal venous system is filled, a guidewire is introduced and manipulated into the main portal vein. The needle is removed, and a catheter is advanced over the guidewire. The initial portal pressure is recorded, and a portal venogram is performed. The

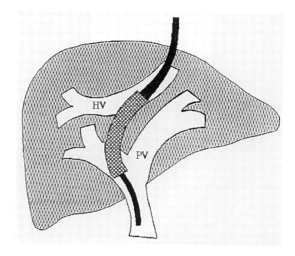

FIGURE 25.1. Schematic representation of a Wallstent forming an intrahepatic shunt between the right hepatic vein and the right portal vein. (Courtesy of JM LaBerge, MD.)

catheter is then exchanged for an 8-mm angioplasty balloon, and the tract between the hepatic and portal veins is dilated. An expandable metallic Wallstent is then deployed across the tract, with care to avoid extension of the stent into the extrahepatic portal vein or inferior vena cava, which might compromise subsequent transplant surgery.

In the treatment of variceal hemorrhage, portal decompression is judged adequate if the portal vein-to-inferior vena cava pressure gradient falls to ≤ 15 mmHg and varices can no longer be demonstrated by hand-injection splenic venography. If the gradient remains elevated or variceal flow persists, the stent is expanded to 10 mm in diameter; if necessary, a second parallel shunt is placed and the varices are embolized with coils or alcohol. The principal endpoint is the absence of variceal flow. In the treatment of refractory ascites, no specific desired portosystemic gradient has been established; typically a single 8-mm stent is placed. After insertion of TIPS, patients are transferred to the intensive care unit for monitoring for 12–24 hours. A Doppler ultrasound examination is performed on the day following TIPS insertion to assess the patency of the shunt.

EARLY EXPERIENCE WITH VARICEAL HEMORRHAGE

It has been demonstrated that varices do not bleed when the portosystemic gradient is < 12 mmHg.[19] However, it is not always possible to

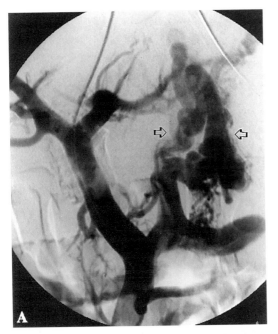

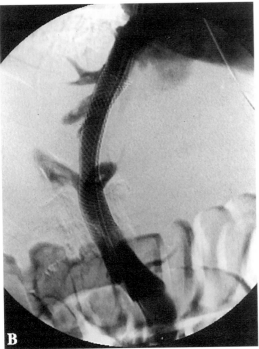

FIGURE 25.2. Total portal diversion after TIPS. *A,* Portal venogram before TIPS demonstrates filling of large esophageal varices (arrows). *B,* After completion of an 8-mm TIPS, flow to varices is eliminated. Intrahepatic portal vein flow is now reversed; the direction of intrahepatic portal flow is now toward the TIPS. (From LaBerge JM, Ring EJ, Lake JR, et al: Transjugular intrahepatic shunts: preliminary results in 25 patients. J Vasc Surg 1992; 16:258–267, with permission.)

achieve this degree of portal decompression with the relatively small stents used in the TIPS procedure. Therefore, most studies have aimed for a fall in the portosystemic pressure gradient to 12–15 mmHg with decreased or absent variceal flow. Four large series of TIPS, predominantly for variceal hemorrhage, have documented that TIPS is an effective means of portal decompression.[20–23] Initial success, defined as creation of an intrahepatic shunt with satisfactory portal pressure reduction, was achieved in 93–96% of cases. Success was associated with cessation of active variceal hemorrhage in 96–100%. Of interest, the reduction in the portal vein-to-vena cava pressure gradient represented a combination of a fall in the portal pressure and a rise in the vena cava pressure. For example, in the report of Rössle et al. the mean inferior vena cava pressure was 6.1 ± 3.6 mmHg before TIPS and 10.7 ± 3.7 mmHg after TIPS insertion.[20] This increase in central venous pressure represented 37% of the decrease in the portosystemic pressure gradient. In addition, Rössle's group estimated portal vein and shunt flow by multiplying mean blood flow velocity by the cross-sectional area of the blood vessel. The investigators observed that mean portal blood flow increased from 800 ± 500 ml/min before TIPS to 1900 ± 800 ml/min after TIPS. Of significance, they estimated TIPS flow at 2200 ± 700 ml/min. The finding of higher flow in the shunt relative to the portal vein suggests that some arterialized sinusoidal flow was diverted through the TIPS. This finding is consistent with the impression that TIPS functions as a side-to-side shunt. Such results suggest that TIPS is able to achieve the hemodynamic goals of a potential treatment for refractory ascites, i.e., improvement in effective blood volume and reduction of portal hypertension.

The initial experience with TIPS for variceal hemorrhage also suggested that it would be effective in the treatment of ascites. LaBerge et al. reported a series of 100 patients at UCSF in whom TIPS was successfully placed in 96.[21] The indication for TIPS was variceal hemorrhage in 92 of the 96 patients, 74 of whom were noted to have ascites before TIPS. Among the 59 patients who were alive without transplantation for longer than 2 weeks after TIPS, 83% showed improvement in ascites control. In the series reported by Rössle and colleagues in Freiburg, TIPS was established successfully in 93 of 100 patients.[20] Fifty-three patients had ascites before TIPS, and improvement

TABLE 25.1. Renal and Humoral Changes Following TIPS[a]

	UCSF n = 5[b]	Pamplona n = 16	Toronto n = 7	Freiberg n = 15
Days post-TIPS	14	30	30	7
Urinary sodium (mEq/24h)[c]	↑ 530%	↑ 239%	↑ 150%	↑ 290%
Urine volume (ml/24h)	↑ 88%[d]	ND[e]	ND	ND
Glomerular filtration rate (ml/min)	↑ 33%[d]	↑ 25%[c]	↓ 8%[d]	↑ 5%[d]
Aldosterone[c]	↓ 67%[f]	↓ 67%	↓ 65%	ND
Plasma renin activity[c]	↓ 90%[f]	↓ 57%	↓ 81%	ND

[a] Expressed as mean percentage differences comparing pre-TIPS and post-TIPS values.
[b] "n" represents the number of patients for whom these values were obtained, which may be fewer than the total number in the study.
[c] p value < 0.05 for each comparison of pre-TIPS and post-TIPS values.
[d] Comparison of pre-TIPS and post-TIPS values represents a trend, p > 0.05.
[e] Not done.
[f] Excludes one patient who developed liver failure after TIPS.

was noted in 89%. None of the patients continued to have severe ascites after the procedure, and only 17% of the patients with ascites required ongoing diuretic therapy. Assessment of ascites in patients with recent variceal hemorrhage, however, is complicated by the fact that the majority of such patients had substantial volume repletion before TIPS. Nevertheless, early results were encouraging.

PHYSIOLOGIC ASSESSMENT IN REFRACTORY ASCITES

Several groups of investigators have initiated studies to assess the physiologic and clinical changes associated with the use of TIPS for refractory ascites (Table 25.1). Although the studies have been small and the duration of follow-up limited, several interesting points have emerged.[24–27] Portosystemic gradient was reduced by a mean of 30–63% with TIPS. The studies in which plasma renin activity (PRA) was assessed in the absence of diuretics showed decreases of 90% and 81% when measured 14–30 days after TIPS.[24,26] One study measured PRA on diuretic therapy and noted a mean fall of 57% one month after TIPS.[25] The plasma aldosterone concentration fell in a similar manner after TIPS, with a mean reduction of two-thirds of the pre-TIPS values. Four of the initial 5 patients reported from UCSF manifested normalization of plasma aldosterone values after TIPS. One patient who developed liver failure after TIPS (and presumably worsened peripheral vasodilatation) had an increase in plasma aldosterone concentration (Fig. 25.3) Improvements in PRA and aldosterone levels have also been observed after peritoneovenous shunts. Blendis and

colleagues demonstrated an almost 50% mean decrease in PRA 2 weeks after peritoneovenous shunt placement.[28] However, the mean value of PRA remained twice the upper limit of normal. In addition, serum aldosterone values fell from 1675 ± 453 to 384 ± 116 pg/ml (upper limit of normal 310 pg/ml; p < 0.025). Such results, compared with those of the aforementioned TIPS studies, suggest that although both TIPS and peritoneovenous shunts reverse some of the hemodynamic abnormalities underlying the development of refractory ascites, the impact of TIPS may be greater.

In the study at UCSF, 24-hour urine sodium excretion was measured after diuretics had been discontinued for 5 days.[24] Patients were avidly retaining sodium, with a mean urinary sodium excretion of only 2.1 mEq/day. Two weeks after the procedure the value increased to 13 mEq/day (p = 0.05; Table 25.2). Of interest, in 2 patients urinary sodium concentration 9 months after TIPS exceeded 125 mEq/L, suggesting progressive natriuresis. In the other studies, increased urinary sodium excretion was a consistent finding after TIPS. There was also a trend toward improvement in glomerular filtration rate, urine volume, and free water clearance. Ochs et al. found a trivial increase in gomerular filtration rate 1 week after TIPS, however, at 6 months the mean glomerular filtration rate had increased by 115%.[27]

CLINICAL EFFICACY IN REFRACTORY ASCITES

The clinical impact of TIPS on refractory ascites has also been reported by these investigators.[24–27] The above studies found improvement in

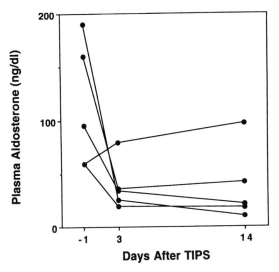

FIGURE 25.3. Plasma aldosterone concentration before TIPS and 3 and 14 days after TIPS. Normal range: 12–36 ng/dl. Excluding the patient who developed liver failure after TIPS, the mean plasma aldosterone concentration fell from 126 ± 29.9 ng/dl before TIPS to 22.8 ± 6.8 ng/dl after TIPS (p = 0.04). (From Somberg KA, Lake JR, Tomlanovich SJ, et al: Transjugular intrahepatic portosystemic shunt for refractory ascites: assessment of clinical and humoral response and renal function. Hepatology 1995;21:709–716, with permission.)

ascites control in 66–100% of patients. In fact, ascites resolved in most patients. This clinical improvement could be maintained for up to 16 months, although revision to treat shunt stenosis was required in many patients.[24] Although ascites typically improves after TIPS, this response is not seen in all patients. Ferral and colleagues reported a prospective study of TIPS for refractory ascites in 14 patients.[29] Treatment success was defined as resolution of ascites or minimal ascites after TIPS. The authors noted success in 50%; however, 4 of 7 patients in the "treatment failure" group had grade 3 hepatic encephalopathy before TIPS, suggesting advanced preexisting liver disease that may have adversely affected results.

A study from Benner et al. of 22 patients who underwent TIPS for refractory ascites also demonstrated that an adverse outcome was associated with more severe liver disease.[30] Thirteen of their patients had a Child-Pugh score > 10. Of this group, 5 died (without improvement in ascites control) within 30 days of TIPS, whereas the remainder underwent subsequent liver transplantation. Conversely, 8 of 9 patients with a Child-Pugh score ≤ 10 survived without transplantation

for a mean of 209 days. Among the 15 patients who survived without liver transplantation for more that 30 days after TIPS, ascites improved in all but one. Similarly, the preliminary report of a randomized controlled trial of TIPS vs. large-volume paracentesis noted improvement in ascites control after TIPS in Child class B but not class C patients.[31] However, TIPS was successful in only 10 of 13 patients in whom it was attempted. Although the results from these studies are preliminary, they suggest that caution should be exercised in using TIPS in patients with more advanced hepatic decompensation.

In a larger group of patients undergoing TIPS for refractory ascites at UCSF, 74% (14 of 19) met the definition of treatment success: resolution of tense ascites and no further requirement of large-volume paracentesis 1 month after TIPS.[24] Diuretic dosages were also dramatically reduced. The mean dose of furosemide was reduced from 145.7 ± 23.2 mg/day before TIPS to 55.7 ± 16.8 mg/day after TIPS (p = 0.001). The mean dose of spironolactone decreased from 203.6 ± 21.3 mg/day before TIPS to 92.6 ± 20.2 mg/day after TIPS (P = 0.001). Although treatment failure did not correlate with Child-Pugh class, nonresponders were characterized by a mean serum creatinine of 2.9 ± 0.7 mg/dl before TIPS vs. 1.8 ± 0.2 mg/dl in the treatment success group (p = 0.02). Patients who did not respond to TIPS also had a trend toward evidence of intrinsic renal disease, such as proteinuria and increased renal parenchymal echogenicity on ultrasonography. Furthermore, the nonresponders included 3 patients who had undergone renal transplantation. This finding of a poor response to TIPS in patients with pre-existing renal disease was confirmed in the study of Ochs et al.[27] Wong and Blendis have also suggested that renal dysfunction of either a parenchymal or a functional nature is associated with a lack of a therapeutic response to TIPS for refractory ascites.[32]

It has often been possible to discontinue diuretics completely after TIPS.[20,24] This result differs from the usual experience with peritoneovenous shunts, in which furosemide is routinely required to maintain diuresis.[33] The major difference between TIPS and peritoneovenous shunts is that, in addition to inducing central hemodynamic changes, TIPS directly reduces portal hypertension.

In addition to being effective in most cases of diuretic refractory ascites, TIPS has been

TABLE 25.2.   Renal Function Before and After TIPS—UCSF Experience*

Parameters	Before TIPS	3 Days After TIPS	14 Days After TIPS	p[†]
Urinary sodium excretion (mEq/24 hr)	2.1 ± 0.6	6.6 ± 3.9	13.0 ± 4.3	0.05
Urine flow (ml/24 hr)	797 ± 148	1077 ± 258	1496 ± 513	0.32
Glomerular filtration rate (ml/min)	68 ± 8	86 ± 14	91 ± 16	0.11
Free water clearance (%)	56 ± 10	60 ± 12	81 ± 11	0.23
Serum creatinine (mg/dl)	1.1 ± 0.1	1.0 ± 0.1	1.0 ± 0.1	0.03

* Data reflect 5 patients who underwent prospective inpatient protocol; all data expressed as means ± SEM
† Comparing before TIPS and 14 days after TIPS values.
(From Somberg KA, Lake JR, Tomlanovich SJ, et al: Transjugular intrahepatic portosystemic shunt for refractory ascites: assessment of clinical and humoral response and renal function. Hepatology 1995;21:709–716, with permission.)

reported to be highly effective in refractory hepatic hydrothorax.[34]

HEPATORENAL SYNDROME

The hepatorenal syndrome (HRS) represents the most advanced stage of renal functional abnormalities in cirrhosis and is reviewed in chapter 3. Although no satisfactory therapy exists, both surgical portacaval shunts and peritoneovenous shunts have been reported to reverse some cases of HRS.[35–37] Schroeder also reported marked improvement in PRA after these operations.[37] However, the limited success and high degree of morbidity and mortality have led to the general abandonment of surgery for HRS.

The less invasive nature of TIPS, as well as the physiologic and clinical improvement noted in patients with refractory ascites, commends it as an attractive potential treatment option for HRS. Ochs and coworkers in Freiburg performed a pilot study in which 5 patients underwent TIPS for HRS.[38] All patients demonstrated significant improvement in serum creatinine and urinary sodium excretion. At UCSF, 4 patients who met the diagnostic criteria for HRS received TIPS. A favorable response was seen in two, one of whom has survived without transplantation for over 1 year.[39] Although such results are preliminary, further study may show that TIPS is an effective therapy for hepatorenal syndrome.

CURRENT ISSUES AND FUTURE DIRECTIONS

In uncontrolled studies, TIPS has demonstrated efficacy in most cases of refractory ascites and some cases of hepatorenal syndrome. However, many questions about the physiology and clinical utility of TIPS remain unanswered.

Mechanism of Response

Possible mechanisms of action of TIPS in relieving ascites, including redistribution of splanchnic blood into the central circulation and reduction of portal hypertension, have been discussed. However, the precise mechanisms by which TIPS is effective in reducing ascites are undefined. In fact, TIPS improves ascites control despite further systemic arterial vasodilatation.[32,42] An interesting finding has been the progressive natriuresis seen in some patients after TIPS, suggesting a persistent mechanism of action in addition to the early changes due to volume distribution.[24] Furthermore, the response to TIPS varies among patients. Some patients manifest a brisk early diuresis, whereas others require weeks or months before diuretic dosage can be reduced.

Possible insights into the mechanism(s) by which TIPS may exert its effects derive from recent studies of endothelin-1, a potent vasoconstrictor. Two groups have presented data suggesting that TIPS reduces endothelin-1 concentrations in the portal and systemic circulations, thereby potentially reversing renal vasoconstriction.[40,41]

Systemic Hemodynamics

In addition to the portal hemodynamic changes described, TIPS has a profound effect on the systemic circulation, as noted above. Azoulay et al. reported a mean decrease in peripheral vascular resistance of 42% and a mean increase in cardiac index of 64% (7.4 vs. 4.5 L/min · m²) 1 month after TIPS compared with pre-TIPS values.[42] Similarly, Wong et al. found a 32% decrease in peripheral vascular resistance and a 74% increase in cardiac output 1 month after TIPS.[26] This persistent worsening of the hyperdynamic circulation of cirrhosis after TIPS has not been fully confirmed in other studies.[43,44] However, such findings suggest the need for a careful evaluation of cardiac status in patients considered for TIPS.

Complications of TIPS

Although TIPS is much less invasive than a surgical portacaval shunt, it is a technically demanding procedure. It is beyond the scope of this chapter to discuss in detail the complications of TIPS. However, procedural complications such as bleeding from capsular rupture or hemobilia, infections, and arrhythmias have been seen.[45] Of greater concern has been the risk of hepatic encephalopathy and liver failure. Hepatic encephalopathy has been been seen in 20–30% of patients after TIPS.[20,46,47] Encephalopathy usually responds to medical therapy, but some cases have been severe. Furthermore, liver failure has been documented after TIPS. One patient in the UCSF study of TIPS for treatment of ascites required liver transplantation 36 days after TIPS for progressive liver failure. No precipitating cause other than TIPS was identifiable.[24] Although changes in liver function after TIPS are not well understood, the risk of rapidly progressive hepatic decompensation must be considered.

Technical Issues

An important issue in creating TIPS for refractory ascites is the optimal size of the shunt. The Wallstent typically used in the United States can be initially dilated to 8, 10, or 12 mm. Refractory ascites is not immediately life-threatening, and no portosystemic pressure gradient is clearly optimal for the treatment of ascites. Wedged hepatic venous pressure gradients have been shown to correlate with elevations in PRA, aldosterone, norepinephrine and antidiuretic hormone.[48,49] However, the UCSF group demonstrated that an excellent response can be achieved with 8-mm stents, regardless of the drop in portosystemic pressure gradient.[24] Therefore, it is preferable to provide the minimal degree of portal diversion that is necessary to achieve the desired clinical outcome. TIPS can be electively dilated to 10 mm if ascites does not improve. Research should be directed toward optimizing the hemodynamic outcome of TIPS in individual patients to improve ascites without leading to excessive risk of encephalopathy.

A significant problem with TIPS over the long term is the risk of stenosis and occlusion. Most studies show cumulative rates of stenosis and occlusion at 1 year of 30–60%.[20,21,50] A stenotic or occluded TIPS can typically be revised on an outpatient basis. However, the need for frequent revisions may make TIPS a less attractive option for patients in whom liver transplantation is not anticipated.

Appropriate Use in Refractory Ascites

TIPS appears to be an attractive option for treating refractory ascites. However, as yet no published data from randomized controlled studies compare TIPS with any other standard form of therapy for refractory ascites. Clearly, studies of TIPS vs. large-volume paracentesis and peritoneovenous shunts are necessary to develop an understanding of the true relative efficacy and safety of TIPS. In the absence of such data, TIPS may be appropriate in selected cases. Clinical features that favor the insertion of TIPS may include failure of or contraindications to peritoneovenous shunting, the need for frequent therapeutic paracentesis, a history of recurrent variceal hemorrhage, and the availability of liver transplantation if hepatic decompensation occurs. Careful consideration of hepatic reserve, underlying renal abnormalities, and cardiac function are necessary to assess the potential risks and benefits of TIPS.

SUMMARY

TIPS is an important advance in the treatment of refractory ascites. Uncontrolled data demonstrate that TIPS improves ascites in the vast majority of patients and allows significant reduction of diuretic usage. TIPS also reverses some of the underlying neurohumoral abnormalities considered to be important in the pathophysiology of refractory ascites. However, TIPS has several drawbacks, including a high degree of technical difficulty, significant risk of encephalopathy, and frequent shunt stenosis. Although TIPS can be very useful in the management of patients with refractory ascites and possibly hepatorenal syndrome, randomized controlled trials are needed to define its optimal role in the management of both disorders.

REFERENCES

1. Ginès P, Arroyo V, Quintero E, et al: Comparison of paracentesis and diuretics in the treatment of cirrhotics with tense ascites. Gastroenterology 1987;93:234–241.

2. Kao, HW, Rakov NE, Savage E, Reynolds TB: The effect of large-volume paracentesis on plasma volume—a cause of hypovolemia? Hepatology 1985;5:403–407.

3. Runyon BA, Antillon MR, Montano AA: Effect of diuresis versus therapeutic paracentesis on ascitic fluid opsonic activity and serum complement. Gastroenterology 1989;97:158–162.

4. Ginès P, Arroyo V, Vargas V, et al: Paracentesis with intravenous infusion of albumin as compared with peritoneovenous shunting in cirrhosis with refractory ascites. N Engl J Med 1991;325:829–835.

5. Smart HL, Triger DR: A randomised prospective trial comparing daily paracentesis and intravenous albumin with recirculation in diuretic refractory ascites. J Hepatol 1990;10:191–197.

6. Bruno S, Borzio M, Romagnoni M, et al: Comparison of spontaneous ascites filtration and reinfusion with total paracentesis with intravenous albumin infusion in cirrhotic patients with tense ascites. BMJ 1992;304:1655–1658.

7. Burchell AR, Rousselot LM, Panke WF: A seven-year experience with side-to-side portacaval shunt for cirrhotic ascites. Ann Surg 1968;168:655–670.

8. Franco D, Vons C, Traynor O, de Smadja C: Should portosystemic shunt be reconsidered in the treatment of intractable ascites in cirrhosis? Arch Surg 1988;123:987–991.

9. Witte MH, Witte CL, Dumont AE: Progress in liver disease: physiological factors involved in the causation of cirrhotic ascites. Gastroenterology 1971;61:742–750.

10. Schrier RW, Arroyo V, Bernardi M, et al: Peripheral arterial vasodilation hypothesis: a proposal for the initiation of renal sodium and water retention in cirrhosis. Hepatology 1988;8:1151–1157.

11. Lieberman FL, Denison EK, Reynolds TB: The relationship of plasma volume, portal hypertension, ascites, and renal sodium retention in cirrhosis: the overflow theory of ascites formation. Ann NY Acad Sci 1970;170:202–212.

12. Lang F, Tschernko E, Schulze E, et al. Hepatorenal reflex regulating kidney function. Hepatology 1991;14:590–594.

13. Rösch J, Hanafee WN, Snow H: Transjugular portal venography and radiologic portacaval shunt: An experimental study. Radiology 1969;92:1112–1114.

14. Palmaz JC, Garcia F, Sibbitt RR, et al: Expandable intrahepatic portacaval shunt stents in dogs with chronic portal hypertension. AJR 1986;147:1251–1254.

15. Richter GM, Noeldge G, Palmaz JC, et al: Transjugular intrahepatic portacaval stent shunt : preliminary clinical results. Radiology 1990; 174:1027–1030.

16. Richter GM, Noeldge G, Palmaz JC, Roessle M: The transjugular intrahepatic portosystemic stent-shunt (TIPSS): Results of a pilot study. Cardiovasc Intervent Radiol 1990;13:200–207.

17. Zemel G, Katzen BT, Becker GJ, et al: Percutaneous transjugular portosystemic shunt. JAMA 1991;266:390–393.

18. Ring EJ, Lake JR, Roberts JP, et al: Using transjugular intrahepatic portosystemic shunts to control variceal bleeding before liver transplantation. Ann Intern Med 1992;116:304–309.

19. Garcia-Tsao G, Groszmann RJ, Fisher RL, et al: Portal pressure, presence of gastroesophageal varices and variceal bleeding. Hepatology 1985;5:419–424.

20. Rössle M, Haag K, Ochs A, et al: The transjugular intrahepatic portosystemic stent-shunt procedure for variceal bleeding. N Engl J Med 1994;330:165–171.

21. LaBerge JM, Ring EJ, Gordon RL, et al:. Creation of transjugular intrahepatic portosystemic shunts with the Wallstent endoprosthesis: Results in 100 patients. Radiology 1993;187:413–420.

22. Martin M, Zajko AB, Orons PD, et al: Transjugular intrahepatic portosystemic shunt in the management of variceal bleeding: Indications and clinical results. Surgery 1993;114:719–727.

23. Helton WS, Belshaw A, Althaus S, et al: Critical appraisal of the angiographic portacaval shunt (TIPS). Am J Surg 1993;165:566–571.

24. Somberg KA, Lake JR, Tomlanovich SJ, et al: Transjugular intrahepatic portosystemic shunt for refractory ascites: Assessment of clinical and humoral response and renal function. Hepatology 1995;21:709–716.

25. Quiroga J, Sangro B, Nunez M, et al: Transjugular intrahepatic portal-systemic shunt in the treatment of refractory ascites: Effect on clinical, renal, humoral, and hemodynamic parameters. Hepatology 1995;21:986–994.

26. Wong F, Sniderman K, Liu P, et al: Transjugular intrahepatic portosystemic stent shunt: Effects on hemodynamics and sodium homeostasis in cirrhosis and refractory ascites. Ann Intern Med 1995;122:816–822.

27. Ochs A, Rössle M, Haag K, et al: The transjugular intrahepatic portosystemic stent-shunt procedure for refractory ascites. N Engl J Med 1995;332:1192–1197.

28. Blendis LM, Greig PD, Langer B, et al: The renal and hemodynamic effects of the peritoneovenous shunt for intractable hepatic ascites. Gastroenterology 1979;77:250–257.

29. Ferral H, Bjarnason H, Wegryn SA, et al: Refractory ascites: early experience in treatment with transjugular intrahepatic portosystemic shunt. Radiology 1993;189:795–801.

30. Benner KG, Sahagun G, Saxon R, et al: Selection of patients undergoing transjugular intrahepatic portosystemic shunt for refractory ascites [abstract]. Hepatology 1994;20:114A.

31. Lebrec D, Giuily N, Hadangue A, et al: Transjugular intrahepatic portosystemic shunt versus paracentesis for refractory ascites. Results of a randomized trial [abstract]. Hepatology 1994;20:201A.

32. Wong F, Blendis L: Transjugular intrahepatic portosystemic shunt for refractory ascites: Tipping the sodium balance. Hepatology 1995;22:358–364.

33. Epstein M: Peritoneovenous shunt in the management of ascites and the hepatorenal syndrome. Gastroenterology 1982;82:790–799.

34. Strauss RM, Martin LG, Kaufman SL, Boyer TD: Transjugular intrahepatic portal systemic shunt for the management of symptomatic cirrhotic hydrothorax. Am J Gastroenterol 1994;89:1520–1522.

35. Ariyan S, Sweeney T, Kerstein MD: The hepatorenal syndrome: recovery after portacaval shunt. Ann Surg 1975;181:847–849.

36. Wapnick S, Grosberg S, Kinney M, LeVeen HH: LeVeen continuous peritoneal-jugular shunt: improvement of renal function in ascitic patients. JAMA 1977;237:131–133.

37. Schroeder ET, Anderson GH Jr, Smulyan H: Effects of a portacaval or peritoneovenous shunt on renin in the hepatorenal syndrome. Kidney Int 1979;15:54–61.

38. Ochs A, Rössle M, Haag K, et al: TIPS for hepatorenal syndrome [abstract]. Hepatology 1994;20:114A.

39. Alam I, Bass NM, LaBerge JM, et al: Treatment of hepatorenal syndrome with the transjugular intrahepatic portosystemic shunt (TIPS) [abstract]. Gastroenterology 1995;108:A1024.

40. Martinet JP, Legault L, Cernacek P, et al: Effect of TIPS on splanchnic and renal production of endothelins [abstract]. Hepatology 1994;20:113A.

41. Sanyal AJ, Gehr T, Freedman AM, et al: Increased splanchnic endothelin-1 plays a role in the pathogenesis of ascites [abstract]. Hepatology 1994;20:113A.

42. Azoulay D, Castaing D, Dennison A, et al: Transjugular intrahepatic portosystemic shunt worsens the hyperdynamic circulatory state of the cirrhotic patient: preliminary report of a prospective study. Hepatology 1994;19:129–132.

43. Colombato LA, Martinet JP, Dufrense MP, et al: Reversal of the initial increase in cardiac index with persistence of worsened vasodilatation two months after TIPS [abstract]. Hepatology 1994;20:101A.

44. Lotterer E, Wengert A, Moosmüller A, et al: Effect of transjugular intrahepatic portal systemic shunt (TIPS) on hepatic and systemic hemodynamics in patients with alcoholic cirrhosis [abstract]. Hepatology 1993;18:102A.

45. Freedman AM, Sanyal AJ, Tisnado J, et al: Complications of transjugular intrahepatic portosystemic shunt: A comprehensive review. RadioGraphics 1993;13:1185–1210.

46. Somberg KA, Riegler JL, Doherty MM, et al: Hepatic encephalopathy following transjugular intrahepatic portosystemic shunts (TIPS): Incidence and risk factors. Am J Gastroenterol 1995;90:549–555.

47. Sanyal AJ, Freedman AM, Shiffman ML, et al: Portosystemic encephalopathy after transjugular intrahepatic portosystemic shunt: results of a prospective controlled study. Hepatology 1994;20:46–55.

48. Bosch J, Arroyo V, Betriu A, et al: Hepatic hemodynamics and the renin-angiotensin-aldosterone system in cirrhosis. Gastroenterology 1980;78:92–99.

49. Henriksen JH, Ring-Larsen H, Kanstrup I-L, Christensen NJ: Splanchnic and renal elimination and release of catecholamines in cirrhosis. Evidence of enhanced sympathetic nervous activity in patients with decompensated cirrhosis. Gut 1984;25:1034–1043.

50. Lind CD, Malisch TW, Chong WK, et al: Incidence of shunt occlusion or stenosis following transjugular intrahepatic portosystemic shunt placement. Gastroenterology 1994;106:1277–1283.

DIALYSIS, HEMOFILTRATION, AND OTHER EXTRACORPOREAL TECHNIQUES IN THE TREATMENT OF THE RENAL COMPLICATIONS OF LIVER DISEASE

GUIDO O. PEREZ, M.D.
THOMAS A. GOLPER, M.D., F.A.C.P.
MURRAY EPSTEIN, M.D., F.A.C.P.
JAMES R. OSTER, M.D.

Management of Intractable Ascites
    Ascites Concentration and Reinfusion into the
      Vascular Compartment
    Dialytic Ultrafiltration of Ascites
    Dialysis and Hemofiltration: Intermittent and
      Continuous Forms
Treatment of Hepatorenal Syndrome
    Peritoneal Dialysis
    Hemodialysis and Hemofiltration
**Role of Extracorporeal Therapies in Patients with
    Fulminant Hepatic Failure and Coma**

Hemodialysis
Hemofiltration
Hemoperfusion
Plasma Exchange
Artificial Liver System
**Potential Advantages and Disadvantages of
    Dialysis or Hemofiltration in Patients with
    Decompensated Liver Disease**
**Maintenance Dialysis in Patients with Chronic
    Liver Disease**
Summary

The role of dialysis, hemofiltration, and other extracorporeal therapies in the management of the renal complications of liver disease, including refractory ascites and the hepatorenal syndrome (HRS), remains controversial. The review in the first edition of this book[1] concluded that these therapies were ineffective in the management of HRS. In the intervening years it has become apparent that such a sweeping condemnation is unwarranted and that in specific instances, especially patients undergoing hepatic transplantation and patients with fulminant hepatic failure, such interventions are justified. In addition, new procedures have been developed to manage intractable ascites. This chapter considers the benefits and drawbacks of dialysis, hemofiltration, and related extracorporeal procedures in the treatment of renal and/or hepatic dysfunction in patients with liver disease.

MANAGEMENT OF INTRACTABLE ASCITES

As noted in chapter 1, patients with cirrhosis manifest a remarkable capacity for sodium chloride retention; indeed, such patients frequently excrete urine that is virtually free of sodium. The result is excessive accumulation of extracellular fluid, which eventually becomes evident as clinically detectable ascites and edema. Although treatment with bed rest, a low sodium diet, and diuretics often suffices to control ascites, an occasional patient may exhibit true refractoriness to convenional therapy. Such patients are usually managed with large volume paracentesis (see chapter 23). Nevertheless, patients who require frequent paracentesis may become candidates for extracorporeal forms of intervention (ascites reinfusion, dialytic ultrafiltration of ascites, or continuous hemofiltration) or for surgical procedures such as peritoneovenous (PV) shunt (see chapter 24), transjugular intrahepatic portosystemic shunt (see chapter 25), or hepatic transplantation (see chapter 27).

Ascites Concentration and Reinfusion into the Vascular Compartment

Because sodium retention in cirrhosis is linked to increased renal tubular sodium reabsorption in response to a contracted effective plasma volume, a physiological approach to its correction has been to expand plasma volume. A profound diuresis occasionally follows infusions of colloid solutions such as albumin or plasma to patients with severe ascites. An alternative and inexpensive way to expand plasma volume is to withdraw ascitic fluid with a peritoneal catheter and to reinfuse it into the systemic circulation. An effective diuresis and relief of ascites is often obtained, especially when ascites reinfusion is used concomitantly with diuretics.[2] This approach, however, is time-consuming, awkward, and occasionally associated with fever, coagulopathy, and bacteremia.

In 1971 the Rhodiascit machine was introduced to facilitate ascites reinfusion in patients with severe ascites. This device consists of sterile disposable intravenous tubing, a pump, and a membrane that concentrates the ascitic fluid 2- to 4-fold prior to its reinfusion into a peripheral vein. This procedure has been used extensively in Europe, but it has not achieved widespread use in the United States.[3,4] No controlled trials have compared treatment with the Rhodiascit machine with conventional diuretic management in terms of morbidity and mortality or cost.

Several practical considerations preclude frequent use of the Rhodiascit machine in patients with refractory ascites. Although this procedure is capable of rendering patients nearly ascites-free and can be repeated at monthly intervals, its use may be attended by an array of complications, including fever, sepsis, congestive heart failure, coagulopathy, and gastrointestinal bleeding.[5,6] The presence of severe heart disease may result in worsening of congestive failure due to the large (200–400 ml/hr) volumes reinfused. Thus, the presence of severe renal failure, which may limit a protective increase in urine flow rate, is a relative contraindication, even in the absence of intrinsic heart disease. Severe hepatic decompensation with prolongation of the prothrombin time (PT) by more than 3–5 seconds or encephalopathy renders the prognosis poor in any event. Thus, ascites must be put in perspective with other aspects of liver failure. Careful assessment of coagulation status, including PT, partial thromboplastin time, platelet count, and bleeding time, is performed as well as a diagnostic paracentesis in the 24–48 hours prior to infusion.

On the morning of the procedure, a pediatric dialysis catheter is placed under local anesthesia, preferably by a surgeon because a secure purse-string suture is advisable to prevent fluid leak. Then the machine is primed with physiologic saline, and the pump is started. Finally, the post-membrane concentrate (when the initial saline has drained through the tubing system) is reinfused via a peripheral intravenous line. Central venous pressure monitoring may be necessary. By means of pressure and resistance adjustments, a hydrostatic head of pressure is maintained in the membrane chamber to effect concentration of the ascitic fluid. Because the pore size permits passage only of molecules with a low molecular weight, the filtrate is a clear fluid with a protein concentration of less than 5 mg/dl. The concentrations of sodium, chloride, and potassium are similar to those of the patient's plasma. The infusion is continued from 4–15 hours, depending on patient need and tolerance of the infusion.

A recent randomized, prospective trial compared daily paracentesis (3-4 L) with ascites recirculation using the Rhodiascit apparatus in 40 consecutive patients with ascites refractory to diuretics.[7] A clinically important diuresis occurred in 14 patients treated with recirculation compared with 4 treated by paracentesis. Complications were more frequent with paracentesis, and the duration of hospitalization was shorter in patients treated by recirculation. Ascites reaccumulation and survival were identical in both groups. The authors concluded that recirculation of ascites with the Rhodiascit apparatus is a reasonable therapeutic alternative to large-volume paracentesis in patients with refractory ascites.

Dialytic Ultrafiltration of Ascites

An alternative approach to the patient with refractory ascites is ultrafiltration of ascitic fluid with reinfusion of the concentrate into the peritoneal cavity.[8–11] This procedure, like that using the Rhodiascit machine, removes salt and water from ascitic fluid without loss of protein. In contrast, volume overload does not occur because the ascitic fluid is not reinfused into the vascular compartment. As shown in Figure 26.1, two catheters (or a single double-lumen catheter) are inserted into the peritoneal cavity. Ascitic fluid is removed through one of the catheters by means of a roller pump and circulated through the ultra-filter. The concentrated protein-rich ascitic fluid is then returned to the abdominal cavity. An alternative method is to use a regular hollow-fiber dialyzer and to connect the outlet dialysate port to wall suction. Otherwise the methodology is the same as in Figure 26.1.

Ultrafiltration of ascites is associated with small but significant increases in cardiac output and stroke volume and an unanticipated fall in plasma renin activity and plasma aldosterone levels.[10] In addition, the patient's responsiveness to diuretics may improve following dialytic ultrafiltration of ascites. Although it was postulated that this procedure induces a net flux of protein from ascitic fluid to plasma,[12] another study[13] showed no change in total protein content of ascitic fluid 7 days after the procedure. Furthermore, the volume of ascites returned to baseline levels, presumably because of the increased intraperitoneal-abdominal oncotic pressure.[13]

Methods for ascites filtration and reinfusion without pump assistance have been reported.[11,14] The ascites flows to a hemofilter located below the patient, wherein the proteins are concentrated by gravity filtration and collected in a sterile bag. When the bag is full, it is raised above the level of the patient, and the partially concentrated ascitic fluid is returned to the peritoneal space. Modest heparinization (approximately 2500 U per procedure) is necessary. In 1–2 hours, 2 or 3 liters of ascites can be filtered and 500–600 ml of concentrated solution reinfused into the abdominal cavity.

Several recent reports[15-23] have described the effectiveness and safety of this procedure in the management of refractory ascites. Three studies[15-17] compared large-volume paracentesis with dialytic ultrafiltration of ascites. One study[15] demonstrated that the incidence of complications was higher with paracentesis; nonetheless, the results are difficult to interpret because the procedure did not include the administration of plasma volume expanders. Another study[16] reported transient increases in the protein concentration of the ascites and in urine output in patients treated with dialytic ultrafiltration of ascites; no serious side effects were observed. Bruno et al.[17] concluded

DIALYTIC ULTRAFILTRATION OF ASCITES

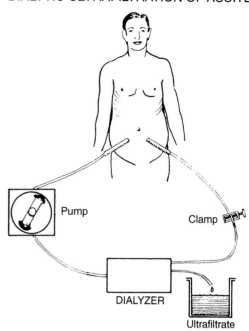

FIGURE 26.1. With dialytic ultrafiltration of ascites, ascitic fluid is removed from the abdomen, passed through a capillary dialyzer, concentrated, and then reinfused into the peritoneal cavity by means of a Teflon catheter. A roller pump allows fluid flow rates through the capillary dialyzer of approximately 150 ml/min. Heparin is usually given intraperitoneally to prevent fibrin clot formation.

that dialytic ultrafiltration of ascites was as effective as paracentesis in the control of tense ascites. Side effects were minor, and the procedure obviated the need for intravenous albumin infusion. Dialytic ultrafiltration of ascites is associated with a parallel fall of both intraperitoneal and hepatic wedge pressure and no changes in mean arterial pressure and central venous pressure.[24]

Dialysis and Hemofiltration: Intermittent and Continuous Forms

Intermittent forms of therapy have constituted the traditional means of support in renal failure, with isolated ultrafiltration used for fluid management and intermittent hemodialysis for electrolyte, acid-base, and azotemic control. Solute removal by ultrafiltration is called convection, and this process more effectively removes molecules up to 10,000 daltons than does diffusion with standard dialyzers. In fact, some hemofiltration membranes may be slightly permeable to

TABLE 26.1. General Categories of Available Extracorporeal Techniques

Modality	Description
Hemodialysis	Dialysate interfacing with blood via a semipermeable membrane results in solute removal by diffusion. Hemodialysis restores fluid, electrolyte, and acid-base balance, and controls azotemia.
Hemofiltration	Solute removal is achieved by convective ultrafiltration. This can be viewed as an exchange of plasma water for a lesser amount of sterile replacement fluid.
Hemodiafiltration	Diffusive and convective techniques are combined.

molecules as large as 50,000 daltons. Nevertheless, the quantity of such molecules removed by convection is small. For most hepatic and uremic toxins the concentration in the filtrate is close to that in plasma water. Hemodiafiltration involves a combination of diffusive and convective techniques. Table 26.1 summarizes the working definitions of these therapeutic variations.

Currently, continuous extracorporeal therapeutic modalities have been applied to various select patients[25,26] (Table 26.2). These methods permit an enhanced level of fluid and solute removal in association with hemodynamic stability and have been applied to the more seriously ill, unstable patient with multiorgan failure. In addition,

TABLE 26.2. Definitions of Available Continuous Extracorporeal Techniques Encompassing Hemofiltration, with or without Dialysis*

Slow continuous ultrafiltration
 The removal of 5 ml/min or less of plasma water for purposes of fluid control only. The ultrafiltration rate is selected based on the desired fluid balance.

Continuous arteriovenous or venovenous hemofiltration (CAVH, CVVH)
 The plasma water exchange is > 5 ml/min. It is used for the management of fluid, electrolyte, and acid-base complications, and for mild azotemia. The rate of ultrafiltration dictates the fluid intake, whereas the clinical and laboratory values dictate substitution fluid composition.

Continuous arteriovenous or venovenous hemodialysis (CAVHD, CVVHD)
 A diffusive-based mode of therapy wherein the purpose is to remove both fluid and solute. This therapy combines dialysis and hemofiltration and is used in patients with higher urea generation.

* See text for explanation of these techniques.

improved fluid balance permits a greater fluid intake with much less risk of fluid overload.

Intermittent hemodialysis has been used for the treatment of fluid overload and ascites. This procedure, however, may be attended by hemodynamic instability and bleeding, and fluid removal is difficult. Slow continuous ultrafiltration (SCUF), continuous arteriovenous or venovenous hemofiltration (CAVH or CVVH), and continuous arteriovenous or venovenous hemodialysis (CAVHD or CVVHD) have been introduced for the removal of fluids and solutes in critically ill patients with liver disease.[27,28] These procedures use small filters with a membrane highly permeable to water and low-molecular-weight solutes. With SCUF, CAVH, and CAVHD, the patient's own blood pressure is usually sufficient to maintain filtration, and high rates of fluid removal (0.4–1.2 L/hr) can be achieved.

We have used CAVH for the treatment of refractory ascites in a patient with advanced liver cirrhosis.[27] The procedure safely induced a negative fluid balance of 4 liters and restored the sensitivity to diuretics without causing hypotension, bleeding, or decreases in renal function. Similarly, in a preliminary communication, Kaplan reported the successful application of CAVH in the management of 2 patients with hepatic insufficiency and concomitant renal failure.[28]

We believe that continuous hemofiltration may prove to have a valuable role in the management of selected patients with massive ascites. Because information concerning the above-mentioned modalities is not yet readily available to clinicians, we provide herein considerable detail, albeit prior to confirmation of their efficacy and safety in this setting.

Continuous arteriovenous hemofiltration requires the use of either temporary access to the circulation (via femoral artery and vein catheters) or a semipermanent Scribner shunt. Blood propelled by the patient's own arterial pressure flows through a low-resistance hemofilter and returns to the patient through the venous limb (Fig. 26.2). Heparinization of the device is necessary to prevent clotting; however, continuous therapy has been successfully performed in patients with liver failure without anticoagulation of the extracorporeal circuit.[29] Pump-assisted CAVH can be used to achieve higher blood flows. In addition, continuous venovenous hemofiltration (CVVH), using a blood pump, has been introduced to eliminate the need of arterial cannulation in CAVH.

Close patient monitoring is necessary when blood pumps are used.

The ultrafiltrate is collected into a plastic bag. According to the need for fluid removal, part of the ultrafiltrate is replaced by intravenous administration of a solution such as isotonic sodium chloride or Ringer's lactate. Replacement fluid can be infused together with heparin through a port that is either proximal to the hemofilter (predilution mode) or distal in the venous limb (postdilution mode).

Treatment is continuous (24 hr/day) until ultrafiltration is no longer needed. It is not unusual for a patient to be treated for several days. Using the postdilution technique with CAVH, urea clearance approximates the amount of filtrate that is removed. Thus, with a fluid removal rate of 500 ml/hr, clearance would be about 12 L/day.

Since their initial introduction in the early 1980s, hemofilters have undergone design modifications that have enhanced their applicability to an increasing patient population. As an example, a second port has been added to the housing of the Diafilter-30 hemofilter. This allows the option of circulating a dialysis solution around its hollow fibers and combining diffusive transport with ultrafiltration for a net gain in blood clearance (CAVHD). The Amicon Diafilter-l0 device, which has a larger number of capillary fibers but a shorter length than the original Amicon Diafilter-20 hemofilter, has a similar membrane area but produces less resistance to blood flow. This design is particularly advantageous in patients with low blood flow due to very low blood pressure or limited vascular access. Alternatively, dialyzers such as the Fresenius F-40 polysulfone dialyzer can be used at lesser cost.

In conclusion, the optimal treatment of truly intractable ascites has not been established. Large-volume paracentesis has achieved widespread use and appears to be effective in the treatment of resistant ascites (see chapter 23). The extracorporeal techniques discussed above are more difficult to institute but may be used in patients requiring frequent paracentesis. A definitive surgical procedure may provide a more permanent solution but entails more risk and expense. The peritoneous-venous shunt has been used several years for this purpose (see chapter 24). The transjugular intrahepatic portosystemic shunt, introduced to decompress the portal system for the treatment of bleeding esophogeal varices, has been shown to be effective in the

CONTINUOUS ARTERIOVENOUS HEMOFILTRATION

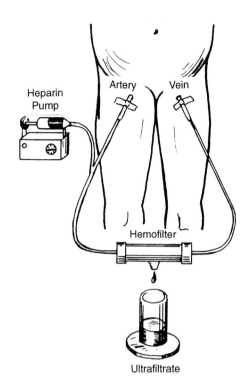

FIGURE 26.2. Schematic view of the procedure used for continuous arteriovenous hemofiltration. Access to the patient's vascular system consists of femoral arterial and venous catheters. The hemofiltration cartidge acts as an ultrafilter, retaining cellular components and proteins in the circulation and allowing water and crystalloids to pass through the pores of hollow fiber membranes. Heparinization of the device is often necessary.

control of ascites[30] (see chapter 25). Finally, because of the poor 1-year survival of patients with diuretic-resistant ascites, it has been suggested that patients who are otherwise good candidates should be considered for hepatic transplantation.

The choice of extracorporeal technique in the management of intractable ascites also remains undefined. Each technique has specific advantages and limitations. As mentioned, ascites infusion with the Rhodiascit machine (or similar devices), although effective in ascites removal, may be accompanied by sepsis, coagulopathy, and fluid overload. Dialytic ultrafiltration of ascites avoids infusion of fluid into the vascular compartment and the expense of albumin infusions but may be ineffective in the long term.

Finally, CAVH or CVVH avoids the insertion of a peritoneal catheter and intravascular infusion of ascites but requires temporary vascular access, anticoagulation, and careful monitoring. It certainly merits further clinical evaluation.

TREATMENT OF HEPATORENAL SYNDROME

As noted in chapter 3, the hepatorenal syndrome (HRS) is a functional disorder characterized by renal hypoperfusion with preferential renal cortical ischemia. The best treatment of acute renal failure is preventive, with prompt attention to contributory factors such as bleeding, sepsis, vomiting, diarrhea (including that induced by lactulose), excessive diuresis or paracentesis, and nephrotoxic agents. The following sections consider the role of extracorporeal techniques in the management of HRS.

Peritoneal Dialysis

There are few published data about the treatment of HRS with peritoneal dialysis.[31–34] Of a total of 47 patients (from four reports) with fulminant hepatic failure and HRS treated with peritoneal dialysis, there were only 4 survivors (Table 26.3). Of patients with cirrhosis and HRS, only 1 of 35 survived. Ring-Larsen et al.[32] reported 12 patients with cirrhosis and 5 with acute hepatic insufficiency and HRS who were treated with peritoneal dialysis to correct hyponatremia. Several patients had hepatic encephalopathy. Despite correction of the electrolyte abnormalities, all of the patients died within a few days. Two recent reports[35,36] describe the successful application of peritoneal dialysis in the setting of acute renal failure associated with liver disease.

Included among the difficulties in instituting peritoneal dialysis in the HRS are (1) coagulopathy requiring surgical rather than percutaneous placement of the catheter, (2) ascites making the exchanges less efficient and augmenting protein losses, and (3) insufficient rates of solute clearance.

Hemodialysis and Hemofiltration

Hemodialysis has been reported to be ineffective in the management of HRS.[37–40] Our own recent experience, however, suggests that such a viewpoint should be qualified. Although most of the published literature indeed suggests a dismal prognosis for patients who are dialyzed, such reports have dealt with patients with chronic end-stage liver disease. Our experience and that of others[34] (Table 26.4) suggest that in carefully selected patients dialytic therapy is indicated. Indications include acute hepatic dysfunction in which there is reason to believe that the underlying liver disease may reverse (making long-term survival and even spontaneous recovery of renal function possible). Thus, sporadic case reports describe prolonged survival and improvement in renal function in selected patients with acute or acute superimposed on chronic liver disease treated by dialysis[41,42] alone or combined with other modalities.[43,44]

Dialysis or hemofiltration may also have a role in the treatment of patients with severe end-stage liver disease with HRS before, during, and after hepatic transplantation. Aside from complicating medical management, the development of acute renal failure in this setting is associated with considerable morbidity and mortality.[45–47] Nevertheless, in one study dialytic therapy was helpful in the life support of patients awaiting liver transplantation, and 4 of 7 patients with HRS experienced recovery of renal function 1–5 weeks after successful hepatic replacement.[40] See chapter 27 for the effect of hepatic transplantation on HRS.

Because many patients undergoing liver transplantation with or without acute renal failure exhibit hemodynamic instability, treatment with continuous hemofiltration may be better tolerated. Fluid removal may facilitate overall management and allow liberal replacement of clotting factors and other fluids during the perioperative period.[48–52] In addition, CAVH or CAVHD may

TABLE 26.3. Peritoneal Dialysis in Hepatorenal Syndrome

	Cirrhosis		Fulminant Hepatic Failure	
	No. Patients	No. Survivors	No. Patients	No. Survivors
Ritt et al., 1969[31]	—	—	3	0
Ring-Larsen et al., 1973[32]	12	0	5	0
Jacobson and Bell, 1973[33]	5	1	—	—
Wilkinson et al., 1977[34]	18	0	39	4

help control hepatic encephalopathy (see below) and the associated increases in intracranial pressure.[53]

EXTRACORPOREAL THERAPIES IN PATIENTS WITH FULMINANT HEPATIC FAILURE AND COMA

Hemodialysis

Because many patients with HRS are in hepatic coma, dialysis with a large pore-size membrane may have a beneficial effect.[54–58] The initial studies suggested that removal of toxic middle-sized molecules with this membrane may have been responsible for the improvement in mental status and possibly survival noted in some patients (Table 26.5). Unfortunately, the number of patients with a clearly established diagnosis of HRS was not specified in most reports.

In 1976 Opolon et al.[54] reported 9 patients with hepatic coma due to fulminant viral hepatitis who underwent hemodialysis with a polyacrylonitrile membrane. Total recovery of consciousness was observed in 5 patients and partial recovery in two. The investigators also compared the effects of conventional hemodialysis with cuprophane or polyacrylonitrile membrane with the effects of cross-hemodialysis in pigs with experimental hepatic coma. Cross-hemodialysis with a healthy donor resulted in prompt but transient recovery of consciousness ,regardless of the type of membrane. Hemodialysis with cuprophane had no effect; polyacrylonitrile dialysis without a donor allowed prolonged clinical and electroencephalographic recovery.

Silk et al.[55] reported their experience with 189 patients with fulminant hepatic failure. Fifty-three patients received conservative treatment alone, whereas 71 were treated with charcoal hemoperfusion and 65 with polyacrylonitrile hemodialysis. Fifteen percent of conservatively treated patients survived. In contrast, the survival rate was 24% in the group treated with charcoal hemoperfusion and 31% in the group treated with hemodialysis. Similar results were obtained by Sakai et al.[56]

Opolon summarized his clinical experience with polyacrylonitrile hemodialysis in the treatment of 39 patients with coma due to fulminant hepatic failure.[57] Despite an overall improvement in neurologic status in 61% of cases, survival was not different from that of untreated patients. Of note, improved survival was noted in patients

TABLE 26.4. Hemodialysis in Hepatorenal Syndrome Associated with Chronic Liver Disease

Author/Year	No. Patients	No. Survivors
Topchiashvili and Sergienko, 1971[37]	8	2
Klingler and Cronin, 1972[38]	5	2
Wilkinson et al., 1977[34]	5	0
Coratelli et al., 1985[39]	8	0
Ellis and Avner, 1986*[40]	12	4

* In patients undergoing hepatic transplantation.

treated by continuous hemofiltration. Similar results were reported by Mathieu et al.[58] It is noteworthy that a study in Italy reported no survivors among 8 patients with chronic liver disease and HRS treated with polyacrylonitrile dialysis.[39]

Hemofiltration

Continuous hemofiltration with membranes with large pores, increased porosity and decreased wall thickness has been introduced.[57,58] Such membranes have been shown to remove substances of middle molecular weight (500–5,000) that are not highly protein bound and to improve the mental status in patients with hepatic encephalopathy.[59–63] Ammonia, mercaptans, fatty acids, and amino acids may fall into this category. Whereas diffusion dialysis can remove these species, hemofiltration has the advantage of less changes in plasma osmolality during the

TABLE 26.5. Hemodialysis with Polyacrylonitrile Membranes in the Treatment of Fulminant Hepatic Failure*

Author/Year	No. Patients	Survival	% Normalization Mental Status
Silk and Williams, 1978[55]	65	31	—
Sakai et al., 1980[56]	9	22	44
Opolon, 1981[57†]	39	23	44
Opolon, 1981[57‡]	10	50	50
Mathieu et al., 1982[58‡]	13	23	54

* Patients treated for advanced hepatic coma. Numbers of patients with hepatorenal syndrome were not specified in most series.
† Among control subjects (n = 117): 22% had an improved level of consciousness; survival was 18%.
‡ Continuous ultrafiltration.

therapy. In addition, convection removes larger molecules than does diffusion. Continuous hemofiltration has been used in conjunction with other forms of artificial liver support such as plasma exchange or charcoal hemoperfusion.[64–68]

Most patients with fulminant hepatic failure ultimately die of brain edema despite artificial liver support. The successful introduction of intracranial pressure monitoring constitutes an important advance in the management of such patients. Davenport et al.[53] described the successful support of patients with fulminant hepatic failure, oliguric renal failure, coma, and cerebral edema with continuous hemofiltration. Osmotic changes were minimized by the use of a continuous (slow) approach and hemofiltration rather than dialysis. Volume and osmolar control were tightly regulated, and intracranial pressure was continuously monitored. Intracranial pressure elevation associated with low systemic blood pressure exacerbates brain ischemia. Continuous hemofiltration appears to be better tolerated than intermittent therapy in this setting. Nevertheless, this form of therapy may be associated with several complications: (1) rebound increases in intracranial pressure after discontinuation of treatment,[67] (2) hyperlactatemia and acidosis associated with lactate-buffered replacement solutions,[68] and (3) bleeding from anticoagulants and decreased platelets.

Venovenous access for continuous therapy has the advantage over arteriovenous access, because an arterial cannulation is avoided (especially important in patients with liver failure and coagulopathy) and because pumped blood flow is faster and more reliable than spontaneous blood flow. The only drawback to venovenous access is the requisite extracorporeal blood pump. Many modern intensive care units now offer or are developing these techniques.

Hemoperfusion

Sorbent systems include activated charcoal and ion exchange resins such as Amberlite XAD-7.[69–71] Charcoal hemoperfusion appeared to be beneficial in early, uncontrolled studies. Nevertheless, clinical trials in 137 patients at King's College Hospital in London[69] revealed no significant improvement in survival over intensive care alone.

Resin columns remove more lipid-soluble/protein-bound toxic substances, whereas charcoal tends to remove smaller-molecular-weight, water-soluble substances[70,71] A column containing 180 gm of albumin-coated Amberlite XAD-7 was used in a pilot study of 19 patients with fulminant hepatic failure and gave encouraging results with removal of bilirubin, bile acids, and middle molecules.[70] Experiments on absorbents to remove cytokines have shown that this resin can remove tumor necrosis factor and interleukin-6.[72]

Plasma Exchange

Plasma exchange can be performed with centrifuges or membranes. Both therapies effectively remove protein-bound toxins because the affinity for the resin may be greater than the affinity for the circulating protein. Plasmapheresis removes circulating proteins, which are exchanged for fresh frozen plasma or purified derivatives. Amino acids, ouabain-like factors (inhibitors of Na+-K+ATPase), and benzodiazepine-like substances are potential central nervous system toxins that are highly protein-bound.

Artificial Liver System

The artificial liver hepatocyte system is still in the experimental stage, but variations may be clinically available by 1996.[73] Such systems resemble artificial kidney dialyzers or sorbent columns, wherein blood perfuses the system and is exposed directly or indirectly to the hepatocytes in the artificial liver. Thus, they are somewhat similar to hemodialysis with blood pumps, air detection devices, extracorporeal circuitry, and anticoagulation.

Because of poor survival with hepatic support systems, hepatic transplantation has matured and is now considered an appropriate therapeutic option in a subset of patients with fulminant hepatic failure[74] (see chapter 27). As mentioned, continuous hemofiltration and other techniques are used to support the patient while awaiting a donor organ for transplantation.

POTENTIAL ADVANTAGES AND DISADVANTAGES OF DIALYSIS OR HEMOFILTRATION IN PATIENTS WITH DECOMPENSATED LIVER DISEASE

The possible benefits of dialysis or hemofiltration in the setting of HRS include (1) correction of fluid, electrolyte, and acid-base abnormalities; (2) correction of the platelet defect of uremia; and (3) removal of toxic metabolites that may contribute to hepatic (e.g., ammonia, mercaptans, amino acids, and octopamine) and/or uremic encephalopathy (Table 26.6).

Dialysis or hemofiltration may correct fluid overload in patients requiring fluids for the treatment of shock or coagulopathy. In addition, the removal of excessive fluid may permit the daily administration of adequate amounts of parenteral nutrition.

It is unlikely that either modality per se improves the renal perfusion defect associated with end-stage liver disease (HRS). One study[39] has shown that hemodialysis with a large-pore membrane is capable of removing endotoxin fragments from the circulation. Because the etiologic role of endotoxemia in the pathogenesis of HRS remains controversial and because all treated patients in the series of Coratelli et al. had a fatal outcome,[39] we do not anticipate that the benefits of dialytic intervention operate through such a mechanism.

There are numerous complications of dialysis in patients with associated severe acute liver disease. The single most frequently encountered problem is sustained hypotension, which is difficult to correct and often limits the effectiveness of treatment. The cardiovascular instability associated with liver disease is due to many factors, including the contracted effective plasma volume, the hemodynamic effects of ascites, and the frequent development of bleeding and sepsis.

Hemodialysis with a synthetic membrane may result not only in higher middle molecule clearances but also in lesser activation of complement and mononuclear cells.[75] In patients with severe coagulopathy, either (1) hemodialysis with minimal or no heparinization or (2) peritoneal dialysis may be necessary. Because of the potential adverse hemodynamic effects of acetate, bicarbonate should be used as the buffer in the dialysate fluid. Constant monitoring of the central venous pressure is advisable, especially in patients receiving crystalloid or colloid infusions. Vasopressor agents can be used in hypotensive patients who do not respond to plasma volume expansion, but they are often ineffective. Alternatively, continuous techniques such as SCUF or CAVH may be used.[28,58]

MAINTENANCE DIALYSIS IN PATIENTS WITH CHRONIC LIVER DISEASE

Many metabolic complications of liver disease are compounded with the onset of uremia. For example, the platelet defect of uremia may

TABLE 26.6. Theoretical Advantages and Disadvantages of Dialysis in Combined Renal and Hepatic Failure

Advantages	Disadvantages
Correction of fluid and electrolyte disturbances	Dialysis-induced hypotension
Improvement in platelet function	Increased risk of infection
Improvement in hepatic coma	Worsening of coagulopathy
Facilitated administration of nutritional supplements	Lack of correction of ascites
Removal of endotoxin fragments	Changes in drug-protein binding

complicate the coagulopathy of liver disease and contribute to worsening of gastrointestinal bleeding. The anemia of cirrhosis, which is multifactorial in origin, may be aggravated by the bone narrow depression associated with renal failure. Likewise, the immunologic defects of uremia and cirrhosis may be additive, and the need for temporary access devices may further increase the susceptibility to infections.

In a previous edition of this book,[1] we discussed the numerous mechanisms by which the onset of uremia may increase the prevalence of encephalopathy in such patients. Although the initiation of maintenance hemodialysis usually results in an improvement in hepatic encephalopathy, altered mental status may be an intermittent problem in patients with chronic liver disease maintained on hemodialysis.[76–79] Of interest, one report[79] describes a patient in whom repeated episodes of hepatic coma during hemodialysis were obviated after switching to chronic ambulatory peritoneal dialysis.

Control of ascites, especially if present before the onset of renal failure, also becomes a difficult management problem. As mentioned, patients often become hypotensive during attempts at fluid removal with hemodialysis. We recently controlled massive ascites with the PV shunt in a regularly dialyzed patient with liver disease associated with chronic active hepatitis (unpublished observations). Fluid overload was avoided by dialytic ultrafiltration and careful control of posture to control the pressure difference between the venous system and the abdominal cavity. Similar experience was reported by Ghandi et al.[80]

In another report,[34] chronic ambulatory peritoneal dialysis (CAPD) was used to maintain 9 patients with end-stage renal disease, preexisting chronic liver disease, and ascites. Five of the 9 survived at least 18 months with adequate control of ascites and uremic symptoms. Two patients developed chronic right-sided pleural effusions and one developed sclerosing peritonitis.

Finally, utmost care should be taken in the use of medications in patients with combined liver and kidney disease. In addition to the accumulation of the parent drug or active metabolites, such patients may exhibit toxic reactions that are mediated by other mechanisms. For example, both renal failure and liver disease alter the protein binding of several drugs.[81] The clinical consequences of this abnormality are difficult to predict because the resultant increase in "free" level of the drug may be negated by its more rapid total body clearance. The free levels of most protein-bound drugs may be increased by heparinization during hemodialysis.[82] Another mechanism of increased drug toxicity is the presence of underlying disease or dysfunction affecting the target organs of the pharmacologic agent. Of note, altered central nervous system sensitivity to sedative-hypnotic agents is a common problem in these patients.[81] This finding may be related to increases in "free" drug levels, altered permeability of the blood-brain barrier, receptor alterations, and preexisting metabolic encephalopathy.

SUMMARY

Extracorporeal techniques have a defined role in the management of renal complications of liver disease. In patients with intractable ascites, ascites reinfusion, dialytic ultrafiltration of ascites, and continuous hemofiltration may be helpful and may obviate the need for repeated paracentesis or surgical procedures such as the PV shunt, TIPS, or hepatic transplantation. Hemodialysis, hemofiltration, and other extracorporeal techniques may be warranted in patients with acute, potentially reversible liver disease and hepatic coma and in patients undergoing hepatic transplantation. Particular attention should be given to the dialysis prescription and to modification of drug usage in such seriously ill patients.

Acknowledgments. The authors thank Elsa V. Reina and Judy Hunter for their secretarial assistance.

REFERENCES

1. Perez GO, Oster JR: A critical review of the role of dialysis in the treatment of liver disease. In Epstein M (ed): The Kidney in Liver Disease. New York: Elsevier/North-Holland, 1978;325–336.

2. Eknoyan G. Martinez-Maldonado M, Yuim JJ, Suki WN: Combined ascitic fluid infusion and furosemide in the management of ascites. N Engl J Med 1970;282:713–717.

3. Wilkinson SP, Henderson J, Davidson AR: Ascites reinfusion using the Rhodiascit apparatus—clinical experience and coagulation abnormalities. Postgrad Med J 1975;51:583–587.

4. Lee WM: Management of massive ascites utilizing ascites reinfusion. J Clin Gastroenterol 1982;4:87–92.

5. Tawes RL, Rydorak GR, Kennedy PA: Coagulation disorder associated with peritoneovenous shunting. Am J Surg 1981;142:51–55.

6. Wilde JT, Cooper P, Kennedy HJ, et al: Coagulation disturbances following ascites recirculation. J Hepatol 1990;10:217–222.

7. Smart HL, Triger DR: A randomized prospective trial comparing daily paracentesis and intravenous albumin with recirculation in diuretic refractory ascites. J Hepatol 1990;10:191–197.

8. Hariprasad MK, Paul PK, Eisinger RP, et al: Extracorporeal dialysis of ascites: A new technique. Arch Intern Med 1981;141:1550–1551.

9. Adler AJ, Feldman J, Friedman EA, Berlyne GM: Use of extracorporeal ascites dialysis in combined hepatic and renal failure. Nephron 1982;30:31–35.

10. Raju SF, Achord JL: The effects of dialytic ultrafiltration and peritoneal reinfusion in the management of diuretic resistant ascites. Am J Gastroenterol 1984;79:308–312.

11. Landini S, Coli U, Fracasso A, et al: Spontaneous ascites filtration and reinfusion (SAFR) in cirrhotic patients. Int J Artif Organs 1985;8:277–280.

12. Hariprassad MK, Timins E, Eisinger RP, Gary NE: Backflow of albumin from ascites to blood. Dialysis Transplantation 1981;10:608.

13. Van Gossum M, Bergmann P, Burelle A, et al: Evaluation du traitement de l'ascite refractaire par ultrafiltration suivi de reinjection intra-abdominale. Acta Gastroenterol Belg 1983;46:232–239.

14. Brendolan A, La Greca G, Fecondini L, et al: New method of extracorporeal concentration of ascitic fluid as a treatment of refractory ascites. Int J Artif Organs 1989;12:339–344.

15. Cadranel JF, Gargot D, Grippon P, et al: Spontaneous dialytic ultrafiltration with intraperitoneal reinfusion of the concentrate versus large paracentesis in cirrhotic patients with intractable ascites: A randomized study. Int J Artif Organs 1992;15:432–435.

16. Lai KN, Li P, Law E, et al: Large volume paracentesis versus dialytic ultrafiltration in the treatment of cirrhotic ascites. Q J Med 1991;78:33–41.

17. Bruno S, Borzio M, Romagnoni M, et al: Comparison of spontaneous ascites filtration and reinfusion with total paracentesis with intravenous albumin infusion in cirrhotic patients with tense ascites. BMJ 1992;304:1655–1658.

18. Lai KN, Leung JW, Swaminathan R, Panesar NS: Treatment of cirrhotic ascites by dialytic ultrafiltration with a hemofilter system. Blood Purif 1987;5:252–255.

19. Valbonesi M, Torre GC, Capra C, et al: Reverse cascade filtration of ascitic fluid—preliminary results. Int J Artif Organs 1988;11:134–138.

20. Landini S, Coli U, Fracasso A, et al: Spontaneous ascites filtration and reinfusion (SAFR) as ambulatory chronic treatment for hepatorenal syndrome. Trans Am Soc Artif Intern Organs 1985;31:439–443.

21. Assadi FK, Gordon D, Kecskes SA, John E: Treatment of refractory ascites by ultrafiltration-reinfusion of ascitic fluid peritoneally. J Pediatr 1985;106:943–946.

22. Cadranel JF, Grippon P, Gargot D, et al: Spontaneous dialytic ultrafiltration with intraperitoneal reinfusion of the concentrate in 15 cirrhotic patients with intractable ascites. Int J Artif Organs 1992;15:168–171.

23. Brendolan A, Ronco C, Feriani M, et al: Extracorporeal treatment of ascitic fluid and intraperitoneal reinfusion in patients with refractory ascites. Contrib Nephrol 1991;93:241–244.

24. Lai KN, Pun CO, Leung JW: Study of hepatic venous wedge and intraperitoneal pressures in cirrhotic patients with refractory ascites treated by dialytic ultrafiltration. J Gastroenterol Hepatol 1989;4:325–330.

25. Lauer A, Saccaggi A, Ronco C, et al: Continuous arteriovenous-hemofiltration in the critically ill patient: Clinical use and operational characteristics. Ann Intern Med 1983;99:455–460.

26. Paganini E: Continuous replacement modalities in acute renal dysfunction. In Paganini E (ed): Acute Continuous Renal Replacement Therapy. Boston: Martinus Nijhoff, 1986;7–50.

27. Epstein M, Perez GO, Bedoya LA, Molina R: Continuous arteriovenous ultrafiltration in cirrhotic patients with ascites or renal failure. Int J Artif Organs 1986;9:253–256.

28. Kaplan AA: Clinical trials with predilution and vacuum suction enchancing the efficiency of the CAVH treatment. Trans Am Soc Artif Intern Organs 1986;32:49–51.

29. Smith D, Paganini EP, Suhoza K, et al: Nonheparin continuous renal replacement therapy is possible. In Nose Y, Kjellstrand C, Ivanovich P (eds): Progress in Artificial Organs. Cleveland: ISAO Press, 1986;226–230.

30. Conn HO: Transjugular intrahepatic portal-systemic shunts: The state of the art. Hepatology 1993;17:148–158.

31. Ritt DJ, Whelan G, Werner DJ, et al: Acute hepatic necrosis with stupor or coma: An analysis of thirty-one patients. Medicine 1969;48:151–172.

32. Ring-Larsen H, Clausen E, Ranek L: Peritoneal dialysis in hyponatremia due to liver failure. Scand J Gastroenterol 1973;8:33–40.

33. Jacobson S, Bell B: Recognition and management of acute and chronic hepatic encephalopathy. Med Clin North Am 1973;57:1569–1577.

34. Wilkinson SP, Weston MJ, Parsons V, Williams R: Dialysis in the treatment of renal failure in patients with liver disease. Clin Nephrol 1977;8:287–292.

35. Marcus RG, Messana J, Swartz R: Peritoneal dialysis in end-stage renal disease patients with preexisting chronic liver disease and ascites. Am J Med 1992;93:35–40.

36. Poulos AM, Howard L, Eisele G, Rodgers JB: Peritoneal dialysis therapy for patients with liver and renal failure with ascites. Am J Gastroenterol 1993;88:109–112.

37. Topchiashvili ZA, Sergienko VS: Hemodialysis in hepatorenal insufficiency. Khirurgiia 1971;47:14–16.

38. Klingler EL Jr, Cronin RJ: Renal failure in cirrhosis of the liver: Observations during intermittent hemodialysis. Abstracts Am Soc Artif Intern Organs 1972;18:26.

39. Coratelli P, Passavanti G, Munno I, et al: New trends in hepatorenal syndrome. Kidney Int 1985;17:S143–S147.

40. Ellis D, Avner ED: Renal failure and dialysis therapy in children with hepatic failure in the perioperative period of orthotopic liver transplantation. Clin Nephrol 1986;25:295–303.

41. Strand V, Mayor G, Ristow G, et al: Concomitant renal and hepatic failure treated by polyacrylonitrile membrane hemodialysis. Int J Artif Organs 1981;4:136–139.

42. Keller F, Wagner K, Lenz T, et al: Hemodialysis in heptorenal syndrome: Report on two cases. Gut 1985;26:208–211.

43. Kearns PJ, Polhemus RJ, Oakes D, Rabkin R: Hepatorenal syndrome managed with hemodialysis then reversed by peritoneovenous shunting. J Clin Gastroenterol 1985;7:341–343.

44. Landini S, Coli U, Lucatello S, et al: Plasma exchange and dialysis. Combined treatment in acute renal insufficiency secondary to severe hepatopathies. Minerva Nefrol 1981;28:179–186.

45. McCauley J, Van Thiel DH, Starzl TE, Puschett JB: Acute and chronic renal failure in liver transplantation. J Nephron 1990;55:121–128.

46. Seu P, Wilkinson AH, Shaked A, Busuttil RW: The hepatorenal syndrome in liver transplant recipients. Am Surgeon 1991;57:806–809.

47. Haller M, Schonfelder R, Briegel J, et al: Renal function in the postoperative period after orthotopic liver transplantation. Transplant Proc 1992;24:2704–2706.

48. Sankary HN, Foster P, Tuman K, et al: Intraoperative continuous arterio-venous hemofiltration (CAVH)—a method to diminish fluid sequestration during liver transplant operations. Transplant Proc 1989;21:2326–2327.

49. Salord F, Bailly MP, Gaussorgues P, et al: Continuous arteriovenous hemodialysis during emergency hepatic retransplantation: Two case reports. Intens Care Med 1990;16:330–331.

50. Pensado Castineiras A, Gomez-Arnau J, Gonzalez Arevalo A, et al: Continuous intraoperative arteriovenous hemodiafiltration in liver transplantation. Rev Esp Anestesiol Reanim 1991;38:271–273.

51. Gomez-Arnau J, Pensado A, Gonzalez A: Continuous arteriovenous hemodialysis during emergency hepatic retransplantation. Intens Care Med 1991;17:241.

52. Legat K, Zimpfer M, Steltzer H, et al: Heparin and prostacyclin in hemofiltration after orthotopic liver transplantation. Transplant Proc 1991;23:1984.

53. Davenport A, Will EJ, Davison AM: Early changes in intracranial pressure during hemofiltration treatment in patients with grade 4 hepatic encephalopathy and acute oliguric renal failure. Nephrol Dialysis Transplant 1990;5:192–198.

54. Opolon P, Rapin JR, Huguet C: Hepatic failure coma treated by polyacrylonitrile membrane and hemodialysis. Trans Am Soc Artif Intern Organs 1976;22:701.

55. Silk DB, Williams R: Experiences in the treatment of fulminant hepatic failure by conservative therapy, charcoal hemoperfusion and polyacrylonitrile hemodialysis. Int J Artif Organs 1978;1:29–33.

56. Sakai K, Suzuki M, Hirashawa Y, Ichida F: Artificial hepatic support device with polyacrylonitrile (PAN) membrane with special reference to hemodiafiltration. Nippon Rinsho 1982;40:890–896.

57. Opolon P: Large pore hemodialysis in fulminant hepatic failure. In Brunner C, Schmidt FW (eds): Artificial Liver Support. New York: Springer Verlag, 1981;141–146.

58. Mathieu D, Gosselin B, Paris JC, et al: Hemofiltration continue dans le traitement de l'encephalopathie hepatique. Nouv Press Med 1982;11:1921–1925.

59. Davenport A, Will EJ, Losowsky MS, Swindells S: Continuous arteriovenous hemofiltration in patients with hepatic encephalopathy and renal failure. BMJ 1987;295:1028.

60. Rakela J, Kurtz SB, McCarthy JT, et al: Postdilution hemofiltration in the management of acute hepatic failure: A pilot study. Mayo Clin Proc 1988;63:113–118.

61. Splendiani G, Tancredi M, Daniele M, Giammaria U: Treatment of acute liver failure with hemodetoxification techniques. Int J Artif Organs 1990;13:370–374.

62. Matsubara S, Okabe K, Ouchi K, et al: Continuous removal of middle molecules by hemofiltration in patients with acute liver failure. Crit Care Med. 1990;18:1331–1338.

63. Ogawa R, Kishikawa T, Kudo J, et al: Effective continuous hemofiltration and plasma exchange for the treatment of subacute type fulminant hepatic failure. Fukuoka Igaku Zasshi-Fukuoka Acta Medica 1992; 83:338–342.

64. Matsubara S, Okabe K, Ouchi K, et al: Temporary metabolic support by extracorporeal blood therapy for liver failure after surgery. ASAIO Trans 1988;34:266–269.

65. Davenport A: Hemofiltration in patients with fulminant hepatic failure. Lancet 1991;338:1604.

66. Yoshiba M, Yamada H, Yoshikawa Y, et al: Hemodiafiltration treatment of deep hepatic coma by protein passing membrane: Case report. Artif Organs 1986;10:417–419.

67. Davenport A, Will EJ, Losowsky MS: Rebound surges of intracranial pressure as a consequence of forced ultrafiltration used to control intracranial pressure in patients with severe hepatorenal failure. Am J Kidney Dis 1989;14:516–519.

68. Davenport A, Aulton K, Payne RB, Will EJ: Hyperlactatemia and increasing metabolic acidosis in hepatorenal failure treated by hemofiltration. Renal Failure 1990;12:99–101.

69. O'Grady JG, Gimson AES. O'Brien CJ, et al: Controlled trials of charcoal hemoperfusion and prognostic factors in fulminant hepatic failure. Gastroenterol 1988;94:1186–1192.

70. Bihari D, Hughes RD, Gimson AES, et al: Effects of serial resin haemoperfusion in fulminant hepatic failure. Int J Artif Organs 1983;6:299–302, 1983.

71. Ash SR, Blake DE, Carr DH, et al: Clinical effects of a sorbent suspension dialysis system in the treatment of hepatic coma (the Biologic-DT). Int J Artif Organs 1992;15:151–161.

72. Hughes RD, Williams R: Use of sorbent columns and haemofiltration in fulminant hepatic failure. Blood Purif 1993;11:163–169.

73. Sussman NL, Kelly JH: Extracorporeal liver assist in the treatment of fulminant hepatic failure. Blood Purif 1993;11:170–174.

74. Chapman RW, Forman D, Peto R, Smallwood R: Liver transplantation for acute hepatic failure. Lancet 1990; 335:32–35.

75. Chatenoud L, Jungers P, Deschamps-Latscha B: Immunological considerations of the uremic and dialyzed patient. Kidney Int 1994;45(Suppl 44):S92–S96.

76. Oster JR, Perez GO, Materson BJ, et al: Exacerbation of hepatic encephalopathy by chronic renal failure: Response to maintenance hemodialysis. Clin Nephrol 1978;9:254–257.

77. Kaneda H, Haruyama T, Chiba S, et al: A patient with recurrent hepatic encephalopathy and chronic renal failure treated successfully with long-term hemodialysis. Nippon Jinzo Gakkai Shi 1977;19:197–208.

78. Zazgornik J. Kreuzer W, Balcke P, Kopsa H, Schmidt P, Marosi L: Portal hypertension and chronic renal insufficiency. Successful treatment with hemodialysis. Fortschr Med 1981;26:407–409.

79. Segaert MF, Carlier B, Verbanck J: Recurrent hepatic coma in a chronic hemodialysis patient: Successful treatment by CAPD. Perit Dial Bull 1984;4:32–34.

80. Gandhi VC, Leehey DJ, Stanley MM, et al: Peritoneo-venous shunting in patients with cirrhotic ascites and end-stage renal failure. Am J Kidney Dis 1985; 6:185–187.

81. Bennett WM: Altering drug dose in patients with diseases of the kidney or liver. In Anderson RJ, Schrier RW (eds): Clinical Use of Drugs in Patients with Kidney and Liver Disease. Philadelphia: W.B. Saunders, 1981;16–29.

82. Kessler KM, Perez GO: Decreases in quinidine plasma protein binding associated with hemodialysis. Clin Pharmacol Exp Ther 1981;30:121–126.

Chapter 27

LIVER TRANSPLANTATION AND RENAL FUNCTION: RESULTS IN PATIENTS WITH AND WITHOUT HEPATORENAL SYNDROME

THOMAS A. GONWA, M.D., F.A.C.P.
ALAN H. WILKINSON, M.D.

Intra- and Perioperative Concerns
Renal Function after Liver Transplantation

Liver Transplantation in Patients with Hepatorenal Syndrome
Combined Liver-Kidney Transplantation

Liver transplantation has moved from the realm of hopeful experimentation to become a successful and accepted treatment for almost all patients with end-stage liver disease. The success is due largely to improvements in surgical technique and immunosuppression combined with practical experience. It is clear that almost all patients with end-stage liver disease have some degree of renal dysfunction, which, as outlined in previous chapters, ranges from functional abnormalities associated with liver disease to hepatorenal syndrome. In addition, multiple acid-base and electrolyte disturbances are associated with liver disease. All of these factors must be taken into account before transplantation in the patient with liver disease; recognition and correction of many abnormalities are possible. In addition, the occasional patient with combined end-stage liver disease and end-stage renal disease must be considered for combined liver-kidney transplantation. This chapter does not address preoperative issues, which are well outlined elsewhere in this textbook. Rather, it addresses four main areas:

1. The intra- and postoperative changes in renal function and fluid and electrolyte status, knowledge of which is crucial for appropriate care to be given to the patient;

2. The effect of liver transplantation on native renal function, including the toxic effect of immunosuppressive agents;

3. The outcome of liver transplantation in patients with hepatorenal syndrome (see previous chapters for the etiology and pathogenesis of hepatorenal syndrome); and

4. Combined liver-kidney transplantation, including indications and results.

Evaluation prior to transplant is aimed at identifying patients with moderate-to-severe renal insufficiency. The major immunosuppressives used after transplant (cyclosporine and FK506) adversely affect renal function with a 30–50% decline in glomerular filtration rate (GFR). It is therefore important to evaluate the pretransplant status of the patient. A determination of GFR by a method other than creatinine clearance is imperative, because the creatinine clearance method may overestimate inulin clearance by a factor of two in patients with severe liver disease.[1] Pretransplant evaluation allows the clinician to identify patients who may benefit from modification of the immunosuppressive protocol in the immediate posttransplant period, patients with hepatorenal syndrome, and patients with intrinsic renal disease who may require combined renal-liver transplant. Evaluation of the patient with intrinsic renal disease is particularly crucial; combined transplant should be reserved for patients with signs of advanced disease in both organ systems. Combined transplant is not indicated for hepatorenal syndrome, as outlined below. The patient suffering from liver disease may have reasons for renal failure other than associated liver disease, such as diabetes, obstruction, or glomerulonephritis. Occasionally, the patient with end-stage renal disease and hepatitis B or C may need a combined transplant. Other etiologies of intrinsic renal disease associated with liver disease are well outlined in previous chapters. Volume status of patients waiting for liver transplantation should be monitored carefully. Because clinical assessment may be misleading, central venous pressure monitoring should be used whenever there is uncertainty. A rapid and irreversible decline in renal function may be caused by reduction in effective plasma volume from overaggressive use of diuretics, aggressive paracentesis, or volume depletion secondary to lactulose therapy. Once a patient is accepted for liver transplantation and the baseline renal function is determined, careful monitoring for deterioration should be maintained. When possible, the use of nephrotoxic antibiotics and nonsteroidal antiinflammatory drugs (NSAIDs) should be avoided before transplantation. Nephrotoxic antibiotics may be more nephrotoxic in patients with liver failure,[2,3] and the NSAIDs may adversely affect the delicate renal dynamic balance in patients with liver disease.

INTRA- AND PERIOPERATIVE CONCERNS

The liver transplant operation is divided into three phases. In phase 1 (the preanhepatic phase), the liver is resected while normal circulation is maintained. The end of phase 1 is characterized by altered hemodynamics, increased sympathetic nerve activity, and suboptimal renal perfusion. All of these changes must be addressed by the anesthesiologist during the operation. The operative technique and intraoperative fluid management have been crucial in decreasing the impact of such changes on renal function. At the end of phase 1, the inferior vena cava is clamped above the renal veins. Clamping by itself may increase renal venous pressure, reduce renal perfusion, and result in hypoperfusion and possible acute renal failure. In phase 2 (the anhepatic phase) the liver is removed. Most surgeons now use venovenous bypass, redirecting blood flow from the inferior vena cava and the portal vein to the central circulation, usually via the subclavian vein. This approach offers three major advantages: (1) renal

congestion is reduced, (2) hemodynamic stability is improved, and (3) the portal circulation drains to the central circulation, thus avoiding build-up of toxic metabolites. Perioperative renal function during liver transplantation with venovenous bypass has been evaluated extensively. During phase 1 clamping, the inferior vena cava pressures become elevated, but mean arterial pressures are also increased so that renal perfusion pressure is maintained. Venovenous bypass improves maintenance of urine output during all three phases of the operation.[4]

A study of 13 patients undergoing venovenous bypass found no significant alteration in systemic hemodynamics and no sustained decrease in blood pressure. Such results emphasize the necessity of superb anesthesiology care. When changes in norepinephrine, epinephrine, and dopamine (used as indirect measures of sympathetic nerve activity) were studied, baseline levels were similar to those reported in cirrhotic patients. The arteriovenous norepinephrine values were not significantly different during any of the three phases of the transplant operation, implying that renal sympathetic nerve activity was constant throughout the procedure.[5] Venovenous bypass thus maintains stability of renal hemodynamics. Furthermore, when the GFR was measured immediately before surgery, on day 1, and 1 week after transplant, no significant change. was found. Therefore, the decline in renal function in most patients at 2–3 months after transplantation is not due to intraoperative factors but may be related to the posttransplant course, particularly the administration of various immunosuppressives.

Phase 3 of the liver transplant operation is the reperfusion phase. Before the introduction of venovenous bypass, this phase was characterized by a marked rise in serum potassium concentration, believed to be due to the release of the portal blood. This rise is less frequent with the use of venovenous bypass but may still occur.

Changes also may occur in calcium, other electrolytes, glucose, and acid-base physiology.[6–13] Many patients with severe liver disease have a reduction in both total and ionized calcium. During the operation ionized calcium may decline further.[6,7] Occasionally, hypercalcemia is found. Gerhardt et al. described a group of 16 patients with advanced liver disease and hypercalcemia. The authors believed that most of the patients had mild-to-moderate renal failure, but neither hyperparathyroidism nor hypervitaminosis D was present.[13] Parathyroidlike hormone may be produced by patients with hepatocellular carcinoma, who thus may develop marked elevations in serum calcium that are not a consequence of skeletal metastatic disease.[14] Such patients occasionally present for liver transplantation if the work-up for metastatic disease is totally negative. The hypercalcemia may be resistant to usual therapy, including mithramycin, calcitonin and other agents. Removal of the tumor by hepatectomy and subsequent liver transplantation control the hypercalcemia. During transplantation and the interim postoperative period, ionized calcium levels must be closely monitored.

During the preanhepatic phase, portal hypertension, coagulation defects, and thrombocytopenia may result in massive blood loss; infusion of large volumes of citrated blood, however, may lead to rapid chelation of calcium and a lowering of the ionized calcium level. In addition, abnormal liver function in a newly transplanted liver impairs the ability to convert citrate to an equivalent amount of bicarbonate, freeing the bound calcium. By the end of phase 1, citrate levels have usually reached a maximum. Vigorous calcium supplementation is not required at this time, although mild hypocalcemia may occur. If the calculated calcium deficit is replaced, profound hypercalcemia may develop when the new liver converts the citrate to bicarbonate, releasing the chelated calcium. Regular intraoperative monitoring using ionized calcium-specific electrodes and empiric replacement is recommended.[6,15,16]

Care must be taken to monitor the ionized calcium during the anhepatic phase. Levels as low as 0.6 mmol/L have been reported, and the risks of myocardial depression and left ventricular dysfunction are increased.[15] Once the old liver has been removed, plasma citrate levels may rise to extremely high levels. The use of venovenous bypass also increases hemodilution and dilutes the level of ionized calcium. Once the new liver is implanted and the reperfusion phase has started, donor liver perfusion fluid is released into the circulation . This fluid, which is usually hypothermic, acidic, and hyperkalemic, is released when the patient is at increased risk for developing systemic hypotension and cardiac arrhythmias. If calcium and fluid replacement are not sufficient, problems may occur. As a result, many centers discard the perfusion fluid rather than allow it to enter the circulation, thus minimizing complications. Occasionally, continuous

arteriovenous hemofiltration (CAVH) or continuous arteriovenous hemodialysis (CAVHD) may be used intraoperatively to maintain electrolyte and volume stability more effectively.

When the donor liver has been reperfused, it metabolizes citrate, releasing bicarbonate and calcium. If it is functioning properly, continued transfusion of blood products does not lower the ionized calcium further. Occasionally, if massive transfusions have been used, the syndrome of metabolic alkalosis and hypercalcemia may develop postoperatively as the metabolism of citrate increases. Such abnormalities usually correct in 36–48 hours in the presence of normal renal function and may be improved by the use of saline diuresis. Dialysis against a calcium-free dialysate may be necessary in the rare patient with abnormal renal function postoperatively.

Munoz et al. described an unusual complication of such derangements in calcium homeostasis. In 7 patients they observed posttransplant calcification in the lungs, liver graft, colon, vascular wall, kidneys, adrenals, and gastric mucosa.[17] Five of the patients had renal failure, emphasizing the importance of correcting hyperphosphatemia. All of the patients had received marked amounts of blood products and showed elevated parathyroid hormone levels, which peaked during the second week. Others have described similar patients.[18]

Most liver transplant recipients are mildly hypokalemic at the time of surgery, unless renal failure has occurred, because of the heavy use of diuretics in the pretransplant phase. During the initial phases of surgery potassium concentrations remain stable.[6,7,10,19] As mentioned above, the serum potassium concentration may rise abruptly if the liver perfusate is allowed into circulation or if venovenous bypass is not used. This rise is transient but may be associated with cardiac arrest. As the new liver begins to function, potassium reenters the hepatocytes. The Mayo Clinic has reported that 56% of patients required some potassium supplementation postoperatively.[8] In addition, changes in glucose concentration may alter the potassium concentration.[9] Many postoperative patients require further potassium supplementation due to losses from nasogastric, biliary, and ascitic drainage. If significant metabolic alkalosis occurs, further renal losses may be magnified. Attention to potassium concentration is necessary to maintain adequate respiratory muscle function in these already weakened patients.

Hyponatremia is common in patients awaiting liver transplantation. During surgery chronic hyponatremia may be corrected over a period of hours.[6] Whether such rapid correction contributes to postoperative neurologic changes is not known. Correlation between preoperative serum sodium concentration or rate of change in serum sodium concentration and postoperative neurologic impairment has not been demonstrated. However, in one case autopsy evidence of pontine myelinolysis was described at autopsy. Whether this is due to rapid correction of chronic hyponatremia is not known.[20]

Hypomagnesemia is common in patients awaiting liver transplants, possibly because of use of diuretics. During surgery levels of magnesium have been noted to decline further.[6,7] Postoperative use of cyclosporine may increase renal magnesium losses. Careful attention must be paid to decreased magnesium levels, which may be associated with convulsions. Furthermore, in patients receiving cyclosporine, seizures and hypertension are more common in hypomagnesemic patients. The effect of hypomagnesemia may be particularly magnified in patients with low serum cholesterol concentrations, which often are due to a malfunctioning graft or preoperative status and have been inversely correlated with seizures.[20–24]

Phosphate levels are usually normal or low in patients awaiting transplantation.[6] Postoperative use of cyclosporine has been known to cause renal phosphate wasting, which may be aggravated by diuretics and extracellular volume expansion. If severe metabolic alkalosis occurs with conversion of citrate to bicarbonate, bicarbonate excretion may increase, further promoting renal phosphate excretion. Antacids are used commonly after surgery to prevent gastric erosions. If aluminum-containing antacids are used with magnesium antacids, phosphate levels may be depleted. Even patients with severe renal failure may have very low levels of phosphate, which impair muscle strength and adversely affect the ability to be weaned from ventilatory support. Furthermore, the risk of rhabdomyolysis may increase with extremely low levels of phosphate.

Potential recipients have mixed respiratory alkalosis and mild metabolic acidosis, particularly those with various degrees of functional renal failure preoperatively. Spironolactone commonly produces a mild renal tubular acidosis and hyperkalemia in such patients. Abnormalities are rapidly corrected during surgery as the patient is transfused with citrate-containing blood and artificially ventilated. Careful measurement of hydrogen ion and lactate concentrations demonstrates an intraoperative rise, and transfusion of bicarbonate is occasionally required to maintain normal pH.[7,10,11] However, as mentioned above, the newly engrafted liver corrects the acidosis as it generates bicarbonate from the accumulated citrate.[6,25] If postoperative metabolic alkalosis is severe, the risk of ventricular arrhythmias is increased, not only because of nasogastric drainage, biliary losses, and metabolism of citrate and lactate, but also because of infusion of excessive acetate in parenteral nutrition solutions and diuretic use. Patients who are extubated early may continue to generate respiratory alkalosis due to decreased diaphragmatic movement and increased respiratory drive. Occasionally, alkalemia may impair cellular metabolism and suppress respiratory drive, thus delaying extubation. Careful attention to ventilator settings must be maintained to adjust concentrations of carbon dioxide. Many programs recommend correction of the elevated arterial pH by constant infusion of hydrochloric acid (150 mmol/L) at a rate that maintains the pH at less than 7.5 or dialysis with a low bicarbonate or sodium chloride dialysate in patients who cannot tolerate further volume expansion. Care must be taken because of experimental evidence that intravenous infusion of 0.3 mol of hydrochloric acid may raise pulmonary artery pressures.[26] This is of theoretical concern because some transplant recipients may have pulmonary hypertension preoperatively.

RENAL FUNCTION AFTER LIVER TRANSPLANTATION

The introduction of cyclosporine improved patient and graft survival after liver transplantation. It was realized early in the experience with cyclosporine that nephrotoxicity was among the major side effects. In an early report using only serum chemistries, severe acute renal dysfunction was seen early in the postoperative course in 21% of adult and 22% of pediatric liver transplant recipients.[27] Attempts to correlate renal dysfunction with pretransplant course demonstrated an increased association of renal impairment with preexisting renal impairment, shock, graft failure, and infection.[27] The authors reported increased mortality in patients with postoperative renal dysfunction. Serum chemistries alone underestimate the severity of renal impairment. Nuclear medicine scanning, which has been used successfully to identify cyclosporine nephrotoxicity, has demonstrated a reduction in renal perfusion prior to the rise in serum creatinine.[28] This reduction, however, is difficult to quantitate, and determination of GFR provides a more accurate measurement of the degree of renal dysfunction after liver transplant. GFR has been quantitated most extensively in patients treated with cyclosporine.[29–33]

The exact mechanism of cyclosporine nephrotoxicity is not known. However, it is known that cyclosporine affects renal hemodynamics and has a direct tubular cell toxicity. An immediate fall in GFR has been seen after introduction of cyclosporine.[29,31] This finding has been well documented in our series from Dallas, which used iothalamate clearance studies.[30] The GFR fell in the first 6 weeks postoperatively by almost 40%. However, up to 4 years after transplantation renal function has been stable despite maintenance of cyclosporine therapy (Figure 27.1). The course is similar to that seen in renal transplant patients maintained on long-term cyclosporine. Other studies have documented stable, but impaired, long-term renal function with measurements of GFR.[31,33] We were unable to correlate use of other nephrotoxic agents (e.g., amphotericin and aminoglycosides), sepsis, shock, infection, intensive care status, or any other factor known to affect renal function with severity of decline in posttransplant kidney function.[29] Evidence of vascular changes, including arterial and arteriolar nephrosclerosis, has been obtained on renal biopsies. In addition, glomerular ischemic changes with mild-to-moderate tubulointerstitial changes have been seen but did not appear to correlate with degree of renal function impairment.[31]

Cyclosporine has been studied extensively in experimental animals and in humans. It is clear that the hallmark of cyclosporine toxicity is renal vasoconstriction, particularly of the afferent arteriole. Cyclosporine has been shown to affect not only the prostaglandin system but also endothelin and renal sympathetic nerve activity,[34–36] all of which play a role in renal vasoconstriction. Increased urinary prostaglandin excretion has been demonstrated in experimental models of cyclosporine nephrotoxicity. Renal production of all major metabolites, including thromboxane B_2, $(TxB)_2$, prostaglandin E_2, and prostacyclin, appears to be increased, as do urinary excretion

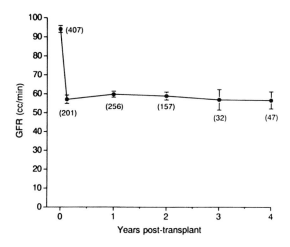

FIGURE 27.1   Average glomerular filtration rate in patients undergoing orthotopic liver transplant. Time points are pretransplant, 4–6 weeks postoperatively, and yearly thereafter.

rates.[37–39] In some experimental models prostaglandin E_1 (a renovasodilator) in the form of its analog misoprostol has been shown to reverse significantly the renal effects of cyclosporine, leading to an increase in GFR and a decrease in renovascular resistance.[40,41] Whether it will be useful in long-term treatment of patients following liver transplant is not currently known. Many such patients cannot tolerate these agents because of associated hypotension. Textor et al.[46] found elevated concentrations of prostacyclin and TXB_2 in pretransplant patients with hepatic cirrhosis. Following liver transplantation the levels of both metabolites decreased, but the concentration of prostacyclin fell below normal, resulting in an increased TXB_2/prostacyclin ratio, which tends to lead to vasoconstriction and may account for decreased renal function. The same group also found transient rises in endothelin, which may contribute to renal vasoconstriction. Studies in rats[35,36] and in humans[38,45,46] demonstrate abnormal renal hemodynamics. Administration of cyclosporine leads to a fall in effective renal plasma flow and a rise in renal vascular resistance. It has been nicely demonstrated in rats that both findings are due to the effect of cyclosporin A on renal sympathetic activity. Such studies indicate that the patient coming to liver transplant is primed to respond adversely to cyclosporine. The introduction of cyclosporine too early or in high amounts may aggravate the abnormal renal function already found in patients awaiting liver transplantation.

Maintenance of adequate volume status, monitoring to avoid excessively high cyclosporine concentrations, and avoidance of potentially nephrotoxic insults are important in preventing early cyclosporine toxicity. Glomerular afferent vasoconstriction has been increased by the use of amphotericin, which may compound the vasoconstrictive effects of cyclosporine. Pharmacologic manipulation to avoid cyclosporine toxicity has met with partial success in renal transplantation. Long-term use of oral misoprostol has improved renal function.[41]

A retrospective study[47] indicated that low-dose dopamine improves renal function as measured by creatinine clearance and urine volumes in the immediate postoperative period, but this finding was not confirmed by a randomized, double-blind, placebo-controlled study.[48] Blood flow may be improved by furosemide, and its use is still recommended in the early phase of acute renal failure and in posttransplant renal dysfunction.[49] Although no good evidence suggests that furosemide ameliorates the long-term decline in renal function associated with liver transplantation, it is useful in the postoperative management of patients who require large volumes of intravenous fluid therapy. Calcium channel blockers, which are approved for treatment of heart failure and hypertension, have been shown to reduce cyclosporine nephrotoxicity in renal transplant recipients.[50,51] A recent controlled, double-blind, randomized trial,[52] however, failed to demonstrate this effect with use of verapamil. Furthermore, a randomized trial of verapamil in liver transplant patients failed to show any amelioration of cyclosporine toxicity.[5] Prophylactic anti–T-cell regimens have been advocated in patients with preoperative renal dysfunction or in all patients undergoing liver transplantation. However, published studies indicate that although such regimens improve serum creatinine at 4 days, they do not maintain renal function at 12 months compared with untreated patients.[53–55] In patients with and without anti–T-cell regimens no difference was found in serum creatinine, rate of rejection, or patient or graft survival. Therefore, such agents should be reserved for the treatment of acute rejection.

The timing and mode of delivery of cyclosporine may also be important. One study of verapamil, in which cyclosporine was administered only after reperfusion of the liver, found no difference in pretransplant, day-1, or day-7 GFR.[5]

In a second study from the same group, however, cyclosporine was administered preoperatively, and verapamil did not prevent a significant fall in GFR from preoperative values.[56]

All of the above findings emphasize the fact that preoperative renal vascular tone is complexly regulated in cirrhotic patients. Studies indicate that prostaglandins, renal sympathetic activity, and endothelin are important factors.[56–67] Derangements of these systems lead to variable pretransplant decreases in GFR, and the patient comes to surgery with abnormal renal vascular regulation. Thus, shifts in the complex balance of vasodilatory and vasoconstrictive regulatory hormones in the posttransplant period, brought about by cyclosporine[37,68°72] or other factors, result in renal dysfunction.

Clearly cyclosporine is nephrotoxic postoperatively. No study indicates that this nephrotoxicity can be avoided, nor is there a clearcut indication of pharmacologic prevention. Patients with worse preoperative (non-HRS) renal function appear to be more sensitive to the effects of cyclosporine and have worse long-term function.[29] When one examines the renal outcome in patients with different degrees of preoperative renal dysfunction, marked differences are seen. Individualizing cyclosporine dosage and using triple therapy with azathioprine in patients with the worst preoperative renal function (GFR = 47 ± 17, n = 100) preserved renal function at 1 year (GFR = 45 ± 15 ml/min). Patients with the best renal function (GFR = 140 ± 20 ml/min, n = 100) had the most dramatic fall in function by 1 year (GFR = 68 ± 17 ml/min). This finding may reflect the aggressive use of cyclosporine and reliance on the measurement of serum creatinine in such patients. Patients with the best renal function had rises in serum creatinine of only 0.8–1.3, leading the physicians to underestimate impairment. There was no difference in patient survival or rejection rate between the two groups.[73]

The introduction of cyclosporine into clinical practice led to major gains in liver transplantation. A new and powerful immunosuppressive agent has come on the scene, the macrolide antibiotic FK506.[74] One prospective study indicates that it may be better than cyclosporine for prevention of rejection.[74] FK506 shares a similar immunosuppressive spectrum with cyclosporine and, unfortunately, also shares many of its toxic features. Nephrotoxicity has been reported to be comparable for both drugs. A number of liver transplant centers participated in prospective, randomized trials of FK506 vs. cyclosporine during the initial postoperative period. Such studies demonstrated similar degrees of posttransplant renal dysfunction as measured by serum creatinine and GFR.[74–76] FK506 has been used for some time at the University of Pittsburgh in liver transplant patients, and results have been conflicting. The invariable perioperative increase in serum creatinine ranged from 0.5–2 mg/dl. However, 76% of patients had values under 2.0 mg/dl at 1 week postoperatively. Of 282 patients, 43 required dialysis in the early or late postoperative period.[77–79] Winkler et al. studied 30 liver transplant patients and found that an increase in serum creatinine of more than 50% was associated with an elevation of FK506 plasma levels. The acute nephrotoxicity was readily reversible, responding rapidly to reduction in the FK506 dosage.[80] The authors found that 10 of 11 patients with clinical toxicity had plasma levels of FK506 above 1 ng/ml. In a recently presented study, reduction in GFR 1 year after transplantation correlated with yearly mean FK506 plasma level but not with dose.[81] In patients with a yearly plasma level less than 0.6 ng/ml, the GFR declined trivially compared with patients with higher mean levels. As in the case of cyclosporine, function of the transplant has important effects on the plasma level profile of FK506. The parent compound and its metabolites are excreted in the bile, and elevations of bilirubin levels are often associated with the accumulation of FK506 and increased toxicity.[82]

In a retrospective study measuring effective renal plasma flow and GFR, Tauxe et al. found significantly less renal dysfunction with FK506 than with cyclosporine.[83] In studies from the University of Pittsburgh, 121 patients were converted from cyclosporine to FK506 because of various toxicities.[77] Levels of serum creatinine. differed according to the reason for conversion. If patients were converted because of presumed renal insufficiency resulting from cyclosporine, there appeared to be a fall in serum creatinine. However, if the patient was treated because of nonresponsive acute allograft rejection, there appeared to be a rise in serum creatinine. The difference may be due to more aggressive treatment with FK506 in the second group of patients. Such studies are relatively short-term, and the long-term effects of FK506 on renal function have yet to be determined. It is not known whether renal function will remain stable after the initial insult and decline in GFR, as has been the case with cyclosporine.

The mechanism for FK506 nephrotoxicity is unknown but appears to be similar to that of cyclosporine. There is an impairment in renal blood flow, which may be reversed with vasodilators. A preliminary study combining FK506 with intravenous prostagalndin E_1 in liver transplant recipients found improved renal function as measured by serum creatinine.[84] To determine whether this strategy will effectively combat renal toxicity in liver transplant recipients requires additional clinical trials. FK506 appears to enhance the production of endothelin in human mesangial and tubular epithelial cells.[85–87] This finding may explain the increased renovascular resistance in transplant patients. In addition, decreased renal cortical blood flow has been demonstrated in mice,[88] but studies in rats have shown no differences in GFR or effective renal plasma flow.[89] Morphologic studies in rat kidneys following FK506 administration demonstrated juxtaglomerular cell transformation and juxtaglomerular cell hyperplasia, both of which are consistent with renal hypoperfusion. In addition, the studies found vacuolization of proximal tubular cells and large granules with a positive periodic acid-Schiff (PAS) reaction.[89]

LIVER TRANSPLANTATION IN PATIENTS WITH HEPATORENAL SYNDROME

The pathogenesis of hepatorenal syndrome is outlined in chapter 3. Before the introduction of liver transplantation it was believed that patients suffering from true hepatorenal syndrome had a uniformly fatal course. Spontaneous recoveries from hepatorenal syndrome were believed to be rare.[90] The true functional nature of hepatorenal syndrome was suggested in studies by Koppel et al., which demonstrated that the transplantation of cadaveric kidneys from patients with hepatorenal syndrome functioned normally in the milieu of a normal liver.[91] Early in 1973 Iwatsuki et al. published the first report of recovery from hepatorenal syndrome after orthotopic liver transplantation.[92] This report offered hope that liver transplantation may treat successfully this previously fatal disease. Later studies in pediatric patients by Wood et al. demonstrated the reversal of hepatorenal syndrome after successful orthotopic liver transplantation.[93]

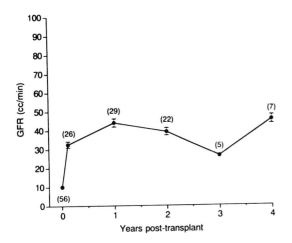

FIGURE 27.2. Average glomerular filtration rate in patients with hepatorenal syndrome undergoing orthotopic liver transplant. Time points are pre-transplant, 4–6 weeks postoperatively, and yearly thereafter.

We previously reported a large series of patients with hepatorenal syndrome.[94] This series now includes 59 patients.[73] When comparing these patients to patients without hepatorenal syndrome (n = 513), we found that they were more likely to be ICU-bound prior to transplant (HRS vs. non-HRS = 61% vs. 12%, p < 0.001) and to require preoperative dialysis (14% vs. 0.4%, p < .0001). Compared with patients without hepatorenal syndrome, patients with HRS had significantly lower preoperative GFRs. In 59 patients with HRS transplanted since 1986, the average GFR has been 14 ± 12 ml/min. Patients without hepatorenal syndrome in our series had a preoperative GFR of 94.1 ± 37 ml/min (see Fig. 27.1). The only other preoperative laboratory value that differed between the two groups has been the bilirubin level (17.2 mg/dl in patients with HRS vs. 9.37 mg/dl in patients without HRS, p = 0.007). Higher hepatic arterial and portal venous resistances were noted in patients with HRS during the intraoperative phase.[95] Whether this finding reflects increased sympathetic tone in hepatic nerves is not known.

Because cyclosporine may increase efferent sympathetic renal nerve activity, vasoconstrictor prostanoids, and endothelin, the renovascular bed in patients with hepatorenal syndrome is primed to respond adversely to early introduction of cyclosporine. The renal vasoconstriction can be demonstrated by duplex Doppler sonography.[96–98] This technique may prove useful in predicting which patients may respond adversely to cyclosporine. As mentioned earlier, all of these renal vascular regulators are increased by cyclosporine.[37,38,68–71] If no cyclosporine is given over the first 48–72 hours following liver transplantation, there is a period for the kidneys to recover from regulatory abnormalities. Some centers recommend withholding cyclosporine until normal renal function has been reestablished. Use of azathioprine or steroid immunosuppression without the addition of T-cell agents has proved successful in our center. In the early postoperative period, anti–T-cell reagents, particularly OKT3, may result in hypotension further aggravating renal dysfunction. These agents may be used if renal function does not improve over 72 hours and patients have regained hemodynamic stability. This protocol usually results in resumption of good renal function within 48–72 hours postoperatively.

Figure 27.2 demonstrates the return of renal function as measured by GFR. Note that the GFR returns toward normal by 6 weeks but does not reach levels in patients without hepatorenal syndrome patients (see Fig. 27.1). Postoperatively, patients with hepatorenal syndrome spend more days in the ICU (17.7 days vs. 6.4, p < .0001) and have a higher rate of postoperative dialysis (nearly 35% vs. 5%). Surprisingly, the incidence of rejection was somewhat lower in our series of patients with hepatorenal syndrome (HRS vs. non-HRS = 31.6% vs. 59.5%, p = 0.02).[94] Whether this finding reflects the immunosuppressive properties of the uremic state is not known. Figure 27.3 outlines the 4-year survival rate in patients with and without hepatorenal syndrome. The 4-year actuarial survival rate of 60% in patients with hepatorenal syndrome is a major step forward in treatment compared with previous results (100% mortality).

In our studies, only 7% of patients with hepatorenal syndrome have progressed to end-stage renal disease during the postoperative period compared with 1.5% of recipients without hepatorenal syndrome.[73] The liver transplant group at U.C.L.A. reported similar results. Postoperative dialysis was required in 46% of patients presenting with hepatorenal syndrome, and another 20% developed reversible episodes of renal dysfunction. Modification of the protocol dropped the overall incidence of postoperative dialysis to 20%. The investigators found no difference in the survival of patients with hepatorenal syndrome who required preoperative dialysis and the group as a whole. Less than 1% of patients with hepatorenal syndrome required long-term dialysis, with no statistical difference between patients with and without hepatorenal syndrome.[99,100] These and similar results from Dallas again stress the excellent prognosis for patients who receive a liver transplant.

Patients with hepatorenal syndrome can be expected to recover renal function. Of over 800 patients undergoing transplantation in Dallas, 59 had hepatorenal syndrome. Of the patients surviving liver transplant, 4 required subsequent renal transplant for nonreturn of function. Of the remaining patients without hepatorenal syndrome (over 650), 2 required subsequent kidney transplant (1 for nonreversible acute renal failure and 1 for progressive polycystic kidney disease). Only 6 other patients have progressed to chronic renal failure or end-stage renal disease: 3 because of chronic cyclosporine toxicity, 1 because of nonrecoverable acute renal failure after a ruptured thoracic aortic aneurysm, 1 because of progressive polycystic kidney disease, and 1 because of progressive chronic interstitial nephritis. The treatment of choice for hepatorenal syndrome, therefore, may be liver transplantation.

The results from Dallas and other centers clearly indicate that patients with HRS have good survival rates following liver transplant but that the rates are statistically inferior compared with patients without HRS. Do other degrees of preoperative renal dysfunction carry the same risk? Early reports of successful liver transplantation emphasized the negative impact of renal impairment on survival following liver transplantation.[101,102] A more recent report confirmed the finding. Baliga et al. at the University of Michigan reviewed their experience in 224 consecutive adult recipients of liver transplant.[103] They found that preoperative renal dysfunction was significantly associated with sepsis and reflected higher hospital mortality rates. They defined renal dysfunction as a serum creatinine of more than 1.7 mg/dl. Similarly, a review of the UNOS database covering over 19,000 liver transplants performed in the U.S. between 1988–1994 demonstrates that patients with preoperative creatinine > 2.0 mg/dl had a 2-year survival rate of 55% compared with 80% in patients with preoperative creatinine < 1 mg/dl.[103a]

In contrast to the above data is our experience in Dallas with over 800 transplants. In patients without HRS, we find no influence of preoperative renal dysfunction on postoperative survival.[73]

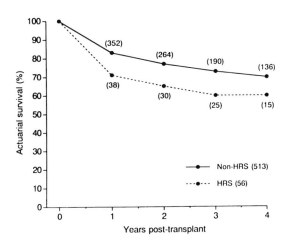

FIGURE 27.3. Actuarial patient survival following orthotopic liver transplantation in patients with and without hepatorenal syndrome.

When we divided patients into those with and without serum creatinines >1.7 mg dl, we found no significant difference in survival rate[73] compared with the data from the University of Michigan.

How can one reconcile such differences? First, one must be careful to exclude patients with HRS from analysis, because they already have a significantly decreased chance of survival. Secondly, preoperative renal dysfunction may not be a risk factor by itself but may be a marker predisposing the patient to another complication that decreases survival. In the Michigan series, preoperative renal dysfunction made patients more likely to develop sepsis. In our stepwise logistic regression analysis of survival in patients with infection and bleeding,[104,105] preoperative renal dysfunction was a risk factor for increased rate of infection and increased bleeding during surgery. Both of these were risk factors for increased mortality. Thus, although renal dysfunction (short of HRS) is not per se a risk factor for increased mortality, it may put patients at increased risk for other complications that increase mortality.

COMBINED LIVER-KIDNEY TRANSPLANTATION

During the pretransplant evaluation of patients with liver disease a reduced GFR is often found. In most cases, this can be attributed to the functional renal failure associated with liver disease or hepatorenal syndrome. However, in some patients the diagnosis is not definite and the possibility of intrinsic or fixed renal disease is entertained. There are also patients who have end-stage renal disease for various reasons and then develop end-stage liver disease, most commonly after necrotic cirrhosis but can take many forms. Previous chapters have outlined the intrinsic renal disease that may be associated with liver disease. The effect of renal failure on the morbidity and cost of liver transplantation has encouraged the development of a combined liver-kidney transplant. This procedure is not indicated in patients with hepatorenal syndrome or acute tubular necrosis who can be expected to recover renal function following liver transplantation. The course of liver transplantation in hepatorenal syndrome is outlined above, and the authors strongly recommend that such patients receive liver transplants only. If a subsequent kidney transplant is needed because of nonrecovery of function (< 10%), it can be entertained after the patient has stabilized. It may take as long as 6–8 weeks after successful liver transplantation for renal function to recover in patients with hepatorenal syndrome.

Primary hyperoxaluria [106–110] is one of the most common indications for combined kidney-liver transplant, which leads to excellent results. Studies have shown reversal of cardiac dysfunction secondary to primary hyperoxaluria.[109] After transplant urinary oxalate excretion is excessive, and care should be taken to maintain optimal urinary output.[106,109] In addition, the oxalate osteopathy that is often severe in such patients while they are on dialysis can be shown to reverse after successful liver-kidney transplantation.[110] Most such transplants occur in the pediatric population but have been reported in adults.

Before 1988, a few centers had presented preliminary results in combined liver-kidney transplantation for various indications.[111–115] The series were small but demonstrated the utility of the procedure. We initially reported results in 7 patients who underwent combined liver-kidney transplantation, all of whom had an excellent course.[116] Encouraged by this initial success, we continued to use the procedure in selected patients. We have now performed 26 combined liver-kidney transplants in 25 patients. The actuarial 4-year survival rate is 59%. Other centers have reported similar results.[117,118] Gil-Vernet et al.[118] in Spain reported 7 patients who underwent combined liver-kidney transplantation with excellent results. The authors recommended the procedure for patients suffering from combined end-organ disease.

In the Baylor and U.C.L.A. programs, 43 combined transplants have been performed. The cause of renal failure was as follows: glomerulonephritis (18), cyclosporine nephrotoxicity in a previously transplanted patient (9), polycystic kidney disease with concomitant polycystic liver disease or hepatitis (4), diabetic nephropathy (5), primary oxaluria (3), chronic interstitial nephritis (3), obstructive uropathy (2), and nonreversible acute tubular necrosis (1). The patient survival rate is not significantly different from that reported for patients undergoing liver transplant alone. The postoperative course is made much easier by a functioning renal transplant. Care should be taken in evaluating patients before transplant to determine that a kidney transplant is indeed needed. When indicated, a biopsy may need to be obtained to confirm the suspicion of significant kidney disease. The use of cyclosporine in patients with severe chronic renal failure (GFR < 15), in addition to other postoperative insults to kidney function, is very likely to lead to further decline in kidney function and the possibility of end-stage renal disease. Therefore, patients with severe chronic renal failure and documented evidence of structural renal disease should be considered for a combined transplant. This procedure is not indicated in patients with hepatorenal syndrome or acute tubular necrosis. Technically, the liver transplant is performed first; after the patient is stable, the renal allograft is performed. For unknown reasons, rejection of the renal allograft is extremely uncommon in this group of patients.[116–118]

A review of the UNOS database indicates that combined liver-kidney transplant may be on the rise. Between 1988 and December 1994, 324 combined liver transplants have been performed in the U.S. (0.61% of all liver transplants). There has been a 48% increase in 1994 compared with 1993 (2.1% of all liver transplants). In contrast to the Baylor and U.C.L.A. experience, the U.S. experience indicates a worse survival for the combined patients.[103a] Obviously, the exact indications for the procedure are still in flux.

Acknowledgment. The expert assistance of Ann Drew in preparation of this manuscript is greatly appreciated.

REFERENCES

1. Papadakis MA, Arieff AI: Unpredictability of clinical evaluation of renal function in cirrhosis. Am J Med 1987;82:945–952.

2. Desai TK, Tsang TK: Aminoglycoside nephrotoxicity in obstructive jaundice. Am J Med 1988;85:47–50.

3. Lietman PS: Liver disease, aminoglycoside antibiotics and renal dysfunction. Hepatology 1988;8:966–968.

4. Brown M, Gunning T, Roberts C, et al: Biochemical markers of renal perfusion are preserved during liver transplantation with venovenous bypass. Transplant Proc 1991;23:1980–1981.

5. Gunning TC, Brown MR, Swygert TH, et al: Peri–operative renal function in patients undergoing orthotopic liver transplantation: A randomized trial of the effects of verapamil. Transplantation 1991;51:422–427.

6. Rettke SR, Janossy TA, Chantigian RC, et al: Hemodynamic and metabolic changes in hepatic transplantation. Mayo Clin Proc 1989;64:232–240.

7. Wu AH, Braccy A, Bryan-Brown CW, et al: Ionized calcium monitoring during liver transplantation. Arch Pathol Lab Med 1987;111:935–938.

8. Atchison SR, Rettke SR, Fromme GA, et al: Plasma glucose concentrations during liver transplantation. Mayo Clin Proc 1989;64:241–245.

9. El Khoury GF, Klandorf H, Brems J, Busuttil RW: Pancreatic hormonal responses to hyperglycemia during orthotopic liver transplantation in man. Transplantation 1989;47:891–893.

10. Fortunato FL, Kang Y, Aggarwal S, et al: Acid-base status during and after orthotopic liver transplantation. Transplant Proc 1987;19:59–60.

11. Gray TA, Buckley BM, Scaley MM, et al: Plasma ionized calcium monitoring during liver transplantation. Transplantation 1986;41:335–339.

12. Ickx B, Walter S, Farman JV: Ionized calcium levels during liver transplantation. Eur J Anaesthesiol 1987; 4:421–427.

13. Gerhardt A, Greenberg A, Reilly JJ, Van Thiel DH: Hypercalcemia. A complication of advanced chronic liver disease. Arch Intern Med 1987;147:274–277.

14. Sealey MM: Severe hypercalcemia due to a parathyroid-type hormone secreting tumour of the liver treated by hepatic transplantation. Anaesthesia 1985;40:170–177.

15. Bertholf RL, Bertholf MF, Brown CM, Riley WJ: Ionized calcium buffering in the transfused anhepatic patient: AB initio calculations of calcium ion concentrations. Ann Clin Lab Sci 1992; 22:40–50.

16. Scheinin B, Orko R, Lalla ML, et al: Significance of ionized calcium during liver transplantation. Acta Anaesthesiol Belg 1989;40:101–105.

17. Munoz SJ, Nagelberg SB, Green PJ, et al: Ectopic soft tissue calcium deposition following liver transplantation. Hepatology 1988;8:476–483.

18. Wachtel MS, Dhettry U, Arkin CF: Tissue calcification after orthotopic liver transplantation. An autopsy study. Arch Pathol Lab Med 1992;116:930–933.

19. El Khoury GF, Foster S, Raybould D, et al: Anesthetic management of severely hypokalemic patients for liver transplantation. Anesthesiology 1990;73:337–340.

20. Vogt DP, Lederman RJ, Carey WD, et al: Neurologic complications of liver transplantation. Transplantation 1988;45:1057–1061.

21. De Groen PC, Aksamit AJ, Rakela J, et al: Central nervous system toxicity after liver transplantation. N Engl J Med 1987;317:861–866.

22. De Groen PC: Cyclosporine, low density lipoprotein and cholesterol. Mayo Clin Proc 1988;63:1012–1021.

23. Deierhoi MH, Kalayoglu M, Sollinger HW, Belzer FO: Cyclosporine neurotoxicity in liver transplant recipients. Transplant Proc 1988;20:116–118.

24. Bennett WM, Porter GA: Cyclosporine associated hypertension. Am J Med 1988;85:131–133.

25. Rettke SR, Chantigian RC, Janossy TA, et al: Anesthesia approach to hepatic transplantation. Mayo Clin Proc 1989;64:224–231.

26. Shirer HW, Erichson DF, Orr JA: Cardiorespiratory responses to HCl vs lactic acid infusion. J Appl Physiol 1988;65:534–540.

27. Iwatsuki S, Esquivel CO, Klintmalm GB, et al: Nephrotoxicity of cyclosporine in liver transplantation. Transplant Proc 1985;17:S191–S195.

28. Keating J, Neuberger J, Clarke M, et al: Renal function and morphology in cyclosporin A-treated liver transplant recipients. Clin Transplant 1988;2:110–116.

29. Poplawski SC, Gonwa TA, Goldstein RM, et al: Renal dysfunction following orthotopic liver transplantation. Clin Transplant 1989;3:94–100.

30. Gonwa TA, Morris CA, Goldstein RM, et al: Long-term survival and renal function following liver transplantation in patients with and without hepatorenal syndrome—experience in 300 patients. Transplantation 1991;51:428–430.

31. Wheatley HC, Datzman M, Williams JW, et al: Long-term effects of cyclosporine on renal function in liver transplant patients. Transplantation 1987;43:641–647.

32. Ayres R, Ismail T, Angrisani L, et al: Long-term renal function in liver transplantation. Transplant Proc 1991; 23:1469–1470.

33. McDiarmid SV, Ettenger RB, Hawkins RA, et al: The impairment of true glomerular filtration rate in long-term cyclosporine-treated paediatric allograft recipients. Transplantation 1990;49:81–85.

34. Winston JA, Feingold R, Safirstein R: Glomerular hemodynamics in cyclosporine nephrotoxicity following uninephrectomy. Kidney Int 1989;35:1175–1182.

35. Murray BM, Paller MS, Ferris TF: Effect of cyclosporine administration on renal hemodynamics in conscious rats. Kidney Int 1985;28:767–774.

36. Moss NG, Powell SL, Falk RJ: Intravenous cyclosporine activates afferent and efferent renal nerves and causes sodium retention in innervated kidneys in rats. Proc Natl Acad Sci USA 1985;82:8222–8226.

37. Bennett WM, Elzinga L, Kelley V: Pathophysiology of cyclosporine nephrotoxcity: Role of eicosanoids. Transplant Proc 1988 20:628–633.

38. Petric R, Freeman D, Wallace C, et al: Effect of cyclosporine on urinary prostanoid excretion, renal blood flow, and glomerulotubular function. Transplantation 1988;45:883–889.

39. Coffman TM, Carr DR, Yarger WE, Klotman PE: Evidence that renal prostaglandin and thromboxane production is stimulated in chronic cyclosporine nephrotoxicity. Transplantation 1987;43:282–285.

40. Paller MS: Effects of the prostaglandin E₁ analog misoprostol on cyclosporine nephrotoxicity. Transplantation 1988;45:1126–1131.

41. Moran M, Mozes MF, Maddux MS: Prevention of acute graft rejection by the prostaglandin E$_1$ analogue misoprostol in renal–transplant recipients treated with cyclosporine and prednisolone. N Engl J Med 1990; 322:1183–1188.

42. Heering P, Strobach H, Schror K, Grabensee B: The role of thromboxane and prostacyclin in cyclosporin-induced nephrotoxicity. Nephron 1992;61:26–31.

43. Olthoff KM, Wasef E, Seu P, Iet al: PGE$_1$ reduces injury in hepatic allografts following preservation. J Surg Res 1991;50:595–601.

44. Greig PD, Woolf GM, Sinclair SB, et al: Treatment of primary liver graft nonfunction with prostaglandin E$_1$. Transplantation 1989;48:447–453.

45. Weir MR, Klassen DK, Shen SY, et al: Acute effects of intravenous cyclosporine on blood pressure, renal hemodynamics, and urine prostaglandin production of healthy humans. Transplantation 1990;49:41–47.

46. Textor SC, Wilson DJ, Lerman A, et al: Renal hemodynamics, urinary eicosanoids, and endothelin after liver transplantation. Transplantation 1992;54:74–80.

47. Polson RJ, Park GR, Lindop MJ, et al: The prevention of renal impairment of patients undergoing orthotopic liver grafting by infusion of low dose dopamine. Anaesthesia 1987;42:15–19.

48. Swygert TH, Roberts LC, Valek TR, et al: Effect of intraoperative low-dose dopamine on renal function in liver transplant recipients. Anesthesiology 1991;75: 571–576.

49. Driscoll DF, Pinson CW, Jenkins RL, Bistrian BR: Potential protective effects of furosemide against early renal injury in liver transplant patients receiving cyclosporine-A. Crit Care Med 1989;17:1341–1343.

50. Dawidson I, Rooth P, Fry WR, et al: Prevention of acute cyclosporine-induced renal blood flow inhibition and improved immunosuppression with verapamil. Transplantation 1989;48:575–580.

51. Kiberd BA: Cyclosporine-induced renal dysfunction in human renal allograft recipients. Transplantation 1989; 48:965–969.

52. Pirsch JD, D'Alessandro AM, Roecker EB, et al: A controlled, double-blind, randomized trial of verapamil and cyclosporine in cadaver renal transplant patients. Am J Kidney Dis 1993;21:189–195.

53. McDiarmid SV, Busuttil RW, Levy P, et al: The long-term outcome of OKT3 compared with cyclosporine prophylaxis after liver transplantation. Transplantation 1991;52:91–97.

54. Farges O, Ericzon BG, Bresson-Hadna S, et al: A randomized trial of OKT3-based versus cyclosporine based immunoprophylaxis after liver transplantation. Long term results of a European and Australian multicentre trial. Transplantation 1994;58:89–898.

55. Gonwa TA, Goldstein RM, Holman M, et al: Orthotopic liver transplantation and renal function. Outcome of hepatorenal syndrome and trial of verapamil for renal protection in non-hepatorenal syndrome. Transplant Proc 1993;25:1891–1982.

56. DiBona GF: Renal neural activity in hepatorenal syndrome. Kidney Int 1984;25:841–853.

57. Lang F, Tschernko E, Häussinger D: Hepatic regulation of renal function. Exp Physiol 1992;77:663–673.

58. Govindarajan S, Nast CC, Smith WL, et al: Immunohistochemical distribution of renal prostaglandin endoperoxide synthase and prostacyclin synthase: Diminished endoperoxide synthase in the hepatorenal syndrome. Hepatology 1987;7:654–659.

59. Zipser RD, Radvan GH, Kronborg IJ, et al: Urinary thromboxane B$_2$ and prostaglandin E$_2$ in hepatrenal syndrome: Evidence for increased vasoconstrictor and decreased vasodilator factors. Gastroenterology 1983; 84:697–703.

60. Moore K, Wendon J, Frazer M, et al: Plasma endothelin immunoreactivity in liver disease and the hepatorenal syndrome. N Engl J Med 1992;327:1774–1778.

61. Uchihara M, Izumi N, Sato C, Marumo F: Clinical significance of elevated plasma endothelin concentration in patients with cirrhosis. Hepatology 1992;16:95–99.

62. Perez-Ayuso RM, Arroyo V, Camps J, et al: Renal kallikrein excretion in cirrhotics with ascites: Relationship to renal hemodynamics. Hepatology 1984;4:247–252.

63. Arroyo V, Planas R, Gaya J, et al: Sympathetic nervous activity, renin angiotensin system and renal excretion of prostaglandin E$_2$ in cirrhotic. Relationship to functional renal failure and sodium and water excretion. Eur J Clin Invest 1983;13:271–278.

64. O'Connor DT, Stone RA: The renal kallikrein-renin system: Description and relationship to liver disease. In Epstein M (ed): The Kidney in Liver Disease, 2nd ed. New York: Elsevier, 1983;469–475.

65. Arroyo V, Rimola V, Gaya J, Rodes J: Prostaglandins and renal function in cirrhosis. Prog Liver Dis 1986; 8:505–523.

66. Ring-Larsen H, Henriksen JH: Pathogenesis of ascites formation: Humoral and hemodynamic factors. Semin Liver Dis 1986;6:341–352.

67. Zipser RD, Kronborg I, Rector W, et al: Therapeutic trial of thromboxane synthesis inhibition in the hepatorenal syndrome. Gastroenterology 1984;87:1228–1232.

68. Stahl RAK, Adler S, Baker PJ, et al: Cyclosporine A inhibits prostaglandin E$_2$ formation by rat mesangial cells in culture. Kidney Int 1989;35:1161–1167.

69. Winston JA, Feingold R, Safirstein R: Glomerular hemodynamics in cyclosporine nephrotoxicity following uninephrectomy. Kidney Int 1989;35:1175–1182.

70. Murray BM, Paller MS, Ferris TF: Effect of cyclosporine administration on renal hemodynamics in conscious rats. Kidney Int 1985;28:767–774.

71. Moss NG, Powell SL, Falk RJ: Intravenous cyclosporine activates afferent and efferent renal nerves and causes sodium retention in innervated kidneys in rats. Proc Natl Acad Sci USA 1985;82:8222–8226.

72. Coffman TM, Carr DR, Yarger WE, Klotman PE: Evidence that renal prostaglandin and thromboxane production is stimulated in chronic cyclosporine nephrotoxicity. Transplantation 1987;43:282–285.

73. Gonwa TA, Klintmalm GB, Jennings LS, et al: The impact of pretransplant renal function on survival following liver transplantation. Transplantation 1995 (in press).

74. The U.S. Multicenter FK506 Liver Study Group: A comparison of tacrolimues (FK506) and cyclosporine for immunosuppression in liver transplantation. N Engl J Med 1994;331:1110–1115.

75. McDiarmid SV, Colonna J, Shaked A, et al: A comparison of renal function in cyclosporine and FK506 treated patients after primary orthotopic liver transplantation. Transplantation 1993;56:847–853.

76. Porayko M, Textor SC, Krom RAF, et al: Nephrotopic effects of primary immunosuppression with FK506 and cyclosporine regimens after liver transplantation. Mayo Clin Proc 1994;64:105–111.

77. McCauley J, Fung JJ, Brown H, et al: Renal function after conversion from cyclosporine to FK506 in liver transplant patients. Transplant Proc 1991;23:3148–3149.

78. McCauley J, Fung JJ, Todo S. et al: Changes in renal function after liver transplantation under FK506. Transplant Proc 1991;23:3143–3145.

79. McCauley J, Takaya S, Fung J, et al: The question of FK506 nephrotoxicity after liver transplantation. Transplant Proc 1991;23:1444–1447.

80. Winkler M, Jost U, Ringe B, et al: Association of elevated FK506 plasma levels with nephrotoxicity in liver–grafted patients. Transplant Proc 1991;23:3153– 3155.

81. Backman L, Nicar M, Levy M, et al: FK506 trough levels in whole blood and plasma in liver transplant recipients: Correlation to clinical events and side effects. Transplantation 1994;57:519–525.

82. Abu-Elmagd K, Fung JJ, Alessiani M, et al: The effect of graft function on FK506 plasma levels, dosages, and renal function, with particular reference to the liver. Transplantation 1991;52:71–77.

83. Tauxe WN, Mochizuki T, McCauley J, et al: A comparison of the renal effects (ERPF, GFR, and FF) of FK506 and cyclosporine in patients with liver transplantation. Transplant Proc 1991;23:3146–3147.

84. Takaya S, Iwaki Y, Starzl TE: Liver transplantation in positive cytotoxic crossmatch cases using FK506, high-dose steroids, and prostaglandin E$_1$. Transplantation 1992;54:927–929.

85. Moutabarrik A, Ishibashi M, Fukunaga M, et al: FK506 mechanism of nephrotoxicity: Stimulatory effect on endothelin secretion by cultured kidney cells and tubular cell toxicity in vitro. Transplant Proc 1991;23:3133–3136.

86. Mountabarrik A, Ishibashi M, Kameoka H, et al: In vitro FK506 kidney tubular cell toxicity. Transplant Proc 1991; 23:3137–3140.

87. Moutabarrik A, Ishibashi M, Fukunaga M, et al: FK506–induced kidney tubular cell injury. Transplantation 1992;54:1041–1047.

88. Ueda D, Tajima A, Ohtawara Y, et al: Influence of FK506 on renal blood flow. Transplant Proc 1991;23: 3121–3122.

89. Perico N, Amuchastegui CS, Zoja C, et al: FK506 does not affect the glomerular filtration rate and plasma flow in the rat. Transplant Proc 1991;23:3123–3125.

90. Goldstein H, Boyle JD: Spontaneous recovery from the hepatorenal syndrome. N Engl J Med 1965;272:895–898.

91. Koppel MH, Coburn JW, Mims MM, et al: Transplantation of cadaveric kidneys from patients with hepatorenal syndrome—evidence for the functional nature of renal failure in advanced liver disease. N Engl J Med 1969;280:1367–1371.

92. Iwatsuki S, Popovtzer MM, Corman JL, et al: Recovery from "hepatorenal syndrome" after orthotopic liver transplantation. N Engl J Med 1973;289:1155–1159.

93. Wood RP, Ellis D, Starzl TE: The reversal of the hepatorenal syndrome in four paediatric patients following successful orthotopic liver transplantation. Ann Surg 1987;205:415–419.

94. Gonwa TA, Morris CA, Goldstein RM, et al: Long-term survival and renal function following liver transplantation in patients with and without hepatorenal syndrome—experience in 300 patients. Transplantation 1991;51:428–430.

95. Gonwa TA, Poplawski S, Paulsen W, et al: Pathogenesis and outcome of hepatorenal syndrome in patients undergoing orthotopic liver transplant. Transplantation 1989;47:395–397.

96. Sacerdoti D, Bolognesi M, Merkel C, et al: Renal vasoconstriction in cirrhosis evaluated by duplex doppler ultrasonography. Hepatology 1993;17:220–224.

97. Maroto A, Gines A, Salo J, et al: Diagnosis of functional kidney failure of cirrhosis with doppler sonography, prognostic value of resistive index. Hepatology 1994; 20:839–844.

98. Platt JF, Ellis JH, Rubin JM, et al: Renal duplex doppler ultrasonography: A noninvasive predictor of kidney dysfunction and hepatorenal failure in liver disease. Hepatology 1994;20:362–369.

99. Seu P, Wilkinson AH, Shaked A, Busuttil RW: The hepatorenal syndrome in liver transplant recipients. Am Surg 1991;57:806–809.

100. Danovitch GM, Wilkinson AH, Colonna JO, Busuttil RW: Determinants of renal failure in patients receiving orthotopic liver transplants. Kidney Int 1987;31:195.

101. Cuervois-Mons V, Millan I, Gavaler JS, et al: Prognostic value of preoperatively obtained clinical and laboratory data in predicting survival following orthotopic liver transplantation. Hepatology 1986;6:922–927.

102. Rimola A, Gavaler JS, Schade RR, et al: Effects of renal impairment on liver transplantation. Gastroenterology 1987;93:148–156.

103. Baliga P, Merion RM, Turcotte JG, et al: Preoperative risk factor assessment in liver transplantation. Surgery 1992;112:704–710.

103a. Breen T, UNOS, personal communication.

104. Mor E, Jennings L, Gonwa TA, et al: The impact of operative bleeding on outcome in transplantation of the liver. Surg Gynecol Obstet 1993;176:219–227.

105. Mora NP, Gonwa TA, Goldstein RM, et al: Risk of postoperative infection after liver transplantation. A univariate and stepwise logistic regression analysis of 150 consecutive patients. Clin Transplant 1992;46:443–449.

106. Watts RW, Danpure CJ, DePauw L, Toussaint C: Combined liver-kidney and isolated transplantations for primary hyperoxaluria type 1: The European experience. The European study group on transplantation in hyperoxaluria type 1. Nephrol Dial Transplant 1991;6:502–511.

107. Lloveras JJ, Durand D, Depre C, et al: Combined liver-kidney transplantation in primary hyperoxaluria type I. Prevention of the recidive of calcium oxalate deposits in the renal graft. Clin Nephrol 1992;38:128–131.

108. Rodby RA, Tyszka TS, Williams JW: Reversal of cardiac dysfunction secondary to type 1 primary hyperoxaluria after combined liver-kidney transplantation. Am J Med 1991;90:498–504.

109. Ruder H, Otto G, Schutgens RB, et al: Excessive urinary oxalate excretion after combined renal and hepatic transplantation for correction of hyperoxaluria type 1. Eur J Pediatr 1990;150:56–58.

110. Toussaint C, DePauw L, Vienne A, et al: Radiological and histological improvement of oxalate osteopathy after combined liver-kidney transplantation in primary hyperoxaluria type 1. Am J Kidney Dis 1993;21:54–63.

111. Rakela J, Kurtz SB, McCarty JT, et al: Fulminant Wilson's disease treated with postdilution hemofiltration and orthotopic liver transplantation. Gastroenterology 1986;90:2004.

112. Margreiter R, Kramar R, Huber C, et al: Combined liver and kidney transplantation. Lancet 1984;1:1077.

113. Fung JJ, Makowka L, Griffin M, et al: Successful sequential liver-kidney transplantation in patients with preformed lymphocytotoxic antibodies. Clin Transplant 1987;1:187.

114. Fung J, Makowka L, Tzakis A, et al: Combined liver kidney transplantation: Analysis of patients with preformed lymphocytotoxic antibodies. Transplant Proc 1988;20:88.

115. Vogel W, Steiner E, Kornberger R, et al: Preliminary results with combined hepatorenal allografting. Transplantation 1988;45:491.

116. Gonwa TA, Nery JR, Husberg BS, Klintmalm GB: Simultaneous liver and renal transplantation in man. Transplantation 1988;46:690–693.

117. Wilkinson AH, Rosenthal T, Shaked A, et al: Combined kidney-liver transplantation: Analysis of indications and outcomes. Presented at the annual meeting of the American Society of Transplant Physicians, May 1, 1993.

118. Gil-Vernet S, Prieto C, Griñó JM, et al: Combined liver-kidney transplantation. Transplant Proc 1992; 24:128–129.

INDEX

Entries in **boldface** type indicate complete chapters.

Abdominal pressure, as cause of hepatorenal syndrome, 83
ACE. *See* Angiotensin-converting enzyme
Acetaminophen, as lactic acidosis cause, 112
Acetate, metabolism of, 109
Acetazolamide
  adverse effects of, 115, 119, 454
  as edema therapy, 451–452
  as hepatic encephalopathy cause, 115
Acetylcholine, nitric oxide-related inhibition of, 376
Acid-base disorders, **109–122**. *See also* Acidosis; Alkalosis
  in acute liver disease, 112–113
  in chronic liver disease, 113–114
  in hyperaldosteronism, 303
  in liver transplantation patients, 114, 530
  effect of mineralocorticoids on, 293–294
  pathophysiology of, 114–118
  therapy for, 118–119
Acidosis
  hyperchloremic, diuretic-related, 455
  lactic, 109, 111–112
    chronic liver disease-related, 113
    D-lactic, 116
    fulminant hepatic failure-related, 112, 113
    pathophysiology of, 115–116
    treatment of, 119
  metabolic
    chronic liver disease-related, 114
    fulminant hepatic failure-related, 112–113
    liver transplantation-related, 114
    pathophysiology of, 115–118
    urea synthesis in, 110
  renal tubular, pathophysiology of, 116–118
  respiratory
    chronic liver disease-related, 113
    fulminant hepatic failure-related, 112–113
    pathophysiology of, 118
    Reye's syndrome-related, 113
Acini, units of liver, 222, 224
Acquired immune deficiency syndrome (AIDS), 138, 139
  false-negative hepatitis serology tests in, 154
Acute tubular necrosis
  differentiated from hepatorenal syndrome, 93–95
  effective arterial blood volume in, 81
Acyclovir, as venoocclusive disease risk factor, 171
Adenosine, in hepatorenal syndrome, 91
Adenosine washout hypothesis, 224–225, 226, 237
Adenylate cyclase, prostaglandin-related activation of, 312
ADH. *See* Antidiuretic hormone
Adhesion proteins, in venoocclusive disease, 173–174
Adrenal cortex, aldosterone secretion by, 291
Adrenergic activity
  in cirrhosis, 19
  hyperreninemia-mediated effects of, 281
Adrenocorticotropic hormone, 365
  aldosterone regulatory activity of, 292

α_1Adrenoreceptors
  in bile duct-ligated animals, 430
  in peripheral vasodilation, 6–7
AIDS. *See* Acquired immune deficiency syndrome
Air embolism, 497
Alanine aminotransferase
  hepatitis-related increase of, 153, 154, 157
  venoocclusive disease-related increase of, 168
Albumin
  in ascites, 185–186, 191–192
  as ascites therapy, 456
  furosemide binding by, 456
  intravenous
    use in outflow dilution studies, 185–186
    as paracentesis plasma volume expander during
      paracentesis, 480–485
  lymph to plasma ratio of, 186
  as metabolic alkalosis therapy, 118
  nonsteroidal antiinflammatory drug binding by, 318
  sinusoidal cell sieving of, 223
Alcoholics, male, feminization of, 23
Alcohol use
  effect on hepatic oxygen uptake, 226
  as mesangial immunoglobulin A deposition cause, 127–128
  effect on renal water excretion, 35–37
  effect on urine osmolality, 42
Aldactone. *See* Spironolactone
Aldosterone, **291–305**. *See also* Aldosteronism, secondary;
  Hyperaldosteronism
  effect on acid-base balance, 293–294
  in advanced liver disease, 4
  angiotensin II-related production of, 269
  in ascites formation, 211
  degradation site of, 294
  hepatic extraction of, 294
  in liver disease, 291, 294–303
  paracentesis-related increase of, 483–486
  peritoneovenous shunting-related decrease of, 495, 496
  physiology of, 291–294
  renal extraction of, 294
  effect on sodium excretion, 13–14
  effect of transjugular intrahepatic shunting on, 511, 512
  effect of water immersion on, 344, 345
Aldosterone antagonists, 454–455, 470–471
Aldosteronism, secondary, 114–115
Alkaline phosphatase, venoocclusive disease-related increase of, 168
Alkaloids, toxic, as venoocclusive disease cause, 167, 168
Alkalosis
  metabolic
    aldosterone-related, 293–294
    chronic liver disease-related, 113
    cirrhosis-related, 114–115
    diuretic-related, 109, 115
    fulminant hepatic failure-related, 112
    in liver transplantation patients, 114, 531, 532

543

Alkalosis *(cont.)*
  metabolic *(cont.)*
    pathophysiology of, 114–115
    severe, therapy for, 118–119
  mixed respiratory-metabolic
    chronic liver disease-related, 114
    fulminant hepatic failure-related, 112
  respiratory
    chronic liver disease-related, 113, 114
    fulminant hepatic failure-related, 112
    in liver transplantation patients, 532
    pathophysiology of, 114
Alkylating agents, as venoocclusive disease risk factor, 168, 172
$Alpha_1$-acid glycoprotein, drug binding by, 462
Amiloride
  pharmacokinetics of, 471
  as spironolactone alternative, 454–455
Amino acids, metabolism of, 109
p-Aminohippuric acid clearance, 495
Aminopeptide of type III collagen, 170
Aminopyrine breath test, 202
Aminopyrine clearance, relationship to sodium excretion, 205
Ammonium
  excretion of, in renal tubular acidosis, 117
  protein metabolism-related production of, 109
  synthesis of, 110
  ureagenesis, acid-base homeostasis and, 109–112
Ammonium chloride, adverse effects of, 119
Amyloidosis, glomerular abnormalities in, 141–142
Anaritide, 347. *See also* Atrial natriuretic factor
Anasarca, 183
Anemia, jaundice-related, 431
Anesthesia, use in jaundiced patients, 433
ANF. *See* Atrial natriuretic factor
Angiotensin [1–7], 366. *See also* Angiotensin I and II
Angiotensinase
  cirrhosis-related increase of, 279
  jaundice-related increase of, 427
Angiotensin-converting enzyme, 269
  cirrhosis-related increase of, 278
Angiotensin-converting enzyme inhibitors (ACE inhibitors), 269, 285
Angiotensin I
  conversion to angiotensin II, 269
  measurement of, 272
Angiotensin II, 267–268, 269
  as angiotensinogen modulator, 268
  cirrhosis-related increase of, 277–278, 279
  conversion to angiotensin III, 268
  effect on proximal tubular reabsorption rate, 15
  hemodynamic effects of, 283
  hepatic clearance of, 280
  in hepatorenal syndrome, 85
  measurement of, 272
  prostaglandin-related inhibition of, 315–316
  pressor responses to, in bile duct-ligated animals, 429, 430
  prostaglandin-stimulated activity of, 310
  relationship to nitric oxide tissue concentration, 377
  in renin release, 270
Angiotensin III, 268, 269
  in control of aldosterone secretion, 300
Angiotensinogen, 267, 268. *See also* Renin substrate
Angiotensin receptors, cirrhosis-related density increase of, 129
Antacids, use in liver transplantation patients, 532
Antibiotics
  contraindication prior to liver transplantation, 530
  as venoocclusive disease risk factor, 171
Antidiuretic hormone. *See also* Arginine vasopressin
  alcohol-related increase of, 35–36

Antidiuretic hormone *(cont.)*
  in ascites formation, 211
  cardiac baroreceptor-related decrease of, 408
  in cirrhosis, 51–52
    indirect assessment of, 42–43
    measurement of, 43–45
    mechanism of increased activity, 45–52
    nonosmotic stimuli-related release of, 45–51
    nonsteroidal antiinflammatory drug-related potentiation of, 467
    relationship to renal water handling, 42–52
    effect of water loading on, 44
  in decompensated cirrhosis, 45–47
    effect of water administration on, 39–40
    nonosmotic stimuli-related release of, 47–51
    water immersion studies of, 45–46, 53
  hepatic metabolism of, 34–35
  in hepatorenal syndrome, 80
  hydroosmotic action of
    atrial natriuretic factor-related inhibition of, 350
    endothelin-related inhibition of, 392–393
    prostaglandin-related enhancement of, 313
    prostaglandin-related inhibition of, 316, 466
  interaction with endothelin, 20
  peritoneovenous shunting-related decrease of, 495
  pharmacologic modulation of, 60
  portal blood osmolality and, increases in, 34
  pressor response to, in bile duct-ligated animals, 429, 430
  prostaglandin synthesis-stimulating activity of, 310, 314
  in renal water handling, in hepatitis, 54
  renin-inhibiting effect of, 271
Antidiuretic hormone, analogs, as hyponatremia therapy, 60
Antidiuretic hormone-like activity, drug-induced, 52, 57
Antiendotoxin therapy, as jaundice-related renal failure prophylaxis, 441
Antiglomerular basement membrane disease, 127
Antilymphocyte globulin, use in hepatitis C virus-infected patients, 161, 162
Antipyrine clearance, correlation with sodium excretion, 3
Antithrombin III, coagulopathy and, 498, 500
Apolipoproteins, in liver disease, 327
Arachidonic acid, 307
  metabolism of, 307–309, 328
  release from phosphoinositol lipids, 310
Arachidonic acid deficiency, 327–328
Arachidonic acid precursors, therapeutic administration of, 327–328
Arginine, hepatic metabolism of, 109–110
L-Arginine salvage pathway, 374
Arginine vasopressin. *See* Antidiuretic hormone
Arterial oxygen saturation, in cirrhosis, 243
Artificial liver hepatocyte system, 524
Ascites
  atrial natriuretic factor in, 340, 341
    arteriovenous extraction of, 342
    renal resistance to, 350–351, 353
    with spontaneous natriuresis, 341–342
    effect of volume expansion on, 344–345, 346
  causes of, 179, 180
  definition of, 179
  exogenous atrial natriuretic factor therapy for, 347, 348
  fluid volume in, 180
  associated with generalized edema, 198
  malignant, 500
  medical management of, 24–25, 447–448, 458
  nonsteroidal antiinflammatory drug nephrotoxicity in, 318–319
  paracentesis management of, **479–490**
    with albumin infusion, 480–485

Ascites *(cont.)*
  paracentesis management of *(cont.)*
    comparison with diuretic therapy, 480–482
    comparison with peritoneovenous shunting, 487–488, 489
    complications of, 480–482, 483, 485,486
    large-volume, 482, 483–485, 489
    total, 482, 487, 488–489
  peritoneovenous shunt management of, **491–506**
    comparison with paracentesis, 487– 488, 489
    complications of, 500
  plasma renin activity in, 273, 274–277
  predominance in liver disease, 24
  prostaglandins in, 314–315
  refractory
    definition of, 507
    extracorporeal treatment techniques for, 517–522, 526
    large-volume paracentesis therapy for, 517–518
    paracentesis versus peritoneovenous shunt management of, 487–488
    transjugular intrahepatic portosystemic shunt therapy for, 507, 511–512, 514
  urinary sodium retention in, 180
Ascites formation, **179–220**
  afferent factors in, 211–212
  causes of, 180–183
  clinical studies of, 207–210
  efferent factors in, 212–213
  nonsplanchnic plasma volume in, 196–197
  pathophysiology of, 192–207
    critical function threshold theory, 201–203
    overfill theory, 5, 7–10, 80–81, 192–201, 210–211, 214, 241, 508
    peripheral arterial vasodilation (revised underfill) theory, 5–7, 45, 80, 508
    peripheral arteriolar dilatation hypothesis, 203–207, 508
    underfill theory, 5, 45, 193, 195, 208–209, 210, 214, 241, 508
  plasma renin activity in, 273, 274–277
  prostaglandins in, 314–315
  restrictive lung disease-related, 118
  effect of sodium restriction on, 2–3
  sodium retention in, 1, 2, 3
    aldosterone levels in, 295, 296, 297
    decreased albumin synthesis, 191–192
    hepatic sinusoids, 185–186
    hepatic venous outflow block, 183–185
    humoral substances, 192
    lymph, 186–187
    myocardial dysfunction, 191
    peritoneal space fluid reabsorption, 187–188
    splanchnic hemodynamics, 188–191
  sympathetic nervous system activity and, 417–418
Ascitic fluid
  intraoperative replacement with saline, 499–500
  precoagulant properties of, 498, 499
  reperfusion into general circulation, 458, 479, 492, 518
Aspartate, metabolism of, 109
Aspartate aminotransferase, venoocclusive disease-related increase of, 168, 171
Aspirin, prostaglandin-inhibiting activity of, 313, 319
Atrial natriuretic factor, **339–358**, 366
  as ADH nonosmotic release mediator, 50
  aldosterone-inhibiting activity of, 292
  in ascites, relationship to aldosterone, 301
  characterization of, 343–344
  in chronic liver disease, dietary sodium challenge response in, 346–347
  in cirrhosis, 241, 248, 339

Atrial natriuretic factor *(cont.)*
  in cirrhosis *(cont.)*
    alterations of, 340–342
    arteriovenous extraction of, 342–343
    circadian patterns of, 348–349
    exogenous peptide infusion responsiveness in, 347–348
    hepatointestinal clearance of, 248
    metabolism of, 342
    during spontaneous natriuresis, 341–342
    volume contraction responsiveness to, 344
    volume expansion responsiveness to, 344–346
  cross-circulation studies of, 359–360
  exogenous infusion of, as cirrhosis therapy, 347–348
  in extracellular fluid volume regulation, 366–367
  in fulminant hepatic failure, 342
  in hepatorenal syndrome, 90–91
  kinetics of, 248
  paracentesis-related increase of, 483– 485
  peptide-enhanced activity of, 351–352
  peritoneovenous shunt-related responsiveness of, 496
  physiologic actions of, 339
  plasma renin activity and, 281
  renal resistance to, 349–351
  in renal sodium excretion, 367
  renal sympathetic nerve activity response to, 415, 416
  renin-inhibiting effect of, 270
  in sodium retention, 17
Atrial natriuretic factor prohormone, 352, 353
Atrial natriuretic factor receptors, 340, 351
Atrial pressure, relationship to sympathetic nerve activity, 408
Auriculin, 17. *See also* Atrial natriuretic factor
Autacoids, 307. *See also* Prostaglandins
Autoimmune liver disease, renal tubular acidosis in, 117
Autoregulation
  of hepatic arterial blood flow, 225
  of renal blood flow, 378–379
Azapropazone
  in cirrhosis, 318
    dosages, 469
  contraindication in liver disease, 467
Azathioprine, as venoocclusive disease risk factor, 167, 168
Azosemide, 453
Azotemia
  acute, differential diagnosis of, 93–95
  in cirrhosis, 201
  drug-induced, 95–96
  peritoneovenous shunt management of, 502–503, 504
  prerenal, effective arterial blood volume in, 81
  uric acid/urea fractional excretion in, 7

Bacteremia, concomitant with endotoxemia, in jaundice, 432
Baroreceptors
  arterial, and sympathetic nerve activity, 407–408, 409–410, 412
  cardiac, and sympathetic nerve activity, 408, 409–410, 412
  of central vascular compartment, 241–242
  intrahepatic
    in cirrhosis, 250, 251, 418
    effect on sympathetic nerve activity, 409–410
  low-pressure
    phrenic nerve pathways of, 260–261, 264–266
    in preascitic sodium retention, 212
    sinusoidal pressure reponse of, 200
    as urinary sodium excretion modulators, 200–201
  in renin release, 269–270
Bartter's syndrome, 469
Beer drinkers, hyponatremia of, 36–37
Beriberi, 111

Beta-blockers
    effect on renin release, 271
    relationship to renal failure, 96
Beta-receptors, in renal sympathetic nerve stimulation,
    270
Bicarbonate
    as lactic acidosis therapy, 119
    protein metabolism-related production of, 109–110
    in ureagenesis, 110–111
Bile acids
    biosynthesis of, 434–435
    digoxin-like immunoreactivity of, 368
    hydrophobicity index of, 436
    nephrotoxicity of, 435–438
    postoperative excretion of, 442
    in renal failure pathogenesis, 433–439
    renoprotective effects of, 435, 438–439
Bile duct-ligated animals
    atrial natriuretic factor levels in, 428
    bilirubin nephrotoxicity in, 440
    cardiovascular system in, 429–431
    comparison with clinical studies, 425– 426
    glomerular filtration rate in, 83
    hemorrhage in, 433
    nitric oxide inhibition in, 380–381
    norepinephrine and epinephrine concentrations in, 427
    plasma renin activity in, 427
    preoperative plasma volume expansion in, 442
    stress response in, 432
    urinary prostaglandin excretion in, 316–317
    vascular overfilling in, 194
    as weight loss cause, 431–432
Bile salts, effect on renal ischemia, 83
Biliary drainage, as jaundice-related renal failure prophylaxis,
    441
Biliary surgery, stress response following, 432
Bilirubin
    biosynthesis of, 439–440
    as jaundice-related renal failure risk factor, 433, 439–440
Bioavailability, of drugs, 460, 463–465
Blood circulation, hepatic, **221–240**
    blood flow in, 221, 222–234
    blood volume in, 222, 234–236
    fluid exchange in, 236–237
    microvasculature in, 222–223
Blood circulation time
    in cirrhosis, 241, 243–244, 245, 247, 252
    in portal hypertension, 241
Blood donors, hepatitis C virus infection seropositivity of, 152,
    159
    screening of, 154
Blood flow
    assessment of, 242–243
    cerebral, in liver disease, 243
    cutaneous, in cirrhosis, 242
    hepatic, 221, 222–234
        arterial regulation of, 223–227
        in chronic liver disease, 294
        hepatic arterial buffer response in, 224–227
        as percentage of cardiac output, 221
        portal venous pressure regulation and, 227–230
        vascular resistance calculation in, 233–234
        venous resistance in, 230–233
    medullary, in cirrhosis, 62, 63
    effect of nitric oxide on, 380
    perfusion coefficient of, 242–243
    portal
        in cirrhosis, 230
        relationship to arterial blood flow, 226, 227

Blood flow *(cont.)*
    renal
        autoregulation of, 378–379
        in cirrhosis, 241, 242
        effect of endothelin on, 399
        in hepatorenal syndrome, 77–78
        in jaundice, 423, 424, 425, 426
        effect of peritoneovenous shunting on, 497
        effect of prostaglandins on, 313, 466, 467
        redistribution of, effect on sodium reabsorption, 21–22
        relationship to cardiac output, 81–82
        effect of sympathetic nerve activity on, 413
    skeletal, in cirrhosis, 242–243
    splanchnic, 242
        in ascites, 45, 188–191
        effect of nitric oxide on, 249
        in transperitoneal solute exchange, 182
Blood pressure
    arterial
        in cirrhosis, 241, 251–252, 413
        effect on sympathetic nerve activity, 407–408, 413, 415
        systemic, in cirrhosis, 251–252
    in cirrhosis
        arterial, 241, 251–252, 413
        relationship to sympathetic nerve activity, 411
        effect of nitric oxide on, 377–378
        effect of nitric oxide synthetase inhibitors on, 380–381
        effect on sympathetic nerve activity, 415
Blood transfusions, hepatitis C virus transmission in, 155–156
Blood volume. *See also* Central blood volume; Effective blood
    volume; Hypovolemia
    and ascites formation, 5–6
    in cirrhosis, 244–246, 247
        correlation with calcitonin gene-related peptide, 250
        relationship to sympathetic nerve activity, 411–412
    hepatic, 182, 222, 234–236
        alterations in, 225
        in liver disease, 235–236
    in jaundice, 431
Body composition, effect of peritoneovenous shunting on, 497
Bone marrow transplantation, hepatic venoocclusive disease
    following. *See* Venoocclusive disease, hepatic, following
    bone marrow transplantation
Borge, Alfred, 448
Bowel obstruction, peritoneovenous shunt-related, 497, 500
Bradykinin
    atrial natriuretic factor interaction of, 352, 353, 354
    in decompensated cirrhosis, 87
    nitric oxide-mediated renal effects of, 376
    in renin release, 272
Brain, hyponatremia adaptation by, 57–58
Brain natriuretic peptide, 18
Bromocriptine, as hyponatremia cause, 59
Brown, John, 1
Budd-Chiari syndrome, 191–192
    distinguished from venoocclusive disease, 167, 170
Bufalin, 364–365
Bufodienolides, 364
Bumetanide, 452, 453
    as furosemide alternative, 456
Busulfan, as venoocclusive disease risk factor, 172
"Buttons," for ascites management, 491

Calcitonin gene-related peptide
    in hepatorenal syndrome, 92
    kinetics of, 248
    systemic vascular resistancecorrelation with, 250, 251
Calcium
    endothelin-mediated release of, 20

Calcium *(cont.)*
in liver transplantation patients, 530, 531
Calcium channel blockers
effect on cyclosporine nephrotoxicity, 534
as hepatorenal syndrome therapy, 100–101
Canrenoate, 454
Canrenone, 454, 470
CAPD (chronic ambulatory peritoneal dialysis), 526
Capillaries. *See also* Sinusoids, hepatic
colonic, in ascites formation, 181–182
Capillarization
hepatic, in cirrhosis, 237
sinusoidal, 191
Capillary permeability, estrogen-related alteration in, 212–213
Captopril, 285–286
Carbicarb, as lactic acidosis therapy, 119
Carbonic anhydrase inhibitors, adverse effects of, 454
Carbon tetrachloride, as fulminant hepatic failure cause, 112
Carbon tetrachloride model, of cirrhosis
excessive nitric oxide formation in, 191
hyperkinetic state in, 207
renal sodium retention in, 201–202, 205–206
Cardiac output
in alcoholic cirrhosis, 204
in cirrhosis, 241, 242, 243, 244, 246, 247
effect of prostaglandins on, 325
hepatic blood flow as percentage of, 221
in hepatorenal syndrome, 81–83
paracentesis-related increase of, 483,484
peritoneovenous shunting-related increase of, 495, 496
in preascitic cirrhotic sodium retention, 203
relationship to renal hemodynamics, 81–82
Cardiomyopathy, jaundice-related, 429–430
Cardiorenal syndrome, 81
Cardiovascular dysfunction, jaundice-related, 424, 428–431
Carprofen
dosage in cirrhosis, 469
pharmacokinetics of, 467–468
Carvedilol, pharmacokinetics of, 463
Catecholamine receptors, in cirrhosis, 19
Catecholamines
in ascites formation, 211
kinetics of, 249
in renal water handling, 65
CAVH. *See* Continuous arteriovenous hemofiltration
CAVHD. *See* Continuous arteriovenous hemodialysis
Cefodizime, pharmacokinetics of, 463
Cefpiramide, pharmacokinetics of, 463
Ceftriaxone, pharmacokinetics of, 463
Central blood volume
in cirrhosis, 209, 244–246, 247
arterial underfilling in, 209–210
atrial natriuretic factor secretion and, 340
correlation with calcitonin gene-related peptide, 250
estimated
in cirrhosis, 10
lack of correlation with atrial natriuretic factor, 341
renin release in, 270
water immersion studies of, 100
Central nervous system
hyponatremia-related dysfunction of, 57–58
in natriuretic hormone regulation, 367
Central pontine myelinosis, 58
Central venous pressure
hepatic modulation of, 232
in lung transplantation candidates, 530
Central volume expansion, water immersion-induced, 7–9
Charcoal hemoperfusion, as hepatorenal syndrome therapy, 100
Chenodeoxycholic acid, 434, 435, 436

Chloramphenicol, as lactic acidosis cause, 112
Chlorthalidone, duration of effects, 472
Choledochocaval shunts, 128–129
Cholestasis
bile acids in, 435
bile constituents disposal in, 423
hypotension in, 429
Cholesterol, in liver disease, 327
Cholic acid, 434, 436
Chronic ambulatory peritoneal dialysis (CAPD), 526
Cimetidine
distribution of, 460
pharmacokinetics of, 463
Circadian rhythms
of atrial natriuretic factor, 348–349
of plasma renin activity, 271, 274
Cirrhosis
active juvenile, 131, 132
alcoholic, 130
acute tubular necrosis in, 93
aldosterone levels in, 296–298
animal model of, 193–194
arterial blood volume depletion in, 210, 211
calcitonin gene-related peptide in, 92
hemodynamic changes in, 189, 204
hepatic lymph protein content in, 186
hepatic venous outflow block in, 213
hepatorenal syndrome associated with, 75–76
myocardial dysfunction in, 191
renal tubular acidosis in, 117–118
source of ascites in, 180–181
water excretion in, 43
aldosterone hepatic clearance in, 294
with ascites. See Ascites
coagulopathy in, 498
compensated
natriuretic hormone abnormalities in, 367–368
prostaglandins in, 314
renal sodium handling abnormalities in, 2–4
decompensated
antidiuretic hormone activity in, 52
atrial stretch in, 341
decreased filtrate delivery in, 52–53
hypernatremia in, 33
renal hemodynamics in, 413
renal vascular resistance in, 130
sympathetic nervous system activity in, 410–411, 419
water administration response in, 37–42
glomerular abnormalities in, 123–130, 131
glomerulonephritis, 125–126
glomerulosclerosis, 124–125
immunoglobulin deposits, 126–128, 129, 130
hepatitis C virus infection-related, 161
Laennec's
renal failure associated with, 76–77
sodium retention in, 1, 2, 4
plasma renin activity in, 273–277
postnecrotic, 54, 55
primary biliary
renal tubular acidosis in, 117
renal water handling in, 55
sodium retention in, 4
renal failure associated with, 2
renal sodium handling in. *See* Sodium handling, renal
renal sodium retention in. *See* Sodium retention, renal
renal vascular tone in, 534
renin secretion increase in, 84
water excretion impairment in, 42–52
Citrate levels, in liver transplantation patients, 531, 532

Clofibrate, pharmacokinetics of, 463
Clonidine
  effect on hepatic hemodynamics, 418–419
  effect on renin release, 271
Coagulopathy, peritoneovenous shunt-related, 498–500
Collagen, as disseminated intravascular coagulopathy risk factor, 499
Collagen disorders, glomerular abnormalities in, 142
Colloid solutions, as pulmonary edema cause, 96–97
Coma, hepatic, 523, 524
Complement
  in cirrhosis, 126, 130
  in hepatitis B-associated nephropathy, 131, 136
  in HIV infection, 139
  in malaria, 141
  in schistosomiasis, 140
  in sickle-cell disease, 142
Compliance, by peritoneovenous shunt patients, 501
Congenital disease, glomerular abnormalities in, 143
Congestive heart failure
  ascites reinfusion in, 518
  atrial natriuretic factor in, 292, 343
  concomitant with venoocclusivedisease, 168
  latent, 96
  low-pressure baroreceptors in, 266
Continuous ambulatory peritoneal dialysis patients, hepatitis C
    virus seropositivity of, 155
Continuous arteriovenous hemodialysis
  as ascites therapy, 520
  use in liver transplantation patients, 531
Continuous arteriovenous hemofiltration
  as ascites therapy, 458, 520–521, 522
  as hepatorenal syndrome therapy, 98
  as hyponatremia therapy, 59
  use in liver transplantation patients, 531
Continuous venovenous hemodialysis, as ascites therapy, 520
Continuous venovenous hemofiltration, as ascites therapy, 520, 522
Convection, in extracorporeal ascites therapy, 519–520
Cordis-Hakim shunt, 492
Cori cycle, 111
Creatinine, as renal function indicator, 76
Creatinine clearance, peritoneovenous shunt-related increase of,
    495, 496, 503, 504
Critical function threshold theory, of sodium retention, 201–203
Cryoglobulinemia, 127, 130
  hepatitis-related
    essential mixed, 163–164
    in hepatitis B virus-associated nephropathy, 133
Cyclic adenosine monophosphate (cAMP), prostaglandin-
    related increase of, 312
Cyclic guanosine monophosphate (cGMP), 208
  interaction with atrial natriuretic factor, 340, 344, 345, 346,
    349, 351, 352
Cyclophosphamide, as venoocclusive disease risk factor, 172
Cyclosporine
  adverse effects of, 529
    in hypomagnesemic patients, 532
    in liver transplantation patients, 532–534, 535, 537
  as venoocclusive disease risk factor, 172, 173
Cysteine, hepatic metabolism of, 109–110
Cystic dysplastic kidneys, 143
Cytochrome P-450 metabolites, of arachidonic acid, 331–332
Cytokines, in venoocclusive disease, 171, 173–174, 176
Cytomegalovirus infections
  in renal transplantation recipients, 162
  as venoocclusive disease risk factor, 172

Demeclocycline
  as azotemia cause, 95
  as renal failure cause, 60

Denervation, renal
  use in renal sympathetic nerve activity evaluation, 406–407
  sodium and water retention following, 417–418
  effect on sympathetic nerve activity-mediated natriuresis, 408
Denver shunt, 492, 494, 495, 500
Deoxycholic acid, 435, 436
  vasorelaxant activity of, 439
1-Des-Asp angiotensin II, 300
Desoxycorticosterone acetate, 13, 14, 200
Dextran-40, as paracentesis plasma volume expander, 487
Dextran-70, as paracentesis plasma volume expander, 484,
    485–486, 487
Dialysis. See also Continuous arteriovenous hemodialysis
  as hepatorenal syndrome therapy, 97–98, 102, 524–525
  as hyponatremia therapy, 59–60
  as maintenance therapy, 525–526
  peritoneal, as hepatorenal syndrome therapy, 522
Diaphragm, hepatic mechanoreceptor phrenic afferents of, 259,
    260, 261–262, 264, 265
Dietary manipulation, in liver disease, 327–328
Diflunisal, 320
Digitalis-like activity, of natriuretic hormone, 361–365
Digitalis-like factors, physiologic significance of, 364–365
Digoxigenin, 363
Digoxin
  absorption of, 459
  in cirrhosis, 367–368
  mammalian production of, 363, 364
Dipyridamole, 225
  renal vasoconstrictive effects of, 91
Disseminated intravascular coagulation, peritoneovenous shunt-
    related, 497, 498, 499–500
Diuresis
  alcohol-related, 35–36
    in decompensated cirrhosis, 42–43
  bile acids-related, 438, 439
  jaundice-related, 428
  peritoneovenous shunting-related, 495–496, 497
  rapid, induction of, 457
Diuretics, 447–458
  as ascites therapy, 447–450, 491
    comparison with paracentesis, 480–482
    complications of, 452–455
    dosage of, 452–456
  choice of, 454–456
  complications of, 447, 448, 452–456, 479
  discontinuation in hyponatremia, 59
  dosages of, 452–455
  as hyponatremia treatment, 59
  indications for, 448–449
  interaction with renal prostaglandins, 310, 321–322
  loop, 453
    classification of, 453
    combined with thiazide diuretics, 456
    dosages of, 452, 455
    as hyponatremia cause, 56–57
    as hyponatremia therapy, 56
    pharmacokinetics of, 472–474
  as metabolic alkalosis cause, 109, 114–115
  nonsteroidal antiinflammatory drug nephrotoxicity and, 319
  pharmacokinetics of, in cirrhosis, 459, 470–474
  potassium-sparing, 453–454
    dosages of, 452
    pharmacokinetics of, 470–471
  effect of prostaglandins on, 310
  for rapid diuresis induction, 456–457
  refractory response to, 455–456, 474
  renal sodium handling and, 450–451
  effect on renin release, 270–271

Diuretics (cont.)
thiazide, 452
combined with loop diuretics, 456
dosages of, 452
pharmacokinetics of, 471–472
Dopamine
as jaundice-related hypotensive crisis therapy, 442
in liver transplantation patients, 530, 534
natriuretic activity of, 366
effect on plasma renin activity, 84–85
Doppler studies
of blood flow, 242
of venooclusive disease, 170
Dosing strategies, 460
for drug accumulation prevention, 465
loading doses, 460–461, 462–463
maintenance doses, 466
Drug absorption, in cirrhosis, 459–460
Drug distribution
in cirrhosis, 460–463
volume of, 460–463
Drug elimination, 463–466
in cirrhosis, 463–466
presystemic, 460, 461, 465
relationship to maintenance dosages, 466
Drugs. See also specific drugs
antidiuresis-inducing, 57, 59
in combined liver and renal disease, 526
Drug serum concentration, 460–462
Duplex sonography, of venooclusive disease, 170

Edema
acetazolamide therapy for, 451–452
atrial natriuretic factor-related, 353
cerebral, fulminant hepatic failure-related, 524
in decompensated cirrhosis, 45
diuretic therapy for, 447, 449, 450
fluid intake in, 448
hepatic protection against, 237
of intestinal wall, 181
medical therapy for, 24–25
peripheral
nonsteroidal antiinflammatory drug-related, 466–467
paracentesis therapy for, 488–489
renal sodium handling impairment-related, 1, 2
renal tubular acidosis associated with, 117
pulmonary
colloid solutions-related, 96–97
peritoneovenous shunt-related, 497
refractory, diuretic therapy for, 455–456
Starling forces and, 198
toxemia-related, 142–143
tubular urine flow in, 54
Effective arterial blood volume
in ascites formation, 203, 214
in hepatorenal syndrome, 81
sodium retention-inducing effect of, 203, 204, 207–208
effect of water immersion on, 207
Effective blood volume
in ascites formation, 508
in cirrhosis, 245–246
definition of, 245
measurement of, 245–246
reduction of
as hepatorenal syndrome risk factor, 76
as left atrial pressure decrease indicator, 88
as renin release determinant, 280
Effective central blood volume, in hepatorenal syndrome, 78–88

Effective plasma volume
definition of, 78
in hepatorenal syndrome, 78
theories of, 5–6
Efferent renal sympathetic nerve activity, 18, 88
Eicosanoids, 307. See also Prostaglandins
in jaundice, 439
Embolism
air, 497
pulmonary, peritoneovenous shunt-related, 500
Encephalopathy
diuretic-related, 480–482
hepatic
acetazolamide-related, 115, 454
acid-base disorders in, 113–114
cerebral blood flow in, 243
continuous arteriovenous hemofiltration/hemodialysis therapy for, 522–523
diuretic-related, 456
drug-induced, 115, 119, 454, 456
renal tubular acidosis-related, 118
transjugular intrahepatic shunt-related, 513–514
paracentesis-related, 480–483
portacaval shunt-related, 508
uremia and, 525
venooclusive disease-related, 174
Endopeptidase inhibitors, effect on atrial natriuretic factor activity, 351–352, 353–354
Endoperoxidases, cyclic, 309
Endorphins, 22, 365. See also Opioids, endogenous
effect on alcohol-induced antidiuretic hormone secretion, 36
Endothelial cells, vascular, effect of endothelin on, 397
Endothelin-converting enzyme, 388
Endothelin-converting enzyme inhibitors, 397
Endothelins, 20–21, **387–404**
in acute renal failure, 398–401
as antidiuretic hormone release mediator, 50
cellular mechanisms of action, 395–398
in cirrhosis, 249–250, 252–253, 399–401
in hepatorenal syndrome, 75, 90, 249, 252–253
isoforms of, 20, 387–388
kinetics of, 249–250
in liver function, 394–395
nitric oxide-releasing activity of, 246
pharmacologic modulation of, 397–398
receptors, 390–392
in renal function, 392–394
synthesis of, 387–390
transhepatic portosystemic shunt-related decrease of, 513
vasoconstricting activity of, 20
Endothelium-derived relaxing factor, 241, 373
Endotoxemia
concomitant with bacteremia, in jaundice, 432
endothelium-derived vasoactive substance, induction of, 400–401
nitric oxide synthesis in, 21
as renal failure risk factor, 88–89
in jaundice, 438–439, 440–441
Endotoxins
in cirrhosis, 241
effect on endothelin synthesis, 390
in hepatorenal syndrome, 88–89
effect on prostaglandin synthesis, 325–326
End-stage renal disease, hepatitis C virus infection in, 151, 154–158
Enkephalins, in cirrhosis, 241

Epinephrine
  plasma levels of in liver transplantation patients, 530
    measurement of, 249
  vasoconstrictive activity of, 246
  vasodilatory activity of, 246
Epoxyeicosatetraenoic acids, natriuretic activity of, 366
Epstein-Barr virus, 141
Erythromycin, pharmacokinetics of, 463
Estrogens, in renal sodium retention, 23, 212–213
Ethacrynic acid, 453
Etodolac, dosage in cirrhosis, 469
Exchange transfusion, as hepatorenal syndrome therapy, 100
Extracellular fluid compartments, in fluid retention, 449
Extracellular fluid volume expansion
    effect on free fatty acids, 367
    in hepatorenal syndrome, 80
    natriuretic hormone-related regulation of, 359–360
      digitalis-like factors in, 361–365
    in mineralocorticoid escape, 293
Extracorporeal techniques. *See also* Dialysis; Hemofiltration
    for liver disease renal complications management, **517–528**

Fatty acids
    effect of extracellular volume on, 367
    in liver disease, 327
Fatty liver of pregnancy, 143
FE$_{Na}$ test (fractional excretion of filtered sodium), 94
Fentanyl, use in jaundiced patients, 433
FE$_{Ur}$ (fractional excretion of urea), 94
Fibrin split product titres, of intraoperative ascitic fluid, 499
Fibrosis, effect on loop vascular resistance, 233
Fick's technique, 242, 247
First-pass effect. *See* Drug elimination, presystemic
Fistulas
    aortoportal, 189, 190
    hepatic artery/portal vein, 189
    portacaval, 183
        end-to-end, 196, 199
        side-to-side, 200
FK506, use in liver transplantation patients, 534–535
Flint, Austin, 75–76
Fluid exchange, hepatic, 236–237
Fluid intake, in edema, 448
Fluid restriction, as hyponatremia treatment, 58–59
Fluid retention. *See also* Water retention
    following bone marrow transplantation, 168
Fractional excretion of filtered sodium (FE$_{Na}$), 94
Fractional excretion of urea (FE$_{Ur}$), 94
Free fatty acids, effect of extracellular fluid volume expansion
    on, 367
Free water clearance
    effect of prostaglandins on, 316, 317
    effect of thromboxane A$_2$ antagonists on, 323, 324
    effect of water immersion on, 46
Fulminant hepatic failure
    acid-base disorders in, 112–113
    atrial natriuretic factor in, 342
    extracorporeal treatment techniques for, 523–524
Fungal disease, concomitant with venoocclusive disease, 168
Furosemide, 453
    absorption of, 459–460
    albumin binding by, 456
    as ascites therapy, comparison with paracentesis, 480–482
    diuresis of, into urine, 473
    dosages of, 455, 474
    in liver transplantation patients, 534
    nonsteroidal antiinflammatory drug nephrotoxicity and,
        318–319
    refractory response to, 455–456

"Galambos' cocktail," 457
Gallbladder, hepatic mechanoreceptor phrenic afferents of, 259,
    261
Gastroesophageal reflux, ascites-related, 447
Gentamicin, interaction with endotoxin, 96
GFR. *See* Glomerular filtration rate
Glomerular abnormalities, in liver disease, **123–150**
    in cirrhosis, 123–130, 131
        as glomerulosclerosis, 124–125
    in hepatitis, 130–138
    in HIV infection, 123, 138–140
    immunoglobulin deposits, 126–128, 129, 130
    in infectious disease, 123, 124, 130–141
    in infectious mononucleosis, 141
    in malaria, 140–141
    in pregnancy, 124, 143
    in schistosomiasis, 140
    in sickle cell disease, 142
    in systemic disease, 123, 124, 141–143
Glomerular filtration rate
    in ascites, 212
    atrial natriuretic factor-related increase of, 271
    bile duct ligation-related increase of, 83
    endothelin-related decrease of, 392
    in hepatorenal syndrome, 76, 80, 85
    immunosuppressive drug-related decrease of, 529
    indomethacin-related decrease of, 318, 319, 320
    in jaundice, 422, 424, 426, 428
    in liver transplantation patients, 530
        effect of cyclosporine on, 533, 534
        effect of FK506 on, 535
        with hepatorenal syndrome, 536
    effect of nitric oxide on, 381
    peritoneal shunt-related increase of, 495, 496, 497
    prostaglandin inhibitor-related decrease of, 86
    prostaglandin-related decrease of, 313
    regulatory systems in, 378–380
    relationship to sodium reabsorption, 22
    renal sodium retention secondary to decrease in, 10
    in saline-loaded alcoholic cirrhosis, 3
Glomeruli, prostaglandin biosynthesis by, 310
Glomerulonephritis
    crescentic, 135
    hepatitis B virus-related, 131, 135–136, 137, 138
    immune-complex, 136, 137–138
        hepatitis C virus-related, 162–163
    membranous, 135–136
        hepatitis B virus-related, 131, 135
    resolution following liver transplantation, 128
Glomerulopressin, in hepatorenal syndrome, 92
Glomerulosclerosis
    lecithin-cholesterol acyltransferase deficiency and, 128–129
    pathogenesis of, 130
Glucagon
    in cirrhosis, 241, 247
    in liver disease-related hypotension, 82
Glucocorticoids, as angiotensinogen modulators, 268
Glucose, formation from lactate, 111
Glutamate, metabolism of, 109
Glycogenolysis, endothelin-related stimulation of, 395
Glycosides, cardiac, 364–365
Graft-versus-host disease, concomitant with venoocclusive
    disease, 168, 172–173, 174
Guanabenz, pharmacokinetics of, 463
Guillain-Barre syndrome, low-pressure baroreceptors in, 266

HABR. *See* Hepatic arterial buffer response
Halothane, use in jaundiced patients, 433
Hangovers, antidiuretic hormone levels in, 35–36

Heart, effect of jaundice on, 429–430

Heart donors, hepatitis C virus seropositivity of, 159

Heart rate, in cirrhosis, 241
  nocturnal, 251–252

Heart transplantation, low-pressure baroreceptor elimination in, 266

Hemaccel, as paracentesis plasma volume expander, 486, 487

Hematocrit, in jaundice, 431

Hemochromatosis, glomerular abnormalities in, 142

Hemodialysis
  as fulminant hepatic failure therapy, 523
  as hepatorenal syndrome therapy, 522

Hemodialysis patients, hepatitis C virus seropositivity of, 152, 154–156, 157–158
  control of, 158, 159

Hemodialysis staff, hepatitis C virus infections in, 156–157

Hemodynamics. *See also* Blood flow; Blood volume; Cerebral blood volume; Effective blood volume; Effective plasma volume; Plasma volume
  in cirrhosis, 241–246
    nitric oxide in, 380
  renal
    in hepatorenal syndrome, 77–83
    effect of nitric oxide on, 381
    effect of renin-angiotensin system on, 283
    effect of sympathetic nerve activity on, 413
    of sodium retention, 411–412
  splanchnic, in ascites, 188–191
  systemic, effect of transjugular intrahepatic shunts on, 513

Hemofiltration
  as ascites therapy, 519–522, 520
  as fulminant hepatic failure therapy, 523–524
  as hepatorenal syndrome therapy, 522–523, 524–525

Hemoperfusion, 524

Hemorrhage
  hepatic blood volume response in, 235–236
  jaundice-related, 433
  variceal
    peritoneovenous shunt-related, 497
    transjugular intrahepatic portosystemic shunt therapy for, 509–511

Heparin, as venoocclusive disease prophylaxis, 175

Hepatic arterial buffer response, 224–226, 231, 236, 237

Hepatic artery
  anatomy of, 222
  blood flow in, 221
    autoregulation of, 225
    regulation of, 223–224
    effect of vasoactive substances on, 226–227
  in cirrhosis, 227

Hepatic artery resistive index, 170

Hepatic disease. *See* Liver disease

Hepatic failure, atrial natriuretic factor natriuretic effects in, 366

Hepatic transplantation. *See* Liver transplantation

Hepatic venous outflow block
  in alcoholic cirrhosis, 213
  in ascites formation, 180–181, 182, 183–185, 214
  as sodium-retaining stimulus, 212

Hepatitis
  autoimmune lupoid, 131
  chronic active, renal tubular acidosis associated with, 117
  as fulminant hepatic failure cause, 112
  non-A, non-B, 151, 154, 158
    posttransplant, 159
  as venoocclusive disease risk factor, 168, 171, 173
  water excretion in, 54

Hepatitis B surface antigen, 132–133, 135, 136, 138

Hepatitis B virus infection
  coinfection with hepatitis C virus, 152, 157, 161

Hepatitis B virus infection *(cont.)*
  in end-stage renal disease, 530
  glomerular abnormalities in, 130–138
  relationship to essential mixed cryoglobulinemia, 163

Hepatitis C virus, biology of, 151–152

Hepatitis C virus infection, **151–166**
  coinfection with hepatitis B virus, 152, 157, 161
  diagnostic tests for, 152–154
  in end-stage renal disease, 154–158, 530
  in renal transplantation recipients, 158–162

Hepatocellular carcinoma, 161, 531

Hepatocytes
  effect of endothelin on, 395
  microvascular environment of, 222

Hepatopulmonary syndrome, 243

Hepatorenal-like syndrome, venoocclusive disease-related, 174

Hepatorenal reflex, 409, 410, 413
  in sodium retention, 202
  effect on sympathetic nerve activity 418, 419

Hepatorenal syndrome, **75–108**, 123
  acute azotemia and, 93–95
  acute renal failure versus, 92–93
  acute tubular necrosis versus, 93–95
  adenosine and renal function in, 91
  angiotensin II increase in, 84–85
  atrial natriuretic factor in, 91
  calcitonin gene-related peptide and, 92
  cardiac output in, 81–83
  clinical features of, 75–77
  as combined transplantation contraindication, 529–530, 538
  in decompensated cirrhosis, water administration response in, 40
  definition of, 75
  diagnostic tests in, 94–95
  differentiated from acute renal failure, 94–95
  diuretic-related, 76
  endothelin levels in, 50, 90, 399–400
  endotoxemia in, 89–90
  glomerulopressin and, 92
  hemodynamic abnormalities in, 77–83
  hepatorenal reflex in, 409
  hyponatremia in, 57
  iatrogenic, 76
  insulinlike growth factor-1, 91–92
  jaundice and, 83, 92–93
  kallikrein-kinin system in, 87–88
  nitric oxide alterations in, 89–90
  overflow theory of, 80–81
  pathogenesis of, 77–92
    afferent events in, 78–83
    efferent events in, 83–92
  peripheral arteriolar dilatation hypothesis of, 80, 203
  platelet activating factor (PAF) and, 92
  prognosis of, relationship to plasma renin activity, 284
  prostaglandins and, 314, 324–325, 86–87
    prostaglandin E_2 decrease in, 326
    prostaglandin E_2 as therapy for, 99, 326
  renal hemodynamics in, 77–78
  renal prostaglandins and, 86–87
  renal venous pressure in, 83
  renin-angiotensin system in, 84–86, 284–285
  renin increase in, 84, 285
  renin substrate decrease in, 85–86, 278
  sympathetic nervous system activity in, 88, 417, 419
  treatment of, 75, 95–102
    arachidonic acid precursor therapy, 327–328
    beta-blockers, 96
    calcium antagonists, 100–101
    dialysis, 97–98, 522–523, 524–525

Hepatorenal syndrome *(cont.)*
  treatment of *(cont.)*
    hemofiltration, 98, 524–525
    nonsteroidal antiinflammatory agents, 86
    ornipressin, 101
    paracentesis, 97
    peritoneovenous shunt, 98, 502–504
    prostaglandin analogues, 99
    thromboxane inhibitors, 99–100, 322–324
    transjugular intrahepatic portosystemic shunt, 99, 507, 512–513
    transplantation, hepatic, 98–99, 529–537
    vasoconstrictor therapy, 101–102
    water immersion, 100
  urinalysis in, 93–95
Histidine, hepatic metabolism of, 109–110
Holmes, Sherlock, 401
Hormones. *See also* specific hormones
  in ascites formation, 192
  hepatic clearance of, 225
Human immune deficiency virus (HIV) infection, glomerular abnormalities in, 123, 138–140
Humoral natriuretic factor, in sodium retention, 16–17
Humoral substances
  in ascites formation, 192, 211–212
  in cholestasis, 426
Hydration, as jaundice-related renal failure prophylaxis, 442
Hydrochlorothiazide, duration of effects, 472
Hydroflumethiazide, duration of effects, 472
Hydrogen ions, hepatic production of, 109–110, 111
Hydrothorax, refractory, 512
Hydroxyepoxyeicosatetraenoic acids, 366
4-Hydroxynonal, 435
Hydroxyzine, pharmacokinetics of, 463
Hyperaldosteronism
  control of, 298–301
  correlation with clinical status, 294–298
  estrogen-related, 212
  in liver disease, 1, 294–303
  plasma aldosterone levels in, 294, 295–303
  sodium retention and, 1, 4, 12–14
Hyperammonemia
  drug-induced, 119
  as hyperventilation cause, 114
Hyperbilirubinemia
  hepatorenal syndrome and, 83, 92–93
  transjugular intrahepatic portosystemic shunt treatment of, 174
  venoocclusive disease-related, 168, 170–171
Hypercalcemia, in liver transplantation patients, 530, 531
Hyperglycemia, diuretics-related, 452
Hyperkalemia, diuretics-related, 454, 455
Hyperlipidemia, diuretics-related, 452
Hypernatremia, 60–61
  in decompensated cirrhosis, 33
Hyperoxaluria, primary, 538
Hypertension
  digitalis-like factors-related, 365
  extracellular fluid volume dysregulation in, 368
  intrahepatic, in ascites formation, 211, 212
  intrasinusoidal
    as sodium retention cause, 353
  mineralocorticoid-related, 374
  portal
    in ascites formation, 45, 213, 182–183, 447
    blood circulation time in, 241
    in cirrhosis, 189, 253
    effect of endothelin on, 394
    hepatic artery/portal vein fistulas in, 189

Hypertension *(cont.)*
  portal *(cont.)*
    as peritoneovenous shunt contraindication, 502
    prostaglandin I_2 in, 325
    splanchnic hemodynamics in, 190–191
    splanchnic hyperemia and, 213
    sympathetic nervous system activity n, 250–251, 409
  toxemia-related, 142–143
Hyperuricemia, diuretics-related, 452
Hyperventilation
  as lactic acidosis cause, 116
  respiratory alkalosis-related, 114
Hypoalbuminemia
  in ascites formation, 191–192
  in hepatitis B virus-related nephropathy, 133
  estrogen-related, 212
Hypocomplementemia, 127, 130. *See also* Complement
Hypokalemia
  decompensated cirrhosis-related, 301
  diuretic-related, 450, 452, 456
  in liver transplantation patients, 531–532
  plasma renin activity and, 280
Hypomagnesemia, in liver transplantation patients, 532
Hyponatremia, 33
  effect on aldosterone secretion, 301
  ascites-related, 211
  in beer drinkers, 36–37
  central nervous system effects of, 57–58
  cirrhosis-related, effect of water administration on, 38
  clinical manifestations of, 55–57
  in decompensated cirrhosis, 55, 57
    effect of water administration on, 56
  development of, 45
  dilutional, 65, 448
  diuretics-related, 56–57, 480, 481, 482
  in liver transplantation patients, 532
  nonsteroidal antiinflammatory drug-related, 466–467
  paracentesis-related, 480, 481, 482, 483, 485, 486
  plasma renin activity and, 281
  prevention of, 58
  treatment of, 58–60, 65
Hypotension
  as antidiuretic hormone release stimulus, 48
  jaundice-related, 429, 431
  peripheral vasodilation in, 82–83
  platelet activating factor-related, 331
Hypotensive crises, jaundice-related, 442
Hypovolemia
  arterial
    as sodium retention mechanism, 411–412
    as sympathetic nervous system activation mechanism, 411–412
  cholestasis-related, 440
  in cirrhosis, 201, 244
    effect of postural change on, 252
    relationship to sympathetic nervous system activity, 250
    relationship to vasodilation, 246
  drug-induced, 95–96
Hypoxemia, as respiratory alkalosis cause, 114
Hypoxia, prostaglandin synthesis-stimulated activity of, 310

Ibuprofen
  dosage in cirrhosis, 469
  effect on angiotensin II pressor response, 325
  effect on creatinine clearance, 319
  pharmacokinetics of, 468
  prostaglandin-inhibiting activity of, 319
  effect on renal plasma flow, 322
Ileoentectomy, 491

Imidazole 2-hydroxybenzoate, 321
Immune complexes
    in AIDS, 139
    in glomerulonephritis, 136, 137–138, 162–163
Immunoglobulins
    in cirrhosis, 126–128, 129, 130
    in hepatitis B-associated nephropathy, 131, 136, 137
    in HIV infection, 139
    in malaria, 141
    in schistosomiasis, 140
    in sickle-cell disease, 142
Immunosuppressive agents, renal effects of, 529
Index of contractility, 230, 231, 232, 234
Indomethacin
    effect on angiotensin II pressor response, 325
    in cirrhosis, 318, 319
    effect on creatinine clearance, 319
    effect on glomerular filtration rate, 130
    nephrotoxicity of, prevention of, 327
    prostaglandin-inhibiting activity of, 313, 319, 320–321, 469–470
    effect on renal plasma flow, 130
Indoramin, pharmacokinetics of, 463
Infection, peritoneovenous shunt-related, 500
Infectious disease, glomerular abnormalities in, 123, 124, 130–141
    in AIDS, 139
Infectious mononucleosis, glomerular abnormalities in, 141
Inferior vena cava, mechanoreceptor phrenic afferents of, 259, 260, 261
Inner medullary collecting duct
    endothelin synthesis by, 389–390
    interaction with endothelins, 20
Inositol triphosphate, synthesis of, 309
Insulin, in jaundice, 432
Insulin deficiency, as ketoacidosis cause, 112
Insulinlike growth factor-1, in hepatorenal syndrome, 91
Interferon a-2b, 158
Interleukin-1, in venoocclusive disease, 171, 173
Interstitial fluid
    capacity of, 6
    in hepatorenal syndrome, 80
Intestinal wall, edema of, 181
Intraperitoneal pressure, effect on ascites reabsorption, 188
Intravenous isotonic infusion, as paracentesis plasma volume expander, 486–487
Ionizing radiation, as venoocclusive disease risk factor, 167, 168, 173
Ischemia, renal
    bile salts in, 83, 436–437
    hepatorenal syndrome-related, 81
    prostaglandin synthesis-stimulated activity of, 310
Isoproterenol, effect on hepatic circulation, 225–226

Jaundice
    catarrhal, 428–429
    in hepatorenal syndrome, 83
    renal failure and, 83, 92–93, **423–446**
        bile constituents in, 433–440
        clinical versus animal studies of, 425–426
        extrarenal and predisposing factors in, 428–433
        postoperative management of, 442
        postoperative mortality rate in, 423
        prophylactic therapy for, 441–442
        renal perfusion effects in, 426–427
        surgery-related stress response and, 432
        tubular function effects in, 427–428
Juxtaglomerular apparatus, 267
    cirrhosis-related changes in, 129
Juxtaglomerular apparatus cell counts,in liver disease, 273
Juxtaglomerular apparatus cells, asstretch receptors, 269
Juxtaglomerular nephrons, sodiumreabsorption in, 22

Kaliuresis. *See also* Potassium
    bile acids-related, 438
    diuretic-related, 456
    jaundice-related, 428
Kaliuretic stimulator, 352, 353
Kallikrein-kinin system
    hepatorenal syndrome and, 87–88
    renin-angiotensin system interactions with, 272
    and sodium retention, 16
Kaposi's sarcoma, 139
Ketansirin, pharmacokinetics of, 463
Ketoacidosis
    diabetic, 112
    hepatic hydrogen ion production in, 109
Ketogenesis, 112
6-Keto-prostaglandin F1a
    biosynthesis of, 311
    in cirrhosis, 314, 316–317, 325, 326
    excretion of
        in cirrhosis, 314, 316–317
        in hepatorenal syndrome, 324
Kidney
    acid-base homeostasis role of, 111
    endothelin synthesis by, 389–390
    failure, 92–93. *See also* Renal failure, acute; Hepatorenal syndrome
    in hyperaldosteronism, 302–303
    in jaundice, 423–424
    natriuretic factors of, 366
    weight of, in cirrhosis, 129–130
Kidney donors, hepatitis C virus seropositivity of, 159–160
Kidney transplantation
    combined with liver transplantation, 529–530, 537–538
    in hepatitis surface antigen carriers, 135
    hepatorenal syndrome donors in, 77
    low-pressure baroreceptor elimination in, 266
    venoocclusive disease following, 167
Kidney transplantation recipients, hepatitis virus C infection in, 158–162
Kininase II. *See* Angiotensin-converting enzyme
Kinins. *See also* Kallikrein-kinin system
    in cirrhosis, 241
    prostaglandin synthesis-stimulated activity of, 310
Kuppfer cells
    endothelin synthesis in, 390, 395
    as endotoxin removal site, 88
    immune complex uptake by, 128

Lactate
    in hepatic metabolism, 111–112
    metabolism of, 109
D-Lactic acidosis syndrome, 109
Lactulose, as jaundice-related renal failure prophylaxis, 441
Lecithin-cholesterol acyltransferase, 327
Lecithin-cholesterol acyltransferase deficiency, 128–129
Left ventricular volume, in cirrhosis, 208–209
Legionnaire's disease, 141
Leg wrapping, in edematous patients, 457
Leukotrienes, 327–330
    cysteinyl, in liver disease, 401
    distribution and functions of, 307
    in hepatorenal syndrome, 329–330
Le Veen shunt, 197–198, 496, 503. *See also* Peritoneovenous shunt
    characteristics of, 492–494

Le Veen shunt *(cont.)*
  comparison with paracentesis, 480, 487–488, 489
  complications of, 497–500
  as hepatorenal syndrome therapy, 98
  patency of, 495
  use in refractory ascites, 189
  thrombotic obstruction of, 487, 488, 489
Lidocaine, pharmacokinetics of, 463
Linoleic acid, 307, 328
Lipids, hepatic synthesis and metabolism of, 327
Lipotropin, 365
Lithium clearance, 11
Liver
  in acid-base homeostasis, 109–112
  as aldosterone degradation site, 294
  as ascitic fluid source, 180
  as blood reservoir, 234. *See also* Blood volume, hepatic
  endothelin receptors in, 391–392
  endothelin synthesis by, 390
  microcirculation in, 182
  water metabolism function of, 33–35
Liver disease. *See also* Cirrhosis
  natriuretic hormone abnormalities in, 367–368
  reversible, 3
  spontaneous diuresis in, 3
    during menstrual cycle, 4
Liver function, endothelin in, 394–395
Liver function testing, of hepatitis C virus infection patients,
    152, 153
Liver perfusion, ex vivo baboon, 100
Liver transplantation, **529–542**
  acid-base abnormalities following, 114, 531, 532
  calcium antagonists as treatment in, 534
  combined liver-kidney, 529–530, 537–538
  cyclosporine and, 532–535
  dopamine, as treatment in, 534
  FK506 and, 534–535
  glomerulonephritis following, 128
  as hepatorenal syndrome therapy, 77, 535–537
  low-pressure baroreceptor elimination in, 266
  metabolic acidosis following, 114, 531, 532
  orthotopic, as hepatorenal syndrome therapy, 75, 78, 98–99,
    102
  perioperative concerns in, 530–532
  as refractory ascites therapy, 507, 17–518
  renal function following, 532–535
Lobar venous pressure, 228–230, 231–232
Lobar venous pressure-central venous pressure gradient, 233
Loop of Henle, sodium chloride absorption in, 18–19
Lymph
  hepatic
    in ascites formation, 183, 187
    in cirrhosis, 237
    flow of, 186–187
    formation of, 182, 183–184, 186, 189–190, 213
    in venous hypertension, 181
  intestinal, 213
Lymphatics, hepatic, 236–237
Lysine, hepatic metabolism of, 109–110
Lysophosphatidyl choline, natriuretic activity of, 365, 367

Macula densa, in renin release, 270, 312–313
Malaria, glomerular abnormalities in, 140–141
Malate, metabolism of, 109
Malnutrition, jaundice-related, 431–432
Malondialdehyde, 435, 437
Mannitol, as jaundice-related renal failure prophylaxis, 442
Mean arterial pressure, in sodium-restricted cirrhosis patients,
    2–3

Mechanoreceptors, hepatic, with phrenic nerve afferents,
    259–266
Medullary cystic disease, 143
Melanocyte-stimulating hormone, 365
Membrane depolarization, endothelin-related, 395–396
Menstrual cycle, spontaneous diuresis during, 4
Mersalyl, 448
Mesangium
  glomerular, nitric oxide synthesis by, 379
  effect of prostaglandins on, 312
Mesenteric vessels, in cirrhosis and ascites, 189
Metaraminol, 101
Methionine, hepatic metabolism of, 109–110
Methionine enkephalin, in cirrhosis, 247
Methotrexate, as venoocclusive disease risk factor, 173
Methyl dopa, effect on renin release, 271
Miconazole, pharmacokinetics of, 463
β_2-Microglobulin, 95
Microsphere method, of blood flow measurement, 242
"Mineralocorticoid escape," 197, 293
Mineralocorticoids, as alkalosis cause, 115
N^GMonomethyl-L-arginine, as nitric oxide inhibitor, 375, 376,
    379
Mucositis, oral, as venoocclusive disease risk factor, 173
Muscles
  blood flow in, 242–243
  sympathetic nerve activity in, 410–411, 412, 416, 417
Muzolimine, 453
Myelinolysis, central pontine, 532
Myocardial dysfunction
  in ascites, 191
  hepatorenal syndrome-related, 96
  renal failure-related, 81

Nabumetone, pharmacokinetics of, 468
Na-K-ATPase. *See* Sodium-potassium-ATPase
Naproxen
  dosage in cirrhosis, 469
  nephrotoxicity of, 318
  pharmacokinetics of, 468
  prostaglandin-inhibiting activity of, 319
Natriuresis. *See also* Sodium excretion; Sodium handling,
    renal
  bile acids-related, 438, 439
  jaundice-related, 428
  nitric oxide-induced, 376–378, 381–382
  nocturnal, atrial natriuretic factor in, 348–349
  peritoneovenous shunting-related increase of, 495–497
  pressure-induced, nitric oxide-mediated, 376–378
  spontaneous, atrial natriuretic factor in, 341–342
Natriuretic hormone, **359–372**
  digitalis-like activity of, 361–365
  in extracellular fluid volume regulation, 359, 366–368
  mineralocorticoid escape-related release of, 293
  sodium pump-inhibiting activity of, 361
Necrosis
  acute tubular, 81, 93–95
  subacute hepatic, 131
Nephritis, HIV-related, 139
Nephrolithiasis, juvenile, 143
Nephrons
  distal
    decreased filrate delivery to, 52–53
    low water flow in, 53–54
    sensitivity to antidiuretic hormone, 52
  diuretics' action sites on, 451
  endothelin receptor distribution in, 391
  prostaglandin synthesis and release by, 309–310
  sodium reabsorption sites of, 10–11

Nephropathy, immunoglobulin A, 127
Nephrotic syndrome, 142, 183
Neuropathy, diabetic, low-pressure baroreceptors in, 266
Nisoldipine, pharmacokinetics of, 463
Nitric oxide, 366, **373–385**
    as antidiuretic hormone release mediator, 50–51
    in arteriolar vasodilation, 7
    in cirrhosis, 248–249, 379–382
        effect on splanchnic arterial inflow, 191
    effect on endothelin receptor binding, 396–397
    in hepatorenal syndrome, 75, 89–90
    kinetics of, 248–249
    in liver disease-related hypotension, 82–83
    renal effects of, 376–382
        glomerular-tubular dynamics regulation, 377–378
        hyperdynamic circulation, 7, 380
        pressure-induced natriuresis, 376–377
        shear stress in, 378, 380
    in sodium retention, 21
    synthesis of, 373–376
        inhibition of, 375
Nitric oxide synthase, 21, 89, 374
    endotoxin induction of, 432
Nitric oxide synthtases, 374
N^{G}Nitro-L-arginine methyl ester (L-NAME), 375–379, 381
Nonsteroidal antiinflammatory drugs
    contraindications to
        in jaundice, 93
        in hepatorenal syndrome, 95
        prior to liver transplantation, 530
    in decompensated cirrhosis, 95, 99
    as edema cause, 313
    interaction with potassium-sparing diuretics, 454
    nephrotoxicity of, in cirrhosis, 318–321
    pharmacokinetics of, 459, 466–470
    prostaglandin-inhibiting action of, 317–318
19-Norbufalin, 363, 364
Norepinephrine
    as antidiuretic hormone nonosmotic release mediator, 48, 49
    in cirrhosis
        in compensated versus decompensated cirrhosis, 410
        in decompensated cirrhosis, 410
        relationship to ascites, 410
        relationship to sympathetic nervous system activity, 19–20, 88, 249
        effect of water immersion on, 281
    hepatic clearance of, 406
    in hepatorenal syndrome, 80
    infusion with exogenous atrial natriuretic factor, 347–348
    in jaundice, 426–427
    in liver transplantation patients, 530
    measurement of plasma levels of, 249, 406
    effect of peritoneovenous shunting on, 250–251
    pressor response to, in bile duct-ligated animals, 429, 430, 431
    prostaglandin synthesis-stimulated activity of, 310
    relationship to creatinine clearance, 97
    as sympathetic nervous system activity indicator, 406, 408, 410–411, 414
        effect of clonidine on, 418–419
        relationship to urinary sodium excretion, 415, 416
    water immersion suppression of, 412

Octapressin, 101
Oliguria
    acute renal failure-related, 94
    antidiuretic hormone mediation of, 43
    in cirrhosis, 93
    hepatorenal syndrome-related, 77
Omentopexy, 491

Opioids, endogenous, in sodium and water retention, 22–23
Organomercurials, 453
Ornipressin, 101–102
Ornithine carbamyl transferase deficiency, 114
Osmoreceptors, hepatic, 33–34
    in cirrhosis, 51
Ouabagenin, 363
Ouabain
    interation with atrial natriuretic factor, 364
    natriuretic action of, 362–363, 368
Ouabain isomer, endogenous, 363–364
Ouabainlike factor, 367
Overfill hypothesis, of ascites, 5, 7–10, 80–81, 192–201, 214, 508
    combined with underfilling theory, 210–211
Oxaprozin
    dosage in cirrhosis, 469
    pharmacokinetics of, 463, 468
Oxidative metabolism dysfunction, relationship to renal sodium retention, 202
Oxygen free radicals, in bile-induced cellular damage, 435, 436–437, 439, 441
Oxygen uptake, hepatic, in pathologic conditions, 226

Paracentesis, 491
    as ascites therapy, 447, **479–490**
        with albumin infusion, 480–485
        comparison with ascites reinfusion, 518
        comparison with diuretic therapy, 480–482
        comparison with peritoneovenous shunting, 487–488, 489
        complications of, 480–482, 483, 485, 486
        large-volume, 482, 483–485, 489, 507, 514, 517–518
        renal function effects of, 83
        total, 482, 487, 488–489
    atrial natriuretic factor levels following, 346
    as hepatorenal syndrome therapy, 97
    large-volume
        as ascites therapy, 482, 483–485, 489
        hyponatremia and, 59
        as refractory ascites therapy, 507, 514, 517–518, 521
        as sodium retention therapy, 25–26
Paracetamol, as fulminant hepatic failure cause, 112
Paracrine factors, renal, 366
Parathyroid hormone, in liver transplantation patients, 531, 532
Parenchyma, hepatic mechanoreceptor phrenic afferents of, 259, 260, 261
Parenteral nutrition, as jaundice-related renal failure prophylaxis, 441
Pentoxifylline, 176
Pericardium, hepatic mechanoreceptor phrenic afferents of, 261–264
Peripheral arterial vasodilation (revised underfill) theory of sodium retention, 5–7, 45, 80, 203–207, 508
Peripheral vascular resistance
    in ascites formation, 197, 211
    in edematous cirrhosis, 6
    in hepatorenal syndrome, 80
    peritoneovenous shunting-related decrease of, 495
    in preascitic cirrhotic sodium retention, 203, 204, 205, 205–207, 209
    in sodium retention, 206–207
Peritoneal space
    ascites sequestration in, 213–214
    ascitic fluid reabsorption in, 187–188
Peritoneo-ureterostomy, 491–492
Peritoneovenous shunting, **491–506**
    as ascites therapy, 199, 447
    atrial natriuretic factor responsiveness to, 345–346
    comparison with paracentesis, 487–488, 489
    complications of, 497–500

Peritoneovenous shunting (cont.)
  Cordis-Hakim shunt, 492
  Denver shunt, 492, 494, 495, 500
  as hepatorenal syndrome therapy, 98, 102, 502–504, 512–513
  Le Veen shunt, 492–494, 495, 496, 503
    complications of, 497–500
  effect on plasma norepinephrine concentration, 250–251
  obstruction of, 487, 488, 489, 507
  physiologic consequences of, 495–500
  as refractory ascites therapy, 507, 514, 517–518, 521
  shunt patency in, 494–495
Peritonitis, peritoneovenous shunt-related, 500
Peroneal nerve, sympathetic nerve activity in, 410
Pharmacokinetics and pharmacodynamics, in liver disease, **459–477**
  principles of, 459–466
  of specific drugs, 466–474
8-Phenyltheophlline, 225
Phenytoin, pharmacokinetics of, 463
Phosphate excretion, effect of water immersion on, 11
Phosphatidyl-choline, 307, 309
Phosphatidyl-ethanolamine, 307, 309
Phosphatidyl-inositol, as arachidonic acid precursor, 309
Phospholipase A_2
  activation of, 309, 312, 313, 330
  in arachidonic acid metabolism, 309
Phospholipase C
  activation of, 312
  in arachidonic acid metabolism, 309
Phospholipids, in liver disease, 327
Phrenic nerve, hepatic mechanoreceptor afferents of, **259–266**
Pinacidil, pharmacokinetics of, 463
Pituitary gland, endothelin synthesis by, 389
Plasma, natriuretic activity of, 360, 361, 368
Plasma exchange, 524
Plasma renin activity
  in advanced liver disease, 4
  age factors as determinant of, 271
  in ascites, 273, 274–277
  assays of, 272–273
  effect of atrial natriuretic factor 270–271, 348
  baroreceptor-related increase of, 270
  in bile duct-ligated animals, 427
  in cirrhosis, 273–276, 298
    relationship to plasma aldosterone levels, 299–301
    relationship to renin secretion, 279–280
  correlation with angiotensin II, 277–278
  in hepatorenal syndrome, 80
  effect of paracentesis on, 483, 484, 485–486
  peritoneovenous shunt-related decrease of, 495, 496
  race factors in, 271
  sympathetic nervous system activity and, 270
  transjugular intrahepatic shunt-related decrease of, 511
  effect of water immersion on, 344–345
Plasma renin concentration (PRC), 272–273
  in cirrhosis, 277–278
Plasma volume. See also Hypovolemia
  in ascites, 5, 7
  in cirrhosis, 244
    effect of intrahepatic pressure on, 201
  nonsplanchnic, in ascites formation, 196–197
  in sodium retention, 7–10
Plasma volume expansion
  and ascites formation, 201
  in cirrhosis, as cause of circulatory abnormalities, 209
  as postoperative renal failure preventive, 442
  in preascitic cirrhotic sodium retention, 194–195, 203, 210
Platelet activating factor, 365
  biochemical and physiologic characteristics of, 330–331

Platelet activating factor (cont.)
  in cirrhosis, 331–332
  in hepatorenal syndrome, 92
  prostaglandin synthesis-stimulated activity of, 310
Platelet aggregating factors, in ascitic fluid, 499
Plethysmography, venous occlusive, 242
PLV-2, as hepatorenal syndrome therapy,101
Pneumothorax, peritoneovenous shunt-related, 497
Polyacrylonitrile dialysis, 523
Polyarteritis nodosa, 137
Polycystic kidney disease, 143
Polymerase chain reaction, use in hepatitis C virus infection diagnosis, 153–154, 155, 158
Polymyxin B, as jaundice-related renal failure prophylaxis, 441
Portacaval collateral channels, 213
Portacaval shunts
  as hepatorenal syndrome therapy, 512–513
  side-to-side, as refractory ascites therapy, 508
Portacaval shunt vessels, 232
Portal vein
  anatomy of, 222
  ascitic fluid pressure on, 213–214
Portal-vein ligation, sodium excretion/peripheral vascular resistance relationship in, 206–207
Portal venous pressure, 222
  in cirrhosis, 232–233, 246, 247
  regulation of, 227–230
  relationship to lobar venous pressure, 228–230, 233
Portal venous pressure-central venous pressure gradient, 233
Portal venous pressure-lobar venous pressure gradient, 233, 228–230
Portal venous resistance, venous distensibility in, 230, 231–232
Posture, effect on renin-aldosterone axis, 271
Potassium
  and aldosterone secretion, 292, 301
  excretion of, mineralocorticoid-related increase of, 293
  effect on renin release, 270, 271, 274
Potassium depletion
  in cirrhosis, hyperaldosteronism-related, 303
  renal, 118
PRA. See Plasma renin activity
Practolol, effect on aldosterone secretion, 299–300
Preanesthesia medications, use in jaundiced patients, 433
Prednisone, as hepatorenal syndrome therapy, 100
Pregnancy, glomerular abnormalities in, 124, 143
Pretanide, 453
Prolactin, in sodium retention, 23–24
Proopiomelanocortin, 365
Propranolol
  effect on aldosterone secretion, 299–300
  pharmacokinetics of, 463
Prorenin, 268
Prostacyclin
  in cirrhosis, 325–326
  cyclosporine-related excretion of, 533
Prostaglandin(s), 366
  biosynthesis of, 307–309
  in cirrhosis, 241
    effects of diuretics on, 321–322
    experimental models of, 316–317
    inhibition of, 317–321
    renal sodium handling effects of, 1– 2, 315–316
    effect on maximal urine osmolality, 63
  as cirrhosis therapy, 326–327
  distribution of, 307, 309–310
  excretion of, 311
  functions of, 307

Prostaglandin(s) *(cont.)*
 half-life of, 311
 in nitric oxide synthesis, 381–382
 nonsteroidal antiinflammatory drug-related inhibition of, 466,
   467, 469–470
 renal
  as antidiuretic hormone nonosmotic release mediator,
    48–50
  biological actions of, 312–313
  in cirrhosis, 313–322
  in hepatorenal syndrome, 86–87
  in jaundice, 427, 428
  metabolism of, 311
  physiologic functions of, 466
  renal perfusion effects of, 466, 467
  in sodium retention, 15–16
  in water handling, 65
 renin-angiotensin system interactions of, 272
 in renin release, 270
 sources of, 309
 systemic, sulindac-related inhibition of, 15–16
 urinary, 311
  in hepatitis, 54
 vasodilator, renal effects of, 312
Prostaglandin A, as prostaglandin deficiency therapy, 99
Prostaglandin A_1, as cirrhosis therapy, 326
Prostaglandin D_2, biosynthesis of, 309
Prostaglandin E, in decompensated cirrhosis, 86
Prostaglandin E_1
 as prostaglandin deficiency therapy, 99
 as venoocclusive disease therapy, 174–175
Prostaglandin E_2
 as antidiuretic hormone nonosmotic release mediator, 48, 49
 biosynthesis of, 309, 310
  correlation with excretion, 311
 excretion of
  in cirrhosis, 63, 313, 314, 316–317
   effect of cyclosporine on, 533
   as estimate of renal PG synthesis, 311
 in hepatorenal syndrome, 324, 325
 as hepatorenal syndrome therapy, 326
 and renal sodium handling, 315–316
 renin-releasing activity of, 313
Prostaglandin E_2 receptors, 311–312
Prostaglandin endoperoxide synthase, 307
 isoenzymes of, 309
 nephronal distribution of, 309–310
 pathway, 308, 309
Prostaglandin $F_2\alpha$
 biosynthesis of, 309, 310
 excretion of, in cirrhosis, 314
Prostaglandin $F_2\alpha$ receptors, 312
Prostaglandin H_2, biosynthesis of, 309
Prostaglandin I_2
 biosynthesis of, 309
  in hepatorenal syndrome, 324–325
 in cirrhosis, 325, 326
 diuretic mediating activity of, 322
 excretion/biosynthesis correlation of, 311
 glomerular production of, 310
 renin-releasing activity of, 313
Prostaglandin I_2 receptors, 312
Prostaglandin receptors, 311–312
Protein
 metabolic oxidation of, 109–111
 reabsorption from ascitic compartment, 188
Protein binding, by drugs, 460–462
Protein C, as venoocclusive disease risk factor, 171–172
Protein kinase C, 351

Protein status, effect of peritoneovenous shunting on, 497
Protein transport, hepatic interstitium in, 186
Proteinuria, 126, 129
 amyloidosis-related, 142
 hepatitis B virus-associated nephropathy-related, 133,
   134–135
 HIV infection-related, 139
 toxemia-related, 142–143
Proximal tubules
 glomerular filtrate absorption by, 451
 inhibition of sodium reabsorption by diuretics, 454
Pseudohepatorenal syndromes, 75, 76, 93
Pulmonary vascular resistance, incirrhosis, 243

Rappaport's zone, 222
Recombinant immunoblot assay, for hepatitis C virus infection
   diagnosis, 154, 156
 in renal transplantation recipients, 160, 161, 162
Recombinant tissue plasminogen factor, 175
Reflex autonomic stimulation, cardiovascular responsiveness to,
   in cirrhosis, 19
Renal dysfunction, cyclosporine-related, in liver transplantation
   patients, 532–534
Renal failure
 acute
  acute tubular necrosis-related, 92
  differentiated from hepatorenal syndrome, 93
  diuretic-related, 456
  endothelin in, 398–399, 400, 401
  myoglobinuria, 95
  postoperative, with jaundice, 92–93, 423, 432
 acute fatty liver of pregnancy-related, 143
 amyloidosis-related, 142
 chronic, hypernatremia in, 60, 61
 functional
  plasma norepinephrine concentration in, 413
  refractory ascites-related, 479
 in hepatitis B virus-associated nephropathy, 134–135
 post-liver transplantation, 532
 post-lung transplantation, 530
 progressive oliguric. *See* Hepatorenal syndrome
 renin-angiotensin system in, 284–285
 venoocclusive disease-related, 174
Renal function
 endothelin in, 392–394
 following liver transplantation, 532–535
 effects of sympathetic nervous system activity on,
   412–419
Renal natriuretic peptide. *See* Urodilatin
Renal perfusion, peritoneovenous shunting-related increase of,
   495
Renal plasma flow, in saline-loadedalcoholic cirrhosis, 3
Renal transplantation. *See* Kidney transplantation
Renal tubular acidosis, 117
Renin. *See also* Plasma renin activity
 active form of, 268–269
  assays of, 273
 in angiotensin II production, 291–292
 angiotensinogen substrate of, 267, 268
 in ascites formation, 211
 cirrhosis-related increase of, 280–281
 discovery of, 267
 factors influencing, 271
 hepatic extraction of, 279–280
 inactive form of, 268–269
  assays of, 273
 release of, 269–271, 312–313
  nitric oxide-mediated, 378–379
 secretion of, 269–271

Renin-angiotensin system, **267–289**, 291–292
  aldosterone regulatory function of, 291–292, 298–301
  in antidiuretic hormone nonosmotic release, 48
  in cirrhosis, 17, 241
    wedged hepatovenous pressure in, 205
  in hepatorenal syndrome, 84–86
  effect of jaundice on, 427
  in liver disease, 273–281
    decreased renin hepatic extraction in, 279–280
    increased renin secretion in, 280–281
    pharmacologic blockade in, 285–286
    relationship to disease prognosis, 283–284
    responsiveness of, 281–283, 301–302
  measurement of components of, 272–273
  physiology of, 267–273
  in renal failure, 284–285
  as renal hemodynamics determinant, 283
  in sodium retention, 14–15, 249
  vasoactive interrelationships of, 271–272
  in water retention, 249
Renin substrate, 267, 268
  hepatorenal syndrome-related decrease of, 85–86
  liver disease-related decrease of, 278
Renin substrate concentration (PRC), 273
Resibufogenin, 363
Respiratory failure, 118
Reye's syndrome
  acid-base abnormalities in, 114
  as fulminant hepatic failure cause, 112, 113
Rhabdomyolysis, in liver transplantation patients, 532
Rhamnose, mammalian production of, 362
Rhodiascit machine, 498, 518, 521
Ro 46-2005, as endothelin receptor antagonist, 398, 399

Saline
  as ascitic fluid replacement, 499–500
  isotonic, as metabolic alkalosis therapy, 118
  volume expansion, atrial natriuretic factor responsiveness to, 345
Saline loading, in compensated alcoholic cirrhosis, 3
Salyrgan, 448
Sarafotoxins, 387
Saralasin, effect on aldosterone secretion, 299
Schistosomiasis, 140, 183, 206
Sedative-hypnotics, central nervous system sensitivity to, 526
Sensory receptors, renal, and sympathetic nerve activity, 408–409
Sepsis, concomitant with venoocclusive disease, 168, 174
Shock
  endotoxic, hypotension during, 374
  hemorrhagic, in jaundice, 433, 440–441
Sickle-cell disease, glomerular abnormalities in, 142
Sinusoidal capillarization, 191
Sinusoidal endothelial cells, 223
Sinusoidal pressure
  hepatic venous outflow block-related increase of, 184–185
  relationship to hepatic venous pressure, 184
Sinusoids, hepatic
  as ascites source, 180, 181, 182
  blood distribution in, 222
  in cirrhosis, 185–186
  filtration function of, 236–237
  fluid exchange across, 182
  hydrostatic pressure increase in, 213
  permeability of, 185, 186
  protein selectivity of, 186
Slow continuous ultrafiltration, as ascites therapy, 520
Smooth muscle, effect of prostaglandins on, 312

Sodium
  effect on aldosterone release, 292–293
  dietary intake of
    atrial natriuretic factor responsiveness in, 346–347
    for cirrhotic ascites management, 25
    effect on sympathetic nervous activity, 409
  prostaglandin-mediated tubular transport of, 313
  relationship to plasma renin activity, 271, 280–281
  urinary concentration of, as sodium retention indicator, 94
Sodium chloride receptors, hepatic, 409
Sodium excretion. *See also* Natriuresis
  aldosterone-related, 12–14, 293
  in cirrhosis, 448
  in decompensated cirrhosis, during water loading, 41–42
  functional, 7
  peritoneovenous shunt-related increase of, 496, 497
  transjugular intrahepatic shunt-related increase of, 511
  relationship to sympathetic nerve activity, 18–20, 414–416, 418–419
Sodium handling, by kidney. *See also* Sodium retention
  effect of Le Veen shunting on, 199, 495–497
  renal, **1–31**
    effect of peritoneovenous shunting on, 496–497
    effect of sympathetic nerve activity on, 414
  in decompensated cirrhosis, following water immersion, 9
  physiology and control of, 315–316
  effect of prostaglandins on, 15–16, 315–316
Sodium ions, renin-inhibiting effect of, 271
Sodium loading, ascites as indicator of, 4
Sodium pentobarbitone, use in jaundiced patients, 433
Sodium-potassium-ATPase
  in acute extracellular fluid volumeexpansion, 367
  in cirrhosis, 367–368
  endothelin-related inhibition of, 392–393
  natriuretic hormone-related inhibition of, 361–362, 363–364
  sodium pump binding inhibitors of, 17
Sodium reabsorption, by kidney
  sites of, 10–12
  in sodium repletion, 450
  in sodium-restricted cirrhosis, 2–3
Sodium-restricted diet
  as cirrhosis therapy, 25, 448
  as hyponatremia therapy, 59
Sodium retention
  without ascites, 198–199
  ascites-related
    afferent factors in, 5–10, 211–212
    clinical studies of, 7–12, 207–208
    critical function threshold theory of, 201–203
    overfill theory of, 5, 7–10, 80–81, 192–201, 210–211, 214, 508
    peripheral arterial vasodilation theory of, 5–7, 45, 80, 203–207, 508
    underfill theory of, 5, 45, 193, 195, 208–209, 210–211, 214, 241, 508
  atrial natriuretic factor in, 17–18, 346–347, 353, 354
  in cirrhosis, 3
    atrial natriuretic factor in, 17–18, 353, 354
    hemodynamic mechanisms of, 411–412
    hyperaldosteronism-related, 12–14, 302–303
  in hepatic disease, 368
  effect of humoral natriuretic factor on, 16–17
  effect of kallikrein-kinin system on, 16
  in liver disease, **1–31**
    afferent events in, 2, 4–10
    clinical features of, 2–4
    efferent events in, 2, 10–24
    factors influencing, 12–24
    management of, 24–26

Sodium retention *(cont.)*
  in liver disease *(cont.)*
    pathogenesis of, 4–24
  in preascitic cirrhosis, 194–201, 203, 210–211
    clinical studies of, 207–210
    peripheral arteriolar dilatation hypothesis of, 5–7, 203–207, 508
  in primary biliary cirrhosis, 4
  effect of prostaglandins on, 15–16
  relationship to hyperaldosteronism, 12–14
  renal sodium reabsorption sites in, 10–12
  resistant, combined diuretic therapy for, 456
  effect on sympathetic nerve activity, 18–20, 417–419
  urine osmolality and, 4
  venoocclusive disease-related, 168
Space of Disse, 236, 237
Space of Mall, 222, 224, 226, 236
Spironolactone
  adverse effects of, 454–455
  in cirrhotic functional renal failure, 479
  dosages of, 454, 458
  furosemide and, as ascites therapy, 480–482
  use in liver transplantation patients, 532
  pharmacokinetics, in cirrhosis, 471–472
  prostaglandin-mediated natriuretic response to, 322
  effect on sodium excretion, 12–13, 14, 454–456
Splanchnic blood vessels. *See also* Blood flow, splanchnic
  in ascites formation, 182
Splenomegaly, portal hypertension and, 189
Staphylococcus aureus infections, in peritoneovenous shunt patients, 500
Starling equation, 236
Starling forces
  in ascites, 5, 6, 7, 180, 192, 193, 214
  in ascitic fluid peritoneal reabsorption, 187
  in cirrhotic edema, 198
  in hepatorenal syndrome, 80
  in renal sodium reabsorption, 22
Steroids
  contraindication in hepatitis, 135
  endogenous ouabain, 363–364
Stress response, jaundice-related impairment of, 432
Substance P
  in cirrhosis, 241, 247
  in liver disease-related hypotension, 82
Sulindac
  dosage in cirrhosis, 469
  effect on diuresis, 322
  interaction with prostaglandins, 15–16, 319–322, 469–460
  effect on natriuresis, 322
  nephrotoxicity of, 318
  pharmacokinetics of, 468
  effect on renal plasma flow, 322
  thromboxane B_2-inhibiting activity of, 469–470
Superior vena cava syndrome, 487
Sympathetic nerve activity, **405–422**
  as atrial natriuretic factor responsiveness determinant, 349–350
  in cirrhosis, 406–419
    cardiac baroreceptors interact with, 408
    effects of, 412–419
    measurement of, 406–407
    mechanisms of, 407–410, 411–412
  in hypovolemia, 250
  in renal sodium handling, 18–20, 416–417
Sympathetic nervous system
  in cirrhosis, 19–20, 250–251
  in hepatorenal syndrome, 88
  in renal vasoconstriction, 424

Sympathetic nervous system *(cont.)*
  in renin release, 270
  in sodium retention, 249
  in water retention, 249
Syndrome of inappropriate antidiuretic hormone secretion, 7, 59
Systemic disease, glomerular abnormalities in, 123, 124, 141–143
Systemic lupus erythematosus, 131, 132
Systemic vascular resistance
  in cirrhosis, 241, 253
  correlation with calcitonin gene-related peptide, 250, 251

Taurocholic acid, 436, 438
Temoxicam, pharmacokinetics of, 468
Thiorphan, 351
Thoracic duct, hepatic lymph flow in, 187
Thromboxane A_2
  as antidiuretic hormone nonosmotic release mediator, 50
  in cirrhosis, 314
    excretion of, 314
    renal functional effects, 322–323
  half-life of, 311
  in hepatorenal syndrome, 87, 324–325
  imidazole 2-hydroxybenzoate-related inhibition of, 321
Thromboxane A_2 receptors, 312
  cyclic endoperoxide binding by, 309
Thromboxane B_2
  excretion of
    in cirrhosis, 314
    in cirrhosis with ascites, 322–323
    correlation with biosynthesis, 311
    cyclosporine-related, 533
  in hepatorenal syndrome, 87
  imidazole 2-hydroxybenzoate-related inhibition of, 321
Thromboxane inhibitors, as hepatorenal syndrome therapy, 99–100
Tolbutamine, pharmacokinetics of, 463
Tolfenamic acid
  dosage in cirrhosis, 469
  pharmacokinetics of, 468
Toxemia. *See also* Endotoxemia
  glomerular abnormalities in, 142–143
Transforming growth factor-β
  effect on endothelin synthesis, 390
  hepatitis-related increase of, 171, 173
Transjugular intrahepatic portosystemic shunting (TIPS), 174, **507–516**
  development of, 508–509
  as hepatorenal syndrome therapy, 75, 99, 507, 512–513
  as refractory ascites therapy, 507, 511–512, 514, 517–518, 521
  techniques of, 510
  theoretical basis of, 508
  as variceal hemorrhage therapy, 509–511
Transplantation, liver, **529–542**
Triamterene
  pharmacokinetics of, 471
  as spironolactone alternative, 454–455
Trichlormethiazide, duration of effects, 472
Tubular function, in jaundice, 427–428, 438
Tubular reabsorption of water, in cirrhosis, 63–64, 65
Tubuloglomerular feedback response, in glomerular filtration, 379–380
Tumor necrosing factor, in venoocclusive disease, 171, 176
Tumor-necrosing factor-α
  in hypertension, 248
  nitric oxide release-inducing activity of, 248

Ultrafiltration
  as ascites therapy, 458
  dialytic, as ascites therapy, 518–520, 521

Ultrasound, hepatic, use in venoocclusive disease evaluation, 170

Underfill theory, of ascites formation, 5, 45, 193, 195, 208–209, 210, 214, 241, 508
  peripheral vascular resistance in, 197

Urate, excretion in biliary cirrhosis, 117

Urea
  excretion of
    in cirrhosis, 40–41, 61–63
    fractional, 94
  hepatic biosynthesis of, 109, 110–111

Uremia, 525

Uric acid, fractional excretion of, 7

Uricosuria, in cirrhosis, 201

Urinary natriuretic factors, 366

Urinary output, peritoneovenous shunt-related increase of, 496

Urinary peptides, natriuretic activity of, 366

Urine
  in jaundice, 423
  kallikrein content measurement in, 87–88
  natriuretic activity of, 360, 368
  osmolality of
    in cirrhosis, 39, 40–41, 61–63
    furosemide-related decrease of, 54
    measurement of, 42–43

Urine-to-plasma creatinine ratio, 95

Urine-to-plasma osmolality ratio, 95

Urine volume, peritoneovenous shunt-related increase of, 496

Urodilatin, 366
  relationship to atrial natriuretic factor activity, 352, 354
  in renal sodium handling, 17–18

Urodiodenone, 366

Ursodeoxycholic acid
  renoprotective effects of, 438–439
  as venoocclusive disease prophylaxis, 175–176

Valproate, pharmacokinetics of, 463

Valsalva maneuver, muscle sympathetic nerve activity response to, 410–411, 412

Vancomycin, as venoocclusive disease risk factor, 171

Vascular bed, hepatic, **221–240**
  blood flow in, 221, 222–234
  blood volume in, 222, 234–236
  fluid exchange in, 236–237
  microvasculature in, 222–223

Vascular resistance
  in cirrhosis, effect of prostaglandins on, 325
  hepatic, calculation of, 233–234

Vasculature, effect of endothelin on, 395–397

Vasculitis, leukocytoclastic, 128, 130

Vasoactive intestinal polypeptide
  in cirrhosis, 241
  in liver disease-related hypotension, 82
  in renal sodium retention, 24

Vasoactive substances, 246–250
  in cirrhosis-related sodium retention, 1–2
  kinetics and disposal of, 246–248
  pressor responses to, in jaundice, 429

Vasoconstriction
  cerebral, effect of bilirubin on, 440
  in cirrhosis
    relationship to norepinephrine concentration, 413
    relationship to vasodilation, 250
  endotoxemia-related, 400–401
  renal, 6
    in hepatorenal syndrome, 80–81
    jaundice-related, 438–439
    relationship to hepatorenal reflex, 409
  effect of sympathetic nervous system on, 424

Vasoconstrictors
  in cirrhosis, 241
  as hepatorenal syndrome therapy, 101–102
  nitric oxide-mediated pressor response to, 381

Vasodilation
  arteriolar, as sodium retention mechanism, 203–207, 411–412, 508
  in cirrhosis, relationship to vasoconstriction, 250
  peripheral, in ascites formation, 5, 6–7
  systemic, in cirrhosis, 246

Vasodilators
  in cirrhosis, 241
  as hepatorenal syndrome therapy, 100
  effect on renin release, 271
  as venoocclusive disease therapy, 174–175

Vasopressin. *See* Antidiuretic hormone

Venoocclusive disease, hepatic
  definition of, 167
  following bone marrow transplantation, **167–178**
    diagnosis of, 168, 170–171
    pathology of, 167–168, 169
    pathophysiology of, 172–173
    predisposing clinical factors in, 171–172
    prophylaxis of, 174–175

Venous pressure
  hepatic, effect on sympathetic nervous activity, 412
  in hepatorenal syndrome, 83
  renal
    in hepatorenal syndrome, 83
    relationship to sympathetic nerve activity, 408

Venous pressure gradient, hepatic, 247

Venous resistance, hepatic, 230–233

Venous sphincters, hepatic, 227–228, 229, 230, 232, 233, 235

Venovenous bypass, in liver transplantation, 530

Verapamil
  effect on cyclosporine nephrotoxicity, 534
  pharmacokinetics of, 463

Vesicocoelomic drainage, of ascitic fluid, 491–493

Volume contraction, atrial natriuretic factor responsiveness to, 344–346

Volume depletion, as hyponatremia cause, 60

Volume expansion. *See also* Extracellular fluid volume expansion
  atrial natriuretic factor responsiveness to, 344
  in cirrhosis-associated hypovolemia, 96
  renin-angiotensin system responsiveness in, 281–282

Volume receptors, location of, 241–242

Wallstent, 509, 514

Water, prostaglandin-mediated tubular transport of, 313

Water conservation, renal, in cirrhosis, 61–64

Water handling, renal, in liver disease, **33–74**
  clinical consequences of, 55–61
  effect of alcohol ingestion on, 35–37
  pathogenetic mechanisms in, 42–54
  water conservation in, 61–64
  water loading response in, 37–42

Water immersion, 7–9
  atrial natriuretic factor response in, 341, 344–345, 349
    with exogenous atrial natriuretic factor, 347
    renal resistance to, 350
  effects of
    on free water clearance, 46–47
    in hyperaldosteronism, 12–14, 301–302
    on norepinephrine levels, 281, 411–412
    on phosphate excretion rate, 10–11
    on plasma aldosterone responsiveness, 301–302
    on plasma renin activity, 282–283

Water immersion *(cont.)*
  effects of *(cont.)*
    on sympathetic nerve activity, 19, 414–415
    of urinary prostaglandins on, 315
  as hepatorenal syndrome therapy, 100
  natriuretic response, by decompensated cirrhotic patients,
    9–10, 207–208
Water metabolism, effect of prostaglandins on, 316
Water retention, effect of sympathetic nerve activity on,
  417–419
Weight gain
  sodium retention-related, in cirrhosis, 2
  venoocclusive disease-related, 168, 170–171

Weight loss, jaundice-related, 431–432
Wilson's disease, 117

Xenobiotic cross-circulation, as hepatorenal syndrome therapy,
  100
Xenon washout studies, 22, 77, 242
  in hepatorenal syndrome, 77
  for renal blood pressure assessment, 22, 77, 82
Ximoprofen
  dosage in cirrhosis, 469
  pharmacokinetics of, 468–469

Zona glomerulosa, aldosterone secretion by, 291